SEVENTH EDITION

ESSENTIALS OF ANATOMY AND PHYSIOLOGY

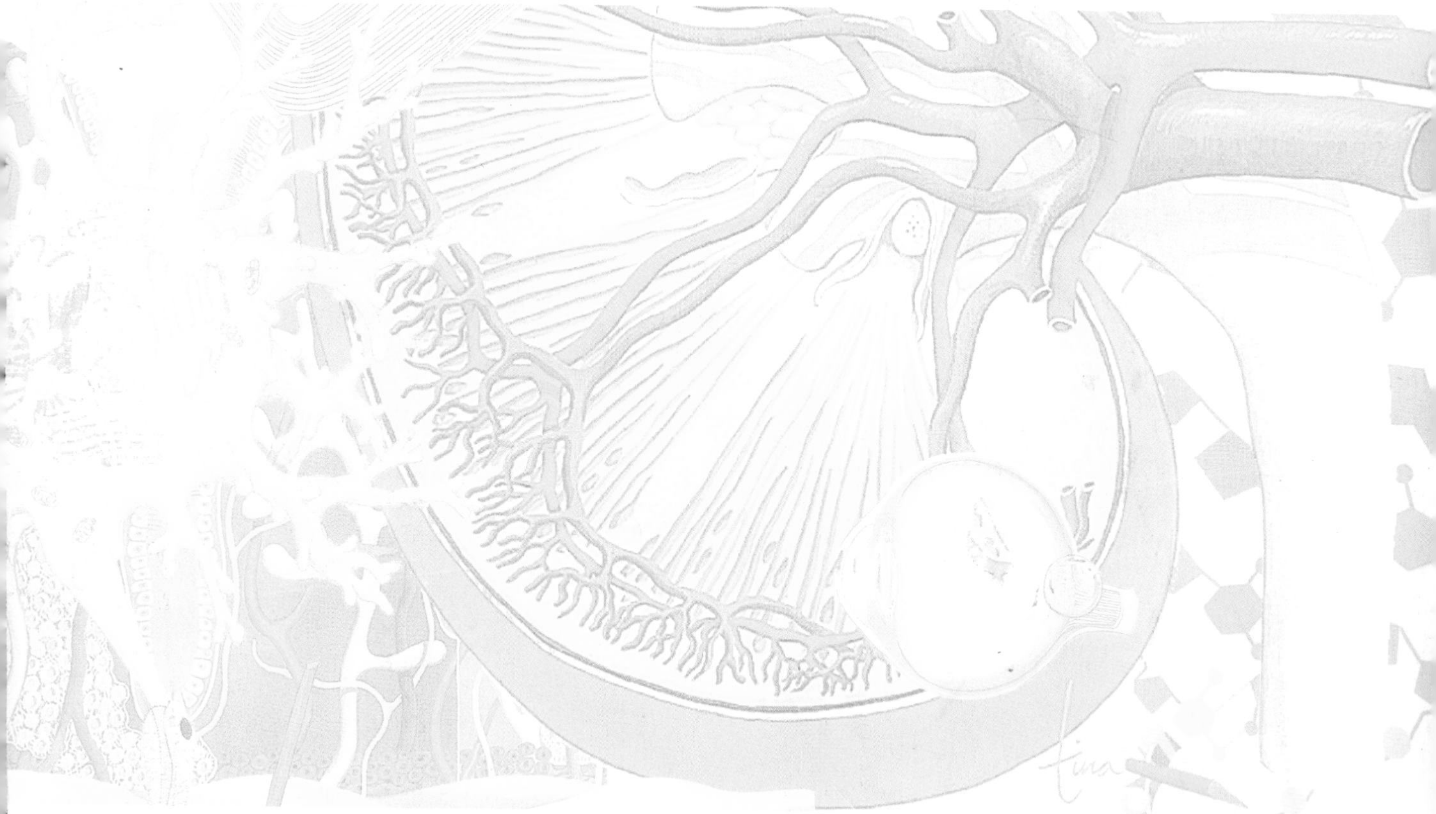

SEVENTH EDITION

ESSENTIALS OF ANATOMY AND PHYSIOLOGY

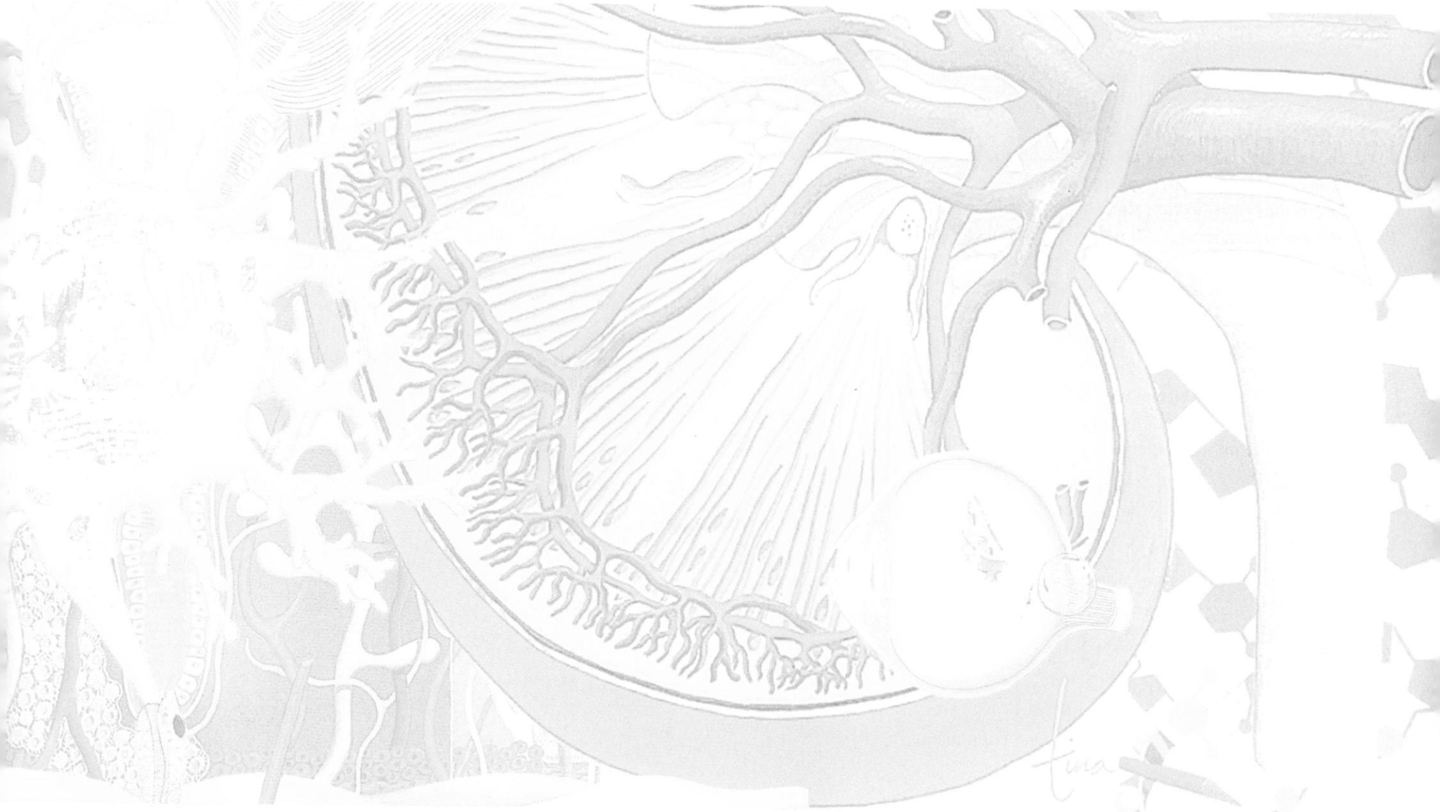

VALERIE C. SCANLON, PhD
College of Mount Saint Vincent
Riverdale, New York

TINA SANDERS
Medical Illustrator
Castle Creek, New York
Formerly Head Graphic Artist
Tompkins Courtland Community College
Dryden, New York

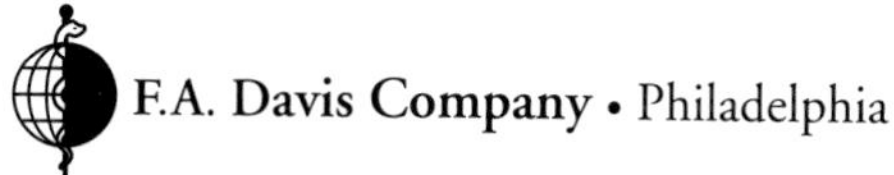

F.A. Davis Company • Philadelphia

F. A. Davis Company
1915 Arch Street
Philadelphia, PA 19103
www.fadavis.com

Printed in the United States of America

Last digit indicates print number: 10 9 8 7 6 5 4 3

Publisher, Nursing: Lisa B. Houck
Director of Content Development: Darlene D. Pedersen
Content Project Manager: Echo Gerhart
Electronic Project Editor: Katherine Crowley
Manager of Design and Illustration: Carolyn O'Brien

Library of Congress Cataloging-in-Publication Data

Scanlon, Valerie C., 1946- author.
Essentials of anatomy and physiology / Valerie C. Scanlon, Tina Sanders. — Seventh edition.
p. ; cm.
Includes index.
ISBN 978-0-8036-3957-7
I. Sanders, Tina, 1943- author. II. Title.
[DNLM: 1. Anatomy. 2. Physiological Phenomena. QS 4]
QP34.5
612—dc23

2014012086

To my students, past and present
VCS

To Brooks, for his encouragement
TS

PREFACE TO THE SEVENTH EDITION

Once again, we extend our gratitude to all of you who have used previous editions of *Essentials of Anatomy and Physiology* and are considering adopting our seventh edition. We are pleased to welcome new readers as well, and we thank you for choosing our book.

The seventh edition remains focused on presenting basic anatomy and physiology with the clarity of the text complemented and enhanced by superb illustrations. The text has been updated in many small ways to remain contemporary. These include brief discussions of our microbiota in Chapter 1 (and appropriate later chapters), the oligosaccharides in breast milk in Chapter 2, epigenetics and primary cilia in Chapter 3, connective tissue disorders in Chapter 4, motor units and the muscle hormone irisin in Chapter 7, celiac disease in Chapter 16, human papillomavirus in Chapter 20, and evaluation of fetal DNA in maternal blood for prenatal testing in Chapter 21. Chapter 12 has been revised and now begins with a description of cardiac muscle tissue, pulling together material from previous chapters.

All of the For Further Thought sections now end with at least one illustration question. New ones include the relationship of organ systems in Chapter 1, the hydrogen bonds formed by water molecules in Chapter 2, effects of sunlight on the skin in Chapter 5, a nerve pathway (to be named by the student) in Chapter 8, the hormones of stressful situations in Chapter 10, a time line of immune responses in Chapter 14, hormones of the duodenum in Chapter 16, regulation of body temperature in Chapter 17, and relationships of the reproductive organs to other organ systems in Chapter 20. When the students have labeled the picture and answered the questions, the whole then becomes an integral part of the chapter. We hope you will consider assigning these questions, and that students will find them enjoyable and helpful.

Colleagues, please keep in mind that the Instructor's Guide contains a full list of these additions in the "New to This Edition" section for each chapter of the textbook, as well as detailed answers to all of the For Further Thought questions.

As always, your comments and suggestions will be most welcome, and they may be sent to us in care of the publisher: F. A. Davis Company, 1915 Arch Street, Philadelphia, PA 19103.

Valerie C. Scanlon
Dobbs Ferry, New York

Tina Sanders
Castle Creek, New York

TO THE INSTRUCTOR

The start of the 21st century has already brought many advances in the science and art of medicine and health care; many of these were made possible by research and discoveries in the basic sciences. Teachers of introductory anatomy and physiology may wish to include some of these discoveries yet will want to maintain their emphasis on the normal structure and function of the human body. Those are the goals of this textbook: to add a little of the new to the foundation of long-standing knowledge and to make all of this material readily accessible to students with diverse backgrounds and varying levels of educational preparation.

No prior knowledge of biology or chemistry is assumed, and even fundamental terms are defined thoroughly. Essential aspects of anatomy are presented clearly and reinforced with excellent illustrations. Essential aspects of physiology are discussed simply yet with accuracy and precision. The illustrations complement the text material and foster comprehension on the part of the student. As you will see, these are images in which detail is readily apparent and all important parts have been labeled. Illustrations of physiology lead the student step-by-step. Wherever appropriate, the legends refer students to the text for further description or explanation. Each illustration also has a question for the student; the illustration questions in each chapter form an ongoing self-test. (The answers are given in Appendix G.)

The text has three unifying themes: the relationship between physiology and anatomy, the interrelations among the organ systems, and the relationship of each organ system to homeostasis. Although each type of cell, tissue, organ, or organ system is discussed simply and thoroughly in itself, applicable connections are made to other aspects of the body or to the functioning of the body as a whole. Our goal is to provide your students with the essentials of anatomy and physiology, and in doing so, to help give them a solid foundation for their future work and an appreciation for the incredible living organism that is the human body.

The sequence of chapters is a very traditional one. Cross-references are used to remind students of what they have learned from previous chapters. Nevertheless, the textbook is very flexible, and, following the introductory four chapters, the organ systems may be covered in almost any order, depending on the needs of your course.

Each chapter is organized from the simple to the more complex, with the anatomy followed by the physiology. The Instructor's Guide presents modifications of the topic sequences that may be used, again depending on the needs of your course. Certain more advanced topics may be omitted from each chapter without losing the meaning or flow of the rest of the material, and these are indicated, for each chapter, in the Instructor's Guide.

Clinical applications are set apart from the text in boxed inserts. These are often aspects of pathophysiology that are related to the normal anatomy or physiology in the text discussion. Each box presents one topic and is referenced at the appropriate point in the text. This material is intended to be an integral part of the chapter but is set apart for ease of reference and to enable you to include or omit as many of these topics as you wish. The use of these boxes also enables students to read the text material without interruption and then to focus on specific aspects of pathophysiology. A comprehensive list of the boxes appears inside the book's back cover, and another list at the beginning of each chapter cites the boxes within that chapter.

Tables are utilized as summaries of structure and function, to present a sequence of events, or additional material that you may choose to include. Each table is referenced in the text and is intended to facilitate your teaching and to help your students learn.

New terms appear in bold type within the text, and all such terms are fully defined in an extensive glossary, with phonetic pronunciations. Bold type may also be used for emphasis whenever one of these terms is used again in a later chapter.

Each chapter begins with a chapter outline and student objectives to prepare the student for the chapter itself. New terminology and related clinical terms are also listed, with phonetic pronunciations. Each of these terms is fully defined in the glossary, with cross-references back to the chapter in which the term is introduced.

At the end of each chapter are review questions and a study outline. The study outline includes all of the essentials of the chapter in a concise form. The review questions may be assigned as homework or used by the students as a review or self-test. Following each question is a page reference in parentheses. This reference cites the page(s) in the chapter on which the content needed to answer the question correctly can be found. The answers themselves are included in the Instructor's Guide. The questions in the sections titled For Further Thought may be used in a variety of ways, and the answers are in the Instructor's Guide.

An important supplementary learning tool for your students is available in the form of a *Student Workbook* that accompanies this text. For each chapter in the textbook, the workbook offers fill-in and matching-column questions, figure-labeling and figure-coloring exercises, and crossword puzzles based on the chapter's vocabulary list. Also included are three comprehensive, multiple-choice chapter tests to provide a thorough review. All answers are provided at the end of the workbook.

Ancillary materials for the teacher using this text are all available on the F.A. Davis website (please contact your F.A. Davis sales representative for access information): a complete Instructor's Guide, a test bank using three formats, an Interactive Teaching Tool presentation of the text illustrations, with related questions for students, podcasts of the chapter study outlines, PowerPoint lecture outlines, and question packages suitable for pre-tests, post-tests, or both. The Instructor's Guide contains notes on each chapter's organization and content (useful for modifying the book to your specific teaching needs), topics for class discussion, answers to the chapter review questions from the textbook, and detailed answers to the For Further Thought questions.

Suggestions and comments from colleagues are always valuable, and yours would be greatly appreciated. When we took on the task of writing and illustrating this textbook, we wanted to make it the most useful book possible for you and your students. Any suggestions that you can provide to help us achieve that goal are most welcome, and they may be sent to us in care of F. A. Davis Company, 1915 Arch Street, Philadelphia, PA 19103.

Valerie C. Scanlon

Dobbs Ferry, New York

Tina Sanders

Castle Creek, New York

TO THE STUDENT

This is your textbook for your course in human anatomy and physiology, a subject that is both fascinating and rewarding. That you are taking such a course says something about you. You may simply be curious as to how the human body functions or you may have a personal goal of making a contribution in one of the health care professions. Whatever your reason, this textbook will help you to be successful in your anatomy and physiology course.

The material is presented simply and concisely yet with accuracy and precision. The writing style is informal yet clear and specific; it is intended to promote your comprehension and understanding.

ORGANIZATION OF THE TEXTBOOK

To use this textbook effectively, you should know the purpose of its various parts. Each chapter is organized in the following way:

Chapter Outline—This presents the main topics in the chapter, which correspond to the major headings in the text.

Student Objectives—These summarize what you should know after reading and studying the chapter. These are not questions to be answered, but are, rather, with the chapter outline, a preview of the chapter contents.

New Terminology and Related Clinical Terminology—These are some of the new terms you will come across in the chapter. Read through these terms before you read the chapter, but do not attempt to memorize them just yet. When you have finished the chapter, return to the list and see how many terms you can define. Note those you may not be sure of and look them up. All of these terms are fully defined in the glossary.

Study Outline—At the end of the chapter, this is a concise summary of the essentials in the chapter. You may find this outline useful as a quick review before an exam.

Review Questions—These are also at the end of the chapter. Your instructor may assign them as homework. If not, the questions may be used as a self-test to evaluate your comprehension of the chapter's content. The page number(s) in parentheses following each question refer you to the page(s) in the chapter on which the content needed to answer the question can be found.

For Further Thought—The heading tells you what these questions are for: thinking. Your instructor may use these for class discussion, and, if so, please do not ever be afraid to be mistaken. Contribute, raise your hand, speak up with your best thoughts, and listen to those of others. Together you will find the answers.

OTHER FEATURES WITHIN EACH CHAPTER

Illustrations—These are an essential part of this textbook. They are intended to help you develop your own mental picture of the body and its parts and processes. You may not have thought of mental pictures as being important, but they are, and each new one you create is a major step in learning. Each illustration is referenced in the text, so you will know when to consult it. With a little concentration, you will have it in your mind for whenever you need it. You will see that each illustration has a question after the legend. These questions provide an ongoing quiz; try to answer each one as you come to it. The answers are given in Appendix G, just before the glossary.

Boxes—Discussions of clinical applications are in separate boxes in the text so that you may find them easily. Your instructor may include all or some of these as required reading. These boxes are an introduction to pathophysiology.

Bold Type—This is used whenever a new term is introduced, or when an old term is especially important. The terms in bold type are fully defined in the glossary, which includes phonetic pronunciations.

Tables—This format is used to present material in a very concise form. Some tables are summaries of text material and are very useful for a quick review. Other tables present additional material that complements the text material.

Glossary—Found at the end of the book, the glossary is your dictionary. All of the terms in bold type in the text, as well as others, are defined here. Make use of it, rather than wonder what a word means. The sooner you have a definition firmly in your mind, the sooner it is truly part of your knowledge.

To make the best use of your study time, a *Student Workbook* is available that will help you to focus your attention on the essentials in each chapter. Also included are comprehensive chapter tests to help you determine which topics you have learned thoroughly and which you may have to review. You will find it very helpful.

SOME FINAL WORDS OF ENCOURAGEMENT

Your success in this course depends to a great extent on you. Try to set aside study time for yourself every day; a little time each day is usually much more productive than trying to cram at the last minute.

Ask questions of yourself as you are studying. What kinds of questions? The simplest ones. If you are studying a part of the body such as an organ, ask yourself: What is its name? Where is it? What is it made of? What does it do? That is: name, location, structure, and function. These are the essentials. If you are studying a process, ask yourself: What is happening here? What is its purpose? That is: What is going on? And what good is it? Again, these are the essentials.

We hope this textbook will contribute to your success in this course and in your education.

Valerie C. Scanlon
Dobbs Ferry, New York

Tina Sanders
Castle Creek, New York

ACKNOWLEDGMENTS

Writing and illustrating are part of a book, yet never the whole, and we thank the editors and production staff of the F. A. Davis Company, especially:

- Lisa B. Houck, Publisher, Nursing
- Echo K. Gerhart, Content Project Manager
- Jean Rodenberger, Editor in Chief, Nursing
- Michael Bailey, Director of Production
- Bob Butler, Production Manager
- Daniel E. Domzalski, Illustration Coordinator
- Production Editors Chris Waller and Kelly Boutross, Tom Klonoski, Allison Repking, and everyone else at Graphic World who participated in this project
- Carolyn O'Brien, Illustration and Design Manager, for designing the layout and the cover
- Neil Kelly, Director of Sales, and all of the F. A. Davis sales representatives

VCS

TS

CONTENTS

SEVENTH EDITION

ESSENTIALS OF ANATOMY AND PHYSIOLOGY

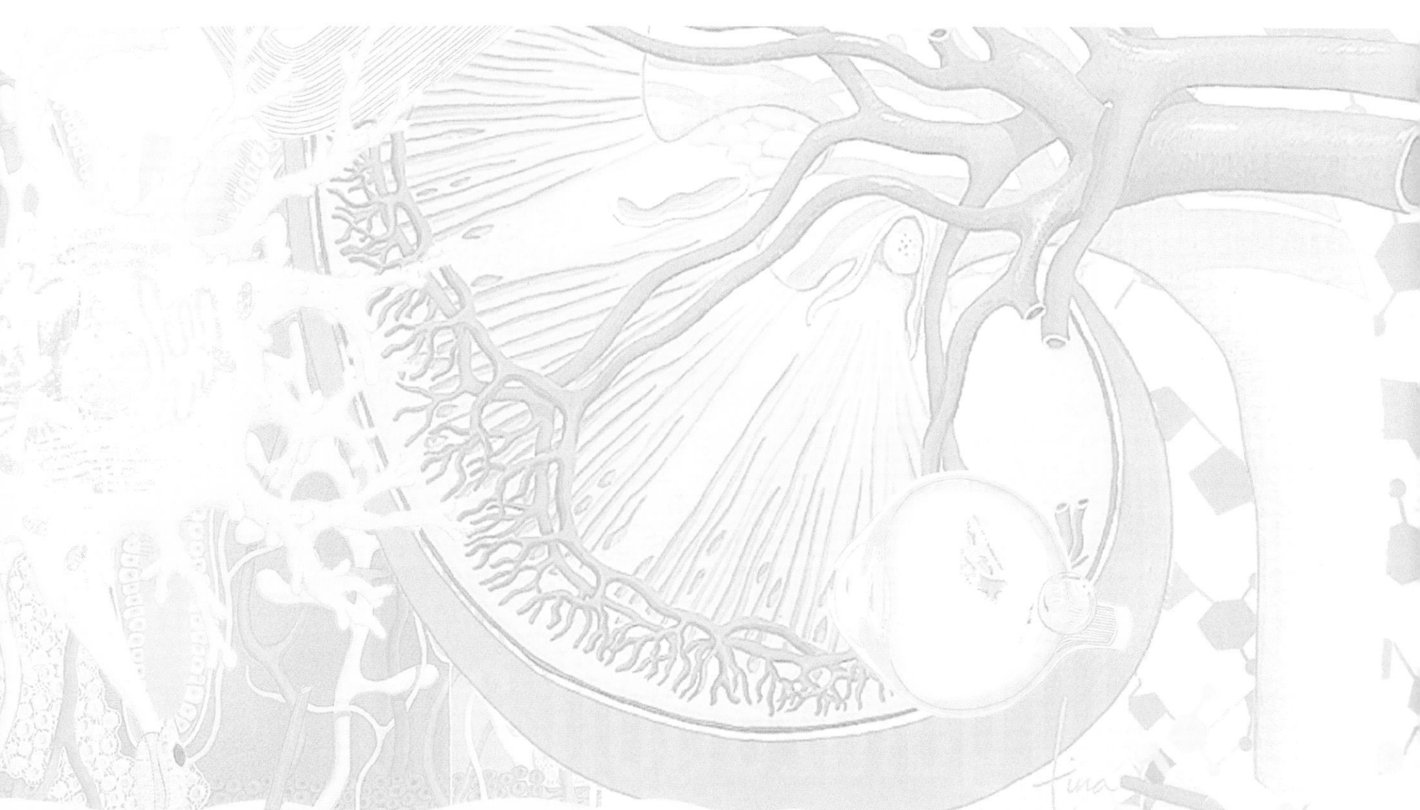

CHAPTER

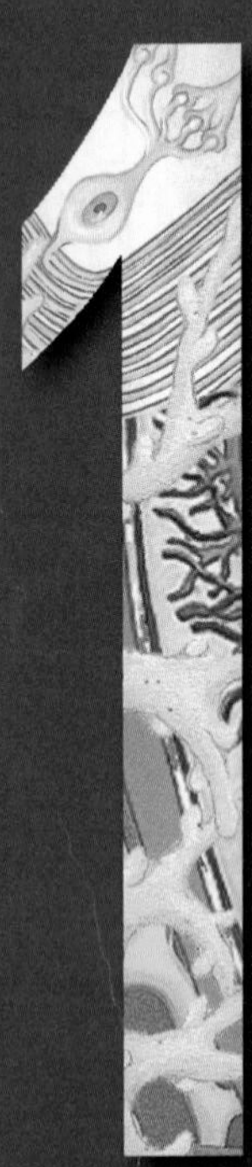

Organization and General Plan of the Body

STUDENT OBJECTIVES

- Define the terms *anatomy*, *physiology*, and *pathophysiology*. Use an example to explain how they are related.
- Name the levels of organization of the body from simplest to most complex, and explain each.
- Define the terms *metabolism*, *metabolic rate*, and *homeostasis*, and use examples to explain each.
- Explain how a negative feedback mechanism works and how a positive feedback mechanism differs.
- Describe the anatomic position.
- State the anatomic terms for the parts of the body.
- Use proper terminology to describe the location of body parts with respect to one another.
- Name the body cavities, their membranes, and some organs within each cavity.
- Describe the possible sections through the body or an organ.
- Explain how and why the abdomen is divided into smaller areas. Be able to name organs in these areas.

CHAPTER OUTLINE

NEW TERMINOLOGY

Anatomy *(uh-**NAT**-uh-mee)*
Body cavity *(**BAH**-dee **KAV**-i-tee)*
Cell *(SELL)*
Homeostasis *(HOH-me-oh-**STAY**-sis)*
Inorganic chemicals *(**IN**-or-GAN-ik **KEM**-i-kuls)*
Meninges *(me-**NIN**-jeez)*
Metabolism *(muh-**TAB**-uh-lizm)*
Microbiota *(MY-kroh-bye-**OH**-ta)*
Microbiome *(MY-kroh-**BYE**-ohm)*
Negative feedback *(**NEG**-ah-tiv **FEED**-bak)*
Organ *(**OR**-gan)*
Organ system *(**OR**-gan **SIS**-tem)*
Organic chemicals *(or-**GAN**-ik **KEM**-i-kuls)*
Pathophysiology *(PATH-oh-FIZZ-ee-**AH**-luh-jee)*
Pericardial membranes *(PER-ee-**KAR**-dee-uhl **MEM**-brayns)*
Peritoneum-mesentery *(PER-i-toh-**NEE**-um **MEZ**-en-TER-ee)*
Physiology *(FIZZ-ee-**AH**-luh-jee)*
Plane *(PLAYN)*
Pleural membranes *(**PLOOR**-uhl **MEM**-brayns)*
Positive feedback *(**PAHS**-ah-tiv **FEED**-bak)*
Section *(**SEK**-shun)*
Tissue *(**TISH**-yoo)*

RELATED CLINICAL TERMINOLOGY

Computed tomography (CT) scan *(kom-**PEW**-ted toh-**MAH**-grah-fee SKAN)*
Diagnosis *(DYE-ag-**NOH**-sis)*
Disease *(di-**ZEEZ**)*
Magnetic resonance imaging (MRI) *(mag-**NET**-ik **REZ**-uh-nanse **IM**-ah-jing)*
Positron emission tomography (PET) *(**PAHZ**-i-tron e-**MISH**-un toh-**MAH**-grah-fee)*

*Terms that appear in **bold type** in the chapter text are defined in the glossary, which begins on page 603.*

The human body is a precisely structured container of chemicals and chemical reactions. Have you ever thought of yourself in this way? Probably not, and yet, in the strictly physical sense, that is what each of us is. The body consists of trillions of atoms in specific arrangements (the chemicals) and thousands of chemical reactions proceeding in a very orderly manner. That literally describes us, and yet it is clearly not the whole story. The keys to understanding human consciousness and self-awareness are still beyond our grasp. We do not yet know what enables us to study ourselves—no other animals do, as far as we know—but we have accumulated a great deal of knowledge about what we are made of and how it all works. Some of this knowledge makes up the course you are about to take, a course in basic human anatomy and physiology.

Anatomy is the study of body structure, which includes size, shape, composition, and perhaps even coloration. **Physiology** is the study of how the body functions. The physiology of red blood cells, for example, includes what these cells do, how they do it, and how this is related to the functioning of the rest of the body. Physiology is directly related to anatomy. For example, red blood cells contain the mineral iron in molecules of the protein called hemoglobin; this is an aspect of their anatomy. The presence of iron enables red blood cells to carry oxygen, which is their function. All cells in the body must receive oxygen in order to function properly, so the physiology of red blood cells is essential to the physiology of the body as a whole.

Pathophysiology is the study of disorders of functioning, and a knowledge of normal physiology makes such disorders easier to understand. For example, you are probably familiar with the anemia called iron-deficiency anemia. With insufficient iron in the diet, there will not be enough iron in the hemoglobin of red blood cells, and hence less oxygen will be transported throughout the body, resulting in the symptoms of the iron-deficiency disorder. This example shows the relationship among anatomy, physiology, and pathophysiology.

The purpose of this text is to enable you to gain an understanding of anatomy and physiology with an emphasis on normal structure and function. Many examples of pathophysiology have been included, however, to illustrate the relationship of **disease** to normal physiology and to describe some of the procedures used in the **diagnosis** of disease. Many of the examples are clinical applications that will help you begin to apply what you have learned. Your knowledge of anatomy and physiology will become the basis for your further study in the health professions.

LEVELS OF ORGANIZATION

The human body is organized into structural and functional levels of increasing complexity. Each higher level incorporates the structures and functions of the previous level, as you will see. We will begin with the simplest level, which is the chemical level, and proceed to cells, tissues, organs, and organ systems. All of the levels of organization are depicted in Fig. 1–1.

CHEMICALS

Recall that the body is a container of chemicals. The chemicals that make up the body may be divided into two major categories: inorganic and organic. **Inorganic chemicals** are usually simple molecules made of one or two elements other than carbon (with a few exceptions). Examples of inorganic chemicals are water (H_2O); oxygen (O_2); one of the exceptions, carbon dioxide (CO_2); and minerals such as iron (Fe) in hemoglobin, sodium (Na) in the salt sodium chloride that makes tears salty, and calcium (Ca) in the calcium salts that make bones hard. **Organic chemicals** are often very complex and always contain the elements carbon and hydrogen. In the category of organic chemicals are carbohydrates, fats, proteins, and nucleic acids. The chemical organization of the body is the subject of Chapter 2.

CELLS

The smallest living units of structure and function are **cells**, and the human body consists of more than 200 different types of cells. Another way to think of the body is as a city of cells. Just as a large city has millions of people with many different jobs, the body contains trillions of cells that perform more than 200 jobs. Despite these different functions, human cells have certain structural similarities. Each type of cell is made of chemicals and carries out specific chemical reactions. Cell structure and function are discussed in Chapter 3.

TISSUES

A **tissue** is a group of cells with similar structure and function. Just as in a city certain groups of individuals work together (in the fire department, for example) to keep the city functioning, groups of similar cells work together in the body. There are four groups of tissues:

Epithelial tissues—cover or line body surfaces; some are capable of producing secretions with specific functions.

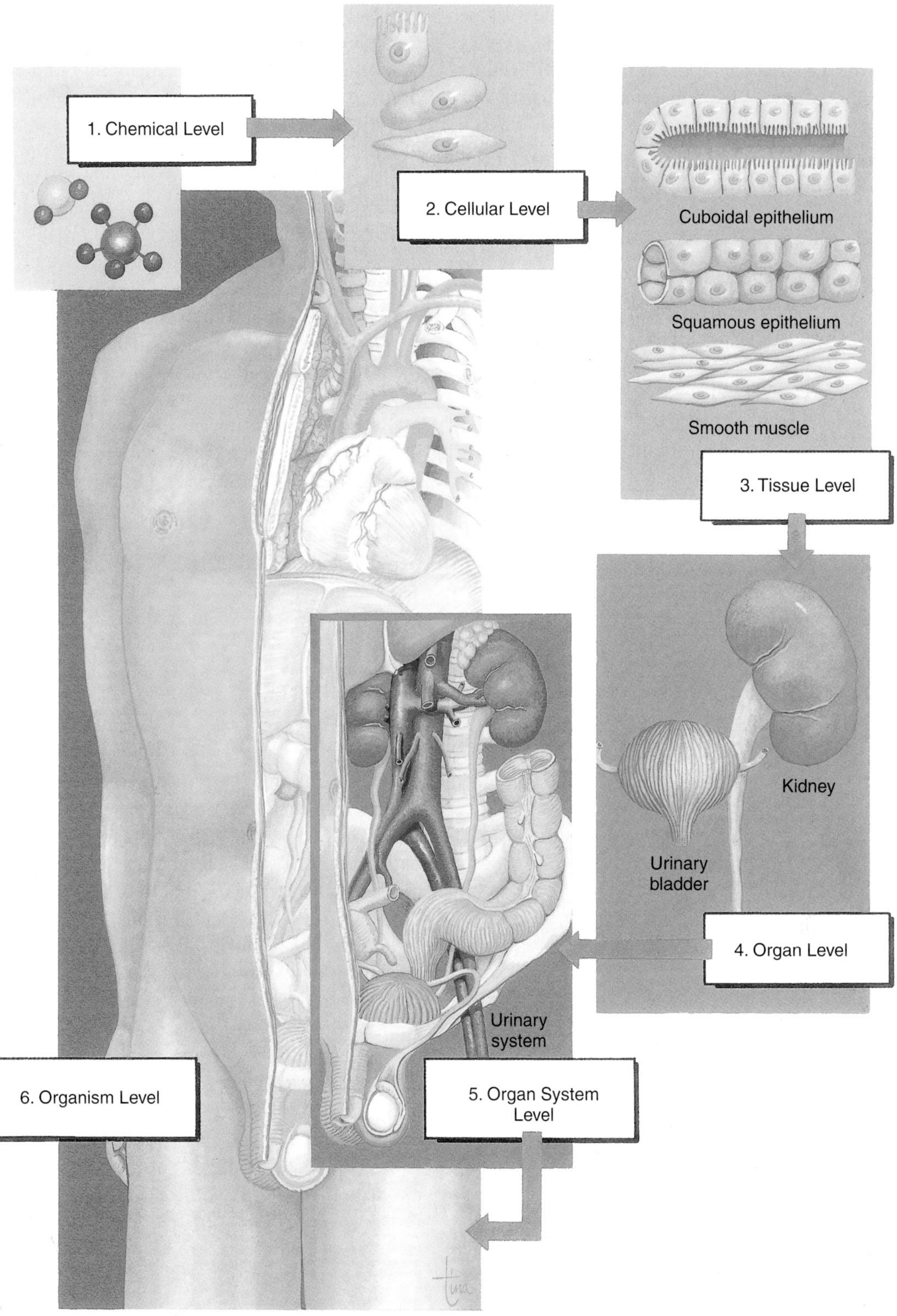

Figure 1–1 Levels of structural organization of the human body, depicted from the simplest (chemical) to the most complex (organism). The organ system shown here is the urinary system.

QUESTION: What other organ system seems to work directly with the urinary system?

The outer layer of the skin and sweat glands are examples of epithelial tissues. Internal epithelial tissues include the walls of capillaries (squamous epithelium) and the kidney tubules (cuboidal epithelium), as shown in Fig. 1–1.

Connective tissues—connect and support parts of the body; some transport or store materials. Blood, bone, cartilage, and adipose tissue are examples of this group.

Muscle tissues—are specialized for contraction, which brings about movement. Our skeletal muscles and the heart are examples of muscle tissue. In Fig. 1–1, you see smooth muscle tissue, which is found in organs such as the urinary bladder and stomach.

Nerve tissues—specialized to generate and transmit electrochemical impulses that regulate body functions. The brain and the optic nerves are examples of nerve tissue.

The types of tissues in these four groups, as well as their specific functions, are the subject of Chapter 4.

ORGANS

An **organ** is a group of tissues precisely arranged so as to accomplish specific functions. Examples of organs are the kidneys, individual bones, the liver, the lungs, and the stomach. The kidneys contain several kinds of epithelial, or surface tissues, for their work of absorption. The stomach is lined with epithelial tissue that secretes gastric juice for digestion, especially of proteins. Smooth muscle tissue in the wall of the stomach contracts to mix food with gastric juice and propel it to the small intestine. Nerve tissue carries impulses that increase or decrease the contractions of the stomach. An organ may be considered a "cooperation of tissues," in which the whole is the anatomic sum of its parts, and much more than the physiologic sum. None of the tissues of the kidney can remove waste products from the blood by itself, but the functioning of all of the kidney tissues does so. Similarly, none of the tissues of the stomach can by itself begin the digestion of protein, but the stomach as a whole can (see Box 1–1: Replacing Tissues and Organs).

ORGAN SYSTEMS

An **organ system** is a group of organs that all contribute to a particular function. Examples are the urinary system, the digestive system, and the respiratory system. In Fig. 1–1 you see the urinary system, which consists of the kidneys, ureters, urinary bladder, and urethra. These organs all contribute to the formation and elimination of urine.

As a starting point, Table 1–1 lists the organ systems of the human body with their general functions and some representative organs, and Fig. 1–2 depicts all of the organ systems. Many of these are already familiar to you. Some organs are part of two organ systems; the pancreas, for example, is both a digestive organ and an endocrine organ, and the diaphragm is part of both the muscular system and the respiratory system. All of the organ systems make up an individual person, and all of them function together; that is, they are interdependent. For now, a few examples will give you an idea of the many interactions among the systems. All cells in the body require oxygen. The respiratory system obtains oxygen from the atmosphere, and the circulatory system distributes the oxygen. All cells need nutrients. The digestive system gets the nutrients, and the circulatory system distributes them. All cells produce waste products. The circulatory system collects the waste products, and the urinary system eliminates them from the blood. The balance of this text discusses each system and its interactions with other systems in more detail.

THE REST OF "US"

We are not alone. Every human being lives with an enormous population of bacteria and other microorganisms, our **microbiota**. It is estimated that the total bacteria that reside on us or inside us, with the most in the intestines, outnumber our own cells about 10 to 1. An older name for this population is **normal flora** (or resident flora, see Table 22–1 for their distribution), and different people have different proportions of the hundreds of species that make us their home. Each site on or inside the body that has bacteria is considered a small ecosystem called a **microbiome.** We have known for years that some intestinal bacteria produce vitamins that we absorb, especially vitamin K. We have also known that these bacteria, in their usual body site (surface of the skin, oral cavity, the vagina in women, among other microbiomes), help to prevent the growth of pathogens. This knowledge has been used lately to try to help those with antibiotic-resistant *Clostridium difficile* intestinal infections, and some people have been cured by "fecal transplants" (in capsule form) of intestinal bacteria from a healthy family member.

Box 1–1 | REPLACING TISSUES AND ORGANS

Blood transfusions are probably the most familiar and frequent form of "replacement parts" for people. Blood is a tissue and, when properly typed and cross-matched (blood types will be discussed in Chapter 11), may safely be given to someone with a blood type that is the same or compatible.

Organs, however, are much more complex structures. When a patient receives an organ transplant, there is always the possibility of rejection (destruction) of the organ by the recipient's immune system (Chapter 14). With the discovery and use of more effective immune-suppressing medications, however, the success rate for many types of organ transplants has increased. Organs that may be transplanted include the corneas, the kidneys, the heart, the liver, and the lungs.

The skin is also an organ, but skin transplanted from another person will not survive very long. Several kinds of artificial skin are now available to temporarily cover large areas of damaged skin. Patients with severe burns, for example, will eventually need skin grafts from their own unburned skin to form permanent new skin over the burn sites. It is possible to "grow" a patient's skin in laboratory culture so that a small patch of skin may eventually be used to cover a large surface. Other cells grown in culture include cartilage, bone, pancreas, liver, and skeletal muscle. Such implants may reduce or eliminate the need for human donors. Tissue engineering is also being used to create tracheas, arteries, urinary bladders, and heart valves.

Many artificial replacement parts have also been developed. These are made of plastic or metal and are not rejected as foreign by the recipient's immune system. Damaged heart valves or sections of arteries may be replaced by grafts made of synthetic materials. Artificial joints are available for every joint in the body, as is artificial bone for reconstructive surgery. Cochlear implants are tiny instruments that convert sound waves to electrical impulses the brain can learn to interpret and have provided some sense of hearing for people with certain types of deafness. A corneal implant is available for a person with age-related macular degeneration (see Chapter 9), in which central vision has been lost. The implant can enable the person to recognize faces and to read large-print books. Work is also progressing on devices that help damaged hearts pump blood more efficiently and on small, self-contained artificial hearts.

Although these new techniques and artificial parts have great promise, we must be realistic: They are very expensive and most will not become the standard of care or be in widespread use for many years.

Recent research suggests that by fermenting the food residues that we do not digest (often fiber, the complex carbohydrates of plants), the intestinal bacteria help nourish the epithelial cells that form the intestinal lining. Not only does this keep the lining intact and prevent leakage of intestinal contents into the tissues of the body, but it also helps suppress inflammation, which in excess can be damaging. Other researchers propose that our microbiota help the immune system to establish itself and contribute to the ability of our white blood cells to distinguish between "self" and "non-self." This is especially important for limiting the development of allergies (mistaken immune responses) and their potentially serious consequences such as asthma. Still other studies are investigating the contribution our microbiota make to weight loss or gain. This is all good but is not the whole story.

The presence of our microbiota has drawbacks as well. Not all bacterial products are beneficial to humans. Some, if absorbed, may be harmful, as is one (made from a chemical called carnitine found in red meat such as beef) that may contribute to heart disease. The total number of genes of all of these bacteria is estimated to be several million (in comparison, the genes of a human cell total about 22,000). Most of the bacterial products

Table 1–1 | **THE ORGAN SYSTEMS**

SYSTEM	FUNCTIONS	ORGANS*
Integumentary	■ Is a barrier to pathogens and chemicals ■ Prevents excessive water loss	skin, subcutaneous tissue
Skeletal	■ Supports the body ■ Protects internal organs and red bone marrow ■ Provides a framework to be moved by muscles	bones, ligaments
Muscular	■ Moves the skeleton ■ Produces heat	muscles, tendons
Nervous	■ Interprets sensory information and decides how to use it ■ Regulates body functions such as movement by means of electrochemical impulses	brain, spinal cord, nerves, eyes, ears
Endocrine	■ Regulates body functions such as growth and reproduction by means of hormones ■ Regulates day-to-day metabolism by means of hormones	thyroid gland, pituitary gland, ovaries or testes, pancreas
Circulatory	■ Transports oxygen and nutrients to tissues and removes waste products	heart, blood, arteries, veins
Lymphatic	■ Returns tissue fluid to the blood ■ Destroys pathogens that enter the body and provides immunity	spleen, lymph nodes, thymus gland
Respiratory	■ Exchanges oxygen and carbon dioxide between the air and blood	lungs, trachea, larynx, diaphragm
Digestive	■ Changes food into simple chemicals that can be absorbed and used by the body	stomach, colon, liver, pancreas
Urinary	■ Removes waste products from the blood ■ Regulates volume and pH of blood and tissue fluid	kidneys, urinary bladder, urethra
Reproductive	■ Produces eggs or sperm ■ *In women*, provides a site for the developing embryo-fetus	Female: ovaries, uterus Male: testes, prostate gland

*These are simply representative organs, not an all-inclusive list.

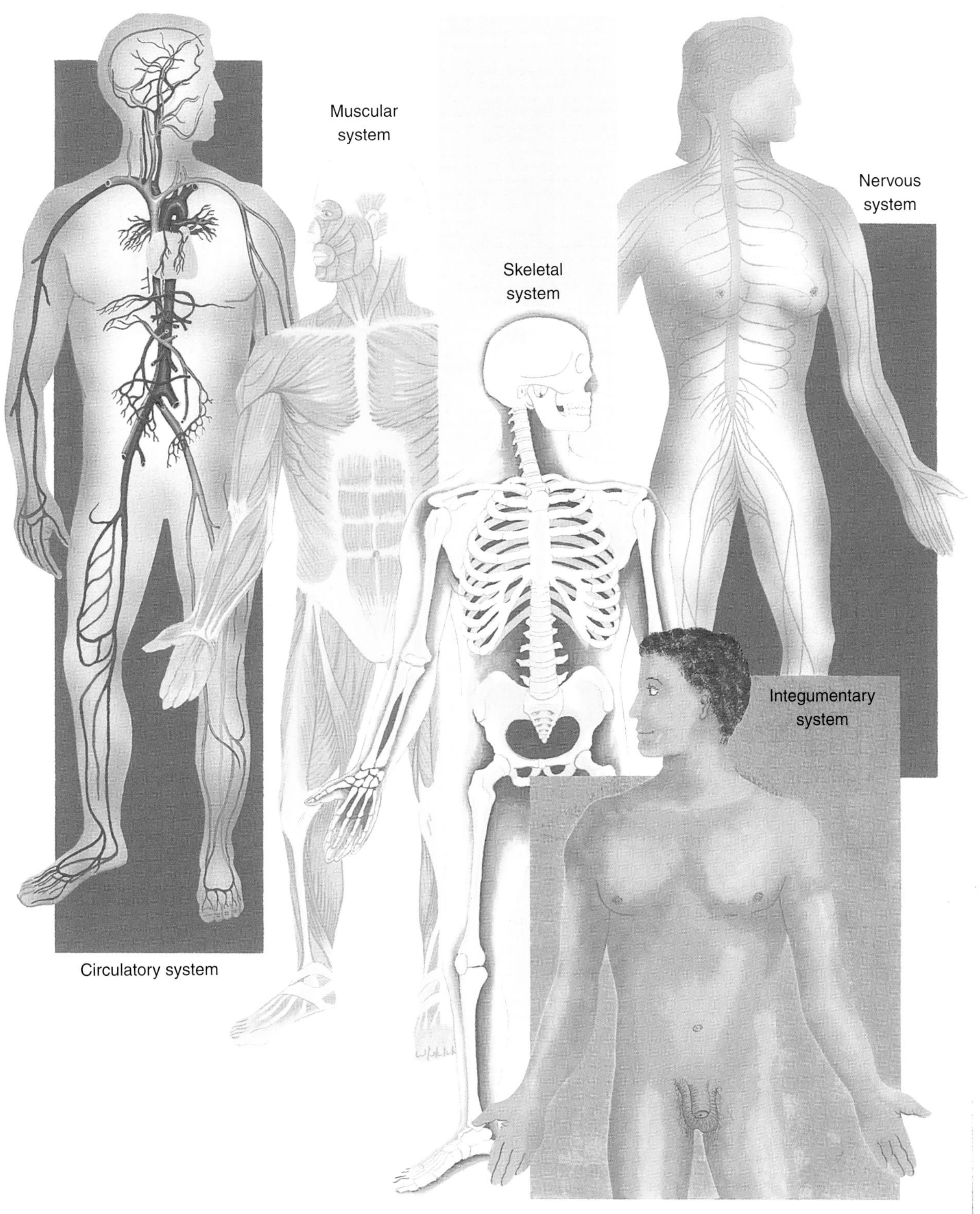

Figure 1–2 Organ systems. Compare the depiction of each system to its description in Table 1–1.

QUESTION: Name at least one organ shown in each system.

Continued

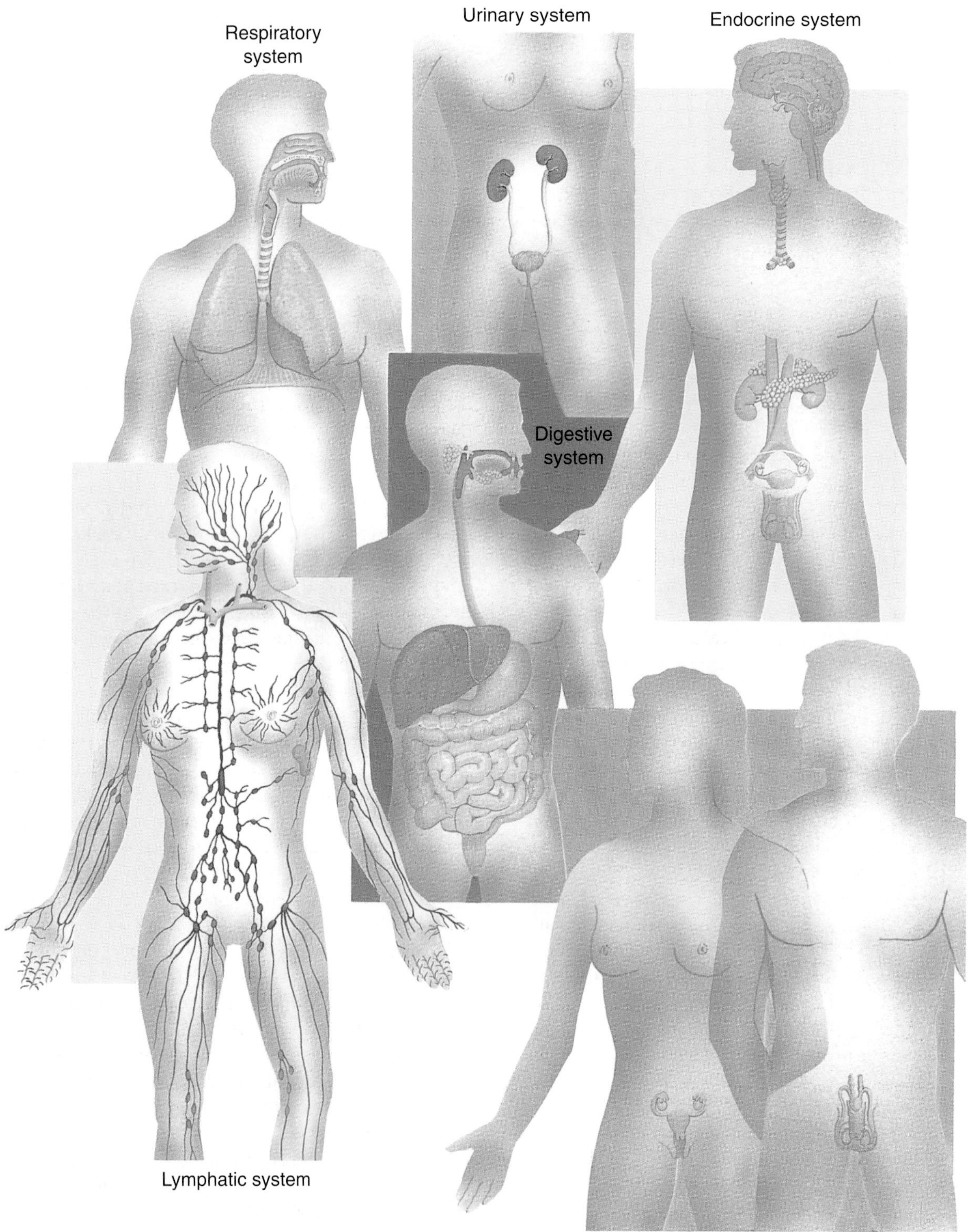

Figure 1–2—cont'd

of these genes have yet to be discovered, and much more work remains to be done before we truly understand the complex relationship we have with our microbiota.

METABOLISM AND HOMEOSTASIS

Metabolism is a collective noun; it is all of the chemical reactions and physical processes that take place within the body. Metabolism includes growing, repairing, reacting, and reproducing—all the characteristics of life. The pumping of the heart, the digestion of food in the stomach, the diffusion of gases in the lungs and tissues, and the production of energy in each cell of the body are just a few of the thousands of aspects of metabolism. *Metabolism* comes from a Greek word meaning "change," and the body is always changing in visible ways (walking down the street), microscopic ways (cells dividing in the skin to produce new epidermis) and submicroscopic or molecular ways (RNA and enzymes constructing new proteins). A related concept, **metabolic rate**, is most often used to mean the speed at which the body produces energy and heat or, put another way, energy production per unit of time, such as 24 hours. Metabolic rate, therefore, is one aspect of metabolism.

A person who is in good health may be said to be in a state of **homeostasis**. Good health is a product of normal metabolism, and homeostasis reflects the ability of the body to maintain a relatively stable metabolism and to function normally despite many constant changes. The changes that are part of normal metabolism may be internal or external, and the body must respond appropriately.

Eating breakfast, for example, brings about an internal change. Suddenly there is food in the stomach, and something must be done with it. What happens? The food is digested or broken down into simple chemicals that the body can use. The protein in a hard-boiled egg is digested into amino acids, its basic chemical building blocks; these amino acids can then be used by the cells of the body to produce their own specialized proteins.

An example of an external change is a rise in environmental temperature. On a hot day, the body temperature would also tend to rise. However, body temperature must be kept within its normal range of about 97° to 99°F (36° to 38°C) to support normal functioning. What happens? One of the body's responses to the external temperature rise is to increase sweating so that excess body heat can be lost by the evaporation of sweat on the surface of the skin. This response, however, may bring about an undesirable internal change, dehydration. What happens? As body water decreases, we feel the sensation of thirst, and we drink fluids to replace the water lost in sweating. Notice that when certain body responses occur, they reverse the event that triggered them. In the preceding example a rising body temperature stimulates increased sweating, which lowers body temperature, which in turn decreases sweating. Unnecessary sweating that would be wasteful of water is prevented. This is an example of a **negative feedback mechanism**, in which the body's response reverses the stimulus (in effect, turning it off for a while) and keeps some aspect of the body metabolism within its normal range.

Look at Fig. 1–3 for another negative feedback mechanism, one in which the hormone thyroxine regulates the metabolic rate of the body. As metabolic rate decreases, the hypothalamus (a part of the brain) and the pituitary gland detect this decrease and secrete hormones to stimulate the thyroid gland (on the front of the neck, just below the larynx) to secrete the hormone thyroxine. Thyroxine stimulates the cellular enzyme systems that produce energy from food, which increases the metabolic rate. The rise in energy and heat production is detected by the brain and pituitary gland. They then decrease secretion of their hormones, which in turn inhibits any further secretion of thyroxine until the metabolic rate decreases again. Metabolic rate does rise and fall, but it is kept within normal limits.

You may be wondering if there is such a thing as a positive feedback mechanism. There is, but such mechanisms are rare in the body and quite different from negative feedback mechanisms. In a **positive feedback mechanism**, the response to the stimulus does not stop or reverse the stimulus, but instead keeps the sequence of events going until it is interrupted by some external event. A good example is childbirth, in which the sequence of events, simply stated, is as follows: Stretching of the uterine cervix stimulates secretion of the hormone oxytocin by the posterior pituitary gland. Oxytocin stimulates contraction of the uterine muscle, which causes more stretching of the cervix as the baby is pushed through, which stimulates the secretion of more oxytocin and, hence, more contractions. The mechanism stops with the delivery of the baby and the placenta. This is the "brake," the interrupting event.

Any positive feedback mechanism requires an external "brake," something to interrupt it. Blood clotting is such a mechanism, and without external controls, clotting may become a vicious cycle of clotting and more clotting, doing far more harm than good (clotting is discussed in Chapter 11). Inflammation, the body's response to

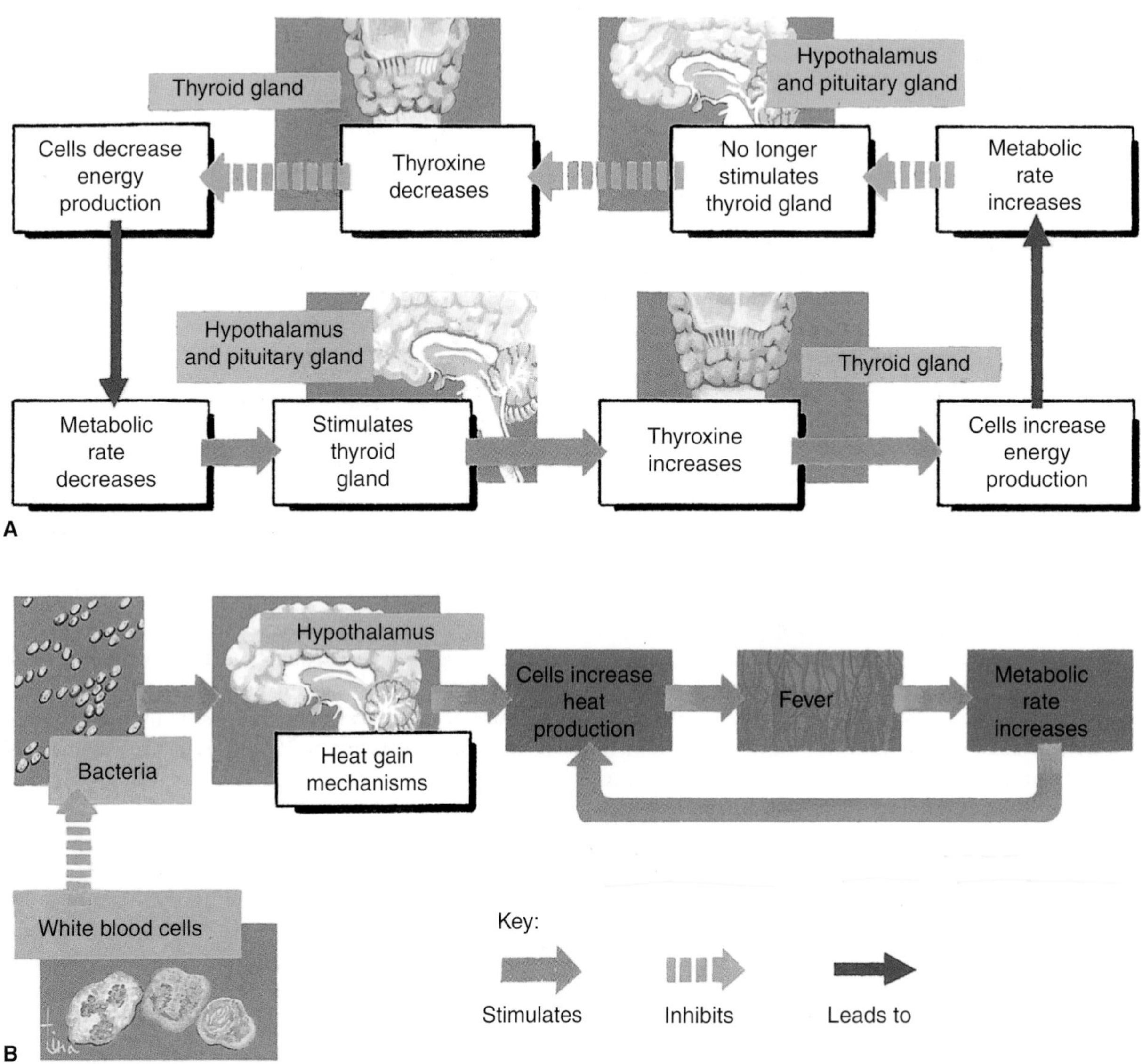

Figure 1–3 Feedback mechanisms. (**A**) The negative feedback mechanism of regulation of metabolic rate by thyroxine. (**B**) The positive feedback mechanism triggered by a fever. See text for description.

QUESTION: For each mechanism, where is the source of the "brake" or inhibition?

damage of any sort, is beneficial and necessary for tissue repair to begin, but the process may evolve into a cycle of damage and more damage, and it requires an external control to stop it. The rise of a fever may also trigger a positive feedback mechanism. Notice in Fig. 1–3 that bacteria have affected the body's thermostat in the hypothalamus and caused a fever. The rising body temperature increases the metabolic rate, which increases body temperature even more, becoming a cycle. Where is the inhibition, the brake? For this infection, the brake is white blood cells destroying the bacteria that caused the fever. An interruption from outside the cycle is necessary.

It is for this reason, because positive feedback mechanisms have the potential to be self-perpetuating and cause harm, that they are rare in the body.

Negative feedback mechanisms, however, contain their own brakes, in that inhibition is a natural part of these cycles, and the body has many such mechanisms. The secretion of most hormones (Chapter 10) is regulated by negative feedback mechanisms. The regulation of heart rate (Chapter 12) and of blood pressure (Chapter 13) involves several negative feedback mechanisms. The result of all of these mechanisms working together is that all aspects of body functioning, that is, of metabolism, are kept within normal limits, a steady state or equilibrium. This is homeostasis.

In the chapters to come, you will find many more examples of homeostasis. As you continue your study of the human body, keep in mind that the proper functioning of each organ and organ system contributes to homeostasis. Keep in mind as well that what we call the normal values of metabolism are often ranges, not single numbers. Recall that normal body temperature is a range: 97° to 99°F (36° to 38°C). Normal pulse rate, another example, is 60 to 80 beats per minute; a normal respiratory rate is 12 to 20 breaths per minute. Variations within the normal range are part of normal metabolism.

TERMINOLOGY AND GENERAL PLAN OF THE BODY

As part of your course in anatomy and physiology, you will learn many new words or terms. At times you may feel that you are learning another language, and indeed you are. Each term has a precise meaning, which is understood by everyone else who has learned the language. Mastering the terminology of your profession is essential to communicating effectively with your coworkers and your future patients. Although the number of new terms may seem a bit overwhelming at first, you will find that using these terms will soon become second nature to you.

The terminology presented in this chapter will be used throughout the text in the discussion of the organ systems. This will help to reinforce the meanings of these terms and will transform these new words into knowledge.

BODY PARTS AND AREAS

Each of the terms listed in Table 1–2 and shown in Fig. 1–4 refers to a specific part or area of the body. For example, the term *femoral* always refers to the thigh, and *brachial* always refers to the upper arm. The femoral

Table 1–2 | DESCRIPTIVE TERMS FOR BODY PARTS AND AREAS

TERM	DEFINITION (REFERS TO)	TERM	DEFINITION (REFERS TO)
Antebrachial	forearm	Gluteal	buttocks
Antecubital	front of elbow	Hepatic	liver
Axillary	armpit	Iliac	hip
Brachial	upper arm	Inguinal	groin
Buccal (oral)	mouth	Lumbar	small of back
Cardiac	heart	Mammary	breast
Cervical	neck	Nasal	nose
Cranial	head	Occipital	back of head
Cutaneous	skin	Orbital	eye
Deltoid	shoulder	Parietal	crown of head
Femoral	thigh	Patellar	kneecap
Frontal	forehead	Pectoral	chest
Gastric	stomach	Pedal	foot

Continued

Table 1–2 | **DESCRIPTIVE TERMS FOR BODY PARTS AND AREAS—cont'd**

TERM	DEFINITION (REFERS TO)	TERM	DEFINITION (REFERS TO)
Perineal	pelvic floor	Scapular	shoulder blade
Plantar	sole of foot	Sternal	breastbone
Popliteal	back of knee	Temporal	side of head
Pulmonary	lungs	Umbilical	navel
Renal	kidney	Volar (palmar)	palm
Sacral	base of spine		

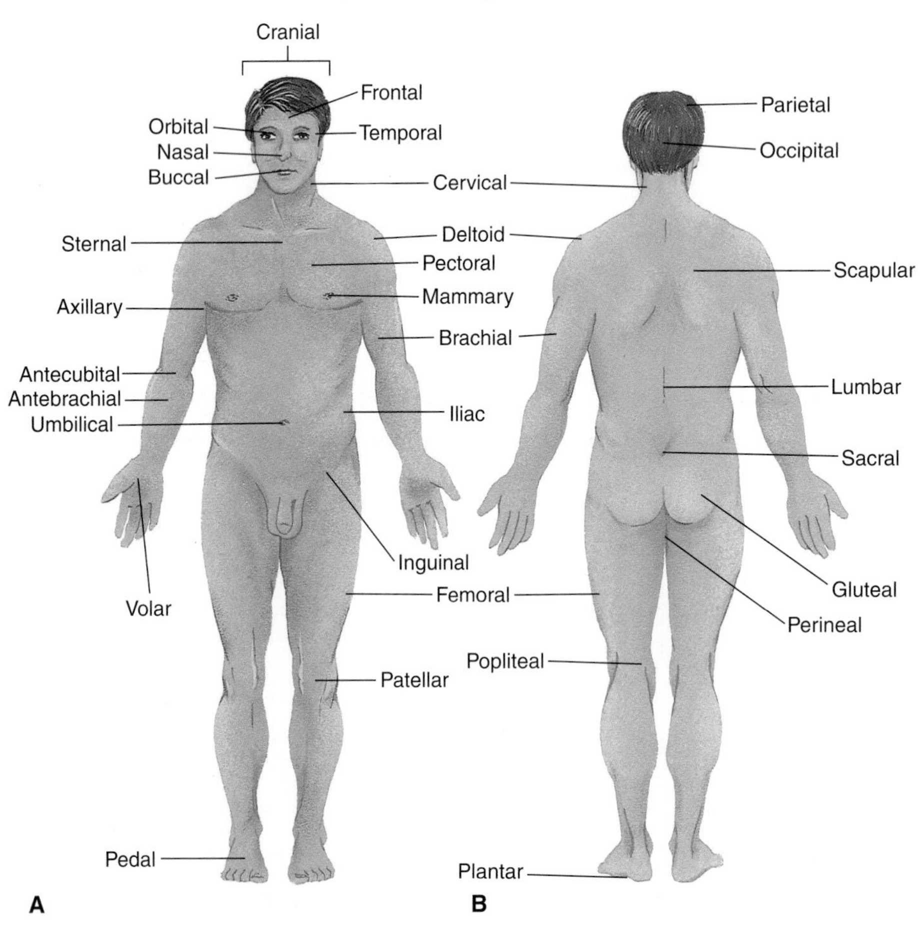

Figure 1–4 Body parts and areas. The body is shown in anatomic position. (**A**) Anterior view. (**B**) Posterior view. (Compare with Table 1–2.)

QUESTION: Name a body area that contains a bone with a similar name. Can you name two more?

artery is a blood vessel that passes through the thigh, and the quadriceps femoris is a large muscle group of the thigh. The brachial artery passes through the upper arm, and the biceps brachii and triceps brachii are the major muscles of the upper arm.

Another example is *pulmonary*, a term that always refers to the lungs, as in pulmonary artery, pulmonary edema, and pulmonary embolism. Although you may not know the exact meaning of each of these terms now, you do know that each has something to do with the lungs.

TERMS OF LOCATION AND POSITION

When describing relative locations, the body is always assumed to be in anatomic position: standing upright facing forward, arms at the sides with palms forward, and the feet slightly apart. The terms of location are listed in Table 1–3, with a definition and example for each. As you read each term, find the body parts used as examples in Figs. 1–4 and 1–5. Notice also that these are pairs of terms and that each pair is a set of opposites. This will help you recall the terms and their meanings.

BODY CAVITIES AND THEIR MEMBRANES

The closed cavities of the body are found in the skull, the vertebral column, and the trunk; each contains specific organs and membranes. These cavities are the cranial, spinal, thoracic, abdominal, and pelvic, and they are shown in Fig. 1–5.

Cranial and spinal cavities

The cranial and spinal cavities contain the central nervous system and are completely enclosed by protective bone. These two cavities are continuous; that is, no wall or

Table 1–3 | TERMS OF LOCATION AND POSITION

TERM	DEFINITION	EXAMPLE
Superior	above, or higher	The heart is superior to the liver.
Inferior	below, or lower	The liver is inferior to the lungs.
Anterior	toward the front	The chest is on the anterior side of the body.
Posterior	toward the back	The lumbar area is posterior to the umbilical area.
Ventral	toward the front	The mammary area is on the ventral side of the body.
Dorsal	toward the back	The buttocks are on the dorsal side of the body.
Medial	toward the midline	The heart is medial to the lungs.
Lateral	away from the midline	The shoulders are lateral to the neck.
Internal	within, or interior to	The brain is internal to the skull.
External	outside, or exterior to	The ribs are external to the lungs.
Superficial	toward the surface	The skin is the most superficial organ.
Deep	within, or interior to	The deep veins of the legs are surrounded by muscles.
Central	the main part	The brain is part of the central nervous system.
Peripheral	extending from the main part	Nerves in the arm are part of the peripheral nervous system.
Proximal	closer to the origin	The knee is proximal to the foot.
Distal	farther from the origin	The palm is distal to the elbow.
Parietal	pertaining to the wall of a cavity	The parietal pleura lines the chest cavity.
Visceral	pertaining to the organs within a cavity	The visceral pleura covers the lungs.

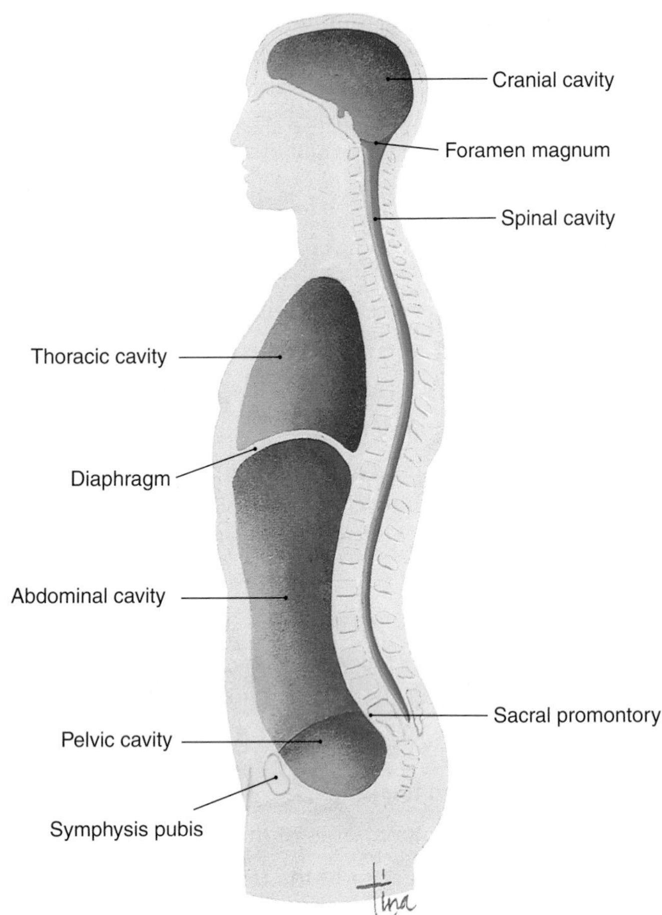

Figure 1–5 Body cavities (lateral view from the left side).

QUESTION: Which of these cavities are surrounded by bone?

boundary separates them. The cranial cavity is formed by the skull and contains the brain. The spinal (or vertebral) cavity is formed by the backbone (vertebral column or spine) and contains the spinal cord. The membranes that line these cavities and cover the brain and spinal cord are called the **meninges**.

Thoracic, Abdominal, and Pelvic Cavities

The thoracic, abdominal, and pelvic cavities are within the trunk of the body, and their contents are at least partially protected by bone. The thoracic (or chest) cavity is the most superior and is separated from the abdominal cavity below by the diaphragm. The diaphragm is a large, dome-shaped respiratory muscle. It has openings for the esophagus and for large blood vessels but otherwise is a wall between the thoracic and abdominal cavities. The pelvic cavity is the most inferior and may be considered a subdivision of the abdominal cavity (there is no wall between the two) or as a separate cavity.

Organs in the **thoracic cavity** include the heart and lungs. The membranes of the thoracic cavity are serous membranes called the **pleural membranes**. The parietal pleura lines the chest wall, and the visceral pleura covers the lungs. The heart has its own set of serous membranes called the **pericardial membranes**. The parietal pericardium lines the fibrous pericardial sac, and the visceral pericardium covers the heart muscle.

Organs in the **abdominal cavity** include the liver, the stomach, and the intestines. The membranes of the abdominal cavity are also serous membranes called the peritoneum and mesentery. The **peritoneum** is the membrane that lines the entire abdominal wall, and the **mesentery** (or visceral peritoneum) is the continuation of this membrane, folded around and covering the outer surfaces of the abdominal organs.

The **pelvic cavity** is inferior to the abdominal cavity. Although the peritoneum does not line the pelvic cavity, it covers the free surfaces of several pelvic organs. Within the pelvic cavity are the urinary bladder and reproductive organs such as the uterus in women and the prostate gland in men.

PLANES AND SECTIONS

When internal anatomy is described, the body, or an organ, is often cut or sectioned in a specific way so as to make particular structures easily visible. A **plane** is an imaginary flat surface that separates two portions of the body or an organ. These planes and **sections** are shown in Fig. 1–6.

Frontal (coronal) section—a plane from side to side separates the body into front and back portions.

Sagittal section—a plane from front to back separates the body into right and left portions. A midsagittal section creates equal right and left halves.

Cross-section—a plane perpendicular to the long axis of an organ. A cross-section of the small intestine (which is a tube) would look like a circle with the cavity of the intestine in the center.

Longitudinal section—a plane along the long axis of an organ. A longitudinal section of the intestine is shown in Fig. 1–6B, and a frontal section of the femur (thigh bone) would also be a longitudinal section (see Fig. 6–1 in Chapter 6).

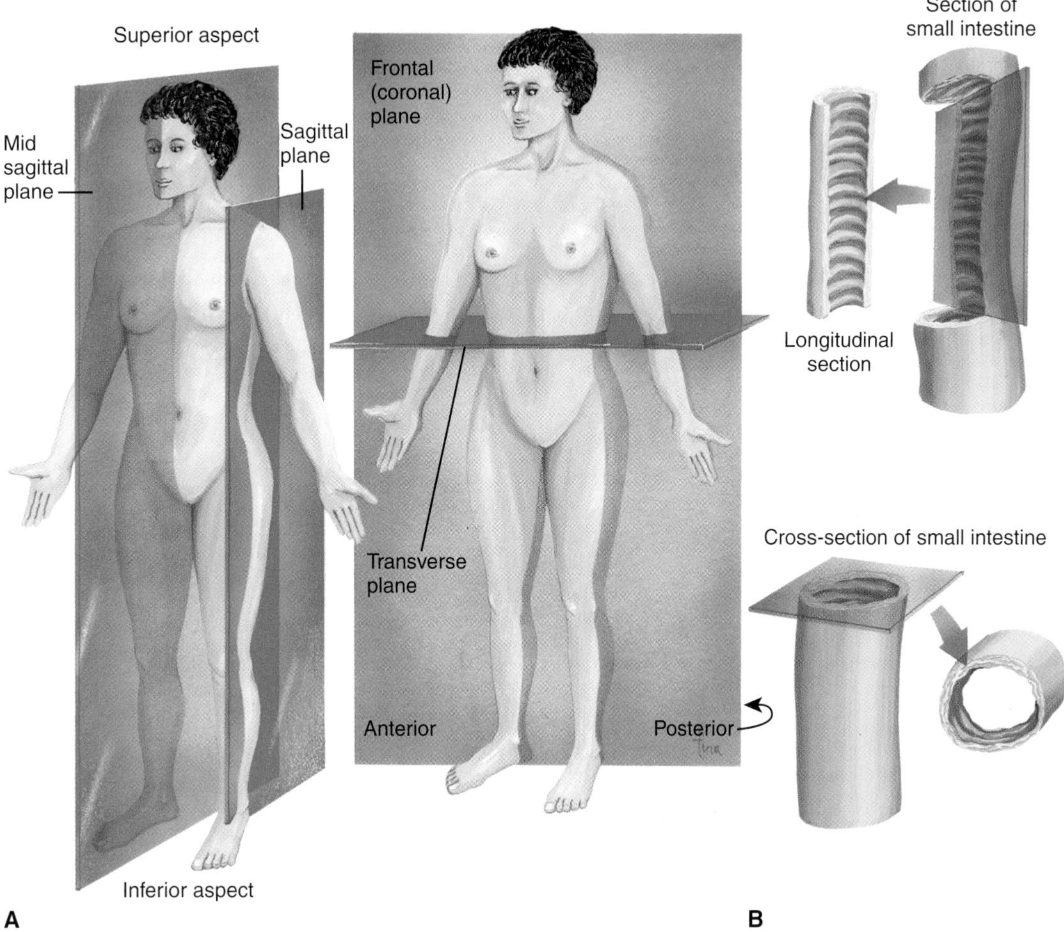

Figure 1–6 (**A**) Planes and sections of the body. (**B**) Cross-section and longitudinal section of the small intestine.

QUESTION: What other organs would have sections that look like those of the small intestine?

Continued

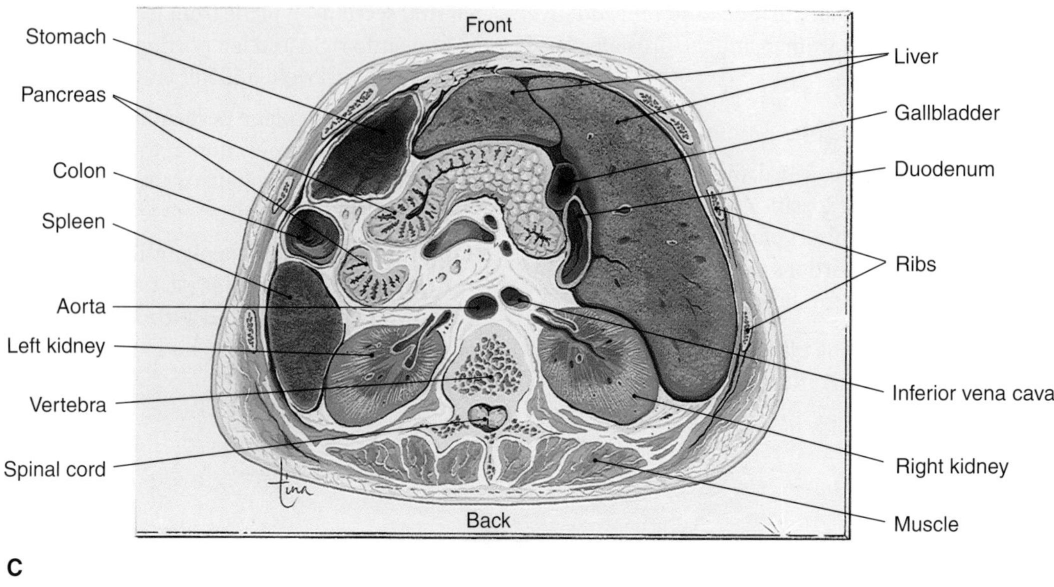

Figure 1–6—cont'd (**C**) Transverse section through the upper abdomen.

Transverse section—a horizontal plane separates the body (or a part) into upper and lower portions. Look at part C of Fig. 1–6; this is a transverse section of the upper abdomen. If you are looking at this picture with the book in front of you, the body in the picture is oriented just the way yours is. The anterior or front is at the top of the illustration, away from you. Place your right hand at the lower edge of your rib cage; that is where this section is taken. Notice all the organs at this level and how they "fit" with one another in the abdominal cavity. Find the aorta; this is a main blood vessel and must be protected. Where is it? Right in front of the backbone, almost in the center of the body, very well protected.

Many pictures in later chapters will be sectional views of organs or body parts. Such sections are often very helpful in learning the spatial relationship of organs or other kinds of parts to one another (see also Box 1–2: Visualizing the Interior of the Body and Box 1–3: Watching the Brain at Work).

AREAS OF THE ABDOMEN

The abdomen is a large area of the lower trunk of the body. If a patient reported abdominal pain, the physician or nurse would want to know more precisely where the pain was. To determine this, the abdomen can be divided into smaller regions or areas, which are shown in Fig. 1–7.

Quadrants—a transverse plane and a midsagittal plane that cross at the umbilicus divide the abdomen into four quadrants. Clinically, this is probably the division used more frequently. The pain of gallstones might then be described as in the right upper quadrant.

Nine areas—two transverse planes and two sagittal planes divide the abdomen into nine areas:

Upper areas—above the lower level of the rib cartilages are the left hypochondriac, epigastric, and right hypochondriac.

Middle areas—the left lumbar, umbilical, and right lumbar.

Lower areas—below the level of the top of the pelvic bone are the left iliac, hypogastric, and right iliac.

These divisions are often used in anatomic studies to describe the location of organs. The liver, for example, is located in the epigastric and right hypochondriac areas.

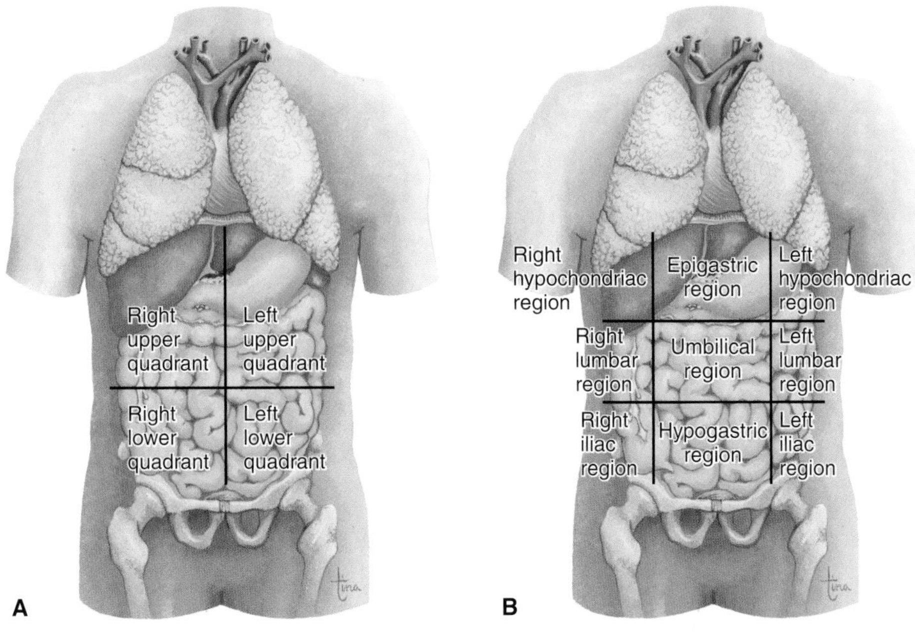

Figure 1–7 Areas of the abdomen. (**A**) Four quadrants. (**B**) Nine regions.

QUESTION: Are there any organs found in all four abdominal quadrants?

Box 1–2 | VISUALIZING THE INTERIOR OF THE BODY

Imaging technologies can often replace exploratory surgery as diagnostic tools. Although expensive, these tools provide great benefits to patients: Highly detailed images of the body are obtained without the risks of surgery and with virtually no discomfort in the procedures themselves.

Computed tomography (CT) scanning uses a narrowly focused x-ray beam that circles rapidly around the body. A detector then measures how much radiation passes through different tissues, and a computer constructs an image of a thin slice through the body. Several images may be made at different levels—each takes only a few seconds—to provide a more complete picture of an organ or part of the body. The images are much more detailed than are those produced by conventional x-rays (Box Figure 1–A, part A).

Magnetic resonance imaging (MRI) is especially useful for visualizing soft tissues, including the brain, spinal cord, and individual nerves. The patient is placed inside a strong magnetic field, and the body's tissues are pulsed with radio waves. Because each tissue has different proportions of various atoms, which resonate or respond differently, each tissue emits a characteristic signal. A computer then translates these signals into an image (part B).

Positron emission tomography (PET) scanning creates images that depict the rates of physiologic processes such as blood flow, oxygen usage, or glucose metabolism. The comparative rates are depicted by colors: Red represents the highest rate, followed by yellow, then green, and finally blue, representing the lowest rate (part C).

Continued

Box 1–2 | VISUALIZING THE INTERIOR OF THE BODY *(Continued)*

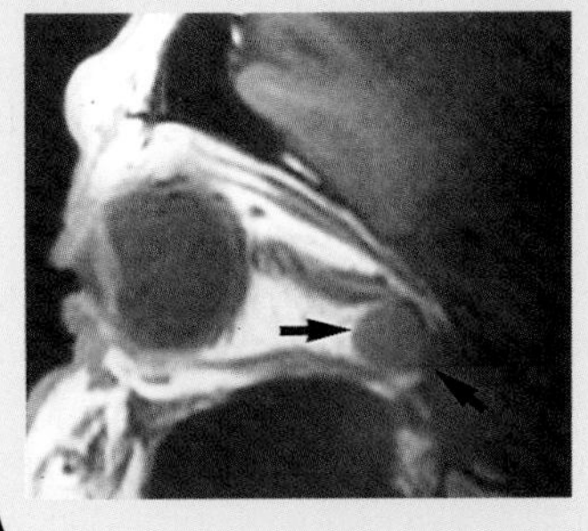
A

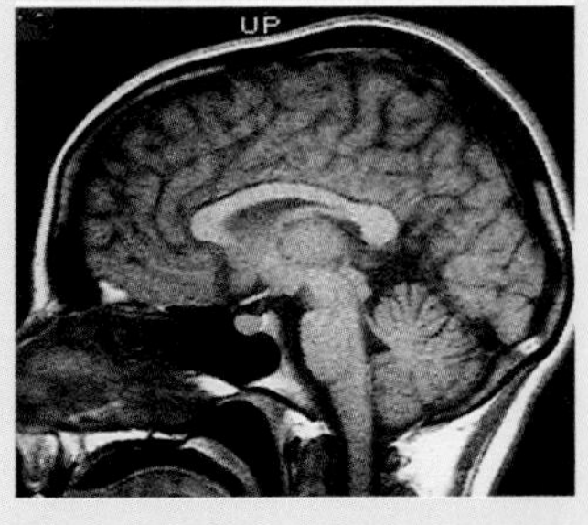

B

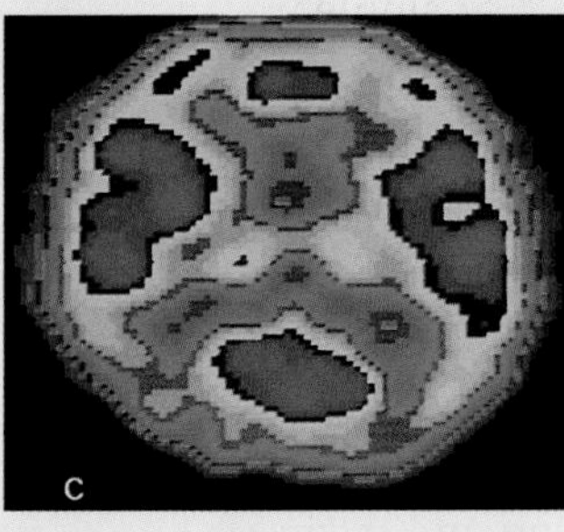

C

Box Figure 1–A Imaging techniques. (**A**) CT scan of eye in lateral view, showing a tumor *(arrow)* below the optic nerve. (**B**) MRI of midsagittal section of head (compare with Figs. 8–6 in Chapter 8 and 15–1 in Chapter 15). (**C**) PET scan of brain in transverse section (frontal lobes at top) showing glucose metabolism. (From Mazziotta, JC, and Gilman, S: Clinical Brain Imaging: Principles and Applications. Philadelphia: FA Davis, 1992, pp 27 and 298, with permission.)

Box 1–3 | WATCHING THE BRAIN AT WORK

Functional magnetic resonance imaging (fMRI) is similar to a PET scan in that it portrays activity within the brain. An fMRI depicts blood flow, and colors to make the gradations of flow distinct are assigned by a computer. An actual fMRI is more of a video than a photograph, and it illustrates physiology and anatomy. In Box Fig. 1–B, each part (A or B) is similar to a

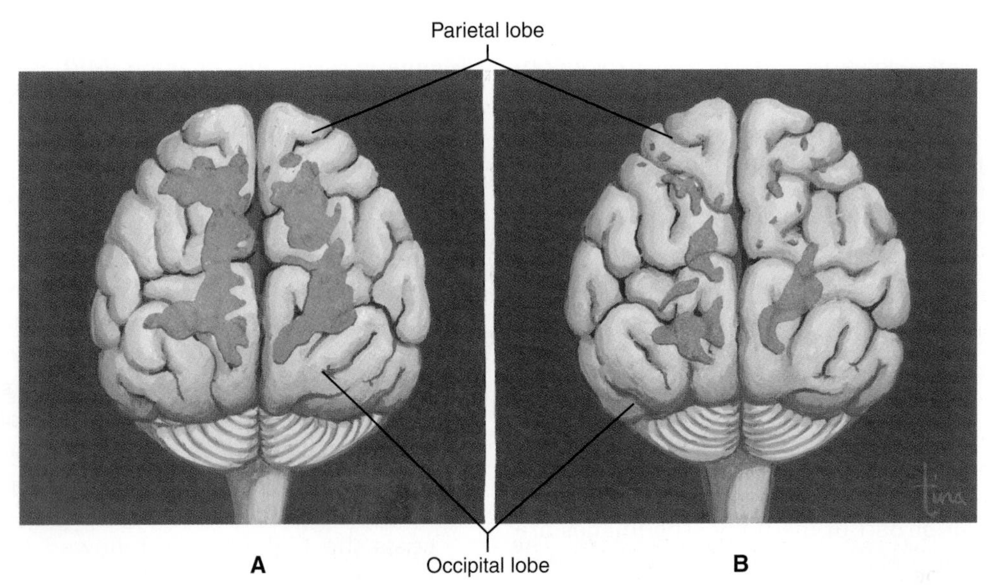

Box Figure 1–B Depiction of a functional MRI, with increased brain activity shown in orange. (**A**) The posterior cerebrum engaged in driving a car. (**B**) The posterior cerebrum, driving and talking on a phone.

Box 1-3 | WATCHING THE BRAIN AT WORK *(Continued)*

"still," or single frame from a movie, and shows what an fMRI would look like in two posterior views of the parietal and occipital lobes of the cerebrum (the pink structure below the occipital lobes is the cerebellum).

Increased brain activity while driving a car (in a simulator) is depicted in part A; this activity is in areas devoted to vision and to analyzing spatial relationships. Part B shows a brain that is driving and talking on a cell phone. You can see that brain activity devoted to driving is diminished. Why might this happen? Because when we talk on a phone we form mental images of the person to whom we are speaking, and we are probably thinking about what we are going to say next. Therefore, those parts of the brain busy with the phone call are not available to look at and analyze the road ahead. Much of driving requires thinking such as "What does what I am seeing mean, and what will I do with that information?" The human brain does best when it focuses on one task; a brain that is distracted by another task is not at all efficient at interpretation or reacting to sudden hazards, and it does neither task well. Evaluations of brain activity such as these can tell us a great deal about how the parts of the brain work together and may also be very useful in the diagnosis or monitoring of certain types of brain damage or disease.

SUMMARY

As you will see, the terminology presented in this chapter is used throughout the text to describe the anatomy of organs and the names of their parts. All organs of the body contribute to homeostasis, the healthy state of the body that is maintained by constant and appropriate responses to internal and external changes. In the chapters that follow, you will find detailed descriptions of the physiology of each organ and organ system, and how the metabolism of each is necessary to homeostasis. We will now return to a consideration of the structural organization of the body and to more extensive descriptions of its levels of organization. The first of these, the chemical level, is the subject of the next chapter.

STUDY OUTLINE

Introduction

1. Anatomy—the study of structure.
2. Physiology—the study of function.
3. Pathophysiology—the study of disorders of functioning.

Levels of Organization

1. Chemical—inorganic and organic chemicals make up all matter, both living and non-living. The body is a container of chemicals.
2. Cells—the smallest living units of the body. The body may be likened to a city of cells.
3. Tissues—groups of cells with similar structure and function.
4. Organs—groups of tissues (a cooperation of tissues) that contribute to specific functions.
5. Organ systems—groups of organs that work together to perform specific functions (see Table 1–1 and Fig. 1–2).
6. Person—all the organ systems functioning properly.
7. The Rest of "Us"—our microbiota, the bacterial population that resides on and inside each human being and contributes to health in many ways, most of which we have yet to discover.

Metabolism and Homeostasis

1. Metabolism is the sum of all of the chemical and physical changes that take place in the body. Metabolic rate is the amount of energy and heat production per unit of time.
2. Homeostasis is a state of good health maintained by the normal metabolism (functioning) of the organ systems.
3. The body constantly responds to internal and external changes yet remains stable; its many aspects of metabolism are kept within normal limits (usually a range of values, not a single value).
4. Negative feedback mechanism—a control system in which a stimulus initiates a response that reverses or reduces the stimulus, thereby stopping the response until the stimulus occurs again and there is a need for the response (see Fig. 1–3).
5. Positive feedback mechanism—a control system that requires an external interruption or brake. Has the potential to become a self-perpetuating and harmful cycle, therefore is rare in the body (see Fig. 1–3).

Terminology and General Plan of the Body

1. Body parts and areas—see Table 1–2 and Fig. 1–4.
2. Terms of location and position—used to describe relationships of position (see Table 1–3 and Figs. 1–4 and 1–5).
3. Body cavities and their membranes (see Fig. 1–5).
   a. Cranial and spinal cavities—within the skull and backbone; lined with membranes called meninges; enclosed by bone to protect the central nervous system.
      - Cranial cavity contains the brain.
      - Spinal (vertebral) cavity contains the spinal cord.

   b. Thoracic, abdominal, and pelvic cavities—within the trunk; the diaphragm separates the thoracic and abdominal cavities; the pelvic cavity is inferior to the abdominal cavity.
      - Thoracic cavity—contains the lungs and heart.
        1) Pleural membranes line the chest wall and cover the lungs.
        2) Pericardial membranes surround the heart.
      - Abdominal cavity—contains many organs including the stomach, liver, and intestines.
        1) The peritoneum lines the abdominal cavity; the mesentery covers the abdominal organs.
      - Pelvic cavity—contains the urinary bladder and reproductive organs.
4. Planes and sections—cutting the body or an organ in a specific way (see Fig. 1–6).
   a. Frontal or coronal—separates front and back parts.
   b. Sagittal—separates right and left parts.
   c. Transverse—separates upper and lower parts.
   d. Cross—a section perpendicular to the long axis.
   e. Longitudinal—a section along the long axis.
5. Areas of the abdomen—permits easier description of locations:
   a. Quadrants—see Fig. 1–7.
   b. Nine areas—see Fig. 1–7.

REVIEW QUESTIONS

1. Explain how the physiology of a bone is related to its anatomy. Explain how the physiology of the hand is related to its anatomy. (p. 4)
2. Describe anatomic position. Why is this knowledge important? (p. 15)
3. Name the organ system that accomplishes each of the following functions: (p. 8)
   a. Moves the skeleton
   b. Regulates body functions by means of hormones
   c. Covers the body and prevents entry of pathogens
   d. Destroys pathogens that enter the body
   e. Exchanges oxygen and carbon dioxide between the air and blood
4. Name the closed body cavities. Name the cavity lined by the peritoneum, meninges, and parietal pleura. (pp. 15–16)
5. Name the four quadrants of the abdomen. Name at least one organ in each quadrant. (pp. 18–19)
6. Name the section through the body that would result in each of the following: equal right and left halves, anterior and posterior parts, superior and inferior parts. (pp. 17–18)
7. Review Table 1–2 and try to find each external area on your own body. (pp. 13–14)
8. Define *cell*. When similar cells work together, what name are they given? (p. 4)
9. Define *organ*. When a group of organs works together, what name is it given? (p. 6)
10. Define *metabolism, metabolic rate,* and *homeostasis.* (p. 11)
    a. Give an example of an external change and explain how the body responds to maintain homeostasis.
    b. Give an example of an internal change and explain how the body responds to maintain homeostasis.
    c. Briefly explain how a negative feedback mechanism works and how a positive feedback mechanism differs.

FOR FURTHER THOUGHT

1. The human foot is similar to the human hand, but it does have anatomic differences. Describe two of these differences, and explain how they are related to the physiology of the hand and the foot.
2. If a person has appendicitis (inflammation of the appendix caused by bacteria), pain is felt in which abdominal quadrant? (If you're not sure, take a look at Fig. 16–1 in Chapter 16.) Surgery is usually necessary to remove an inflamed appendix before it ruptures and causes peritonitis. Using your knowledge of the location of the peritoneum, explain why peritonitis is a very serious condition.
3. Keep in mind your answer to Question 3, and explain why bacterial meningitis can be a very serious infection.
4. Use a mental picture to cut the following sections. Then describe in simple words what each section looks like, and give each a proper anatomic name.

   First: a tree trunk cut top to bottom, then cut side to side.

   Second: a grapefruit cut top to bottom (straight down from where the stem was attached), then sliced through its equator.
5. Look at Question Figure 1–A. This is a transverse section through the middle of the right upper arm; the front of the arm is at the top of the picture, away from you, oriented the same way you would see your own right arm. Can you name the labeled structures? Need help? Go back to the section *Body Parts and Areas* or look ahead to Fig. 7–11 in Chapter 7.

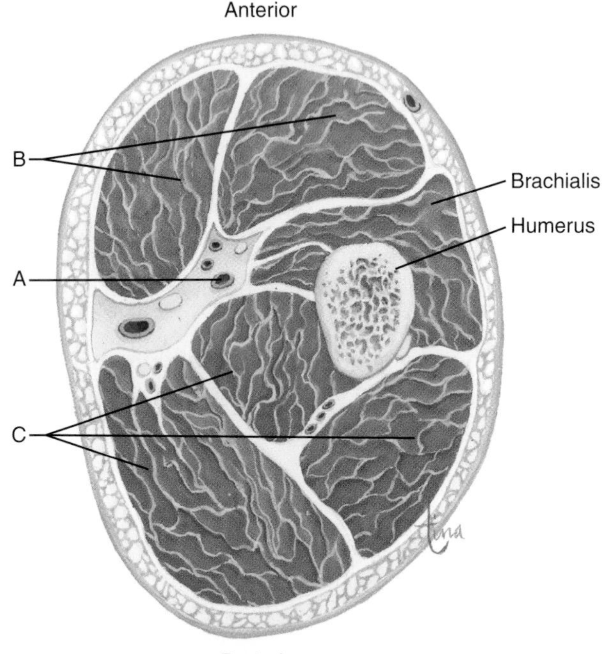

QUESTION FIGURE 1–A: A midtransverse section of right upper arm.

6. Question Figure 1–B is a schematic representation of the interdependency of several of the body's organ systems depicted in a rectangular organism. The lettered arrows represent interactions of the body with the environment. The number arrows represent internal interactions. Label each arrow with what is moving.

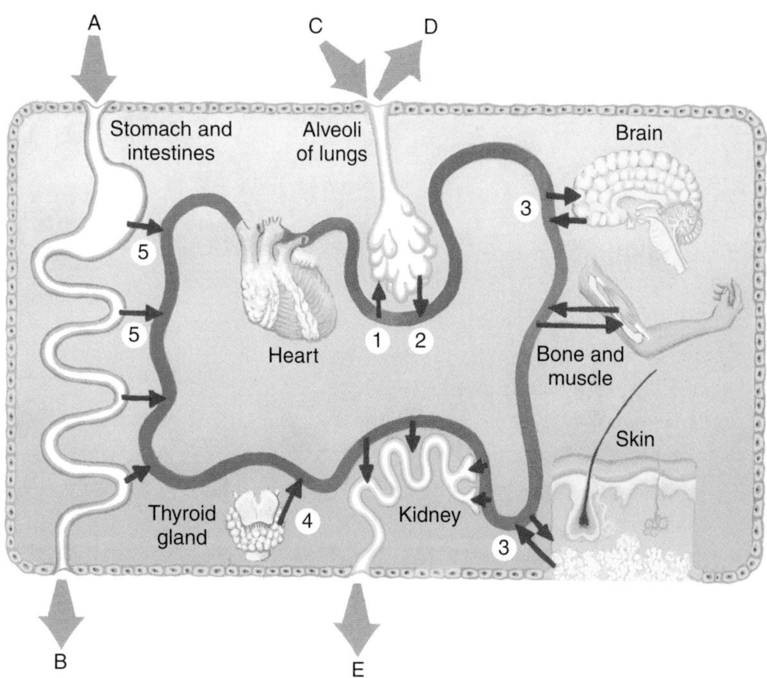

QUESTION FIGURE 1–B: Relationships of organ systems.

CHAPTER

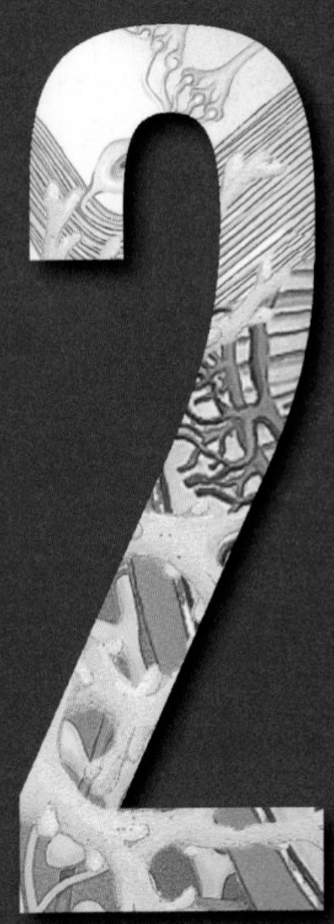

Some Basic Chemistry

STUDENT OBJECTIVES

- Define the terms *element, atom, proton, neutron,* and *electron.*
- Describe the formation and purpose of ionic bonds, covalent bonds, disulfide bonds, and hydrogen bonds.
- Describe what happens in synthesis and decomposition reactions.
- Explain the importance of water to the functioning of the human body.
- Name and describe the water compartments.
- Explain the roles of oxygen and carbon dioxide in cell respiration.
- State what trace elements are and name some, with their functions.
- Explain the pH scale. State the normal pH ranges of body fluids.
- Explain how a buffer system limits great changes in pH.
- Describe the functions of monosaccharides, disaccharides, oligosaccharides, and polysaccharides.
- Describe the functions of true fats, phospholipids, and steroids.
- Describe the functions of proteins, and explain how enzymes function as catalysts.
- Describe the functions of DNA, RNA, and ATP.

NEW TERMINOLOGY

Acid *(**ASS**-sid)*
Amino acid *(ah-**MEE**-noh **ASS**-sid)*
Atom *(**A**-tum)*
Base *(BAYSE)*
Buffer system *(**BUFF**-er **SIS**-tem)*
Carbohydrates *(KAR-boh-**HIGH**-drayts)*
Catalyst *(**KAT**-ah-list)*
Cell respiration *(SELL RES-pi-**RAY**-shun)*
Covalent bond *(ko-**VAY**-lent)*
Dissociation/ionization *(dih-SOH-see-**AY**-shun/EYE-uh-nih-**ZAY**-shun)*
Element *(**EL**-uh-ment)*
Enzyme *(**EN**-zime)*
Extracellular fluid *(EKS-trah-**SELL**-yoo-ler)*
Intracellular fluid *(IN-trah-**SELL**-yoo-ler)*
Ion *(**EYE**-on)*
Ionic bond *(eye-**ON**-ik)*
Lipids *(**LIP**-ids)*
Matter *(**MAT**-ter)*
Molecule *(**MAHL**-e-kuhl)*
Nucleic acids *(new-**KLEE**-ik **ASS**-sids)*
pH and pH scale *(pee-H SKALE)*
Protein *(**PROH**-teen)*
Salt *(SAWLT)*
Solvent/solution *(**SAHL**-vent/suh-**LOO**-shun)*
Steroid *(**STEER**-oyd)*
Theory *(**THEER**-ree)*
Trace elements *(TRAYSE **EL**-uh-ments)*

RELATED CLINICAL TERMINOLOGY

Acidosis *(ASS-i-**DOH**-sis)*
Atherosclerosis *(ATH-er-oh-skle-**ROH**-sis)*
Hypoxia *(high-**POK**-see-ah)*
Saturated *(**SAT**-uhr-ay-ted)*
Unsaturated *(un-**SAT**-uhr-ay-ted)*

*Terms that appear in **bold type** in the chapter text are defined in the glossary, which begins on page 603.*

CHAPTER OUTLINE

When you hear or see the word "chemistry," you may think of test tubes and beakers in a laboratory experiment. For our study of the human body, however, let us think of our laboratory as a kitchen with pots and pans and good food simmering on the stove or baking in the oven. The scents of that food are carried in the air, which is a mixture of gaseous chemicals that we inhale and exhale. The pots and pans, as well as the paper of a cookbook (once the wood of a tree), are solid chemicals. Water is a liquid chemical, and all of our foods are chemicals. Recall from Chapter 1 that the simplest level of organization is the chemical level. Our bodies are complex arrangements of thousands of chemicals. Where do we obtain new chemicals to make new body parts or supply energy? That's right: from food. Good cooking is a science and as an art. And eating? It's all chemistry.

This chapter covers some very basic aspects of chemistry as they are related to living organisms and most especially as they are related to our understanding of the human body. So try to think of chemistry not as a complicated science, but as the air, water, and food we need, and every substance that is part of us. Before we get to food groups, however, we must begin with the fundamentals of chemical structure: the atoms of elements and the bonds that hold them together.

ELEMENTS

All **matter**, both living and not living, is made of elements, the simplest chemicals. An **element** is a substance made of only one type of atom (therefore, an atom is the smallest part of an element). There are 92 naturally occurring elements in the world around us. Examples are hydrogen (H), iron (Fe), oxygen (O), calcium (Ca), nitrogen (N), and carbon (C). In nature, an element does not usually exist by itself but rather combines with the atoms of other elements to form compounds. Examples of some compounds important to our study of the human body are water (H_2O), in which two atoms of hydrogen combine with one atom of oxygen; carbon dioxide (CO_2), in which an atom of carbon combines with two atoms of oxygen; and glucose ($C_6H_{12}O_6$), in which six carbon atoms and six oxygen atoms combine with 12 hydrogen atoms.

The elements carbon, hydrogen, oxygen, nitrogen, phosphorus, and sulfur are found in all living things. If calcium is included, these seven elements make up approximately 99% of the human body (weight).

More than 20 different elements are found, in varying amounts, in the human body. Some of these are listed in Table 2–1. As you can see, each element has a standard chemical symbol. This is simply the first (and sometimes the second) letter of the element's English or Latin name. You should know the symbols of the elements in this table because they are used in textbooks, articles, hospital lab reports, and so on. Notice that if a two-letter symbol is used for an element, the second letter is always lowercase, not a capital. For example, the symbol for calcium is Ca, not CA. CA is an abbreviation often used for cancer.

Table 2–1 | **ELEMENTS IN THE HUMAN BODY**

ELEMENTS	SYMBOL	ATOMIC NUMBER*	PERCENT OF THE BODY BY WEIGHT
Hydrogen	H	1	9.5
Carbon	C	6	18.5
Nitrogen	N	7	3.3
Oxygen	O	8	65.0
Fluorine	F	9	Trace
Sodium	Na	11	0.2
Magnesium	Mg	12	0.1
Phosphorus	P	15	1.0
Sulfur	S	16	0.3
Chlorine	Cl	17	0.2
Potassium	K	19	0.4
Calcium	Ca	20	1.5
Manganese	Mn	25	Trace
Iron	Fe	26	Trace
Cobalt	Co	27	Trace
Copper	Cu	29	Trace
Zinc	Zn	30	Trace
Iodine	I	53	Trace

*Atomic number is the number of protons in the nucleus of the atom. It is also the number of electrons that orbit the nucleus.

ATOMS

Atoms are the smallest parts of an element that have the characteristics of that element. An atom consists of three major subunits or particles: protons, neutrons, and electrons (Fig. 2–1). A **proton** has a positive electrical charge and is found in the nucleus (or center) of the atom. A **neutron** is electrically neutral (has no charge) and is also found in the nucleus. An **electron** has a negative electrical charge and is found outside the nucleus orbiting in what may be called an electron cloud or shell around the nucleus.

The number of protons in an atom gives it its **atomic number**. Protons and neutrons have mass and weight; they give an atom its **atomic weight**. In an atom, the number of protons (+) equals the number of electrons (−); therefore, an atom is electrically neutral. The electrons, however, are important in that they may enable an atom to connect or **bond** to other atoms to form **molecules**. A molecule is a combination of atoms (usually of more than one element) that are so tightly bound together that the molecule behaves as a single unit.

Each atom is capable of bonding in only very specific ways. This capability depends on the number and the arrangement of the electrons of the atom. Electrons orbit the nucleus of an atom in shells or **energy levels**. The first, or innermost, energy level can contain a maximum of two electrons and is then considered stable. The second energy level is stable when it contains its maximum of eight electrons. The remaining energy levels, more distant from the nucleus, are also most stable when they contain eight electrons, or a multiple of eight.

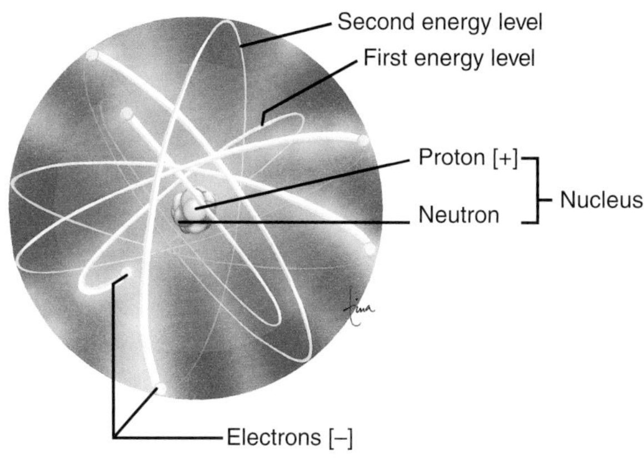

Figure 2–1 An atom of carbon. The nucleus contains six protons and six neutrons (not all are visible here). Six electrons orbit the nucleus, two in the first energy level and four in the second energy level.

QUESTION: What is the electrical charge of this atom as a whole?

A few atoms (elements) are naturally stable, or uninterested in reacting, because their outermost energy level already contains the maximum number of electrons. The gases helium and neon are examples of these stable atoms, which do not usually react with other atoms. Most atoms are not stable, however, and tend to gain, lose, or share electrons in order to fill their outermost shell. By doing so, an atom is capable of forming one or more chemical bonds with other atoms. In this way, the atom becomes stable because its outermost shell of electrons has been filled. It is these reactive atoms that are of highest interest in our study of anatomy and physiology.

CHEMICAL BONDS

A chemical bond is not a structure, but rather a force or attraction between positive and negative electrical charges. A chemical bond keeps two or more atoms closely associated with each other to form a molecule. By way of comparison, think of gravity. We know that gravity is not a "thing," but rather the force that keeps our feet on the floor and allows us to pour coffee with consistent success. Molecules formed by chemical bonding often have physical characteristics different from those of the atoms of the original elements. For example, the elements hydrogen and oxygen are gases, but atoms of each may chemically bond to form molecules of water, which is a liquid.

The type of chemical bonding depends on the tendencies of the electrons of atoms involved, as you will see. Four kinds of bonds are very important to the chemistry of the body: ionic bonds, covalent bonds, disulfide bonds, and hydrogen bonds.

IONIC BONDS

An **ionic bond** involves the loss of one or more electrons by one atom and the gain of the electron(s) by another atom or atoms. Refer to Fig. 2–2 as you read the following.

An atom of sodium (Na) has one electron in its outermost shell, and, in order to become stable, it tends to lose that electron. When it does so, the sodium atom has one more proton than it has electrons. Therefore, it now has an electrical charge (or **valence**) of +1 and is called a sodium **ion** (Na^+). An atom of chlorine has seven electrons in its outermost shell, and in order to become stable it tends to gain one electron. When it does so, the chlorine atom has one more electron than it has protons and now has a charge (valence) of −1. It is called a chloride ion (Cl^-).

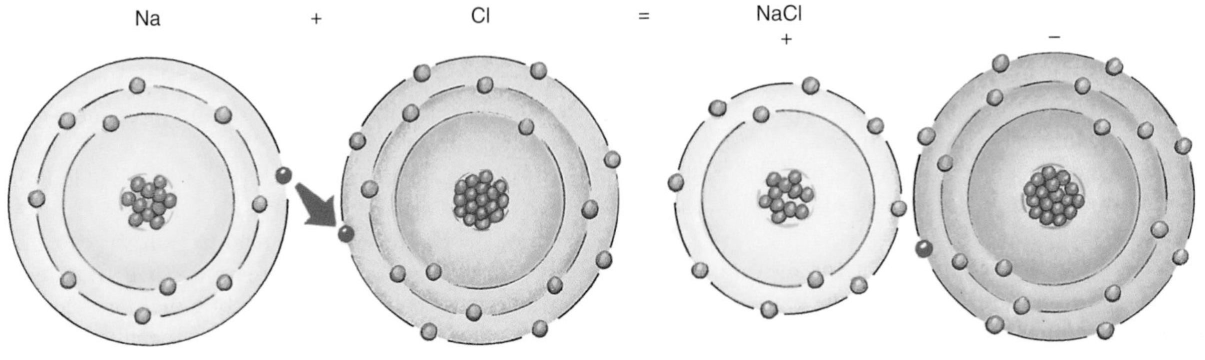

Figure 2–2 Formation of an ionic bond. An atom of sodium loses an electron to an atom of chlorine. The two ions formed have unlike charges, are attracted to one another, and form a molecule of sodium chloride.

QUESTION: Why is the charge of a sodium ion +1?

When an atom of sodium loses an electron to an atom of chlorine, their ions have unlike charges (positive and negative) and are thus attracted to one another. The result is the formation of a molecule of sodium chloride: NaCl, or common table salt. The bond that holds these ions together is called an ionic bond.

Another example is the bonding of chlorine to calcium. An atom of calcium has two electrons in its outermost shell and tends to lose those electrons in order to become stable (a calcium ion, Ca^{+2}). If two atoms of chlorine each gain one of those electrons, they become chloride ions. The positive and negative ions are then attracted to one another, forming a molecule of calcium chloride, $CaCl_2$, which is also a salt. A **salt** is a molecule made of ions other than hydrogen (H^+) ions or hydroxyl (OH^-) ions.

Ions with positive charges are called **cations**. These include Na^+, Ca^{+2}, K^+, Fe^{+2}, and Mg^{+2}. Ions with negative charges are called **anions**, which include Cl^-, SO_4^{-2} (sulfate), and HCO_3^- (bicarbonate). The types of compounds formed by ionic bonding are inorganic salts, acids, and bases. (Acids and bases are discussed later in this chapter.)

In the solid state, ionic bonds are relatively strong. Our bones, for example, contain the salt calcium carbonate ($CaCO_3$), which helps give bone its strength. In an **aqueous** (water) **solution**, however, many ionic bonds are weakened. The bonds may become so weak that the bound ions of a molecule separate, creating a solution of free positive and negative ions. For example, if sodium chloride is put in water, it dissolves and then **ionizes**. The water now contains Na^+ ions and Cl^- ions. Ionization, also called **dissociation**, is important to living organisms because the ions produced are free to take part in other chemical reactions within the body. Cells in the stomach lining must have Cl^- ions to produce hydrochloric acid (HCl). The chloride in NaCl would not be free to take part in another reaction because it is tightly bound to the sodium atom. However, the Cl^- ions available from ionized NaCl in the cellular water can be used for the **synthesis**, or chemical manufacture, of HCl in the stomach.

COVALENT BONDS

Covalent bonds involve the sharing of electrons between atoms. As shown in Fig. 2–3, an atom of oxygen needs two electrons to become stable. It may share two of its electrons with another atom of oxygen, also sharing two electrons. Together they form a molecule of oxygen gas (O_2), which is the form in which oxygen exists in the atmosphere.

An atom of oxygen may also share two of its electrons with two atoms of hydrogen, each sharing its single electron (see Fig. 2–3). Together they form a molecule of water (H_2O). When writing structural formulas for chemical molecules, a pair of shared electrons is indicated by a single line, as shown in Fig. 2–3, the formula for water; this is a single covalent bond. A double covalent bond is indicated by two lines, as in the formula for oxygen; this represents two pairs of shared electrons.

The element carbon always forms covalent bonds; an atom of carbon has four electrons to share with other atoms. If these four electrons are shared with four atoms

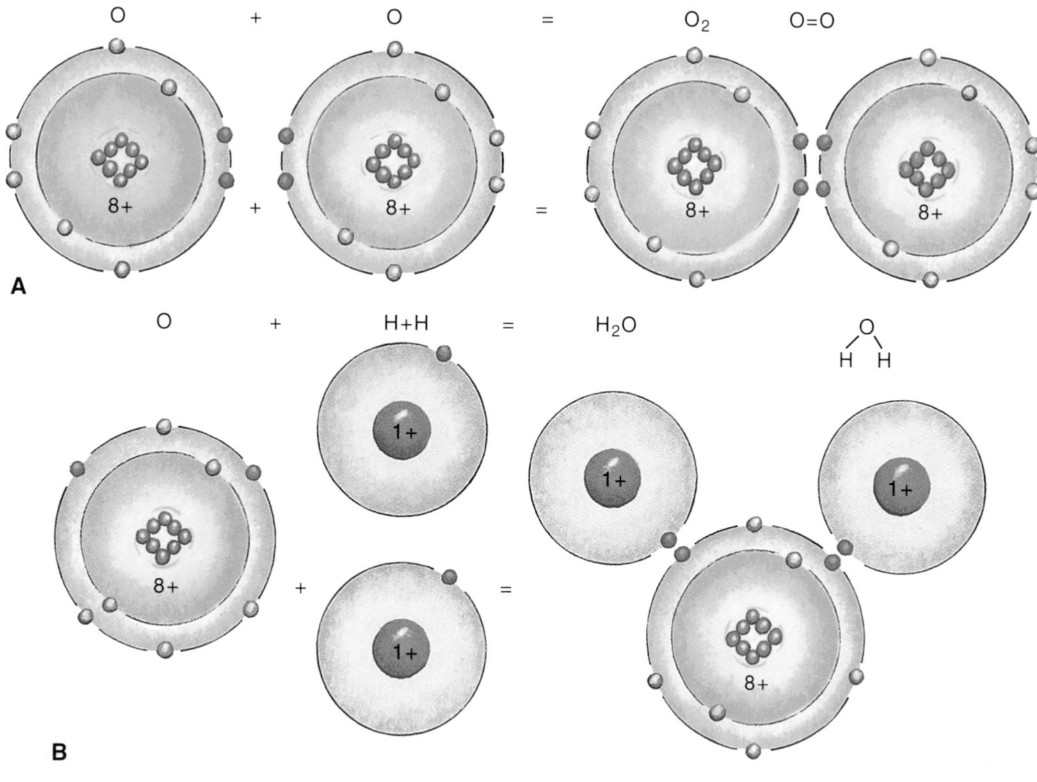

Figure 2–3 Formation of covalent bonds. (**A**) Two atoms of oxygen share two electrons each, forming a molecule of oxygen gas. (**B**) An atom of oxygen shares one electron with each of two hydrogen atoms, each sharing its electron. A molecule of water is formed.

QUESTION: Which of the bonds shown here is a double covalent bond?

of hydrogen, each sharing its one electron, a molecule of methane gas (CH_4) is formed. Carbon may form covalent bonds with other carbons, hydrogen, oxygen, nitrogen, or other elements. Organic compounds such as proteins and carbohydrates are complex and precise arrangements of these atoms, covalently bonded to one another. Covalent bonds are relatively strong and are not weakened in an aqueous solution. This is important because the proteins produced by the body, in muscle and skin, for example, must remain intact in order to function properly in the water of our cells and blood. The functions of organic compounds will be considered later in this chapter.

DISULFIDE BONDS AND HYDROGEN BONDS

Two other types of bonds that are important to the chemistry of the body are disulfide bonds and hydrogen bonds. Disulfide bonds are found in some proteins. Hydrogen bonds are part of many different molecules.

A **disulfide bond** (also called a disulfide bridge) is a covalent bond formed between two atoms of sulfur, usually within the same large protein molecule. The hormone insulin, for example, is a protein that must have a very specific three-dimensional shape in order to function properly to regulate the blood glucose level. Each molecule of insulin has two disulfide bonds that help maintain its proper shape and function (see Box Fig. 10–A in Chapter 10). Other proteins with shapes that depend upon disulfide bonds are antibodies of the immune system (see Fig. 14–8 in Chapter 14) and keratin of the skin and hair.

A strand of hair maintains its shape (a genetic characteristic) because of disulfide bonds. When naturally curly hair is straightened, the disulfide bonds in the keratin molecules are broken. When naturally straight hair is "permed" or curled, the disulfide bonds in the keratin are first broken, then re-formed in the curled hair. Neither process affects the living part of the hair, the hair root, so the hair will grow out in its original shape. We would not want such a process affecting our insulin or antibody molecules, for that would destroy their functioning.

A **hydrogen bond** does not involve the sharing or exchange of electrons, but rather results from a property of hydrogen atoms. When a hydrogen atom shares its one electron in a covalent bond with another atom, its proton has a slight positive charge and may then be attracted to a nearby oxygen or nitrogen atom, which has a slight negative charge.

Although they are weak bonds, hydrogen bonds are important in several ways. Large organic molecules such as proteins and the DNA in our chromosomes have very specific functions that depend upon their three-dimensional shapes (see Fig. 2–10). The shapes of these molecules, so crucial to their proper functioning, are often maintained by hydrogen bonds.

Hydrogen bonds also make water cohesive. **Cohesion** is the tendency of similar molecules to "stick to" one another. In a glass of water, for example, each water molecule is attracted to nearby water molecules. One water molecule forms up to four hydrogen bonds, one with each of four other water molecules. Each of those four molecules can form four hydrogen bonds, and so on, making all of the water cohesive. Water can also be adhesive with other molecules. **Adhesion** is the tendency of unlike molecules to be attracted to one another. Both the cohesion and adhesion of water molecules is what keeps the grains of a sand castle together. The cohesiveness of water itself can be seen if water is dropped onto clean glass; the surface tension created by the hydrogen bonds makes the water form three-dimensional beads. Within the body, the cohesiveness of water helps keep blood a continuous stream as it flows within the blood vessels and also keeps tissue fluid continuous around cells. These hydrogen bonds are also responsible for the other important characteristics of water, which are discussed in a later section.

CHEMICAL REACTIONS

A chemical reaction is a change brought about by the formation or breaking of chemical bonds. Two general types of reactions are synthesis reactions and decomposition reactions.

In a **synthesis reaction**, bonds are formed to join two or more atoms or molecules to make a new compound. The production of the protein hemoglobin in potential red blood cells is an example of a synthesis reaction. Proteins are synthesized by the bonding of many amino acids, their smaller subunits. Synthesis reactions require energy for the formation of bonds.

In a **decomposition reaction**, bonds are broken, and a large molecule is changed to two or more smaller ones. One example is the digestion of large molecules of starch into many smaller glucose molecules. Some decomposition reactions release energy; this is described in a later section on cell respiration.

Within cells, synthesis is often coupled with decomposition. When membranes or other cell parts break down, they must be replaced. The old or damaged structures may be recycled for their smaller parts or subunits. These parts can be minerals (such as iron) or organic molecules (such as amino acids) and can be used in subsequent synthesis reactions. When older hemoglobin breaks down, for example, its iron can be used over and over to synthesize new hemoglobin for red blood cells (this will be covered in Chapter 11).

In this and future chapters, keep in mind that the term *reaction* refers to the making or breaking of chemical bonds and thus to changes in the physical and chemical characteristics of the molecules involved.

INORGANIC COMPOUNDS OF IMPORTANCE

Inorganic compounds are usually simple molecules that often consist of only one or two different elements. Despite their simplicity, however, some inorganic compounds are essential to normal structure and functioning of the body.

WATER

Water makes up 55% to 70% of the human body and is essential to life for several reasons:

1. *Water is a **solvent**;* that is, many substances (called solutes) can dissolve in water. Nutrients such as glucose are dissolved in blood plasma (which is largely water) to be transported to cells throughout the body. The excretion of waste products is possible because the products are dissolved in the water of urine produced by the kidneys. The senses that enable us to enjoy our food, taste and smell, both depend upon the solvent ability of water. Food molecules dissolved in saliva stimulate receptors in taste buds on the tongue. Vaporized food molecules

(especially from hot foods) are sniffed into the upper nasal cavities, where they dissolve in the thin film of water and stimulate olfactory receptors. Hot foods often seem more tasty than cold foods because the sense of smell contributes more to our perception of them.

2. *Water is a lubricant*, which prevents friction where surfaces meet and move. In the digestive tract, swallowing depends on the presence of saliva, and mucus is a slippery fluid that permits the smooth passage of food through the intestines. Synovial fluid within joint cavities prevents friction as bones move.
3. *Water changes temperature slowly.* Water has a high heat capacity, which means that it will absorb a great deal of heat before its temperature rises significantly, or it must lose a great deal of heat before its temperature drops significantly. This is one of the factors that helps the body maintain a constant temperature. Water also has a high heat of vaporization, the heat needed to change water from a liquid to a gas. This is important for the process of sweating. Excess body heat evaporates sweat on skin surfaces, rather than overheating the body's cells, and because of water's high heat of vaporization, a great deal of heat can be given off with the loss of a relatively small amount of water.

WATER COMPARTMENTS

All water within the body is continually moving, but water is given different names when it is in specific body locations, which are called compartments (Fig. 2–4):

Intracellular fluid (ICF)—the water within cells; about 65% of the total body water

Extracellular fluid (ECF)—all the rest of the water in the body; about 35% of the total. More specific compartments of extracellular fluid include the following:

- **Plasma**—water found in blood vessels
- **Lymph**—water found in lymphatic vessels
- **Tissue fluid or interstitial fluid**—water found in the small spaces between cells
- **Specialized fluids**—synovial fluid in joints, cerebrospinal fluid around the brain and spinal cord, aqueous humor in the eye, and others

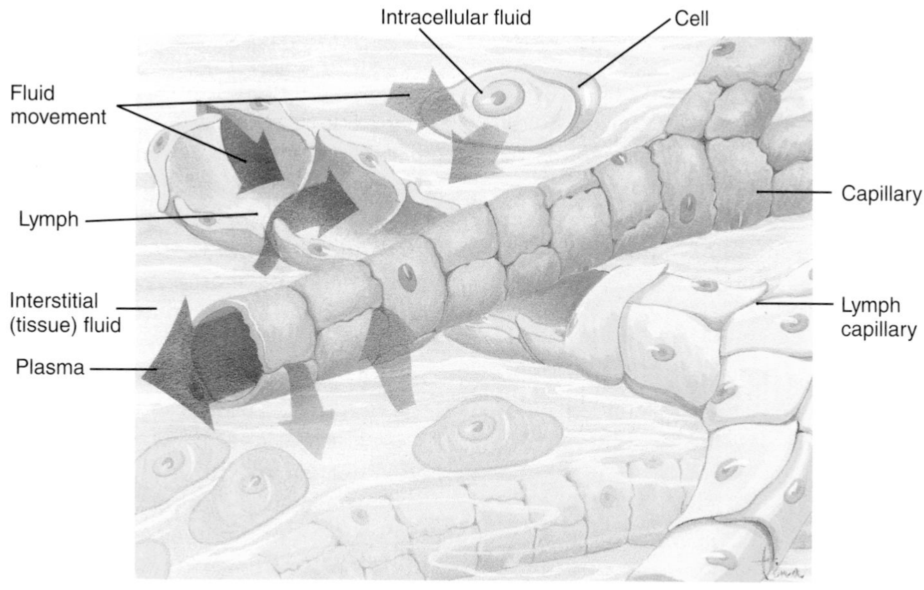

Figure 2–4 Water compartments, showing the names that water is given in its different locations and the ways in which water moves between compartments.

QUESTION: Which of the fluids shown are extracellular fluids?

The movement of water between compartments in the body and the functions of the specialized fluids will be discussed in later chapters.

OXYGEN

Oxygen in the form of a gas (O_2) is approximately 21% of the atmosphere, which we inhale. We all know that without oxygen we wouldn't survive very long, but exactly what does oxygen do? Oxygen is important to us because it is essential for a process called cell respiration, in which cells break down simple nutrients such as glucose in order to release energy. The reason we breathe is to obtain oxygen for cell respiration and to exhale the carbon dioxide produced in cell respiration (this will be discussed in the next section). Biologically useful energy that is released by the reactions of cell respiration is trapped in a molecule called ATP (adenosine triphosphate). ATP can then be used for cellular processes that require energy.

CARBON DIOXIDE

Carbon dioxide (CO_2) is produced by cells as a waste product of cell respiration. You may ask why a waste product is considered important. Keep in mind that "important" does not always mean "beneficial"; instead, it can mean "significant." If the amount of carbon dioxide in the body fluids increases, it causes these fluids to become too acidic. Therefore, carbon dioxide must be exhaled as rapidly as it is formed to keep the amount in the body within normal limits. Normally this is just what happens, but severe pulmonary diseases such as pneumonia or emphysema decrease gas exchange in the lungs, resulting in the accumulation of carbon dioxide in the blood. When this happens, a person is said to be in a state of **acidosis**, which may seriously disrupt body functioning (see the sections on pH and enzymes later in this chapter; see also Box 2–1: Blood Gases).

CELL RESPIRATION

Cell respiration is the name for energy production within cells and involves both respiratory gases, oxygen and carbon dioxide. Many chemical reactions are involved, some of which take place in cell organelles called **mitochondria**. In its simplest form, cell respiration may be summarized by the following equation:

$$\text{Glucose } (C_6H_{12}O_6) + 6O_2 \rightarrow 6CO_2 + 6H_2O + \text{ATP} + \text{heat}$$

Box 2–1 | BLOOD GASES

A patient is admitted to the emergency department with a possible heart attack, and the doctor in charge orders "blood gases." Another patient hospitalized with pneumonia has "blood gases" monitored at frequent intervals. What are blood gases, and what does measurement of them tell us? The blood gases are oxygen and carbon dioxide, and their levels in arterial blood provide information about the functioning of the respiratory and circulatory systems. Arterial blood normally has a high concentration of oxygen and a low concentration of carbon dioxide. These levels are maintained by gas exchange in the lungs and by the proper circulation of blood.

A pulmonary disease such as pneumonia interferes with efficient gas exchange in the lungs. As a result, blood oxygen concentration may decrease, and blood carbon dioxide concentration may increase. Either of these changes in blood gases may become life threatening for the patient, so monitoring of blood gases is important. If blood oxygen falls below the normal range, oxygen will be administered; if blood carbon dioxide rises above the normal range, blood pH will be corrected to prevent serious acidosis.

Damage to the heart may also bring about a change in blood gases, especially oxygen. Oxygen is picked up by red blood cells as they circulate through lung capillaries; as red blood cells circulate through the body, they release oxygen to tissues. What keeps the blood circulating or moving? The pumping of the heart.

A mild heart attack, when heart failure is unlikely, is often characterized by a blood oxygen level that is low but still within normal limits. A more severe heart attack that seriously impairs the pumping of the heart will decrease the blood oxygen level to less than normal; this is called **hypoxemia**. A consequence is **hypoxia**, which means that too little oxygen is reaching tissues. When this is determined by measurement of blood gases, appropriate oxygen therapy can be started to correct the hypoxia and prevent tissue death.

This reaction shows us that glucose and oxygen combine to yield carbon dioxide, water, ATP, and heat. Food, represented here by glucose, in the presence of oxygen is broken down into the simpler molecules carbon dioxide and water. The potential energy in the glucose molecule is released in two forms: ATP and heat. Each of the four products of this process has a purpose or significance in the body. The carbon dioxide is a waste product that moves from the cells into the blood, which carries it to the lungs where it is eventually exhaled. The water formed is useful and becomes part of the intracellular fluid. The heat produced contributes to normal body temperature. ATP is used for cell processes such as mitosis, protein synthesis, and muscle contraction, all of which require energy and will be discussed a bit further on in the text.

We will also return to cell respiration in later chapters and to mitochondria in Chapter 3. For now, the brief description just given will suffice to show that eating and breathing are interrelated; both are essential for energy production.

TRACE ELEMENTS

Trace elements are those that are needed by the body in very small amounts. When they are present in food or nutritional supplements, we often call them minerals. Examples are iron (found in meat and legumes), cobalt (found only in animal foods such as liver and fish), magnesium (found in green vegetables because it is part of chlorophyll), and iodine (found in seafood and iodized salt). Although trace elements may not be as abundant in the body as carbon, hydrogen, and oxygen, they are nonetheless essential. Table 2–2 lists some of these trace elements and their functions. Calcium and phosphorus (found in milk, cheese, meat, and fish) are included in this table, though they are needed in somewhat larger amounts than are the others. (See also Box 2–2: Nitric Oxide.)

ACIDS, BASES, AND PH

An **acid** may be defined as a substance that increases the concentration of hydrogen ions (H^+) in a water solution. A **base** is a substance that decreases the concentration of H^+ ions, which, in the case of water, has the same effect as increasing the concentration of hydroxyl ions (OH^-).

The acidity or alkalinity (basicity) of a solution is measured on a scale of values called **pH** (parts hydrogen). The values on the **pH scale** range from 0 to 14, with 0 indicating the most acidic level and 14 the most alkaline. A solution with a pH of 7 is neutral because it

Table 2–2 | TRACE ELEMENTS

ELEMENT	FUNCTION
Calcium	■ Provides strength in bones and teeth ■ Necessary for blood clotting ■ Necessary for muscle contraction
Phosphorus	■ Provides strength in bones and teeth ■ Part of DNA, RNA, and ATP ■ Part of cell membranes in phospholipids
Iron	■ Part of hemoglobin in red blood cells; transports oxygen ■ Part of myoglobin in muscles; stores oxygen ■ Part of mitochondria in cells; necessary for cell respiration
Copper	■ Part of mitochondria in cells; necessary for cell respiration ■ Necessary for hemoglobin synthesis
Magnesium	■ Necessary for energy production and bone formation
Sodium and potassium	■ Necessary for muscle contraction and nerve impulse transmission ■ Necessary for proper movement of water (osmosis) among its compartments
Sulfur	■ Part of some proteins such as insulin, keratin, and antibodies
Cobalt	■ Part of vitamin B_{12}
Iodine	■ Part of thyroid hormones (thyroxine); essential for normal mental and physical development

Box 2–2 | NITRIC OXIDE

Nitric oxide is a gas with the molecular formula NO (N=O, a double covalent bond). You have probably heard of it as a component of air pollution and cigarette smoke, but it is synthesized by several human tissues, and this deceptively simple molecule has important functions.

Nitric oxide is produced by the endothelium (lining) of blood vessels and promotes vasodilation of arterioles, permitting greater blood flow and oxygen delivery to tissues. It is involved in nerve impulse transmission in the brain, and it may contribute to memory storage. Some immune system cells produce nitric oxide as a cytotoxic (cell-poisoning) agent to help destroy foreign cells such as bacteria.

Nitric oxide is also being used therapeutically. It has been found useful in the treatment of pulmonary hypertension to relax abnormally constricted arteries in the lungs to permit normal gas exchange. Other studies show that nitric oxide helps some premature babies breathe more easily and efficiently. With short-term treatment, serious side effects have not yet been found.

contains the same number of H^+ ions and OH^- ions. Pure water has a pH of 7. A solution with a higher concentration of H^+ ions than OH^- ions is an acidic solution with a pH below 7. An alkaline solution, therefore, has a higher concentration of OH^- ions than H^+ ions and has a pH above 7.

The pH scale, with the relative concentrations of H^+ ions and OH^- ions, is shown in Fig. 2–5. A change of one pH unit is a 10-fold change in H^+ ion concentration. This means that a solution with a pH of 4 has 10 times as many H^+ ions as a solution with a pH of 5 and 100 times as many H^+ ions as a solution with a pH of 6. Figure 2–5 also shows the pH of some body fluids and other familiar solutions. Notice that gastric juice has a pH of 1 and coffee has a pH of 5. This means that gastric juice has 10,000 times as many H^+ ions as coffee has. Although coffee is acidic, it is a weak acid and does not have the corrosive effect of gastric juice, a strong acid.

The cells and internal fluids of the human body have a pH close to neutral. The pH of intracellular fluid is around 6.8 to 7.0, and the normal pH range of blood is 7.35 to 7.45. Fluids such as gastric juice and urine are technically external fluids because they are in body tracts that open to the environment. The pH of these fluids may be more strongly acidic or alkaline without harm to the body.

The pH of blood, however, must be maintained within its very narrow, slightly alkaline range. A decrease of only one pH unit, which is 10 times as many H^+ ions, would disrupt the chemical reactions of the blood and cause the death of the individual. Normal metabolism tends to make body fluids more acidic, and this tendency to acidosis must be continually corrected. Normal pH of internal fluids is maintained by the kidneys, respiratory system, and buffer systems. Although acid–base balance will be a major topic of Chapter 19, we will briefly mention buffer systems here.

Buffer Systems

A **buffer system** is a chemical or pair of chemicals that minimizes changes in pH by reacting with strong acids or strong bases to transform them into substances that will not drastically change pH. Expressed in another way, a buffer may bond to H^+ ions when a body fluid is becoming too acidic, or release H^+ ions when a fluid is becoming too alkaline.

We will use the bicarbonate buffer system as a specific example. This system consists of carbonic acid (H_2CO_3), a weak acid, and sodium bicarbonate ($NaHCO_3$), a weak base. This pair of chemicals is present in all body fluids but is especially important to buffer blood and tissue fluid.

Carbonic acid ionizes as follows (but remember, because it is a weak acid it does not contribute many H^+ ions to a solution):

$$H_2CO_3 \rightarrow H^+ + HCO_3^-$$

Sodium bicarbonate ionizes as follows:

$$NaHCO_3 \rightarrow Na^+ + HCO_3^-$$

If a strong acid, such as HCl, is added to extracellular fluid, the following reaction will occur:

$$HCl + NaHCO_3 \rightarrow NaCl + H_2CO_3$$

What has happened here? Hydrochloric acid, a strong acid that would greatly lower pH, has reacted with sodium

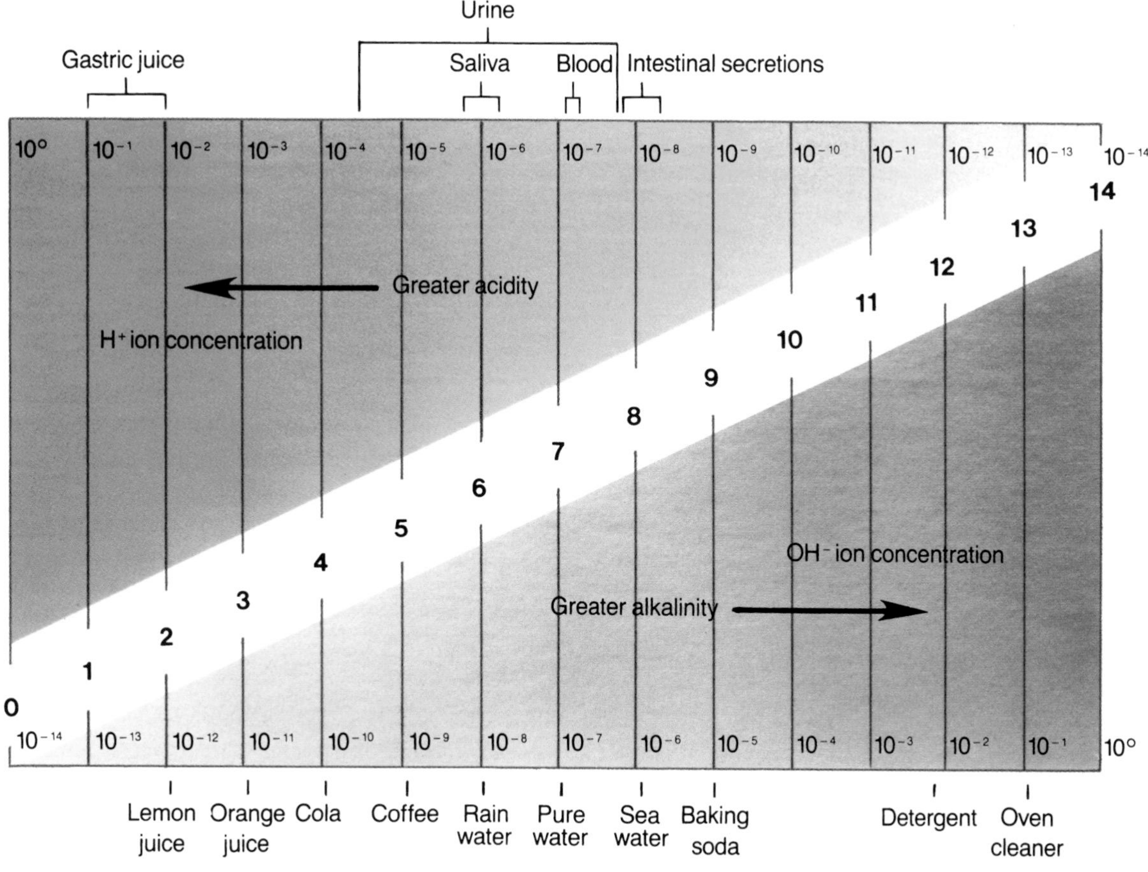

Figure 2–5 The pH scale. The pH values of several body fluids are indicated above the scale. The pH values of some familiar solutions are indicated below the scale.

QUESTION: Describe the pH range of blood compared with the pH range of urine.

bicarbonate. The products of this reaction are NaCl, a salt that has no effect on pH, and H_2CO_3, a weak acid that lowers pH only slightly. This prevents a drastic change in the pH of the extracellular fluid.

If a strong base, such as sodium hydroxide, is added to the extracellular fluid, this reaction will occur:

$$NaOH + H_2CO_3 \rightarrow H_2O + NaHCO_3$$

Sodium hydroxide, a strong base that would greatly raise pH, has reacted with carbonic acid. The products of this reaction are water, which has no effect on pH, and sodium bicarbonate, a weak base that raises pH only slightly. Again, this prevents a drastic change in the pH of the extracellular fluid.

In the body, such reactions take place in less than a second whenever acids or bases are formed that would greatly change pH. Because of the body's tendency to become more acidic, the need to correct acidosis is more frequent. With respect to the bicarbonate buffer system, this means that more $NaHCO_3$ than H_2CO_3 is needed. For this reason, the usual ratio of these buffers is 20:1 ($NaHCO_3$:H_2CO_3).

ORGANIC COMPOUNDS OF IMPORTANCE

Organic compounds all contain covalently bonded carbon and hydrogen atoms and perhaps other elements as well. In the human body there are four major groups of organic compounds: carbohydrates, lipids, proteins, and nucleic acids.

CARBOHYDRATES

A primary function of **carbohydrates** is to serve as sources of energy in cell respiration. All carbohydrates contain carbon, hydrogen, and oxygen and are classified as monosaccharides, disaccharides, oligosaccharides, and polysaccharides. *Saccharide* means "sugar," and the prefix indicates how many are present.

Monosaccharides, or single-sugar compounds, are the simplest sugars. Glucose is a **hexose**, or six-carbon, sugar with the formula $C_6H_{12}O_6$ (Fig. 2–6). Fructose and galactose also have the same formula, but the physical arrangement of the carbon, hydrogen, and oxygen atoms in each differs from that of glucose. This gives each hexose sugar a different three-dimensional shape. The honey produced by bees contains fructose and glucose. Sweet fruits contain fructose (glucose does not taste very sweet to us). Galactose is usually part of the disaccharide lactose in milk. The liver is able to change fructose and galactose to glucose, which is then used by cells in the process of cell respiration to produce ATP.

Another type of monosaccharide is the **pentose**, or five-carbon, sugar. These are not involved in energy production but rather are structural components of the nucleic acids. Deoxyribose ($C_5H_{10}O_4$) is part of DNA, which is the genetic material of chromosomes. Ribose ($C_5H_{10}O_5$) is part of RNA, which is essential for protein synthesis. We will return to the nucleic acids later in this chapter.

Disaccharides are double sugars, made of two monosaccharides linked by a covalent bond. When that bond is formed, a molecule of water (H–O–H) is removed, so the general formula of a disaccharide is not quite twice that of a glucose molecule; it is $C_{12}H_{22}O_{11}$. Sucrose, or cane sugar, for example, is made of one glucose and one fructose; it is also found in beets and other vegetables. Lactose is made

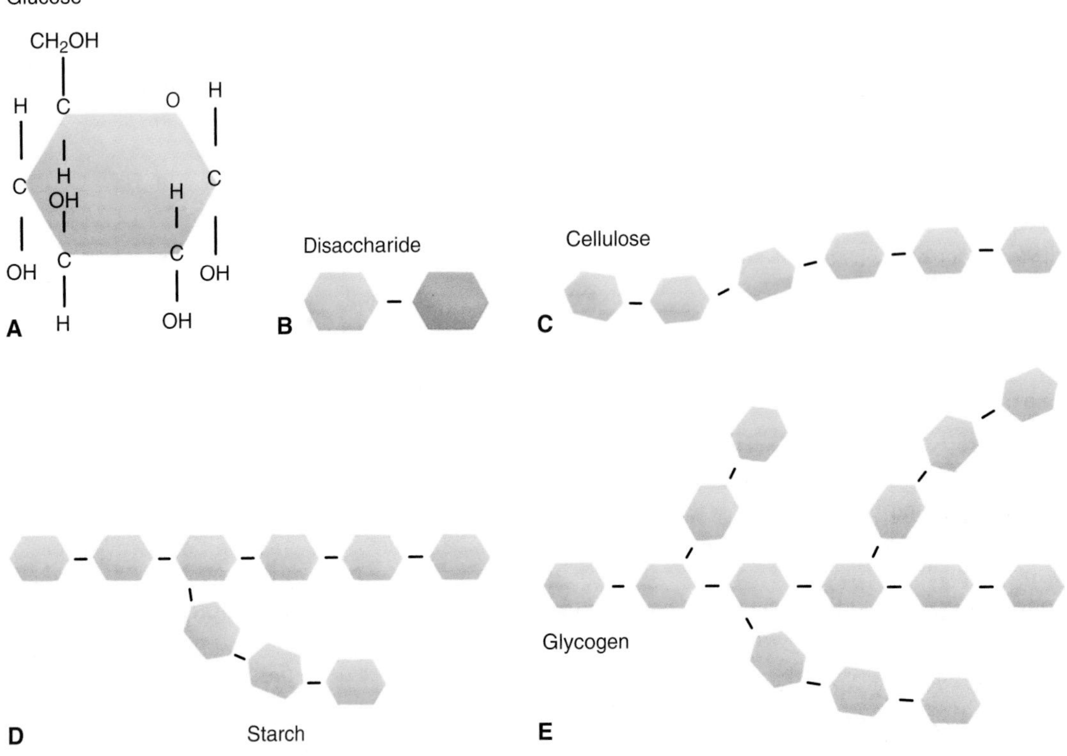

Figure 2–6 Carbohydrates. (**A**) Glucose, depicting its structural formula. (**B**) A disaccharide such as sucrose. (**C**) Cellulose, a polysaccharide. (**D**) Starch, a polysaccharide. (**E**) Glycogen, a polysaccharide. Each hexagon represents a hexose sugar such as glucose.

QUESTION: What is the chemical formula for glucose?

of one glucose and one galactose; it is found in milk, ice cream, yogurt, and other milk products. The grain sugar maltose is made of two glucose molecules. Disaccharides in our food are digested into monosaccharides that are then used for energy production.

The prefix *oligo* means "few"; **oligosaccharides** consist of from 3 to 20 monosaccharides. Unlike other carbohydrates, oligosaccharides are not sources of energy for us because we cannot digest them. In human cells, oligosaccharides are found on the outer surface of cell membranes. Here they serve as **antigens**, which are chemical markers (or "signposts") that identify cells. The A, B, and AB blood types, for example, are the result of oligosaccharide antigens on the outer surface of red blood cell membranes. All of our cells have "self" antigens, which identify the cells that belong in an individual. The presence of "self" antigens on our own cells provides a comparison for the white blood cells of the immune system to use with foreign material; the white blood cells are then able to recognize antigens that are "non-self." Such foreign antigens include bacteria and viruses, and immunity will be a major topic of Chapter 14.

Different oligosaccharides are produced by the cells of the mammary glands and become part of breast milk. These carbohydrates are not meant to nourish the breast-fed infant (milk contains lactose for the baby), but rather to encourage the growth of beneficial bacteria in the infant's intestines (the newborn's intestines are sterile, but bacteria arrive with every swallow). Recall from Chapter 1 that such bacteria, our microbiota or normal flora, are believed to contribute to the health of the intestinal tract throughout life, as well as to aspects of immunity. (See also Box 2–3: Vegetables: Tears and Gas.)

Polysaccharides are made of thousands of glucose molecules, bonded in different ways, resulting in different shapes (see Fig. 2–6). **Starches** are branched chains of glucose and are produced by plant cells to store energy. Potatoes, rice, corn, and wheat all contain useful starches. Nearly every human culture has learned to cultivate a major crop to be a source of starch. We consume starches as part of bread, pasta, pizza crust, noodles, French fries, and dumplings, as well as cookies, cakes, and pies. Humans have the digestive enzymes that split the bonds of starch molecules, releasing glucose. The glucose is then absorbed and used by cells to produce ATP.

Glycogen, a highly branched chain of glucose molecules, is our own storage form for glucose. After a meal high in carbohydrates, the blood glucose level rises. If the level were to remain high, glucose would be lost as the kidneys excreted it in urine (this is what happens in diabetes). But with the presence of the hormone insulin, excess glucose in the blood is quickly changed to glycogen and stored in the liver and skeletal muscles. When the blood glucose level decreases between meals, the glycogen is converted back to glucose, which is released into the blood (these reactions are regulated by other hormones). The blood glucose level is kept within normal limits, and cells can take in this glucose to produce energy.

Cellulose is a nearly straight chain of glucose molecules produced by plant cells as part of their cell walls. We have

Box 2-3 | VEGETABLES: TEARS AND GAS

Chopping onions often makes the cook cry. Vegetables that are part of a healthful diet, such as beans, cabbage, broccoli, and cauliflower, give many people the discomfort of intestinal gas and bloating. Why does this happen? By now you know; it's all in their chemistry.

Some of the amino acids in onion cells contain sulfur. Chopping an onion ruptures cells and releases a sulfur compound that vaporizes easily. When this sulfur compound comes in contact with the water that covers the surface of the eye (tears), it dissolves and forms a very dilute sulfuric acid, which stings. The lacrimal (tear) glands are stimulated to produce tears more rapidly, and blinking increases to spread the tears. Both of these responses may help to wash the irritating acid away.

Among many other vegetables, beans and broccoli contain oligosaccharides that we cannot digest. Our intestinal bacteria, however, which are part of our normal flora, especially in the colon, produce enzymes that ferment oligosaccharides. One of the fermentation products is gas (actually several gases, some with unpleasant odors). You may be wondering if "gas-relief" products work. Any that contain the enzyme alpha-galactosidase will prevent this type of gas formation. This enzyme will digest oligosaccharides before they reach the colon bacteria. The oligosaccharides are not fermented, and so gas is not produced.

no enzyme to digest the cellulose we consume as part of vegetables (such as beans, broccoli, and peas), grains, and nuts, so it passes through the digestive tract unchanged. Many raw vegetables and nuts, such as carrots or walnuts, are crunchy; what we are crunching is cellulose. Even fruits that are not especially crunchy, such as peaches or strawberries, contain quite a bit of cellulose. Another name for dietary cellulose is "fiber," and although we cannot use its glucose for energy, it does have a function. **Fiber** provides bulk within the cavity of the large intestine. This promotes efficient **peristalsis**, the waves of contraction that propel undigested material through the colon. A diet low in fiber does not give the colon much exercise, and the muscle tissue of the colon will contract weakly, just as our skeletal muscles will become flabby without exercise. A diet high in fiber provides exercise for the colon muscle and may help prevent chronic constipation. Plant fiber also provides food for our intestinal bacteria; they do have enzymes to break down these complex carbohydrates.

The structure and functions of the carbohydrates are summarized in Table 2–3.

LIPIDS

Lipids contain the elements carbon, hydrogen, and oxygen; some also contain phosphorus. This group of organic compounds includes different types of substances with very

Table 2–3 | **CARBOHYDRATES**

NAME	STRUCTURE	FUNCTION
MONOSACCHARIDES: SINGLE SUGARS		
Glucose	Hexose sugar	■ Most important energy source for cells
Fructose and galactose	Hexose sugar	■ Converted to glucose by the liver and then used for energy production
Deoxyribose	Pentose sugar	■ Part of DNA, the genetic code in the chromosomes of cells
Ribose	Pentose sugar	■ Part of RNA, needed for protein synthesis within cells
DISACCHARIDES: DOUBLE SUGARS		
Sucrose, lactose, and maltose	Two hexose sugars	■ Present in food; digested to monosaccharides, which are then used for energy production
OLIGOSACCHARIDES: FEW SUGARS		
	3 to 20 monosaccharides	■ Form "self" antigens on cell membranes; important to permit the immune system to distinguish "self" from foreign antigens (pathogens) ■ Produced by cells of the mammary glands; encourage growth of beneficial bacteria in the infant's intestinal tract
POLYSACCHARIDES: MANY SUGARS (THOUSANDS)		
Starches	Branched chains of glucose molecules	■ Found in plant foods; digested to monosaccharides and used for energy production
Glycogen	Highly branched chains of glucose molecules	■ Storage form for excess glucose in the liver and skeletal muscles
Cellulose	Straight chains of glucose molecules	■ Part of plant cell walls; provides fiber to promote peristalsis, especially by the colon, and to nourish intestinal microbiota

different functions. We will consider three types: true fats, phospholipids, and steroids (Fig. 2–7).

True fats (also called neutral fats) are made of one molecule of glycerol and one, two, or three fatty acid molecules. Glycerol is a small 3-carbon molecule ($C_3H_8O_3$). A fatty acid is a long molecule that has an even number of carbons, from 12 to 24, bonded to hydrogens, with the first carbon a carboxyl group: COOH. If three fatty acid molecules are bonded to a single glycerol, a **triglyceride** is formed. Two fatty acids and a glycerol form a **diglyceride**, and one fatty acid and a glycerol form a **monoglyceride**.

The fatty acids in a true fat may be **saturated** or **unsaturated**. Refer to Fig. 2–7 and notice that one of the fatty acids has single covalent bonds between all of its carbon atoms. Each of these carbons is then bonded to the maximum number of hydrogens; this is a saturated fatty acid, meaning saturated with hydrogen. The other fatty acids shown have one or more (poly) double covalent bonds between their carbons and less than the maximum number of hydrogens; these are unsaturated fatty acids. Many triglycerides contain both saturated and unsaturated fatty acids, and although not as precise, it is often easier to speak of saturated and unsaturated *fats*,

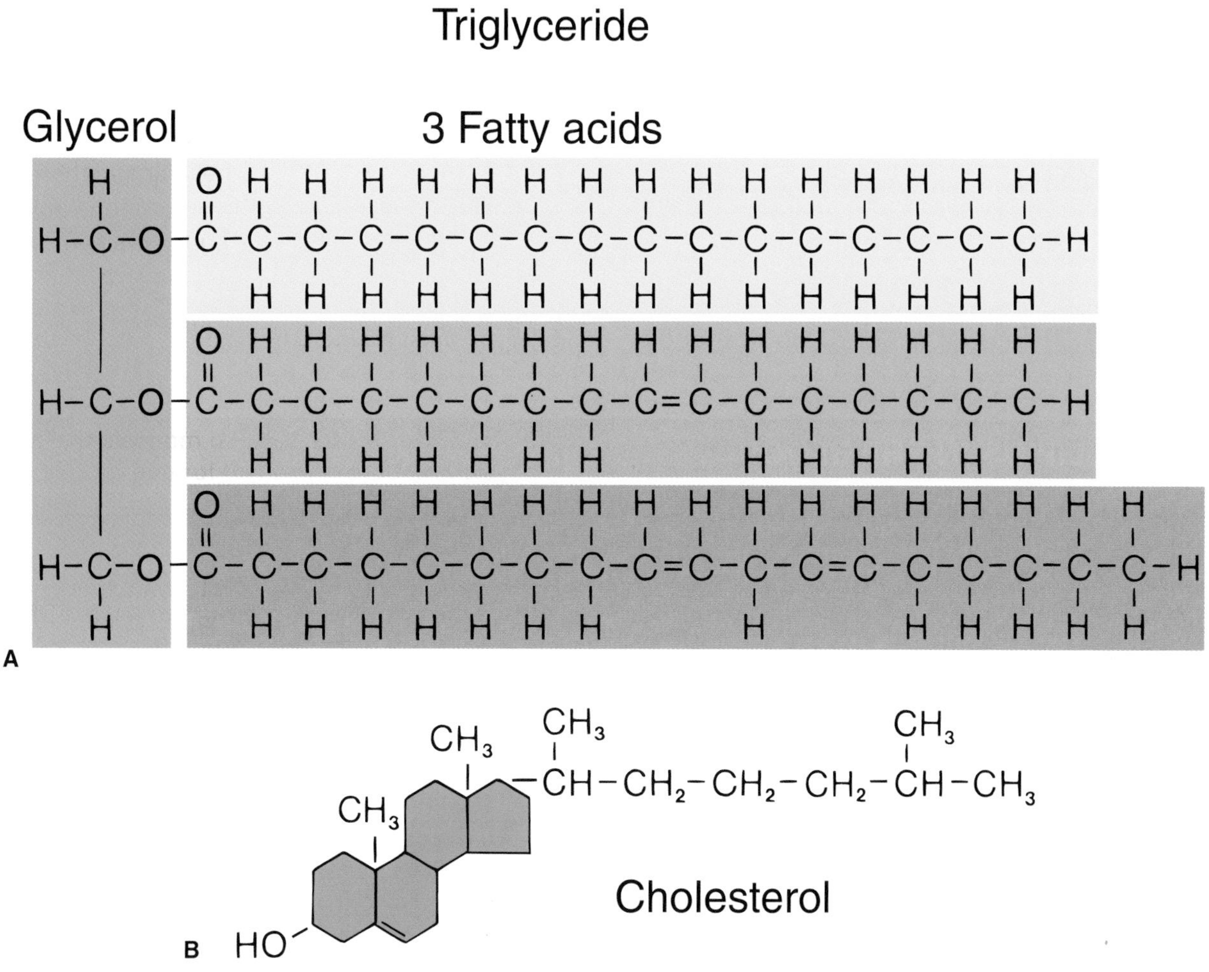

Figure 2–7 Lipids. (**A**) A triglyceride made of one glycerol and three fatty acids. (**B**) The steroid cholesterol. The hexagons and pentagon represent rings of carbon and hydrogen.

QUESTION: What would a diglyceride look like?

indicating the predominance of one or the other type of fatty acid.

At room temperature, saturated fats are often in solid form, whereas unsaturated fats are often (not always) in liquid form. Saturated fats tend to be found in animal-based foods such as beef, pork, chicken, eggs, and cheese, but palm oil and coconut oil are also saturated. Unsaturated fats are found in other plant oils such as corn oil, sunflower oil, and safflower oil, but certain fish oils are also unsaturated, and even pork contains some unsaturated fatty acids.

Unsaturated fats may be changed to saturated fats in order to give packaged foods a more pleasing texture or taste, or to allow them to be stored longer without refrigeration (a longer shelf life). These are hydrogenated fats (meaning that hydrogens have been added), also called trans fats. Trans fats contribute significantly to **atherosclerosis** of arteries; that is, abnormal cholesterol deposits in the lining that may clog arteries, especially the coronary arteries of the heart. As of early 2014, the Food and Drug Administration was considering banning the use of trans fats in prepared foods. (See also Box 2–4: Lipids in the Blood.)

The triglyceride forms of true fats are a storage form for excess food; that is, they are stored energy (potential energy). Any type of food consumed in excess of the body's caloric needs will be converted to fat and stored in adipose tissue. Most adipose tissue is subcutaneous, between the skin and muscles. Some organs, however, such as the eyes and kidneys, are enclosed in a layer of fat that acts as a cushion to absorb shock. (We will consider the other functions of adipose tissue in Chapter 4.)

Phospholipids are diglycerides with a phosphate group (PO_4) in the third bonding site of glycerol. Although similar in structure to the true fats, phospholipids are not stored energy but rather structural components of cells. Lecithin is a phospholipid that is part of our **cell membranes** (see Fig. 3–1 in Chapter 3; each phospholipid molecule looks like a sphere with two tails; the sphere is the glycerol and phosphate, the tails are the two fatty acids). Another phospholipid is **myelin**, which forms the myelin sheath around nerve cells and provides electrical insulation for nerve impulse transmission.

The structure of **steroids** is very different from that of the other lipids. **Cholesterol** is an important steroid; it is made of four rings of carbon and hydrogen (not fatty acids and glycerol) and is shown in Fig. 2–7. The liver synthesizes cholesterol, in addition to the cholesterol we eat in food. Only animal foods such as beef, pork, milk products, and egg yolks contain cholesterol. Vegetarians do not have cholesterol in their diet and depend upon synthesis by the liver. Cholesterol is

Box 2–4 | LIPIDS IN THE BLOOD

Triglycerides and cholesterol are transported in the blood in combination with proteins. Such molecules made by the small intestine are called chylomicrons. Those made by the liver are called lipoproteins and are categorized by their density, which reflects the proportion of protein to cholesterol.

Low-density lipoproteins (LDLs, which are low in protein and high in cholesterol) transport cholesterol to the tissues, where it is used to synthesize cell membranes or secretions. LDLs are also called "bad cholesterol" because in this form the cholesterol is more likely to be deposited in the walls of blood vessels, leading to atherosclerosis.

High-density lipoproteins (HDLs, which are higher in protein and lower in cholesterol than LDLs) transport cholesterol from the tissues to the liver. HDLs are also called "good cholesterol" because in this form cholesterol is more easily removed from the blood by the liver and excreted in bile.

A diet low in total fat, with most of it unsaturated fat, tends to raise HDL levels and lower LDL levels. These levels are believed to delay the development of atherosclerosis and coronary artery disease. A simple blood test called a lipid profile (or lipid panel) can determine levels of total cholesterol, triglycerides, HDLs, and LDLs. A high HDL level, above 50 mg/dL, is considered good (above 60 mg/dL is considered even more protective), as is a low LDL level, below 100 mg/dL.

Other factors contribute to coronary artery disease, such as heredity, smoking, being overweight, and lack of exercise. Diet alone cannot prevent atherosclerosis. However, a diet low in total fat and high in polyunsaturated fats is a good start.

another significant component of cell membranes and is the precursor (raw material) for the synthesis of other steroids. In the ovaries or testes, cholesterol is used to synthesize the steroid hormones estrogen or testosterone, respectively. A form of cholesterol in the skin is changed to vitamin D on exposure to sunlight. Liver cells use cholesterol for the synthesis of bile salts, which emulsify fats in digestion. Despite its link to coronary artery disease and heart attacks, cholesterol is an essential substance for human beings.

The structure and functions of lipids are summarized in Table 2–4.

PROTEINS

Proteins are made of smaller subunits or building blocks called **amino acids**, which all contain the elements carbon, hydrogen, oxygen, and nitrogen. Some amino acids contain sulfur, which permits the formation of disulfide bonds in proteins such as insulin and antibodies. There are about 20 amino acids that make up human proteins. We obtain these amino acids from animal proteins such as beef, chicken, pork, and fish, and from plant proteins such as those found in beans, peas, nuts, corn, and other grains.

The structure of amino acids is shown in Fig. 2–8, and you will notice that they all have several parts in common. Each amino acid has a central carbon atom covalently bonded to an atom of hydrogen, an amino group (NH_2), and a carboxyl group (COOH). At the fourth bond of the central carbon is the variable portion of the amino acid, represented by R. The R group may be a single hydrogen atom, or a CH_3 group, or a more complex configuration of carbon and hydrogen and perhaps sulfur. This gives each of the 20 amino acids a slightly different physical shape. A bond between two amino acids is called a **peptide bond**, and a short chain of amino acids linked by peptide bonds is a **polypeptide**.

A protein may consist of from 50 to thousands of amino acids. The sequence of the amino acids is specific and unique for each protein and is called its primary structure. This unique sequence, and the hydrogen bonds and disulfide bonds formed within the amino acid chain, determines how the protein will be folded to complete its synthesis. The folding may be simple, a helix (coil) or pleated sheet called the secondary structure, or more complex folding may occur to form a globular protein called the tertiary structure. Myoglobin, found in muscles, is a globular protein (Fig. 2–8E). When complete, each protein has a characteristic three-dimensional shape, which in turn determines its function. Some proteins consist of more than one amino acid chain (quaternary structure). Hemoglobin, for example, has four amino acid chains (see Box 3–2 in Chapter 3). Notice that myoglobin contains an atom of iron (a hemoglobin molecule has four iron atoms). Some proteins require a trace element such as iron or zinc to complete their structure and permit them to function properly.

Table 2–4 | LIPIDS

NAME	STRUCTURE	FUNCTION
True fats	A triglyceride consists of three fatty acid molecules bonded to a glycerol molecule (some are monoglycerides or diglycerides)	■ Storage form for excess food molecules in subcutaneous tissue ■ Cushion organs such as the eyes and kidneys
Phospholipids	Diglycerides with a phosphate group bonded to the glycerol molecule	■ Part of cell membranes (lecithin) ■ Form the myelin sheath to provide electrical insulation for neurons
Steroids (cholesterol)	Four carbon–hydrogen rings	■ Part of cell membranes ■ Converted to vitamin D in the skin on exposure to UV rays of the sun ■ Converted by the liver to bile salts, which emulsify fats during digestion ■ Precursor for the steroid hormones such as estrogen in women (ovaries) or testosterone in men (testes)

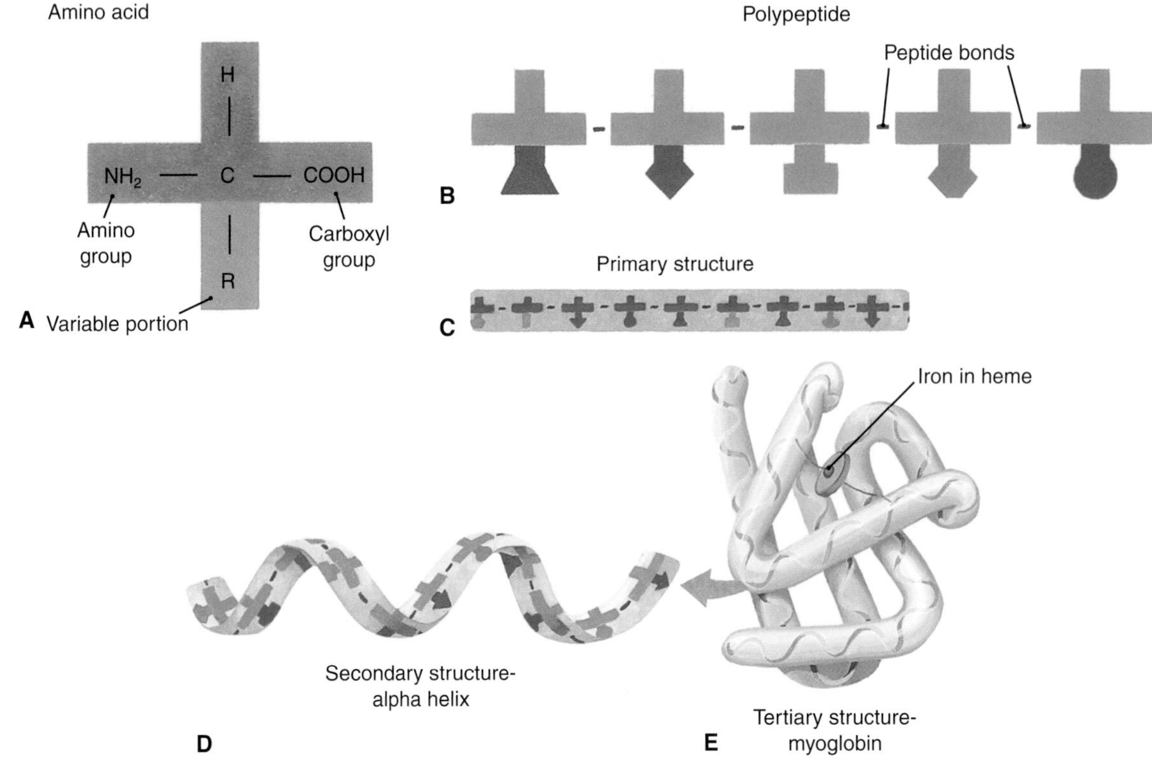

Figure 2–8 Amino acid and protein structure. (**A**) The structural formula of an amino acid. The "R" represents the variable portion of the molecule. (**B**) A polypeptide. Several amino acids, represented by different shapes, are linked by peptide bonds. (**C**) The primary structure of a protein. (**D**) The secondary structure of a protein. (**E**) The tertiary structure of the protein myoglobin. See text for further description.

QUESTION: What mineral is part of myoglobin, and what is its function?

Our body proteins have many functions; some of these are listed in Table 2–5 and will be mentioned again in later chapters. Although we usually do not think of protein as an energy food, if our diet includes more amino acids than are necessary for our protein synthesis, those excess amino acids will be converted to simple carbohydrates, or even to fat, to be stored as potential energy. (See Box 2–5: A Protein Mystery: Prions for a discussion of disease-causing proteins.) One very important function of proteins will be discussed further here: the role of proteins as enzymes.

Enzymes

Enzymes are **catalysts**, which means that they speed up chemical reactions without the need for an external source of energy such as heat. The many reactions that take place within the body are catalyzed by specific enzymes; all of these reactions must take place at body temperature.

The way in which enzymes function as catalysts is called the **active site theory**. Keep in mind that a "theory" is not a guess; a scientific theory is the best explanation for all the available evidence. All the evidence of enzyme functioning supports the active site theory, which states that the shape of an enzyme determines its function. The specific function also includes the shapes of the reacting molecules, called **substrates**. A simple synthesis reaction is depicted in Fig. 2–9A. Notice that the enzyme has a specific shape, as do the substrate molecules. The active site of the enzyme is the

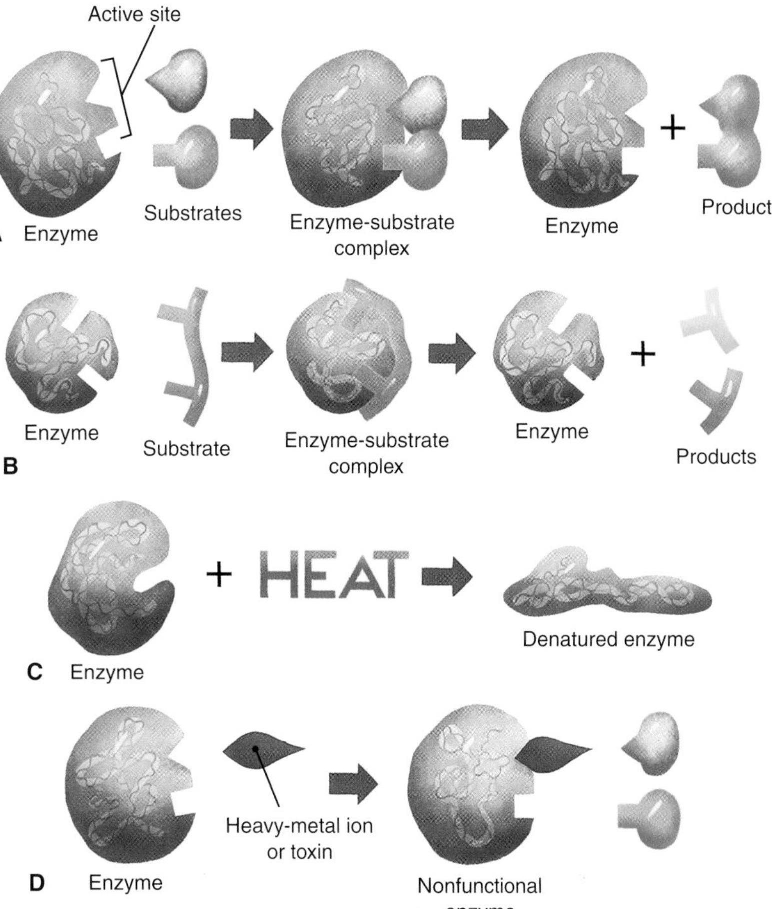

Figure 2–9 Active site theory. (**A**) Synthesis reaction. (**B**) Decomposition reaction. (**C**) The effect of heat. (**D**) The effect of poisons. See text for description.

QUESTION: Which of these four pictures best represents the effect of an acidic pH on an enzyme, and why?

Table 2–5 | **FUNCTIONS OF PROTEINS**

TYPE OF PROTEIN	FUNCTION
Structural proteins	■ Form channels, transporters, intercellular junctions, and receptor sites in cell membranes ■ Keratin—part of hair, nails, and the epidermis of the skin ■ Collagen—part of tendons, ligaments, and the dermis of the skin
Hormones	■ Insulin—enables cells to take in glucose; lowers blood glucose level ■ Growth hormone—increases protein synthesis and cell division
Hemoglobin	■ Enables red blood cells to carry oxygen
Myoglobin	■ Stores oxygen in muscle cells
Antibodies	■ Produced by lymphocytes (white blood cells); label pathogens for destruction
Myosin and actin	■ Muscle structure and contraction ■ Part of the cytoskeleton that gives shape to cells and permits movement
Enzymes	■ Catalyze reactions: synthesis, decomposition, energy production, cellular reproduction

Box 2–5 | A PROTEIN MYSTERY: PRIONS

Prions are proteinaceous infectious particles, the cause of lethal diseases of the nervous system in people and animals. Besides Creutzfeldt-Jakob disease (CJD), mad-cow disease is perhaps the best known; its formal name is bovine spongiform encephalopathy (BSE). The name tells us about the disease: *Encephalopathy* means that the brain is affected, and *spongiform* indicates that brain tissue becomes spongy, or full of holes. People may acquire BSE by eating beef contaminated with infected cow brain tissue. They develop what is called variant Creutzfeldt-Jakob disease. Variant CJD is characterized by loss of coordination, loss of memory and personality, and death within a few months. There is no treatment.

How do prions cause this disease? We do not yet have the entire answer. We do know that prions are natural proteins; they function in nerve tissue and seem to be involved in creating myelin sheaths and contributing to memory. But just like any other part of a living organism, they can malfunction. Malfunctioning prions are believed to change the structure of other brain proteins, causing misfolding. Misfolded proteins are treated like old or damaged proteins: The cell uses cleanup enzymes and mechanisms to get rid of them, but the excess of faulty proteins overburdens these mechanisms and brings about deterioration of brain tissue.

Unfortunately, we do not know how to destroy prions. Prions are not living; they do not contain genetic material or carry out processes that might be disrupted by antibiotics or antiviral medications. Cooking does not seem to affect them. Standard sterilization practices that kill bacteria and viruses do not seem to inactivate prions.

Prevention of prion disease depends on keeping animal brain tissue from contaminating meat destined for human or animal consumption. In Great Britain, where the human form of mad-cow disease emerged and killed nearly 100 people, butchering practices are now stringently regulated. As of this writing, infected cattle have been found in North America, but no cases of variant CJD have occurred in people.

part that matches the shapes of the substrates. The substrates must "fit" into the active site of the enzyme, and temporary bonds may form between the enzyme and the substrate. This is called the enzyme–substrate complex. In this case, two substrate molecules are thus brought close together so that chemical bonds are formed between them, creating a new compound. The product of the reaction, the new compound, is then released, leaving the enzyme itself unchanged and able to catalyze another reaction of the same type.

The reaction shown in Fig. 2–9B is a decomposition reaction. As the substrate molecule bonds to the active site of the enzyme, strain is put on its internal bonds, which break, forming two product molecules and again leaving the enzyme unchanged. Each enzyme is specific in that it will catalyze only one type of reaction. An enzyme that digests the protein in food, for example, has the proper shape for that reaction but cannot digest starches. For starch digestion, another enzyme with a differently shaped active site is needed. Thousands of chemical reactions take place within the body, and therefore we have thousands of enzymes, each with its own shape and active site.

The ability of enzymes to function may be limited or destroyed by changes in the intracellular or extracellular fluids in which they are found. Changes in pH and temperature are especially crucial. Recall that the pH of intracellular fluid is approximately 6.8 to 7.0 and that a decrease in pH means that more H^+ ions are present. If pH decreases significantly, the excess H^+ ions will react with the active sites of cellular enzymes, change their shapes, and prevent them from catalyzing reactions. This is why a state of acidosis may cause the death of cells—the cells' enzymes are unable to function properly.

With respect to temperature, most human enzymes have their optimum functioning in the normal range of body temperature: 97° to 99°F (36° to 38°C). A temperature of 106°F, a high fever, may break the chemical bonds that maintain the shapes of enzymes (see Fig. 2–9C). If an enzyme loses its shape, it is said to be **denatured**, and a denatured enzyme is unable to function as a catalyst. Some human enzymes, when denatured by a high fever, may revert to their original shapes if the fever is lowered quickly. Others, however, will not. (An example of irreversible denaturation is a hard-boiled egg; the proteins in the egg white and yolk will never revert to what they were in the original egg.) A high fever may cause brain damage or death because enzymes in the brain have become permanently denatured.

You already know that metals such as lead and mercury are harmful to humans and that both may cause serious damage to the nervous system and other body tissues. These heavy metals are harmful to us because they are very reactive and block the actions of our enzymes. Fig. 2–9D depicts what happens. Notice that the heavy metal ion bonds with part of the active site of the enzyme and changes its shape. The substrate molecule cannot fit, and the enzyme is useless. Many other chemicals are poisonous to us for the very same reason: They destroy the functioning of our enzymes, and essential reactions cannot take place.

NUCLEIC ACIDS

DNA and RNA

The **nucleic acids**, **DNA** (deoxyribonucleic acid) and **RNA** (ribonucleic acid), are large molecules made of smaller subunits called nucleotides. A **nucleotide** consists of a pentose sugar, a phosphate group, and one of several nitrogenous bases. In DNA nucleotides, the sugar is deoxyribose, and the bases are adenine, guanine, cytosine, or thymine. In RNA nucleotides, the sugar is ribose, and the bases are adenine, guanine, cytosine, or uracil. DNA and RNA molecules are shown in Fig. 2–10. Notice that DNA looks somewhat like a twisted ladder; this ladder is two strands of nucleotides called a double helix (two coils). Alternating phosphate and sugar molecules form the uprights of the ladder, and pairs of nitrogenous bases form the rungs. The size of the bases and the number of hydrogen bonds each can form the complementary base pairing of the nucleic acids. In DNA, adenine is always paired with thymine (with two hydrogen bonds), and guanine is always paired with cytosine (with three hydrogen bonds).

DNA makes up the chromosomes of cells and is therefore the **genetic code** for hereditary characteristics. The sequence of bases in the DNA strands is actually a code for the many kinds of proteins living things produce; the code is the same in plants, other animals, and microbes. The sequence of bases for one protein is called a gene. Human genes are the codes for the proteins produced by human cells (though many of these genes are also found in all other forms of life—we are all very much related). The functioning of DNA will be covered in more detail in the next chapter.

RNA is often a single strand of nucleotides (see Fig. 2–10), with uracil nucleotides in place of thymine nucleotides. RNA is synthesized from DNA in the nucleus of a cell, and there are several forms. All carry out their functions in the cytoplasm. RNA copies the genetic code from DNA and helps assemble amino acids into proteins. Protein synthesis will also be discussed in the following chapter.

ATP

ATP (adenosine triphosphate) is a specialized nucleotide that consists of the base adenine, the sugar ribose, and three phosphate groups (see Fig. 2–11). Mention has already been made of ATP as a product of cell respiration that contains biologically useful energy. ATP is one of several "energy transfer" molecules within cells, transferring the potential energy in food molecules to cell processes. When a molecule of glucose is broken down into carbon dioxide and water with the release of energy, the cell uses some of this energy to synthesize ATP. Present in cells are molecules of ADP (adenosine diphosphate) and free phosphate groups. The energy released from glucose is used to loosely bond a third phosphate to ADP, forming ATP (moving right to left in Fig. 2–11). When the bond of this third phosphate is again broken and energy is released (moving left to right in Fig. 2–11), ATP then becomes the energy source for cell processes such as mitosis, muscle contraction, or protein synthesis for growth and repair.

All cells have enzymes that can remove the third phosphate group from ATP to release its energy, forming ADP and phosphate. As cell respiration continues, ATP is resynthesized from ADP and phosphate. ATP formation to trap energy from food and ATP breakdown to release energy for cell processes is a continuing cycle in cells.

The structure and functions of the nucleic acids are summarized in Table 2–6.

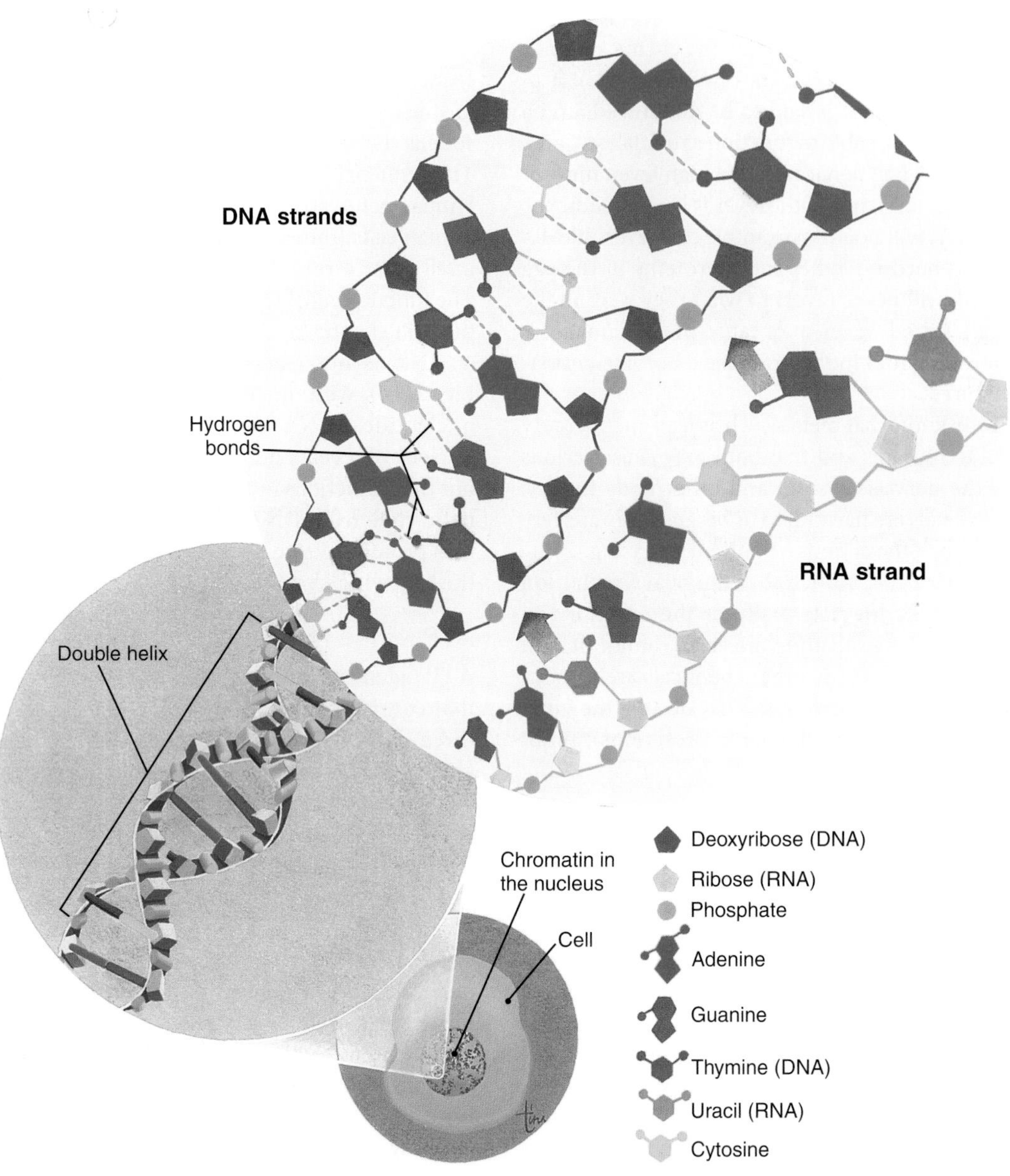

Figure 2–10 DNA and RNA. Both molecules are shown, with each part of a nucleotide represented by its shape and in a different color. Note the complementary base pairing of DNA (A–T and G–C). When RNA is synthesized, it is a complementary copy of half the DNA molecule (with U in place of T).

QUESTION: Why can't adenine pair with guanine to form a rung of the DNA ladder?

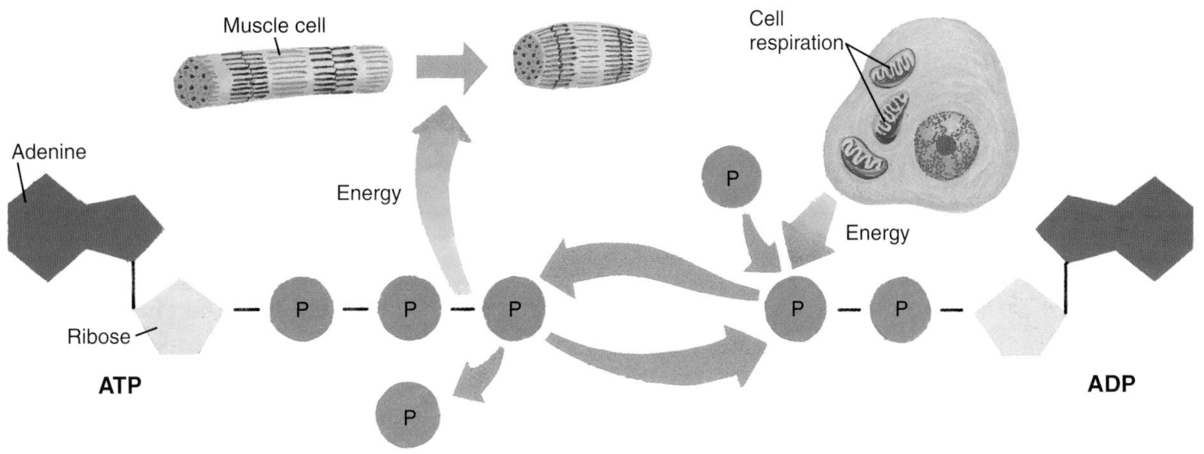

Figure 2–11 ATP. A molecule of ATP is shown on the left, and ADP + phosphate is shown on the right. Notice that this is a cycle.

QUESTION: The energy from ATP is being used here for contraction of a muscle cell. What else may such energy be used for?

Table 2–6 | **NUCLEIC ACIDS**

NAME	STRUCTURE	FUNCTION
DNA (deoxyribonucleic acid)	A double helix of nucleotides; adenine paired with thymine, and guanine paired with cytosine; the two strands of the helix are connected by hydrogen bonds	■ Found in the chromosomes in the nucleus of a cell ■ The sequence of bases is the genetic code for hereditary characteristics
RNA (ribonucleic acid)	A single strand of nucleotides; adenine, guanine, cytosine, and uracil	■ Copies the genetic code of DNA to direct protein synthesis in the cytoplasm of cells ■ Contributes to the assembly of amino acids into proteins
ATP (adenosine triphosphate)	A single adenine nucleotide with three phosphate groups	■ An energy-transferring molecule ■ Formed when cell respiration releases energy from food molecules ■ Used for energy-requiring cellular processes

SUMMARY

Chemicals may be inorganic, such as water, oxygen, and iron, or organic, such as carbohydrates, lipids, proteins, and nucleic acids. All of the chemicals we have just described are considered to be nonliving, even though they are essential parts of all living organisms. The cells of our bodies are precise arrangements of these nonliving chemicals and yet are considered living matter. The cellular level, therefore, is the next level of organization we will examine.

STUDY OUTLINE

Elements

1. Elements are the simplest chemicals, which make up all matter.
2. Carbon, hydrogen, oxygen, nitrogen, phosphorus, sulfur, and calcium make up 99% of the human body.
3. Elements combine in many ways to form molecules, both inorganic and organic.

Atoms (see Fig. 2–1)

1. An atom is the smallest part of an element that still retains the characteristics of the element.
2. Atoms consist of positively and negatively charged particles and neutral (or uncharged) particles.
   a. Protons have a positive charge and are found in the nucleus of the atom.
   b. Neutrons have no charge and are found in the nucleus of the atom.
   c. Electrons have a negative charge and orbit the nucleus.
3. The number and arrangement of electrons give an atom its bonding capabilities.

Chemical Bonds

1. An ionic bond involves the loss of electrons by one atom and the gain of these electrons by another atom: Ions are formed that attract one another (see Fig. 2–2).
   a. Cations are ions with positive charges: Na^+, Ca^{+2}.
   b. Anions are ions with negative charges: Cl^-, HCO_3^-.
   c. Inorganic salts, acids, and bases are formed by ionic bonding.
   d. In water, many ionic bonds break; dissociation releases ions for other reactions.
2. A covalent bond involves the sharing of electrons between two atoms (see Fig. 2–3).
   a. Oxygen gas (O_2) and water (H_2O) are covalently bonded molecules.
   b. Carbon always forms covalent bonds; these are the basis for the organic compounds.
   c. Covalent bonds are not weakened in an aqueous solution.
3. A disulfide bond is a covalent bond between two sulfur atoms in a protein; it helps maintain the three-dimensional shape of proteins such as insulin and antibodies.
4. A hydrogen bond is the attraction of a covalently bonded hydrogen (slightly positive) to a nearby oxygen or nitrogen atom (slightly negative).
   a. The three-dimensional shape of proteins and nucleic acids is maintained by hydrogen bonds.
   b. Water is cohesive and adhesive because of hydrogen bonds.

Chemical Reactions

1. A change brought about by the formation or breaking of chemical bonds.
2. Synthesis—bonds are formed to join two or more molecules.
3. Decomposition—bonds are broken within a molecule.
4. Within cells, the products of decomposition reactions are often recycled for synthesis reactions.

Inorganic Compounds of Importance

1. Water—makes up 55% to 70% of the body.
   a. Solvent—for transport of nutrients in the blood and excretion of wastes in urine.
   b. Lubricant—mucus in the digestive tract.
   c. Temperature stabilizer—changes temperature slowly, preventing sudden changes in body temperature; absorbs body heat in evaporation of sweat.
   d. Water compartments—the locations of water within the body (see Fig. 2–4).
      - Intracellular—within cells; 65% of total body water.
      - Extracellular—35% of total body water
         1) Plasma—in blood vessels.
         2) Lymph—in lymphatic vessels.
         3) Tissue fluid—in tissue spaces between cells.
         4) Specialized fluids in joints, the eyes, and the central nervous system.
2. Oxygen—21% of the atmosphere.
   a. Essential for cell respiration: the breakdown of food molecules to release energy.
3. Carbon dioxide
   a. Produced as a waste product of cell respiration.
   b. Must be exhaled; excess CO_2 in body fluids causes acidosis.
4. Cell respiration—the energy-producing processes of cells.
   a. Glucose + O_2 → CO_2 + H_2O + ATP + heat
   b. This is why we breathe: to take in oxygen to break down food to produce energy, and to exhale the CO_2 produced.
5. Trace elements—minerals needed in small amounts (see Table 2–2).
6. Acids, bases, and pH
   a. The pH scale ranges from 0 to 14; 7 is neutral. Below 7 is acidic, and above 7 is alkaline.
   b. An acid increases the H^+ ion concentration of a solution; a base decreases the H^+ ion concentration (or increases the OH^- ion concentration) (see Fig. 2–5).
   c. The pH range within cells is about 6.8 to 7.0. The normal pH range of blood is 7.35 to 7.45. Normal metabolism tends to make body fluids more acidic.
   d. Buffer systems maintain normal pH by reacting with strong acids or strong bases to change them to substances that do not greatly change pH.
   e. The bicarbonate buffer system consists of $NaHCO_3$ to react with strong acids and H_2CO_3 to react with strong bases (ratio about 20:1).

Organic Compounds of Importance

1. Carbohydrates (see Table 2–3 and Fig. 2–6).
   a. Monosaccharides are simple sugars. Glucose, a hexose sugar ($C_6H_{12}O_6$), is the primary energy source for cell respiration. Fructose and galactose have the same chemical formula.
      - Pentose sugars are part of the nucleic acids DNA and RNA.
   b. Disaccharides are made of two hexose sugars. Sucrose, lactose, and maltose are digested to monosaccharides and used for cell respiration.
   c. Oligosaccharides consist of from 3 to 20 monosaccharides.
      - On cell membranes they are antigens that identify cells as "self."
      - In breast milk they nourish an infant's beneficial intestinal bacterial population.
   d. Polysaccharides are made of thousands of glucose molecules.
      - Starches are plant products broken down in digestion to glucose.
      - Glycogen is the form in which glucose is stored in the liver and muscles to help regulate the blood glucose level.
      - Cellulose, the fiber of plant cells, cannot be digested but promotes efficient peristalsis in the colon.

2. Lipids (see Table 2–4 and Fig. 2–7).
   a. True fats are made of fatty acids and glycerol; triglycerides are a storage form for potential energy in adipose tissue. The eyes and kidneys are cushioned by fat. Fatty acids may be saturated (maximum number of hydrogens) or unsaturated (less than the maximum number of hydrogens). Saturated fats and hydrogenated or trans fats contribute to atherosclerosis.
   b. Phospholipids are diglycerides such as lecithin that are part of cell membranes. Myelin is a phospholipid that provides electrical insulation for nerve cells.
   c. Steroids consist of four rings of carbon and hydrogen. Cholesterol, produced by the liver and consumed in food, is the basic steroid from which the body manufactures others: steroid hormones, vitamin D, and bile salts.
3. Proteins
   a. Amino acids are the subunits of proteins; 20 amino acids make up human proteins. Peptide bonds join amino acids to one another (see Fig. 2–8).
   b. A protein consists of from 50 to thousands of amino acids in a specific sequence (primary structure) that is folded into a specific shape (secondary and tertiary structures). Some proteins are made of two or more amino acid chains (quaternary structure); some proteins contain trace elements.
   c. Protein functions—see Table 2–5.
   d. Amino acids in excess of the need for protein synthesis are converted to simple carbohydrates or to fat, for energy production.
   e. Enzymes are catalysts, which speed up reactions without additional energy. The active site theory is based on the shapes of the enzyme and the substrate molecules: These must "fit" (see Fig. 2–9). The enzyme remains unchanged after the product of the reaction is released. Each enzyme is specific for one type of reaction. The functioning of enzymes may be disrupted by changes in pH or body temperature, or by the presence of a poison, which changes the shape of the active sites of enzymes.
4. Nucleic acids (see Table 2–6 and Fig. 2–10).
   a. Nucleotides are the subunits of nucleic acids. A nucleotide consists of a pentose sugar, a phosphate group, and a nitrogenous base.
   b. DNA is a double strand of nucleotides, coiled into a double helix, with complementary base pairing: A–T and G–C. DNA makes up the chromosomes of cells and is the genetic code for the synthesis of proteins.
   c. RNA is a single strand of nucleotides, synthesized from DNA, with U in place of T. RNA functions in protein synthesis; several forms function in the process of protein synthesis in the cytoplasm of a cell.
   d. ATP is a nucleotide that is specialized to trap and transfer energy (see Fig. 2–11). Energy released from food in cell respiration is used to synthesize ATP from ADP + P. When cells need energy, ATP is broken down to ADP + P and the energy is transferred to cell processes.

REVIEW QUESTIONS

1. State the chemical symbol for each of the following elements: sodium, potassium, iron, calcium, oxygen, carbon, hydrogen, copper, and chlorine. (p. 28)
2. Explain, in terms of their electrons, how an atom of sodium and an atom of chlorine form a molecule of sodium chloride. (p. 30)
3. a. Explain, in terms of their electrons, how an atom of carbon and two atoms of oxygen form a molecule of carbon dioxide. (p. 34)
   b. Explain the functions of hydrogen bonds.
   c. Explain the function of disulfide bonds.
4. Name the subunits (smaller molecules) of which each of the following is made: DNA, glycogen, a true fat, and a protein. (pp. 47, 39, 41, 43)
5. State precisely where in the body each of these fluids is found: plasma, intracellular water, lymph, and tissue fluid. (p. 33)
6. Explain why it is important to the body that water changes temperature slowly. (p. 33)
7. Describe two ways in which the solvent ability of water is important to the body. (pp. 32–33)
8. Name the organic molecule with each of the following functions: (p. 40)
   a. The genetic code in chromosomes
   b. "Self" antigens in our cell membranes
   c. The storage form for glucose in the liver
   d. The storage form for excess food in adipose tissue
   e. The precursor molecule for the steroid hormones
   f. The undigested part of food that promotes peristalsis
   g. The sugars that are part of the nucleic acids
9. State the summary equation of cell respiration. (p. 34)
10. State the role or function of each of the following in cell respiration: CO_2, glucose, O_2, heat, and ATP. (p. 35)
11. State a specific function of each of the following in the human body: Ca, Fe, Na, I, and Co. (p. 35)
12. Explain, in terms of relative concentrations of H^+ ions and OH^- ions, each of the following: acid, base, and neutral substance. (pp. 36–37)
13. State the normal pH range of blood. (p. 36)
14. Complete the following equation, and state how each of the products affects pH: (pp. 36–37)

    $HCl + NaHCO_3 \rightarrow$ ______ + ______
15. Explain the active site theory of enzyme functioning. (p. 44)
16. Explain the difference between a synthesis reaction and a decomposition reaction. (pp. 44–46)

FOR FURTHER THOUGHT

1. Orange juice usually has a pH of around 4. How does this compare with the pH of human blood? Why is it possible for us to drink orange juice without disrupting the pH of our blood?
2. Estrela, age 7, has hot cereal with milk and sugar for breakfast and then walks to school. Explain the relationship between eating and walking; keep in mind that Estrela is breathing.
3. The body is able to store certain nutrients. Name the storage forms, and state an advantage and a disadvantage.
4. Many "vitamin pills" also contain minerals. Which minerals are likely to be found in such dietary supplements? What purposes do these minerals have; that is, what are their functions?
5. Lead is an element that is poisonous to people; it is toxic because it reacts readily with sulfur. Which group of organic molecules is most likely to be damaged by lead and why?
6. Look at the organic molecule depicted in Question Figure 2–A. Begin by naming the major category (one of the four), and then see how specific you can be. Even if you are not sure, give reasons for the possible molecules you can eliminate.

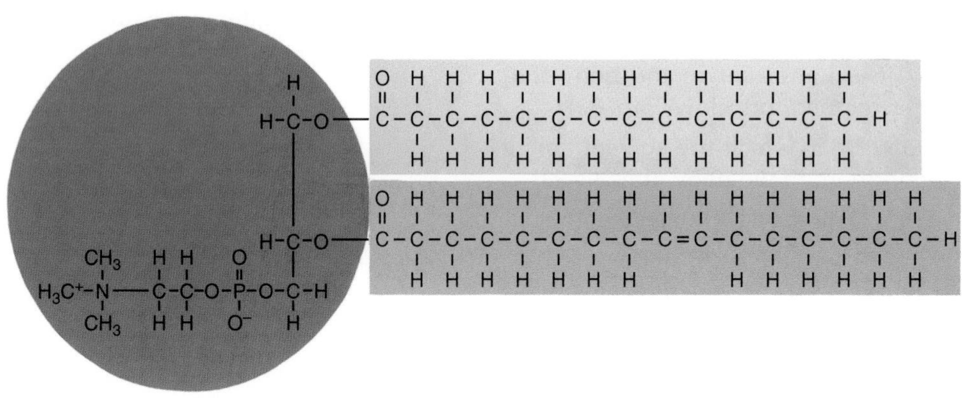

QUESTION FIGURE 2–A: Organic molecule.

7. Look at the inorganic molecules depicted in Question Figure 2–B; they are all the same. What are these five molecules? What kind of bond holds each one together? What kind of bond (shown by dotted lines) holds the five of them together? (The lowercase Greek letter delta [δ^+ or δ^-] indicates that a partial positive or negative charge is present.) What physical property does this type of bond provide to this substance?

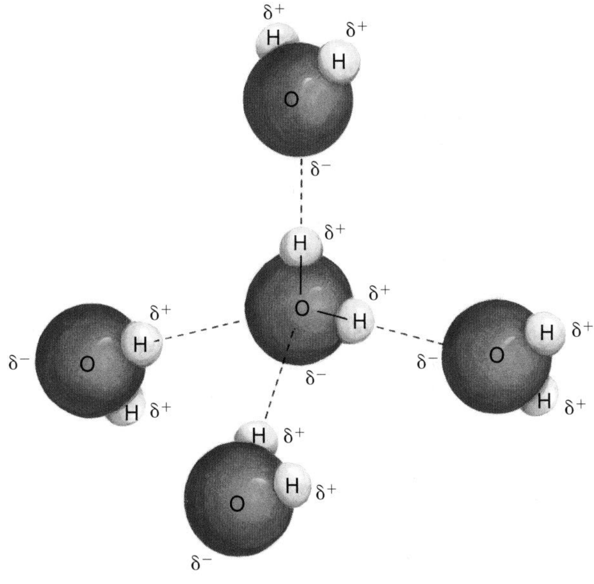

QUESTION FIGURE 2–B: Inorganic molecules.

CHAPTER

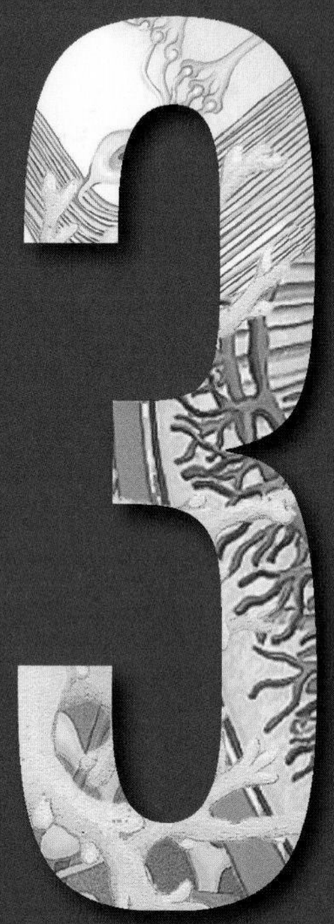

Cells

STUDENT OBJECTIVES

- Name the organic molecules that make up cell membranes and state their functions.
- State the functions of the nucleus and chromosomes.
- Describe the functions of the cell organelles.
- Define each of these cellular transport mechanisms and give an example of the role of each in the body: diffusion, osmosis, facilitated diffusion, active transport, filtration, phagocytosis, and pinocytosis.
- Describe the triplet code of DNA.
- Explain how the triplet code of DNA is transcribed and translated in the synthesis of proteins.
- Describe what happens in mitosis and in meiosis.
- Use examples to explain the importance of mitosis.
- Explain the importance of meiosis.

NEW TERMINOLOGY

Absorption *(ab-**ZORB**-shun)*
Active transport *(**AK**-tiv **TRANS**-port)*
Aerobic *(air-**ROH**-bik)*
Apoptosis *(ap-oh-**TOH**-sis)*
Autophagy *(aw-**TOFF**-uh-jee)*
Autosomes *(**AW**-toh-sohms)*
Cell membrane *(SELL **MEM**-brayn)*
Chromosomes *(**KROH**-muh-sohms)*
Cilia *(**SILLY**-ah)*
Cytoplasm *(**SIGH**-toh-plazm)*
Cytoskeleton *(SIGH-toh-**SKEL**-e-ton)*
Diffusion *(di-**FEW**-zhun)*
Diploid number *(**DIH**-ployd)*
Epigenetics *(EP-i-je-**NET**-iks)*
Filtration *(fill-**TRAY**-shun)*
Gametes *(**GAM**-eets)*
Gene *(JEEN)*
Haploid number *(**HA**-ployd)*
Meiosis *(my-**OH**-sis)*
Microvilli *(MY-kro-**VILL**-eye)*
Mitochondria *(MY-toh-**KAHN**-dree-ah)*
Mitosis *(my-**TOH**-sis)*
Nucleus *(**NEW**-klee-us)*
Organelles *(OR-gan-**ELLS**)*
Osmosis *(ahs-**MOH**-sis)*
Phagocytosis *(FAG-oh-sigh-**TOH**-sis)*
Pinocytosis *(PIN-oh-sigh-**TOH**-sis)*
Selectively permeable *(se-**LEK**-tiv-lee **PER**-me-uh-buhl)*

RELATED CLINICAL TERMINOLOGY

Benign *(bee-**NINE**)*
Carcinogen *(kar-**SIN**-oh-jen)*
Chemotherapy *(KEE-moh-**THER**-uh-pee)*
Genetic disease *(je-**NET**-ik di-**ZEEZ**)*
Hypertonic *(HIGH-per-**TAHN**-ik)*
Hypotonic *(HIGH-poh-**TAHN**-ik)*
Isotonic *(EYE-soh-**TAHN**-ik)*
Malignant *(muh-**LIG**-nunt)*
Metastasis *(muh-**TASS**-tuh-sis)*
Mutation *(mew-**TAY**-shun)*

CHAPTER OUTLINE

*Terms that appear in **bold type** in the chapter text are defined in the glossary, which begins on page 603.*

Recall in Chapter 1 that we suggested that the body may be considered a "city of cells" and a "container of chemicals." Chemicals are nonliving. Cells are living. What is it that can change a particular assortment of nonliving chemicals into a living cell capable of reproducing itself? We don't know. We do know that such a transformation occurred at least once several billion years ago—and these billions of years later, here we are, each of us a fine city with a population of trillions of cells.

Cells are the smallest living subunits of a multicellular organism such as a human being. A cell is a complex and precise arrangement of the organic and inorganic chemicals discussed in the previous chapter, and it carries out specific activities. Microorganisms, such as amoebas and bacteria, are single cells that function independently. Human cells, however, must work together and function interdependently. Homeostasis depends on the contributions of all of the different kinds of cells.

Human cells vary in size, shape, and function. Most human cells are so small they can be seen only with the aid of a microscope and are measured in units called **micrometers** (formerly called microns). One micrometer = 1/1,000,000 of a meter or 1/25,000 of an inch (see Appendix A: Units of Measure). One exception is the human ovum or egg cell, which is about 1 millimeter in diameter, just visible to the unaided eye. Some nerve cells, although microscopic in diameter, may be quite long. Those in our arms and legs, for example, are at least 2 feet (60 cm) long.

With respect to shape, human cells vary greatly. Some are round or spherical, others are rectangular, and still others are irregular. White blood cells even change shape as they move.

Cell functions also vary, and because our cells do not act independently, we will cover specialized cell functions as part of tissue functions in Chapter 4. On the basis of function, there are more than 200 different kinds of human cells. This chapter is concerned with the basic structure of cells and the cellular activities common to all or most of our cells.

CELL STRUCTURE

Despite their many differences, human cells have several similar structural features: a cell membrane, a nucleus, and cytoplasm and cell organelles. Red blood cells are an exception because they have no nuclei when mature. The cell membrane forms the outer boundary of the cell and surrounds the cytoplasm, organelles, and nucleus.

CELL MEMBRANE

Also called the **plasma membrane**, the **cell membrane** is the outer boundary of a cell and is made of phospholipids, cholesterol, and proteins. The arrangement of these organic molecules is shown in Fig. 3–1. The phospholipids are diglycerides, and they form a bilayer, or double layer, which makes up most of the membrane. Phospholipids permit lipid-soluble materials to easily enter or leave the cell by diffusion through the cell membrane. The presence of cholesterol decreases the fluidity of the membrane, thus making it more stable. The proteins have several functions: Some form **channels** to permit passage of materials such as water or ions; others are carrier enzymes or **transporters** that also help substances enter the cell. Still other proteins, with oligosaccharides on their outer surface, are **antigens**, markers that identify the cells of an individual as "self." These self-antigens are used by the white blood cells of the immune system to distinguish pathogens (foreign antigens) from the cells that belong in the body. Other membrane proteins form intercellular junctions, attachment points with neighboring cells; this contributes to the strength and resistance to tearing of some tissues. Yet another group of proteins serves as **receptor sites** for hormones, growth factors, and other signaling chemicals. These chemicals bring about their specific effects by first bonding to a particular receptor on the cell membrane, a receptor with the proper shape. This bonding, or fit, then triggers chemical reactions within the cell membrane or the interior of the cell (see Box 10–3 in Chapter 10 for an illustration involving the hormone insulin). The cell membrane of a single human cell has hundreds of different receptors.

All of these molecules that bond to cell membranes are part of the chemical communication networks our cells have. An unavoidable consequence of having so many receptors for chemical communication is that some pathogens have evolved shapes to match certain receptors. For example, HIV, the virus that causes AIDS, just happens to fit a particular surface receptor on our white blood cells. When the virus fits in, the receptor becomes a gateway into the cell, which begins the takeover of the cell by the virus.

Most often, however, the cell membrane is a beneficial structure. Although the cell membrane is the outer boundary of the cell, it should already be apparent to you that it is not a static or wall-like boundary, but rather an active, dynamic one. It is much more like a line of tollbooths than a concrete barrier. The cell membrane is **selectively permeable**; that is, certain substances are permitted to

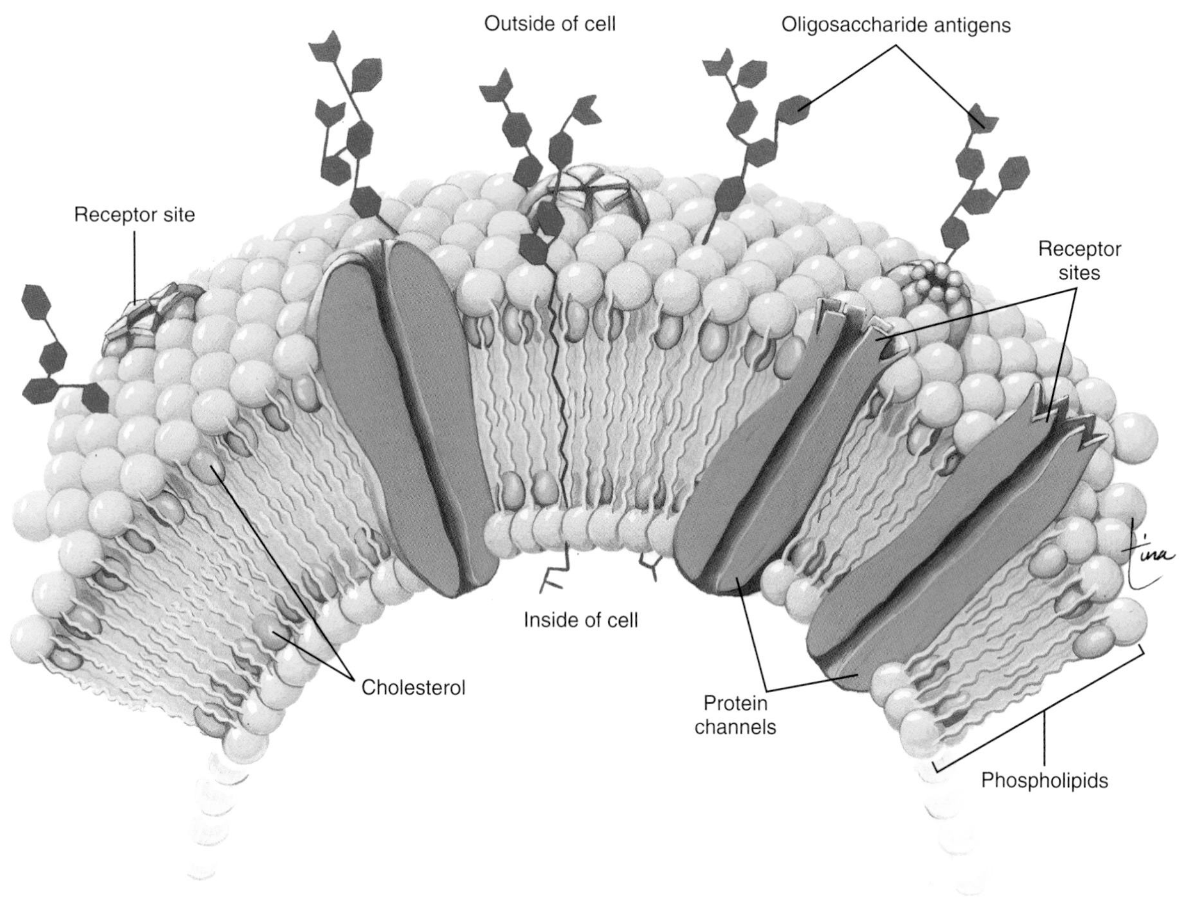

Figure 3–1 The cell (plasma) membrane depicting the types of molecules present.

QUESTION: The receptor sites shown are probably what type of organic molecule?

pass through and others are not. These mechanisms of cellular transport will be covered later in this chapter. The cell membrane is of particular importance for muscle cells and nerve cells because it carries electrical impulses. This topic will be covered in Chapters 7 and 8.

NUCLEUS

With the exception of mature red blood cells, all human cells have a nucleus. The **nucleus** is within the cytoplasm and is bounded by a double-layered **nuclear membrane** with many pores. It contains one or more nucleoli and the chromosomes of the cell (Fig. 3–2).

A **nucleolus** is a small sphere made of DNA, RNA, and protein. The nucleoli form a type of RNA called ribosomal RNA, which is assembled with protein to become ribosomes (a cell organelle) and is involved in protein synthesis.

The nucleus is the control center of the cell because it contains the chromosomes. The chromosome number for humans is 46, and these are in 23 pairs (maternal and paternal). Pairs 1 through 22 are called **autosomes**; the remaining pair consists of the sex chromosomes, designated XX for women and XY for men. Even with a microscope, the chromosomes of a human cell are usually not visible; they are long threads called **chromatin** (it is estimated that the DNA of a cell's 46 chromosomes, if uncoiled and placed end to end, would be about 6 feet long). Before a cell divides, however, the chromatin coils extensively into visible chromosomes. Chromosomes are made of DNA and protein. Some chromosomal proteins

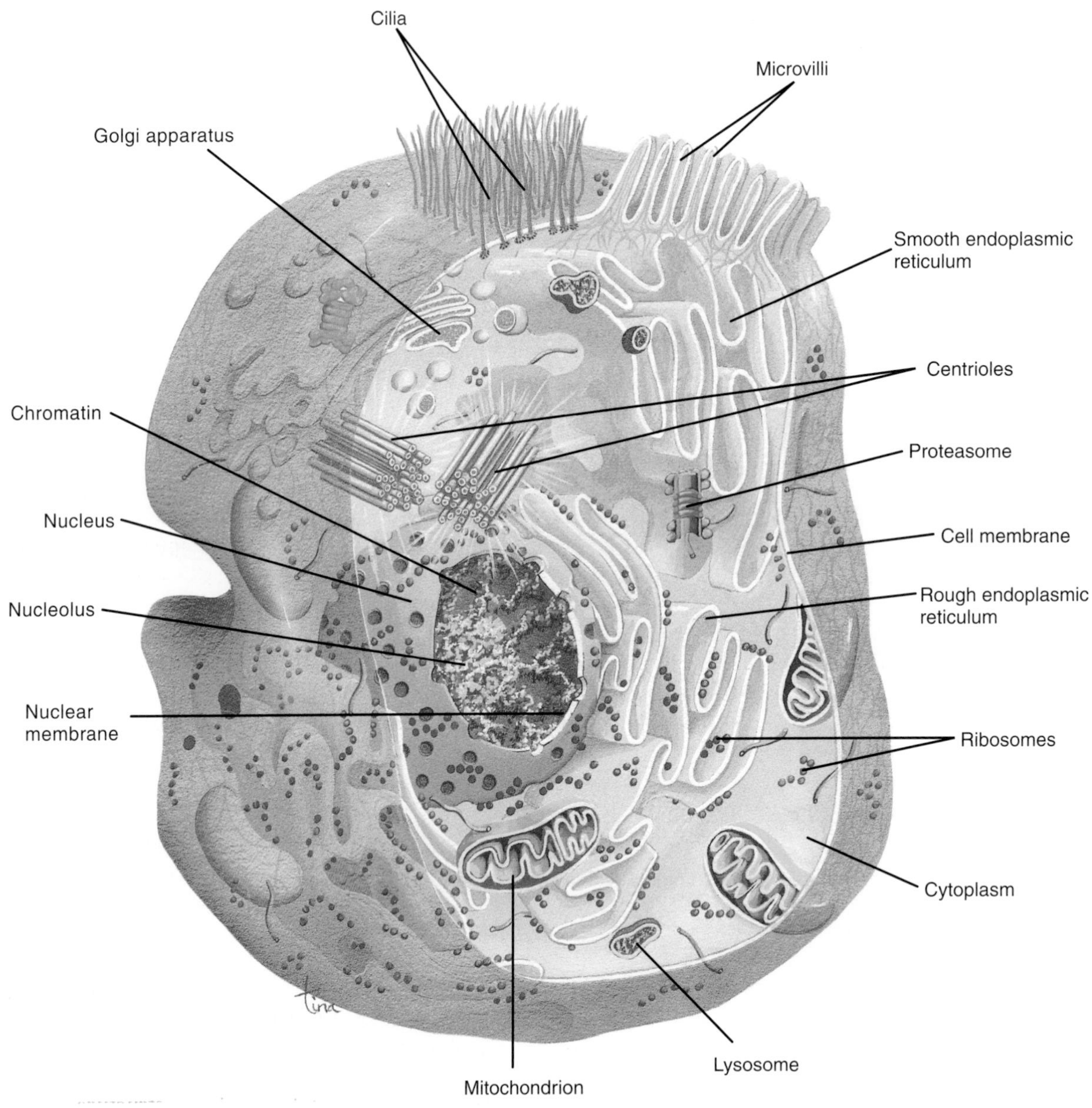

Figure 3–2 Generalized human cell depicting the structural components. See text and Table 3–1 for descriptions.

QUESTION: How do cilia differ in structure from microvilli?

provide the structural framework for the coiling of the chromatin into chromosomes so that cell division can take place. Other chromosomal proteins are enzymes that help regulate the activity of the DNA. Remember from our earlier discussion that the DNA is the genetic code for the characteristics and activities of the cell. Although the DNA in the nucleus of each cell contains all of the genetic information for all human traits, only a small number of genes (a **gene** is the genetic code for one protein) are actually active, or "switched on," in a particular cell. These active genes are the codes for the proteins necessary for the specific cell type and its functions. For example, the gene for insulin is present in all human cells, but only in certain islet cells of the pancreas is the gene active or switched on. Only in these cells is insulin produced. Similarly, the genes for antibody production are present in all human cells, but only in certain lymphocytes are these genes active; only these lymphocytes produce antibodies. How the genetic code in chromosomes is translated into proteins will be covered in a later section.

CYTOPLASM AND CELL ORGANELLES

Cytoplasm is a watery solution of minerals, gases, organic molecules, and cell organelles that is found between the cell membrane and the nucleus. **Cytosol** is the water portion of cytoplasm, and many chemical reactions take place within it. Cell **organelles** (from the Latin for "little tools") are intracellular structures, often bounded by their own membranes, that have specific functions in cellular metabolism. They are shown in Fig. 3–2.

The **endoplasmic reticulum** (ER) is an extensive network of membranous tubules that extend from the nuclear membrane to the cell membrane. Rough ER has numerous ribosomes on its surface, whereas smooth ER has no ribosomes. As a network of interconnected tunnels, the ER is a passageway for the transport of the materials necessary for cell function within the cell. These include proteins synthesized by the ribosomes on the rough ER and lipids synthesized by the smooth ER.

Ribosomes are very small structures made of protein and ribosomal RNA. Some are found on the surface of rough ER, while others float freely within the cytoplasm. Ribosomes are the site of protein synthesis. The proteins produced may be structural proteins such as collagen in the skin, enzymes, or hormones such as insulin that regulate cellular processes. These proteins may function within the cell or be secreted from the cell to be used elsewhere in the body.

Our protein molecules are subject to damage, and some cellular proteins, especially regulatory proteins, may be needed just for a very short time. All such proteins must be destroyed, and this is the function of proteasomes. A **proteasome** is a barrel-shaped organelle made of enzymes that cut protein molecules apart (protease enzymes). Proteins that are to be destroyed; that is, those no longer needed or those that are damaged or misfolded, are tagged by a protein called **ubiquitin** (sort of a cellular mop or broom) and carried into a proteasome. The protein is snipped into peptides or amino acids, which may be used again for protein synthesis on ribosomes. Proteasomes are particularly important during cell division and during embryonic development, when great changes are taking place very rapidly as cells become specialized.

Many of our cells have secretory functions; that is, they produce specific products to be used elsewhere in tissues. Secretion is one task of the **Golgi apparatus**, a series of flat, membranous sacs, somewhat like a stack of saucers. Carbohydrates are synthesized within the Golgi apparatus and are packaged, along with other materials, for secretion from the cell. Proteins from the ribosomes or lipids from the smooth endoplasmic reticulum may also be secreted in this way. To secrete a substance, small sacs of the Golgi membrane break off and fuse with the cell membrane, releasing the substance to the exterior of the cell. This is **exocytosis**, *exo* meaning "to go out" of the cell.

Mitochondria are oval or spherical organelles bounded by a double membrane. The inner membrane has folds called cristae. Within the mitochondria, the **aerobic** (oxygen-requiring) reactions of cell respiration take place. Therefore, mitochondria are the site of ATP (and hence energy) production. Cells that require large amounts of ATP, such as muscle cells, have many mitochondria to meet their need for energy. Athletic training increases the number of mitochondria within a muscle cell. Brown adipose tissue has abundant mitochondria because it is a heat-producing tissue (see Chapter 4).

Mitochondria contain their own genes (37 of them) in a single circular DNA molecule. They duplicate themselves when a cell divides. An individual's mitochondrial DNA (mDNA) is of maternal origin; that is, from the mitochondria that were present in the ovum, or egg cell, which was then fertilized by a sperm cell. The mitochondria of the sperm cell usually do not enter the ovum during fertilization because they are not found in the head of the sperm with the chromosomes (see Fig. 20–1 in Chapter 20).

Lysosomes are single-membrane structures that contain digestive enzymes. When certain white blood cells engulf bacteria, the bacteria are digested and destroyed by these lysosomal enzymes. Worn-out cell parts, old proteins, and dead cells are also digested by these enzymes; the products, simple chemicals, may then be recycled. This is **autophagy** ("self-eating"), a beneficial process that is necessary to keep cells healthy. Autophagy also cleans up damaged parts after injury so that tissue repair can begin. But it does have a disadvantage in that lysosomal digestion contributes to inflammation in damaged tissues. An excess of inflammation can start a vicious cycle, actually a positive feedback mechanism, that results in even more extensive tissue damage. The opposite, impaired autophagy, can result in the accumulation of damaged proteins or cell parts within cells. Some degenerative diseases of the nervous system and cardiovascular system are believed to be in part the result of lysosomal malfunctioning, as are some autoimmune diseases and the aging process.

Many of our cells are capable of dividing, or reproducing, themselves. **Centrioles** are a pair of rod-shaped structures perpendicular to one another, located just outside the nucleus. Their function is to organize the spindle fibers during cell division. The spindle fibers are contracting proteins that pull the two sets of chromosomes apart, toward the ends of the original cell as it divides into two new cells. Each new cell then has a full set of chromosomes.

Flagella and **cilia** are threadlike projections through the cell membrane; each is anchored by a basal body just within the membrane. Flagella are usually long; cilia are shorter. Many species of bacteria and protozoa have one or several flagella to enable them to move. The only human cell with a flagellum is the sperm cell, and the flagellum provides for **motility**, or movement.

Human cells may have two kinds of cilia. **Motile cilia** occur in bunches or swaths on the free surface of one type of epithelial cell; they resemble small fields of wheat. These cilia beat (bend) in unison and sweep materials across the cell surface. Cells lining the trachea, for example, have cilia to sweep mucus and trapped dust up toward the pharynx. In women, the cells lining the fallopian tubes have cilia to sweep the egg cell toward the uterus.

Most human cells have a sensory cilium called a **primary cilium**; this single cilium is part of a cell's communication system and has been likened to an antenna. Just as the antenna of a radio can pick up signals from hundreds of stations, a primary cilium can detect many different kinds of changes. Some of these changes are chemicals produced by other cells; other changes are mechanical, such as the flow of blood or tissue fluid in the cell's environment. Primary cilia seem to be essential to proper mitosis and development of an embryo (including the left-right asymmetry of thoracic and abdominal organs) and for many functions in established tissues as well. For example, the rods and cones of the retina of the eye, the receptors for light, are primary cilia.

Microvilli are folds of the cell membrane on the free surface of a cell. These folds greatly increase the surface area of the membrane and are part of the cells lining organs that absorb materials. The small intestine, for example, requires a large surface area for the **absorption** of nutrients, and many of its lining cells have microvilli. Some cells of the kidney tubules also have microvilli (see Fig. 1–1 in Chapter 1) that provide for the efficient reabsorption of useful materials back to the blood.

The **cytoskeleton** is just what its name suggests: the framework or support of a cell. Microfilaments made of the protein actin help support the cell membrane (and microvilli if they are present), give shape to the cell, and contribute to the movement of the cell. When you think of movement you may rightly think of muscle cells; as you will see in Chapter 7, actin is one of a muscle cell's contracting proteins. Other protein filaments provide for the support of organelles within the cell and help form junction or linkage sites between adjacent cells.

The functions of the cell organelles are summarized in Table 3–1.

CELLULAR TRANSPORT MECHANISMS

Living cells constantly interact with the blood or tissue fluid around them, taking in some substances and secreting or excreting others. Several mechanisms of transport enable cells to move materials into or out of the cell: diffusion, osmosis, facilitated diffusion, active transport, filtration, phagocytosis, and pinocytosis. Some of these take place without the expenditure of energy by the cells. Others, however, *do* require energy, often in the form of ATP. Each of these mechanisms is described in the following sections, and an example is included to show how each is important to the body.

DIFFUSION

Diffusion is the movement of molecules from an area of greater concentration to an area of lesser concentration (that is, with or along a **concentration gradient**). Diffusion occurs because molecules have free energy; that is, they are always in motion. The molecules in a solid move very slowly; those in a liquid move faster; and those in a gas move faster still, such as when ice absorbs heat energy, melts, and then evaporates. Imagine at the bottom of a glass of water a green sugar cube (green so that we can see it). As the sugar dissolves, the sugar molecules collide with one another or the water molecules, and the green color seems to rise in the glass. These collisions spread out the sugar molecules until they are evenly dispersed among the water molecules (this would take a very long time), and the water eventually becomes entirely green. The molecules are still moving, but as some go to the top, others go to the

Table 3–1 | FUNCTIONS OF CELL ORGANELLES

ORGANELLE	FUNCTION
Endoplasmic reticulum (ER)	■ Passageway for transport of materials within the cell ■ Synthesis of lipids
Ribosomes	■ Site of protein synthesis
Proteasomes	■ Site of destruction of misfolded or damaged proteins
Golgi apparatus	■ Synthesis of carbohydrates ■ Packaging of materials for secretion from the cell
Mitochondria	■ Site of aerobic cell respiration—production of ATP and heat
Lysosomes	■ Containers for enzymes that digest ingested foreign material (such as bacteria) or digest and recycle damaged tissue or cellular parts (autophagy)
Centrioles	■ Organizer of the spindle fibers for the distribution of chromosomes during cell division
Cilia	■ Motile cilia sweep materials across the cell surface. ■ A sensory or primary cilium detects chemical or mechanical signals from other cells or the tissue environment.
Flagellum	■ Long appendage that enables a cell to move (sperm cells)
Microvilli	■ Folds of the cell membrane that increase a cell's surface area for absorption
Cytoskeleton	■ Protein microfilaments that give shape to a cell, support the membrane and microvilli, and provide for attachment and movement

bottom, and so on. Thus, an equilibrium (or steady state) is reached.

Diffusion is a very slow process, but it can be an effective transport mechanism across microscopic distances. Within the body, the gases oxygen and carbon dioxide move by diffusion. In the lungs, for example, there is a high concentration of oxygen in the alveoli (air sacs) and a low concentration of oxygen in the blood in the surrounding pulmonary capillaries (see Fig. 3–3A). The opposite is true for carbon dioxide: a low concentration is in the air in the alveoli and a high concentration is in the blood in the pulmonary capillaries. These gases diffuse in opposite directions, each moving from where there is more to where there is less. Oxygen diffuses from the air to the blood to be circulated throughout the body. Carbon dioxide diffuses from the blood to the air to be exhaled.

OSMOSIS

Osmosis may be defined simply as the diffusion of water through a selectively permeable membrane. That is, water will move from an area with more water to an area with less water. Another way to say this is that water will naturally tend to move to an area where there is more dissolved material, such as salt or sugar. If a 2% salt solution and a 6% salt solution are separated by a membrane allowing water but not salt to pass through it, water will diffuse from the 2% salt solution to the 6% salt solution. The result is that the 2% solution will become more concentrated, and the 6% solution will become more dilute, until the concentrations reach equilibrium.

In the body, the cells lining the small intestine absorb water from digested food by osmosis. These cells have first absorbed salts and have become more "salty," and water follows salt into the cells (see Fig. 3–3B). The process of osmosis also takes place in the kidneys, which reabsorb large amounts of water (many gallons each day) to prevent its loss in urine. Box 3–1: Terminology of Solutions lists some terminology we use when discussing solutions and the effects of various solutions on cells.

FACILITATED DIFFUSION

The word *facilitate* means "to help or assist." In **facilitated diffusion**, molecules move through a membrane from an

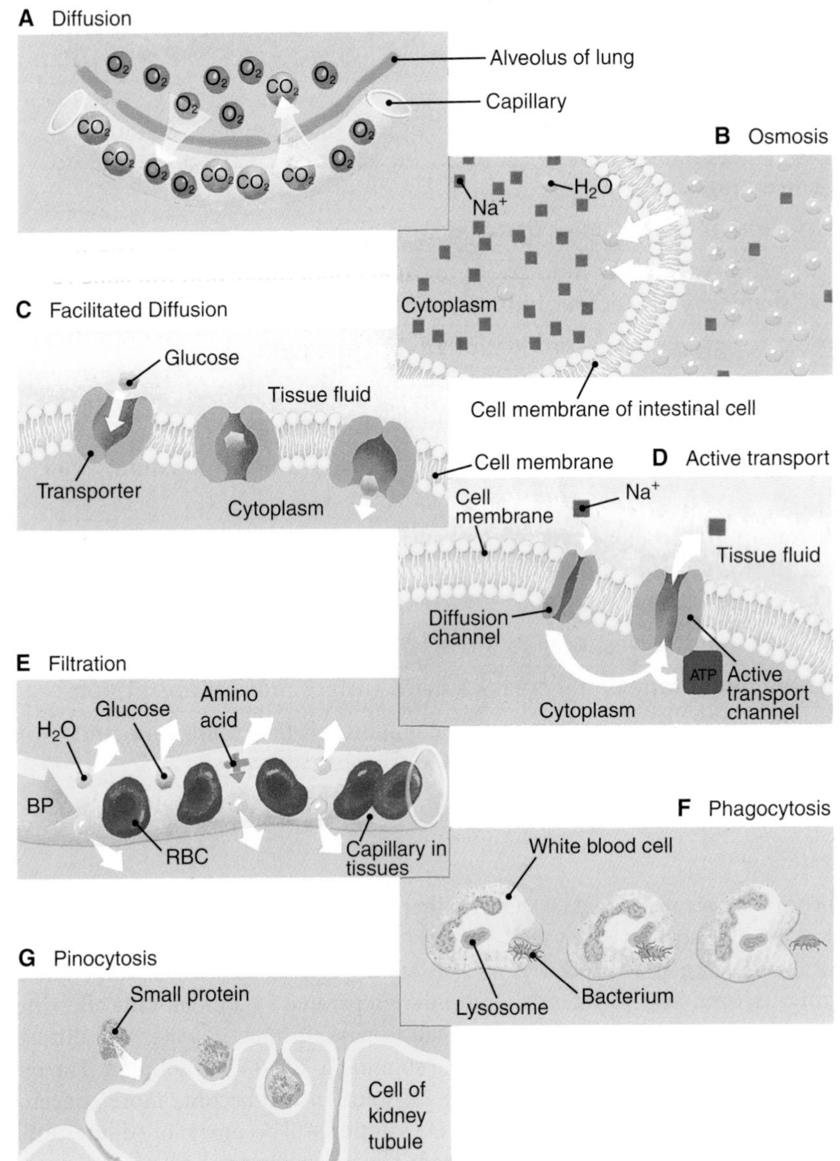

Figure 3–3 Cellular transport mechanisms. (**A**) Diffusion in an alveolus in the lung. (**B**) Osmosis in the small intestine. (**C**) Facilitated diffusion in a muscle cell. (**D**) Active transport in a muscle cell. (**E**) Filtration in a capillary. (**F**) Phagocytosis by a white blood cell. (**G**) Pinocytosis by a cell of the kidney tubules. See text for description.

QUESTION: Which mechanism depends on blood pressure? Which depends on the movement of a cell?

area of greater concentration to an area of lesser concentration, but they need some help to do this.

In the body, our cells must take in glucose to use for ATP production. Glucose, however, will not diffuse through most cell membranes by itself, even if there is more outside the cell than inside. Diffusion of glucose into most cells requires a glucose **transporter**, which may also be called a **carrier enzyme**. These transporters are proteins that are part of the cell membrane. Glucose bonds to the transporter (see Fig. 3–3C) and, by doing so, changes the shape of the protein. This physical change propels the glucose into the interior of the cell. Other transporters are specific for other organic molecules such as amino acids.

ACTIVE TRANSPORT

Active transport requires the energy of ATP to move molecules from an area of lesser concentration to an area of greater concentration. Notice that this is the opposite of diffusion, in which the free energy of molecules causes

Box 3–1 | TERMINOLOGY OF SOLUTIONS

Human cells or other body fluids contain many dissolved substances (called **solutes**) such as salts, sugars, acids, and bases. The concentration of solutes in a fluid creates the **osmotic pressure** of the solution, which in turn determines the movement of water through membranes.

As an example here, we will use sodium chloride (NaCl). Human cells have an NaCl concentration of 0.9%. With human cells as a reference point, the relative NaCl concentrations of other solutions may be described with the following terms:

Isotonic—a solution with a salt concentration equal to that in cells.

The blood plasma is isotonic to red blood cells.

Hypotonic—a solution with a salt concentration lower than that in cells.

Distilled water (0% salt) is hypotonic to human cells.

Hypertonic—a solution with a salt concentration higher than that in cells.

Seawater (3% salt) is hypertonic to human cells.

Refer now to the diagrams shown in Box Figure 3–A of red blood cells (RBCs) in each of these different types of solutions, and note the effect of each on osmosis:

- When RBCs are in plasma, water moves into and out of them at equal rates, and the cells remain normal in size and water content.
- If RBCs are placed in distilled water, more water will enter the cells than leave, and the cells will swell and eventually burst.
- If RBCs are placed in seawater, more water will leave the cells than enter, and the cells will shrivel and die.

This knowledge of osmotic pressure is used when replacement fluids are needed for a patient who has become dehydrated. Isotonic solutions are usually used; normal saline and Ringer's solution are examples. These will provide rehydration without causing osmotic damage to cells or extensive shifts of fluid between the blood and tissues.

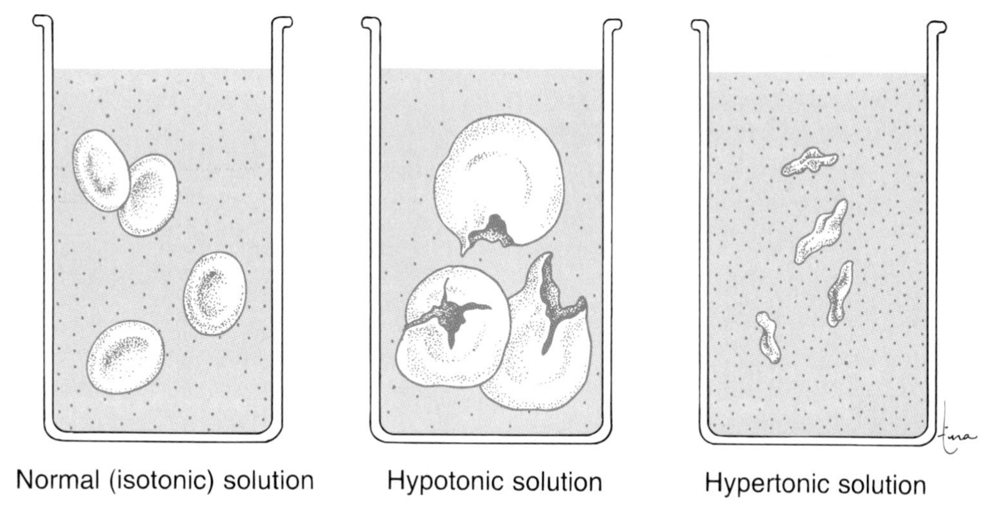

Box Figure 3–A Red blood cells in different solutions and the effect of osmosis in each.

them to move to where there are fewer of them. Active transport is therefore said to be movement against a concentration gradient.

In the body, nerve cells and muscle cells have "sodium pumps" to move sodium ions (Na^+) out of the cells. Sodium ions are more abundant outside the cells, and (through specific diffusion channels) they constantly diffuse into the cell, their area of lesser concentration (see Fig. 3–3D). Without the sodium pumps to return them outside, the incoming sodium ions would bring about an unwanted nerve impulse or muscle contraction. Nerve and muscle cells constantly produce ATP to keep their sodium pumps (and similar potassium pumps) working and prevent spontaneous impulses.

Another example of active transport is the absorption of glucose and amino acids by the cells lining the small intestine. The cells use ATP to absorb these nutrients from digested food, even when their intracellular concentration becomes greater than their extracellular concentration.

FILTRATION

The process of **filtration** also requires energy, but the energy needed does not come directly from ATP. It is the energy of mechanical pressure. Filtration means that water and dissolved materials are forced through a membrane from an area of higher pressure to an area of lower pressure.

In the body, **blood pressure** is created by the pumping of the heart. Filtration occurs when blood flows through capillaries, whose walls are only one cell thick and very permeable. The blood pressure in capillaries is higher than the pressure of the surrounding tissue fluid. In capillaries throughout the body, blood pressure forces plasma (water) and dissolved materials through the capillary membranes into the surrounding tissue spaces (see Fig. 3–3E). This creates more tissue fluid and is how cells receive glucose, amino acids, and other nutrients. Blood pressure in the capillaries of the kidneys also brings about filtration, which is the first step in the formation of urine.

PHAGOCYTOSIS AND PINOCYTOSIS

These two processes are similar in that both involve a cell engulfing something, and both are forms of **endocytosis**, *endo* meaning "to take into" a cell. An example of **phagocytosis** is a white blood cell engulfing bacteria. The white blood cell flows around the bacterium (see Fig. 3–3F), taking it in and eventually digesting it. Digestion is accomplished by the enzymes in the cell's lysosomes.

Other cells that are stationary may take in small molecules that become adsorbed or attached to their membranes. The cells of the kidney tubules reabsorb small proteins by **pinocytosis** (see Fig. 3–3G) so that the protein is not lost in urine.

Table 3–2 summarizes the cellular transport mechanisms.

Table 3–2 | CELLULAR TRANSPORT MECHANISMS

MECHANISM	DEFINITION	EXAMPLE IN THE BODY
Diffusion	Movement of molecules from an area of greater concentration to an area of lesser concentration	Exchange of gases in the lungs or body tissues
Osmosis	The diffusion of water	Absorption of water by the small intestine or kidneys
Facilitated diffusion	Transporters and carrier enzymes move molecules across cell membranes.	Intake of glucose by most cells
Active transport	Movement of molecules from an area of lesser concentration to an area of greater concentration (requires ATP)	Absorption of amino acids and glucose from food by the cells of the small intestine Sodium and potassium pumps in muscle and nerve cells
Filtration	Movement of water and dissolved substances from an area of higher pressure to an area of lower pressure (blood pressure)	Formation of tissue fluid in capillaries throughout the body; the first step in the formation of urine in the capillaries of the kidneys
Phagocytosis	A moving cell engulfs something.	White blood cells engulf bacteria.
Pinocytosis	A stationary cell engulfs something.	Cells of the kidney tubules reabsorb small proteins.

THE GENETIC CODE AND PROTEIN SYNTHESIS

The structure of DNA, RNA, and protein was described in Chapter 2. We will review some of the essentials here and go a step further with a simple description of how all of these organic molecules are involved in the process of protein synthesis.

DNA AND THE GENETIC CODE

DNA consists of two strands of nucleotides in the form of a **double helix**, very much like a spiral ladder. The uprights of the ladder are made of alternating phosphate groups and deoxyribose sugar molecules. The rungs of the ladder are made of the four nitrogenous bases, always found in complementary pairs: adenine with thymine (A–T) and guanine with cytosine (G–C). Although DNA contains just these four bases, the bases may be arranged in many different sequences (reading up or down the ladder). It is the sequence of bases, the sequence of A, T, C, and G, that is the **genetic code**. The DNA of our 46 chromosomes may also be called our **genome**, which is the term for the total genetic information in a particular species. The human genome is believed to contain about 3.2 billion base pairs, and the number of our genes is estimated to be about 22,000.

Recall that in Chapter 2 you read that a **gene** is the genetic code for one protein. This is a simplification, and the functioning of genes is often much more complex. We have genes with segments that may be shuffled or associated in many combinations, or that function as networks, with the potential for coding for many more proteins. A full explanation is beyond the scope of our book, so for the sake of simplicity, and in the following discussion, we will say that a gene is the DNA code for one protein. Recall too that a protein is a specific sequence of amino acids. Therefore, a gene, or segment of DNA, is the code for the sequence of amino acids in a particular protein.

The code for a single amino acid consists of three bases in the DNA molecule; this **triplet** of bases may be called a **codon** (see Fig. 3–4). There is a triplet of bases in the DNA for each amino acid in the protein. If a protein consists of 100 amino acids, the gene for that protein would consist of 100 triplets, or 300 bases. Some of the triplets will be the same because the same amino acid may be present in several places within the protein. Also part of the gene are other triplets that start and stop the process of making the protein, rather like the way that capital letters or punctuation marks start and stop sentences. Genes may also be influenced by chemical activity that has come to be called **epigenetics**, and we will consider this briefly before discussing the synthesis of proteins.

Epigenetics

The prefix *epi* means "upon, outer, on top of, or in addition to." *Epigenetics,* therefore, means "something in addition to genetics, the DNA in chromosomes." This something may be changes in cellular structure or chemistry, or changes in the chromosomes themselves when certain genes are switched on or off. These are not mutations; the DNA genes remain unchanged. But the activity of genes is altered; **gene expression** is affected. The expression of a gene means that the product of the gene is somehow apparent to us, in a way we can see or measure, or is not apparent when it should be. Examples would be having brown eyes or blue eyes, or producing or not producing the intestinal enzyme lactase to digest milk sugar.

Gene expression can be altered in several ways. Certain types of RNA molecules can suppress the activity of DNA genes. Parts of the chromosomes that are *not* codes for proteins, called **noncoding DNA**, also act as switches for the genes for proteins (this noncoding DNA was once called "junk" DNA, before its function was discovered). Gene expression can also be affected by the attachment of simple chemicals to a chromosome. For example, methyl groups (CH_3) are switches that inactivate genes, and acetyl groups (C_2H_5) are switches that activate genes. Recent research suggests that environmental factors may influence these modifications of gene activity. Factors such as smoking or obesity are believed to affect gene expression in harmful ways, permitting lipid buildup in arteries, for example, while a factor such as regular exercise will alter gene expression in a beneficial way, preventing such buildup. We have so much more to learn about how diet, exercise, and even the air we breathe can affect our genes, but let us return now to the synthesis of proteins.

RNA AND PROTEIN SYNTHESIS

RNA has been found to have many functions; it contributes to the repair of DNA, and it is involved in gene expression. Although these functions of RNA are essential for us, the details are beyond the scope of our book, so the roles of RNA in the process of protein synthesis will be our focus.

The transcription and translation of the genetic code in DNA into proteins require several types of RNA. DNA is found in the chromosomes in the nucleus of the cell, but

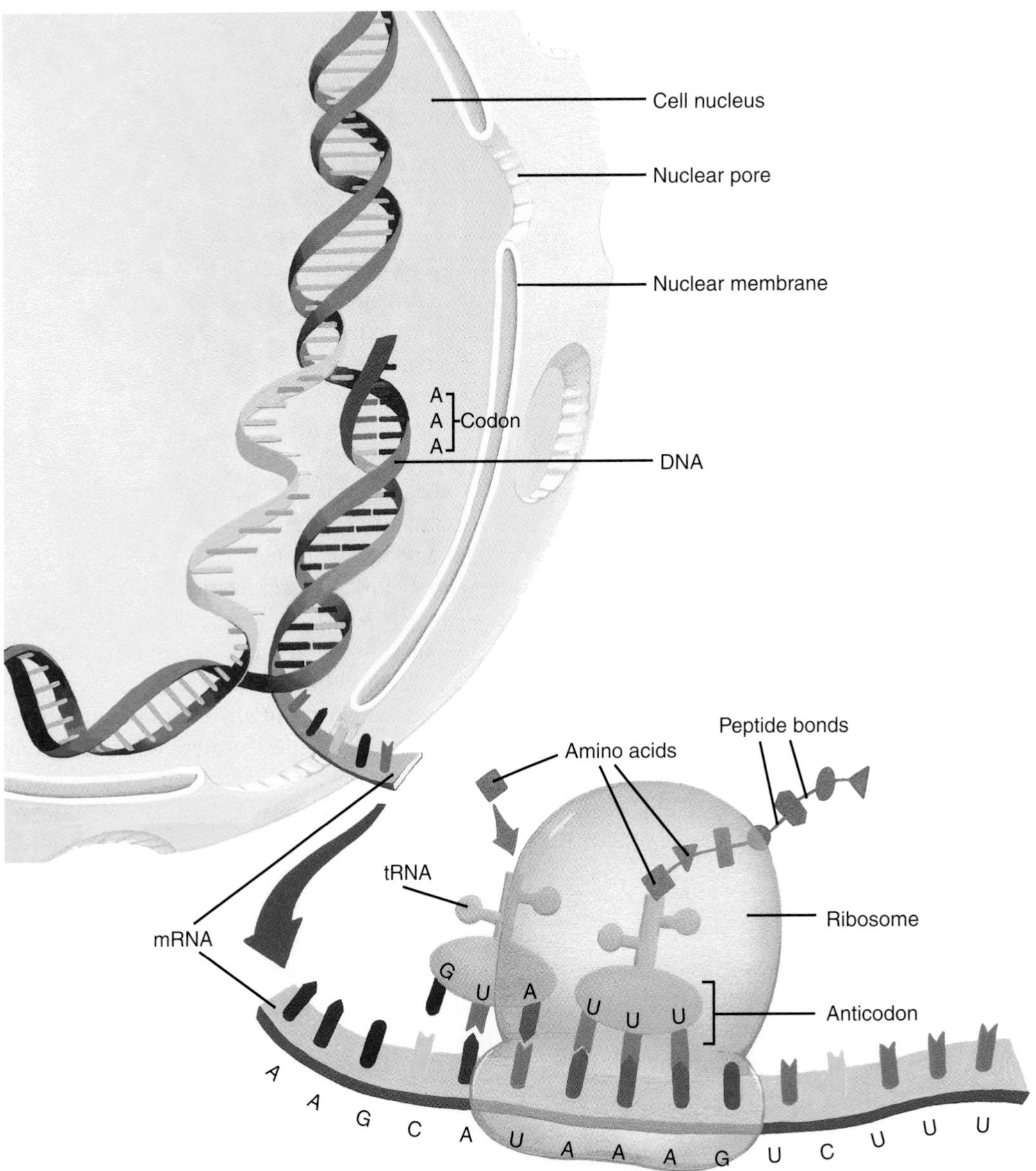

Figure 3–4 Protein synthesis. The mRNA is formed as a copy of a portion of the DNA in the nucleus of a cell. In the cytoplasm, the mRNA becomes attached to ribosomes. See text for further description.

QUESTION: A tRNA molecule has two attachment sites; what is each for?

protein synthesis takes place on the ribosomes in the cytoplasm. **Messenger RNA (mRNA)** is the intermediary molecule between these two sites.

When a protein is to be made, the segment of DNA that is its gene uncoils, and the hydrogen bonds between the base pairs break (see Fig. 3–4). Within the nucleus are RNA nucleotides (A, C, G, U) and enzymes to construct a single strand of nucleotides that is a complementary copy of half the DNA gene (with uracil in place of thymine). This process is **transcription**, or copying, and the copy of the gene is mRNA, which now has the codons for the amino acids of the protein, and will then separate from the DNA. The gene coils back into the double helix, and the mRNA leaves the nucleus, enters the cytoplasm, and becomes attached to ribosomes.

As the copy of the gene, mRNA is a series of triplets of bases; each triplet is a codon, the code for one amino acid. Another type of RNA, called **transfer RNA (tRNA)**, is also found in the cytoplasm. Each tRNA molecule has an **anticodon**, a triplet complementary to a triplet on the mRNA. The tRNA molecules pick up specific amino acids (which have come from protein in our food) and bring them to their proper triplets on the mRNA. This process is **translation**; that is, it is as if we are translating from one language to another—the language of nucleotide bases to that of amino acids. The ribosomes contain structural proteins and ribosomal RNA (rRNA) that functions as an enzyme, called a **ribozyme**, to catalyze the formation of **peptide bonds** between the amino acids. When an amino acid has been brought to each triplet on the mRNA, and all peptide bonds have been formed, the protein is finished.

The protein then leaves the ribosomes and may be transported by the endoplasmic reticulum to wherever it is needed in the cell, or it may be packaged by the Golgi apparatus for secretion from the cell. A summary of the process of protein synthesis is found in Table 3–3.

Thus, the expression of the genetic code may be described by the following sequence:

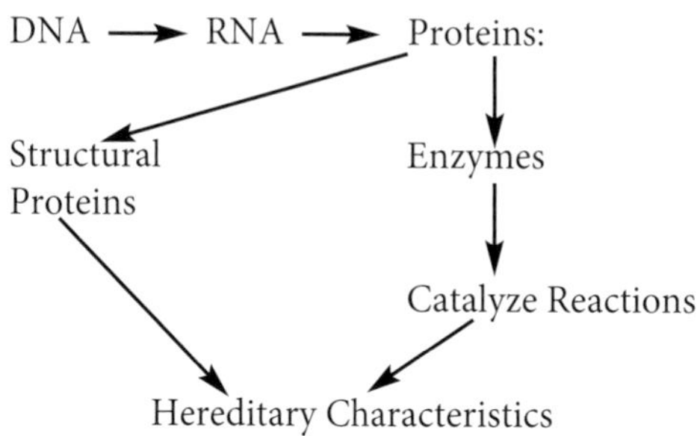

Each of us is the sum of our genetic characteristics. Blood type, hair color, muscle proteins, nerve cells, and thousands of other aspects of our structure and functioning have their basis in the genetic code of DNA.

If there is a "mistake" in the DNA, that is, incorrect bases or triplets of bases, this mistake will be copied by the mRNA. The result is the formation of a malfunctioning or nonfunctioning protein. This is called a **genetic** or **hereditary disease**, and a specific example is described in Box 3–2: Genetic Disease—Sickle-Cell Anemia.

Table 3–3 | PROTEIN SYNTHESIS

MOLECULE OR ORGANELLE	FUNCTION
DNA	■ A double strand (helix) of nucleotides that is the genetic code in the chromosomes of cells ■ A gene is the sequence of bases (segment of DNA) that is the code for one protein.
mRNA (messenger RNA)	■ A single strand of nucleotides that is formed as a complementary copy of a gene in the DNA ■ Contains the triplet code: three bases is the code for one amino acid (a codon) ■ Leaves the DNA in the nucleus, enters the cytoplasm of the cell, and becomes attached to ribosomes
Ribosomes	■ The cell organelles that are the site of protein synthesis ■ Attach to the mRNA molecule ■ Contain rRNA, a ribozyme that forms peptide bonds between amino acids
tRNA (transfer RNA)	■ Picks up amino acids (from food) in the cytoplasm and transports them to their proper sites (triplets) along the mRNA molecule; has anticodons to match mRNA codons

Box 3–2 | GENETIC DISEASE—SICKLE-CELL ANEMIA

A **genetic disease** is a hereditary disorder, one that may be passed from generation to generation. Although there are hundreds of genetic diseases, they all have the same basis: a mistake in DNA. Because DNA makes up the chromosomes that are found in eggs and sperm, this mistake may be passed from parents to children.

Sickle-cell anemia is the most common genetic disorder among people of African descent and affects the hemoglobin in red blood cells. Normal hemoglobin, called hemoglobin A (HbA), is a protein made of two alpha chains (141 amino acids each) and two beta chains (146 amino acids each). In sickle-cell hemoglobin (HbS), the sixth amino acid in each beta chain is incorrect; it is valine instead of the glutamic acid found in HbA. This difference seems minor—only 2 incorrect amino acids out of more than 500—but the consequences for the person are very serious.

HbS has a great tendency to crystallize when oxygen levels are low, as is true in capillaries. When HbS crystallizes, the red blood cells are deformed into crescents (sickles) and other irregular shapes. These irregular, rigid red blood cells clog and rupture capillaries, causing internal bleeding and severe pain. These cells are also fragile and break up easily, leading to anemia and hypoxia (lack of oxygen). Treatment of this disease has improved greatly, but it is still incurable.

What has happened to cause the formation of HbS rather than HbA? Hemoglobin is a protein; the gene for its beta chain is in DNA (chromosome 11). One amino acid in the beta chains is incorrect; therefore, one triplet in its DNA gene must be, and is, incorrect. This mistake is copied by mRNA in the cells of the red bone marrow, and HbS is synthesized in red blood cells.

Sickle-cell anemia is a recessive genetic disease, which means that a person with one gene for HbS and one gene for HbA will have "sickle-cell trait." Such a person usually will not have the severe effects of sickle-cell anemia but may pass the gene for HbS to children. It is estimated that 9% of African Americans have sickle-cell trait and about 1% have sickle-cell anemia.

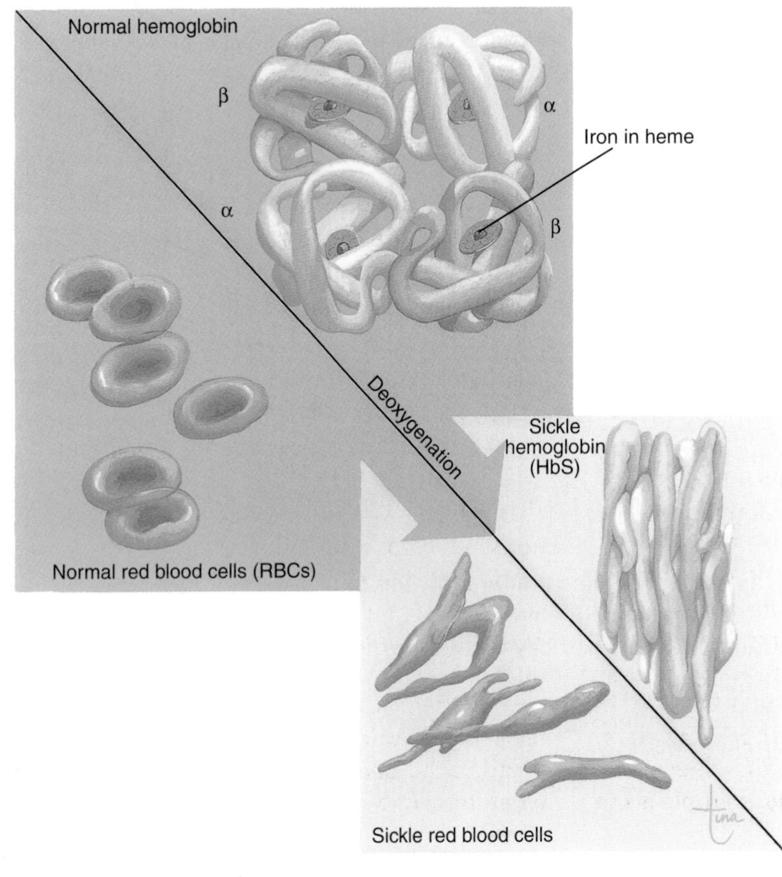

Box Figure 3–B Structures of hemoglobin A and sickle-cell hemoglobin and their effect on red blood cells.

CELL DIVISION

Cell division is the process by which a cell reproduces itself. There are two types of cell division, mitosis and meiosis. Although both types involve cell reproduction, their purposes are very different.

MITOSIS AND THE CELL CYCLE

Each of us began life as one cell, a fertilized egg. Each of us now consists of trillions of cells produced by the process of mitosis. In **mitosis**, one cell with the **diploid number** of chromosomes (the usual number, 46 for humans) divides into two identical cells, each with the diploid number of chromosomes. This production of identical cells is necessary for the growth of the organism and for repair of tissues (see also Box 3–3: Abnormal Cellular Functioning—Cancer).

Before mitosis can take place, a cell must have two complete sets of chromosomes, because each new cell must have the diploid number. The process of **DNA replication** enables each chromosome (in the form of chromatin) to make a copy of itself. This takes place during **interphase**, the time between mitotic divisions. Although interphase is sometimes referred to as the resting stage, resting means "not dividing" rather than "inactive." The cell is quite actively producing a second set of chromosomes and storing energy in ATP.

The long, thin, and invisible chromatin molecules then begin to coil very precisely and extensively, and if we were

Box 3–3 | ABNORMAL CELLULAR FUNCTIONING—CANCER

There are more than 200 different types of **cancer**, all of which are characterized by abnormal cellular functioning. Normally our cells undergo mitosis only when necessary and stop when appropriate. A cut in the skin, for example, is repaired by mitosis, usually without formation of excess tissue. The new cells fill in the damaged area, and mitosis slows when the cells make contact with surrounding cells. This is called contact inhibition, which limits the new tissue to just what is needed. **Malignant** (cancer) cells, however, are characterized by uncontrolled cell division. Our cells are genetically programmed to have particular life spans and to divide or die. Malignant cells simply keep dividing, and they tend to spread.

A malignant tumor begins in a primary site, such as the colon, then may spread or metastasize. The malignant cells are carried by the lymph or blood to other organs, such as the liver, where secondary tumors develop. **Metastasis** is characteristic only of malignant cells; **benign** tumors do not metastasize but remain localized in their primary site.

What causes normal cells to become malignant? At present, we have only partial answers. A malignant cell is created by a **mutation**, a genetic change that brings about abnormal cell functions or responses and often leads to a series of mutations. Environmental substances that cause mutations are called **carcinogens**. One example is the tar found in cigarette smoke, which is a cause of lung cancer. Ultraviolet light may also cause mutations, especially in skin that is overexposed to sunlight.

Mutations in the genes for proteins that correct the "mistakes" that occur naturally during DNA replication result in the synthesis of other faulty proteins. A protein called p53 has several critical functions. Among these, p53 activates genes that prevent excessive mitosis, and it contributes to the triggering of apoptosis in damaged cells. Many cancers involve some malfunction of the p53 gene and its protein.

For a few specific kinds of cancer, the trigger is believed to be infection with certain viruses that cause cellular mutations. Carriers of hepatitis B virus, for example, are more likely to develop primary liver cancer than are people who have never been exposed to this virus. Human herpesvirus 8 causes Kaposi's sarcoma, a malignancy of blood vessels.

Once cells have become malignant, their functioning cannot return to normal, and though the immune system will often destroy such cells, sometimes it does not, especially as we get older. Some cancer cells have been found to produce a barrier of proteins that clogs the receptors a lymphocyte (a type of white blood cell) uses to recognize a malignant cell and initiate its destruction. Because malignant cells do not die when they should, the treatments for cancer are

Continued

Box 3–3 | ABNORMAL CELLULAR FUNCTIONING—CANCER *(Continued)*

directed at removing or destroying the abnormal cells. Surgery to remove tumors, radiation to destroy cells, and **chemotherapy** to stop cell division or interfere with other aspects of cell metabolism are all aspects of cancer treatment.

New chemotherapy drugs are becoming more specific, with very precise targets. For example, medications that target altered cell-membrane receptors for growth factors may limit uncontrolled cell division. Immunotherapy is also undergoing clinical trials. The use of synthetic antibodies to increase white blood cell activity has resulted in shrinkage of brain tumors in some children. And "vaccines" of a person's own cancer cells have stimulated the immune system of the person to destroy the malignant cells. These individualized therapies do have promise, but they are very expensive, and much more testing is required.

looking at the nucleus of a living cell under a microscope, we would see the duplicated chromosomes appear. Each would look somewhat like the letter X because the original DNA molecule and its copy (now called chromatids) are still attached.

The stages of mitosis are **prophase**, **metaphase**, **anaphase**, and **telophase**. What happens in each of these stages is described in Table 3–4. As you read the events of each stage, refer to Fig. 3–5, which depicts mitosis in a cell with a diploid number of four.

As mentioned previously, mitosis is essential for repair of tissues because it replaces damaged or dead cells. Some examples may help illustrate this. In several areas of the body, mitosis takes place constantly. These sites include the epidermis of the skin, the stomach lining, and the red bone marrow. For each of these sites, there is a specific reason why this constant mitosis is necessary.

What happens to the surface of the skin? The dead, outer cells flake off or are worn off by contact with the environment. Mitosis of the epidermal cells in the lower living layer replaces these cells, and the epidermis maintains its normal thickness.

The stomach lining, although internal, is also constantly worn away. Gastric juice, especially hydrochloric

Table 3–4 | STAGES OF MITOSIS

STAGE	EVENTS
Prophase	1. The chromosomes coil up and become visible as short rods. Each chromosome is really two chromatids (original DNA plus its copy) still attached at a region called the centromere. 2. The nuclear membrane disappears. 3. The centrioles move toward opposite poles of the cell and organize the spindle fibers, which extend across the equator of the cell.
Metaphase	1. The pairs of chromatids line up along the equator of the cell. The centromere of each pair is attached to a spindle fiber. 2. The centromeres now divide.
Anaphase	1. Each chromatid is now considered a separate chromosome; there are two complete and separate sets. 2. The spindle fibers contract and pull the chromosomes, with one set pulled toward each pole of the cell.
Telophase	1. The sets of chromosomes reach the poles of the cell and become indistinct as their DNA uncoils to form chromatin. 2. A nuclear membrane re-forms around each set of chromosomes.
Cytokinesis	1. The cytoplasm divides; new cell membrane is formed.

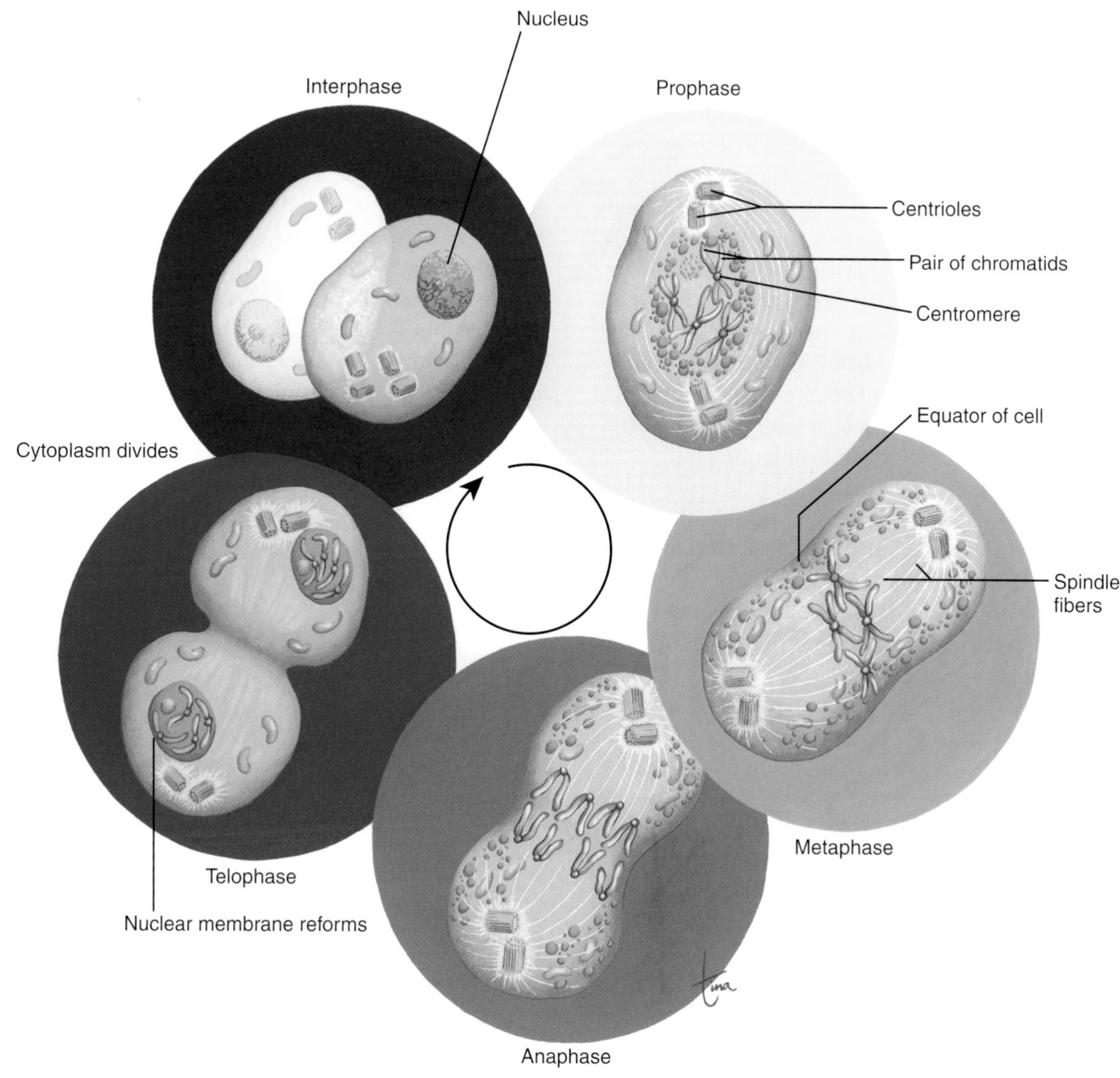

Figure 3–5 Stages of mitosis in a cell with the diploid number of four. See Table 3–4 for description.

QUESTION: In prophase, what is a pair of chromatids made of?

acid, is very damaging to cells. Rapid mitosis of the several kinds of lining cells replaces damaged cells and keeps the stomach lining intact.

One of the functions of red bone marrow is the production of red blood cells. Because red blood cells have a life span of only about 120 days, new ones are needed to replace the older ones that die. Very rapid mitosis in the red bone marrow produces approximately 2 million new red blood cells every second. These dividing cells in the red bone marrow are among the stem cells present in the body. A **stem cell** is an unspecialized cell that may develop into several different kinds of cells. Stem cells in the red bone marrow may become red blood cells, white blood cells, or platelets. These marrow stem cells are often called adult stem cells, and many, if not all, of the body's organs have such cells. Embryonic stem cells will be described in a later chapter; these are cells in which all of the DNA still has the potential to be active. They may become any of the more than 200 different kinds of human cells. The stem cells found in the umbilical cords of newborns are between the adult and embryonic cells in terms of their potential.

It is also important to be aware of the areas of the body where mitosis does not take place. In an adult, most muscle cells and neurons (nerve cells) do not reproduce themselves. If the cells die, their functions are also lost. Someone whose spinal cord has been severed will have paralysis and loss of sensation below the level of the injury. The spinal cord neurons do not undergo mitosis to replace the ones that were lost, and such an injury is permanent.

Skeletal muscle cells are capable of limited mitosis for repair. The heart is made of cardiac muscle cells, which, like many neurons, do not *seem* to be capable of mitosis. A heart attack (myocardial infarction) means that a portion of cardiac muscle dies because of lack of oxygen. These cells are not replaced, and the heart becomes a less effective pump. If a large enough area of the heart muscle dies, the heart attack is fatal.

Research has found evidence for ongoing mitosis in the heart and the potential for mitosis after damage in both the central nervous system and the heart. Such cell division may be that of neurons or muscle cells that were stimulated to divide by chemicals from the adjacent damaged tissue. Or the dividing cells may be stem cells that are among the specialized cells. (A region of the brain that does have cells capable of division is the hippocampus—a structure that is found in both sides of the brain and that is necessary to form new memories and keep old ones.) At present we do know that for most people with heart damage or central nervous system injury, mitosis does not take place rapidly or at least not sufficiently fast enough to replace the cells that have died and preserve or restore normal functioning of the organ. Research is continuing and may eventually find the stimulus necessary to produce extended mitosis that would bring about true tissue repair.

The Cell Cycle

The life span of a cell is specific and is genetically programmed. Some cells divide as part of their life cycle. Others do not; they simply carry out their functions. At the end of a cell's life span, the death of the cell is programmed as well. Chemical signals (which may be internal or come from other cells) cause a cell to produce enzymes that destroy its own nucleus. The nucleus-damaged cell begins to shrivel and is detected by phagocytic white blood cells, which clean up the cellular remains. This self-destruction or programmed cell death is called **apoptosis** and is essential for the normal functioning of tissues, organs, and ultimately the entire body.

Some examples will be helpful. As you probably know, hair grows in tubular structures called follicles. A hair root in the follicle is active for a certain length of time and then becomes inactive. The cells at the root of the hair die by apoptosis; the old hair falls out and a new hair begins to grow. An example of greater importance is the development of the brain. The brain of an infant contains many "extra" neurons. The neurons that do not make connections with other nerve cells die by apoptosis and are removed. This process "prunes" the nerve pathways of the brain for the most efficient functioning. A third example, also of great importance, is the fetal immune system, which will have to distinguish "nonself" pathogens from the cells that are "self;" that is, part of the body. White blood cells (the lymphocytes) that do not learn to "recognize" the body's own cells must be destroyed, and they are triggered into apoptosis.

One other aspect of apoptosis is significant: Although the process damages cells and attracts phagocytes, inflammation does not occur, as it would if those same cells were damaged by infection or physical trauma such as a burn. As mentioned earlier, inflammation is a beneficial process, but excessive inflammation can damage healthy surrounding tissue. No such damage occurs around cells that die of apoptosis.

MEIOSIS

Meiosis is a more complex process of cell division that results in the formation of **gametes**, which are egg and sperm cells. In a cell about to undergo meiosis, DNA replication takes place, and then the cell divides into two cells. Each of these cells still has the diploid number of chromosomes, and each divides into two cells. DNA replication does *not* take place before this second division, so each of the four new cells will have half the usual number of chromosomes. Stated most simply, in meiosis, one cell with the diploid number of chromosomes divides twice to form four cells, each with the **haploid number** (half the usual number) of chromosomes. In women, meiosis takes place in the ovaries and is called **oogenesis**. In men, meiosis takes place in the testes and is called **spermatogenesis**. The differences between oogenesis and spermatogenesis will be discussed (and illustrated) in Chapter 20, The Reproductive Systems.

The egg and sperm cells produced by meiosis have the haploid number of chromosomes, which is 23 for humans. Meiosis is sometimes called reduction division because the division process reduces the chromosome number in the egg or sperm. Then, during **fertilization**, in which the egg unites with the sperm, the 23 chromosomes of the sperm plus the 23 chromosomes of the egg will restore the diploid number of 46 in the fertilized egg. Thus, the proper chromosome number is maintained in the cells of the new individual.

AGING AND CELLS

Multicellular organisms, including people, age and eventually die; our cells do not have infinite life spans. It has been proposed that some cells capable of mitosis are limited to a certain number of divisions; that is, every division is sort of a tick-tock of a biological clock. We do not yet know exactly what this cellular biological countdown is. There is evidence that the ends of chromosomes, short sequences of DNA called **telomeres**, may be an aspect of it. With each cell division, part of the telomeres is lost (rather like a piece of rope fraying at both ends), and eventually the telomeres are gone. With the next division, the ends of the chromosomes, actual genes, begin to be lost. This may be one signal that a cell's life span has come to an end (there are probably many different kinds of signals).

Cellular aging also involves the inevitable deterioration of membranes and cell organelles. Just as the parts of a car break down in time, so too will cells. Unlike cars or machines, however, cells can often repair themselves, but they do have limits. As cells age, structural proteins break down and are not replaced, or necessary enzymes are not synthesized. Proteins called **chaperones**, which are responsible for the proper folding of many other proteins and for the repair or disposal of damaged proteins, no longer function as well as cells age. Without chaperones, damaged proteins accumulate within cells and disrupt normal cellular processes. Clinical manifestations of impaired chaperones include cataracts (see Box 9–1 in Chapter 9) and neurodegenerative diseases such as Alzheimer's disease, Parkinson's disease (see Boxes 8–6 and 8–7 in Chapter 8), and Huntington's disease (see Table 21–4 in Chapter 21).

Much about the chemistry of the aging process remains a mystery, though we can describe what happens to organs and to the body as a whole. Each of the following chapters on body systems provides a brief discussion of how aging affects the system. Keep in mind that a system is the sum of its cells, in tissues and organs, and that all aging is ultimately at the cellular level.

SUMMARY

As mentioned at the beginning of this chapter, human cells work closely together and function interdependently. Each type of human cell makes a contribution to the body as a whole. Usually, however, cells do not function as individuals, but rather in groups. Groups of cells with similar structure and function form a tissue, which is the next level of organization.

STUDY OUTLINE

Human cells vary in size, shape, and function. Our cells function interdependently to maintain homeostasis.

Cell Structure—the major parts of a cell are the cell membrane, the nucleus (except mature RBCs), the cytoplasm, and the cell organelles

1. Cell membrane—the selectively permeable boundary of the cell (see Fig. 3–1).
   a. Phospholipids permit diffusion of lipid-soluble materials.
   b. Cholesterol provides stability.
   c. Proteins form channels, transporters, "self" antigens, junctions, and receptor sites for hormones or other signaling molecules.
2. Nucleus—the control center of the cell; has a double-layer membrane.
   a. Nucleolus—forms ribosomal RNA and assembles ribosomes.
   b. Chromosomes—made of DNA and protein. DNA is the genetic code for the structure and functioning of the cell. A gene is a segment of DNA that is the code for one protein. Human cells have 46 chromosomes in 23 pairs (22 pairs of autosomes and one pair of sex chromosomes), and the total of their genetic information is called the genome. Human cells have the same chromosomes, and the activity of certain genes (and not others) creates the different kinds of cells.

3. Cytoplasm—a watery solution of minerals, gases, and organic molecules; contains the cell organelles; site for many chemical reactions.
4. Cell organelles—intracellular structures with specific functions (see Table 3–1 and Fig. 3–2).

Cellular Transport Mechanisms—the processes by which cells take in or secrete or excrete materials through the selectively permeable cell membrane (see Fig. 3–3 and Table 3–2).

1. Diffusion—movement of molecules from an area of greater concentration to an area of lesser concentration; it occurs because molecules have free energy: they are constantly in motion. Oxygen and carbon dioxide are exchanged by diffusion in the lungs and tissues.
2. Osmosis—the diffusion of water. Water diffuses to an area of less water, that is, to an area of more dissolved material. The small intestine absorbs water from digested food by osmosis. For isotonic, hypertonic, and hypotonic solutions, see Box 3–1.
3. Facilitated diffusion—transporters (carrier enzymes) that are part of the cell membrane permit cells to take in materials that would not diffuse by themselves. Most cells take in glucose by facilitated diffusion.
4. Active transport—a cell uses ATP to move substances from an area of lesser concentration to an area of greater concentration. Nerve cells and muscle cells have sodium pumps to return Na^+ ions to the exterior of the cells; this prevents spontaneous impulses. Cells of the small intestine absorb glucose and amino acids from digested food by active transport.
5. Filtration—pressure forces water and dissolved materials through a membrane from an area of higher pressure to an area of lower pressure. Tissue fluid is formed by filtration: Blood pressure forces plasma and dissolved nutrients out of capillaries and into tissues. Blood pressure in the kidney capillaries creates filtration, which is the first step in the formation of urine.
6. Phagocytosis—(a form of endocytosis) a moving cell engulfs something; white blood cells phagocytize bacteria to destroy them.
7. Pinocytosis—(another form of endocytosis) a stationary cell engulfs small molecules; kidney tubule cells reabsorb small proteins by pinocytosis.

The Genetic Code and Protein Synthesis (see Fig. 3–4 and Table 3–3)

1. DNA and the genetic code
   a. DNA is a double helix of nucleotides with complementary base pairing: A–T and G–C.
   b. The sequence of bases in the DNA is the genetic code for proteins; when a gene is switched on, its protein is synthesized; when a gene is switched off, its protein is not produced.
   c. The triplet code: three bases (a codon) is the code for one amino acid.
   d. A gene consists of all the triplets that code for a single protein.
   e. Epigenetics is a change in gene expression that occurs without any change in the DNA sequence of bases; noncoding DNA, some RNA molecules, and simple chemical attachments to chromosomes all may act as switches for gene activity. Factors such as diet, exercise, obesity, and exposure to pollution may bring about changes in gene expression by influencing the switching on or switching off of genes.

2. RNA and protein synthesis
   a. Transcription—mRNA is formed as a complementary copy of the sequence of bases in a gene (DNA).
   b. mRNA moves from the nucleus to the ribosomes in the cytoplasm.
   c. tRNA molecules (in the cytoplasm) have anticodons for the triplets on the mRNA.
   d. Translation—tRNA molecules bring amino acids to their proper triplets on the mRNA.
   e. Ribosomes contain rRNA, which acts as an enzyme (a ribozyme) to form peptide bonds between the amino acids.
3. Expression of the genetic code
   a. DNA → RNA → proteins (structural proteins and enzymes that catalyze reactions) → hereditary characteristics.
   b. A genetic disease is a "mistake" in the DNA, a mutation that is copied by mRNA and results in a malfunctioning protein.

Cell Division

1. Mitosis—one cell with the diploid number of chromosomes divides once to form two cells, each with the diploid number of chromosomes (46 for humans).
   a. DNA replication forms two sets of chromosomes during interphase.
   b. Stages of mitosis (see Fig. 3–5 and Table 3–4): prophase, metaphase, anaphase, and telophase. Cytokinesis is the division of the cytoplasm following telophase.
   c. Mitosis is essential for growth and for repair and replacement of damaged cells.
   d. Most adult nerve and muscle cells are not able to divide sufficiently to bring about repair of damaged tissue; their loss may involve permanent loss of function.
   e. Apoptosis is genetically programmed cell death, which occurs at the end of a cell's life span or when a cell is damaged.
2. Meiosis—one cell with the diploid number of chromosomes divides twice to form four cells, each with the haploid number of chromosomes (23 for humans).
   a. Oogenesis in the ovaries forms egg cells.
   b. Spermatogenesis in the testes forms sperm cells.
   c. Fertilization of an egg by a sperm restores the diploid number in the fertilized egg.

REVIEW QUESTIONS

1. State the functions of the organic molecules of cell membranes: cholesterol, proteins, and phospholipids. (p. 58)
2. Describe the function of each of these cell organelles: mitochondria, lysosomes, Golgi apparatus, ribosomes, proteasomes, motile cilia, primary cilia, flagella, and endoplasmic reticulum. (pp. 61–62)
3. Explain why the nucleus is the control center of the cell. (pp. 59–61)
4. What part of the cell membrane is necessary for facilitated diffusion? Describe one way this process is important within the body. (pp. 63–64)
5. What provides the energy for filtration? Describe one way this process is important within the body. (p. 66)
6. What provides the energy for diffusion? Describe one way this process is important within the body. (pp. 62–63)
7. What provides the energy for active transport? Describe one way this process is important within the body. (pp. 64–66)
8. Define osmosis, and describe one way this process is important within the body. (p. 63)
9. Explain the difference between *hypertonic* and *hypotonic,* using human cells as a reference point. (p. 65)
10. In what way are phagocytosis and pinocytosis similar? Describe one way each process is important within the body. (p. 66)
11. How many chromosomes does a human cell have? What are these chromosomes made of? (p. 67)
12. Name the stage of mitosis in which each of the following takes place: (p. 72)
    a. The two sets of chromosomes are pulled toward opposite poles of the cell.
    b. The chromosomes become visible as short rods.
    c. A nuclear membrane re-forms around each complete set of chromosomes.
    d. The pairs of chromatids line up along the equator of the cell.
    e. The centrioles organize the spindle fibers.
    f. Cytokinesis takes place after this stage.
13. Compare mitosis and meiosis in terms of: (p. 74)
    a. Importance within the body
    b. Number of divisions
    c. Number of cells formed
    d. Chromosome number of the cells formed
14. Explain the triplet code of DNA. Name the molecule that copies the triplet code of DNA. Name the organelle that is the site of protein synthesis. What other function does this organelle have in protein formation? (p. 67)

FOR FURTHER THOUGHT

1. Antibiotics are drugs used to treat bacterial infections. Some antibiotics disrupt the process of protein synthesis within bacteria. Others block DNA synthesis and cell division by the bacteria. Still others inhibit cell wall synthesis by the bacteria. If all antibiotics worked equally well against bacteria, would any of those mentioned here be better than the others, from the patient's perspective? Explain your answer.
2. A new lab instructor wants his students to see living cells. He puts a drop of his own blood on a glass slide, adds two drops of distilled water "so the cells will spread out and be easier to see," puts on a cover glass, and places the slide under a microscope on high power. He invites his students to see living red blood cells. The students claim that they cannot see any cells. Explain what has happened. How could this have been prevented?
3. A bacterial toxin is found to cause harm by first fitting into a receptor on human cell membranes; once the toxin fits, the cell will be destroyed. A medication is going to be made to stop this toxin, and it can work in one of two ways: The drug can block the receptors to prevent the toxin from fitting in, or the drug can act as decoy molecules shaped like the receptors. Which one of these might be better and why?
4. Look at Question Figure 3–A, Cells with organelles. Can you identify the prominent organelles in cell A on the left? In cell B on the right? (See Fig. 3–2 if you need a reminder.) Give a brief, general explanation of what each cell does, based on the functions of the main organelles you identified.

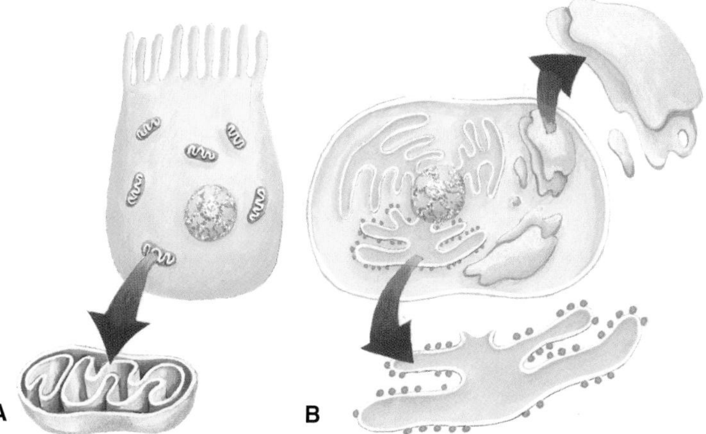

QUESTION FIGURE 3–A: Cells with organelles.

CHAPTER

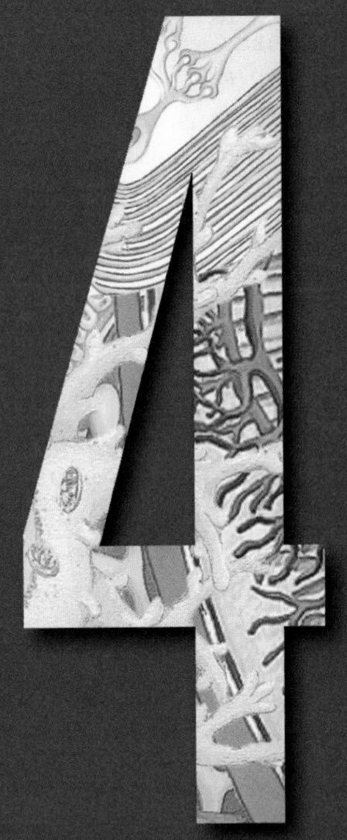

Tissues and Membranes

STUDENT OBJECTIVES

- Describe the general characteristics of each of the four major categories of tissues.
- Describe the functions of the types of epithelial tissues with respect to the organs in which they are found.
- Describe the functions of the connective tissues, and relate them to the functioning of the body or a specific organ system.
- Explain the difference between exocrine and endocrine glands, and give an example of each.
- Explain the differences, in terms of location and function, among skeletal muscle, smooth muscle, and cardiac muscle.
- Name the three parts of a neuron and state the function of each. Name the organs made of nerve tissue.
- Describe the locations of the pleural membranes, the pericardial membranes, and the peritoneum-mesentery. State the function of serous fluid in each of these locations.
- State the locations of mucous membranes and the functions of mucus.
- Name some membranes made of connective tissue.

NEW TERMINOLOGY

Bone *(BOWNE)*
Cartilage *(**KAR**-ti-lidj)*
Chondrocyte *(**KON**-droh-sight)*
Collagen *(**KAH**-lah-jen)*
Connective tissue *(kah-**NEK**-tiv **TISH**-yoo)*
Elastin *(eh-**LAS**-tin)*
Endocrine gland *(**EN**-doh-krin GLAND)*
Epithelial tissue *(EP-i-**THEE**-lee-uhl **TISH**-yoo)*
Exocrine gland *(**EK**-so-krin GLAND)*
Hemopoietic *(HEE-moh-poy-**ET**-ik)*
Matrix *(**MAY**-triks)*
Mucous membrane *(**MEW**-kuss **MEM**-brayn)*
Muscle tissue *(**MUSS**-uhl **TISH**-yoo)*
Myocardium *(MY-oh-**KAR**-dee-um)*
Myocyte *(**MYE**-oh-sight)*
Nerve tissue *(NERV **TISH**-yoo)*
Neuron *(**NYOOR**-on)*
Neurotransmitter *(NYOOR-oh-**TRANS**-mih-ter)*
Osteocyte *(**AHS**-tee-oh-sight)*
Plasma *(**PLAZ**-mah)*
Secretion *(si-**KREE**-shun)*
Serous membrane *(**SEER**-us **MEM**-brayn)*
Synapse *(**SIN**-aps)*
Thermogenic *(THER-moh-**JEN**-ik)*

*Terms that appear in **bold type** in the chapter text are defined in the glossary, which begins on page 603.*

CHAPTER OUTLINE

In our city of cells that is the human body, similar cells work together and have the same function. A group of cells with similar structure and function is called a **tissue**. Think for a moment of a hospital and its groups of workers: nurses, aides, lab techs, cooks, janitors, doctors, and many others. If each nurse equals a cell, then all the nurses in the hospital could be considered a tissue, as could all the aides, and all the cooks, and so on. Each tissue would contribute to the proper functioning of the hospital. What, then, would the hospital be? Right—the hospital would be an organ, a cooperation of tissues.

Recall from Chapter 1 that there are four major groups of tissues: epithelial, connective, muscle, and nerve tissue. An organ may (and usually does) contain tissues from all four groups. This chapter presents more detailed descriptions of the tissues in these four categories. You will notice that the function of a tissue is most often a description of what the tissue contributes to the functioning of an organ of which it is a part. Also in this chapter is a discussion of **membranes**, which are sheets of tissues. Some of these were mentioned in Chapter 1 with the body cavities. As you might expect, each type of membrane has its specific locations and functions.

EPITHELIAL TISSUE

Epithelial tissues are found on surfaces as either coverings (outer surfaces) or linings (inner surfaces). Because they have no capillaries of their own, epithelial tissues receive oxygen and nutrients from the blood supply of the connective tissue beneath them. Many epithelial tissues are capable of secretion and may be called glandular epithelium, or more simply, **glands**.

Classification of the epithelial tissues is based on the type of cell of which the tissue is made, the characteristic shape of the cell, and the number of layers of cells. There are three distinctive shapes: **squamous** cells are flat, **cuboidal** cells are cube shaped, and **columnar** cells are tall and narrow. **Simple** is the term for a single layer of cells, and **stratified** means that many layers of cells are present (Fig. 4–1).

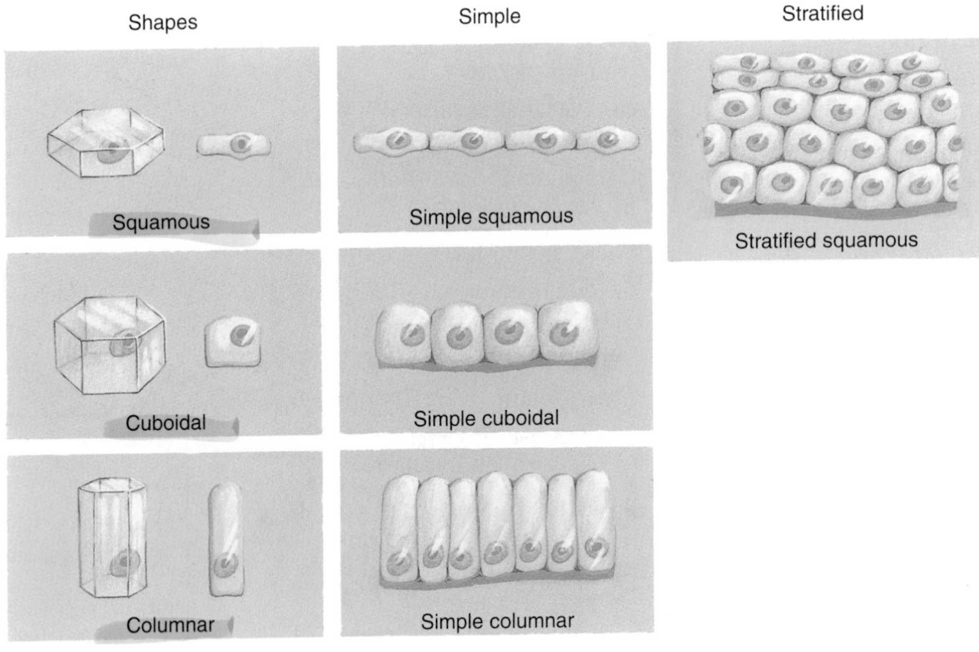

Figure 4–1 Classification of epithelial tissues based on the shape of the cells and the number of layers of cells.

QUESTION: Which of these might be best for efficient diffusion, and why?

SIMPLE SQUAMOUS EPITHELIUM

Simple squamous epithelium is a single layer of flat cells (Fig. 4–2). These cells are very thin and very smooth—these are important physical characteristics. The alveoli (air sacs) of the lungs are simple squamous epithelium. The thinness of the cells permits the diffusion of gases between the air and blood.

Another location of this tissue is capillaries, the smallest blood vessels. Capillary walls are only one cell thick, which permits the exchange of gases, nutrients, and waste products between the blood and the tissue fluid. The interior surface of capillaries is also very smooth (and these cells continue as the lining of the arteries, veins, and heart); this is important because the smooth surface prevents abnormal blood clotting within blood vessels.

STRATIFIED SQUAMOUS EPITHELIUM

Stratified squamous epithelium consists of many layers of mostly flat cells, although lower cells are rounded. In the lowest layer, mitosis takes place to continually produce new cells to replace those worn off the surface (see Fig. 4–2). This type of epithelium makes up the epidermis of the skin, where it is called "keratinizing" because the protein keratin is produced, and the surface cells are dead. Stratified squamous epithelium of the non-keratinizing type lines the oral cavity, the esophagus, and, in women, the vagina. In these locations the surface cells are living and make up the mucous membranes of these organs. In all of its body locations, this tissue is a barrier to microorganisms because the cells of which it is made are very close together. The more specialized functions of the epidermis will be covered in the next chapter.

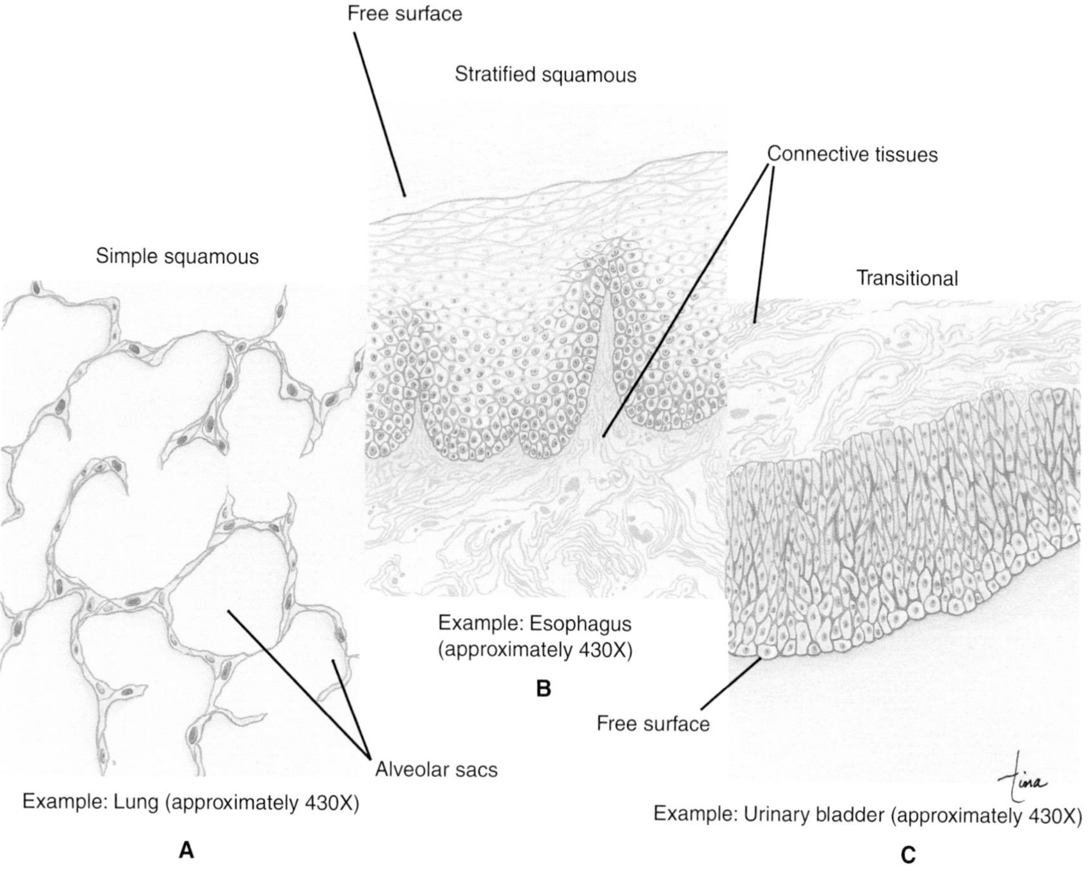

Figure 4–2 Epithelial tissues. (**A**) Simple squamous. (**B**) Stratified squamous. (**C**) Transitional.

QUESTION: Which two of these tissues seem to be most related in structure?

TRANSITIONAL EPITHELIUM

Transitional epithelium is a type of stratified epithelium in which the surface cells change shape from round to squamous. The urinary bladder is lined with transitional epithelium. When the bladder is empty, the surface cells are rounded (see Fig. 4–2). As the bladder fills, these cells become flattened. Transitional epithelium enables the bladder to fill and stretch without tearing the lining.

SIMPLE CUBOIDAL EPITHELIUM

Simple cuboidal epithelium is a single layer of cube-shaped cells (Fig. 4–3). This type of tissue makes up the functional units of the thyroid gland and salivary glands. These are examples of **glandular epithelium**; their function is **secretion**. In these glands the cuboidal cells are arranged in small spheres and secrete into the cavity formed by the sphere. In the thyroid gland, the cuboidal epithelium secretes the thyroid hormones; thyroxine is an example. In the salivary glands, the cuboidal cells secrete saliva. Cuboidal epithelium also makes up portions of the kidney tubules. Here the cells have microvilli (see Fig. 1–1 in Chapter 1), and their function is the reabsorption of useful materials back to the blood.

SIMPLE COLUMNAR EPITHELIUM

Columnar cells are taller than they are wide and are specialized for secretion and **absorption**. The stomach lining is made of **columnar epithelium** that secretes gastric juice for digestion. The lining of the small intestine (see Fig. 4–3) secretes digestive enzymes, but these cells also absorb the end products of digestion from the cavity of the intestine into the blood and lymph. To absorb efficiently, the columnar cells of the small intestine have **microvilli**, which you may recall are folds of the cell membrane on their free surfaces (see Fig. 3–2 in Chapter 3). These microscopic folds greatly increase the surface area for absorption.

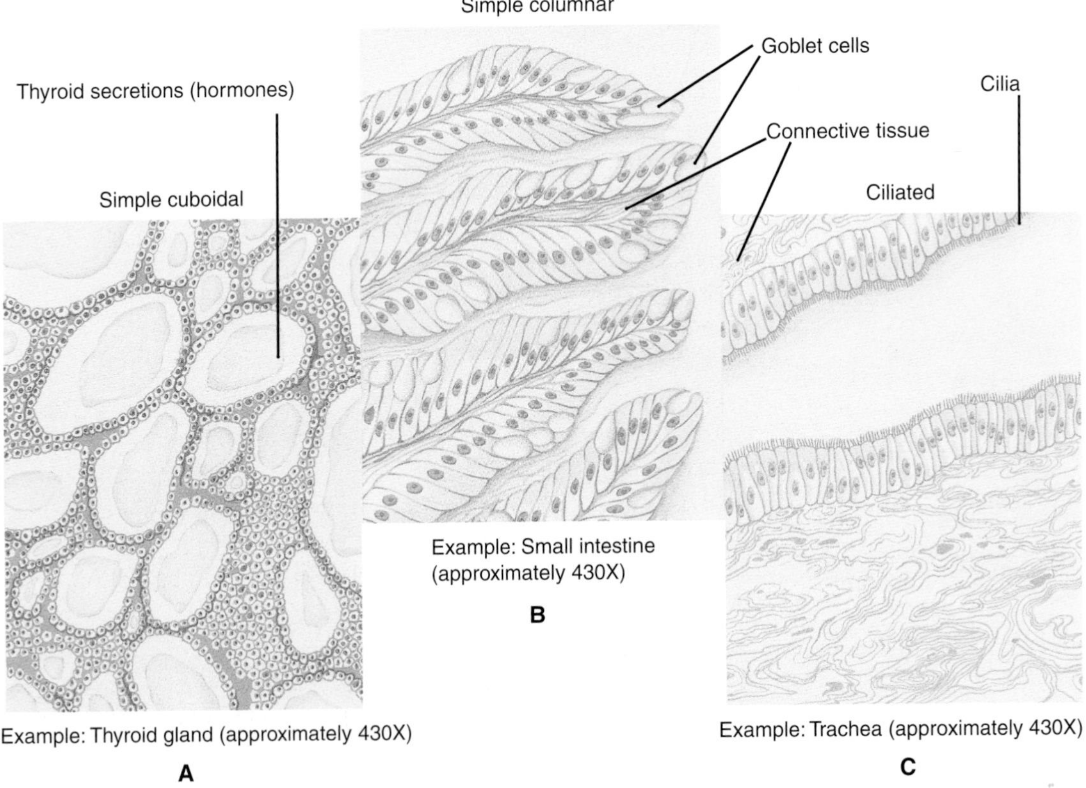

Figure 4–3 Epithelial tissues. (**A**) Simple cuboidal. (**B**) Simple columnar. (**C**) Ciliated.

QUESTION: What is the function of the cilia that line the trachea?

Yet another type of columnar cell is the **goblet cell**, which is a unicellular gland. Goblet cells secrete **mucus** and are found in the lining of the intestines and the lining of parts of the respiratory tract such as the trachea. Mucous membranes will be described in a later section.

CILIATED EPITHELIUM

Ciliated epithelium consists of columnar cells that have swaths ("wheat fields") of motile **cilia** on their free surfaces (see Fig. 4–3). Recall from Chapter 3 that the function of these motile cilia is to sweep materials across the cell surface. Ciliated epithelium lines the nasal cavities, larynx, trachea, and large bronchial tubes. The cilia sweep mucus, including trapped dust and bacteria from inhaled air, toward the pharynx to be swallowed. Bacteria are then destroyed by the hydrochloric acid in the stomach. The air that reaches the lungs is almost entirely free of pathogens and particulate pollution.

Another location of ciliated epithelium in women is the lining of the fallopian tubes. The cilia here sweep the ovum, which has no means of self-locomotion, toward the uterus.

The epithelial tissues are summarized in Table 4–1.

GLANDS

Glands are cells or organs that secrete something; that is, they produce a substance that has a function either at that site or at a more distant site.

Unicellular Glands

Unicellular means "one cell." Goblet cells are an example of unicellular glands. As mentioned earlier, goblet cells are found in the lining of the respiratory and digestive tracts. Their secretion is mucus (see also Box 4–1: Cystic Fibrosis).

Multicellular Glands

Most glands are made of many similar cells or of a variety of cells with their secretions mingled into a collective

Table 4–1 | TYPES OF EPITHELIAL TISSUE

TYPE	STRUCTURE	LOCATION AND FUNCTION
Simple squamous	One layer of flat cells	■ Alveoli of the lungs—thin to permit diffusion of gases ■ Capillaries—thin to permit exchanges of materials; smooth to prevent abnormal blood clotting
Stratified squamous	Many layers of cells; surface cells flat; lower cells rounded; lower layer undergoes mitosis	■ Epidermis—surface cells are dead; a barrier to pathogens ■ Lining of esophagus, vagina—surface cells are living; a barrier to pathogens
Transitional	Many layers of cells; surface cells change from rounded to flat	■ Lining of urinary bladder—permits expansion without tearing the lining
Cuboidal	One layer of cube-shaped cells	■ Thyroid gland—secretes thyroxine ■ Salivary glands—secrete saliva ■ Kidney tubules—permit reabsorption of useful materials back to the blood
Columnar	One layer of column-shaped cells	■ Lining of stomach—secretes gastric juice ■ Lining of small intestine—secretes enzymes and absorbs end products of digestion (microvilli present)
Ciliated	One layer of columnar cells with motile cilia on their free surfaces	■ Lining of trachea—sweeps mucus and dust to the pharynx ■ Lining of fallopian tube—sweeps ovum toward uterus

Box 4–1 | CYSTIC FIBROSIS

Cystic fibrosis (CF) is a genetic disorder (there are many forms) of certain exocrine glands including the salivary glands, the sweat glands, the pancreas, and the mucous glands of the respiratory tract.

In the pancreas, thick mucus clogs the ducts and prevents pancreatic enzymes from reaching the small intestine, thus impairing digestion, especially of fats. But the most serious effects of CF are in the lungs. The genetic mistake in CF often involves a gene called CFTR, which codes for chloride ion channels (proteins) in the membranes of epithelial cells. In the lungs, the defective channels are destroyed (by protease enzymes of proteasomes), which causes a change in the composition of the tissue fluid around the cells. This change inactivates defensin, a natural antibiotic produced by lung tissue. In the absence of defensin, a bacterium called *Pseudomonas aeruginosa* stimulates the lung cells to produce copious thick mucus, an ideal growth environment for bacteria. Defensive white blood cells cannot get through the thick mucus, and their activity mistakenly destroys lung tissue. A person with CF has clogged bronchial tubes, frequent episodes of pneumonia, and, ultimately, lungs that cannot carry out gas exchange. CF is a chronic, progressive disease that is eventually fatal unless a lung transplant is performed.

CF is a recessive disease; a child must inherit the gene from both parents. CF is the most common genetic disease among people of Caucasian ancestry. CF is one of the disorders that may be correctable with gene therapy, but because it involves human subjects, this kind of work proceeds very slowly. Medications to improve chloride ion transport (which would thin the mucus and thereby decrease the chance of bacterial infection) are being developed.

secretion. **Multicellular** glands may be divided into two major groups: exocrine glands and endocrine glands.

Exocrine glands have **ducts** (tubes) to take the secretion away from the gland to the site of its function. Salivary glands, for example, secrete saliva that is carried by ducts to the oral cavity. Sweat glands secrete sweat that is transported by ducts to the skin surface, where the sweat can be evaporated by excess body heat. The gastric glands of the stomach lining contain different kinds of cells (see Fig. 16–5 in Chapter 16), which produce hydrochloric acid and the enzyme pepsin. Both of these secretions are part of gastric juice.

Endocrine glands are ductless glands. The secretions of endocrine glands are a group of chemicals called **hormones**, which enter capillaries and are circulated throughout the body. Hormones then bring about specific effects in their target organs. These effects include aspects of growth, use of minerals and other nutrients, and regulation of blood pressure, and they will be covered in more detail in Chapter 10. Examples of endocrine glands are the thyroid gland, the adrenal glands, and the pituitary gland.

The pancreas is an organ that is both an exocrine and an endocrine gland. The exocrine portions secrete digestive enzymes that are carried by ducts to the duodenum of the small intestine, their site of action. The endocrine portions of the pancreas, called pancreatic islets or islets of Langerhans, secrete the hormones insulin and glucagon directly into the blood.

CONNECTIVE TISSUE

There are several kinds of **connective tissue**, some of which may at first seem more different than alike. The types of connective tissue include areolar, adipose, fibrous, and elastic tissue, as well as blood, bone, and cartilage; these are summarized in Table 4–2. A characteristic that all connective tissues have in common is the presence of a matrix in addition to cells. The **matrix** is a structural network or solution of nonliving intercellular material. Each connective tissue has its own specific kind of matrix. The matrix of blood, for example, is blood plasma, which is mostly water. The matrix of bone is made primarily of calcium salts, which are hard and strong. As each type of connective tissue is described in the following sections, mention will be made of the types of cells present, as well as the kind of matrix.

BLOOD

Although **blood** is the subject of Chapter 11, a brief description will be given here. Blood consists of cells and plasma; cells are the living portion. The matrix of blood is

Table 4–2 | TYPES OF CONNECTIVE TISSUE

TYPE	STRUCTURE	LOCATION AND FUNCTION
Blood	Plasma (matrix) and red blood cells, white blood cells, and platelets	Within blood vessels ■ Plasma—transports materials ■ RBCs—carry oxygen ■ WBCs—destroy pathogens ■ Platelets—prevent blood loss
Areolar (loose)	Fibroblasts and a matrix of tissue fluid, collagen, and elastin fibers	Subcutaneous ■ Connects skin to muscles; WBCs destroy pathogens Below lining of mucous membranes (digestive, respiratory, urinary, reproductive tracts) ■ WBCs destroy pathogens
Adipose	Adipocytes that store fat (little matrix)	Subcutaneous (white) adipose ■ Stores excess energy ■ Produces chemicals that influence appetite, use of nutrients, and inflammation Around eyes and kidneys ■ Cushions Brown fat generates heat ■ In infants maintains body temperature ■ Amount increases in adults who exercise
Fibrous	Mostly collagen fibers (matrix) with few fibroblasts	Tendons and ligaments (regular, with parallel fibers) ■ Strong to withstand forces of movement of joints Dermis (irregular, with criss-cross fibers) ■ The strong inner layer of the skin
Elastic	Mostly elastin fibers (matrix) with few fibroblasts	Within the walls of large arteries ■ Helps maintain blood pressure Around alveoli in lungs ■ Promotes normal exhalation
Bone	Osteocytes in a matrix of calcium salts and collagen	Bones ■ Support the body and attach muscles ■ Protect internal organs from mechanical injury ■ Store excess calcium ■ Contain and protect red bone marrow
Cartilage	Chondrocytes in a flexible protein matrix	Within the wall of the trachea ■ Keeps airway open On joint surfaces of bones ■ Smooth to prevent friction Tip of nose and outer ear ■ Support, maintain shape Between vertebrae ■ Absorb shock, permit movement

plasma, which is about 52% to 62% of the total blood volume in the body. The water of plasma contains dissolved salts, nutrients, gases, and waste products. As you might expect, one of the primary functions of plasma is transport of these materials within the body.

Blood cells are produced from stem cells in the red bone marrow, the body's primary **hemopoietic tissue** (blood-forming tissue), which is found in flat and irregular bones such as the hip bone and vertebrae. The blood cells are red blood cells, platelets, and the five kinds of white blood cells: neutrophils, eosinophils, basophils, monocytes, and lymphocytes (see Fig. 4–4 and also Fig. 11–2 in Chapter 11). Lymphocytes mature and divide in lymphatic tissue, which makes up the spleen, the lymph nodes, and the thymus gland. The thymus also contains stem cells, but they produce only lymphocytes. Stem cells are present in the spleen and lymph nodes as well, though the number of lymphocytes they produce is a small fraction of the total.

The blood cells make up 38% to 48% of the total blood, and each type of cell has its specific function. **Red blood cells** (RBCs) carry oxygen bonded to the iron in their hemoglobin. **White blood cells** (WBCs) destroy pathogens by phagocytosis, the production of antibodies, or other chemical methods, and provide us with immunity to some diseases. **Platelets** prevent blood loss; the process of blood clotting involves platelets.

AREOLAR CONNECTIVE TISSUE

The cells of **areolar** (or **loose**) **connective tissue** are called **fibroblasts**. A *blast* cell is a "producing" cell, and fibroblasts produce protein fibers. The most abundant fibers are **collagen** and **elastin.** Collagen fibers are very strong; elastin fibers are elastic; that is, they are able to return to their original length, or recoil, after being stretched. Fibroblasts are able to migrate to sites of damage and produce these protein fibers as part of the repair

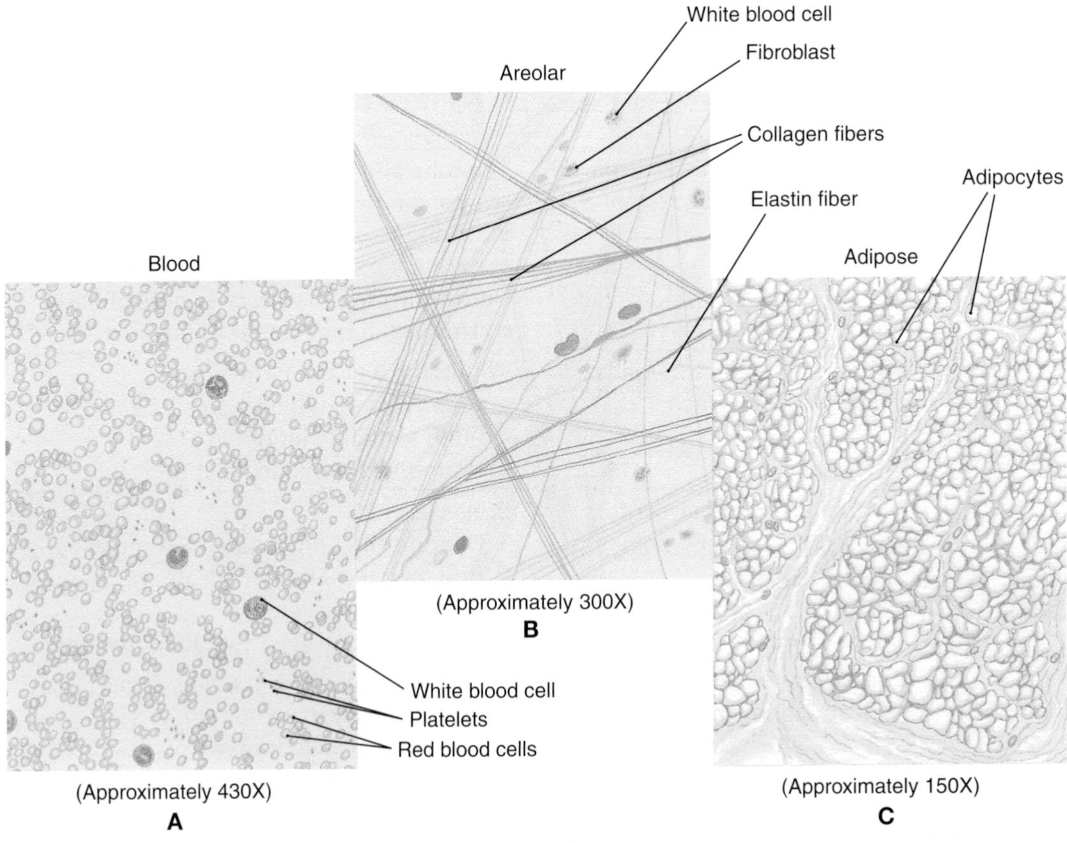

Figure 4–4 Connective tissues. (**A**) Blood. (**B**) Areolar. (**C**) Adipose.

QUESTION: What is the matrix of blood, and what is found in adipocytes?

process. Collagen, elastin, and tissue fluid make up the matrix, or nonliving portion, of areolar connective tissue (see Fig. 4–4). Also within the matrix are mast cells that release inflammatory chemicals when tissue is damaged and many white blood cells, which are capable of self-locomotion. Their importance here is related to the locations of areolar connective tissue.

Areolar tissue is found beneath the dermis of the skin and beneath the epithelial tissue of all the body systems that have openings to the environment. Recall that one function of white blood cells is to destroy pathogens. How do pathogens enter the body? Many do so through breaks in the skin. Bacteria and viruses also enter with the air we breathe and the food we eat, and some may get through the epithelial linings of the respiratory and digestive tracts and cause tissue damage. Areolar connective tissue with its mast cells and many white blood cells is strategically placed to intercept pathogens before they get to the blood and circulate throughout the body.

ADIPOSE TISSUE

Humans have two kinds of **adipose tissue**. The more familiar and more abundant kind is white adipose tissue (which we will call "adipose tissue" or "white fat"). The less familiar and less abundant kind is brown adipose tissue (which we will call "brown fat"). The cells of both kinds are called **adipocytes**. The adipocytes of adipose tissue are specialized to store fat in microscopic droplets, and the true fats are the chemical form of long-term energy storage. Excess nutrients have calories that are not wasted but are converted to fat to be stored for use when food intake decreases. Any form of excess calories, whether in fats, carbohydrates, or amino acids from protein, may be changed to triglycerides and stored. The amount of matrix in adipose tissue is small and consists of tissue fluid and a few collagen fibers (see Fig. 4–4).

Most fat is stored subcutaneously in the areolar connective tissue between the dermis and the muscles. This layer varies in thickness among individuals; the more excess calories consumed and stored, the thicker the layer. Adipocytes can be replaced by mitosis, and the body's number of adipocytes is believed to remain relatively constant throughout the life of an individual. Each adipocyte, however, may change in size, becoming larger if there is more fat to be stored or smaller if the fat is used to supply cellular energy. As mentioned in Chapter 2, adipose tissue also cushions organs such as the eyes and kidneys.

Adipose tissue is also considered an endocrine tissue, because it produces at least one hormone. Leptin is an appetite-suppressing hormone secreted by adipocytes to signal the hypothalamus in the brain that fat storage is sufficient (see also Chapter 17). When leptin secretion diminishes, appetite increases. Leptin also stimulates the formation of bone matrix by cells called osteoblasts and has other effects on bone tissue. Adipocytes secrete at least two chemicals that help regulate the use of insulin in glucose and fat metabolism. Adipose tissue is also involved in inflammation, the body's first response to injury, in that it produces cytokines, chemicals that activate white blood cells. Our adipose tissue is not simply an inert depository of fat; rather, it is part of the complex systems that ensure we are nourished properly and that protect us from pathogens that get through the skin.

Brown fat is found in abundance in infants and to a lesser extent in adults. Unlike white adipose tissue, brown fat is not an energy-storage tissue; it is instead a **thermogenic** (heat-generating) tissue in which the cells rapidly break down glucose (or fat) in cell respiration. In these cells, however, the decomposition of glucose is uncoupled from the synthesis of ATP, and most of the energy is released as heat. When do we need more heat? When we are chilled by a cool environment. One automatic response to external cold is that we shiver. The shivering reflex in infants is not efficient, and a chill to the body stimulates the mitochondria in brown fat to become very active.

As an infant gets older, shivering becomes more effective, and the amount of brown fat diminishes. In adults, brown fat may be found in the neck and shoulder areas and along the backbone. Lean adults seem to have more brown fat than do those who are overweight, and the amount in human adults does not seem to be a constant. It is still a heat-generating tissue, however, and may contribute to a person's ability to maintain a normal body weight. Regular exercise or exposure to cold stimulates muscle cells to release the hormone **irisin**, which transforms white adipocytes to brown adipocytes. The heart also secretes hormones, the natriuretic peptides, that promote the conversion of white fat cells to brown fat cells. Brown fat cells use up more energy nutrients (*not* storing them as triglycerides), thereby using more calories and producing heat. You may be wondering what gives brown fat its color. The numerous mitochondria contain iron, which colors the fat tissue a reddish-brown the same way it colors muscle tissue.

FIBROUS CONNECTIVE TISSUE

Fibrous connective tissue consists mainly of parallel (regular) collagen fibers with a few fibroblasts scattered among them (Fig. 4–5). This parallel arrangement of collagen provides great strength yet is flexible. The locations of this

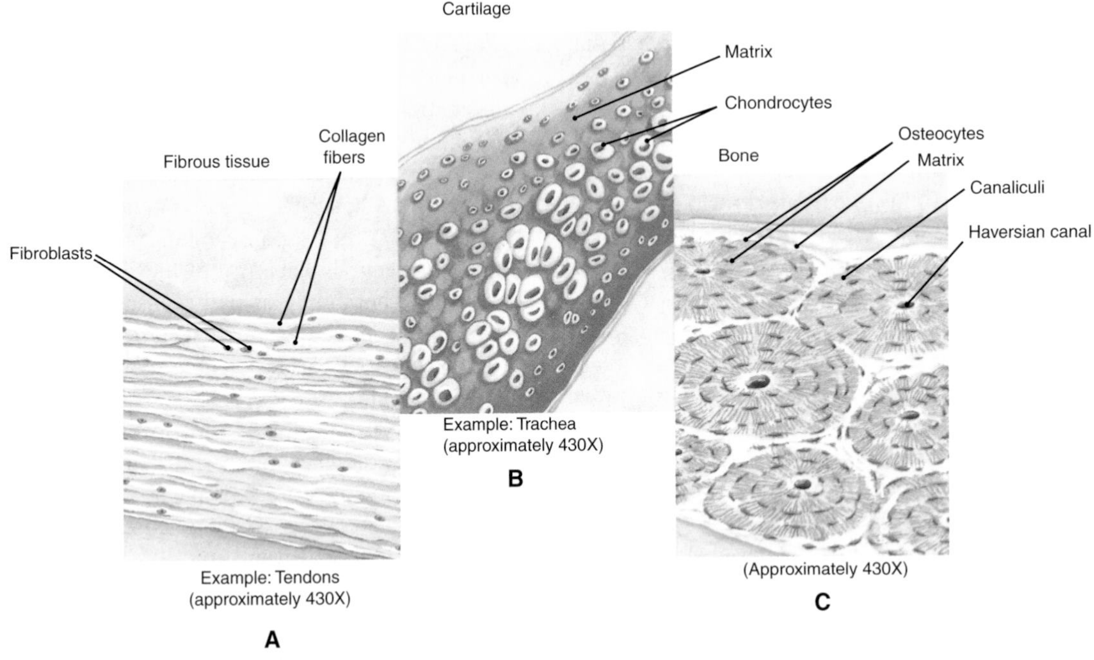

Figure 4–5 Connective tissues. (**A**) Fibrous. (**B**) Cartilage. (**C**) Bone.

QUESTION: What is the matrix of fibrous tissue, and of bone?

tissue are related to the need for flexible strength. The outer walls of arteries are reinforced with fibrous connective tissue because the blood in these vessels is under high pressure. The strong outer wall prevents rupture of the artery (see also Box 4–2: Missed Connections). Tendons and ligaments are made of fibrous connective tissue. Tendons connect muscle to bone; ligaments connect bone to bone. When the skeleton is moved, these structures must be able to withstand the great mechanical forces exerted on them.

Fibrous connective tissue has a relatively poor blood supply, which makes repair a slow process. If you have ever had a severely sprained ankle (which means the ligaments have been overly stretched), you know that complete healing may take several months.

An irregular type of fibrous connective tissue forms the dermis of the skin and the fasciae (membranes) around muscles. Although the collagen fibers here are not parallel to one another (instead they are criss-cross at many angles), the tissue is still strong. The dermis is different from other fibrous connective tissue in that it has a good blood supply.

ELASTIC CONNECTIVE TISSUE

As its name tells us, **elastic connective tissue** is made primarily of elastin fibers; also important are stabilizing fibers of the protein **fibrillin**. One of the locations of this tissue is the walls of large arteries such as the aorta (which emerges from the left ventricle of the heart) and its branches. These vessels are stretched when the heart contracts and pumps blood, and then they recoil, or snap back, when the heart relaxes. This recoil helps keep the blood moving away from the heart and is important to maintain normal blood pressure.

Elastic connective tissue is also found surrounding the alveoli of the lungs. The elastic fibers are stretched during inhalation and then recoil during exhalation to squeeze air out of the lungs. If you pay attention to your breathing for a few moments, you will notice that normal exhalation does not require "work" or energy. This is because of the normal elasticity of the lungs.

BONE

The prefix that designates bone is "osteo," so bone cells are called **osteocytes**. The matrix of **bone** is made of calcium salts and collagen and is strong, hard, and not flexible. In the shafts of long bones such as the femur, the osteocytes, matrix, and blood vessels are in very precise arrangements called **haversian systems** or **osteons** (see Fig. 4–5). Bone has a good blood supply, which enables it

Box 4–2 | MISSED CONNECTIONS

Some connective tissues make literal connections. Collagen and elastin are proteins that do so. Let us see what happens if these connections are weak or absent, as they are in scurvy (a nutritional deficiency of vitamin C) and Marfan syndrome (a genetic disease).

Many people take extra vitamin C, for various reasons. Vitamin C has several functions, and an important one is the synthesis of collagen. Collagen is the protein that makes tendons, ligaments, and other connective tissues strong. Imagine the protein collagen as a ladder with three uprights and rungs that connect adjacent uprights. Vitamin C is essential for forming the "rungs," without which the uprights will not stay together as a strong unit. Collagen formed in the absence of vitamin C is weak, and the effects of weak collagen are dramatically seen in the disease called scurvy, which had been known (though not its cause) for centuries.

Scurvy is characterized by bleeding gums and loss of teeth, poor healing of wounds, fractures, and bleeding in the skin, joints, and elsewhere in the body. In 1753 James Lind, a Scottish surgeon, recommended to the British Navy that lime juice be taken on long voyages to prevent scurvy among the sailors (whose diet was mainly bread and salt pork or beef). The lime juice did prevent this potentially fatal disease, as did consumption of fresh fruits and vegetables, although at the time no one knew why. Vitamin C was finally isolated in the laboratory in 1928.

Marfan syndrome is a genetic disorder; the mutated gene is the code for the protein fibrillin, the stabilizing protein of elastic connective tissue. A person with Marfan syndrome is often tall and thin, with joints that are overly flexible (hyperextension of elbows or knees, for example) because tendons and ligaments stretch too much and do not recoil as they should. A very serious possible consequence is overstretching and tearing of the wall of the aorta; rupture of our largest artery with hemorrhage into the chest cavity can be rapidly fatal. Correcting this genetic mistake is not yet possible, and Marfan syndrome is a dominant genetic condition, meaning that inheriting only one gene is sufficient to produce the disease.

to serve as a storage site for calcium and to repair itself relatively rapidly after a simple fracture. Some bones, such as the sternum (breastbone) and pelvic bone, contain red bone marrow, the primary hemopoietic tissue that produces blood cells.

Other functions of bone tissue are related to the strength of bone matrix. The skeleton supports the body, and some bones protect internal organs from mechanical injury. A more complete discussion of bone is found in Chapter 6.

CARTILAGE

The protein–carbohydrate matrix of **cartilage** does not contain calcium salts, and it also differs from that of bone in that it contains more water, which makes it resilient. It is firm yet smooth and flexible. Cartilage is found on the joint surfaces of bones, where its smooth surface helps prevent friction. The tip of the nose and the external ear are supported by flexible cartilage. The wall of the trachea, the airway to the lungs, contains firm rings of cartilage to maintain an open passageway for air. Discs of cartilage are found between the vertebrae of the spine. Here the cartilage is a firm cushion; it absorbs shock and permits movement.

Within the cartilage matrix are the **chondrocytes**, or cartilage cells (see Fig. 4–5). There are no capillaries within the cartilage matrix, so these cells are nourished by diffusion through the matrix, a slow process. This becomes clinically important when cartilage is damaged because repair will take place very slowly or not at all. Athletes sometimes damage cartilage within the knee joint. Such damaged cartilage is usually surgically removed in order to preserve as much joint mobility as possible.

MUSCLE TISSUE

Muscle tissue is specialized for contraction. When muscle cells (also called muscle fibers or **myocytes**) contract, they shorten and bring about some type of movement. There are three types of muscle tissue: skeletal, smooth, and cardiac (Table 4–3). The movements that each can produce have very different purposes.

SKELETAL MUSCLE

Skeletal muscle may also be called **striated** muscle or **voluntary** muscle. Each name describes a particular aspect of this tissue, as you will see. The skeletal muscle cells are

Table 4–3 | TYPES OF MUSCLE TISSUE

TYPE	STRUCTURE	LOCATION AND FUNCTION	EFFECT OF NERVE IMPULSES
Skeletal	Large cylindrical cells with striations and several nuclei each	Attached to bones ■ Moves the skeleton and produces heat	Essential to cause contraction (voluntary)
Smooth	Small tapered cells with no striations and one nucleus each	Within walls of arteries ■ Maintain blood pressure Within walls of stomach and intestines ■ Peristalsis Iris of eye ■ Regulates size of pupil	Bring about contraction or regulate the rate of contraction (involuntary)
Cardiac	Branched cells with faint striations and one nucleus each	Forms the walls of the chambers of the heart ■ Pumps blood	Regulate only the rate of contraction (involuntary)

cylindrical, have several nuclei each, and appear striated, or striped (Fig. 4–6). The striations are the result of the precise arrangement of the contracting proteins within the cells.

Skeletal muscle tissue makes up the muscles that are attached to bones. These muscles are supplied with motor nerves and thus move the skeleton. An important exception is the diaphragm, which does not move bones, but rather enlarges the thoracic cavity and brings about inhalation. Skeletal muscles also produce a significant amount of heat, which is important to help maintain the body's constant temperature. Each muscle cell has its own motor nerve ending. The nerve impulses that can then travel to the muscles are essential to cause contraction. Although we do not have to consciously plan all our movements, the nerve impulses for them originate in the cerebrum, the "thinking" part of the brain.

Let us return to the three names for this tissue: *skeletal* describes its location, *striated* describes its appearance, and *voluntary* describes how it functions. The skeletal muscles and their functioning are the subject of Chapter 7.

SMOOTH MUSCLE

Smooth muscle may also be called **involuntary** muscle or **visceral** muscle. The cells of smooth muscle have tapered ends, a single nucleus, and no striations (see Fig. 4–6). Although nerve impulses do bring about contractions, this is not something most of us can control, hence the name *involuntary*. The term *visceral* refers to internal organs, many of which contain smooth muscle. The functions of smooth muscle are actually functions of the organs in which the muscle is found.

In the stomach and intestines, smooth muscle contracts in waves called peristalsis to propel food through the digestive tract. In the walls of arteries and veins, smooth muscle constricts or dilates the vessels to maintain normal blood pressure. The iris of the eye has two sets of smooth muscle fibers to constrict or dilate the pupil, which regulates the amount of light that strikes the retina.

Other functions of smooth muscle are mentioned in later chapters. This is an important tissue that you will come across again and again in our study of the human body.

CARDIAC MUSCLE

The cells of the heart, **cardiac muscle**, are shown in Fig. 4–6. They are branched, have one nucleus each, and have faint striations. The cell membranes at the ends of these cells are extensively folded and fit into matching folds of the membranes of the next cells (see Fig. 12–1 in Chapter 12). These interlocking folds are called **intercalated discs** and permit the electrical impulses of muscle contraction to pass swiftly from cell to cell. This enables the heart to beat in a very precise wave of contraction from the upper chambers to the lower chambers. Cardiac muscle as a whole is called the **myocardium** and forms the walls of the atria and ventricles, the four chambers of the heart. Its function, therefore, is the function of the heart: to pump blood. The contractions of the myocardium create blood pressure and keep blood circulating

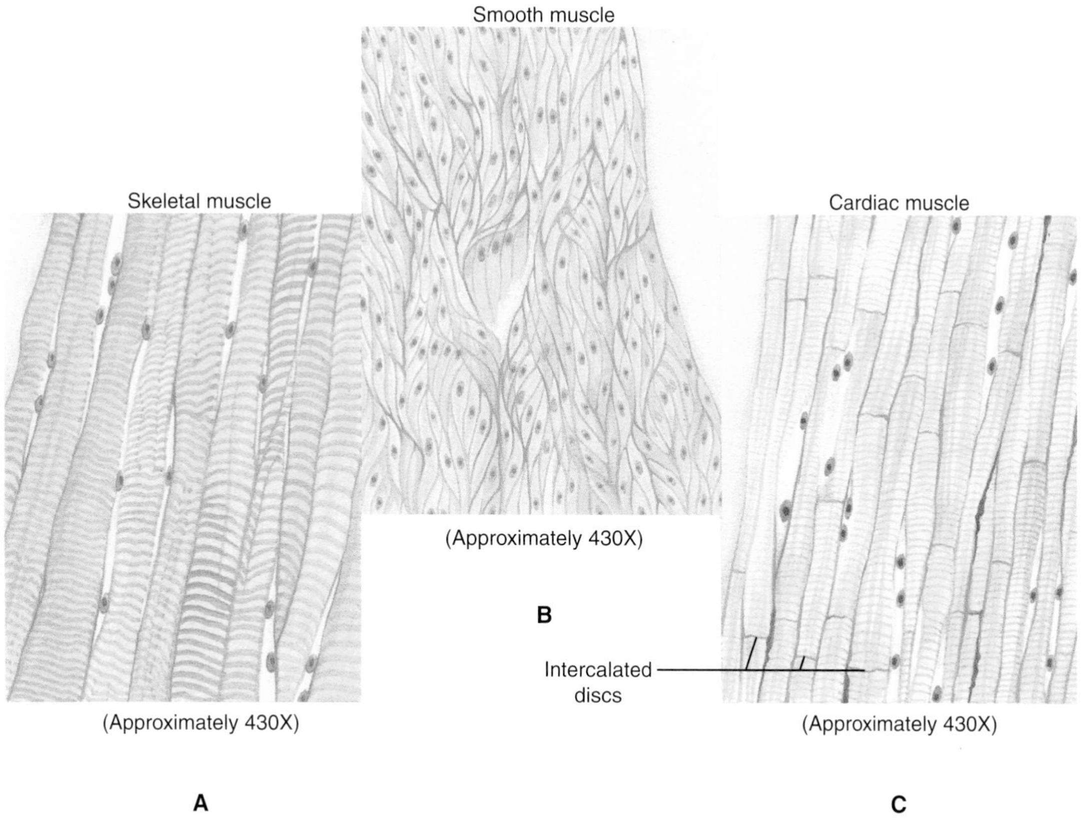

Figure 4–6 Muscle tissues. (**A**) Skeletal. (**B**) Smooth. (**C**) Cardiac.

QUESTION: Which kinds of muscle cells have striations? What forms these striations?

throughout the body so that the blood can carry out its many functions.

Cardiac muscle cells have the ability to contract by themselves. Thus the heart maintains its own beat. The role of nerve impulses is to increase or decrease the heart rate, depending on whatever is needed by the body in a particular situation. We will return to the heart in more detail in Chapter 12.

NERVE TISSUE

Nerve tissue consists of nerve cells called **neurons** and some specialized cells found only in the nervous system. The nervous system has two divisions: the central nervous system (CNS) and the peripheral nervous system (PNS). The brain and the spinal cord are the organs of the CNS. They are made of neurons and specialized cells called neuroglia. The CNS and the neuroglia are discussed in detail in Chapter 8. The PNS consists of all of the nerves that emerge from the CNS and supply the rest of the body. These nerves are made of neurons and specialized cells called Schwann cells. The Schwann cells form the myelin sheath (myelin is a phospholipid) to electrically insulate neurons.

Neurons are capable of generating and transmitting electrochemical impulses. There are many different kinds of neurons, but they all have the same basic structure (Fig. 4–7). The **cell body** contains the nucleus and is essential for the continuing life of the neuron. An **axon** is a process (the term *process* here means "something that sticks out," a cellular extension) that carries electrical impulses away from the cell body; a neuron has only one axon. **Dendrites** are processes that carry impulses toward the cell body; a neuron may have several or even many dendrites. An electrical nerve impulse travels along the cell membrane of a neuron. Where neurons meet, however, there is a small space called a **synapse**, which an electrical impulse cannot cross. At a synapse, between the axon of one neuron and the dendrite or cell body of

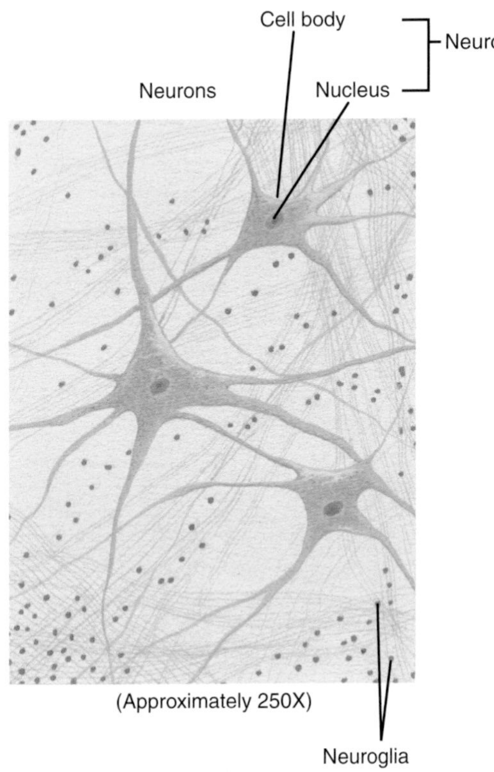

Figure 4–7 Nerve tissue of the central nervous system (CNS).

QUESTION: How many processes does the central neuron have, and what are they called?

the next neuron, impulse transmission depends on chemicals called **neurotransmitters**. A summary of nerve tissue is found in Table 4–4.

Nerve tissue makes up the brain, spinal cord, and peripheral nerves (see also Box 4–3: Tay-Sachs Disease). The nervous system is one of the control systems of the body, and each organ of the system has very specific functions. These aspects of the nervous system are covered in more detail in Chapter 8. For now, we will mention only the categories of the functions of nerve tissue. These include feeling and interpreting sensation, the initiation of movement, the rapid regulation of body functions such as heart rate and breathing, and the organization of information for learning and memory.

MEMBRANES

Membranes are sheets of tissue that cover or line surfaces or that separate organs or parts (lobes) of organs from one another. Many membranes produce secretions that have specific functions. The two major categories of membranes are epithelial membranes and connective tissue membranes.

EPITHELIAL MEMBRANES

There are two types of epithelial membranes, serous and mucous. Each type is found in specific locations within the body and secretes a fluid. These fluids are called serous fluid and mucus.

Serous Membranes

Serous membranes are sheets of simple squamous epithelium that line some closed body cavities and cover the organs in these cavities (Fig. 4–8). The **pleural membranes** are the serous membranes of the thoracic cavity. The parietal pleura lines the chest wall, and the visceral pleura covers the lungs. (Notice that *line* means "on the inside" and *cover* means "on the outside." These terms cannot be used interchangeably because each indicates a different location.) The pleural membranes secrete **serous fluid**, which prevents friction between them as the lungs expand and recoil during breathing.

The heart, in the thoracic cavity between the lungs, has its own set of serous membranes. The parietal **pericardium** lines the fibrous pericardium (a connective tissue membrane), and the visceral pericardium, or **epicardium**, is on the surface of the heart muscle (see also Fig. 12–1 in Chapter 12). Serous fluid is produced to prevent friction as the heart beats.

In the abdominal cavity, the **peritoneum** is the serous membrane that lines the cavity. The **mesentery**, or visceral peritoneum, is folded over and covers the abdominal organs. Here, the serous fluid prevents friction as the stomach and intestines contract and slide against other organs (see also Fig. 16–4 in Chapter 16).

Mucous Membranes

Mucous membranes line the body tracts (systems) that have openings to the environment. These are the respiratory, digestive, urinary, and reproductive tracts. The epithelium of a mucous membrane (**mucosa**) varies with the different organs involved. The mucosa of the esophagus and of the vagina is stratified squamous epithelium, the mucosa of the trachea is ciliated epithelium, and the mucosa of the stomach is columnar epithelium.

The **mucus** secreted by these membranes keeps the lining epithelial cells wet. Remember that these are living cells, so if they dry out, they will die. In the digestive tract, mucus also lubricates the surface to permit the smooth passage of food. In the respiratory tract the mucus traps

Table 4–4 | NERVE TISSUE

PART	STRUCTURE	FUNCTION
Neuron (nerve cell)		
Cell body	Contains the nucleus	Regulates the functioning of the neuron
Axon	Cellular process (extension)	Carries electrical impulses away from the cell body
Dendrites	Cellular process (extension)	Carry electrical impulses toward the cell body
Synapse	Space between axon of one neuron and the dendrite or cell body of the next neuron	Transmits impulses from one neuron to others by means of chemicals
Neurotransmitters	Chemicals released by axons	Transmit impulses across synapses
Neuroglia	Specialized cells in the central nervous system	Form myelin sheaths and other functions
Schwann cells	Specialized cells in the peripheral nervous system	Form the myelin sheaths around neurons

Box 4–3 | TAY-SACHS DISEASE

In Chapter 3 you learned about the function of lysosomes; these cell organelles dispose of damaged or worn-out parts of a cell. The importance of lysosomal cleanup can be seen in Tay-Sachs disease. One of the lysosomal enzymes is missing, and the lipids of old membranes, such as myelin sheaths, accumulate in cells and nerve tissue. Imagine replacing the damaged parts of a car's engine but leaving the old parts in the engine—very soon the engine will be clogged with old parts and will not function. The damage caused by accumulating lipids in cells has profound effects in the cells of the nervous system.

A baby with Tay-Sachs disease usually shows symptoms by 6 months of age: regression of acquired motor skills and loss of mental acuity and personality. These losses progress to complete physical and mental deterioration, a vegetative (unresponsive) state, and death within a few years. There is no treatment.

What causes this devastating disease? Perhaps you already know, or if not, you can figure it out. The problem is a missing lysosomal enzyme. Enzymes are proteins. Why does a cell make certain proteins and not others? Because of its DNA. Protein synthesis depends on DNA, the genetic code for proteins.

Tay-Sachs is a recessive genetic disorder (the mutated gene is on chromosome 15), meaning that a child must have two genes for it (like cystic fibrosis). It is the most common genetic disease among people of Jewish ancestry, but genetic testing on the part of potential parents who know they may have a Tay-Sachs gene has made this disease rare in the United States.

dust and bacteria, which are then swept to the pharynx by ciliated epithelium.

CONNECTIVE TISSUE MEMBRANES

Many membranes are made of connective tissue. You may recall that the meninges were mentioned in Chapter 1; the meninges line the cranial and spinal cavities and cover the brain and spinal cord. Again, notice that *line* and *cover* have very precise meanings. The connective tissue membranes will be covered with the organ systems of which they are a part, so for now their locations and functions are summarized in Table 4–5.

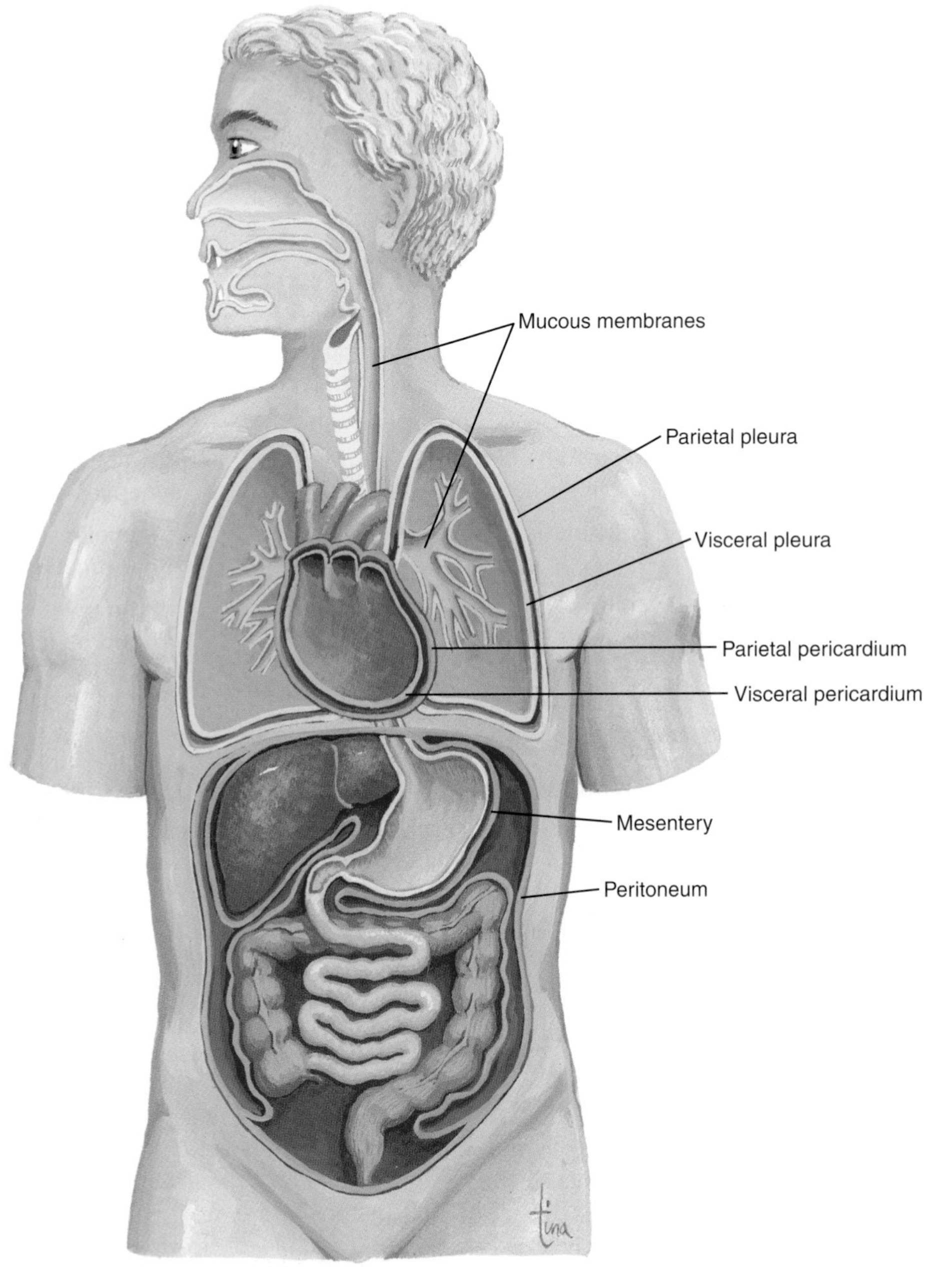

Figure 4–8 Epithelial membranes. Mucous membranes line body tracts that open to the environment. Serous membranes are found within closed body cavities such as the thoracic and abdominal cavities. See text for further description.

QUESTION: Name the organs covered by mesentery.

Table 4–5 | CONNECTIVE TISSUE MEMBRANES

MEMBRANE	LOCATION AND FUNCTION
Superficial fascia	Between the skin and muscles; adipose tissue stores fat; WBCs destroy pathogens that enter breaks in the skin
Periosteum	Covers each bone; contains blood vessels that enter the bone Anchors tendons from muscles and ligaments from other bones
Perichondrium	Covers cartilage; contains capillaries, the only blood supply for cartilage
Synovial	Lines joint cavities; secretes synovial fluid to prevent friction when joints move
Deep fascia	Covers each skeletal muscle; anchors tendons
Meninges	Cover the brain and spinal cord (line the cranial and spinal cavities); contain cerebrospinal fluid
Fibrous pericardium	Forms a sac around the heart; lined by the serous parietal pericardium

AGING AND TISSUES

As mentioned in the previous chapter, aging takes place at the cellular level, but it is of course apparent in the groups of cells we call tissues. In muscle tissue, for example, the proteins that bring about contraction deteriorate and are not repaired or replaced. The same is true of collagen and elastin, the proteins of connective tissue such as the dermis of the skin. Other aspects of the aging of tissues will be more meaningful to you in the context of the functions of organs and systems, so we will save those for the following chapters.

SUMMARY

The tissues and membranes described in this chapter are more complex than the individual cells of which they are made. We have reached only an intermediate level, however, with respect to the structural and functional complexity of the body as a whole. The following chapters are concerned with the organ systems, the most complex level. In the descriptions of the organs of these systems, you will find mention of the tissues and their contributions to each organ and organ system.

STUDY OUTLINE

A tissue is a group of cells with similar structure and function. The four main groups of tissues are epithelial, connective, muscle, and nerve.

Epithelial Tissue–found on surfaces; have no capillaries; some are capable of secretion; classified as to shape of cells and number of layers of cells (see Table 4–1 and Figs. 4–1, 4–2, and 4–3)

1. Simple squamous—one layer of flat cells; thin and smooth. Sites: alveoli (to permit diffusion of gases); capillaries (to permit exchanges between blood and tissues).
2. Stratified squamous—many layers of mostly flat cells; mitosis takes place in lowest layer. Sites: epidermis, where surface cells are dead (a barrier to pathogens); lining of mouth; esophagus; and vagina (surface cells are living, but still a barrier to pathogens).
3. Transitional—stratified, yet surface cells are rounded and flatten when stretched. Site: urinary bladder (to permit expansion without tearing the lining).

4. Simple cuboidal—one layer of cube-shaped cells. Sites: thyroid gland (to secrete thyroid hormones); salivary glands (to secrete saliva); kidney tubules (to reabsorb useful materials back to the blood).
5. Simple columnar—one layer of column-shaped cells. Sites: stomach lining (to secrete gastric juice); small intestinal lining (to secrete digestive enzymes and absorb nutrients–microvilli increase surface area for absorption).
6. Ciliated—columnar cells with swaths of motile cilia on free surfaces. Sites: trachea (to sweep mucus and bacteria to the pharynx); fallopian tubes (to sweep ovum to uterus).
7. Glands—epithelial tissues that produce secretions.
   a. Unicellular—one-celled glands. Goblet cells in the lining of the respiratory and digestive tracts secrete mucus.
   b. Multicellular–many-celled glands.
      - Exocrine glands have ducts; salivary glands secrete saliva into ducts that carry it to the oral cavity.
      - Endocrine glands secrete hormones directly into capillaries (no ducts); thyroid gland secretes thyroxine.

Connective Tissues–all have a nonliving intercellular matrix and specialized cells (see Table 4–2 and Figs. 4–4 and 4–5)

1. Blood—the matrix is plasma, which is mostly water; it transports materials in the blood. Red blood cells carry oxygen; white blood cells destroy pathogens and provide immunity. Platelets prevent blood loss, as in clotting. Blood cells are made in red bone marrow.
2. Areolar (loose)—cells are fibroblasts, which produce protein fibers: collagen is strong, and elastin is elastic; the matrix is collagen, elastin, and tissue fluid. White blood cells and mast cells are also present. Sites: below the dermis and below the epithelium of tracts that open to the environment (to destroy pathogens that enter the body).
3. Adipose—cells are adipocytes; little matrix. White adipocytes store fat. Sites: between the skin and muscles (to store energy); around the eyes and kidneys (to cushion). Also involved in appetite, use of insulin, and inflammation. Brown fat (adipocytes) is a heat-generating tissue and is of importance in infants to maintain body temperature. In adults, exercise or exposure to cold (by way of hormones from skeletal muscle and the heart) promotes conversion of white adipocytes to brown adipocytes.
4. Fibrous—mostly matrix, strong collagen fibers; cells are fibroblasts. Sites of regular fibrous (with parallel fibers): tendons (to connect muscle to bone); ligaments (to connect bone to bone); poor blood supply, slow healing. Sites of irregular fibrous (with criss-cross fibers): dermis of the skin and the fascia around muscles.
5. Elastic—mostly matrix, elastin fibers that recoil after being stretched; cells are fibroblasts. Sites: walls of large arteries (to maintain blood pressure); around alveoli (to promote normal exhalation).
6. Bone—cells are osteocytes; matrix is calcium salts and collagen, strong and not flexible; good blood supply, rapid healing. Sites: bones of the skeleton (to support the body and protect internal organs from mechanical injury).
7. Cartilage—cells are chondrocytes; protein matrix is firm yet flexible; no capillaries in matrix, very slow healing. Sites: joint surfaces of bones (to prevent friction); tip of nose and external ear (to support); wall of trachea (to keep air passageway open); disks between vertebrae (to absorb shock).

Muscle Tissue–specialized to contract and bring about movement (see Table 4–3 and Fig. 4–6)

1. Skeletal—also called striated or voluntary muscle. Cells are cylindrical, have several nuclei, and have striations. Each cell has a motor nerve ending; nerve impulses are essential for contraction. Site: skeletal muscles attached to bones (to move the skeleton and produce heat).

2. Smooth—also called visceral or involuntary muscle. Cells have tapered ends, one nucleus each, and no striations. Contraction is not under voluntary control. Sites: stomach and intestines (peristalsis); walls of arteries and veins (to maintain blood pressure); iris (to constrict or dilate pupil).
3. Cardiac—cells are branched, have one nucleus each, and faint striations. Site: walls of the four chambers of the heart (to pump blood and thereby circulate oxygen and maintain BP); nerve impulses regulate the rate of contraction.

Nerve Tissue–neurons are specialized to generate and transmit electrochemical impulses (see Table 4–4 and Fig. 4–7)

1. Cell body contains the nucleus; axon carries electrical impulses away from the cell body; dendrites carry impulses toward the cell body.
2. A synapse is the space between two neurons; a chemical neurotransmitter carries the impulse across a synapse.
3. Specialized cells in nerve tissue are neuroglia in the CNS and Schwann cells in the PNS.
4. Sites: brain; spinal cord; and peripheral nerves (to provide sensation, movement, regulation of body functions, learning, and memory).

Membranes–sheets of tissue on surfaces, or separating organs or lobes

1. Epithelial membranes (see Fig. 4–8)
   a. Serous membranes–in closed body cavities of the trunk; the serous fluid prevents friction between the two layers of the serous membrane.
      - Thoracic cavity–parietal pleura lines chest wall; visceral pleura covers the lungs.
      - Pericardial sac–parietal pericardium lines fibrous pericardium; visceral pericardium (epicardium) covers the heart muscle.
      - Abdominal cavity–peritoneum lines the abdominal cavity; mesentery covers the abdominal organs.

   b. Mucous membranes–line body tracts that open to the environment: respiratory, digestive, urinary, and reproductive. Mucus keeps the living epithelium wet; provides lubrication in the digestive tract; traps dust and bacteria in the respiratory tract.
2. Connective tissue membranes–see Table 4–5.

REVIEW QUESTIONS

1. Explain the importance of each tissue in its location: (pp. 83, 85, 91)
   a. Simple squamous epithelium in the alveoli of the lungs
   b. Ciliated epithelium in the trachea
   c. Cartilage in the trachea
2. Explain the importance of each tissue in its location: (pp. 89–91)
   a. Bone tissue in bones
   b. Cartilage on the joint surfaces of bones
   c. Fibrous connective tissue in ligaments
3. State the functions of red blood cells, white blood cells, and platelets. (p. 88)
4. Name two organs made primarily of nerve tissue, and state the general functions of nerve tissue. (pp. 93–94)
5. State the location and function of cardiac muscle. (pp. 92–93)
6. Explain the importance of each of these tissues in the small intestine: smooth muscle and columnar epithelium. (pp. 92, 84)
7. State the precise location of each of the following membranes: (p. 94)
   a. Peritoneum
   b. Visceral pericardium
   c. Parietal pleura
8. State the function of: (pp. 94–95, 86–88)
   a. Serous fluid
   b. Mucus
   c. Blood plasma
9. State two functions of skeletal muscles. (p. 92)
10. Name three body tracts lined with mucous membranes. (p. 94)
11. Explain how endocrine glands differ from exocrine glands. (p. 86)
12. State the function of adipose tissue: (p. 89)
    a. Around the eyes
    b. Between the skin and muscles
13. State the location of the meninges and synovial membranes. (p. 97)
14. State the important physical characteristics of collagen and elastin, and name the cells that produce these protein fibers. (pp. 88–89)

FOR FURTHER THOUGHT

1. A friend suffers a knee injury involving damage to bone, cartilage, and ligaments. What can you tell your friend about the healing of these tissues?
2. Stratified squamous keratinizing epithelium is an excellent barrier to pathogens in the epidermis of the skin. Even though this tissue is such a good barrier, it would not be suitable for the lining of the trachea or small intestine. Explain why.
3. Many tissues have protective functions, but it is important to be specific about the kind of protection provided. Name at least three tissues with a protective function, and state what each protects the body (or parts of the body) against.
4. Why is blood classified as a connective tissue? What does it connect? What kinds of connections does it make?
5. Look at Question Fig. 4–A; this is a microscopic section of a human organ (magnification: 250×). What tissue seems to be most abundant? Choose one of the four major categories first (with a reason), and then see if you can be even more precise.

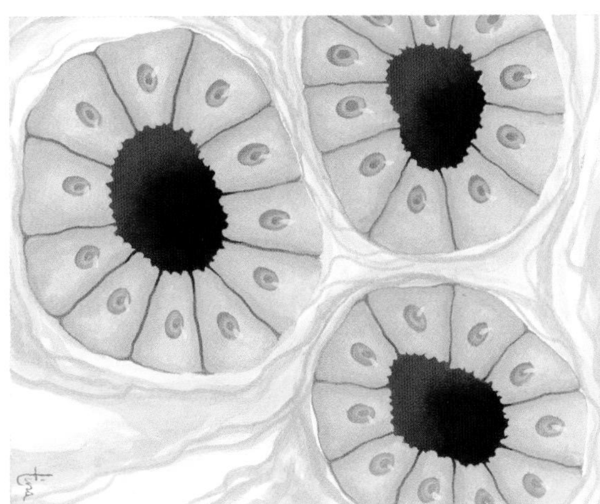

QUESTION FIGURE 4–A

CHAPTER

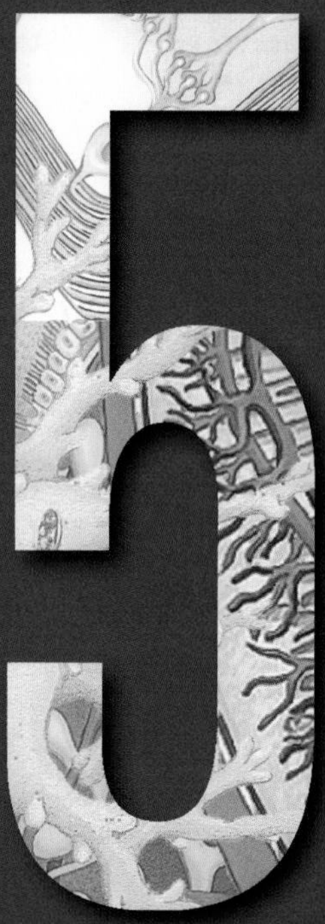

The Integumentary System

STUDENT OBJECTIVES

- Name the two major layers of the skin and the tissue of which each is made.
- State the locations and describe the functions of the stratum germinativum and stratum corneum.
- Describe the function of Langerhans cells.
- Describe the function of melanocytes and melanin.
- Describe the functions of hair and nails.
- Name the cutaneous senses and explain their importance.
- Describe the functions of the secretions of sebaceous glands, ceruminous glands, and eccrine sweat glands.
- Describe how the arterioles in the dermis respond to heat, cold, and stress.
- Name the tissues that make up the subcutaneous tissue, and describe their functions.

NEW TERMINOLOGY

Arterioles *(ar-**TEER**-ee-ohls)*
Ceruminous gland/cerumen *(suh-**ROO**-mi-nus GLAND/suh-**ROO**-men)*
Dermis *(**DER**-miss)*
Eccrine sweat gland *(**EK**-rin SWET GLAND)*
Epidermis *(EP-i-**DER**-miss)*
Hair follicle *(HAIR **FAH**-li-kull)*
Keratin *(**KER**-uh-tin)*
Melanin *(**MEL**-uh-nin)*
Melanocyte *(muh-**LAN**-oh-sight)*
Nail follicle *(NAIL **FAH**-li-kull)*
Papillary layer *(**PAP**-i-LAR-ee **LAY**-er)*
Receptors *(ree-**SEP**-turs)*
Sebaceous gland/sebum *(suh-**BAY**-shus GLAND/**SEE**-bum)*
Stratum corneum *(**STRA**-tum **KOR**-nee-um)*
Stratum germinativum *(**STRA**-tum JER-min-ah-**TEE**-vum)*
Subcutaneous tissue *(SUB-kew-**TAY**-nee-us **TISH**-yoo)*
Vasoconstriction *(VAY-zoh-kon-**STRIK**-shun)*
Vasodilation *(VAY-zoh-dye-**LAY**-shun)*

RELATED CLINICAL TERMINOLOGY

Acne *(**AK**-nee)*
Alopecia *(AL-oh-**PEE**-she-ah)*
Biopsy *(**BYE**-op-see)*
Carcinoma *(KAR-sin-**OH**-mah)*
Circulatory shock *(**SIR**-kew-lah-TOR-ee SHAHK)*
Decubitus ulcer *(dee-**KEW**-bi-tuss **UL**-ser)*
Dehydration *(DEE-high-**DRAY**-shun)*
Eczema *(**EK**-zuh-mah)*
Erythema *(ER-i-**THEE**-mah)*
Histamine *(**HISS**-tah-meen)*
Hives *(**HIGHVZ**)*
Inflammation *(IN-fluh-**MAY**-shun)*
Melanoma *(MEL-ah-**NOH**-mah)*
Nevus *(**NEE**-vus)*
Pruritus *(proo-**RYE**-tus)*

*Terms that appear in **bold type** in the chapter text are defined in the glossary, which begins on page 603.*

CHAPTER OUTLINE

An itchy mosquito bite . . . a painful sunburn . . . a really *good* hair day. Despite its unfamiliar name, the **integumentary system** is an organ system that is very familiar to us. This system includes structures we can see: the skin, hair, and nails. Parts of the system we cannot see are glands such as sweat glands, the sensory receptors, and the subcutaneous tissue below the skin. An integument is a covering; the integumentary system covers the body and is a barrier between the external environment and internal environment of the body. The skin is made of several different tissue types and is considered an organ. In part nonliving, the skin prevents the entry of many harmful substances. The living parts of the skin have several very different roles in the maintenance of homeostasis. The subcutaneous tissue directly underneath the skin connects it to the muscles and has other functions as well.

THE SKIN

The two major layers of the skin are the outer **epidermis** and the inner **dermis**. Each of these layers is made of different tissues and has very different functions.

EPIDERMIS

The **epidermis** is made of stratified squamous keratinizing epithelial tissue and is thickest on the palms of the hands and the soles of the feet. The cells that are most abundant are called **keratinocytes**, and there are no capillaries present between them. Rather, the keratinocytes are bound to one another in what are called "tight junctions" made of proteins of their cell membranes (picture sheets of flat cells all zippered together along their sides). Although the epidermis may be further subdivided into four or five sublayers, two of these are of greatest importance: the innermost layer, the stratum germinativum, and the outermost layer, the stratum corneum (Fig. 5–1).

Stratum Germinativum

The **stratum germinativum** may also be called the stratum basale. Each name tells us something about this layer. To *germinate* means to "sprout" or "grow." *Basal* means "the base" or "the lowest part." The stratum germinativum is the base of the epidermis, the innermost layer, in which **mitosis** takes place. New cells are continually being produced, pushing the older cells toward the skin surface. These cells produce the protein **keratin**, and as they get farther away from the capillaries in the dermis, they die. As dead cells are worn off the skin's surface, they are replaced by cells from the lower layers. Scattered among the keratinocytes of the stratum germinativum are very different cells called Merkel cells (or Merkel discs); these are receptors for the sense of touch (Fig. 5–2).

The living keratinocytes are able to synthesize antimicrobial peptides called **defensins**; these and other chemicals are produced following any injury to the skin, as part of the process of inflammation. Defensins rupture the membranes of pathogens such as bacteria that may enter by way of breaks in the skin.

The living portion of the epidermis also produces a vitamin; the cells have a form of cholesterol that, on exposure to ultraviolet light, is changed to vitamin D (a form then modified by the liver and converted by the kidneys to its most active form, called 1,25-D, or calcitriol, which is considered a hormone). This is why vitamin D is sometimes referred to as the "sunshine vitamin." People who do not get much sunlight depend more on nutritional sources of vitamin D, such as fortified milk. But sunlight is probably the best way to get vitamin D, and 15 minutes a day a few times a week is often enough. Excess vitamin D is stored in the liver (vitamin D is fat soluble, and if taken in excessive amounts can become toxic).

Vitamin D is important for the absorption of calcium and phosphorus from food in the small intestine, and these minerals are used to build the matrix of bones and teeth; this function has been known for years. Recent research indicates that vitamin D also contributes to other important body processes. It is involved in maintaining muscle strength, especially in elderly people, and in the functioning of insulin for the regulation of blood glucose level. Vitamin D may provide protection against some types of cancer and against infections caused by certain bacteria or viruses. For example, people with a vitamin D deficiency seem more susceptible to tuberculosis and influenza. Vitamin D stimulates skin cells and white blood cells to produce **cathelicidin**, a natural antimicrobial that punctures the membranes or outer coverings of pathogens. We still have much to learn about this vitamin.

Stratum Corneum

The **stratum corneum**, the outermost epidermal layer, consists of many layers of dead cells; all that is left is their **keratin**. The protein keratin is relatively waterproof, and though the stratum corneum should not be thought of as a plastic bag encasing the body, it does prevent most evaporation of body water. Also of importance, keratin prevents the entry of water. Without a waterproof stratum corneum, it would be impossible to swim in a pool or even take a shower without damaging our cells.

The stratum corneum is also a barrier to chemicals and pathogens. Most chemicals, unless they are corrosive, like

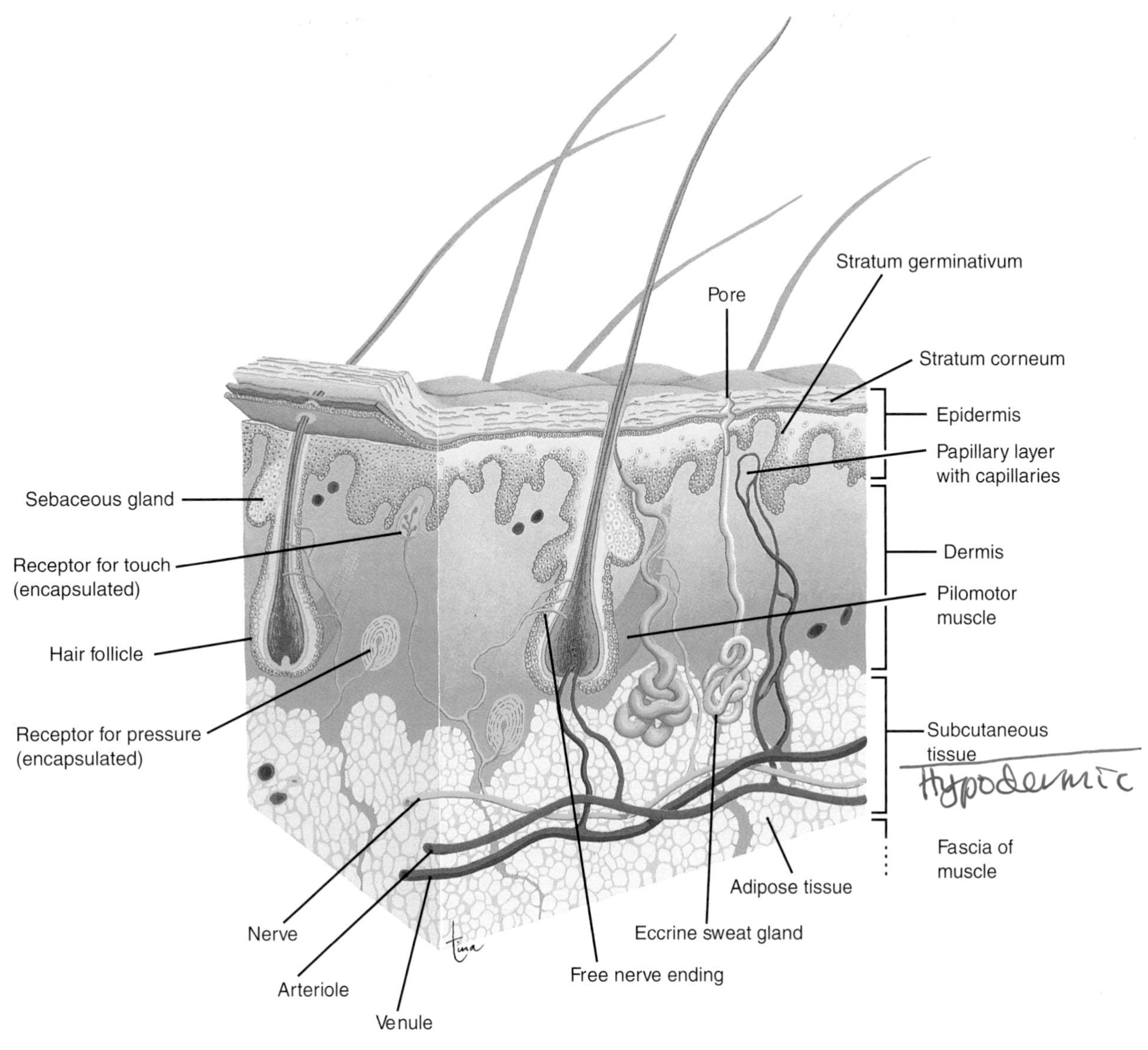

Figure 5–1 Skin. Structure of the skin and subcutaneous tissue.

QUESTION: Which layers of the integumentary system have blood vessels?

acids, will not get through unbroken skin to the living tissue within. One painful exception is the sap of poison ivy. This resin does penetrate the skin and initiates an allergic reaction in susceptible people. The welts we call **hives** are an inflammatory response characteristic of allergies. The hives of poison ivy become blisters and itch severely.

Recall from Chapter 1 that our skin surface is a **microbiome**, an environment for the bacteria we call our **microbiota** (or normal flora). Hundreds of species of bacteria make their home on the surface of the skin; they are not harmful as long as they remain outside the body. An intact stratum corneum helps keep them outside, as do the tight junctions between keratinocytes. Most bacteria and other microorganisms cannot penetrate unbroken skin. Some species of our microbiota are actively beneficial; by their simple presence and perhaps by the chemicals they secrete, they help to prevent most pathogenic bacteria and fungi from colonizing the skin enough to cause an infection. The

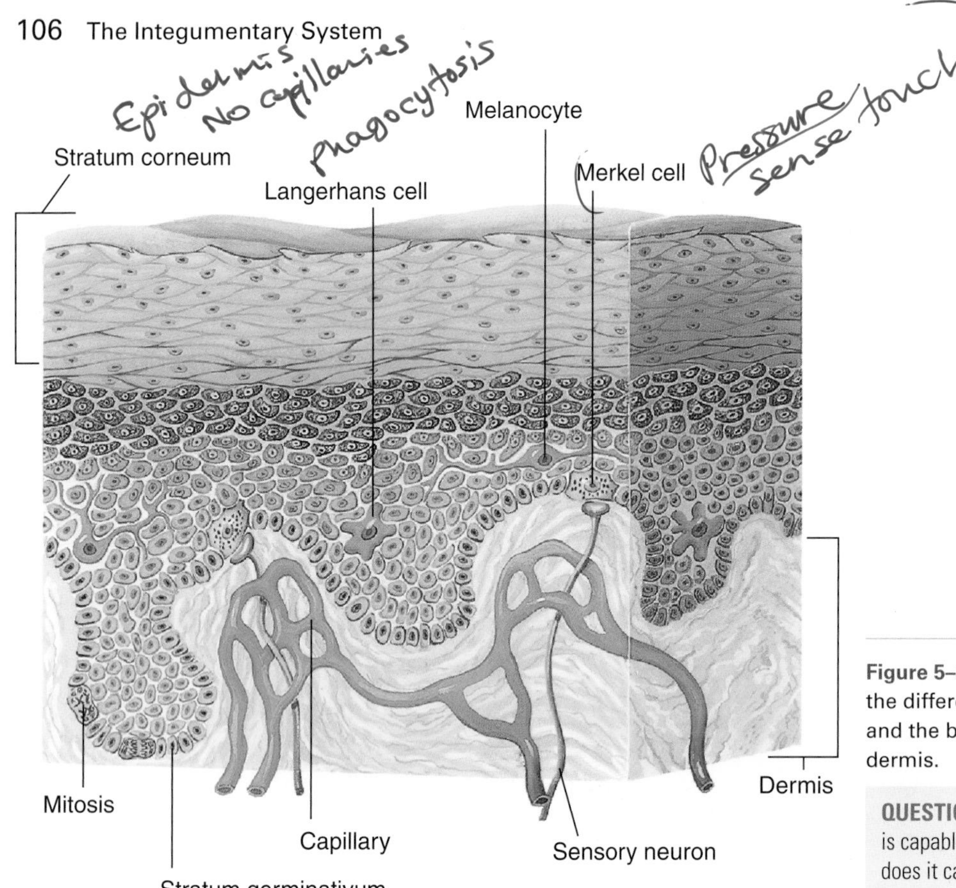

Figure 5–2 The epidermis, showing the different kinds of cells present and the blood supply in the upper dermis.

QUESTION: Which type of cell shown is capable of self-locomotion, and what does it carry?

epidermis does its part to keep the bacterial population in check, in that the flaking of dead cells from the skin surface helps remove microorganisms; the fatty acids in sebum also help inhibit microbial growth. The importance of the stratum corneum becomes especially apparent when it is lost (see Box 5–1: Burns).

Certain minor changes in the epidermis are undoubtedly familiar to you. When a person wears new shoes, for example, the skin of the foot may be subjected to friction. This will separate layers of the epidermis, or separate the epidermis from the dermis, and tissue fluid may collect, causing a **blister**. If the skin is subjected to pressure, the rate of mitosis in the stratum germinativum will increase and create a thicker epidermis; we call this a **callus**. Although calluses are more common on the palms and soles, they may occur on any part of the skin.

Also familiar to you on the palms and soles are what we call prints. The ridges of the epidermal junction with the dermis are most apparent as fingerprints and footprints. The function of these whorls and loops and lines is not known with certainty. Some biologists suggest that prints help with gripping; others propose that prints make fingertips more sensitive to the texture of objects. Although each person's fingerprints are unique, they are not unchangeable. As we age, our epidermal ridges become less distinct, and new lines or wrinkles form on the fingertip surfaces.

Langerhans Cells

Within the epidermis are **Langerhans cells**, which are also called **dendritic cells** because of their branched appearance when they move (see Fig. 5–2 and also Fig. 14–6 and Box 14–5 in Chapter 14). These cells originate in the red bone marrow and are quite mobile. They are able to phagocytize foreign material, such as bacteria that enter the body through breaks in the skin. With such ingested pathogens, the Langerhans cells migrate to lymph nodes and present the pathogen to lymphocytes, a type of white blood cell. This triggers an immune response such as the production of antibodies (antibodies are proteins that label foreign material for destruction). Because the skin is positioned adjacent to the external environment, it is an important component of the body's protective responses, though many of the exact aspects of this have yet to be determined. Langerhans cells are part of innate (inborn) immune mechanisms, our most rapid response to pathogens (immunity is covered in detail in Chapter 14).

Box 5–1 | BURNS

Burns of the skin may be caused by flames, hot water or steam, sunlight, electricity, or corrosive chemicals. The severity of burns ranges from minor to fatal, and the classification of burns is based on the extent of damage (see Box Figure 5–A).

First-Degree Burn—(also called "superficial") only the superficial epidermis is burned and is painful but not blistered. Light-colored skin will appear red (**erythema**) due to localized **vasodilation** in the damaged area. Vasodilation is part of the inflammatory response that brings more blood to the injured site.

Second-Degree Burn—(partial-thickness burn) deeper layers of the epidermis are affected. Another aspect of **inflammation** is that damaged cells release **histamine**, which makes capillaries more permeable. More plasma leaves these capillaries and becomes tissue

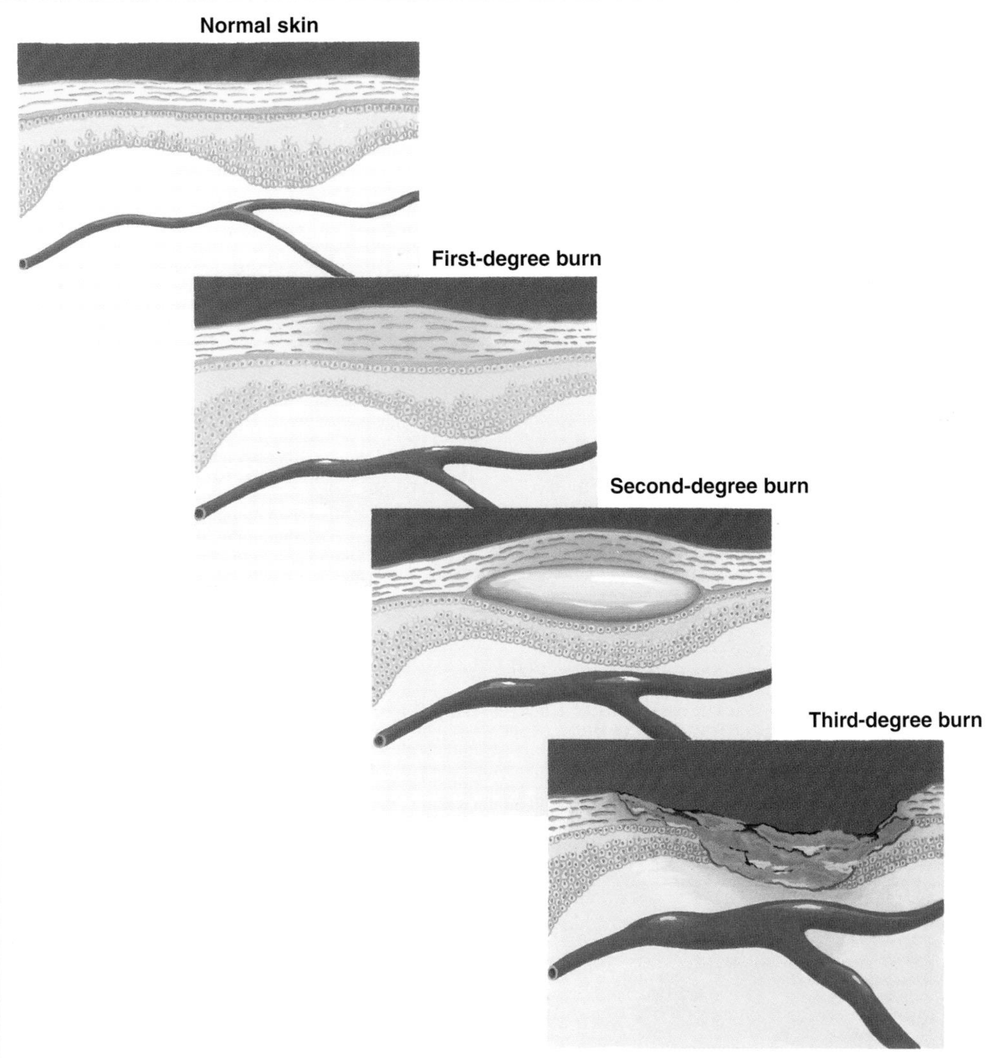

Box Figure 5–A Normal skin section and representative sections showing first-degree, second-degree, and third-degree burns.

Continued

Box 5–1 | BURNS *(Continued)*

fluid, which collects at the burn site, creating blisters. The burned skin is often very painful.

Third-Degree Burn—(full-thickness burn) the entire epidermis is charred or burned away, and the burn may extend into the dermis or subcutaneous tissue. Often such a burn is not painful at first if the receptors in the dermis have been destroyed.

Extensive third-degree burns are potentially life-threatening because of the loss of the stratum corneum. Without this natural barrier, living tissue is exposed to the environment and is susceptible to infection and dehydration.

Fourth-Degree Burn—(deep full-thickness burn) the burn has reached the underlying muscle tissue or bone.

Bacterial infection is a serious problem for burn patients; the pathogens may get into the blood (**septicemia**) and quickly spread throughout the body. Dehydration may also be fatal if medical intervention does not interrupt and correct the following sequence: Tissue fluid evaporates from the burned surface, and more plasma is pulled out of capillaries into the tissue spaces. As more plasma is lost, blood volume and blood pressure decrease. This is called **circulatory shock**; eventually the heart simply does not have enough blood to pump, and heart failure is the cause of death. To prevent these serious consequences, third-degree and fourth-degree burns are covered with donor skin or artificial skin until skin grafts of the patient's own skin can be put in place.

Melanocytes

Another type of cell found in the lower epidermis is the melanocyte, which is also shown in Fig. 5–2. **Melanocytes** produce a pigment called **melanin**, which is made primarily from the amino acid tyrosine. People of the same size have approximately the same number of melanocytes, though these cells may differ in their level of activity. In people with dark skin, the melanocytes continuously produce large amounts of melanin. The melanocytes of light-skinned people produce less melanin. The activity of melanocytes is genetically regulated; skin color is one of our hereditary characteristics.

In all people, melanin production is increased by exposure of the skin to ultraviolet rays, which are part of sunlight and are damaging to living cells. As more melanin is produced, it is taken in by the epidermal cells as they are pushed toward the surface. This gives the skin a darker color, which acts as a barrier and reduces exposure of the living stratum germinativum and the roaming Langerhans cells to ultraviolet rays. People with light skin do not have much natural protection against ultraviolet rays, and exposure to sun will tan the epidermis and form a temporary shield (see Box 5–2: Preventing Skin Cancer: Common Sense and Sunscreens). People with dark skin already have good protection against the damaging effects of ultraviolet rays, but unfortunately they produce less vitamin D.

Melanin also gives color to hair, though its protective function is confined to the hair of the head. Two parts of the eye obtain their color from melanin: the iris and the interior choroid layer of the eyeball (the eye is discussed in Chapter 9).The functions of the epidermis and its cells are summarized in Table 5–1.

DERMIS

The **dermis** is made of an irregular type of fibrous connective tissue, irregular meaning that the fibers are not parallel but criss-cross and run in all directions. Fibroblasts produce both **collagen** and **elastin** fibers. Recall that collagen fibers are strong, and elastin fibers are able to recoil after being stretched. Strength and elasticity are two characteristics of the dermis. With increasing age, however, the deterioration of the elastin fibers causes the skin to lose its elasticity. We can all look forward to at least a few wrinkles as we get older.

The uneven junction of the dermis with the epidermis is called the **papillary layer** (see Fig. 5–1). Capillaries are abundant here to nourish not only the dermis but also the stratum germinativum. The epidermis has no capillaries of its own, and the lower, living cells depend on the blood supply in the dermis for oxygen and nutrients.

Within the dermis are the accessory skin structures: hair and nail follicles, sensory receptors, and several types of glands. Some of these structures project through the epidermis to the skin surface, but their active portions are in the dermis.

Hair Follicles

Hair follicles are made of epidermal tissue, and the growth process of hair is very similar to the growth of the

Box 5–2 | PREVENTING SKIN CANCER: COMMON SENSE AND SUNSCREENS

Anyone can get skin cancer, and the most important factor is exposure to sunlight. Light-skinned people are, of course, more susceptible to the effects of ultraviolet (UV) rays, which may trigger **mutations** in living epidermal cells.

Squamous cell **carcinoma** and basal cell carcinoma (see A in Box Fig. 5–B) are the most common forms of skin cancer. The lesions are visible as changes in the normal appearance of the skin, and a **biopsy** (microscopic examination of a tissue specimen) is used to confirm the diagnosis. These lesions usually do not **metastasize** rapidly and can be completely removed using simple procedures.

Malignant **melanoma** (see B in Box Fig. 5–B) is a more serious form of skin cancer, which begins in melanocytes. Any change in a pigmented spot or mole (**nevus**) should prompt a person to see a doctor. Melanoma is serious not because of its growth in the skin but because it may **metastasize** very rapidly to the lungs, liver, or other vital organ. Researchers are testing individualized vaccines for people who have had melanoma. The purpose of the vaccine is to stimulate the immune system strongly enough to prevent a second case, because such recurrences are often fatal.

Although the most common forms of skin cancer are readily curable, prevention is a better strategy. We cannot, and we would not want to, stay out of the sun altogether (because sunlight may be the best way to get sufficient vitamin D), but we may be able to do so when sunlight is most damaging. During the summer months, UV rays are especially intense between 10 a.m. and 2 p.m. If we are or must be outdoors during this time, dermatologists recommend use of a sunscreen.

Sunscreens contain chemicals that block UV rays and prevent them from damaging the epidermis. A "broad spectrum" sunscreen is protective against both UVA (the carcinogenic rays) and UVB (the burning rays), and an SPF (sun protection factor) between 15 and 50 is considered good protection if the sunscreen is applied often. Use of a sunscreen on exposed skin not only helps prevent skin cancer but also prevents sunburn and its painful effects. It is especially important to prevent children from getting severely sunburned, because such burns have been linked to the development of skin cancer years later.

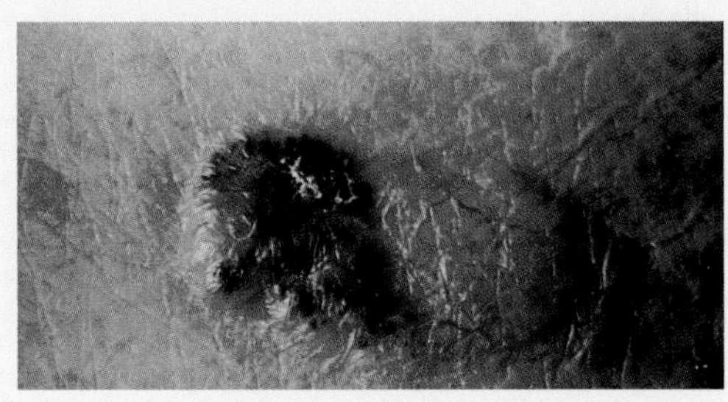

A

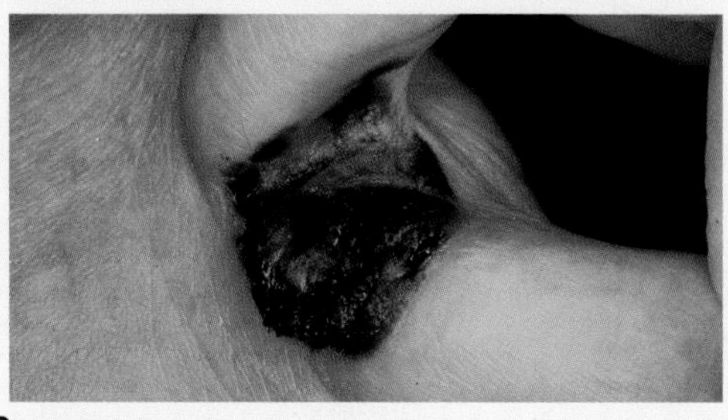

B

Box Figure 5–B (A) Classic basal-cell carcinoma on face. (**B**) Melanoma in finger web. (From Goldsmith, LA, Lazarus, GS, and Tharp, MD: Adult and Pediatric Dermatology: A Color Guide to Diagnosis and Treatment. FA Davis, 1997, pp 137 and 144, with permission.)

epidermis. At the base of a follicle is the dermal papilla, a projection of connective tissue of the dermis; it contains blood vessels. Just above the dermal papilla is the **hair root**, which contains cells called the **matrix**, where mitosis takes place (Fig. 5–3). The new cells produce keratin, get their color from melanin, and then die and become incorporated into the **hair shaft**, which is pushed toward the surface of the skin. The hair that we comb and brush every day consists of dead, keratinized cells. The monthly rate of hair growth averages 0.3 to 0.4 in. (8 to 10 mm), and eventually a follicle will become dormant before starting to grow a new hair that pushes the old hair out.

Table 5–1 | EPIDERMIS

PART	FUNCTION
Stratum corneum (keratin)	■ Prevents loss or entry of water ■ If unbroken, prevents entry of pathogens and most chemicals
Stratum germinativum (stratum basale)	■ Continuous mitosis produces new cells to replace worn-off surface cells ■ Produces antimicrobial defensins ■ Cholesterol is changed to vitamin D on exposure to UV rays
Langerhans cells	■ Phagocytize foreign material and stimulate an immune response by lymphocytes
Merkel cells	■ Receptors for sense of touch
Melanocytes	■ Produce melanin on exposure to UV rays
Melanin	■ Protects living skin layers from further exposure to UV rays

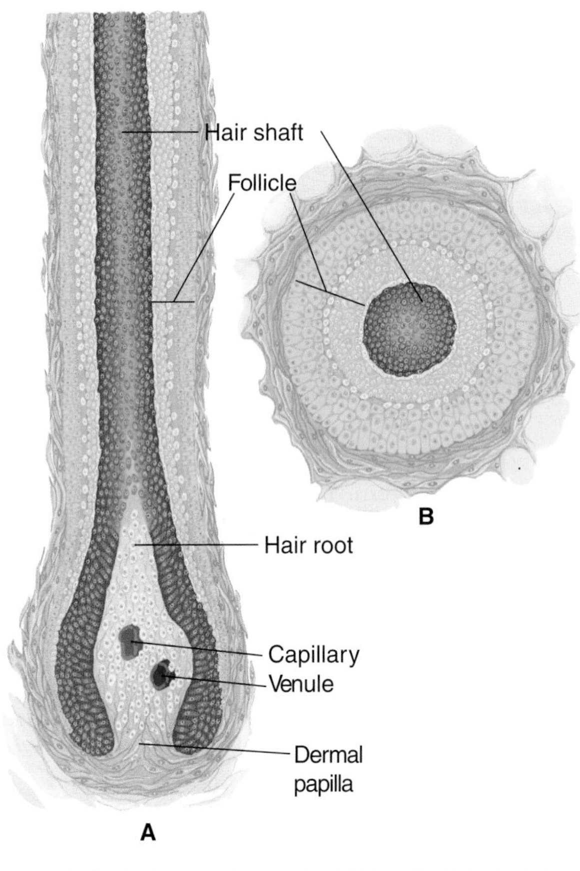

Figure 5–3 Structure of a hair follicle. (**A**) Longitudinal section. (**B**) Cross-section.

QUESTION: What is the hair shaft made of?

We lose hair from the scalp every day; estimates range from 50 to 100 hairs lost per day.

Compared with some other mammals, humans do not have very much hair. The actual functions of human hair are few. Eyelashes and eyebrows help to keep dust and perspiration out of the eyes, and the hairs just inside the nostrils help to keep dust out of the nasal cavities. Hair of the scalp does provide insulation from cold for the head. The hair on our bodies, however, no longer serves this function, but we have the evolutionary remnants of it. Attached to each hair follicle is a small, smooth muscle called the **pilomotor** or arrector pili muscle. When stimulated by cold or emotions such as fear, these muscles pull the hair follicles upright (piloerection). For an animal with fur, this would trap air and provide greater insulation. Because people do not have thick fur, all this does is give us "goose bumps."

Nail Follicles

Found on the ends of fingers and toes, **nail follicles** produce nails, just as hair follicles produce hair. Mitosis takes place in the **nail root** at the base of the nail (Fig. 5–4), and the new cells produce keratin (a stronger form of this protein than is found in hair) and then die. Although the nail itself consists of keratinized dead cells, the flat nail bed is living epidermis and dermis. This is why cutting a nail too short can be quite painful. Nails protect the ends of the fingers and toes from mechanical injury and give the fingers greater ability to pick up small objects. Fingernails are also good for scratching. This is more important than it may seem at first. An itch might mean the presence of an arthropod parasite: a mosquito, tick, flea, or louse. These parasites (all but the tick are insects) feed on blood, and all are potential vectors of diseases caused by bacteria, viruses, or protozoa. A quick

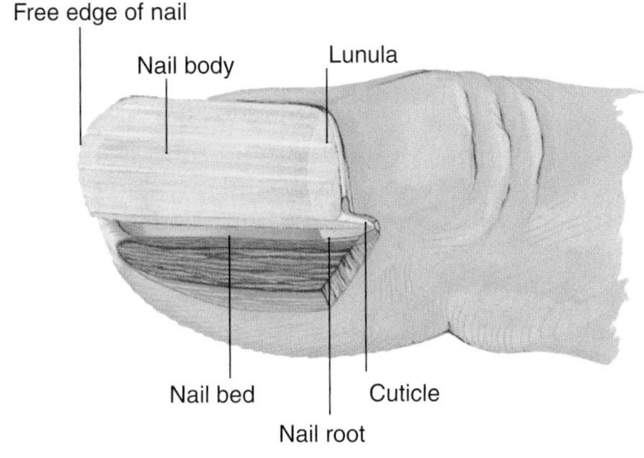

Figure 5–4 Structure of a fingernail shown in longitudinal section.

QUESTION: The nail bed is which part of the skin?

and vigorous scratch may kill or at least dislodge the arthropod and prevent the transmission of the disease. Fingernails grow at a monthly rate of about 0.12 in. (3 mm), and growth is a little faster during the summer months.

Receptors

Most sensory **receptors** for the cutaneous senses are found in the dermis (Merkel cells are in the stratum germinativum, as are some nerve endings). The cutaneous senses are touch, pressure, heat, cold, itch, and pain. For each sensation there is a specific type of receptor, which is a structure that will detect a particular change. For heat, cold, itch, and pain the receptors are **free nerve endings**. For touch and pressure, the receptors are called **encapsulated nerve endings**, which means there is a cellular structure around the sensory nerve ending (see Fig. 5–1). The purpose of these receptors and sensations is to provide the central nervous system with information about the external environment and its effect on the skin. This information may stimulate responses, such as washing a painful cut finger, scratching an insect bite, or responding to a feeling of cold by putting on a sweater.

The sensitivity of an area of skin is determined by how many receptors are present, that is, the spatial density of the receptors. Think for a moment of the density of houses in a city compared with the spacing of farmhouses in the countryside. If a meteorite were to fall on a city, it would very likely strike a house. But if it fell in the countryside, the meteorite would likely strike between houses. The skin of the fingertips is like the city in that it is very sensitive to touch because there are many receptors per square inch. The skin of the upper arm, with few touch receptors per square inch, is more like the countryside and is less sensitive.

When receptors detect changes, they generate nerve impulses that are carried to the brain, which interprets the impulses as a particular sensation. Sensation, therefore, is actually a function of the brain (we will return to this in Chapters 8 and 9).

Glands

Glands are made of epithelial tissue. The exocrine glands of the skin have their secretory portions in the dermis. Some of these are shown in Fig. 5–1.

Sebaceous Glands. The ducts of **sebaceous glands** open into hair follicles or directly to the skin surface. Their secretion is **sebum**, a lipid substance that we commonly refer to as oil. As mentioned previously, the fatty acids of sebum inhibit the growth of bacteria on the skin surface. Another function of sebum is to prevent the drying out of skin and hair. The importance of this may not be readily apparent, but skin that is dry tends to crack more easily. Even very small breaks in the skin are potential entryways for bacteria. Decreased sebum production is another consequence of getting older, and elderly people often have dry and more fragile skin.

Adolescents may have the problem of overactive sebaceous glands and the inflammatory condition called **acne**. Too much sebum may trap bacteria within hair follicles and create small infections. Because sebaceous glands are more numerous around the nose and mouth, these are common sites of pimples in young people (see also Box 5–3: Common Skin Disorders).

Ceruminous Glands. These glands are located in the dermis of the ear canals. Their secretion is called **cerumen** or earwax (which includes the sebum secreted in the ear canals). Cerumen keeps the outer surface of the eardrum pliable and prevents drying. However, if excess cerumen accumulates in the ear canal, it may become impacted against the eardrum. This might diminish the acuity of hearing by preventing the eardrum from vibrating properly.

Sweat Glands. There are two types of sweat glands, apocrine and eccrine. Sweat is mostly water and contains sodium chloride, making sweat salty. Also found in sweat are very small amounts of hundreds of other chemicals, many of them volatile, meaning that they readily evaporate at moderate temperatures. Each individual produces a slightly different combination of these chemicals, which gives each person a unique scent. Animals such as dogs can easily distinguish among people (even identical twins) because of their individual scents.

Box 5-3 | COMMON SKIN DISORDERS

Impetigo—a bacterial infection often caused by streptococci or staphylococci (Box Fig. 5–C), with characteristic pustules (pus-containing lesions); the infection is contagious to others.

Eczema—a symptom of what is more properly called atopic dermatitis. This is an allergic reaction with a genetic component that changes the chemistry and structure of the skin. The antimicrobial chemical cathelicidin is often deficient. A protein of the tight junctions between epidermal cells is weak and makes the epidermis more permeable, or "leaky," allowing water to evaporate through the skin, and bacteria or other irritants to enter the skin. The resulting itchy rash (**pruritus**) may blister or ooze, and flare-ups can be triggered by allergens that enter the body in places other than the skin. Eczema may be related to foods such as fish, eggs, or milk products, or to inhaled allergens such as dust, pollens, or animal dander. More common in children than adults (the allergic reaction often diminishes as a child gets older), prevention depends on determining what the child is allergic to and eliminating or at least limiting exposure.

Warts—caused by a virus that makes epidermal cells divide abnormally, producing a growth that is often raised and has a rough or pitted surface. Warts are most common on the hands, but they may be anywhere on the skin.

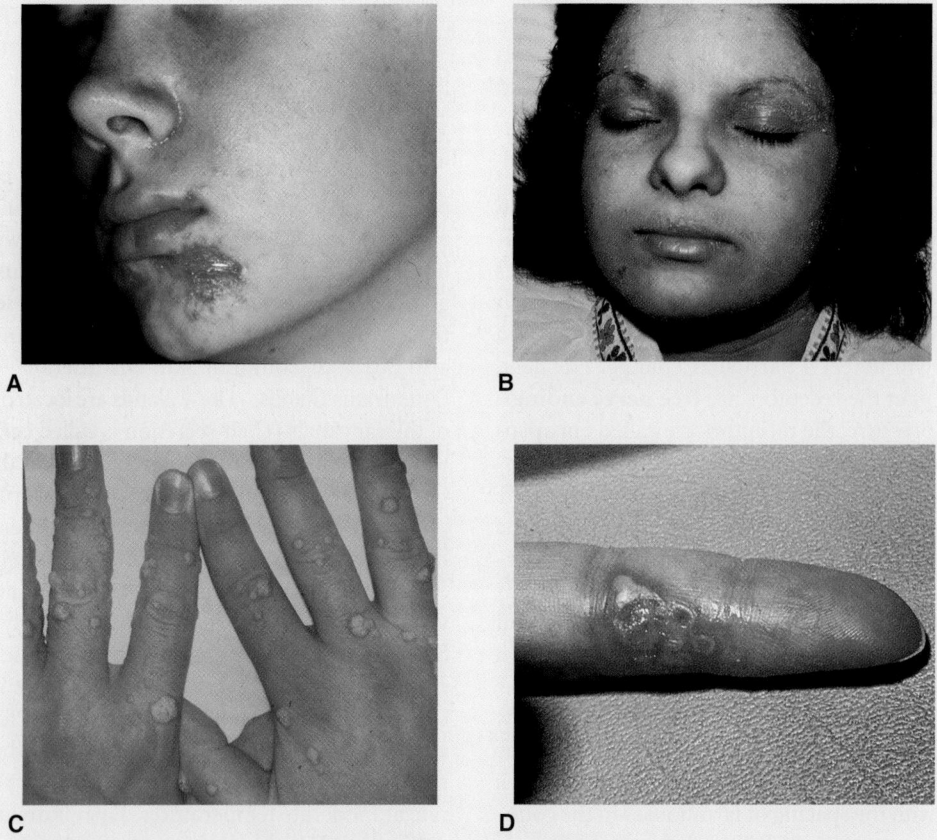

Box Figure 5–C (A) Impetigo. (**B**) Eczema of atopic dermatitis. (**C**) Warts on back of hands. (**D**) Fever blister on finger, localized but severe. (From Goldsmith, LA, Lazarus, GS, and Tharp, MD. *Adult and Pediatric Dermatology: A Color Guide to Diagnosis and Treatment.* Philadelphia: FA Davis, 1997, pp 80, 241, 306, and 317, with permission.)

Box 5–3 | COMMON SKIN DISORDERS *(Continued)*

Plantar warts on the sole of the foot may become quite painful because of the constant pressure of standing and walking.

Fever blisters (cold sores)—caused by the herpes simplex virus, to which most people are exposed as children. An active lesion, usually at the edge of the lip (but may be anywhere on the skin), is painful and oozes. If not destroyed by the immune system, the virus "hides out" and becomes dormant in nerves of the face. Another lesion, weeks or months later, may be triggered by stress or another illness.

Apocrine glands are most numerous in the axillae (underarm) and genital areas and are most active in stressful and emotional situations. Although their secretion does have an odor, it is barely perceptible to other people. If the apocrine secretions are allowed to accumulate on the skin, however, bacteria metabolize the chemicals in the sweat and produce waste products that have distinct odors that many people find unpleasant.

Eccrine glands are found all over the body but are especially numerous on the forehead, upper lip, palms, and soles. The secretory portion of these glands is simply a coiled tube in the dermis. The duct of this tube extends to the skin's surface, where it opens into a **pore**.

The sweat produced by eccrine glands is important in the maintenance of normal body temperature. In a warm environment, or during exercise, more sweat is secreted onto the skin surface, where it is then evaporated by excess body heat. Recall that water has a high heat of vaporization, which means that a great deal of heat can be lost in the evaporation of a relatively small amount of water. Although this is a very effective mechanism of heat loss, it has a potentially serious disadvantage. Loss of too much body water in sweat may lead to **dehydration**, especially after exercise on a hot and humid day. Increased sweating during exercise or on warm days should always be accompanied by increased fluid intake.

Those who exercise know that they must replace salt, as well as water. Sodium chloride is also lost in sweat, as are small amounts of **urea** (a nitrogenous waste product of amino acid metabolism). This excretory function of the skin is very minor, however; the kidneys are primarily responsible for removing waste products from the blood and for maintaining the body's proper salt-to-water proportion.

Blood Vessels

Besides the capillaries in the dermis, the other blood vessels of great importance are the arterioles. **Arterioles** are small arteries, and the smooth muscle in their walls permits them to constrict (close) or dilate (open). This is important in the maintenance of body temperature because blood carries heat, which is a form of energy.

In a warm environment the arterioles dilate (**vasodilation**), which increases blood flow through the dermis and brings excess heat close to the body surface to be radiated to the environment. In a cold environment, however, body heat must be conserved if possible, so the arterioles constrict. This **vasoconstriction** decreases the flow of blood through the dermis and keeps heat within the core of the body. This adjusting mechanism is essential for maintaining homeostasis. Regulation of the diameter of the arterioles in response to external temperature changes is controlled by the nervous system. These changes can often be seen in light-skinned people. Flushing, especially in the face, may be observed in hot weather. In cold, the skin of the extremities may become even paler as blood flow through the dermis decreases. In people with dark skin, such changes are not as readily apparent because the changes are masked by melanin in the epidermis.

Vasoconstriction in the dermis may also occur during stressful situations. For our ancestors, stress usually demanded a physical response: either stand and fight or run away to try to reach a safe place. This is called the "fight-or-flight response." Our nervous systems are still programmed to respond as if physical activity were necessary to cope with the stress situation. Vasoconstriction in the dermis will shunt, or redirect, blood to more vital organs such as the muscles, heart, and brain. In times of stress, the skin is a relatively unimportant organ and can function temporarily with a minimal blood flow. You have probably heard the expression "broke out in a cold sweat" and may even have felt this way in a stressful situation. Such sweating feels cold because vasoconstriction in the dermis makes the skin relatively cool.

Blood flow in the dermis may be interrupted by prolonged pressure on the skin. For example, hospital patients who cannot turn over by themselves may develop **decubitus ulcers**, also called pressure ulcers or pressure sores. The skin is compressed between the object outside, such as a bed, and a bony prominence within, such as the heel bone or the sacrum in the lower back. Without its blood supply the skin dies, and the dead tissue is a potential site for bacterial infection.

The functions of dermal structures are summarized in Table 5–2.

SUBCUTANEOUS TISSUE

The **subcutaneous tissue** may also be called the **superficial fascia**, one of the connective tissue membranes. Made of areolar connective tissue and adipose tissue, the superficial fascia connects the dermis to the underlying muscles. Its other functions are those of its tissues, as you may recall from Chapter 4.

Table 5–2 | DERMIS

PART	FUNCTION
Papillary layer	■ Contains capillaries that nourish the stratum germinativum
Hair (follicles)	■ Eyelashes and nasal hair keep dust out of eyes and nasal cavities ■ Scalp hair provides insulation from cold for the head
Nails (follicles)	■ Protect ends of fingers and toes from mechanical injury
Receptors	■ Detect changes that are felt as the cutaneous senses: touch, pressure, heat, cold, itch, and pain
Sebaceous glands	■ Produce sebum, which prevents drying of skin and hair and inhibits growth of bacteria
Ceruminous glands	■ Produce cerumen, which prevents drying of the eardrum
Eccrine sweat glands	■ Produce watery sweat that is evaporated by excess body heat to cool the body
Arterioles	■ Dilate in response to warmth to increase heat loss ■ Constrict in response to cold to conserve body heat ■ Constrict in stressful situations to shunt blood to more vital organs

Areolar connective tissue, or loose connective tissue, contains collagen and elastin fibers and many white blood cells that have left capillaries to wander around in the tissue fluid between skin and muscles. These migrating white blood cells destroy pathogens that enter the body through breaks in the skin. Also present are **mast cells**. These cells are produced in the red bone marrow and found in connective tissue throughout the body. They are especially numerous in areolar tissue, where they produce histamine, leukotrienes, and other chemicals that help bring about inflammation, the body's response to damage (inflammation is described in Chapters 10 and 14).

The cells (adipocytes) of adipose tissue are specialized to store fat, and our subcutaneous layer of fat stores excess nutrients as a potential energy source. This layer also cushions bony prominences, such as those during sitting, and provides some insulation from cold. For people, this last function is relatively minor because we do not have a thick layer of fat, as do animals such as whales and seals. As mentioned in Chapter 4, adipose tissue is involved in the onset or cessation of eating and in the use of insulin by body cells, and it contributes to inflammation by producing cytokines, chemicals that activate white blood cells.

Just as the epidermis forms a continuous sheet that covers the body, the subcutaneous tissue is a continuous layer, though it is internal. If we consider the epidermis as a first line of defense against pathogens, we can consider the subcutaneous tissue as a secondary line of defense. There is, however, a significant anatomic difference. The cells of the epidermis are very closely and tightly packed, but the cells and protein fibers of subcutaneous tissue are farther apart, and there is much more tissue fluid. If we imagine the epidermis as a four-lane highway during rush hour with bumper-to-bumper traffic, the superficial fascia would be that same highway at three o'clock in the morning, when it is not crowded and cars can move much faster. This is an obvious benefit for the migrating white blood cells but may become a disadvantage because some bacterial pathogens, once established, can spread even more rapidly throughout subcutaneous tissue.

Group A streptococcus, for example, is a cause of **necrotizing fasciitis**. *Necrotizing* means "to cause death," and *fasciitis* is the inflammation of a fascia, in this case the superficial fascia and the deep fasciae around muscles. Necrotizing fasciitis is an **acute** infection in both meanings of *acute*: "sudden onset" and "extremely serious." It requires surgical removal of the infected tissue, or even amputation of an infected limb, to try to stop the spread of the bacteria. The body's defenses have been overwhelmed because what is usually an anatomic benefit, the "looseness" of areolar connective tissue, has become a detriment.

The functions of subcutaneous tissue are summarized in Table 5–3. Box 5–4: Administering Medications describes ways in which we give medications through the skin.

Table 5–3 | SUBCUTANEOUS TISSUE

PART	FUNCTION
Areolar connective tissue	■ Connects skin to muscles ■ Contains many WBCs to destroy pathogens that enter breaks in the skin ■ Contains mast cells that release histamine, leukotrienes, and other chemicals involved in inflammation
Adipose tissue	■ Contains stored energy in the form of true fats ■ Cushions bony prominences ■ Provides some insulation from cold ■ Contributes to appetite ■ Contributes to use of insulin ■ Produces cytokines that activate WBCs

AGING AND THE INTEGUMENTARY SYSTEM

The effects of age on the integumentary system are often quite visible. Both layers of skin become thinner and more fragile as mitosis in the epidermis slows and fibroblasts in the dermis die and are not replaced; repair of even small breaks or cuts is slower. The skin becomes wrinkled as collagen and elastin fibers in the dermis deteriorate.

Sebaceous glands and sweat glands become less active; the skin becomes dry, and temperature regulation in hot weather becomes more difficult. Hair follicles become inactive and hair on the scalp and body thins. A marked loss of hair is called **alopecia** and is often genetically regulated (women and men may be affected). Melanocytes die and are not replaced; the hair that remains becomes white. The remaining melanocytes may not be enough to create an efficient barrier of melanin, and the skin becomes more susceptible to sunburn. The ability to produce vitamin D also decreases, as much as 50% to 70%, and older people must rely more on diet for this essential nutrient.

There is often less fat in the subcutaneous tissue, which may make an elderly person more sensitive to cold. It is important for elderly people (and those who care for them) to realize that extremes of temperature may be harmful and to take special precautions in very hot or very cold weather.

Box 5–4 | ADMINISTERING MEDICATIONS

You have probably seen advertisements for skin patches that supply medications. This method of supplying a drug is called *transdermal administration*. The name is a little misleading because the most difficult part of cutaneous absorption of a drug is absorption through the stratum corneum of the epidermis. Because such absorption is slow, skin patches are useful for medications needed in small but continuous amounts and over a prolonged period of time.

You would expect that such patches should be worn where the epidermis is relatively thin. These sites include the upper arm and the chest. The recommended site for a patch to prevent motion sickness is the skin behind the ear. Also available in patch form are medications for birth control, overactive bladder, high blood pressure, smoking cessation (nicotine patches), and both systemic and localized pain relief. Elderly people and those who care for them should be aware that the skin becomes much thinner with age and therefore more permeable, and the absorption of medication from a patch may become so rapid as to cause an overdose.

Medications may also be injected through the skin. Some injections are given subcutaneously,

Continued

Box 5-4 | ADMINISTERING MEDICATIONS *(Continued)*

that is, into subcutaneous tissue (see Box Fig. 5–D). Subcutaneous adipose tissue has a moderate blood supply, so the rate of absorption of the drug will be moderate, but predictable. Insulin is given subcutaneously. Other injections are intramuscular, and absorption into the blood is rapid because muscle tissue has a very good blood supply. Most injectable vaccines are given intramuscularly to promote rapid absorption to stimulate antibody production.

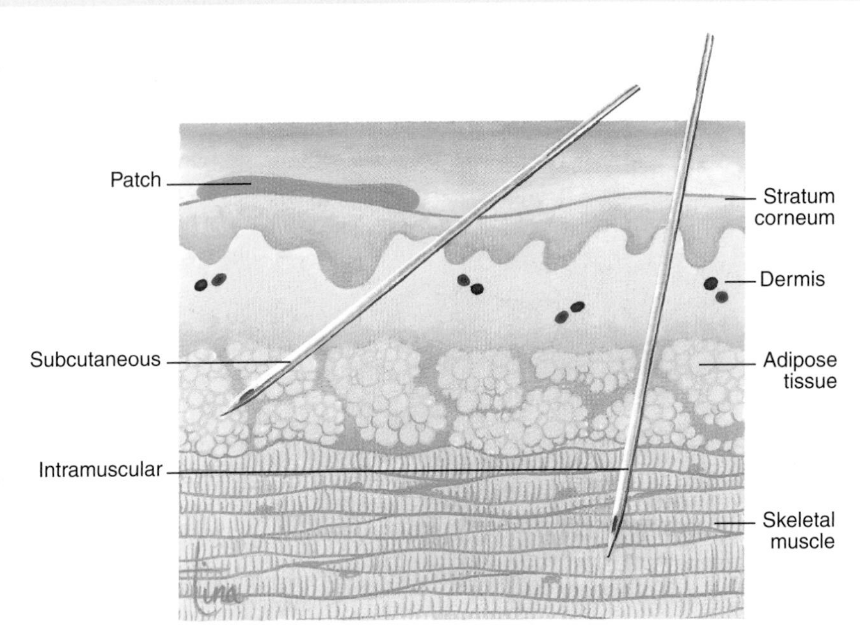

Box Figure 5–D The skin, subcutaneous tissue, and muscle sites for the delivery of medications.

SUMMARY

The integumentary system is the outermost organ system of the body. You have noticed that many of its functions are related to this location. The skin protects the body against pathogens and chemicals, minimizes loss or entry of water, blocks the harmful effects of sunlight, and produces vitamin D. Sensory receptors in the skin provide information about the external environment, and the skin helps regulate body temperature in response to environmental changes. The subcutaneous tissue is a secondary line of defense against pathogens and a site of fat storage and of the other metabolic functions of adipose tissue.

STUDY OUTLINE

The integumentary system consists of the skin and its accessory structures and the subcutaneous tissue. The two major layers of the skin are the outer epidermis and the inner dermis.

Epidermis—made of stratified squamous epithelium; no capillaries; cells are called keratinocytes, have tight junctions between them, and are a first line of defense (see Figs. 5–1 and 5–2 and Table 5–1)

1. Stratum germinativum—the innermost layer where mitosis takes place; new cells produce keratin and die as they are pushed toward the surface. Defensins are antimicrobial peptides produced when the skin is injured. Vitamin D is formed from cholesterol on exposure to the UV rays of sunlight; it is converted to its most active form by the kidneys, and any excess is stored in the liver.
2. Stratum corneum—the outermost layers of dead cells; keratin prevents loss and entry of water and, if unbroken, resists entry of chemicals and pathogens. The microbiota of the skin surface help to prevent the growth of pathogenic bacteria and fungi.
3. Langerhans cells—phagocytize foreign material, take it to lymph nodes, and stimulate an immune response by lymphocytes.
4. Melanocytes—in the lower epidermis, produce the protein melanin. UV rays stimulate melanin production; melanin prevents further exposure of the stratum germinativum to UV rays by darkening the skin.

Dermis—made of irregular fibrous connective tissue; collagen provides strength, and elastin provides elasticity; capillaries in the papillary layer nourish the stratum germinativum (see Fig. 5–1 and Table 5–2)

1. Hair follicles—mitosis takes place in the hair root; new cells produce keratin, die, and become the hair shaft. Hair of the scalp provides insulation from cold for the head; eyelashes help keep dust out of eyes; nostril hairs keep dust out of nasal cavities (see Figs. 5–1 and 5–3).
2. Nail follicles—at the ends of fingers and toes; mitosis takes place in the nail root; the nail itself consists of dead, keratinized cells. Nails protect the ends of the fingers and toes, enable the fingers to pick up small objects, and provide for efficient scratching (see Fig. 5–4).
3. Receptors—detect changes on or in the skin: touch, pressure, heat, cold, itch, and pain; provide information about the external environment that initiates appropriate responses; sensitivity of the skin depends on the number of receptors present.
4. Sebaceous glands—secrete sebum into hair follicles or to the skin surface; the fatty acids of sebum inhibit the growth of some bacteria and prevent drying of skin and hair.
5. Ceruminous glands—secrete cerumen in the ear canals; cerumen prevents drying of the eardrum.
6. Apocrine sweat glands—modified scent glands in axillae and genital area; activated by stress and emotions.
7. Eccrine sweat glands—most numerous on face, palms, soles. Activated by high external temperature or exercise; sweat on skin surface is evaporated by excess body heat; potential disadvantage is dehydration. Excretion of small amounts of NaCl and urea is a very minor function.
8. Arterioles—smooth muscle in their walls permits constriction or dilation. Vasoconstriction in cold temperatures decreases dermal blood flow to conserve heat in the body core. Vasodilation in warm temperatures increases dermal blood flow to bring heat to the surface to be lost. Vasoconstriction during stressful situations shunts blood away from the skin to more vital organs, such as muscles, to permit a physical response, if necessary.

Subcutaneous Tissue—also called the superficial fascia; connects skin to muscles and is a secondary line of defense (see Fig. 5–1 and Table 5–3)

1. Areolar tissue—also called loose connective tissue; the matrix contains tissue fluid and WBCs that destroy pathogens that get through breaks in the skin; mast cells produce chemicals that bring about inflammation (the body's response to any type of damage).
2. Adipose tissue—stores fat as potential energy; cushions bony prominences; provides some insulation from cold. Other functions: contributes to appetite, the use of insulin, and the activation of WBCs.

REVIEW QUESTIONS

1. Name the parts of the integumentary system. (p. 104)
2. Name the two major layers of skin, the location of each, and the tissue of which each is made. (pp. 104,108)
3. In the epidermis: (pp. 104,106)
   a. Where does mitosis take place?
   b. What protein do the new cells produce?
   c. What happens to these cells?
   d. What is the function of Langerhans cells?
4. Describe the functions of the stratum corneum. (pp. 104–105)
5. Name the cells that produce melanin. What is the stimulus? Describe the function of melanin (p. 108)
6. Where, on the body, does human hair have important functions? Describe these functions. (p. 110)
7. Describe the functions of nails. (pp. 110–111)
8. Name the cutaneous senses. Describe the importance of these senses. (p. 111)
9. Explain the functions of sebum and cerumen. (p. 111)
10. Explain how sweating helps maintain normal body temperature. (p. 113)
11. Explain how the arterioles in the dermis respond to cold or warm external temperatures and to stress situations. (p. 113)
12. What vitamin is produced in the skin? What is the stimulus for the production of this vitamin? (p. 104)
13. Name the tissues of which the superficial fascia is made. Describe the functions of these tissues. (pp. 114–115)

FOR FURTHER THOUGHT

1. The epidermis has no capillaries of its own; the stratum corneum is made of dead cells and doesn't need a blood supply at all. Explain why the epidermis is affected by a decubitus ulcer. Name another group of people, besides hospital or nursing home patients, that is especially susceptible to developing pressure ulcers.
2. Ringworm is a skin condition characterized by scaly red patches, often circular or oval in shape. It is caused not by a worm but rather by certain fungi. What is the food of these fungi; that is, what are they digesting?
3. Wearing a hat in winter is a good idea. What happens to the arterioles in the dermis in a cold environment? How does this affect heat loss? Is the head an exception? Explain.
4. The responses of the skin to sunlight are depicted in Question Figure 5–A. Label the parts indicated.

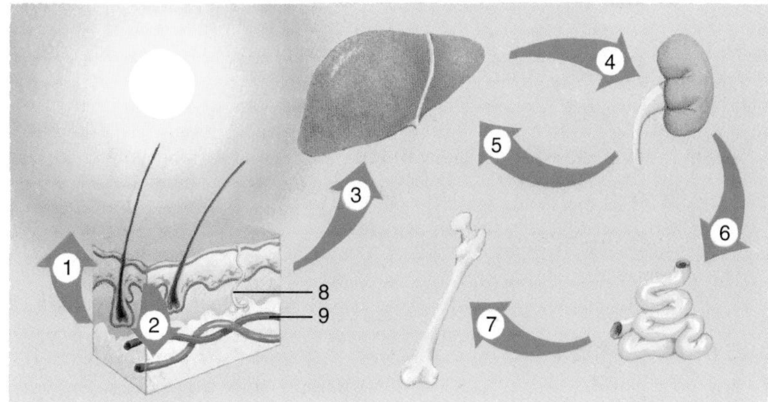

QUESTION FIGURE 5–A Responses of the skin to sunlight.

CHAPTER

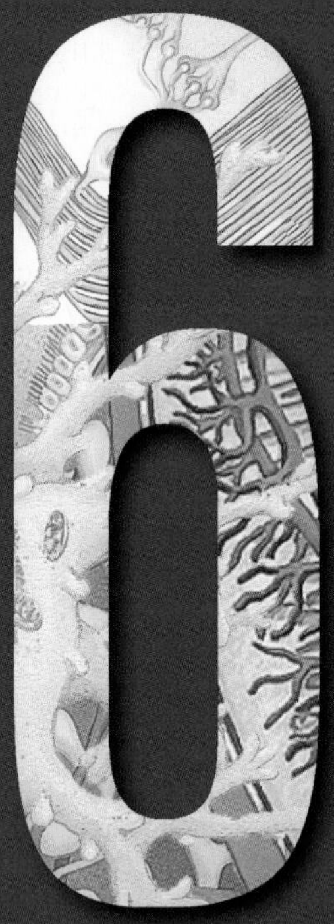

The Skeletal System

STUDENT OBJECTIVES

- Describe the functions of the skeleton.
- Explain how bones are classified, and give an example of each type.
- Describe how the embryonic skeleton model is replaced by bone.
- Name the nutrients necessary for bone growth, and explain their functions.
- Name the hormones involved in bone growth and maintenance, and explain their functions.
- Explain what is meant by "exercise" for bones, and explain its importance.
- Name all the bones of the human skeleton (be able to point to each on diagrams, skeleton models, or yourself).
- Describe the functions of the skull, vertebral column, rib cage, scapula, and pelvic bone.
- Explain how joints are classified. For each type, give an example, and describe the movement possible.
- Describe the parts of a synovial joint, and explain their functions.

NEW TERMINOLOGY

Appendicular *(AP-en-**DIK**-yoo-lar)*
Articulation *(ar-TIK-yoo-**LAY**-shun)*
Axial *(**AK**-see-uhl)*
Bursa *(**BURR**-sah)*
Diaphysis *(dye-**AFF**-i-sis)*
Epiphyseal disc *(e-**PIFF**-i-SEE-al DISK)*
Epiphysis *(e-**PIFF**-i-sis)*
Fontanel *(FON-tah-**NELL**)*
Haversian system *(ha-**VER**-zhun **SIS**-tem)*
Ligament *(**LIG**-uh-ment)*
Ossification *(AHS-i-fi-**KAY**-shun)*
Osteoblast *(**AHS**-tee-oh-BLAST)*
Osteoclast *(**AHS**-tee-oh-KLAST)*
Paranasal sinus *(PAR-uh-**NAY**-zuhl **SIGH**-nus)*
Periosteum *(PER-ee-**AHS**-tee-um)*
Suture *(**SOO**-cher)*
Symphysis *(**SIM**-fi-sis)*
Synovial fluid *(sin-**OH**-vee-al **FLOO**-id)*

RELATED CLINICAL TERMINOLOGY

Autoimmune disease *(AW-toh-im-**YOON** di-**ZEEZ**)*
Bursitis *(burr-**SIGH**-tiss)*
Fracture *(**FRAK**-chur)*
Herniated disc *(**HER**-nee-ay-ted DISK)*
Kyphosis *(kye-**FOH**-sis)*
Lordosis *(lor-**DOH**-sis)*
Osteoarthritis *(AHS-tee-oh-ar-**THRY**-tiss)*
Osteomyelitis *(AHS-tee-oh-my-uh-**LYE**-tiss)*
Osteoporosis *(AHS-tee-oh-por-**OH**-sis)*
Rheumatoid arthritis *(**ROO**-muh-toyd ar-**THRY**-tiss)*
Rickets *(**RIK**-ets)*
Scoliosis *(SKOH-lee-**OH**-sis)*

*Terms that appear in **bold type** in the chapter text are defined in the glossary, which begins on page 603.*

CHAPTER OUTLINE

Imagine for a moment that people did not have skeletons. What comes to mind? Probably that each of us would be a little heap on the floor, much like a jellyfish out of water. Such an image is accurate and reflects the most obvious function of the skeleton: to support the body. Although it is a framework for the body, the skeleton is not at all like the wooden beams that support a house. Bones are living organs that actively contribute to the maintenance of the internal environment of the body.

The **skeletal system** consists of bones and other structures that make up the joints of the skeleton. The types of tissue present are bone tissue, cartilage, and the fibrous connective tissue that forms the ligaments to connect bone to bone.

FUNCTIONS OF THE SKELETON

1. Provides a framework that supports the body; the muscles that are attached to bones move the skeleton.
2. Protects some internal organs from mechanical injury; the rib cage protects the heart and lungs, for example.
3. Contains and protects the red bone marrow, the primary hemopoietic (blood-forming) tissue.
4. Provides a storage site for excess calcium. Calcium may be removed from bone to maintain a normal blood calcium level, which is essential for blood clotting and proper functioning of muscles and nerves.

TYPES OF BONE TISSUE

Bone was described as a tissue in Chapter 4. Recall that bone cells are called **osteocytes**, and the **matrix** of bone is made of **calcium salts** and collagen. The calcium salts are calcium carbonate ($CaCO_3$) and calcium phosphate ($Ca_3(PO_4)_2$), which give bone the strength required to perform its supportive and protective functions. Bone matrix is non-living, but it changes constantly, with calcium that is taken from bone into the blood replaced by calcium from the diet. In normal circumstances, the amount of calcium that is removed is replaced by an equal amount of calcium deposited. This is the function of osteocytes. The primary cilia of osteocytes detect changes in the calcium content of the tissue fluid that surrounds them, which enables the cells to regulate the amount of calcium that is deposited in, or removed from, the bone matrix.

In bone as an organ, two types of bone tissue are present (Fig. 6–1). **Compact bone** looks solid but is very precisely structured. Compact bone is made of **osteons** or **haversian systems**, microscopic cylinders of bone matrix with osteocytes in concentric rings around central **haversian canals.** You can see that the osteocytes look somewhat like spiders, with the "legs" of adjacent spiders in contact. These "legs" are cytoplasmic extensions of osteocytes through microscopic **canaliculi**, or "little canals" in the matrix. In the haversian canals are blood vessels; the innermost osteocytes are in contact with these blood vessels and receive nutrients and oxygen. These useful materials are then passed to the osteocytes in the outer rings.

The second type of bone tissue is **spongy bone**, which does look rather like a sponge with its visible holes or cavities. Osteocytes, matrix, and blood vessels are present but are not arranged in haversian systems. The cavities in spongy bone often contain **red bone marrow**, which produces red blood cells, platelets, and the five kinds of white blood cells.

CLASSIFICATION OF BONES

1. **Long bones**—the bones of the arms, legs, hands, and feet (but not the wrists and ankles). The shaft of a long bone is the **diaphysis**, and the ends are called **epiphyses** (see Fig. 6–1). The diaphysis is made of compact bone and is hollow, forming a canal within the shaft. This **marrow canal** (or medullary cavity) contains **yellow bone marrow**, which is mostly adipose tissue. The epiphyses are made of spongy bone covered with a thin layer of compact bone. Although red bone marrow is present in the epiphyses of children's bones, it is largely replaced by yellow bone marrow in adult bones.
2. **Short bones**—the bones of the wrists and ankles.
3. **Flat bones**—the ribs, shoulder blades, hipbones, and cranial bones.
4. **Irregular bones**—the vertebrae and facial bones.

Short, flat, and irregular bones are all made of spongy bone covered with a thin layer of compact bone. Red bone marrow is found within the spongy bone.

The joint surfaces of bones are covered with **articular cartilage**, which provides a smooth surface. Covering the rest of the bone is the **periosteum**, a fibrous connective tissue membrane whose collagen fibers merge with those of the tendons and **ligaments** that are attached to the bone. The periosteum anchors these structures and contains both the blood vessels that enter the bone itself and osteoblasts that will become active if the bone is damaged.

EMBRYONIC GROWTH OF BONE

During embryonic development, the skeleton is first made of cartilage and fibrous connective tissue, which are gradually replaced by bone. Bone matrix is produced by cells

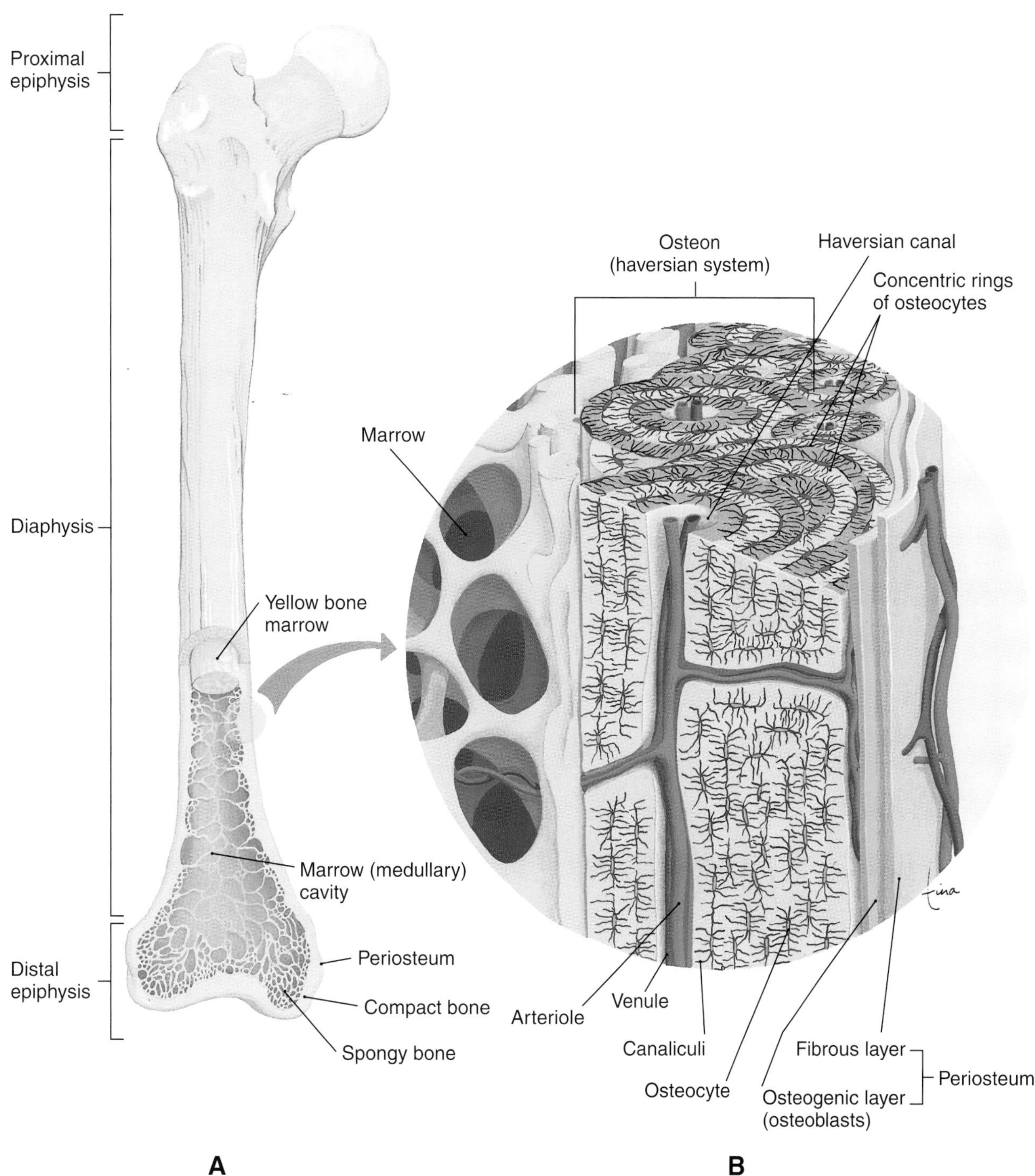

Figure 6–1 Bone tissue. (**A**) Femur with distal end cut in longitudinal section. (**B**) Compact bone showing haversian systems (osteons).

QUESTION: What is the purpose of the blood vessels in bone tissue?

called **osteoblasts** (a *blast* cell is a "growing" or "producing" cell, and *osteo* means "bone"). In the embryonic model of the skeleton, osteoblasts differentiate from the fibroblasts that are present. The production of bone matrix, called **ossification**, begins in a **center of ossification** in each bone.

The cranial and facial bones are first made of fibrous connective tissue. In the third month of fetal development, fibroblasts (spindle-shaped connective tissue cells) become more specialized and differentiate into osteoblasts, which produce bone matrix. From each center of ossification, bone growth radiates outward as calcium salts are deposited in the collagen of the model of the bone. This process is not complete at birth; a baby has areas of fibrous connective tissue remaining between the bones of the skull. These are called **fontanels** (Fig. 6–2), which permit compression of the baby's head during

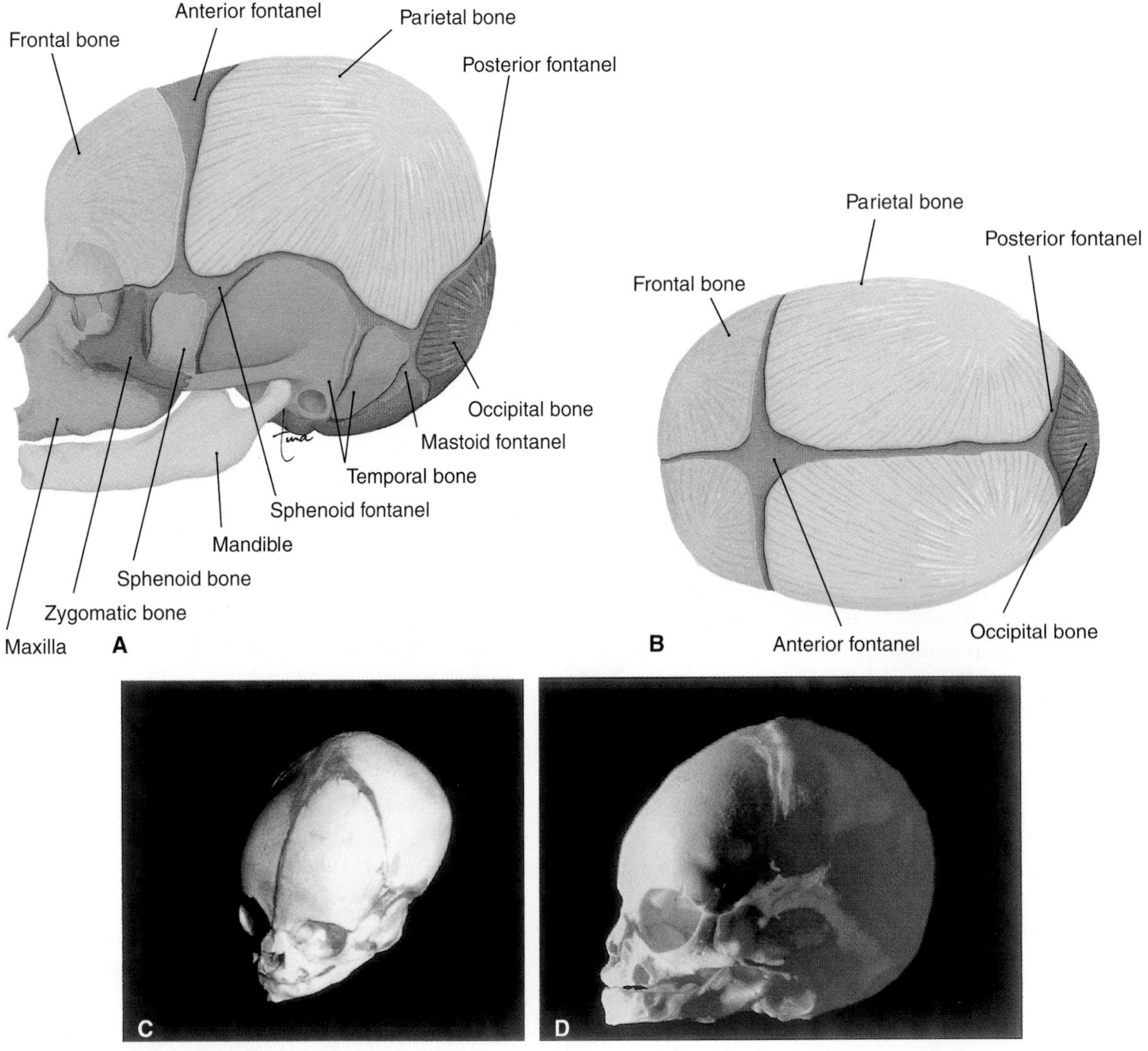

Figure 6–2 Infant skull with fontanels. (**A**) Lateral view of left side. (**B**) Superior view. (**C**) Fetal skull in anterior superior view. (**D**) Fetal skull in left lateral view. Try to name the bones; use part A as a guide. The fontanels are translucent connective tissue. (C and D photographs by Dan Kaufman.)

QUESTION: What is the difference between the frontal bone of the infant skull and that of the adult skull?

birth without breaking the still thin cranial bones. The fontanels also permit the growth of the brain after birth. You may have heard fontanels referred to as "soft spots," and indeed they are. A baby's skull is quite fragile and must be protected from trauma. By the age of 2 years, all the fontanels have become ossified, and the skull becomes a more effective protective covering for the brain.

The rest of the embryonic skeleton is first made of cartilage, and ossification begins in the third month of gestation in the long bones. Osteoblasts produce bone matrix in the center of the diaphyses of the long bones and in the center of short, flat, and irregular bones. Bone matrix gradually replaces the original cartilage (Fig. 6–3).

The long bones also develop centers of ossification in their epiphyses. At birth, ossification is not yet complete and continues throughout childhood. In long bones, growth occurs in the **epiphyseal discs** at the junction of the diaphysis with each epiphysis. An epiphyseal disc is still cartilage, and the bone grows in length as more cartilage is produced on the epiphysis side (see Fig. 6–3). On the diaphysis side, osteoblasts produce bone matrix to replace the cartilage. Some osteoblasts become surrounded by bone and settle down to become maintenance cells, the osteocytes. As long as cartilage is produced, some osteoblasts will follow and replace the cartilage. Between the ages of 16 and 25 years (influenced by estrogen or testosterone), all of the cartilage matrix of the epiphyseal discs is replaced by bone matrix. This is called closure of the epiphyseal discs (or we say the discs are closed), and the bone lengthening process stops.

Also in bones, and shown in Fig. 6–3, are the specialized cells called **osteoclasts** (a *clast* cell is a "destroying" cell), which are large cells with several nuclei and a "ruffled skirt" appearance. An osteoclast secretes acid and enzymes to dissolve and digest a microscopic bit of bone matrix, and then absorbs the minerals and amino acids; this process is called **resorption**. Osteoclasts are very active in embryonic long bones, and they reabsorb bone matrix in the center of the diaphysis to form the **marrow canal**. Blood vessels grow into the marrow canals of embryonic long bones, and red bone marrow is established. After birth, the red bone marrow is replaced by yellow bone marrow. Red bone marrow remains in the spongy bone of short, flat, and irregular bones.

Bone tissue and bones as organs are never really "finished." Throughout life, bone matrix undergoes a process called **remodeling**. Calcium is removed by osteoclasts to raise the blood calcium level, or calcium salts are made and deposited by osteoblasts to lower the blood calcium level. These cells also respond to environmental factors such as the body's bearing extra weight. For the functions of osteoclasts and osteoblasts following bone injury, see Box 6–1: Fractures and Their Repair.

FACTORS THAT AFFECT BONE GROWTH AND MAINTENANCE

1. Heredity—each person has a genetic potential for height, that is, a maximum height, with genes inherited from both parents. Many genes are involved, and their interactions are not well understood. Some of these genes are probably those for the enzymes involved in cartilage and bone production because this is how bones grow.
2. Nutrition—nutrients are the raw materials of which bones are made. Calcium, phosphorus, and protein become part of the bone matrix itself. Vitamin D is needed for the efficient absorption of calcium and phosphorus by the small intestine. Vitamin D deficiency in children causes **rickets**; bones are soft and weight-bearing bones often bend. Vitamins A and C do not become part of bone but are necessary for the process of bone matrix formation (ossification or calcification). Without these and other nutrients, bones cannot grow properly. Children who are malnourished grow very slowly and may not reach their genetic potential for height.
3. Hormones—endocrine glands produce hormones that stimulate specific effects in certain cells. Several hormones make important contributions to bone growth and maintenance. These include growth hormone, thyroxine, parathyroid hormone, and insulin, which help regulate cell division, protein synthesis, calcium metabolism, and energy production. The sex hormones estrogen or testosterone help bring about the cessation of bone growth. The hormones and their specific functions are listed in Table 6–1.
4. Chemical communication from other tissues—as mentioned in Chapter 4, adipose tissue produces leptin that stimulates osteoblasts to produce bone matrix. The body's energy-storage tissue communicates with the body's weight-bearing tissue. Bone tissue communicates in return. Osteoblasts produce a protein called **osteocalcin**, which decreases fat storage by adipose tissue and increases insulin production by the pancreas. Both of these responses are believed to help the body maintain a normal weight.

   The small intestine also communicates with bone tissue. Cells in the small intestine produce serotonin

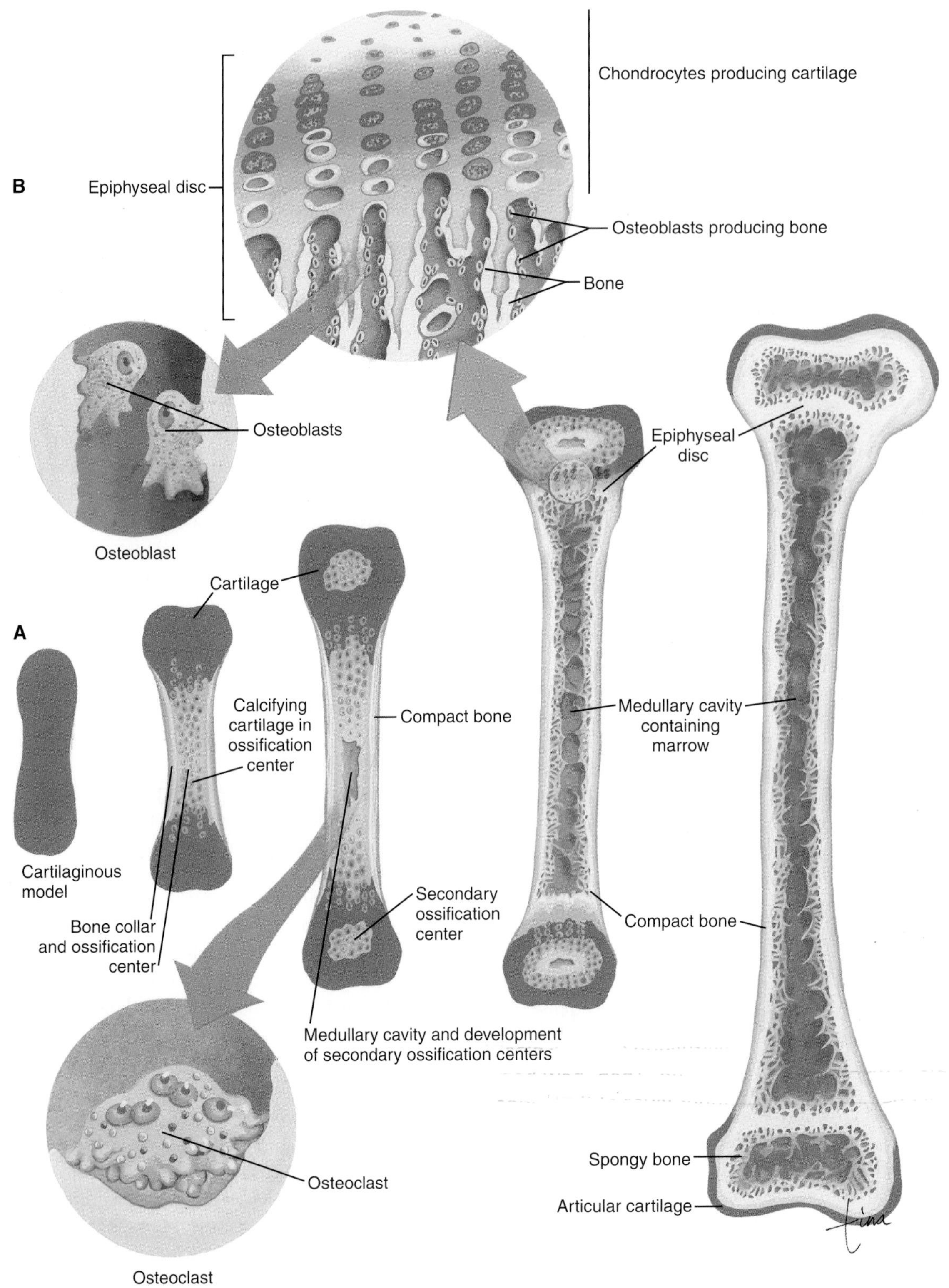

Figure 6–3 The ossification process in a long bone. (**A**) Progression of ossification from the cartilage model of the embryo to the bone of a young adult. (**B**) Microscopic view of an epiphyseal disc showing cartilage production and bone replacement.

QUESTION: The epiphyseal discs of the bone on the far right are closed. What does that mean?

Box 6–1 | FRACTURES AND THEIR REPAIR

A **fracture** means that a bone has been broken. There are different types of fractures classified as to extent of damage (Box Fig. 6–A):

Simple (closed)—the broken parts are still in normal anatomic position; surrounding tissue damage is minimal (skin is not pierced).

Compound (open)—the broken end of a bone has been moved, and it pierces the skin; there may be extensive damage to surrounding blood vessels, nerves, and muscles. The break in the skin permits the entry of bacteria, which may cause **osteomyelitis**, an infection of bone.

Greenstick—the bone splits longitudinally. The bones of children contain more collagen than do adult bones and tend to splinter rather than break completely.

Comminuted—two or more intersecting breaks create several bone fragments.

Impacted—the broken ends of a bone are forced into one another; many bone fragments may be created.

Pathologic (spontaneous)—a bone breaks without apparent trauma; may accompany bone disorders such as osteoporosis.

THE REPAIR PROCESS

Even a simple fracture involves significant bone damage that must be repaired if the bone is to resume its normal function. Fragments of dead or damaged bone must first be removed. This is accomplished by osteoclasts, which dissolve and reabsorb the calcium salts of bone matrix. Imagine a building that has just collapsed; the rubble must be removed before reconstruction can take place. This is what the osteoclasts do. Then, new bone must be produced. The inner layer of the periosteum contains osteoblasts that are activated when bone is damaged. The osteoblasts produce bone matrix to knit the broken ends of the bone together.

Because most bone has a good blood supply, the repair process is usually relatively rapid, and a simple fracture often heals within 6 weeks. Some parts of bones, however, have a poor blood supply, and repair of fractures takes longer. These areas are the neck of the femur (the site of a "fractured hip") and the lower third of the tibia.

Other factors that influence repair include the age of the person, general state of health, and nutrition. The elderly and those in poor health often have slow healing of fractures. A diet with sufficient calcium, phosphorus, vitamin D, and protein is also important. If any of these nutrients is lacking, bone repair will be a slower process.

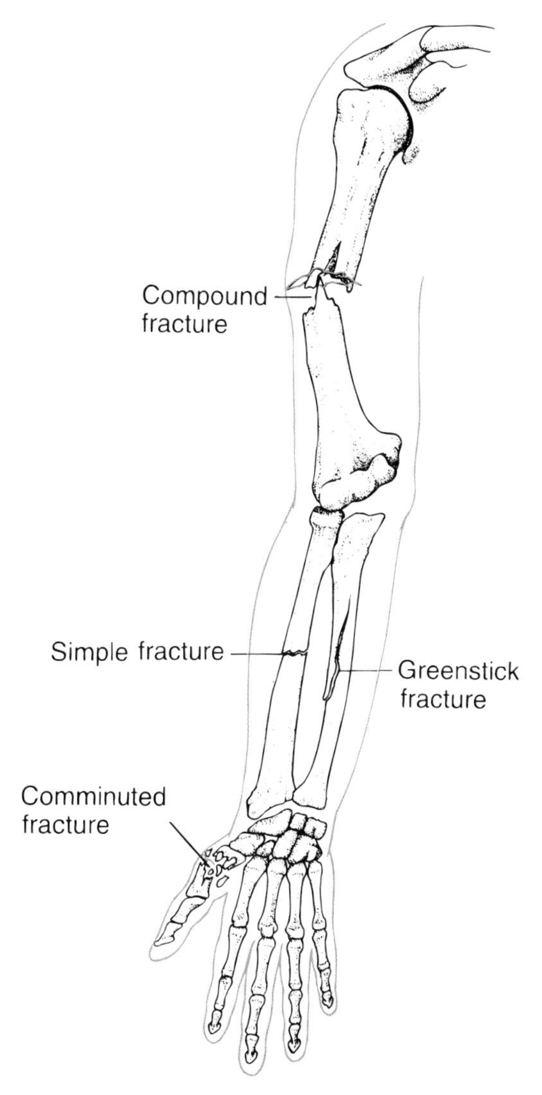

Box Figure 6–A Types of fractures. Several types of fractures are depicted in the right arm.

Table 6–1 | HORMONES INVOLVED IN BONE GROWTH AND MAINTENANCE

HORMONE (GLAND)	FUNCTIONS
Growth hormone (anterior pituitary gland)	■ Increases the rate of mitosis of chondrocytes and osteoblasts ■ Increases the rate of protein synthesis (collagen, cartilage matrix, and enzymes for cartilage and bone formation)
Thyroxine (thyroid gland)	■ Increases the rate of protein synthesis ■ Increases energy production from all food types
Insulin (pancreas)	■ Increases energy production from glucose
Parathyroid hormone (parathyroid glands)	■ Increases the reabsorption of calcium from bones to the blood (raises blood calcium level) ■ Increases the absorption of calcium by the small intestine and kidneys (to the blood)
Calcitonin (thyroid gland)	■ Decreases the reabsorption of calcium from bones (lowers blood calcium level)
Estrogen (ovaries) or testosterone (testes)	■ Promotes closure of the epiphyses of long bones (growth stops) ■ Helps retain calcium in bones to maintain a strong bone matrix

(gut serotonin); you may have heard of serotonin as a CNS neurotransmitter that affects mood (brain serotonin). Gut serotonin is much more abundant than brain serotonin, but gut serotonin does not affect the brain. It does, however, inhibit osteoblasts from producing bone matrix, the opposite of the effect of leptin. We have much more to learn, but for now we can say that bone tissue is also influenced by the organ most responsible for absorption of nutrients, the small intestine.

5. Exercise or "stress"—for bones, exercise means bearing weight, which is just what bones are specialized to do. Without this stress (which is normal and necessary), bones will lose calcium faster than it is replaced. Exercise need not be strenuous; it can be as simple as the walking involved in everyday activities. Strenuous exercise that includes bearing more than the body's own weight will remodel bones; they will become thicker and stronger as more matrix is deposited (given sufficient calcium and phosphorus in the diet). Bones that do not get even minimal exercise, such as those of patients confined to bed, will be remodeled as well, but they will lose matrix and become thinner and more fragile. This condition is discussed further in Box 6–2: Osteoporosis.

THE SKELETON

The human skeleton has two divisions: the **axial skeleton**, which forms the axis of the body, and the **appendicular skeleton**, which supports the appendages or limbs. The axial skeleton consists of the skull, vertebral column, and rib cage. The bones of the arms and legs and the shoulder and pelvic girdles make up the appendicular skeleton. Many bones are connected to other bones across joints by ligaments, which are strong cords or sheets of fibrous connective tissue. The importance of ligaments becomes readily apparent when a joint is sprained. A sprain is the stretching or even tearing of the ligaments of a joint, and though the bones are not broken, the joint is weak and unsteady. We do not often think of our ligaments, but they are necessary to keep our bones in the proper positions to keep us upright or to bear weight.

The body has 206 bones in total. The complete skeleton is shown in Fig. 6–4.

SKULL

The **skull** consists of 8 cranial bones and 14 facial bones. Also in the head are three small bones in each middle ear cavity and the hyoid bone that supports the base of the tongue. The **cranial bones** form the braincase (lined with

Box 6–2 | OSTEOPOROSIS

Bone is an active tissue; calcium is constantly being removed to maintain normal blood calcium levels. Usually, however, calcium is replaced in bones at a rate equal to its removal, and the bone matrix remains strong.

Osteoporosis is characterized by excessive loss of calcium from bones without sufficient replacement (Box Fig. 6–B). Research has suggested that a certain gene for bone buildup in youth is an important factor; less buildup would mean earlier bone thinning. Contributing environmental factors include smoking, insufficient dietary intake of calcium, inactivity, and lack of the sex hormones. Osteoporosis is most common among elderly women because estrogen secretion decreases sharply at menopause (in older men, testosterone is still secreted in significant amounts). Factors such as bed rest or inability to get even minimal exercise will make calcium loss even more rapid.

As bones lose calcium and become thin and brittle, fractures are much more likely to occur. Among elderly women, a fractured hip (the neck of the femur) may be a consequence of this degenerative bone disorder. Such a serious injury is not inevitable, however, and neither is the thinning of the vertebrae that bows the spines of some elderly people. After menopause, women may wish to have a bone density test to determine the strength of their bone matrix. Several medications are available that diminish the rate of bone loss, and some claim to increase matrix production. A diet high in calcium and vitamin D is essential for both men and women, as is moderate exercise. Young women and teenagers should make sure they get adequate dietary calcium to form strong bone matrix because this will delay the serious effects of osteoporosis later in life.

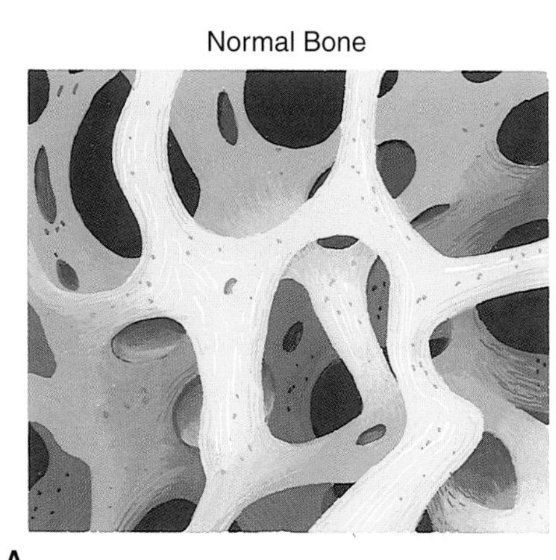

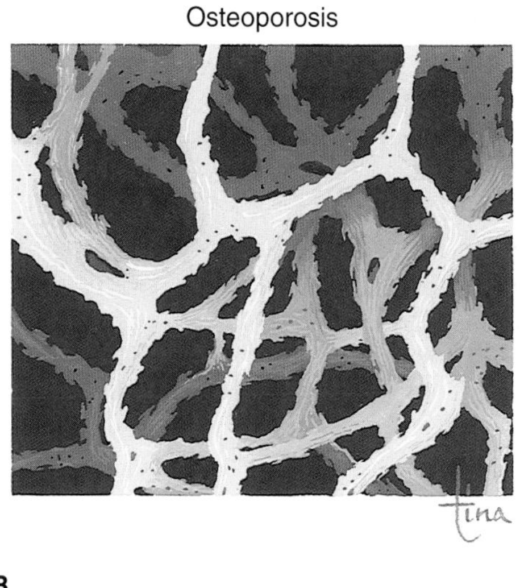

Box Figure 6–B (A) Normal spongy bone, as in the body of a vertebra. (**B**) Spongy bone thinned by osteoporosis.

the meninges) that encloses and protects the brain, eyes, and ears. The names of some of these bones will be familiar to you; they are the same as the terminology used (see Chapter 1) to describe areas of the head. These are the frontal bone, parietal bones (two), temporal bones (two), and occipital bone. The sphenoid bone and ethmoid bone are part of the floor of the braincase and the orbits (sockets) for the eyes. The **frontal bone** forms the forehead and the anterior part of the top of the skull. *Parietal* means "wall," and the two large **parietal bones** form the posterior top and

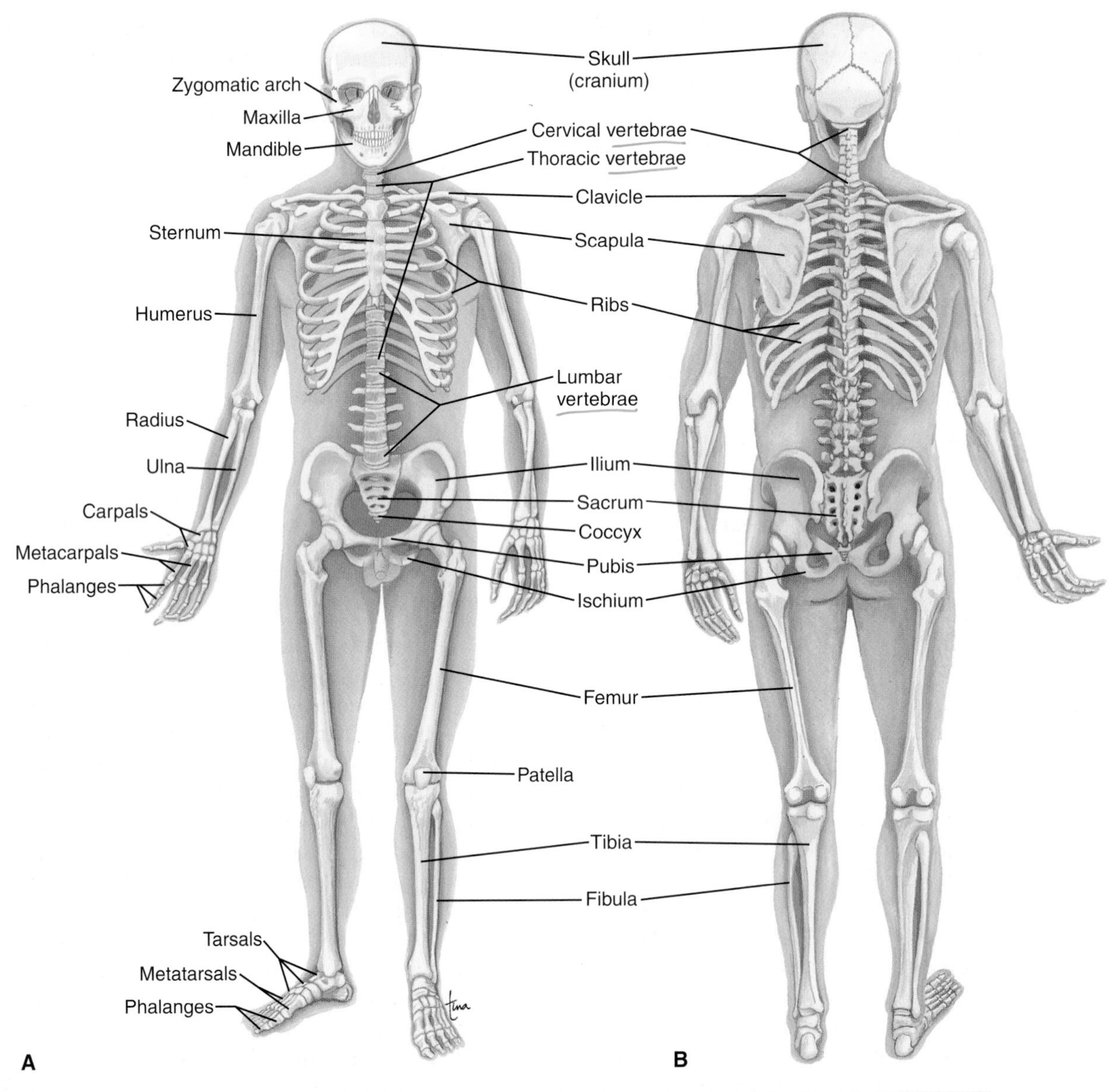

Figure 6–4 Skeleton. (**A**) Anterior view. (**B**) Posterior view.

QUESTION: Which of the bones shown here are classified as irregular bones?

much of the side walls of the skull. Each **temporal bone** on the side of the skull contains an external auditory meatus (ear canal), a middle ear cavity, and an inner ear labyrinth. The **occipital bone** forms the lower, posterior part of the braincase. Its foramen magnum is a large opening for the spinal cord, and the two condyles (rounded projections) on either side articulate with the atlas, the first cervical vertebra. The **sphenoid bone** is said to be shaped like a bat, and the greater wing is visible on the side of the skull between the frontal and temporal bones. The body of the bat has a depression called the sella turcica, which encloses the pituitary gland. The **ethmoid bone** has a vertical projection called the crista galli ("rooster's comb") that anchors the cranial meninges. The rest of the ethmoid bone forms the roof and upper walls of the nasal cavities, and its perpendicular plate forms the upper part of the nasal septum.

All of the joints between cranial bones are immovable joints called **sutures**. It may seem strange to refer to a joint without movement, but the term *joint* (or **articulation**) is used for any junction of two bones. (The classification of joints will be covered later in this chapter.) In a suture, the serrated, or sawtooth, edges of adjacent bones fit into each other. These interlocking projections prevent sliding or shifting of the bones if the skull is subjected to a blow or pressure. In Fig. 6–5 you can see the coronal suture between the frontal and parietal bones, the squamosal suture between the parietal and temporal bones, and the lambdoidal suture between the occipital and parietal bones. Not visible is the sagittal suture, where the two parietal bones articulate along the midline of the top of the skull. All the bones of the skull, as well as the large sutures, are shown in Figs. 6–5 through 6–8. Their anatomically important parts are described in Table 6–2.

Of the 14 **facial bones**, only the **mandible** (lower jaw) is movable; it forms a **condyloid joint** with each temporal bone. The other joints between facial bones are all sutures. The **maxillae** are the two upper jawbones, which also form the anterior portion of the hard palate (roof of the mouth). Sockets for the roots of the teeth are found in the maxillae and the mandible. The two **nasal bones** form the bridge of the nose where they articulate with the frontal bone (the rest of the nose is supported by cartilage). There is a **lacrimal bone** at the medial side of each orbit; the lacrimal canal contains the lacrimal sac, a passageway for tears. Each of the two **zygomatic bones** forms the point of a cheek and articulates with the maxilla, frontal bone, and temporal bone. The two **palatine bones** are the posterior portion of the hard palate. The plow-shaped **vomer** forms the lower part of the nasal septum; it articulates with the perpendicular plate of the ethmoid bone. On either side of the vomer are the **conchae**, six scroll-like bones that curl downward from the sides of the nasal cavities; they help increase the surface area of the nasal mucosa. These facial bones are included in Table 6–2.

Paranasal sinuses are air cavities located in the maxillae and frontal, sphenoid, and ethmoid bones (Fig. 6–9). As the name *paranasal* suggests, they open into the nasal cavities and are lined with **ciliated epithelium** continuous with the mucosa of the nasal cavities. We are aware of our sinuses only when they become “stuffed up,” which means that the mucus they produce cannot drain into the nasal cavities. This may happen during upper respiratory infections such as colds, or with allergies such as hay fever. These sinuses, however, do have functions: They make the skull lighter in weight because air is lighter than bone, and they provide resonance for the voice, meaning more air to vibrate and thus deepen the pitch of the voice.

The **mastoid sinuses** are air cavities in the mastoid process of each temporal bone; they open into the middle ear. Before the availability of antibiotics, middle ear infections often caused mastoiditis, infection of these sinuses.

Within each middle ear cavity are three **auditory bones**: the malleus, incus, and stapes. As part of the hearing process (discussed in Chapter 9), these bones transmit vibrations from the eardrum to the receptors in the inner ear (see Fig. 9–9 in Chapter 9).

VERTEBRAL COLUMN

The **vertebral column** (spinal column or backbone) is made of individual bones called **vertebrae**. The names of vertebrae indicate their location along the length of the spinal column. There are 7 cervical vertebrae, 12 thoracic, 5 lumbar, 5 sacral fused into 1 sacrum, and 4 to 5 small coccygeal vertebrae fused into 1 coccyx (Fig. 6–10).

The seven **cervical vertebrae** are those within the neck. The first vertebra is called the **atlas**, which articulates with the occipital bone to support the skull and forms a **pivot joint** with the odontoid process of the **axis**, the second cervical vertebra. This pivot joint allows us to turn our heads from side to side. The remaining five cervical vertebrae do not have individual names.

The **thoracic vertebrae** articulate (form joints) with the ribs on the posterior side of the trunk. The **lumbar vertebrae**, the largest and strongest bones of the spine, are found in the small of the back. The **sacrum** permits the articulation of the two hipbones: the **sacroiliac joints**. The **coccyx** is the remnant of tail vertebrae, and some muscles of the perineum (pelvic floor) are anchored to it.

All of the vertebrae articulate with one another in sequence, connected by ligaments, to form a flexible backbone that supports the trunk and head. They also form the **vertebral canal**, a continuous tunnel (lined with the meninges) that contains the spinal cord and protects it from mechanical injury. The spinous and transverse processes are projections for the attachment of the muscles that bend the vertebral column. The facets of some vertebrae are small flat surfaces for articulation with other bones, such as the ribs with the facets of the thoracic vertebrae.

The supporting part of a vertebra is its body; the bodies of adjacent vertebrae are separated by **discs** of fibrous cartilage. These discs cushion and absorb shock and permit some movement between vertebrae (**symphysis joints**).

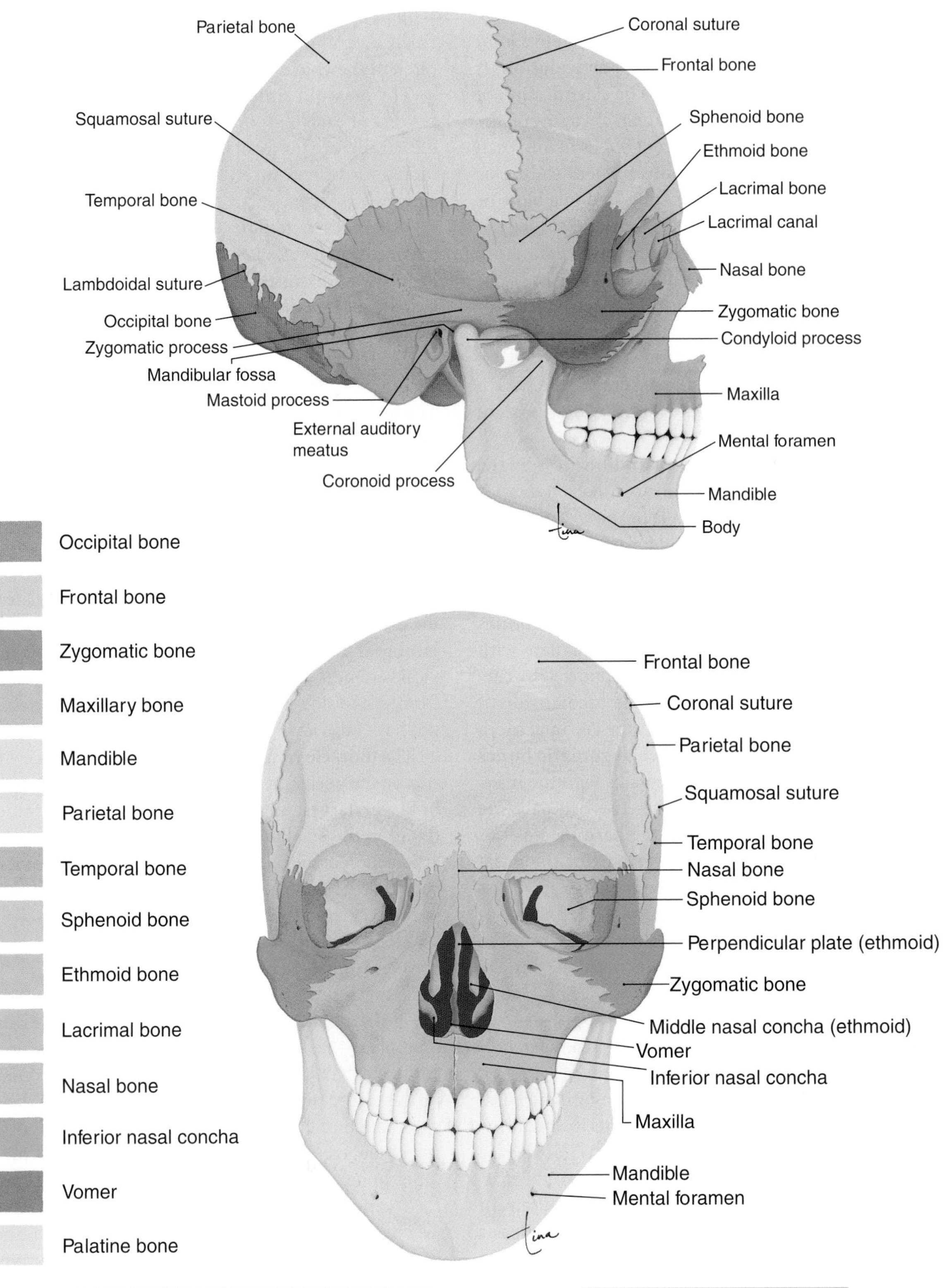

Figure 6–5 Skull. Lateral view of right side.

Figure 6–6 Skull. Anterior view.

QUESTION: What might be the purpose of the openings at the back of the eye sockets?

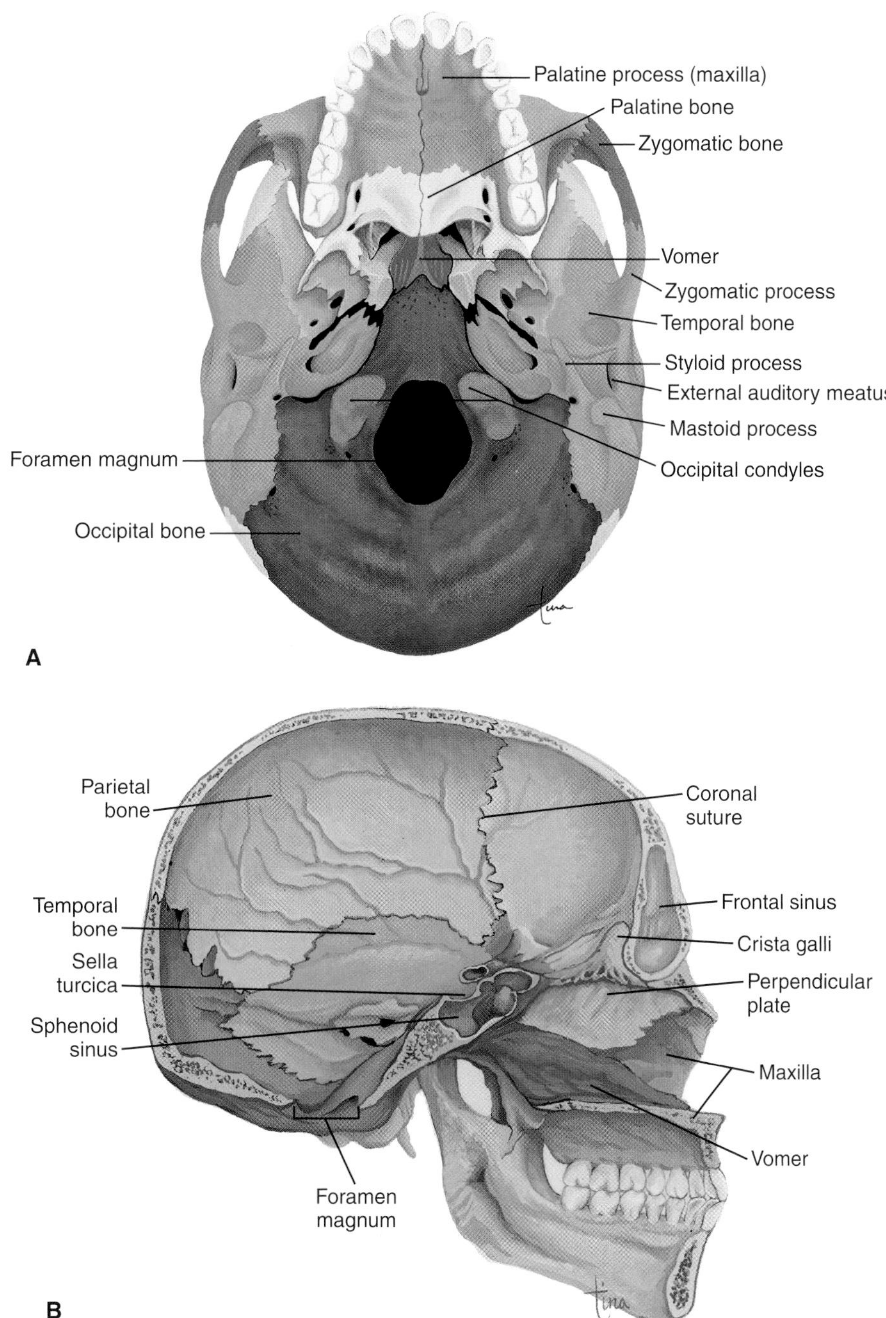

Figure 6–7 Skull. (**A**) Inferior view with mandible removed. (**B**) Midsagittal section showing interior of left side.

QUESTION: What is the purpose of the foramen magnum?

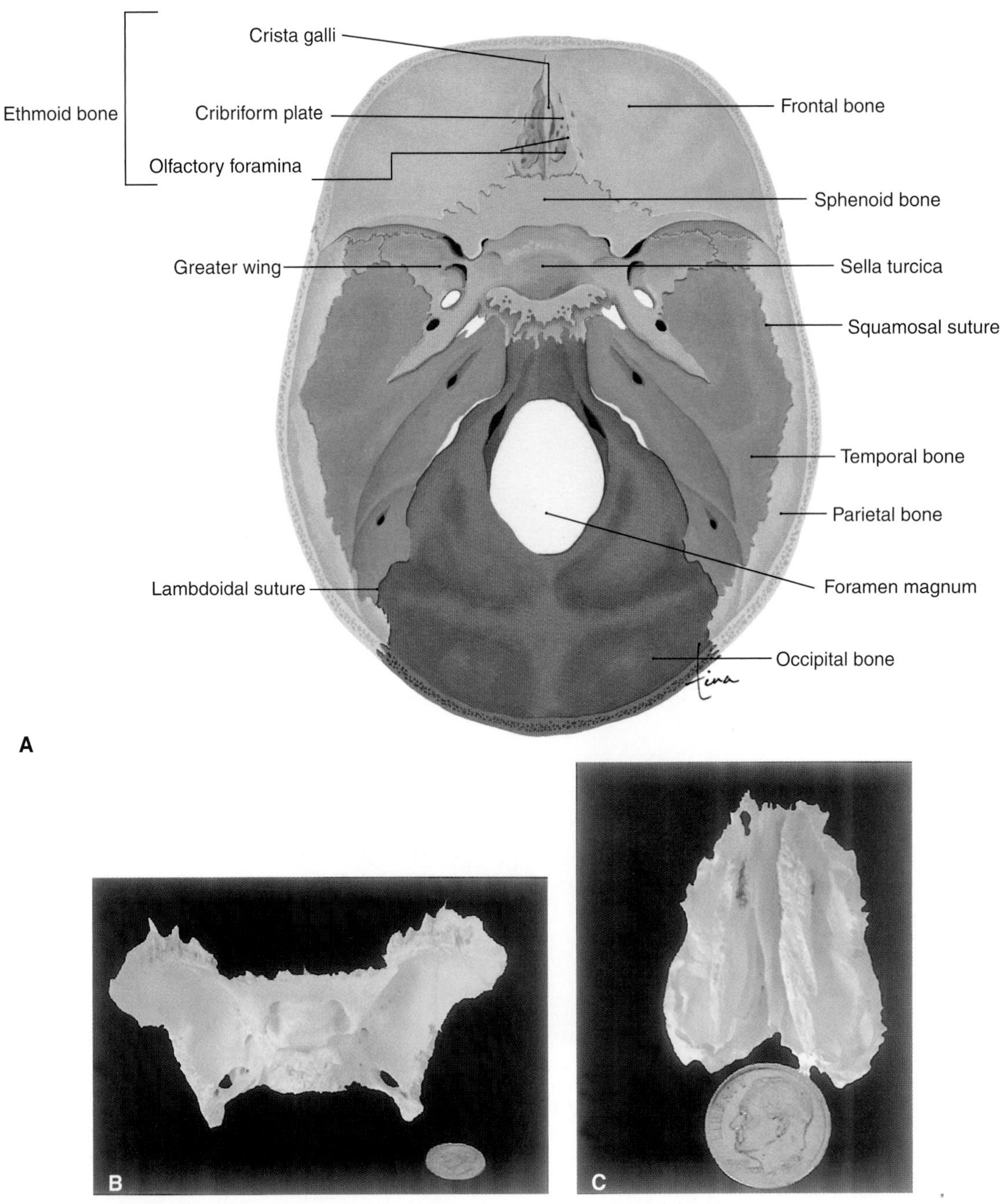

Figure 6–8 (**A**) Skull. Superior view with the top of cranium removed. (**B**) Sphenoid bone in superior view. (**C**) Ethmoid bone in superior view. (B and C photographs by Dan Kaufman.)

QUESTION: What are the olfactory foramina of the ethmoid bone for?

Table 6–2 | **BONES OF THE SKULL—IMPORTANT PARTS**

TERMINOLOGY OF BONE MARKINGS		
Foramen—a hole or opening	Meatus—a tunnel-like cavity	Condyle—a rounded projection
Fossa—a depression	Process—a projection	Plate—a flat projection
Crest—a ridge or edge	Facet—a flat projection	Tubercle—a round projection

BONE	PART	DESCRIPTION
Frontal	Frontal sinus Coronal suture	■ Air cavity that opens into nasal cavity ■ Joint between frontal and parietal bones
Parietal (2)	Sagittal suture	■ Joint between the 2 parietal bones
Temporal (2)	Squamosal suture External auditory meatus Mastoid process Mastoid sinus Mandibular fossa Zygomatic process	■ Joint between temporal and parietal bone ■ The tunnel-like ear canal ■ Oval projection behind the ear canal ■ Air cavity that opens into middle ear ■ Oval depression anterior to the ear canal; articulates with mandible ■ Anterior projection that articulates with the zygomatic bone
Occipital	Foramen magnum Condyles Lambdoidal suture	■ Large opening for the spinal cord ■ Oval projections on either side of the foramen magnum; articulate with the atlas ■ Joint between occipital and parietal bones
Sphenoid	Greater wing Sella turcica Sphenoid sinus	■ Flat, lateral portion between the frontal and temporal bones ■ Central depression that encloses the pituitary gland ■ Air cavity that opens into the nasal cavity
Ethmoid	Ethmoid sinus Crista galli Cribriform plate and olfactory foramina Perpendicular plate Conchae (4 are part of ethmoid; 2 inferior are separate bones)	■ Air cavity that opens into nasal cavity ■ Superior projection for attachment of meninges ■ On either side of base of crista galli; olfactory nerves pass through foramina ■ Upper part of nasal septum ■ Shelf-like projections into nasal cavities that increase surface area of nasal mucosa
Mandible	Body Condyles Sockets	■ U-shaped portion with lower teeth ■ Oval projections that articulate with the temporal bones ■ Conical depressions that hold roots of lower teeth

Continued

Table 6–2 | **BONES OF THE SKULL—IMPORTANT PARTS—cont'd**

BONE	PART	DESCRIPTION
Maxilla (2)	Maxillary sinus Palatine process Sockets	■ Air cavity that opens into nasal cavity ■ Projection that forms anterior part of hard palate ■ Conical depressions that hold roots of upper teeth
Nasal (2)	—	■ Form the bridge of the nose
Lacrimal (2)	Lacrimal canal	■ Opening for nasolacrimal duct to take tears to nasal cavity
Zygomatic (2)	—	■ Form point of cheek; articulate with frontal, temporal, and maxillae
Palatine (2)	—	■ Form the posterior part of hard palate
Vomer	—	■ Lower part of nasal septum

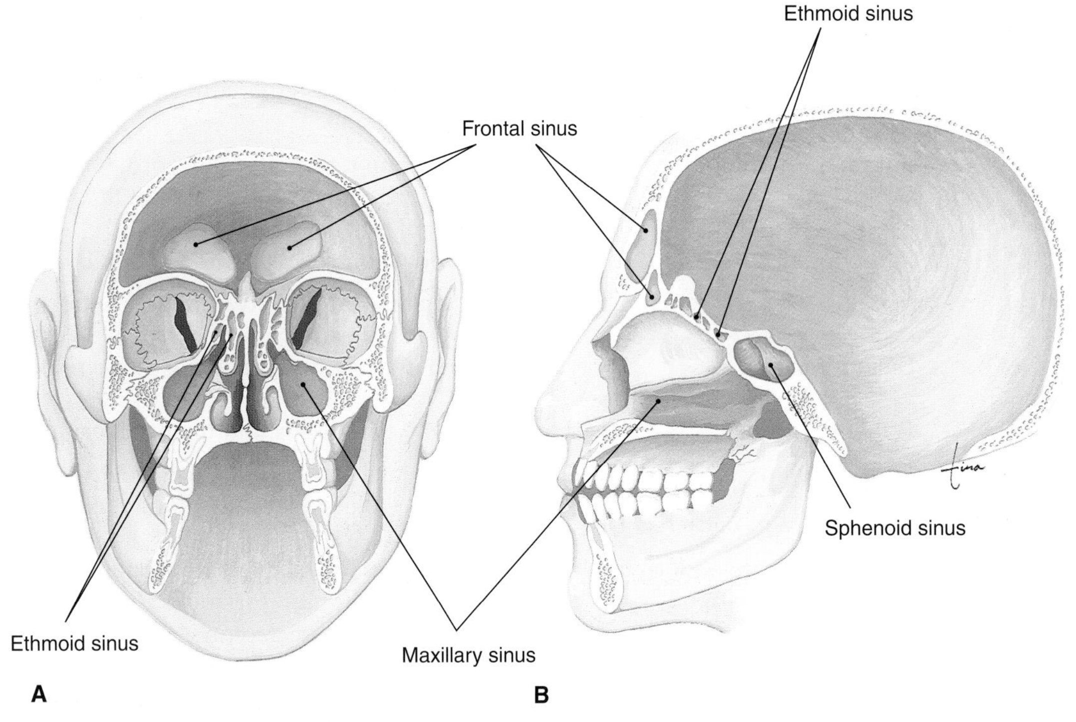

Figure 6–9 Paranasal sinuses. (**A**) Anterior view of the skull. (**B**) Left lateral view of skull.

QUESTION: Which of these sinuses often cause the pain of a sinus headache?

Because there are so many joints, the backbone as a whole is quite flexible (see also Box 6–3: Herniated Disc).

The normal spine in anatomic position has four natural curves, which are named after the vertebrae that form them. Refer to Fig. 6–10, and notice that the cervical curve is forward, the thoracic curve backward, the lumbar curve forward, and the sacral curve backward. These curves center the skull over the rest of the body, which enables a person to more easily walk upright (see Box 6–4: Abnormalities of the Curves of the Spine).

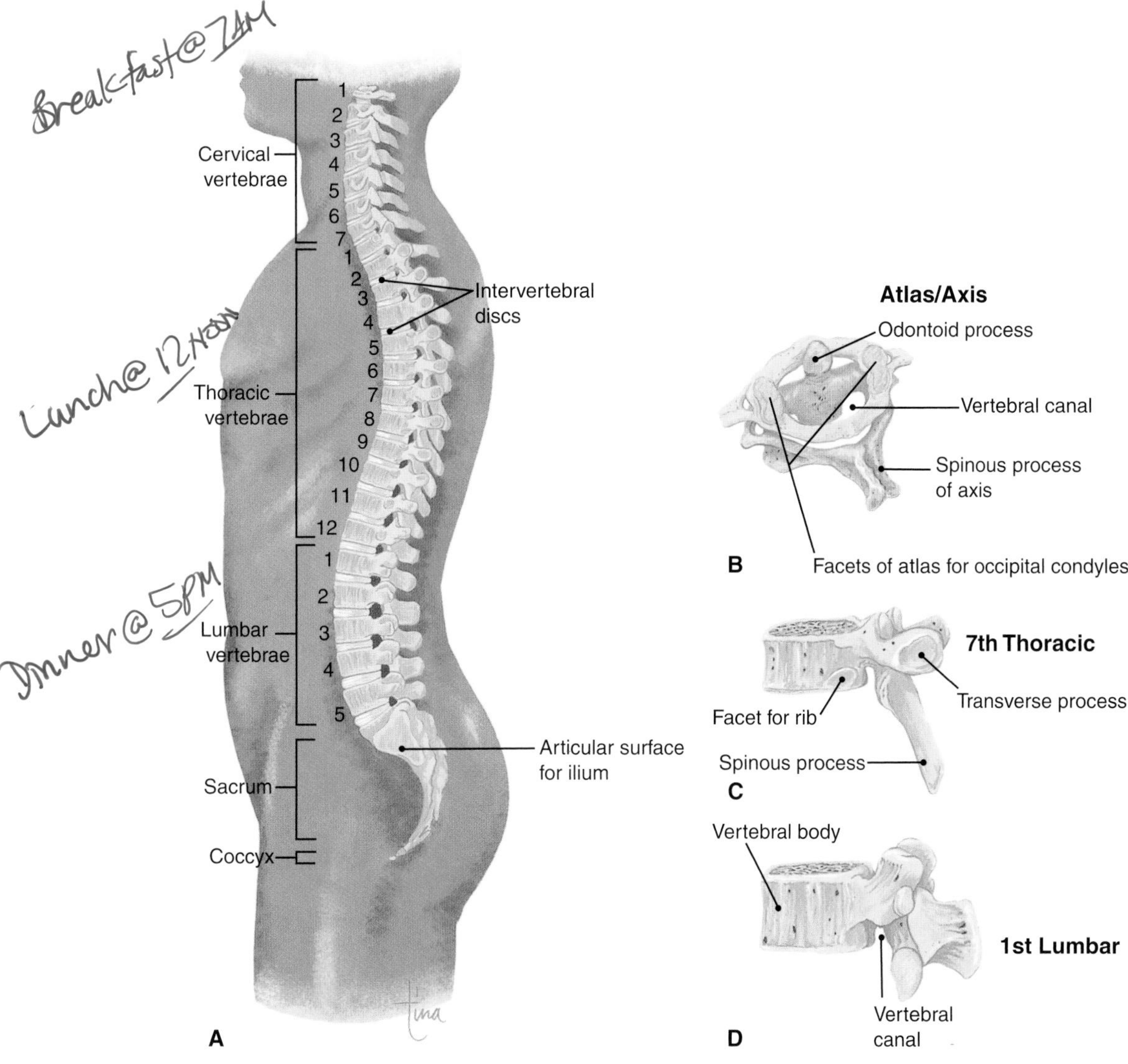

Figure 6–10 Vertebral column. (**A**) Lateral view of left side. (**B**) Atlas and axis, superior view. (**C**) 7th thoracic vertebra, left lateral view. (**D**) 1st lumbar vertebra, left lateral view.

QUESTION: Compare the size of the individual thoracic and lumbar vertebrae. What is the reason for this difference?

RIB CAGE

The **rib cage** consists of the 12 pairs of ribs and the sternum, or breastbone. The three parts of the sternum are the upper **manubrium**, the central **body**, and the lower **xiphoid process** (Fig. 6–11). Notice in Fig. 6–4 that the manubrium articulates with the clavicles.

All of the **ribs** articulate posteriorly with the thoracic vertebrae. The first seven pairs of ribs are called **true ribs**; they articulate directly with the manubrium and body of the sternum by means of costal cartilages. The next three pairs are called **false ribs**; their cartilages join the 7th rib cartilage. The last two pairs are called **floating ribs** because they do not articulate with the sternum at all (see Fig. 6–11).

An obvious function of the rib cage is that it encloses and protects the heart and lungs. Keep in mind, though, that the rib cage also protects organs in the upper abdominal cavity, such as the liver and spleen. The other important function of the rib cage depends on its flexibility: The ribs are pulled upward and outward by the external intercostal muscles. This enlarges the chest cavity, which expands the lungs and contributes to inhalation.

Box 6–3 | HERNIATED DISC

The vertebrae are separated by discs of fibrous cartilage that act as cushions to absorb shock. An intervertebral disc has a tough outer covering and a soft center called the nucleus pulposus. Extreme pressure on a disc may rupture the outer layer and force the nucleus pulposus out. This may occur when a person lifts a heavy object improperly, that is, using the back rather than the legs and jerking upward, which puts sudden, intense pressure on the spine. Most often this affects discs in the lumbar region.

Although often called a "slipped disc," the affected disc is usually not moved out of position. The terms **herniated disc** or **ruptured disc** more accurately describe what happens. The nucleus pulposus is forced out, often posteriorly, where it puts pressure on a spinal nerve (Box Fig. 6–C). For this reason a herniated disc may be very painful or impair function in the muscles supplied by the nerve.

Healing of a herniated disc may occur naturally if the damage is not severe and the person rests and avoids activities that would further compress the disc. Surgery may be required, however, to remove the portion of the nucleus pulposus that is out of place and disrupting nerve functioning.

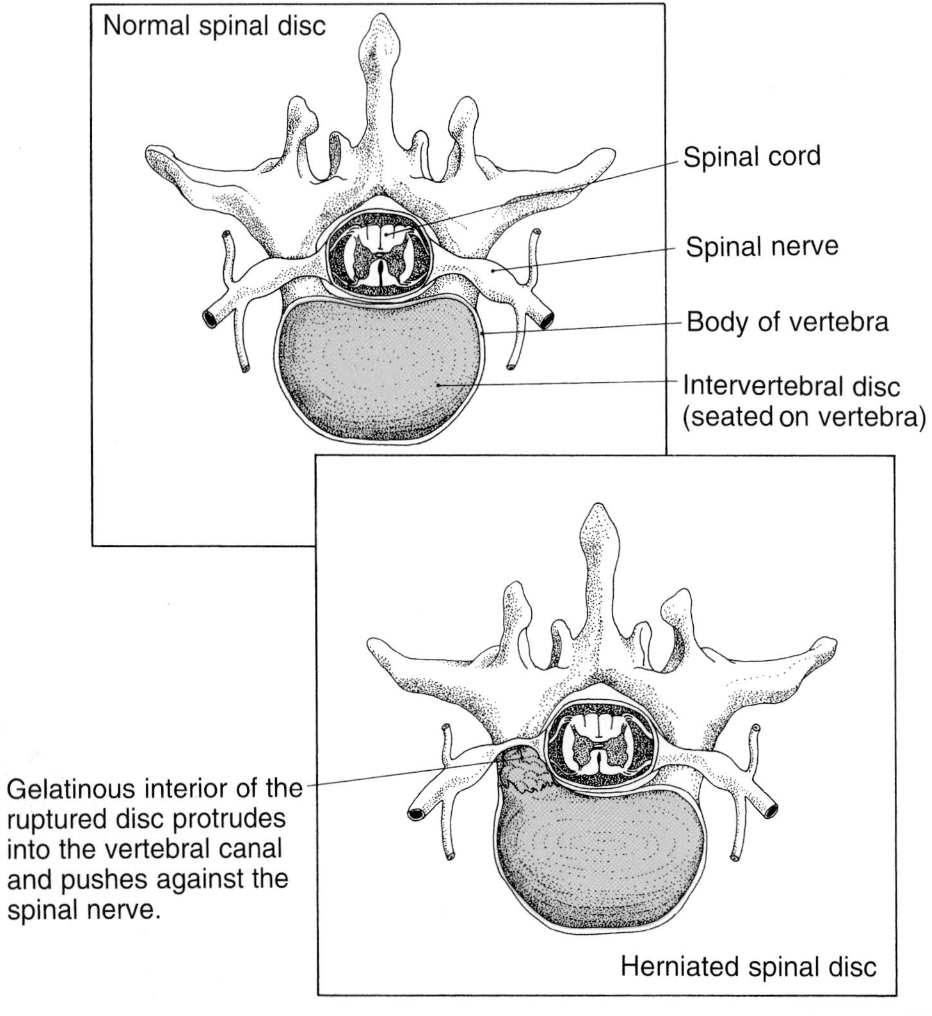

Box Figure 6–C Herniated disc. As a result of compression, a ruptured intervertebral disc puts pressure on a spinal nerve.

Box 6–4 | ABNORMALITIES OF THE CURVES OF THE SPINE

Scoliosis—an abnormal lateral curvature, which may be congenital, the result of having one leg longer than the other, or the result of chronic poor posture during childhood while the vertebrae are still growing. Usually the thoracic vertebrae are affected, which displaces the rib cage to one side. In severe cases, the abdominal organs may be compressed, and the expansion of the rib cage during inhalation may be impaired.

Kyphosis*—an exaggerated thoracic curve; sometimes referred to as hunchback.

Lordosis*—an exaggerated lumbar curve; sometimes referred to as swayback.

These abnormal curves are usually the result of degenerative bone diseases such as osteoporosis or tuberculosis of the spine. If osteoporosis, for example, causes the bodies of the thoracic vertebrae to collapse, the normal thoracic curve will be increased. Most often the vertebral body "settles" slowly (rather than collapses suddenly) and there is little, if any, damage to the spinal nerves. The damage to the vertebrae, however, cannot be easily corrected, so these conditions should be thought of in terms of prevention rather than cure.

*Although descriptive of normal anatomy, the terms *kyphosis* and *lordosis*, respectively, are commonly used to describe the abnormal condition associated with each.

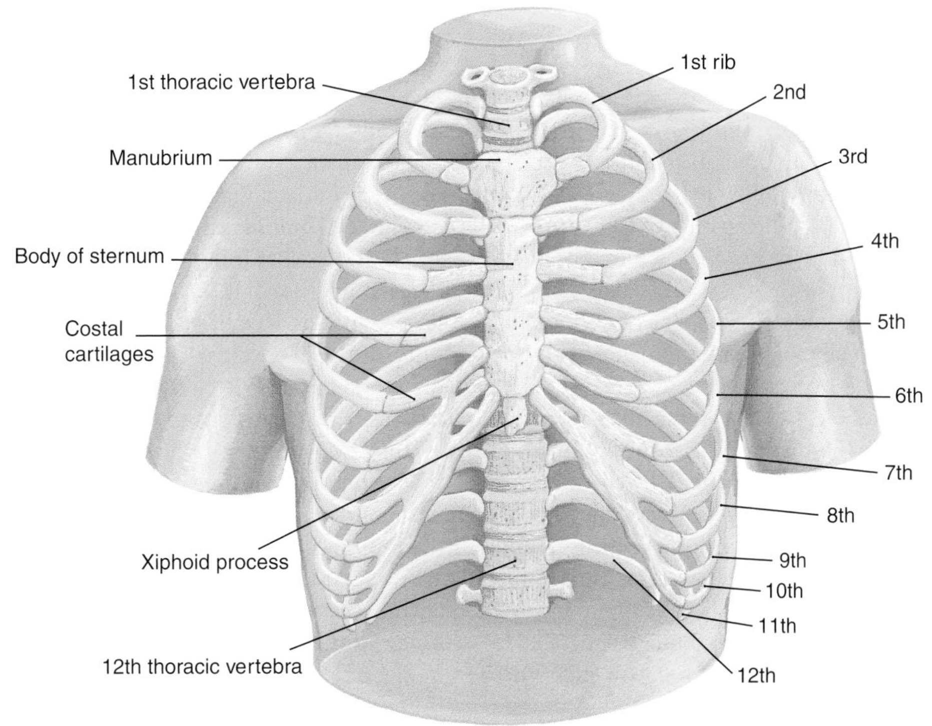

Figure 6–11 Rib cage. Anterior view.

QUESTION: With what bones do all of the ribs articulate?

THE SHOULDER AND ARM

The shoulder girdles attach the arms to the axial skeleton. Each consists of a scapula (shoulder blade) and clavicle (collarbone). The **scapula** is a large, flat bone with several projections (the spine of the scapula, the coracoid process) that anchor some of the muscles that move the upper arm and the forearm. A shallow depression called the glenoid fossa forms a **ball-and-socket joint** with the humerus, the bone of the upper arm (Fig. 6–12). If you look at the posterior view of the skeleton in Fig. 6–4, you will see that the scapulae do not articulate with the backbone, but seem to be resting on the rib cage. Each scapula is held in place on the rib cage by many muscles that are anchored to the backbone and to the humerus.

The medial end of each **clavicle** articulates with the manubrium of the sternum. At the base of your neck, you can feel the space between the two clavicles; this is the interclavicular notch, also called the suprasternal notch. The lateral end of each clavicle articulates with the scapula on its own side. In their position between the scapulae and the sternum, the clavicles act as braces for the scapulae and prevent the shoulders from coming too far forward. Although the shoulder joint is capable of a wide range of movement, the shoulder itself must be relatively stable if these movements are to be effective.

The **humerus** is the long bone of the upper arm. In Fig. 6–12, notice the deltoid tubercle (or tuberosity); the triangular deltoid muscle that caps the shoulder joint is anchored here. Proximally, the head of the humerus forms a ball-and-socket joint with the scapula. Distally, the humerus forms a **hinge joint** with the ulna of the forearm. This hinge joint, the elbow, permits movement in one plane, that is, back and forth with no lateral movement.

The forearm bones are the **ulna** on the little finger side and the **radius** on the thumb side. The semilunar notch of the ulna is part of the hinge joint of the elbow; it articulates with the trochlea of the humerus. The radius and ulna articulate proximally to form a **pivot joint**, which permits turning the hand palm up to palm down. You can demonstrate this yourself by holding your arm palm up in front of you, and noting that the radius and ulna are parallel to each other. Then turn your hand palm down, and notice that your upper arm does not move. The radius crosses over the ulna, which permits the hand to perform a great variety of movements without moving the entire arm.

The **carpals** are eight small bones in the wrist; **gliding joints** between them permit a sliding movement. The carpals also articulate with the distal ends of the ulna and radius, and with the proximal ends of the **metacarpals**, the five bones of the palm of the hand. All of the joints formed by the carpals and metacarpals make the hand very flexible at the wrist (try this yourself: flexion to extension should be almost 180 degrees), but the thumb is more movable than the fingers because of its carpometacarpal joint. This is a **saddle joint**, which enables the thumb to cross over the palm, and permits gripping.

The **phalanges** are the bones of the fingers. There are two phalanges in each thumb and three in each of the fingers. Between phalanges are **hinge joints**, which permit movement in one plane. Important parts of the shoulder and arm bones are described in Table 6–3.

THE HIP AND LEG

The pelvic girdle (or pelvic bone) consists of the two **hipbones** (coxae or innominate bones), which articulate with the axial skeleton at the sacrum. Each hipbone has three major parts: the ilium, ischium, and pubis, and these are shown in Fig. 6–13, which depicts both a male and a female pelvis. The **ilium** is the flared, upper portion that forms the sacroiliac joint. The **ischium** is the lower, posterior part that we sit on. The **pubis** is the lower, most anterior part. The two pubic bones articulate with one another at the **pubic symphysis**, with a disc of fibrous cartilage between them. Notice the pubic angle of both the male and female pelvises in Fig. 6–13. The wider female angle is an adaptation for childbirth, in that it helps make the pelvic outlet larger.

The **acetabulum** is the socket in the hipbone that forms a **ball-and-socket joint** with the femur. Compared with the glenoid fossa of the scapula, the acetabulum is a much deeper socket. This has great functional importance because the hip is a weight-bearing joint, whereas the shoulder is not. Because the acetabulum is deep, the hip joint is not easily dislocated, even by activities such as running and jumping (landing), which put great stress on the joint.

The **femur** is the long bone of the thigh. As mentioned, the femur forms a very movable ball-and-socket joint with the hipbone. At the proximal end of the femur are the greater and lesser trochanters, large projections that are anchors for muscles. At its distal end, the femur forms a **hinge joint**, the knee, with the tibia of the lower leg. Notice in Fig. 6–14 that each bone has condyles, which are the rounded projections that actually form the joint. The **patella**, or kneecap, is anterior to the knee joint, enclosed in the tendon of the quadriceps femoris, a large muscle group of the anterior thigh.

The **tibia** is the weight-bearing bone of the lower leg. You can feel the tibial tuberosity (a bump) and anterior crest (a ridge) on the front of your own leg. The medial malleolus, what we may call the "inner ankle bone," is at

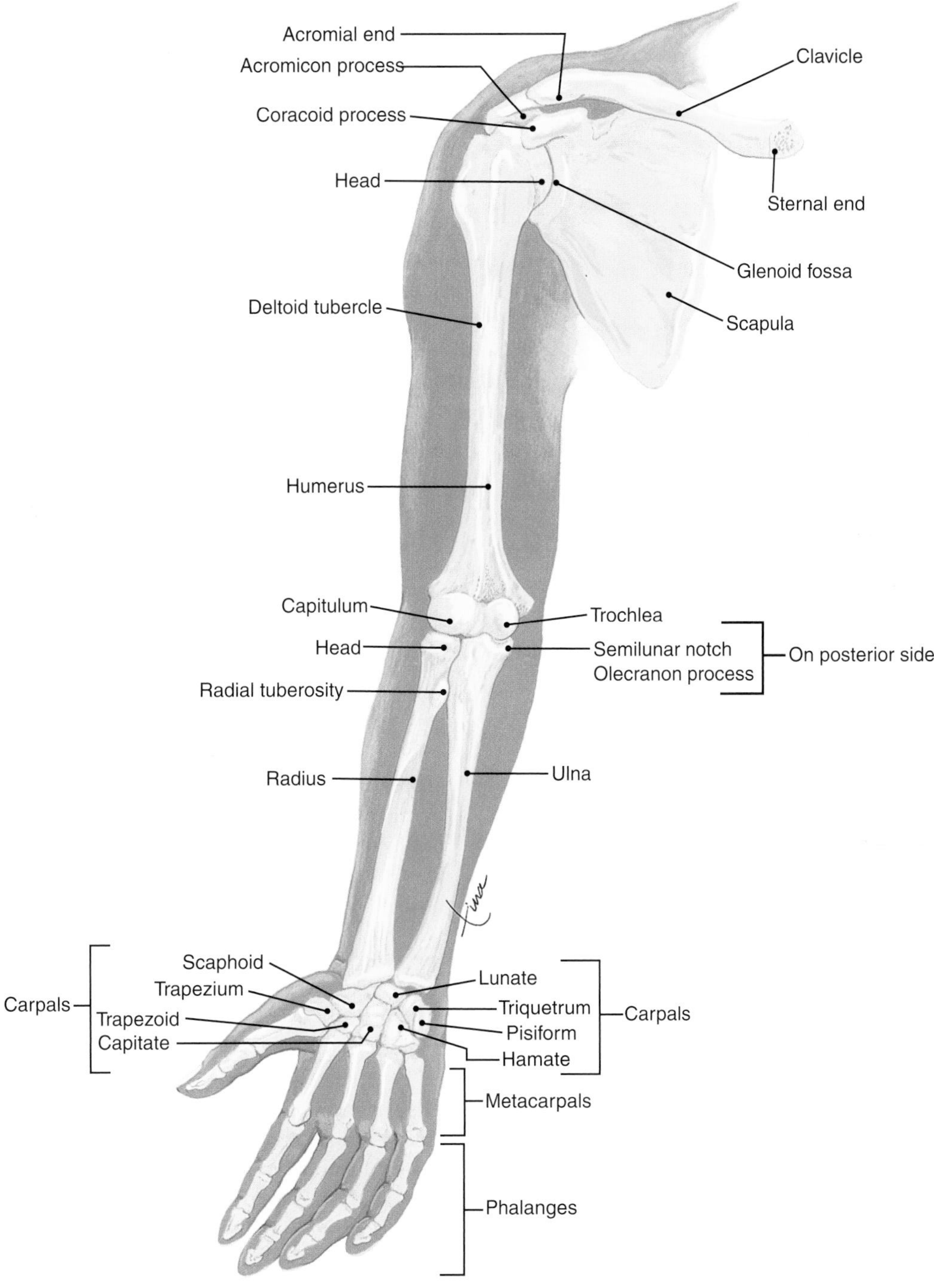

Figure 6–12 Bones of arm and shoulder girdle. Anterior view of right arm.

QUESTION: What types of joints are found in the arm? Begin at the shoulder and work downward.

Table 6–3 | BONES OF THE SHOULDER AND ARM—IMPORTANT PARTS

BONE	PART	DESCRIPTION
Scapula	Glenoid fossa	■ Depression that articulates with humerus
	Spine	■ Long, posterior process for muscle attachment
	Acromion process	■ Articulates with clavicle
Clavicle	Acromial end	■ Articulates with scapula
	Sternal end	■ Articulates with manubrium of sternum
Humerus	Head	■ Round process that articulates with scapula
	Deltoid tubercle	■ Round process for the deltoid muscle
	Olecranon fossa	■ Posterior, oval depression for the olecranon process of the ulna
	Capitulum	■ Round process superior to radius
	Trochlea	■ Concave surface that articulates with ulna
Radius	Head	■ Articulates with the ulna
Ulna	Olecranon process	■ Fits into olecranon fossa of humerus
	Semilunar notch	■ "Half-moon" depression that articulates with the trochlea of ulna
Carpals (8)	Scaphoid, Lunate, Triquetrum, Pisiform	■ Proximal row
	Trapezium, Trapezoid, Capitate, Hamate	■ Distal row

the distal end. Notice in Fig. 6–14 that the **fibula** is not part of the knee joint and does not bear much weight. The lateral malleolus of the fibula is the "outer ankle bone" you can find just above your foot. Though not a weight-bearing bone, the fibula is important in that leg muscles are attached and anchored to it, and it helps stabilize the ankle. Two bones on one is a much more stable arrangement than one bone on one, and you can see that the malleoli of the tibia and fibula overlap the sides of the talus. The tibia and fibula do not form a pivot joint as do the radius and ulna in the forearm; this also contributes to the stability of the lower leg and foot and the support of the entire body.

The **tarsals** are the seven bones in the ankle. As you would expect, they are larger and stronger than the carpals of the wrist, and their gliding joints do not provide nearly as much movement. The largest is the **calcaneus**, or heel bone; the **talus** transmits weight between the calcaneus and the tibia. **Metatarsals** are the five long bones of each foot, and **phalanges** are the bones of the toes. There are two phalanges in the big toe and three in each of the other toes. The phalanges of the toes form hinge joints with each other. Because there is no saddle joint in the foot, the big toe is not as movable as the thumb. The foot has two major arches, longitudinal and transverse, which are supported by ligaments. These are adaptations for walking completely upright, in that arches provide for spring or bounce in our steps. Important parts of hip and leg bones are described in Table 6–4.

JOINTS—ARTICULATIONS

A joint is where two bones meet, or articulate.

THE CLASSIFICATION OF JOINTS

The classification of joints is based on the amount of movement possible. A synarthrosis is an immovable joint, such as a suture between two cranial bones. An amphiarthrosis is a slightly movable joint, such as the symphysis joint between adjacent vertebrae. A diarthrosis is a freely movable joint. This is the largest category of joints and includes the ball-and-socket joint, the pivot, hinge, and others. Examples of each type of joint are described in Table 6–5, and many of these are illustrated in Fig. 6–15.

SYNOVIAL JOINTS

All diarthroses, or freely movable joints, are synovial joints because they share similarities of structure. A typical synovial

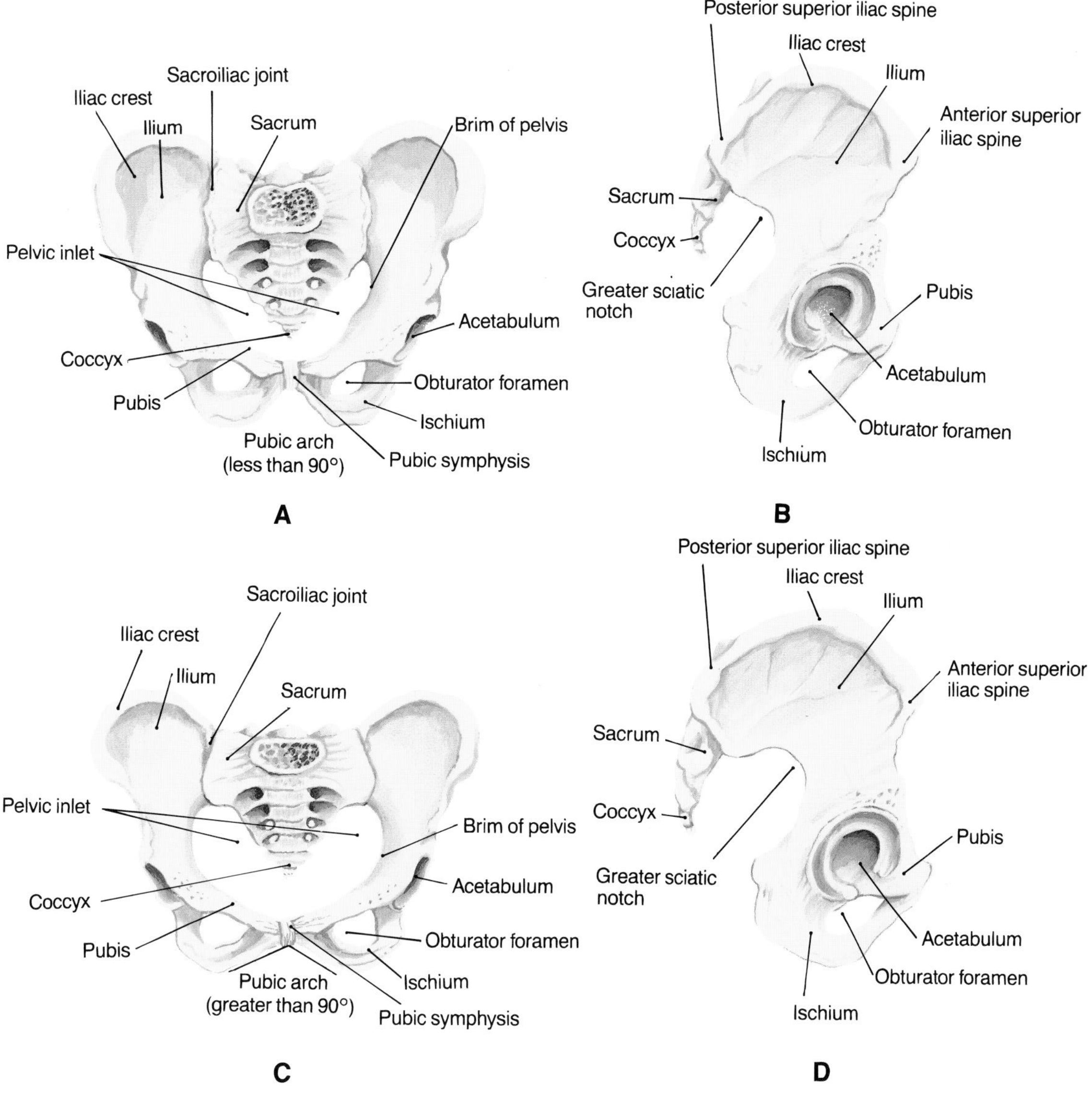

Figure 6–13 Hipbones and sacrum. (**A**) Male pelvis, anterior view. (**B**) Male pelvis, lateral view of right side. (**C**) Female pelvis, anterior view. (**D**) Female pelvis, lateral view of right side.

QUESTION: Compare the male and female pelvic inlets. What is the reason for this difference?

joint is shown in Fig. 6–16. On the joint surface of each bone is the **articular cartilage**, which provides a smooth surface. The **joint capsule**, made of fibrous connective tissue, encloses the joint in a strong sheath, like a sleeve. This capsule contributes to the stability of a joint. At the hip, for example, the joint capsule extends from the neck of the femur to the rim of the acetabulum and fits snugly, like a tight sleeve. The joint capsule at the shoulder has a more loose fit, which permits the shoulder joint greater range of motion. Lining the joint capsule is the synovial membrane, which secretes **synovial fluid** into the joint cavity. Synovial fluid is thick and slippery and prevents friction as the bones move.

Many synovial joints also have **bursae** (or bursas), which are small sacs of synovial fluid between the joint and the tendons that cross over the joint. Bursae permit the tendons to slide easily as the bones are moved. If

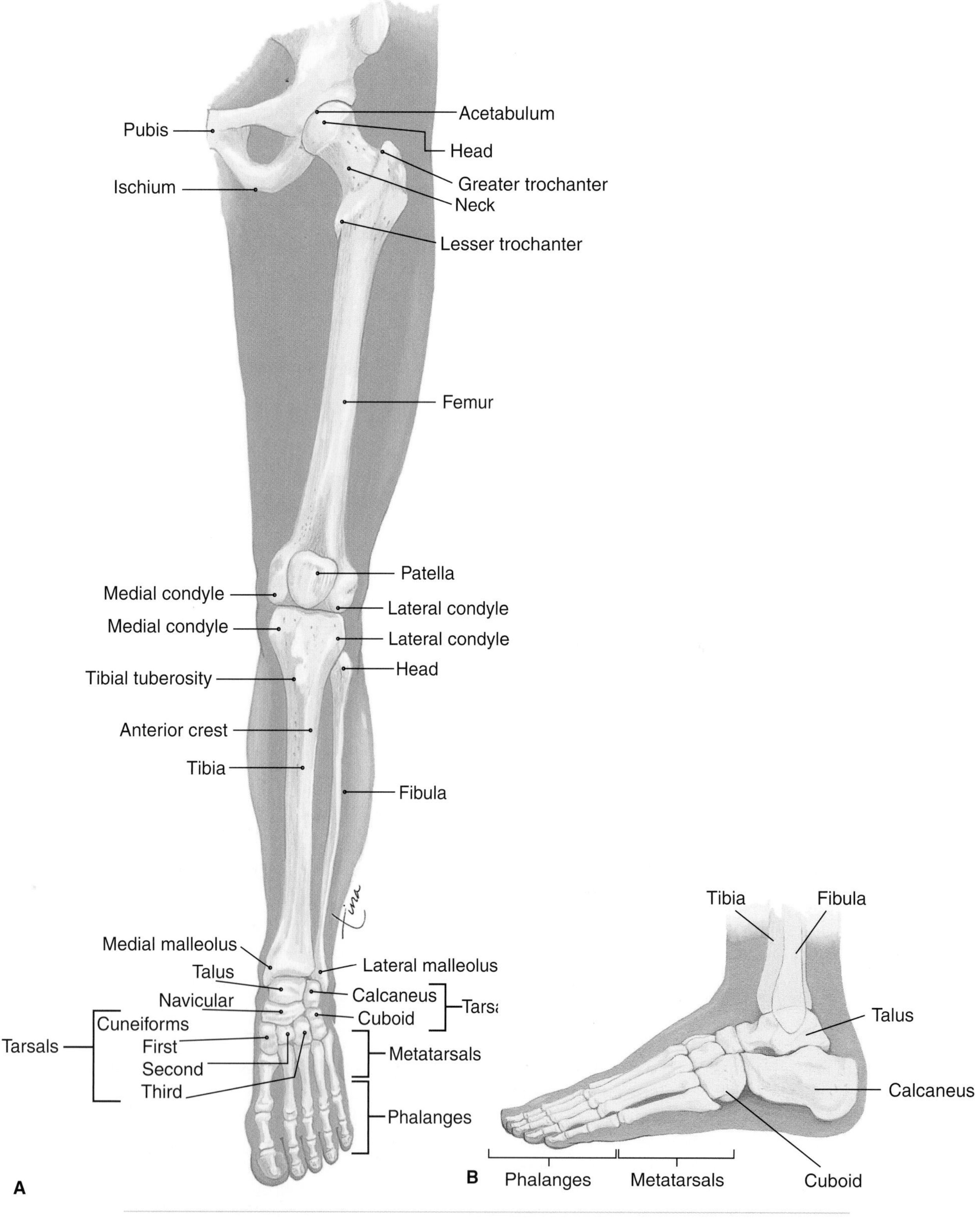

Figure 6–14 (**A**) Bones of the leg and portion of hipbone, anterior view of left leg. (**B**) Lateral view of left foot.

QUESTION: What types of joints found in the arm do not have counterparts in the leg?

Table 6–4 | **BONES OF THE HIP AND LEG—IMPORTANT PARTS**

BONE	PART	DESCRIPTION
Pelvic (2 hip bones)	Ilium Iliac crest Posterior superior iliac spine Ischium Pubis Pubic symphysis Acetabulum	■ Flared, upper portion ■ Upper edge of ilium ■ Posterior continuation of iliac crest ■ Lower, posterior portion ■ Anterior, medial portion ■ Joint between the 2 pubic bones ■ Deep depression that articulates with femur
Femur	Head Neck Greater trochanter Lesser trochanter Condyles	■ Round process that articulates with hip bone ■ Constricted portion distal to head ■ Large lateral process for muscle attachment ■ Medial process for muscle attachment ■ Rounded processes that articulate with tibia
Tibia	Condyles Tibial tuberosity Anterior crest Medial malleolus	■ Articulate with the femur ■ Round process for the patellar ligament ■ Vertical ridge ■ Distal process; medial "ankle bone"
Fibula	Head Lateral malleolus	■ Articulates with tibia ■ Distal process; lateral "ankle bone"
Tarsals (7)	Calcaneus Talus Cuboid, navicular Cuneiform: 1st, 2nd, 3rd	■ Heel bone ■ Articulates with calcaneus and tibia — —

Table 6–5 | **TYPES OF JOINTS**

CATEGORY	TYPE AND DESCRIPTION	EXAMPLES
Synarthrosis (immovable)	Suture—fibrous connective tissue between bone surfaces	■ Between cranial bones ■ Between facial bones
Amphiarthrosis (slightly movable)	Symphysis—disc of fibrous cartilage between bones	■ Between vertebrae ■ Between pubic bones
Diarthrosis (freely movable)	Ball and socket—movement in all planes	■ Scapula and humerus ■ Pelvic bone and femur
	Hinge—movement in one plane	■ Humerus and ulna ■ Femur and tibia ■ Between phalanges
	Condyloid—movement in one plane with some lateral movement	■ Temporal bone and mandible
	Pivot—rotation	■ Atlas and axis ■ Radius and ulna
	Gliding—side-to-side movement	■ Between carpals ■ Sacrum and ilium
	Saddle—movement in several planes	■ Carpometacarpal of thumb

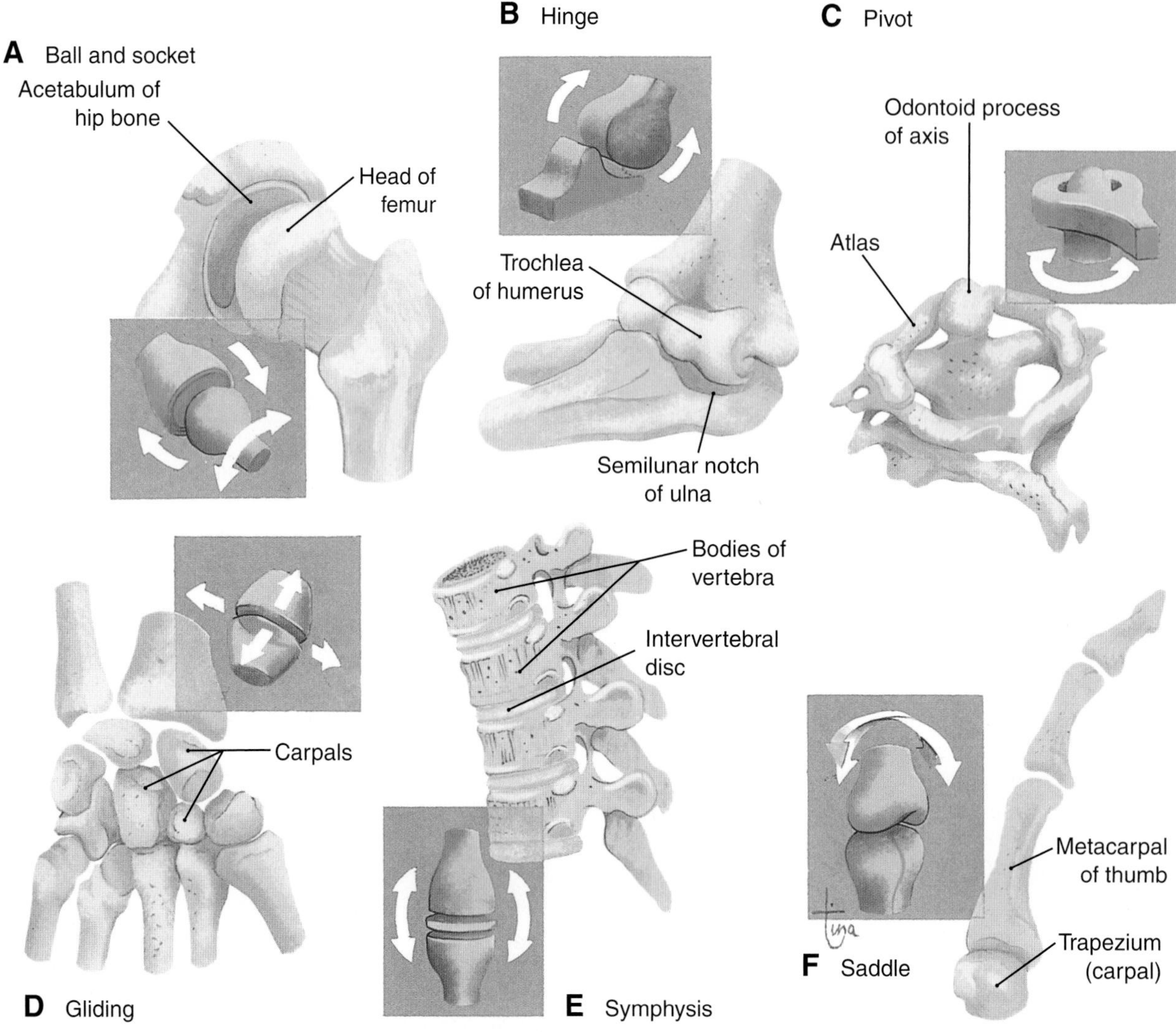

Figure 6–15 Types of joints. For each type, a specific joint is depicted, and a simple diagram shows the position of the joint surfaces. (**A**) Ball and socket. (**B**) Hinge. (**C**) Pivot. (**D**) Gliding. (**E**) Symphysis. (**F**) Saddle.

QUESTION: Which of these types of joints is most movable? Which is least movable?

a joint is used excessively, the bursae may become inflamed and painful; this condition is called **bursitis**. Some other disorders of joints are described in Box 6–5: Arthritis.

AGING AND THE SKELETAL SYSTEM

With age, bone tissue tends to lose more calcium than is replaced. Bone matrix becomes thinner, the bones themselves become more brittle, and fractures are more likely to occur with mild trauma.

Erosion of the articular cartilages of joints is also a common consequence of aging. Joints affected include weight-bearing joints such as the knees and active, small joints such as those of the fingers.

Although the normal wear and tear of joints cannot be prevented, elderly people can preserve their bone matrix with exercise (dancing counts) and diets high in calcium and vitamin D.

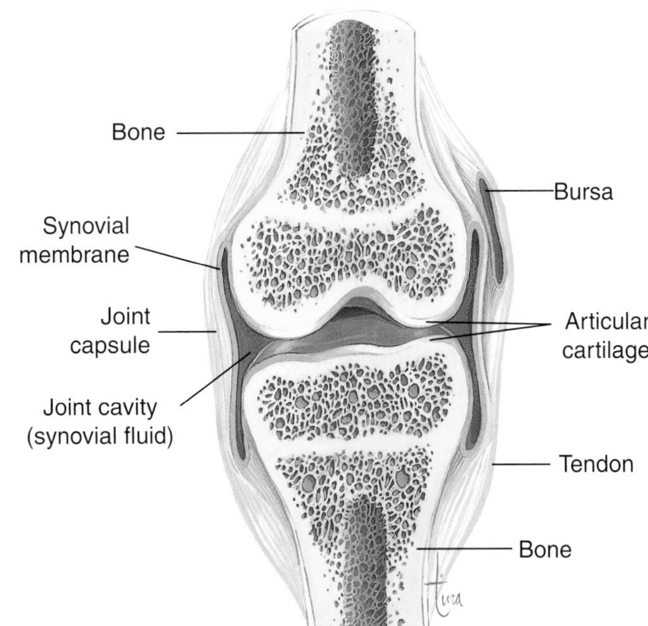

Figure 6–16 Structure of a synovial joint. See text for description.

QUESTION: How can you tell that this is a joint between two long bones? Give an example of two such bones.

Box 6–5 | ARTHRITIS

The term **arthritis** means "inflammation of a joint." Of the many types of arthritis, we will consider two: osteoarthritis and rheumatoid arthritis.

Osteoarthritis is a natural consequence of getting older. In joints that have borne weight for many years, the articular cartilage is gradually worn away. The once smooth joint surface becomes rough, and the affected joint is stiff and painful. As you might guess, the large, weight-bearing joints are most often subjected to this form of arthritis. If we live long enough, most of us can expect some osteoarthritis in knees, hips, or ankles.

Rheumatoid arthritis (RA) can be a truly crippling disease that may begin in early middle age or, less commonly, during adolescence. It is an **autoimmune disease**, which means that the immune system mistakenly directs its destructive capability against part of the body. Exactly what triggers this abnormal response by the immune system is not known with certainty, but certain bacterial and viral infections have been suggested as possibilities.

Rheumatoid arthritis often begins in joints of the extremities, such as those of the fingers. The autoimmune activity seems to affect the synovial membrane, and joints become painful and stiff. Sometimes the disease progresses to total destruction of the synovial membrane and calcification of the joint. Such a joint is then fused and has no mobility at all. Autoimmune damage may also occur in the heart and blood vessels, and those with RA are more prone to heart attacks and strokes (RA is a systemic, not a localized, disease).

Treatment of rheumatoid arthritis is directed at reducing inflammation as much as possible, because it is the inflammatory process that causes the damage. Therapies being investigated involve selectively blocking specific aspects of the immune response, such as antibody production. At present there is no cure for autoimmune diseases.

SUMMARY

Your knowledge of the bones and joints will be useful in the next chapter as you learn the actions of the muscles that move the skeleton. It is important to remember, however, that bones have other functions as well. As a storage site for excess calcium, bones contribute to the maintenance of a normal blood calcium level. The red bone marrow found in flat and irregular bones produces the blood cells: red blood cells, white blood cells, and platelets. Some bones protect vital organs such as the brain, heart, and lungs. As you can see, bones themselves may also be considered vital organs.

STUDY OUTLINE

The skeleton is made of bone and cartilage and has these functions:

1. Is a framework for support, connected by ligaments, moved by muscles.
2. Protects internal organs from mechanical injury.
3. Contains and protects red bone marrow.
4. Stores excess calcium; important to regulate blood calcium level.

Bone Tissue (see Fig. 6–1)

1. Osteocytes (cells) are found in the matrix of calcium phosphate, calcium carbonate, and collagen.
2. Compact bone—haversian systems are present.
3. Spongy bone—no haversian systems; red bone marrow present.
4. Articular cartilage—smooth, on joint surfaces.
5. Periosteum—fibrous connective tissue membrane; anchors tendons and ligaments; has blood vessels that enter the bone.

Classification of Bones

1. Long—arms, legs; shaft is the diaphysis (compact bone) with a marrow cavity containing yellow bone marrow (fat); ends are epiphyses (spongy bone) (see Fig. 6–1).
2. Short—wrists, ankles (spongy bone covered with compact bone).
3. Flat—ribs, pelvic bone, cranial bones (spongy bone covered with compact bone).
4. Irregular—vertebrae, facial bones (spongy bone covered with compact bone).

Embryonic Growth of Bone

1. The embryonic skeleton is first made of other tissues that are gradually replaced by bone. Ossification begins in the third month of gestation; osteoblasts differentiate from fibroblasts and produce bone matrix.
2. Cranial and facial bones are first made of fibrous connective tissue; osteoblasts produce bone matrix in a center of ossification in each bone; bone growth radiates outward; fontanels remain at birth to permit compression of the infant skull during birth; fontanels are calcified by age 2 (see Fig. 6–2).
3. All other bones are first made of cartilage. In a long bone the first center of ossification is in the diaphysis; other centers develop in the epiphyses. After birth a long bone grows at the epiphyseal discs: Cartilage is produced on the epiphysis side, and bone replaces cartilage on the diaphysis side. Osteoclasts form the marrow cavity by reabsorbing bone matrix in the center of the diaphysis (see Fig. 6–3).

Factors That Affect Bone Growth and Maintenance

1. Heredity—many pairs of genes contribute to genetic potential for height.
2. Nutrition—calcium, phosphorus, and protein become part of the bone matrix; vitamin D is needed for absorption of calcium in the small intestine; vitamins C and A are needed for bone matrix production (calcification).
3. Hormones—produced by endocrine glands; concerned with cell division, protein synthesis, calcium metabolism, and energy production (see Table 6–1).

4. Other tissues—leptin from adipose tissue stimulates bone growth; serotonin from the small intestine inhibits bone growth.
5. Exercise or stress—weight-bearing bones must bear weight or they will lose calcium and become brittle.

The Skeleton—206 bones (see Fig. 6–4); bones are connected by ligaments

1. Axial—skull, vertebrae, rib cage.
   a. Skull—see Figs. 6–5 through 6–8 and Table 6–2.
      - Eight cranial bones form the braincase, which also protects the eyes and ears; 14 facial bones make up the face; the immovable joints between these bones are called sutures.
      - Paranasal sinuses are air cavities in the maxillae, frontal, sphenoid, and ethmoid bones; they lighten the skull and provide resonance for voice (see Fig. 6–9).
      - Three auditory bones in each middle ear cavity transmit vibrations for hearing.

   b. Vertebral column—see Fig. 6–10.
      - Individual bones are called vertebrae: 7 cervical, 12 thoracic, 5 lumbar, 5 sacral (fused into one sacrum), 4 to 5 coccygeal (fused into one coccyx). Supports trunk and head, encloses and protects the spinal cord in the vertebral canal. Discs of fibrous cartilage absorb shock between the bodies of adjacent vertebrae, also permit slight movement. Four natural curves center head over body for walking upright (see Table 6–5 for joints).

   c. Rib cage—see Fig. 6–11.
      - Sternum and 12 pairs of ribs; protects thoracic and upper abdominal organs from mechanical injury and is expanded to contribute to inhalation. Sternum consists of manubrium, body, and xiphoid process. All ribs articulate with thoracic vertebrae; true ribs (first seven pairs) articulate directly with sternum by means of costal cartilages; false ribs (next three pairs) articulate with 7th costal cartilage; floating ribs (last two pairs) do not articulate with the sternum.

2. Appendicular—bones of the arms and legs and the shoulder and pelvic girdles.
   a. Shoulder and arm—see Fig. 6–12 and Table 6–3.
      - Scapula—shoulder muscles are attached; glenoid fossa articulates with humerus.
      - Clavicle—braces the scapula.
      - Humerus—upper arm; articulates with the scapula and the ulna (elbow).
      - Radius and ulna—forearm—articulate with one another and with carpals.
      - Carpals (8)—wrist; metacarpals (5)—hand; phalanges (14)—fingers (for joints, see Table 6–5).

   b. Hip and leg—see Figs. 6–13 and 6–14 and Table 6–4.
      - Pelvic bone—two hipbones; ilium, ischium, pubis; acetabulum articulates with femur.
      - Femur—thigh; articulates with pelvic bone and tibia (knee).
      - Patella—kneecap; in tendon of quadriceps femoris muscle.
      - Tibia and fibula—lower leg; tibia bears weight; fibula does not bear weight, but does anchor muscles and stabilizes ankle.
      - Tarsals (7)—ankle; calcaneus is heel bone.
      - Metatarsals (5)—foot; phalanges (14)—toes (see Table 6–5 for joints).

Joints—Articulations

1. Classification based on amount of movement:
   a. Synarthrosis—immovable.
   b. Amphiarthrosis—slightly movable.
   c. Diarthrosis—freely movable (see Table 6–5 for examples; see also Fig. 6–15).
2. Synovial joints—all diarthroses have similar structure (see Fig. 6–16):
   a. Articular cartilage—smooth on joint surfaces.
   b. Joint capsule—strong fibrous connective tissue sheath that encloses the joint.
   c. Synovial membrane—lines the joint capsule; secretes synovial fluid that prevents friction.
   d. Bursae—sacs of synovial fluid that permit tendons to slide easily across joints.

REVIEW QUESTIONS

1. Explain the differences between compact bone and spongy bone, and state where each type is found. (p. 122)
2. State the locations of red bone marrow, and name the blood cells it produces. (p. 122)
3. Name the tissue of which the embryonic skull is first made. Explain how ossification of cranial bones occurs. (p. 124)
4. State what fontanels are, and explain their function. (pp. 124–125)
5. Name the tissue of which the embryonic femur is first made. Explain how ossification of this bone occurs. Describe what happens in epiphyseal discs to produce growth of long bones. (p. 125)
6. Explain what is meant by "genetic potential" for height, and name the nutrients a child must have in order to attain genetic potential. (p. 125)
7. Explain the functions of calcitonin and parathyroid hormone with respect to bone matrix and to blood calcium level. (p. 128)
8. Explain how estrogen or testosterone affects bone growth and when. (p. 125)
9. State one way each of the following hormones helps promote bone growth: insulin, thyroxine, growth hormone. (p. 128)
10. Name the bones that make up the braincase. (pp. 129–130)
11. Name the bones that contain paranasal sinuses and explain the functions of these sinuses. (p. 131)
12. Name the bones that make up the rib cage, and describe two functions of the rib cage. (p. 137)
13. Describe the functions of the vertebral column. State the number of each type of vertebra. (p. 131)
14. Explain how the shoulder and hip joints are similar and how they differ. (pp. 140–142)
15. Give a specific example (name two bones) for each of the following types of joints: (p. 145)
    a. Hinge
    b. Symphysis
    c. Pivot
    d. Saddle
    e. Suture
    f. Ball and socket
16. Name the part of a synovial joint with each of the following functions: (p. 143)
    a. Fluid within the joint cavity that prevents friction
    b. Encloses the joint in a strong sheath
    c. Provides a smooth surface on bone surfaces
    d. Lines the joint capsule and secretes synovial fluid
17. Refer to the diagram of the full skeleton (Fig. 6–4), and point to each bone on yourself. (p. 130)

FOR FURTHER THOUGHT

1. Following a severe spinal cord injury in the lumbar region, the voluntary muscles of the legs and hips will be paralyzed. Describe the effects of paralysis on the skeleton.
2. Without looking at any of the illustrations, try to name all the bones that form the orbits, the sockets for the eyes. Check your list with Figs. 6–5 and 6–6.
3. In an effort to prevent sudden infant death syndrome (SIDS), parents were advised to put their infants to sleep lying on their backs, not their stomachs. Since then (1994), the number of SIDS deaths has decreased markedly. What do you think has happened to the skulls of many of those infants? Explain.
4. A 5-month-old infant is brought to a clinic after having diarrhea for 2 days. The nurse checks the baby's anterior fontanel and notices that it appears sunken. What has caused this?
5. Look at the lateral view of the adult skull in Fig. 6–5 and notice the size of the face part in proportion to the braincase part. Compare the infant skull in Fig. 6–2, and notice how small the infant face is relative to the size of the braincase. There is a very good reason for this. What do you think it is?
6. Look at the photograph here, Question Fig. 6–A. Name the bone and the type of section in which it is cut. What are the large arrows indicating? What are the smaller arrows indicating? Look carefully at this site, describe it, and explain possible consequences.

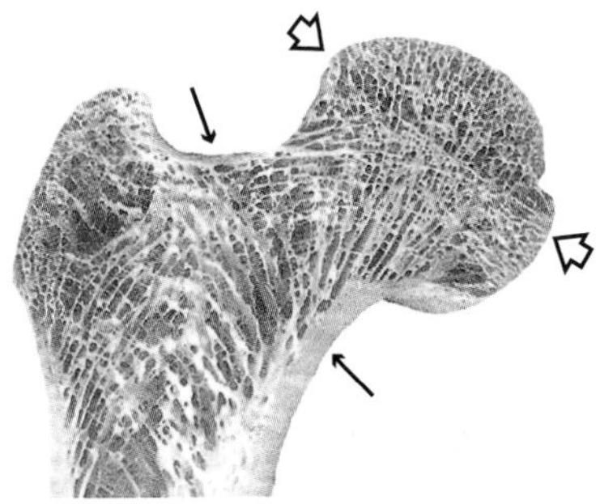

QUESTION FIGURE 6–A (Photograph by Dan Kaufman.)

CHAPTER

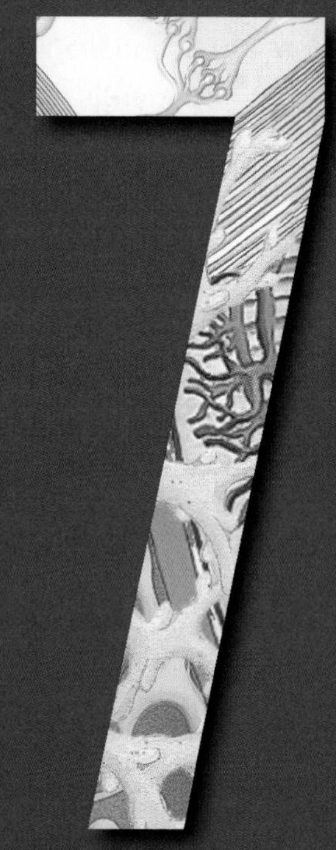

The Muscular System

STUDENT OBJECTIVES

- Name the organ systems directly involved in movement, and state how they are involved.
- Describe muscle structure in terms of muscle cells, tendons, and bones.
- Describe the difference between antagonistic and synergistic muscles, and explain why such arrangements are necessary.
- Explain the role of the brain with respect to skeletal muscle.
- Define muscle tone and explain its importance.
- Explain the difference between isotonic and isometric exercise.
- Define muscle sense and explain its importance.
- Name the energy sources for muscle contraction, and state the simple equation for cell respiration.
- Explain the importance of hemoglobin and myoglobin, oxygen debt, and lactic acid.
- Describe the neuromuscular junction and state the function of each of its parts.
- Describe the structure of a sarcomere.
- Explain the following in terms of ions and charges: polarization, depolarization, and repolarization.
- Describe the sliding filament mechanism of muscle contraction.
- Describe some of the body's responses to exercise and explain how each maintains homeostasis.
- Learn the major muscles of the body and their functions.

CHAPTER OUTLINE

NEW TERMINOLOGY

Actin *(**AK**-tin)*
Antagonistic muscles *(an-**TAG**-on-ISS-tik **MUSS**-uhls)*
Creatine phosphate *(**KREE**-ah-tin **FOSS**-fate)*
Depolarization *(DE-poh-lahr-i-**ZAY**-shun)*
Fascia *(**FASH**-ee-ah)*
Insertion *(in-**SIR**-shun)*
Isometric *(EYE-so-**MEH**-trik)*
Isotonic *(EYE-so-**TAHN**-ik)*
Lactic acid *(**LAK**-tik **ASS**-id)*
Muscle fatigue *(**MUSS**-uhl fah-**TEEG**)*
Muscle sense *(**MUSS**-uhl SENSE)*
Muscle tone *(**MUSS**-uhl TONE)*
Myoglobin *(**MYE**-oh-GLOW-bin)*
Myosin *(**MYE**-oh-sin)*
Neuromuscular junction *(NYOOR-oh-**MUSS**-kyoo-ler **JUNK**-shun)*
Origin *(**AHR**-i-jin)*
Oxygen debt *(**AHKS**-ah-jen DET)*
Polarization *(POH-lahr-i-**ZAY**-shun)*
Prime mover *(PRIME **MOO**-ver)*
Sarcolemma *(SAR-koh-**LEM**-ah)*
Sarcomeres *(**SAR**-koh-meers)*
Synergistic muscles *(**SIN**-er-JIS-tik **MUSS**-uhls)*
Tendon *(**TEN**-dun)*

*Terms that appear in **bold type** in the chapter text are defined in the glossary, which begins on page 603.*

RELATED CLINICAL TERMINOLOGY

Anabolic steroids *(an-a-**BAHL**-ik **STEER**-oyds)*

Atrophy *(**AT**-ruh-fee)*

Botulism *(**BAHT**-chu-lizm)*

Hypertrophy *(high-**PER**-truh-fee)*

Intramuscular injection *(IN-trah-**MUSS**-kyoo-ler in-**JEK**-shun)*

Muscular dystrophy *(**MUSS**-kyoo-ler **DIS**-truh-fee)*

Myalgia *(my-**AL**-jee-ah)*

Myasthenia gravis *(MY-ass-**THEE**-nee-yuh **GRAH**-viss)*

Myopathy *(my-**AH**-puh-thee)*

Paralysis *(pah-**RAL**-i-sis)*

Range-of-motion exercises *(RANJE-of-**MOH**-shun **EKS**-err-sigh-zez)*

Sex-linked trait *(SEX-LINKED TRAYT)*

Tetanus *(**TET**-uh-nus)*

Do you like to dance? Most of us do, or we may simply enjoy watching good dancers. The grace and coordination involved in dancing result from the interaction of many of the organ systems, but the one you think of first is probably the muscular system.

There are more than 600 muscles in the human body. Most of these muscles are attached to the bones of the skeleton by tendons, although a few muscles are attached to the undersurface of the skin. The primary function of the **muscular system** is to move the skeleton. The muscle contractions required for movement also produce heat, which contributes to the maintenance of a constant body temperature. The other body systems directly involved in movement are the nervous, respiratory, and circulatory systems. The nervous system, by way of motor neurons, transmits the electrochemical impulses that cause muscle cells to contract. The respiratory system exchanges oxygen and carbon dioxide between the air and blood. The circulatory system brings oxygen to the muscles and takes carbon dioxide away.

These interactions of body systems are covered in this chapter, which focuses on the **skeletal muscles**. You may recall from Chapter 4 that there are two other types of muscle tissue: smooth muscle and cardiac muscle. These types of muscle tissue will be discussed in other chapters in relation to the organs of which they are part. Before you continue, you may find it helpful to go back to Chapter 4 and review the structure and characteristics of skeletal muscle tissue. In this chapter we will begin with the gross (large) anatomy and physiology of muscles, then discuss the microscopic structure of muscle cells and the biochemistry of muscle contraction.

MUSCLE STRUCTURE

All muscle cells are specialized for contraction. When these cells contract, they shorten and pull a bone to produce movement. Each skeletal muscle is made of thousands of individual muscle cells, which also may be called **myocytes** or **muscle fibers** (see Fig. 7–3 later in this chapter). Depending on the work a muscle is required to do, variable numbers of muscle fibers contract. When finger muscles grip to pick up a pencil, for example, only a small portion of the muscle fibers in each finger-flexing muscle will contract. If the muscle has more work to do, such as picking up a book, more muscle fibers will contract to accomplish the task.

Muscles are anchored firmly to bones by **tendons**. Most tendons are rope-like, but some are flat; a flat tendon is called an **aponeurosis**. (See Fig. 7–9 later in this chapter for the epicranial aponeurosis, but before you look, decide what *epicranial* means.) Tendons are made of fibrous connective tissue, which, you may remember, is very strong and merges with the **fascia** that covers the muscle and with the **periosteum**, the fibrous connective tissue membrane that covers bones. A muscle usually has at least two tendons, each attached to a different bone. The more immobile or stationary attachment of the muscle is its **origin**; the more movable attachment is called the **insertion**. The muscle itself crosses the joint of the two bones to which it is attached, and when the muscle contracts it pulls on its insertion to move the bone in a specific direction.

MUSCLE ARRANGEMENTS

Muscles are arranged around the skeleton so as to bring about a variety of movements. The two general types of arrangements are the opposing **antagonists** and the cooperative **synergists**.

Antagonistic Muscles

Antagonists are opponents, so we use the term **antagonistic muscles** for muscles that have opposing or opposite functions. An example will be helpful here—refer to Fig. 7–1 as you read the following. The biceps brachii is the muscle on the front of the upper arm. The origin of the biceps is on the scapula (there are actually two tendons, hence the name *biceps*), and the insertion is on the radius. When the biceps contracts, it **flexes** the forearm, that is, bends the elbow (see Table 7–4 later in this chapter). Recall that when a muscle contracts, it gets shorter and pulls. Muscles cannot push, because when they relax, they exert no force. Therefore, the biceps can bend the elbow but cannot straighten it; another muscle is needed. The triceps brachii is located on the back of the upper arm. Its origins (the prefix *tri* tells you that there are three of them) are on the scapula and humerus, and its insertion is on the ulna. When the triceps contracts and pulls, it **extends** the forearm, that is, straightens the elbow.

Joints that are capable of a variety of movements have several sets of antagonists. Notice how many ways you can move your upper arm at the shoulder, for instance. Abducting (laterally raising) the arm is the function of the deltoid. Adducting the arm is brought about by the pectoralis major and latissimus dorsi. Flexion of the arm (across the chest) is also a function of the pectoralis major, and extension of the arm (behind the back) is also a function of the latissimus dorsi. All of these muscles are described and depicted in the tables and figures later in the chapter. Without antagonistic muscles, this variety of movements would not be possible.

You may be familiar with **range-of-motion** (or ROM) **exercises**, which are often recommended for patients confined to bed. Such exercises are designed to stretch and contract the antagonistic muscles of a joint to preserve as much muscle function and joint mobility as possible.

Synergistic Muscles

Synergistic muscles are those with the same function, or those that work together to perform a particular function. Recall that the biceps brachii flexes the forearm. The brachioradialis, with its origin on the humerus and insertion on the radius, also flexes the forearm. There is even a third flexor of the forearm, the brachialis. You may wonder why we need three muscles to perform the same function, and the explanation lies in the great mobility of the hand. If the hand is palm up, the biceps does most of the work of flexing and may be called the **prime mover**. When the hand is thumb up, the brachioradialis is in position to be the prime mover, and when the hand is palm down, the brachialis becomes the prime mover. If you have ever tried to do chin-ups, you know that it is much easier with your palms toward you than with palms away from you. This is because the biceps is a larger, and usually much stronger, muscle than is the brachialis.

Muscles may also be called synergists if they help to stabilize or steady a joint to make a more precise movement possible. If you drink a glass of water, the biceps brachii may be the prime mover to flex the forearm. At the same time, the muscles of the shoulder keep that joint stable, so that the water gets to your mouth, not over your shoulder

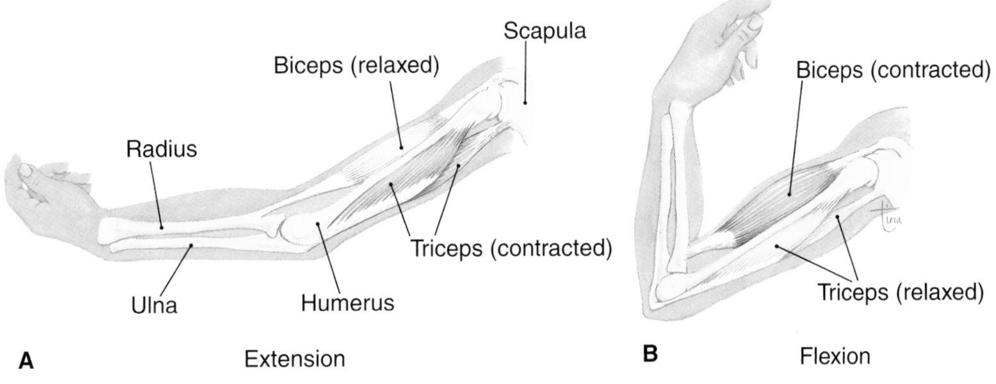

Figure 7–1 Antagonistic muscles. (**A**) Extension of the forearm. (**B**) Flexion of the forearm.

QUESTION: When the biceps contracts, what happens to its length, and what kind of force does it exert?

or down your chin. The shoulder muscles are considered synergists for this movement because their contribution makes the movement effective.

THE ROLE OF THE BRAIN

Even our simplest movements require the interaction of many muscles, and the contraction of skeletal muscles depends on the brain. The nerve impulses for movement come from the **frontal lobes** of the **cerebrum**. The cerebrum is the largest part of the brain; the frontal lobes are beneath the frontal bone. The **motor areas** of the frontal lobes generate electrochemical impulses that travel along motor neurons (grouped in nerves) to muscle fibers, causing the muscle fibers to contract.

The single axon of a motor neuron may branch extensively, and one neuron may therefore innervate from a few to hundreds of muscle fibers; this is called a **motor unit**. Small motor units, with 2 to 100 muscle fibers per neuron, are found in muscles that perform small, precise movements, such as those that move the fingers or eyes. Large motor units, with several hundred or more muscle fibers per neuron, are found in muscles where the need is usually for powerful movements rather than precise movements, such as the large muscles of the legs and hips.

For a movement to be effective, some muscles must contract while others relax. When we are walking, for example, antagonistic muscles on the front and back of the thigh or the lower leg will alternate their contractions and relaxations, and our steps will be smooth and efficient. This is what we call *coordination*, and we do not have to think about making it happen. Coordination takes place below the level of conscious thought and is regulated by the **cerebellum**, which is located below the occipital lobes of the cerebrum.

MUSCLE TONE

Except during certain stages of sleep, most of our muscles are in a state of slight contraction; this is what is known as **muscle tone**. When sitting upright, for example, the tone of your neck muscles keeps your head up, and the tone of your back muscles keeps your back straight. This is an important function of muscle tone for human beings because it helps us to maintain an upright posture. For a muscle to remain slightly contracted, only a few of the muscle fibers in that muscle must contract. Alternate fibers (different motor units) contract so that the muscle as a whole does not become fatigued. This is similar to a pianist continuously rippling her fingers over the keys of the piano—some notes are always sounding at any given moment, but the notes that are sounding are always changing. This contraction of alternate fibers, muscle tone, is also regulated by the cerebellum of the brain.

Muscle fibers need the energy of **ATP** (adenosine triphosphate) in order to contract. When they produce ATP in the process of cell respiration, muscle fibers also produce heat. The heat generated by normal muscle tone is approximately 25% of the total body heat at rest. During exercise, of course, heat production increases significantly.

EXERCISE

Good muscle tone improves coordination. When muscles are slightly contracted, they can react more rapidly if and when greater exertion is necessary. Muscles with poor tone are usually soft and flabby, but exercise will improve muscle tone.

There are two general types of exercise: isotonic and isometric. In **isotonic exercise**, muscles contract and bring about movement. Jogging, swimming, weight lifting, and walking are examples. Isotonic exercise improves muscle tone, muscle strength, and, if done repetitively against great resistance (as in weight lifting), muscle size. This type of exercise also improves cardiovascular and respiratory efficiency because movement exerts demands on the heart and respiratory muscles. If done for 30 minutes or longer, such exercise may be called *aerobic*, because it strengthens the heart and respiratory muscles, as well as the muscles attached to the skeleton.

Isotonic contractions are of two kinds, concentric or eccentric. A **concentric contraction** is the shortening of a muscle as it exerts force. An **eccentric contraction** is the lengthening of a muscle as it still exerts force. Imagine lifting a book straight up (or try it); the triceps brachii contracts and shortens to straighten the elbow and raise the book, a concentric contraction. Now imagine slowly lowering the book. The triceps brachii is still contracting even as it is lengthening, exerting force to oppose gravity (which would make the book drop quickly). This is an eccentric contraction.

Isometric exercise involves contraction without movement. If you put your palms together and push one hand against the other, you can feel your arm muscles contracting. If both hands push equally, there will be no movement; this is isometric contraction. Such exercises will increase muscle tone and muscle strength but are not considered aerobic. When the body is moving, the brain receives sensory information about this movement from the joints involved and responds with reflexes that increase heart rate and respiration. Without movement, the brain does not get this sensory information, and heart rate and breathing do not increase nearly as much as they would during an equally strenuous isotonic exercise.

Many of our actions involve both isotonic and isometric contractions. Pulling open a door requires isotonic contractions of arm muscles, but if the door is then held open for someone else, those contractions become isometric. Picking up a pencil is isotonic; holding it in your hand is isometric. Walking uphill involves concentric isotonic contractions and may be quite strenuous. Walking downhill seems easier, but is no less complex. The eccentric isotonic contractions involved make each step a precisely aimed and controlled fall against gravity. Without such control (which we do not have to think about) a downhill walk would quickly become a roll. These various kinds of contractions are needed for even the simplest activities. (With respect to increasing muscle strength, see Box 7–1: Anabolic Steroids.)

Exercise also brings out another aspect of skeletal muscle, this one more recently discovered. Striated muscle is also an endocrine tissue, and exercise stimulates the secretion of the hormone **irisin**. This hormone (a myokine; *myokine* means "muscle-signaler") affects adipose tissue, and converts white adipocytes to brown adipocytes. Recall from Chapter 4 that white fat cells store fat, but brown fat cells are thermogenic—that is, heat-producing. They metabolize fat to CO_2 and H_2O, and the energy is released as heat. In part, this is why regular and consistent exercise can contribute to weight loss.

MUSCLE SENSE

When you walk up a flight of stairs, do you have to look at your feet to be sure each will get to the next step? Most of us don't (an occasional stumble doesn't count), and for this freedom we can thank our muscle sense. **Muscle sense** (**proprioception**) is the brain's ability to know where our muscles are and what they are doing, without our having to look at them and be aware of them.

Within muscles are receptors called **stretch receptors** (or proprioceptors or muscle spindles). The general function of all sensory receptors is to detect changes. The function of stretch receptors is to detect changes in the length of a muscle as it is stretched. The sensory impulses generated by these receptors are interpreted by the brain as a mental "picture" of where the muscle is.

We can be aware of muscle sense if we choose to be, but usually we can safely take it for granted. In fact, that is what we are meant to do. Imagine what life would be like if we had to watch every move to be sure that a hand or foot performed its intended action. Even simple activities such as walking or eating would require our constant attention.

At times, we may become aware of our muscle sense. Learning a skill such as typing or playing the guitar involves very precise movements of the fingers, and beginners will often watch their fingers to be sure they are moving properly. With practice, however, the movements simply "feel" right, which means that the brain has formed a very good mental picture of the task. Muscle sense again becomes unconscious, and the experienced typist or guitarist need not watch every movement.

All sensation is a function of brain activity, and muscle sense is no exception. The impulses for muscle sense are integrated in the **parietal lobes** of the cerebrum (conscious muscle sense) and in the cerebellum (unconscious muscle sense) and are used to promote coordination.

Box 7–1 | ANABOLIC STEROIDS

Anabolic steroids are synthetic drugs very similar in structure and action to the male hormone **testosterone**. Normal secretion of testosterone, beginning in males at puberty, increases muscle size and is the reason men usually have larger muscles than do women.

Some athletes, both male and female, both amateur and professional, take anabolic steroids to build muscle mass and to increase muscle strength. There is no doubt that the use of anabolic steroids will increase muscle size, but there are hazards, some of them very serious. Side effects of such self-medication include liver damage, kidney damage, disruption of reproductive cycles, and mental changes such as irritability and aggressiveness.

Female athletes may develop increased growth of facial and body hair and may become sterile as a result of the effects of a male hormone on their own hormonal cycles.

As drug testing has improved, steroid manufacturers have tried to make chemicals that are less detectable. A synthetic form of testosterone cannot be distinguished from natural testosterone by current testing methods. However, this synthetic is not as easily metabolized by the liver, and its use may cause tumors of the liver or liver failure.

ENERGY SOURCES FOR MUSCLE CONTRACTION

Before discussing the contraction process itself, let us look first at how muscle fibers obtain the energy they need to contract. The direct source of energy for muscle contraction is ATP. ATP, however, is not stored in large amounts in muscle fibers and in contracting fibers is depleted in a few seconds.

The secondary energy sources are creatine phosphate and glycogen. **Creatine phosphate** is, like ATP, an energy-transferring molecule. When it is broken down (by an enzyme) to creatine, phosphate, and energy, the energy is used to synthesize more ATP. Most of the creatine formed is used to resynthesize creatine phosphate, but some is converted to **creatinine**, a nitrogenous waste product that is excreted by the kidneys.

The most abundant energy source in muscle fibers is **glycogen**. When glycogen is needed to provide energy for sustained contractions (more than a few seconds), it is first broken down into the **glucose** molecules of which it is made. Glucose is then further broken down in the process of cell respiration to produce ATP, and muscle fibers may continue to contract.

Recall from Chapter 2 our simple reaction for cell respiration:

$$\text{Glucose} + O_2 \rightarrow CO_2 + H_2O + \text{ATP} + \text{heat}$$

Look first at the products of this reaction. ATP will be used by the muscle fibers for contraction. The heat produced will contribute to body temperature and, if exercise is strenuous, will increase body temperature. The water becomes part of intracellular water, and the carbon dioxide is a waste product that will be exhaled.

Now look at what is needed to release energy from glucose: oxygen. If oxygen is present, cell respiration is said to be an **aerobic** process. Muscles have two sources of oxygen. The blood delivers a continuous supply of oxygen from the lungs; the oxygen is carried by the **hemoglobin** in red blood cells. Within muscle fibers themselves there is another protein called **myoglobin** (depicted in Fig. 2–8 part E), which stores some oxygen within the muscle cells. Both hemoglobin and myoglobin contain the mineral iron, which enables them to bond to oxygen. (Iron also makes both molecules red, and it is myoglobin that gives muscle tissue a red or dark color.)

During strenuous exercise, the oxygen stored in myoglobin is quickly used up, and normal circulation may not deliver oxygen fast enough to permit the completion of aerobic cell respiration. Even though the respiratory rate increases, the muscle fibers may literally run out of oxygen. This state is called **oxygen debt**, and in this case, glucose cannot be completely broken down into carbon dioxide and water. If oxygen is not present (or not present in sufficient amounts), the cell respiration process becomes **anaerobic**, and glucose is converted to an intermediate molecule called **lactic acid** (or lactate: $C_3H_5O_3$). Lactic acid lowers the pH of the intracellular fluid and contributes to **muscle fatigue**.

In a state of fatigue, muscle fibers cannot contract efficiently, and contraction may become painful. To be in oxygen debt means that we owe the body some oxygen. Lactic acid from muscles enters the blood and circulates to the liver, where it is converted to pyruvic acid (or pyruvate, also three carbons: $C_3H_3O_3$), a simple carbohydrate that can later be used for energy. This conversion of lactic acid to pyruvic acid requires ATP, and oxygen is needed to produce the necessary ATP in the liver. This is why, after strenuous exercise, the respiratory rate and heart rate remain high for a time and only gradually return to normal. Another name for this state is **recovery oxygen uptake**, which is a little longer but also makes sense. Oxygen uptake means a faster and deeper respiratory rate. What is this uptake for? For recovery from strenuous exercise.

MUSCLE FIBER—MICROSCOPIC STRUCTURE

We will now look more closely at a muscle fiber, keeping in mind that there are thousands of these cylindrical cells in one muscle. Each muscle fiber has its own motor nerve ending; the **neuromuscular junction** is where the motor neuron terminates on the muscle fiber (Fig. 7–2 and Table 7–1). The **axon terminal** is the enlarged tip of the motor neuron; it contains sacs of the neurotransmitter **acetylcholine** (ACh). The membrane of the muscle fiber is the **sarcolemma**, which contains receptor sites for acetylcholine, and an inactivator called **cholinesterase**. The **synapse** (or synaptic cleft) is the small space between the axon terminal and the sarcolemma.

Within the muscle fiber are thousands of individual contracting units called **sarcomeres**, which are arranged end to end in cylinders called **myofibrils**. The structure of a sarcomere is shown in Fig. 7–3: The Z lines are the end boundaries of a sarcomere. Thick filaments made mainly of the protein **myosin** are in the center of the sarcomere, and thin filaments that contain the protein **actin** are at the ends, attached to the Z lines. Myosin filaments are anchored to the Z lines by the protein **titin**.

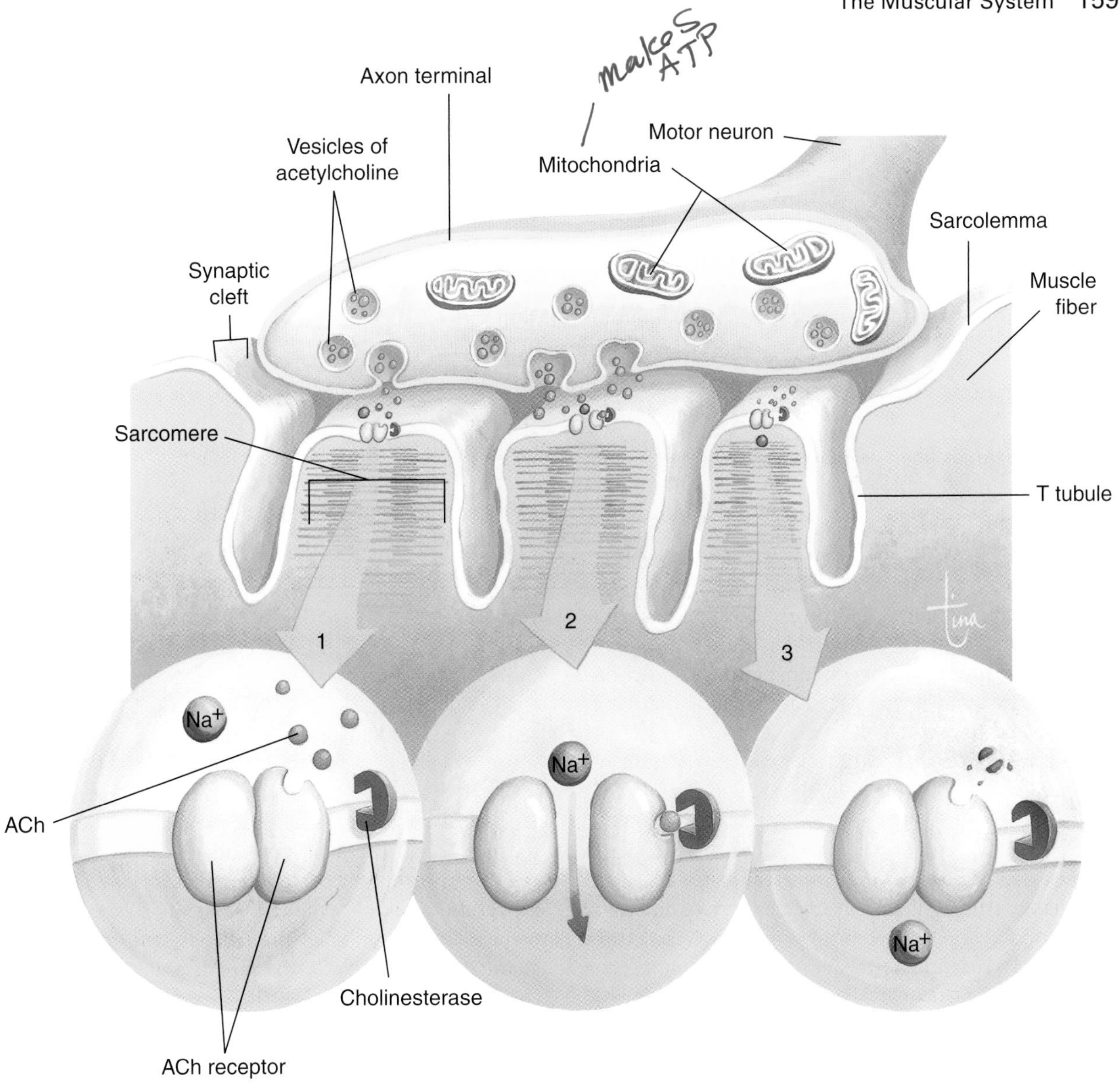

Figure 7–2 Structure of the neuromuscular junction, showing an axon terminal adjacent to the sarcolemma of a muscle fiber. Schematic of events: (1) Acetylcholine is about to bond to the ACh receptor in the sarcolemma. (2) Channel opens to allow Na+ ions into the muscle cell. (3) Cholinesterase inactivates acetylcholine.

QUESTION: What event opens a sodium channel in the sarcolemma?

Myosin and actin are the contractile proteins of a muscle fiber. Their interactions produce muscle contraction. Also present are two inhibitory proteins, **troponin** and **tropomyosin**, which are part of the thin filaments and prevent the sliding of actin and myosin when the muscle fiber is relaxed.

Surrounding the sarcomeres is the **sarcoplasmic reticulum**, the endoplasmic reticulum of muscle cells. The sarcoplasmic reticulum is a reservoir for calcium ions (Ca^{+2}), which are essential for the contraction process.

All of these parts of a muscle fiber are involved in the contraction process. Contraction begins when a nerve

Table 7–1 | THE NEUROMUSCULAR JUNCTION

PART	DESCRIPTION
Axon terminal	The end of a motor neuron; contains vesicles of acetylcholine that are opened by the arrival of a nerve impulse
Sarcolemma	The cell membrane of the muscle fiber; has receptors for acetylcholine
Synaptic cleft	The space between the axon terminal and the sarcolemma
Acetylcholine receptors	Proteins of the sarcolemma that are channels for Na^+ ions; are opened by acetylcholine
Acetylcholine (ACh)	The neurotransmitter released by the axon terminal; it diffuses across the synaptic cleft, bonds to the ACh receptors, and brings about depolarization of the sarcolemma with an influx of Na^+ ions
Cholinesterase	The enzyme that inactivates acetylcholine; prevents continued depolarization and contraction

impulse arrives at the axon terminal and stimulates the release of acetylcholine. Acetylcholine generates electrical changes (the movement of ions) at the sarcolemma of the muscle fiber. These electrical changes initiate a sequence of events within the muscle fiber that is called the **sliding filament mechanism** of muscle contraction. We will begin our discussion with the sarcolemma.

SARCOLEMMA—POLARIZATION

When a muscle fiber is relaxed, the sarcolemma is polarized (has a resting potential), which refers to a difference in electrical charges between the outside and the inside. During **polarization**, the outside of the sarcolemma has a positive charge relative to the inside, which is said to have a negative charge. Sodium ions (Na^+) are more abundant outside the cell, and potassium ions (K^+) and negative ions are more abundant inside the cell (Fig. 7–4).

The Na^+ ions outside tend to diffuse into the cell, and the **sodium pump** transfers them back out. The K^+ ions inside tend to diffuse outside, and the **potassium pump** returns them inside. Both of these pumps are active transport mechanisms, which, you may recall, require ATP. Muscle fibers use ATP to maintain a high concentration of Na^+ ions outside the cell and a high concentration of K^+ inside. The pumps, therefore, maintain polarization and relaxation until a nerve impulse stimulates a change.

SARCOLEMMA—DEPOLARIZATION

When a nerve impulse arrives at the axon terminal, it causes the release of acetylcholine, which diffuses across the synapse and bonds to **ACh receptors** on the sarcolemma. By doing so, acetylcholine makes the sarcolemma very permeable to Na^+ ions, which rush into the cell. This makes the inside of the sarcolemma positive relative to the outside, which is now considered negative. This reversal of charges is called **depolarization**. The electrical impulse thus generated (called an **action potential**) then spreads along the entire sarcolemma of a muscle fiber. The sarcolemma has inward folds called **T tubules** (transverse tubules, shown in Fig. 7–2), which carry the action potential to the interior of the muscle cell. Depolarization initiates changes within the cell that bring about contraction and is followed by **repolarization** to complete the action potential. Repolarization involves the outflow of K^+ ions that will restore the positive charge to the outside of the sarcolemma. The electrical changes that take place at the sarcolemma are summarized in Table 7–2 and shown in Fig. 7–4.

CONTRACTION—THE SLIDING FILAMENT MECHANISM

All of the parts of a muscle fiber and the electrical changes described earlier are involved in the contraction process, which is a precise sequence of events called the sliding filament mechanism. (See Fig. 7–5 and Table 7–3.)

In summary, a nerve impulse causes depolarization of a muscle fiber, and this electrical change enables the myosin filaments to pull the actin filaments toward the center of the sarcomere, making the sarcomere shorter. All of the sarcomeres shorten and the muscle fiber contracts. A more detailed description of this process is the following:

1. A nerve impulse arrives at the axon terminal; acetylcholine is released and diffuses across the synapse to the sarcolemma.

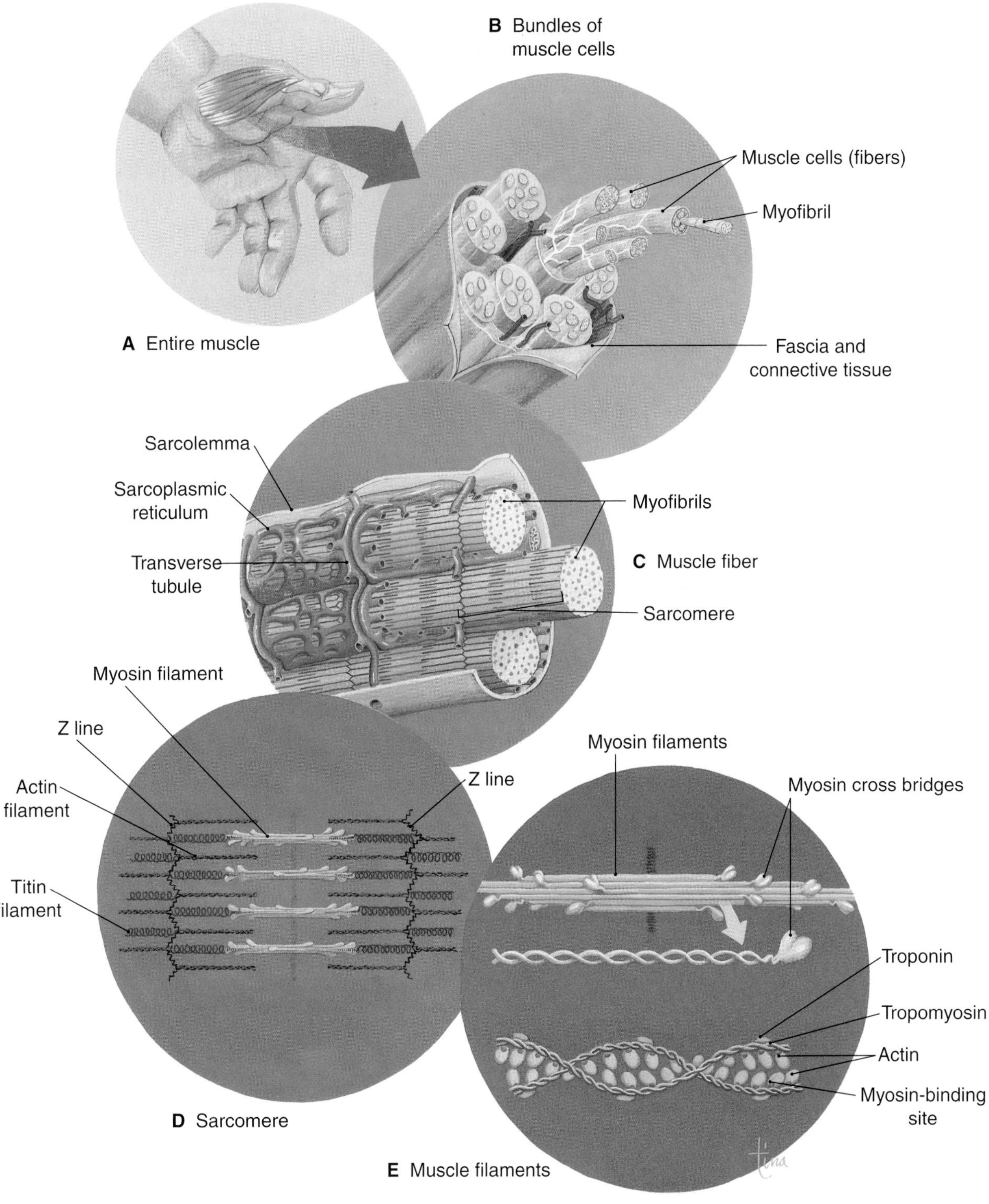

Figure 7–3 Structure of skeletal muscle. (**A**) Entire muscle. (**B**) Bundles of muscle cells within a muscle. **(C)** Single muscle fiber, microscopic structure. (**D**) A sarcomere. (**E**) Structure of muscle filaments.

QUESTION: What is the unit of contraction of a muscle fiber?

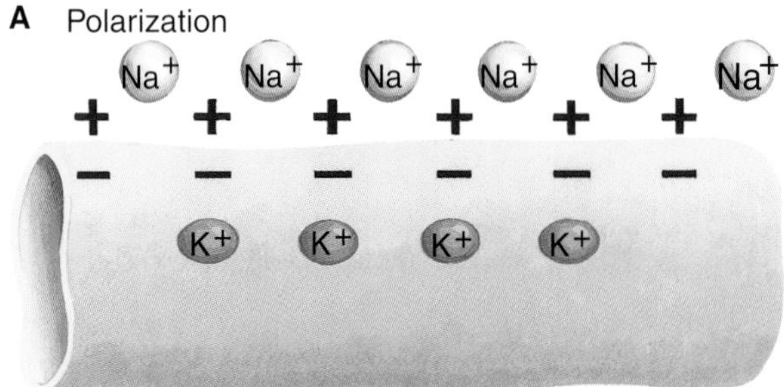

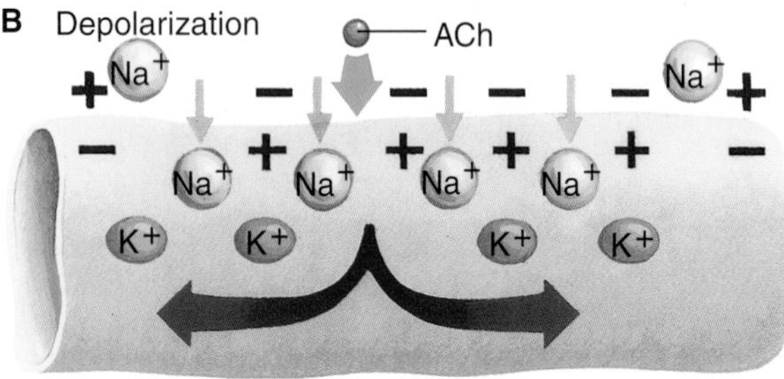

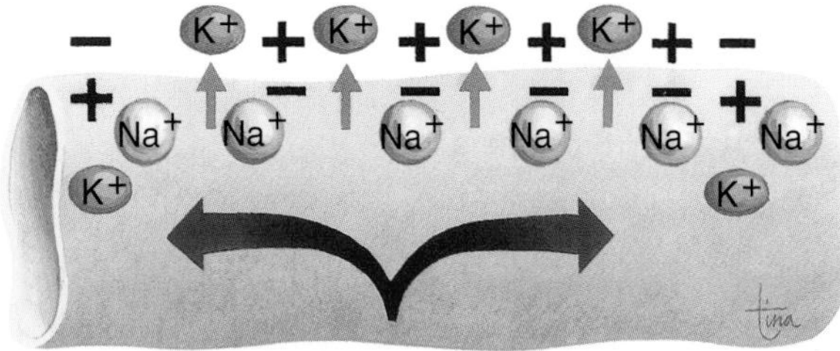

Figure 7–4 Electrical charges and ion concentrations at the sarcolemma. (**A**) Polarization, when the muscle fiber is relaxed. (**B**) Wave of depolarization in response to stimulus of acetylcholine. (**C**) Wave of repolarization.

QUESTION: Which ion enters the cell during depolarization? Which ion leaves during repolarization?

2. Acetylcholine bonds to acetylcholine receptors and makes the sarcolemma more permeable to Na^+ ions, which rush into the cell.
3. The sarcolemma depolarizes, becoming negative outside and positive inside. The T tubules bring the reversal of charges to the interior of the muscle cell.
4. Depolarization stimulates the release of Ca^{+2} ions from the sarcoplasmic reticulum. Ca^{+2} ions bond to the troponin–tropomyosin complex, which shifts it away from the actin filaments.

Table 7–2 | **SARCOLEMMA—ELECTRICAL CHANGES**

STATE OR EVENT	DESCRIPTION
RESTING POTENTIAL	
Polarization	■ Sarcolemma has a positive (+) charge outside and a negative (–) charge inside. ■ Na^+ ions are more abundant outside the cell; as they diffuse inward, the sodium pump returns them outside. ■ K^+ ions are more abundant inside the cell; as they diffuse out, the potassium pump returns them inside.
ACTION POTENTIAL	
Depolarization	■ ACh makes the sarcolemma very permeable to Na^+ ions, which rush into the cell. ■ Reversal of charges on the sarcolemma: now negative (–) outside and positive (+) inside. ■ The reversal of charges spreads along the entire sarcolemma. ■ Cholinesterase at the sarcolemma inactivates ACh.
Repolarization	■ Sarcolemma becomes very permeable to K^+ ions, which rush out of the cell. ■ Restoration of charges on the sarcolemma: positive (+) outside and negative (–) inside. ■ The sodium and potassium pumps return Na^+ ions outside and K^+ ions inside. ■ The muscle fiber is now able to respond to ACh released by another nerve impulse arriving at the axon terminal.

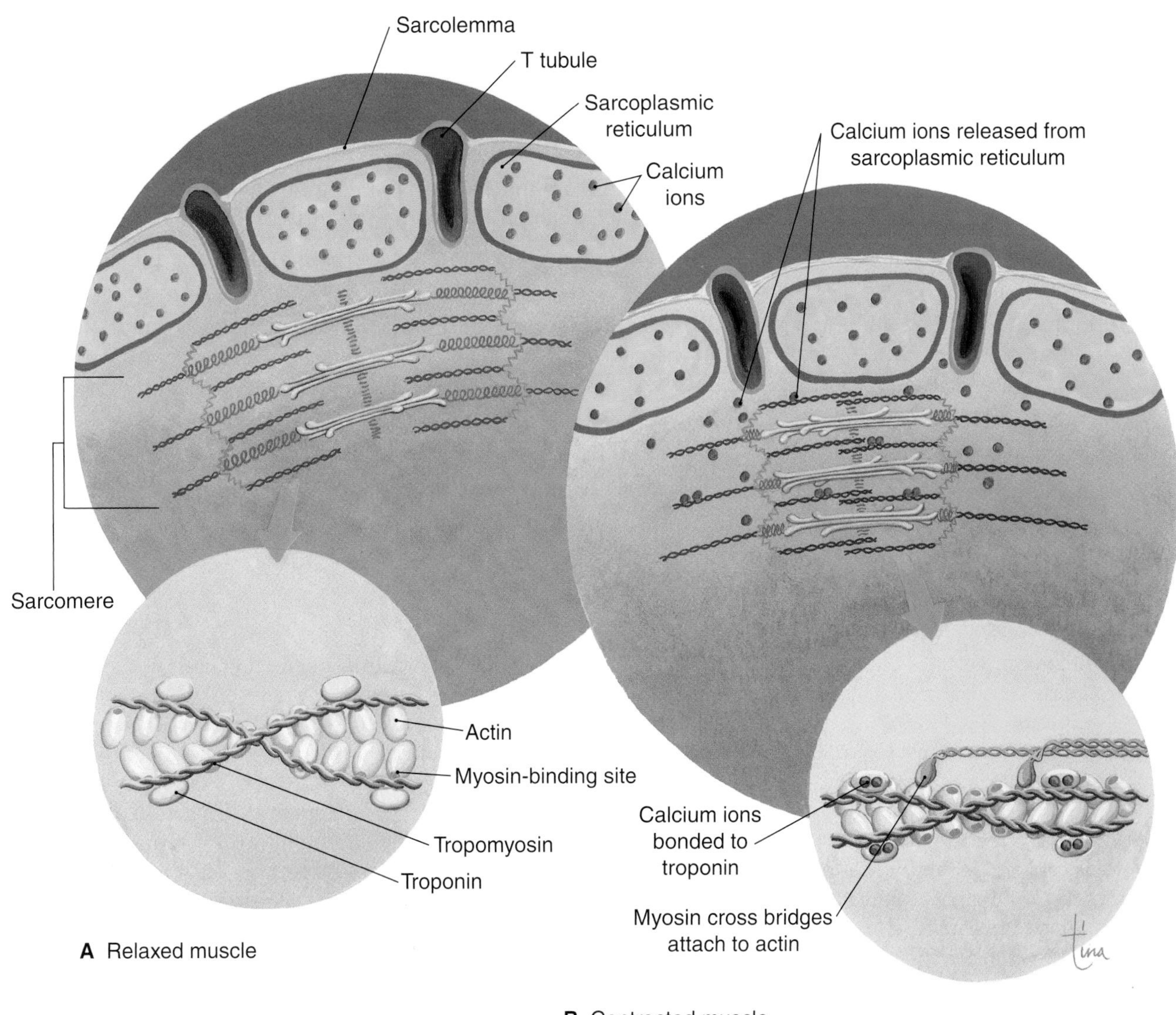

Figure 7–5 Sliding filament mechanism. (**A**) Sarcomere in relaxed muscle fiber. (**B**) Sarcomere in contracted muscle fiber. See text for description.

QUESTION: During contraction, which filaments do the pulling?

5. Myosin splits ATP to release its energy; bridges on the myosin attach to the actin filaments and pull them toward the center of the sarcomere, thus making the sarcomere shorter.
6. All of the sarcomeres in a muscle fiber shorten—the entire muscle fiber contracts.
7. The sarcolemma repolarizes: K^+ ions leave the cell, restoring a positive charge outside and a negative charge inside. The pumps then return Na^+ ions outside and K^+ ions inside.
8. Cholinesterase in the sarcolemma inactivates acetylcholine.
9. Subsequent nerve impulses will prolong contraction (more acetylcholine is released).
10. When there are no further impulses, the muscle fiber will relax and return to its original length.

Table 7–3 | THE SLIDING FILAMENT MECHANISM

PART	DESCRIPTION
Sarcomere	The unit of contraction of a muscle fiber; made of central thick and lateral thin filaments; extends from Z line to Z line
Myosin	A contracting protein of the thick filaments at the center of a sarcomere; it releases energy from ATP and pulls actin filaments toward the center of the sarcomere
Actin	A contracting protein of the thin filaments of a sarcomere; the two sets are pulled by myosin filaments toward the center of the sarcomere
Troponin and tropomyosin	The inhibiting proteins of a sarcomere; prevent the pulling of actin by myosin until the sarcolemma depolarizes
T tubules	Folds of the sarcolemma into the interior of the muscle fiber; carry the action potential to the innermost sarcomeres.
Sarcoplasmic reticulum	The endoplasmic reticulum of a muscle fiber; stores Ca^{+2} ions when the sarcolemma is polarized
Calcium ions (Ca^{+2})	Stored in the sarcoplasmic reticulum; released when the sarcolemma depolarizes; bond to troponin

Steps 1 through 8 of this sequence describe a single muscle fiber contraction (called a *twitch*) in response to a single nerve impulse. Because all of this takes place in less than a second, useful movements would not be possible if muscle fibers relaxed immediately after contracting. Normally, however, nerve impulses arrive in a continuous stream and produce a sustained contraction called a **tetanus**, which is a normal state not to be confused with the disease tetanus (see Box 7–2: Tetanus and Botulism). When in tetanus, muscle fibers remain contracted and are capable of effective movements. In a muscle such as the biceps brachii that flexes the forearm, an effective movement means that many of its thousands of muscle fibers are in tetanus, a sustained contraction.

As you might expect with such a complex process, muscle contraction may be impaired in many different ways. Perhaps the most obvious is the loss of nerve impulses to muscle fibers, which can occur when nerves or the spinal cord are severed, or when a **stroke** (**cerebrovascular accident**) occurs in the frontal lobes of the cerebrum. Without nerve impulses, skeletal muscles become **paralyzed**, unable to contract. Paralyzed muscles eventually **atrophy**, that is, become smaller from lack of use. Other disorders that affect muscle functioning are discussed in Box 7–3: Muscular Dystrophy and Box 7–4: Myasthenia Gravis.

RESPONSES TO EXERCISE—MAINTAINING HOMEOSTASIS

Although entire textbooks are devoted to exercise physiology, we will discuss it only briefly here as an example of the body's ability to maintain homeostasis. Engaging in moderate or strenuous exercise is a physiological stress situation, a change that the body must cope with, yet still maintain a normal internal environment, that is, homeostasis.

Some of the body's responses to exercise are diagrammed in Fig. 7–6; notice how the responses are related to cell respiration. As you can see, the respiratory and cardiovascular systems make essential contributions to exercise. The integumentary system also has a role because it eliminates excess body heat by way of vasodilation and sweating. Although not shown, the nervous system is also directly involved, as we have seen. The brain generates the impulses for muscle contraction, coordinates those contractions, and regulates heart rate, breathing rate, and the diameter of blood vessels. The next time you run up a flight of stairs, hurry to catch a bus, or just go dancing, you might reflect a moment on all of the things that are actually happening to your body . . . after you catch your breath.

AGING AND THE MUSCULAR SYSTEM

With age, muscle cells die and are replaced by fibrous connective tissue or fat. Regular exercise, however, delays atrophy of muscles. Although muscles become slower to contract and their maximal strength decreases, exercise can maintain muscle functioning at a level that meets whatever a person needs for daily activities. The lifting of

Box 7–2 | TETANUS AND BOTULISM

Some bacteria cause disease by producing toxins. A **neurotoxin** is a chemical that in some way disrupts the normal functioning of the nervous system. Because skeletal muscle contraction depends on nerve impulses, the serious consequences for the individual may be seen in the muscular system.

Tetanus is characterized by the inability of muscles to relax. The toxin produced by the tetanus bacteria (*Clostridium tetani*) affects the nervous system in such a way that muscle fibers receive too many impulses, and muscles go into spasms. Lockjaw, the common name for tetanus, indicates one of the first symptoms, which is difficulty opening the mouth because of spasms of the masseter muscles. Treatment requires the antitoxin (an antibody to the toxin) to neutralize the toxin. In untreated tetanus the cause of death is spasm of the respiratory muscles.

Botulism is usually a type of food poisoning, but it is not characterized by typical food poisoning symptoms such as diarrhea or vomiting. The neurotoxin produced by the botulism bacteria (*Clostridium botulinum*) prevents the release of acetylcholine at neuromuscular junctions. Without acetylcholine, muscle fibers cannot contract, and muscles become paralyzed. Early symptoms of botulism include blurred or double vision and difficulty speaking or swallowing. Weakness and paralysis spread to other muscle groups, eventually affecting all voluntary muscles. Without rapid treatment with the antitoxin (the specific antibody to this toxin), botulism is fatal because of paralysis of the respiratory muscles.

Box 7–3 | MUSCULAR DYSTROPHY

Muscular dystrophy is really a group of genetic diseases in which muscle tissue is replaced by fibrous connective tissue or by fat. Neither of these tissues is capable of contraction, and the result is progressive loss of muscle function. The most common form is Duchenne's muscular dystrophy, in which the loss of muscle function affects not only skeletal muscle but also cardiac muscle. Symptoms begin between the ages of 2 and 5. Death usually occurs before the age of 20 due to heart failure, and at present there is no cure.

Duchenne's muscular dystrophy is a **sex-linked** (or X-linked) **trait**, which means that the gene for it is on the X chromosome and is recessive. The female sex chromosomes are XX. If one X chromosome has a gene for muscular dystrophy, and the other X chromosome has a dominant gene for normal muscle function, the woman will not have muscular dystrophy but will be a carrier who may pass the muscular dystrophy gene to her children. The male sex chromosomes are XY, and the Y has no gene at all for muscle function, that is, no gene to prevent the expression of the gene on the X chromosome. If the X chromosome has a gene for muscular dystrophy, the male will have the disease. This is why Duchenne's muscular dystrophy is more common in males; the presence of only one gene means the disease will be present.

The muscular dystrophy gene on the X chromosome has been located, and the protein the gene codes for has been named *dystrophin*. Dystrophin is necessary for the stability of the sarcolemma and the proper movement of ions. Treatments for muscular dystrophy that are being investigated include the injection of normal muscle cells or stem cells into affected muscles, and the insertion (using viruses) of normal genes for dystrophin into affected muscle cells.

small weights is recommended as exercise for elderly people, women as well as men. Such exercise also benefits the cardiovascular, respiratory, and skeletal systems.

The loss of muscle fibers also contributes to a loss of proprioception, because the brain is getting less information about where and how the body is positioned. The loss of muscle sense contributes to unsteadiness in elderly people and to an impaired sense of balance, which in turn may lead to a fall. Simple awareness of this may help an elderly person prevent such accidents. Another preventive measure is

Box 7–4 | MYASTHENIA GRAVIS

Myasthenia gravis is an **autoimmune** disorder characterized by extreme muscle fatigue even after minimal exertion. Women are affected more often than are men, and symptoms usually begin in middle age. Weakness may first be noticed in the facial or swallowing muscles and may progress to other muscles. Without treatment, the respiratory muscles will eventually be affected, and respiratory failure is the cause of death.

In myasthenia gravis, the autoantibodies (self-antibodies) destroy the **acetylcholine receptors** on the sarcolemma. These receptors are the sites to which acetylcholine bonds and stimulates the entry of Na^+ ions. Without these receptors, the acetylcholine released by the axon terminal cannot cause depolarization of a muscle fiber.

Treatment of myasthenia gravis may involve anticholinesterase medications. Recall that cholinesterase is present in the sarcolemma to inactivate acetylcholine and prevent continuous, unwanted impulses. If this action of cholinesterase is inhibited, acetylcholine remains on the sarcolemma for a longer time and may bond to any remaining receptors to stimulate depolarization and contraction.

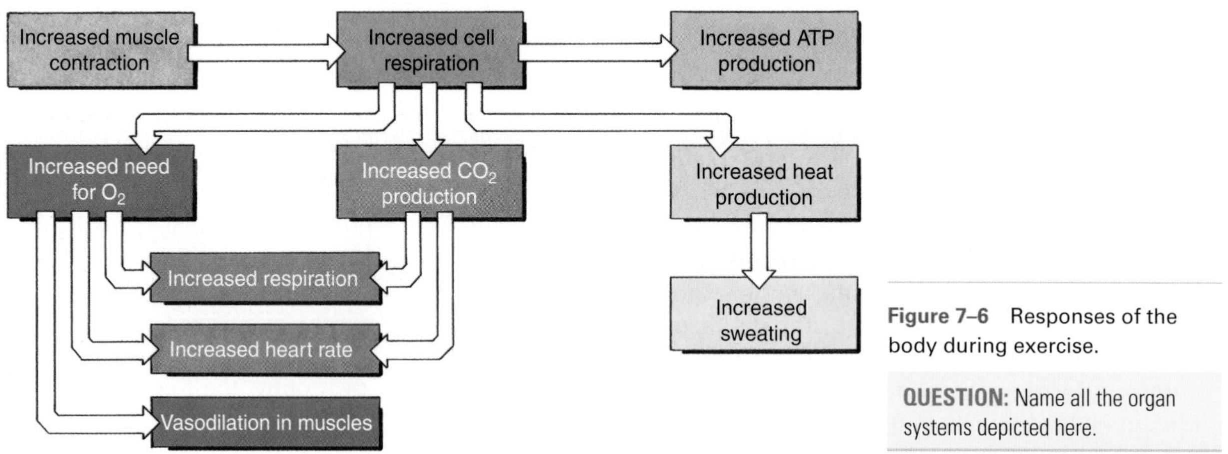

Figure 7–6 Responses of the body during exercise.

QUESTION: Name all the organ systems depicted here.

exercise—yes, exercise benefits sensation. The more that muscles are exercised, the more the brain keeps track of them. Giving the brain such "work" keeps its mental imaging of muscles a full-time job. For older people, exercise to music (or dancing of any kind) seems to be especially beneficial for helping to maintain the sense of balance and muscle strength.

MAJOR MUSCLES OF THE BODY

The actions that muscles perform are listed in Table 7–4 and are shown in Fig. 7–7. Most are in pairs as antagonistic functions.

After the brief summaries of the muscles of each body area that follow, the major muscles are shown in Fig. 7–8. They are listed, according to body area, in Tables 7–5 through 7–9, with associated Figs. 7–9 through 7–13, respectively. When you study the diagrams of these muscles, as well as the tables that accompany them, keep in mind the types of joints formed by the bones of their origins and insertions. Muscles pull bones to produce movement, and if you can remember the joints involved, you can easily learn the locations and actions of the muscles. The name of the muscle may also be helpful, and again, many of the terms are ones you have already learned. Some examples: "abdominis" refers to an abdominal muscle, "femoris" to a thigh muscle, "brachii" to a muscle of the upper arm, "oculi" to an eye muscle, and so on. Other parts of muscle names may be words such as "longus" or "maximus" that tell you about size, and "flexor" or "adductor" that tell you about function.

Muscles that are sites for intramuscular injections are shown in Box 7–5.

Table 7–4 | ACTIONS OF MUSCLES

ACTION	DEFINITION
Flexion	To decrease the angle of a joint
Extension	To increase the angle of a joint
Adduction	To move closer to the midline
Abduction	To move away from the midline
Pronation	To turn the palm down
Supination	To turn the palm up
Dorsiflexion	To elevate the foot
Plantar flexion	To lower the foot (point the toes)
Inversion	To move the sole of the foot medially at the ankle
Eversion	To move the sole of the foot laterally at the ankle
Rotation	To move a bone around its longitudinal axis

Most are grouped in pairs of antagonistic functions.

MUSCLES OF THE HEAD AND NECK

Three general groups of muscles are found in the head and neck: those that move the head or neck, the muscles of facial expression, and the muscles for chewing. The muscles that turn or bend the head, such as the sternocleidomastoids (flexion) and the pair of splenius capitis muscles (extension), are anchored to the skull and to the clavicle and sternum anteriorly or the vertebrae posteriorly. The muscles for smiling or frowning or raising our eyebrows in disbelief are anchored to the bones of the head or to the undersurface of the skin of the face. The masseter is an important chewing muscle in that it raises the mandible (closes the jaw), and you can feel it at the rear edge of your mandible when you clench your teeth.

MUSCLES OF THE TRUNK

The muscles of the trunk cannot be described with one or two general functions. Some form the wall of the trunk and bend the trunk, such as the rectus abdominis (flexion) and the sacrospinalis group (extension). The trapezius (both together form the shape of a trapezoid) is a large muscle that can raise (shrug) the shoulder or pull it back, and it can help extend the head. Other muscles found on the trunk help move the arm at the shoulder. The pectoralis major is a large muscle of the chest that pulls the arm across the chest (flexion and adduction). On the posterior side of the trunk, the latissimus dorsi pulls the arm downward and behind the back (extension and adduction). These muscles have their origins on the bones of the trunk, the sternum, or the vertebrae, which are strong, stable anchors. Another set of muscles forms the pelvic floor, where the muscles support the pelvic organs and assist with urination and defecation. Yet another category is the muscles that are concerned with breathing. These are the intercostal muscles between the ribs and the diaphragm, which separates the thoracic and abdominal cavities (see Fig. 15–6 in Chapter 15).

MUSCLES OF THE SHOULDER AND ARM

The triangular deltoid muscle covers the point of the shoulder like a cap, and can pull the humerus to the side (abduction), forward (flexion), or backward (extension). You already know the functions of the biceps brachii and triceps brachii, the muscles that form the bulk of the upper arm. Other muscles partially in the upper arm help bend the elbow (flexion). The muscles that form the bulk of the forearm are the flexors and extensors of the hand and fingers. You can demonstrate this yourself by clasping the middle of your right forearm with your left hand, then moving your right hand at the wrist and closing and opening a fist; you can both feel and see the hand and finger muscles at work.

MUSCLES OF THE HIP AND LEG

The hip muscles that move the thigh are anchored to the pelvic bone and cross the hip joint to the femur. Among these are the gluteus maximus (extension), gluteus medius (abduction), and iliopsoas (flexion). The muscles that form the thigh include the quadriceps group anteriorly and the hamstring group posteriorly. For most people, the quadriceps is stronger than the hamstrings, which is why athletes more often have a "pulled hamstring" rather than a "pulled quadriceps." The adductor group of muscles is medial and opposes the gluteus medius. Movement of the knee joint depends on thigh muscles and lower leg muscles. Movement of the foot depends on lower leg muscles such as the gastrocnemius (dorsiflexion or flexion) and the tibialis anterior (plantar flexion or extension).

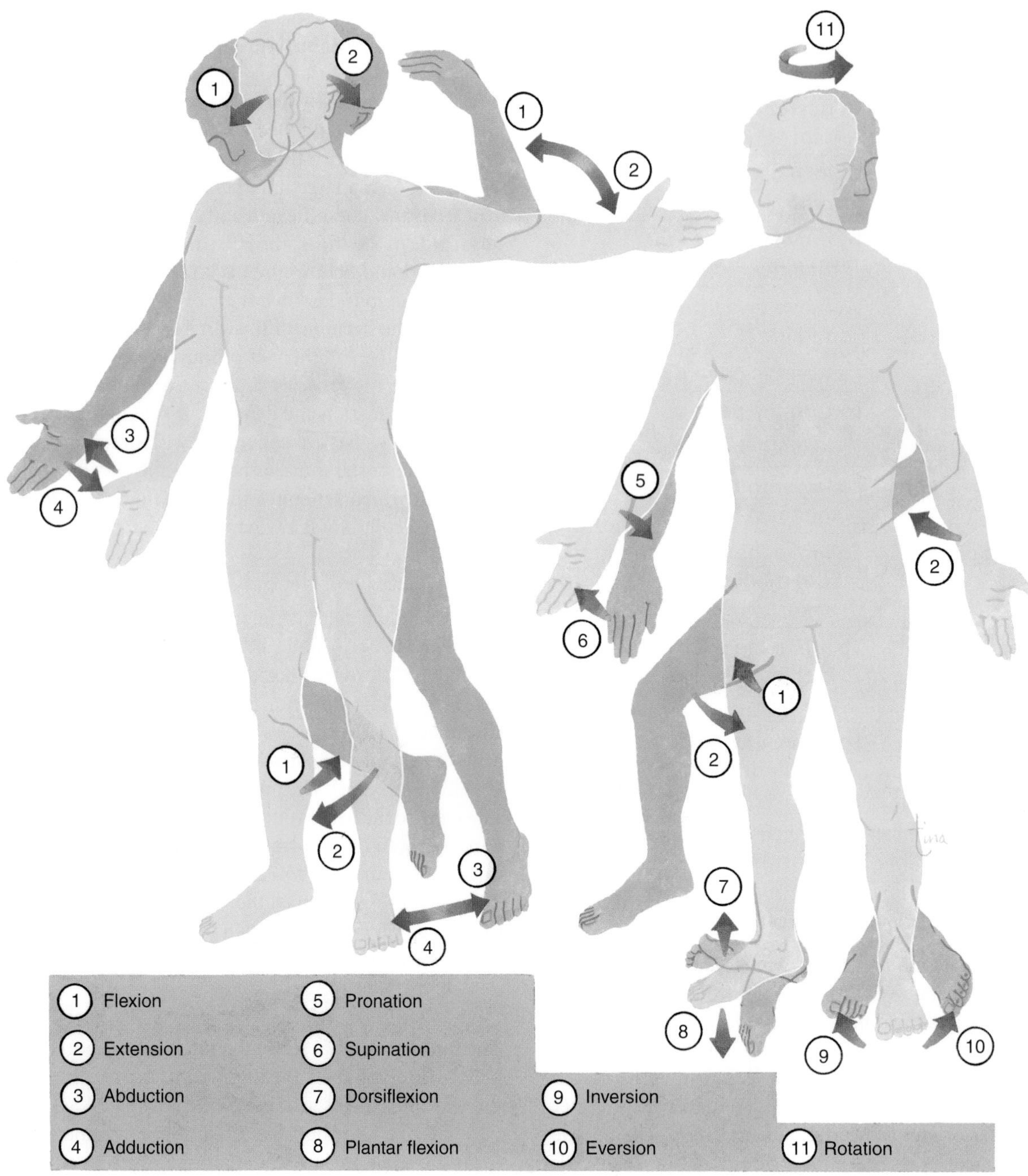

Figure 7–7 Actions of muscles.

QUESTION: Crossing the arm in front of the chest would be which of these actions?

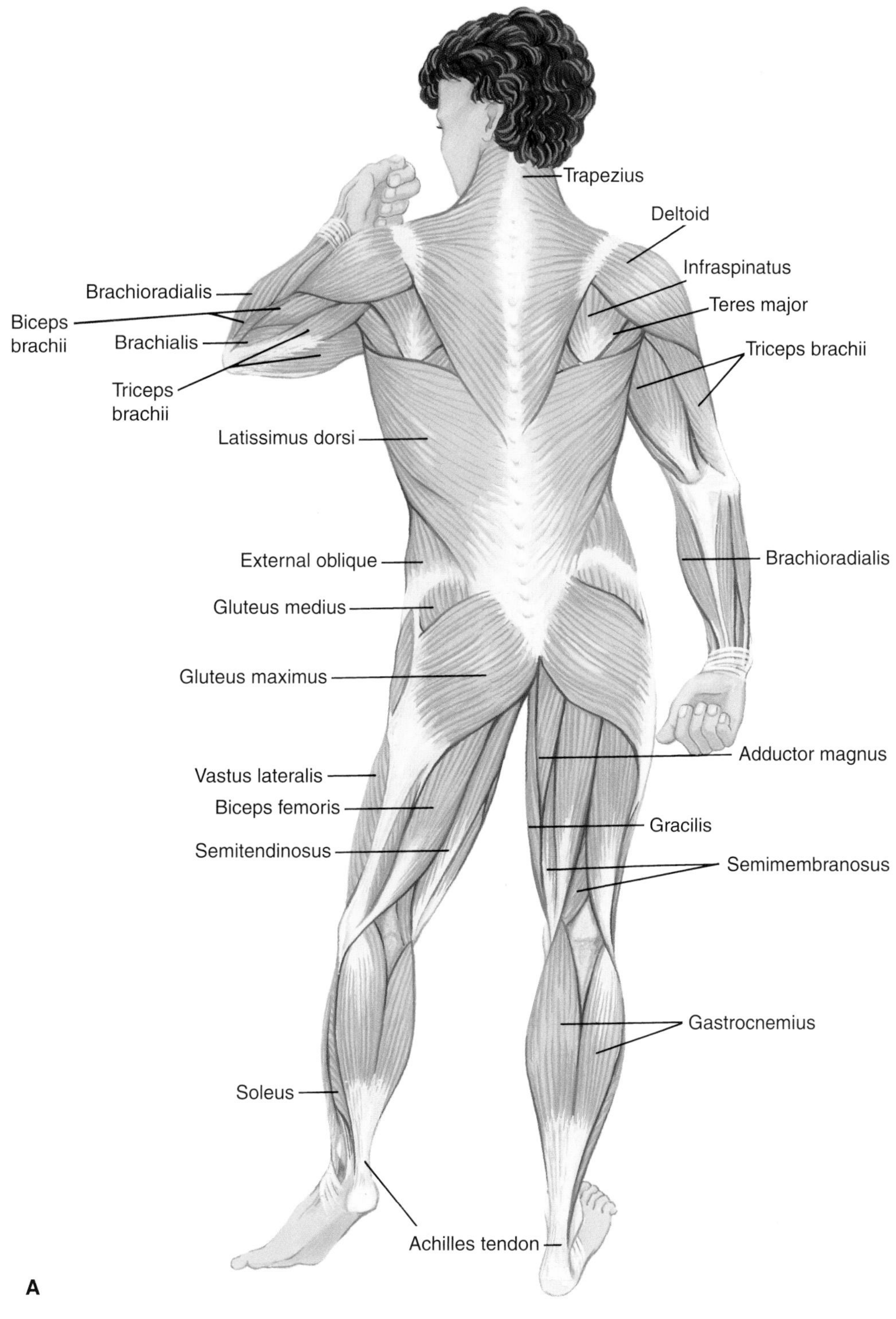

Figure 7–8 Major muscles of the body. (**A**) Posterior view.

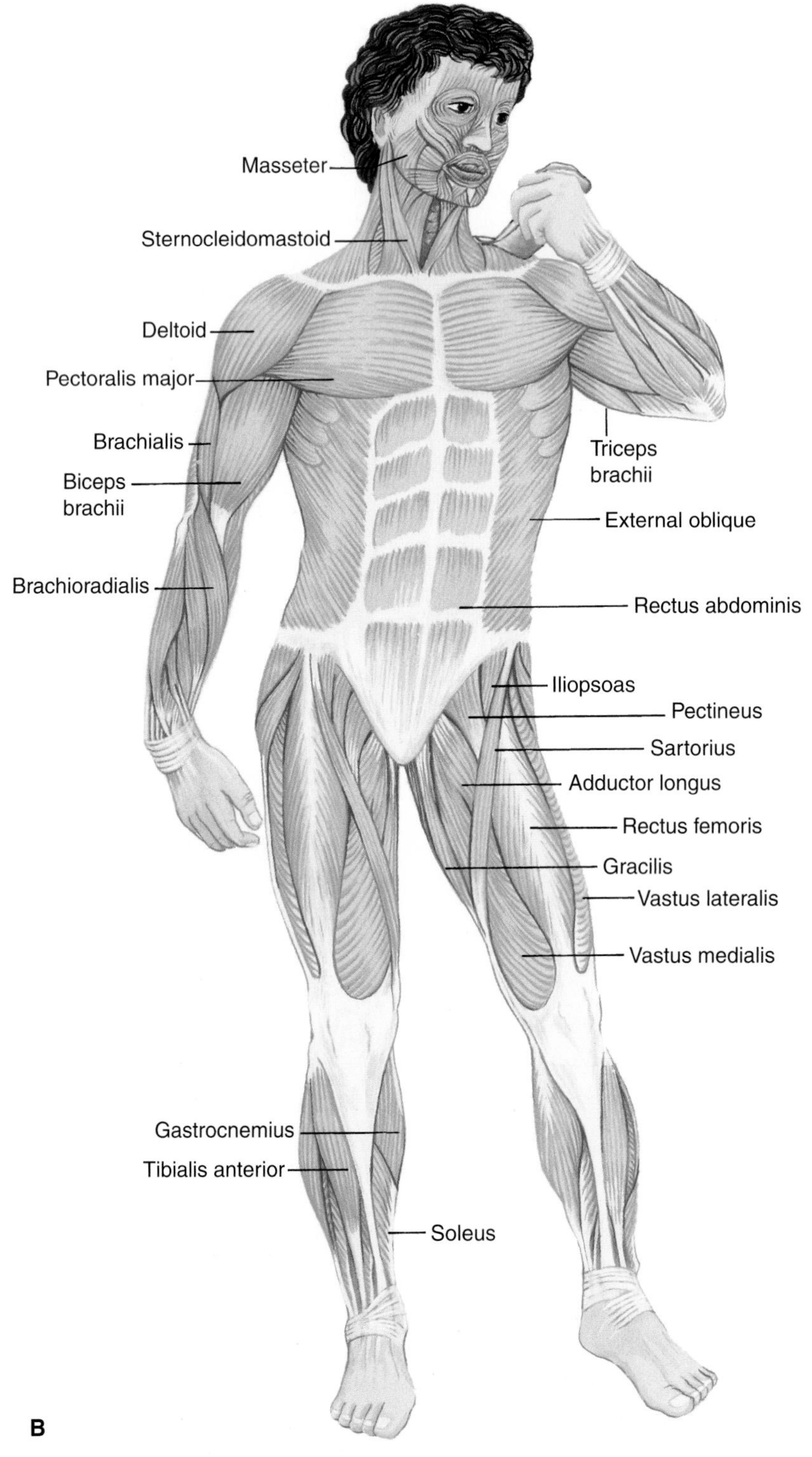

Figure 7–8 Major muscles of the body. (**B**) Anterior view.

QUESTION: Find a muscle named for each of the following: shape, size, location, a bone it is near, and function.

Table 7–5 | MUSCLES OF THE HEAD AND NECK

MUSCLE	FUNCTION	ORIGIN	INSERTION
Frontalis	Raises eyebrows, wrinkles skin of forehead	Epicranial aponeurosis	Skin above supraorbital margin
Orbicularis oculi	Closes eye	Medial side of orbit	Encircles eye
Orbicularis oris	Puckers lips	Encircles mouth	Skin at corners of mouth
Masseter	Closes jaw	Maxilla and zygomatic	Mandible
Buccinator	Pulls corners of mouth laterally	Maxilla and mandible	Orbicularis oris
Sternocleidomastoid	Turns head to opposite side (both—flex head and neck)	Sternum and clavicle	Temporal bone (mastoid process)
Semispinalis capitis (a deep muscle)	Turns head to same side (both—extend head and neck)	7th cervical and first 6 thoracic vertebrae	Occipital bone
Splenius capitis	Turns head to same side (both—extend head)	7th cervical and first 4 thoracic vertebrae	Occipital bone

Table 7–6 | MUSCLES OF THE TRUNK

MUSCLE	FUNCTION	ORIGIN	INSERTION
Trapezius	Raises, lowers, and adducts shoulders	Occipital bone and all thoracic vertebrae	Spine of scapula and clavicle
External intercostals	Pull ribs up and out (inhalation)	Superior rib	Inferior rib
Internal intercostals	Pull ribs down and in (forced exhalation)	Inferior rib	Superior rib
Diaphragm	Flattens (down) to enlarge chest cavity for inhalation	Last 6 costal cartilages and lumbar vertebrae	Central tendon
Rectus abdominis	Flexes vertebral column, compresses abdomen	Pubic bones	5th–7th costal cartilages and xiphoid process
External oblique	Rotates and flexes vertebral column, compresses abdomen	Lower 8 ribs	Iliac crest and linea alba
Sacrospinalis group (deep muscles)	Extends vertebral column	Ilium, lumbar, and some thoracic vertebrae	Ribs, cervical, and thoracic vertebrae

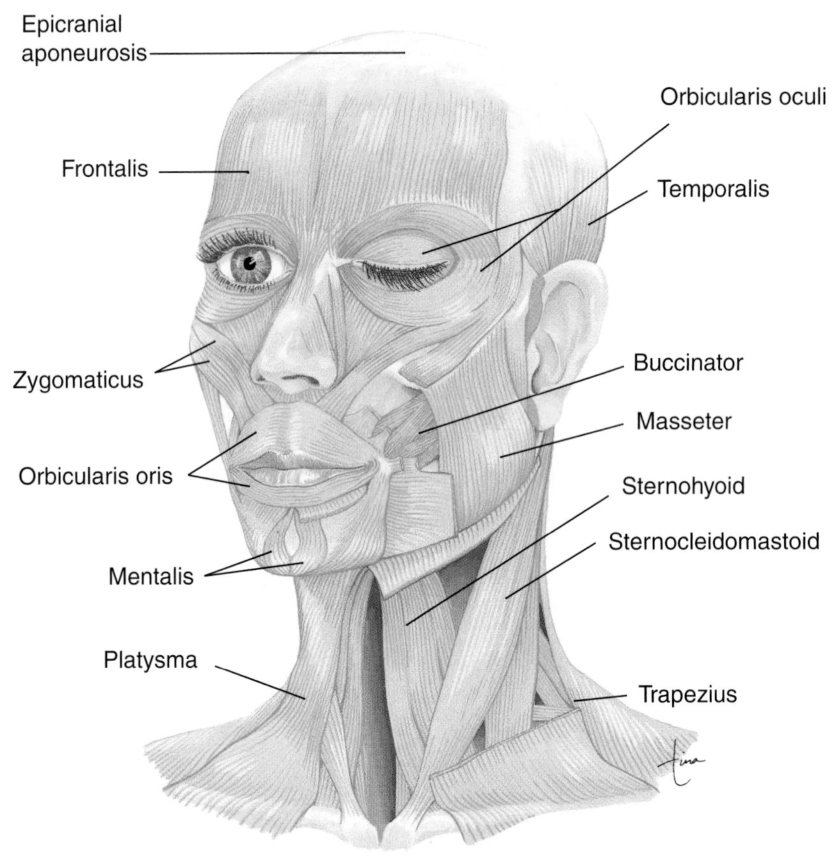

Figure 7–9 Muscles of the head and neck in anterior, left-lateral view.

QUESTION: In what way are both orbicularis muscles similar?

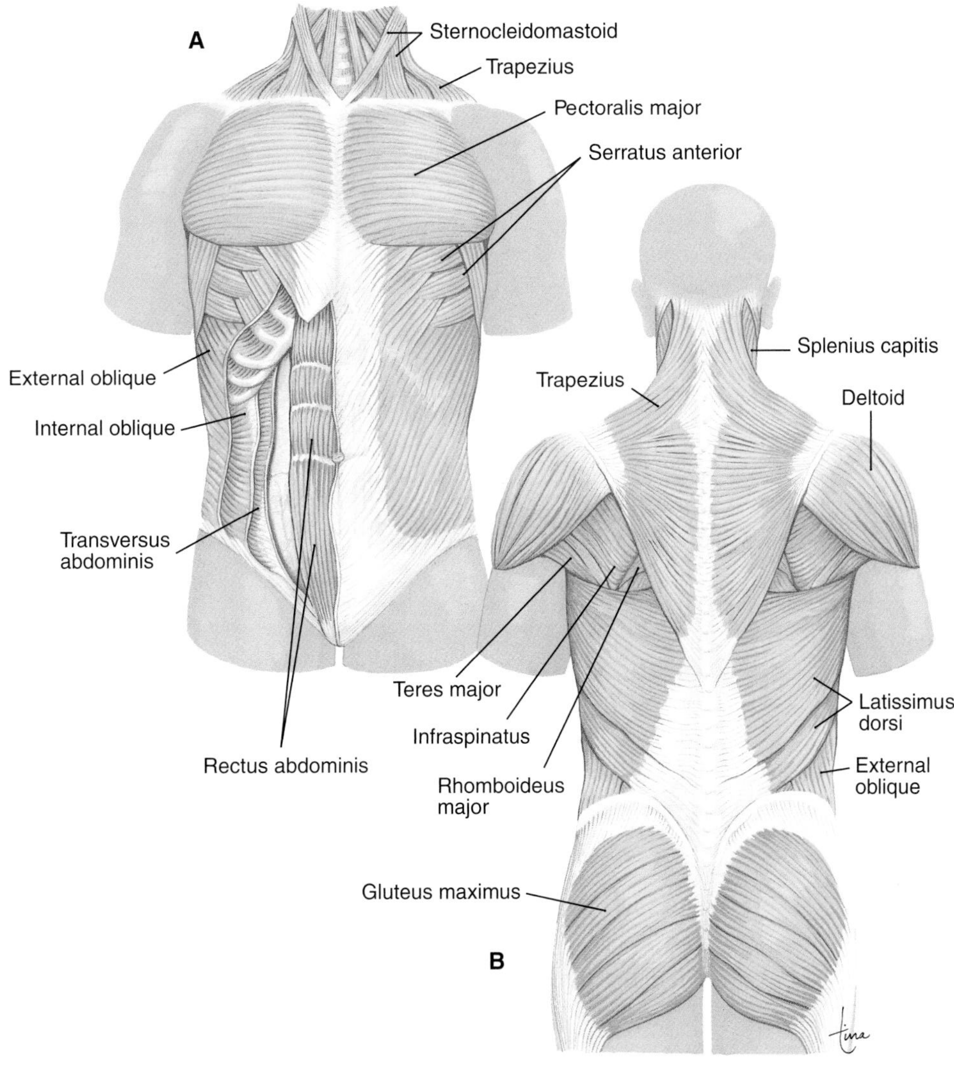

Figure 7–10 Muscles of the trunk. (**A**) Anterior view. (**B**) Posterior view.

QUESTION: Which muscles of the trunk move the arm? Why are they on the trunk?

Table 7–7 | MUSCLES OF THE SHOULDER AND ARM

MUSCLE	FUNCTION	ORIGIN	INSERTION
Deltoid	Abducts the humerus	Scapula and clavicle	Humerus
Pectoralis major	Flexes and adducts the humerus	Clavicle, sternum, 2nd–6th costal cartilages	Humerus
Latissimus dorsi	Extends and adducts the humerus	Last 6 thoracic vertebrae, all lumbar vertebrae, sacrum, iliac crest	Humerus
Teres major	Extends and adducts the humerus	Scapula	Humerus
Triceps brachii	Extends the forearm	Humerus and scapula	Ulna
Biceps brachii	Flexes the forearm	Scapula	Radius
Brachialis	Flexes the forearm	Humerus	Ulna
Brachioradialis	Flexes the forearm	Humerus	Radius

Table 7–8 | MUSCLES OF THE HIP AND LEG

MUSCLE	FUNCTION	ORIGIN	INSERTION
Iliopsoas	Flexes femur	Ilium, lumbar vertebrae	Femur
Pectineus	Flexes and adducts femur	Pubic bone	Femur
Gluteus maximus	Extends femur	Iliac crest, sacrum, coccyx	Femur
Gluteus medius	Abducts femur	Ilium	Femur
Quadriceps femoris group: Rectus femoris Vastus lateralis Vastus medialis Vastus intermedius	Flexes femur and extends lower leg	Ilium and femur	Tibia
Hamstring group Biceps femoris Semimembranosus Semitendinosus	Extends femur and flexes lower leg	Ischium	Tibia and fibula
Adductor group Adductor magnus Adductor longus Gracilis	Adducts femur	Ischium and pubis	Femur

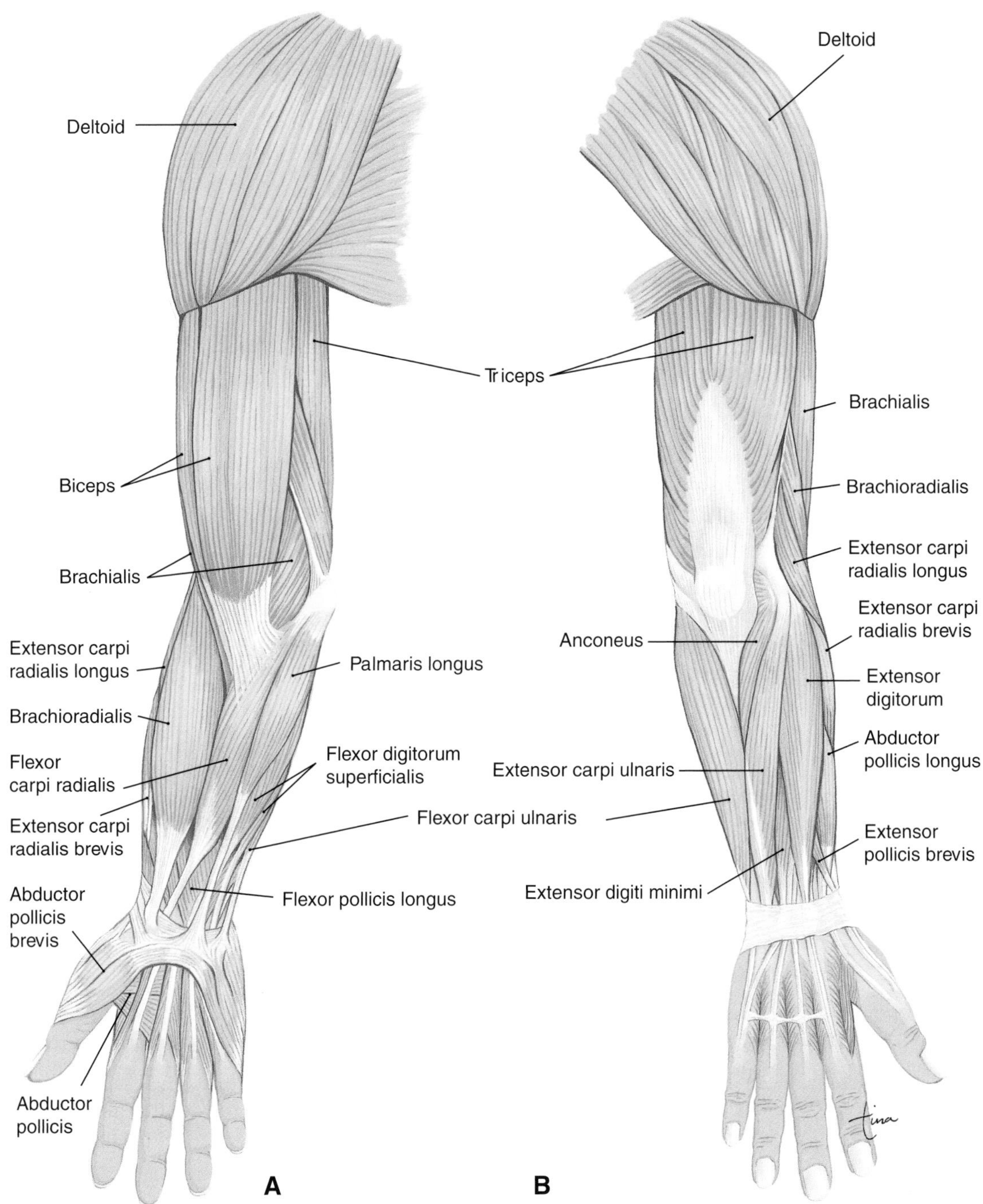

Figure 7–11 Muscles of the arm. (**A**) Anterior view. (**B**) Posterior view.

QUESTION: Where are the muscles that flex the fingers located? How did you know?

Table 7–8 | **MUSCLES OF THE HIP AND LEG—cont'd**

MUSCLE	FUNCTION	ORIGIN	INSERTION
Sartorius	Flexes femur and lower leg	Ilium	Tibia
Gastrocnemius	Plantar flexes foot	Femur	Calcaneus (Achilles tendon)
Soleus	Plantar flexes foot	Tibia and fibula	Calcaneus (Achilles tendon)
Peroneus (fibularis) longus	Plantar flexes and everts foot	Tibia and fibula	1st metatarsal and cuneiform
Tibialis anterior	Dorsiflexes foot	Tibia	Metatarsals

Table 7–9 | **MUSCLES OF THE PELVIC FLOOR**

MUSCLE	FUNCTION	ORIGIN	INSERTION
Levator ani	Supports pelvic organs, especially during defecation, urination, coughing, and forced exhalation; constricts anus, urethra, and vagina	Pubis and ischium	Coccyx, anal canal, urethra
Coccygeus	Supports pelvic organs, especially during defecation, urination, coughing, and forced exhalation	Ischium	Coccyx and sacrum
Ischiocavernosus	Erection of clitoris in female, penis in male	Ischium and pubis	Clitoris or penis
Bulbospongiosus	Assists urination; erection in female; erection and ejaculation in male	Central tendon of perineum	Fasciae, pubic arch, clitoris or penis
Transverse perineus (superficial and deep)	Assists urination in female; urination and ejaculation in male	Ischium	Central tendon of perineum
External anal sphincter	Closes anus	Anococcygeal ligament	Central tendon of perineum

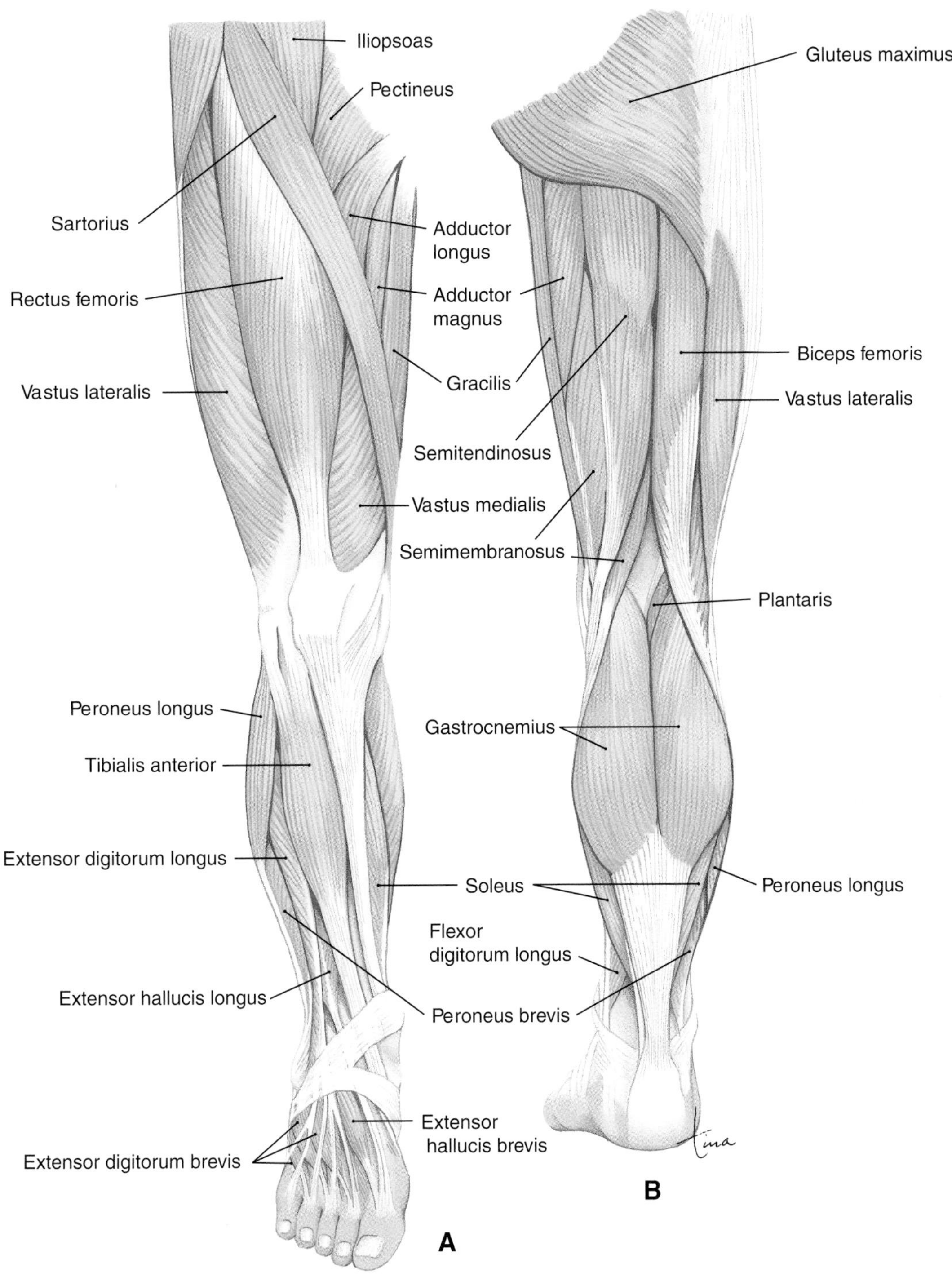

Figure 7–12 Muscles of the leg. (**A**) Anterior view. (**B**) Posterior view.

QUESTION: How does the gastrocnemius compare in size to the tibialis anterior? What is the reason for this difference?

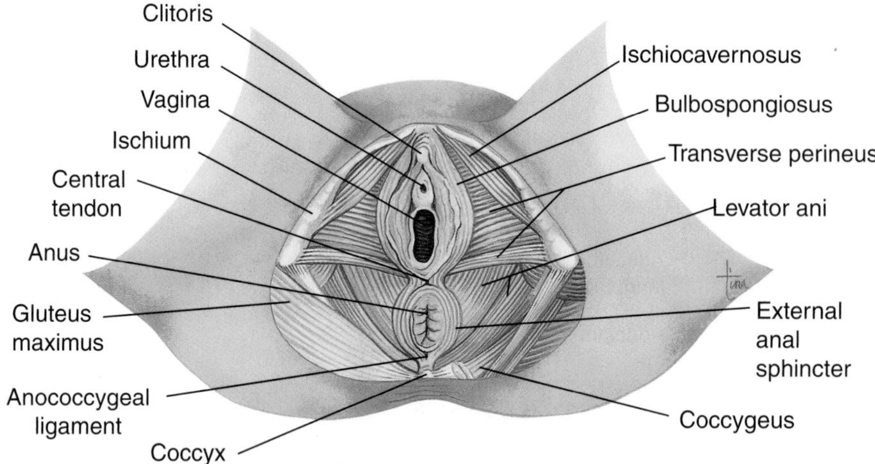

Figure 7–13 Muscles of the female pelvic floor.

QUESTION: In women, what organs are directly supported by this "floor" of muscles?

Box 7–5 | COMMON INJECTION SITES

Intramuscular injections are used when rapid absorption is needed, because muscle has a good blood supply. The safest location for an injection is now considered to be the gluteus medius muscle, in what is called the anterior gluteal site. Alternatives are the vastus lateralis muscle of the lateral thigh and the deltoid muscle of the shoulder. These sites are shown; also shown are the large nerves to be avoided when giving such injections.

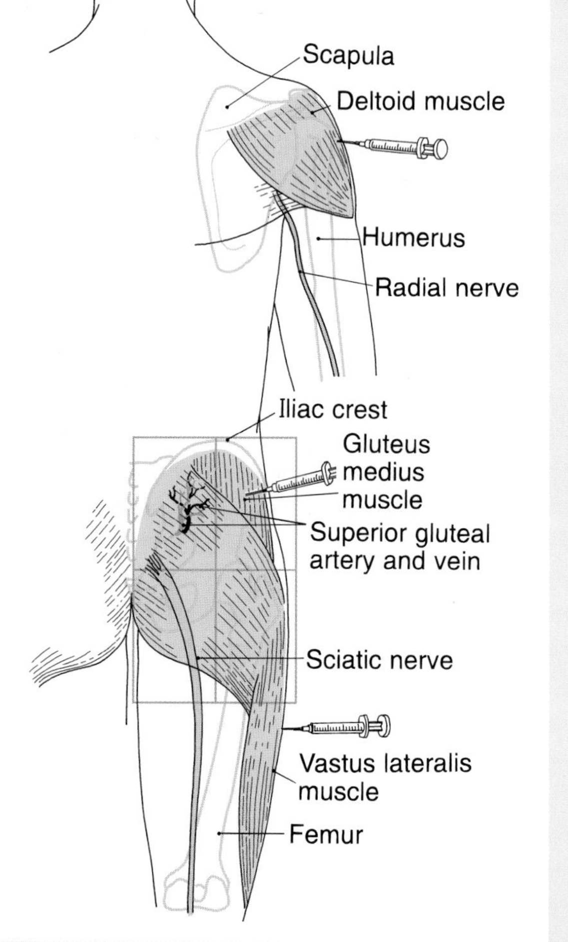

Box Figure 7–A Sites for intramuscular injections. Posterior view of right side of body.

STUDY OUTLINE

Organ Systems Involved in Movement

1. Muscular—moves the bones.
2. Skeletal—bones are moved, at their joints, by muscles.
3. Nervous—transmits impulses to muscles to cause contraction.
4. Respiratory—exchanges O_2 and CO_2 between the air and blood.
5. Circulatory—transports O_2 to muscles and removes CO_2.

Muscle Structure

1. Muscle fibers (cells) are specialized to contract, shorten, and produce movement.
2. A skeletal muscle is made of thousands of muscle fibers. Varying movements require contraction of variable numbers of muscle fibers in a muscle.
3. Tendons attach muscles to bone; the origin is the more stationary bone, the insertion is the more movable bone. A tendon merges with the fascia of a muscle and the periosteum of a bone; all are made of fibrous connective tissue.

Muscle Arrangements

1. Antagonistic muscles have opposite functions. A muscle pulls when it contracts but exerts no force when it relaxes and it cannot push. When one muscle pulls a bone in one direction, another muscle is needed to pull the bone in the other direction (see also Table 7–4 and Fig. 7–1).
2. Synergistic muscles have the same function and alternate as the prime mover depending on the position of the bone to be moved. Synergists also stabilize a joint to make a more precise movement possible.
3. The frontal lobes of the cerebrum generate the impulses necessary for contraction of skeletal muscles. The cerebellum regulates coordination.
4. A motor unit consists of a motor neuron and all of the muscle fibers its branched axon innervates; precise movements require motors units with fewer than 100 muscle fibers.

Muscle Tone and Exercise

1. Muscle tone is the state of slight contraction present in healthy muscles; alternate fibers (different motor units) contract to prevent muscle fatigue; regulated by the cerebellum.
2. Good tone helps maintain posture, produces 25% of body heat (at rest), and improves coordination.
3. Isotonic exercise involves contraction with movement; improves tone and strength and improves cardiovascular and respiratory efficiency (aerobic exercise).
   a. Concentric contraction—muscle exerts force while shortening.
   b. Eccentric contraction—muscle exerts force while lengthening.
4. Isometric exercise involves contraction without movement; improves tone and strength but is not aerobic.

5. Exercise stimulates skeletal muscle cells to secrete the hormone irisin, which converts fat-storing white adipocytes to thermogenic brown adipocytes.

Muscle Sense—proprioception: knowing where our muscles are without looking at them

1. Permits us to perform everyday activities without having to concentrate on muscle position.
2. Stretch receptors (proprioceptors) in muscles respond to stretching and generate impulses that the brain interprets as a mental "picture" of where the muscles are. Parietal lobes: conscious muscle sense; cerebellum: unconscious muscle sense used to promote coordination.

Energy Sources for Muscle Contraction

1. ATP is the direct source; the ATP stored in muscles lasts for only a few seconds of contraction.
2. Creatine phosphate is a secondary energy source; is broken down to creatine + phosphate + energy. The energy is used to synthesize more ATP. Some creatine is converted to creatinine, which must be excreted by the kidneys. Most creatine is used for the resynthesis of creatine phosphate.
3. Glycogen is the most abundant energy source and is first broken down to glucose. Glucose is broken down in cell respiration:

$$\text{Glucose} + O_2 \rightarrow CO_2 + H_2O + \text{ATP} + \text{heat}$$

   ATP is used for contraction; heat contributes to body temperature; H_2O becomes part of intracellular fluid; CO_2 is eventually exhaled.
4. Oxygen is essential for the completion of cell respiration. Hemoglobin in red blood cells carries oxygen to muscles; myoglobin stores oxygen in muscles; both of these proteins contain iron, which enables them to bond to oxygen.
5. Oxygen debt (recovery oxygen uptake): Muscle fibers run out of oxygen during strenuous exercise, and glucose is converted to lactic acid, which lowers cellular pH and contributes to fatigue. Breathing rate remains high after exercise to deliver more oxygen to the liver, which converts lactic acid to pyruvic acid, a simple carbohydrate (ATP required).

Muscle Fiber—microscopic structure

1. Neuromuscular junction: axon terminal and sarcolemma; the synapse is the space between. The axon terminal contains acetylcholine (a neurotransmitter), and the sarcolemma contains cholinesterase (an inactivator) (see Fig. 7–2 and Table 7–1).
2. Sarcomeres are the contracting units of a muscle fiber. Myosin and actin filaments are the contracting proteins of sarcomeres. Troponin and tropomyosin are proteins that inhibit the sliding of myosin and actin when the muscle fiber is relaxed (see Figs. 7–3 and 7–5).
3. The sarcoplasmic reticulum surrounds the sarcomeres and is a reservoir for calcium ions.
4. Polarization (resting potential): When the muscle fiber is relaxed, the sarcolemma has a positive (+) charge outside and a negative (–) charge inside. Na^+ ions are more abundant outside the cell and K^+ ions are more abundant inside the

cell. The Na^+ and K^+ pumps maintain these relative concentrations on either side of the sarcolemma (see Table 7–2 and Fig. 7–4).

5. Depolarization: This process is started by a nerve impulse. Acetylcholine released by the axon terminal makes the sarcolemma very permeable to Na^+ ions, which enter the cell and cause a reversal of charges to negative (–) outside and positive (+) inside. The depolarization spreads along the entire sarcolemma and initiates the contraction process. Folds of the sarcolemma called T tubules carry the depolarization into the interior of the muscle cell. Repolarization is the exit of K^+ ions and the restoration of a positive (+) charge outside. An action potential (or impulse) is depolarization followed by repolarization.

Contraction—the sliding filament mechanism (see Fig. 7–5 and Table 7–3)

1. Depolarization stimulates a sequence of events that enables myosin filaments to pull the actin filaments to the center of the sarcomere, which shortens.
2. All of the sarcomeres in a muscle fiber contract in response to a nerve impulse; the entire cell contracts.
3. Tetanus is a sustained contraction brought about by continuous nerve impulses; all our movements involve tetanus.
4. Paralysis: Muscles that do not receive nerve impulses are unable to contract and will atrophy. Paralysis may be the result of nerve damage, spinal cord damage, or brain damage.

Responses to Exercise—maintaining homeostasis

See section in chapter and Fig. 7–6.

Major Muscles

See Tables 7–4 through 7–9 and Figs. 7–7 through 7–13.

REVIEW QUESTIONS

1. Name the organ systems directly involved in movement, and for each state how they are involved. (p. 154)
2. State the function of tendons. Name the part of a muscle and a bone to which a tendon is attached. (p. 154)
3. State the term for: (p. 155)
   - a. Muscles with the same function
   - b. Muscles with opposite functions
   - c. The muscle that does most of the work in a movement
4. Explain why antagonistic muscle arrangements are necessary. Give two examples. (p. 155)
5. State three reasons why good muscle tone is important. (p. 156)
6. Explain why muscle sense is important. Name the receptors involved and state what they detect. (p. 157)
7. With respect to muscle contraction, state the functions of the cerebellum and the frontal lobes of the cerebrum. (p. 156)
8. Name the direct energy source for muscle contraction. Name the two secondary energy sources. Which of these is more abundant? (p. 158)
9. State the simple reaction of cell respiration and what happens to each of the products of this reaction. (p. 158)
10. Name the two sources of oxygen for muscle fibers. State what the two proteins have in common. (p. 158)
11. Explain what is meant by oxygen debt. What is needed to correct oxygen debt, and where does it come from? (p. 158)
12. Name these parts of the neuromuscular junction: (p. 158)
    - a. The membrane of the muscle fiber
    - b. The end of the motor neuron
    - c. The space between neuron and muscle cell

    State the locations of acetylcholine and cholinesterase. (p.158)
13. Name the contracting proteins of sarcomeres, and describe their locations in a sarcomere. Where is the sarcoplasmic reticulum and what does it contain? (pp. 158–159)
14. In terms of ions and charges, describe: (pp. 160, 162)
    - a. Polarization
    - b. Depolarization
    - c. Repolarization
15. With respect to the sliding filament mechanism, explain the function of: (pp. 160–163)
    - a. Acetylcholine
    - b. Calcium ions
    - c. Myosin and actin
    - d. Troponin and tropomyosin
    - e. Cholinesterase
16. State three of the body's physiological responses to exercise, and explain how each helps maintain homeostasis. (pp. 164–166)
17. Find the major muscles on yourself, and state a function of each muscle. (pp. 169–178)

FOR FURTHER THOUGHT

1. In an accident with farm machinery, Mr. R. had his left arm severed just below the elbow. Mrs. R. stopped the bleeding, called for an ambulance, and packed the severed arm in ice for the EMTs to take to the hospital. Will Mr. R. ever be able to move the fingers of his left hand again? What structures must be reattached, and what has to happen?
2. Muscle contraction is important for posture. Muscles oppose each other, contracting equally to keep us upright. Picture the body in anatomic position, and describe what would happen if each of these muscles *relaxed* completely:
   - Semispinalis capitis
   - Masseter
   - Rectus abdominis
   - Sacrospinalis
   - Quadriceps femoris
   - Gluteus maximus
3. An exercise for skiers involves sitting against a wall as if you were sitting in a chair, but without a chair. Thighs should be parallel to the floor and the knees should make a 90° angle. Try it. What kind of exercise is this? Which muscles are doing most of the work (which ones begin to hurt)? Which do you think would be easier: 3 minutes of this exercise or 3 minutes of jogging? Can you think of an explanation?
4. Can you juggle? Don't just say "no"—have you ever tried? Find some old tennis balls and try juggling two balls with one hand, or three balls with two hands. Explain how muscle sense is involved in juggling.

   Now try to imagine what it would be like to be without muscle sense. Some people do not have muscle sense in certain parts of their bodies. Who are these people, and what has happened that cost them their muscle sense (and muscle contraction)?
5. Look at Question Figure 7–A. This is a transverse section of the right thigh. If you are seated, put your right hand on the middle of your own right thigh; that is the site of the section, and the front of the thigh is at the top of the picture. The sartorius is labeled for you. Can you name the other groups of muscles, labeled A, B, and C?

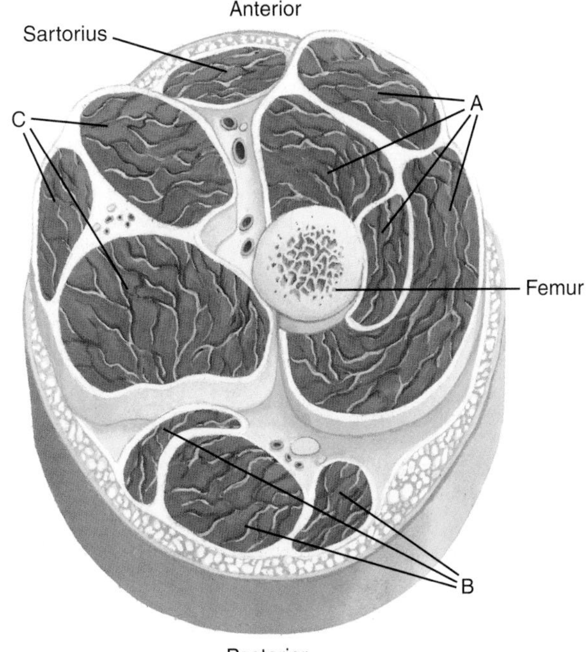

QUESTION FIGURE 7–A Transverse section of right thigh.

CHAPTER

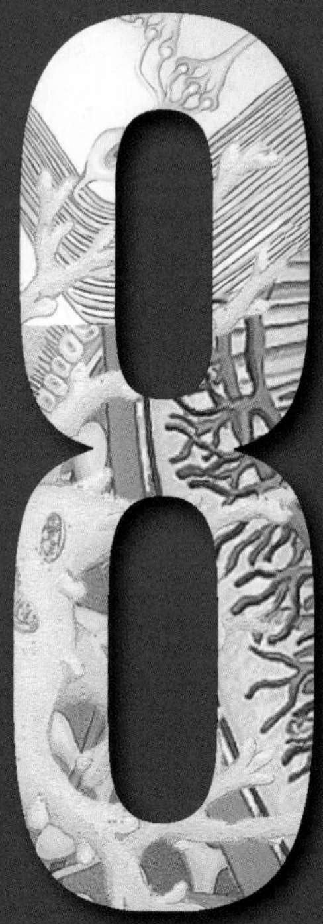

The Nervous System

STUDENT OBJECTIVES

- Name the divisions of the nervous system and the parts of each, and state the general functions of the nervous system.
- Name the parts of a neuron and state the function of each.
- Explain the importance of Schwann cells in the peripheral nervous system and neuroglia in the central nervous system.
- Describe the electrical nerve impulse, and describe impulse transmission at synapses.
- Describe the types of neurons, nerves, and nerve tracts.
- State the names and numbers of the spinal nerves, as well as their destinations.
- Explain the importance of stretch reflexes and flexor reflexes.
- State the functions of the parts of the brain; be able to locate each part on a diagram.
- Name the meninges and describe their locations.
- State the locations and functions of cerebrospinal fluid.
- Name the cranial nerves, and state their functions.
- Explain how the sympathetic division of the autonomic nervous system enables the body to adapt to a stress situation.
- Explain how the parasympathetic division of the autonomic nervous system promotes normal body functioning in relaxed situations.

NEW TERMINOLOGY

Afferent *(**AFF**-uh-rent)*

Autonomic nervous system *(AW-toh-**NOM**-ik)*

Cauda equina *(**KAW**-dah ee-**KWHY**-nah)*

Cerebral cortex *(se-**REE**-bruhl **KOR**-teks)*

Cerebrospinal fluid *(se-**REE**-broh-**SPY**-nuhl)*

Choroid plexus *(**KOR**-oid **PLEK**-sus)*

Corpus callosum *(**KOR**-pus kuh-**LOH**-sum)*

Cranial nerves *(**KRAY**-nee-uhl NERVS)*

Efferent *(**EFF**-uh-rent)*

Gray matter *(GRAY **MA**-TUR)*

Neuroglia *(new-**ROG**-lee-ah)*

Neurolemma *(NYOO-ro-**LEM**-ah)*

Parasympathetic *(PAR-uh-SIM-puh-**THET**-ik)*

Reflex *(**REE**-fleks)*

Somatic *(soh-**MA**-tik)*

Spinal nerves *(**SPY**-nuhl NERVS)*

Sympathetic *(SIM-puh-**THET**-ik)*

Ventricles of brain *(**VEN**-trick'ls)*

Visceral *(**VISS**-er-uhl)*

White matter *(WIGHT **MA**-TUR)*

*Terms that appear in **bold type** in the chapter text are defined in the glossary, which begins on page 603.*

CHAPTER OUTLINE

RELATED CLINICAL TERMINOLOGY

Alzheimer's disease *(**ALZ**-high-mer's duh-ZEEZ)*

Aphasia *(ah-**FAY**-zhuh)*

Blood–brain barrier *(BLUHD BRAYNE-BARE-ee-ur)*

Cerebrovascular accident (CVA) *(se-**REE**-broh-**VAS**-kyoo-lur AX-uh-dent)*

Lumbar puncture *(**LUM**-bar **PUNK**-chur)*

Meningitis *(MEN-in-**JIGH**-tis)*

Multiple sclerosis (MS) *(**MULL**-ti-puhl skle-**ROH**-sis)*

Neuralgia *(new-**RAL**-juh)*

Neuritis *(new-**RYE**-tis)*

Neuropathy *(new-**RAH**-puh-thee)*

Parkinson's disease *(**PAR**-kin-sonz duh-ZEEZ)*

Remission *(ree-**MISH**-uhn)*

Spinal shock *(**SPY**-nuhl SHAHK)*

Most of us can probably remember being told, when we were children, not to touch the stove or some other source of potential harm. Because children are curious, such warnings often go unheeded. The result? Touching a hot stove brings about an immediate response of pulling away and a vivid memory of painful fingers. This simple and familiar experience illustrates the functions of the **nervous system**:

1. To detect changes and feel sensations
2. To initiate appropriate responses to changes
3. To organize information for immediate use and store it for future use

The nervous system is one of the regulating systems (the endocrine system is the other and is discussed in Chapter 10). The electrochemical impulses of the nervous system make it possible to obtain information about the external or internal environment and do whatever is necessary to maintain homeostasis. Some of this activity is conscious, but much of it happens without our awareness.

NERVOUS SYSTEM DIVISIONS

The nervous system has two divisions. The **central nervous system** (**CNS**) consists of the brain and spinal cord. The **peripheral nervous system** (**PNS**) consists of cranial nerves and spinal nerves. The PNS includes nerves to and from skin and skeletal muscles. It also includes the autonomic nervous system (ANS), with nerves to visceral effectors, and the enteric nervous system, which is located in the wall of the alimentary tube (and will be covered in Chapter 16).

The peripheral nervous system relays information to and from the central nervous system, and the brain is the center of activity that integrates this information, initiates responses, and makes us the individuals we are.

NERVE TISSUE

Nerve tissue was briefly described in Chapter 4, so we will begin by reviewing what you already know and then add to it.

Nerve cells are called **neurons**, or **nerve fibers**. Whatever their specific functions, all neurons have the same physical parts. The **cell body** contains the nucleus (Fig. 8–1) and is essential for the continued life of the neuron. As you will see, neuron cell bodies are found in the central nervous system or close to it in the trunk of the body. In these locations, cell bodies are protected by bone. There are no cell bodies in the arms and legs, which are much more subject to injury.

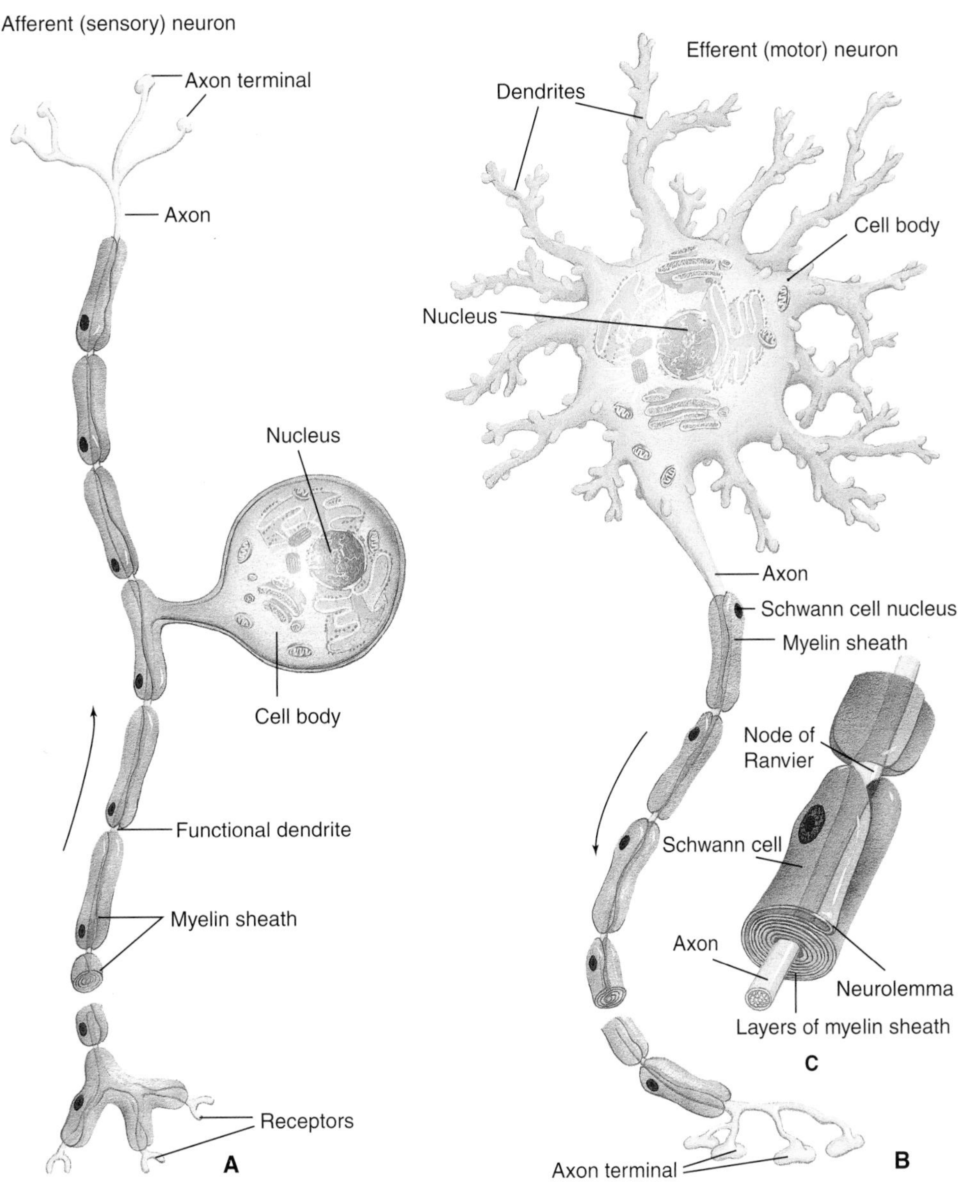

Figure 8–1 Neuron structure. (**A**) A typical sensory neuron. (**B**) A typical motor neuron. The arrows indicate the direction of impulse transmission. (**C**) Details of the myelin sheath and neurolemma formed by Schwann cells.

QUESTION: The axon terminal of the motor neuron would be found at what kinds of effectors?

Dendrites are processes (extensions) that transmit electrical impulses toward the cell body. The one **axon** of a neuron transmits impulses away from the cell body, perhaps to another neuron, or to an effector cell of muscle or glandular tissue. It is the cell membrane of the dendrites, cell body, and axon that carries the electrical nerve impulse.

In the peripheral nervous system, axons and dendrites are "wrapped" in specialized cells called **Schwann cells** (see Fig. 8–1). During embryonic development, Schwann cells grow to surround the neuron processes, enclosing them in several layers of Schwann cell membrane. These layers are the **myelin sheath**; myelin is a phospholipid that electrically insulates neurons from one another. Without the myelin sheath, neurons would short-circuit, just as electrical wires would if they were not insulated (see Box 8–1: Multiple Sclerosis).

The spaces between adjacent Schwann cells, or segments of the myelin sheath, are called nodes of Ranvier (neurofibril nodes). These nodes are the parts of the neuron cell membrane that depolarize when an electrical impulse is transmitted (see "saltatory conduction" in the next section).

The nuclei and cytoplasm of the Schwann cells are wrapped around the outside of the myelin sheath and are called the **neurolemma** (or neurilemma), which becomes very important if nerves are damaged. If a peripheral nerve is severed and reattached precisely by microsurgery, the axons and dendrites may regenerate through the tunnels formed by the neurolemmas. The Schwann cells are also believed to produce a chemical growth factor that stimulates regeneration. Although this regeneration may take months, the nerves may eventually reestablish their proper connections, and the person may regain some sensation and movement in the once-severed limb.

In the central nervous system, the myelin sheaths are formed by **oligodendrocytes**, one of the **neuroglia** (**glial cells**), the specialized cells found only in the brain and spinal cord. Because no Schwann cells are present, however, there is no neurolemma, and regeneration of neurons does not occur. This is why severing of the spinal cord, for example, results in permanent loss of function. **Microglia** are another kind of neuroglia; these cells are phagocytes and are constantly moving. They clean up cellular debris and damaged cells and phagocytize pathogens.

Yet another type of glial cell is the **astrocyte** (literally, "star cell"). In the embryo, these cells provide a framework for the migrating neurons that will form the brain. Thereafter, the extensions of astrocytes are wrapped around neurons and around brain capillaries (see Table Fig. 8–A in Table 8–1), and these cells are not passive supports. Astrocytes help regulate localized blood flow within the brain. They are believed to detect the release of neurotransmitters by neurons, and to increase blood flow when their neurons become more active. Astrocytes also contribute to the **blood–brain barrier**, which prevents potentially harmful waste products in the blood from diffusing out into brain tissue. These waste products are normal in the blood and tissue fluid, but brain tissue is much more sensitive to even low levels of them than are other tissues such as muscle tissue or connective tissue. The capillaries of the brain also contribute to this barrier because their cells are tightly packed edge

Box 8–1 | MULTIPLE SCLEROSIS

Multiple sclerosis (MS) is a demyelinating disease; that is, it involves deterioration of the myelin sheath of neurons in the central nervous system. Without the myelin sheath, the impulses of these neurons are short-circuited and do not reach their proper destinations; hence, the neuron axons are damaged and gradually die.

Multiple sclerosis is an **autoimmune** disorder that is brought on by both genetic and environmental factors. Exactly how genes increase a person's susceptibility to an autoimmune disease is still unknown. Environmental factors that increase the risk for MS include infection with the Epstein-Barr virus and a deficiency of vitamin D. In MS, the autoantibodies that are produced destroy the oligodendrocytes, the myelin-producing neuroglia of the central nervous system, which results in the formation of scleroses, or plaques of scar tissue, that do not provide electrical insulation or protect the axon. Because loss of myelin may occur in many parts of the central nervous system, the symptoms vary, but they usually include muscle weakness or paralysis, numbness or partial loss of sensation, double vision, and loss of spinal cord reflexes, including those for urination and defecation.

The first symptoms usually appear between the ages of 20 and 40 years, and the disease may progress either slowly or rapidly. Some MS patients have **remissions**, periods of time when their symptoms diminish, but remissions and progression of the disease are not predictable. There is still no cure for MS, but therapies include suppression of the immune response, and interferon, which seems to prolong remissions in some patients. The possibility of stimulating remyelination of neurons is also being investigated.

Table 8–1 | NEUROGLIA

NAME	FUNCTION
Oligodendrocytes	Produce the segments of the myelin sheath to electrically insulate neurons of the CNS.
Microglia	Capable of movement and phagocytosis of pathogens and damaged tissue.
Astrocytes	Provide a framework for the developing fetal brain and support established neurons Regulate localized blood flow in response to brain activity Help maintain K^+ level Contribute to the blood–brain barrier.
Ependyma	Line the ventricles of the brain and central canal of the spinal cord; many of the cells have cilia; involved in circulation of cerebrospinal fluid.

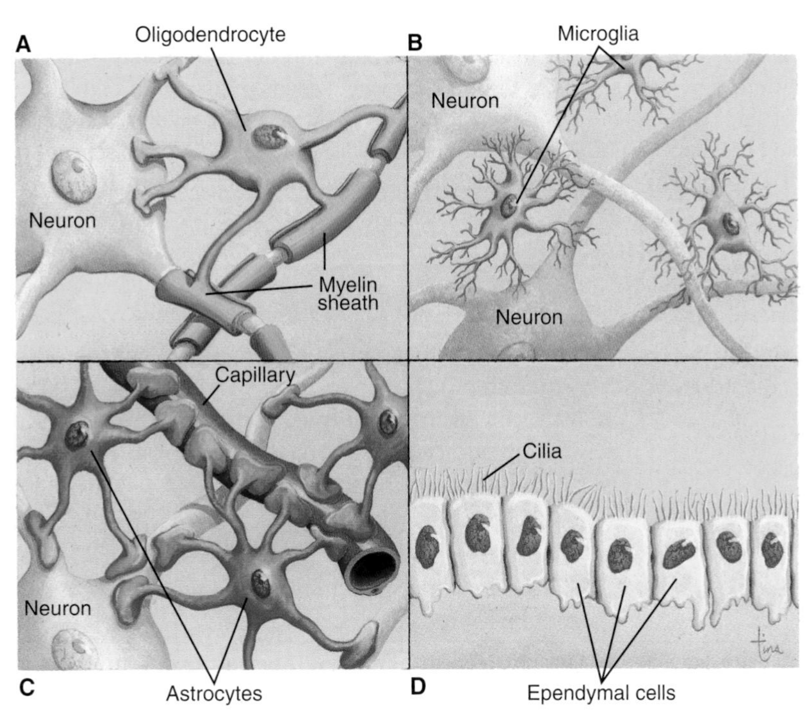

Table Figure 8–A Neuroglia. (A) Oligodendrocyte. (B) Microglia. (C) Astrocytes. (D) Ependymal cells.

QUESTION: Which of these CNS cells is the counterpart of Schwann cells in the PNS, and why?

to edge, making brain capillaries less permeable than other capillaries. Some harmful chemicals, such as alcohol and nicotine, do cross the blood–brain barrier, and the rabies virus is a pathogen that can cross it. A disadvantage of the blood–brain barrier is that some useful medications cannot cross it, and the antibodies produced by lymphocytes cross only with difficulty. This becomes an important consideration when treating brain infections or other diseases or disorders (Table 8–1 summarizes the functions of the neuroglia).

THE NERVE IMPULSE

The events of an electrical nerve impulse are the same as those of the electrical impulse generated in muscle fibers, which is discussed in Chapter 7. Stated simply, a neuron not carrying an impulse is in a state of **polarization**, with Na^+ ions more abundant outside the cell and K^+ ions and negative ions more abundant inside the cell. The neuron has a positive charge on the outside of the cell membrane and a relative negative charge inside. A stimulus (such as a neurotransmitter) makes the membrane very permeable to Na^+ ions, which rush into the cell. This brings about **depolarization**, a reversal of charges on the membrane. The outside now has a negative charge, and the inside has a positive charge.

As soon as depolarization takes place, the neuron membrane becomes very permeable to K^+ ions, which rush out of the cell. This restores the positive charge outside and the negative charge inside and is called **repolarization**. (The term *action potential* refers to depolarization followed by repolarization.) Then the sodium and potassium pumps return Na^+ ions outside and K^+ ions inside, and the neuron is ready to respond to another stimulus and transmit another impulse. An action potential in response to a stimulus takes place very rapidly and is measured in milliseconds. An individual neuron is capable of transmitting hundreds of action potentials (impulses) each second. A summary of the events of nerve impulse transmission is given in Table 8–2.

Transmission of electrical impulses is very rapid. The presence of an insulating myelin sheath increases the velocity of impulses, since only the nodes of Ranvier depolarize. This is called **saltatory conduction**. Many of our neurons are capable of transmitting impulses at a speed of many meters per second. Imagine a person 6 feet (about 2 meters) tall who stubs a toe; sensory impulses travel from the toe to the brain in less than a second (crossing a few synapses along the way, and although diffusion across synapses is slow, the synapses are so small that this does not significantly affect the velocity of impulses in a living person). Electrical impulses enable the nervous system to communicate very rapidly with all parts of the body, making it such an important regulatory system.

You may have read or heard that nerve impulses can be called "messages," as in, "sensory neurons send messages to the brain," or "the brain sends messages to muscles." To

Table 8–2 | THE NERVE IMPULSE

STATE OR EVENT	DESCRIPTION
Polarization (the neuron is not carrying an electrical impulse)	■ Neuron membrane has a positive (+) charge outside and a negative (−) charge inside. ■ Na^+ ions are more abundant outside the cell. ■ K^+ ions and negative ions are more abundant inside the cell. Sodium and potassium pumps maintain these ion concentrations.
Depolarization (generated by a stimulus)	■ Neuron membrane becomes very permeable to Na^+ ions, which rush into the cell. ■ The neuron membrane then has a negative (−) charge outside and a positive (+) charge inside.
Propagation of the impulse from point of stimulus	■ Depolarization of part of the membrane makes adjacent membrane very permeable to Na^+ ions, and subsequent depolarization, which similarly affects the next part of the membrane, and so on. ■ The depolarization continues along the membrane of the neuron to the end of the axon.
Repolarization (immediately follows depolarization to complete the action potential)	■ Neuron membrane becomes very permeable to K^+ ions, which rush out of the cell. This restores the positive (+) charge outside and negative (−) charge inside the membrane. ■ The Na^+ ions are returned outside and the K^+ ions are returned inside by the sodium and potassium pumps. ■ The neuron is now able to respond to another stimulus and generate another impulse.

understand how the nervous system works, however, this may not be the best analogy. A message says something; e-mails, letters, or phone calls say something specific and rarely the same. Nerve impulses, however, are all exactly the same—the same electrical action potentials. The effect of a nerve impulse is not a quality of the impulse itself, but rather of its destination. For example, when a person takes a step, nerve impulses from the left foot arrive in the cutaneous area for the left foot in the right parietal lobe of the cerebrum, and the person feels the left foot hit the floor. If those impulses could be routed to the area for the right foot in the left parietal lobe (this type of experiment has been done with rats), we would feel as if the right foot were hitting the floor instead of the left.

Destination is all that matters; the recipient is all that matters. Just as the electricity (all the same) carried by the wires of a house can enable different appliances to fulfill their purposes (from refrigerators to hair dryers to light bulbs), so too can nerve impulses enable bodily functions. Impulses arriving at sweat glands bring about secretion of sweat, because that is what these glandular cells do. Impulses arriving in the visual area of the occipital lobe bring about a sensation of seeing something, because that is what these neurons do. Impulses arriving at skeletal muscle cells bring about contraction, because that is what muscle cells do. Therefore, a nerve impulse is not in itself a message. If anything, a nerve impulse may be considered more like a switch or simple signal, in that it activates (or inhibits) the cell, tissue, or organ of its destination.

In keeping with this idea, the brain may be likened to the conductor of an orchestra. And let us say the musicians are the skeletal muscles (of the legs, trunk, and arms) needed to climb a mountain. Each muscle is structured so as to do a particular job, as each musician is trained on a specific instrument. The conductor does not play the bassoon or trumpet or timpani or cello but will cue the musicians to play their parts. These cues will also signal the proper time for each, and in the proper sequence; for muscle activity, this would be coordination. The cues by the conductor—the signals—are very much the same. The signals are not the effect; the recipients of the signals create the effect.

On their way to their recipient (or effector) cells, electrical nerve impulses cross one or more synapses. You may recall from Chapter 4 that at the synapses, nerve impulse transmission changes from electrical to chemical and depends on the release of neurotransmitters.

SYNAPSES

Neurons that transmit impulses to other neurons (or to effector cells) do not actually touch one another. The small gap or space between the axon of one neuron and the dendrites or cell body of the next neuron is called the **synapse**. Within the synaptic knob (terminal end) of the presynaptic axon is a chemical **neurotransmitter** that is released into the synapse by the arrival of an electrical nerve impulse (Fig. 8–2). The neurotransmitter diffuses across the synapse, combines with specific receptor sites on the cell membrane of the postsynaptic neuron, and there generates an electrical impulse that is, in turn, carried by this neuron's axon to the next synapse, and so forth. A chemical **inactivator** at the cell body or dendrite of the postsynaptic neuron quickly inactivates the neurotransmitter. This prevents unwanted, continuous impulses, unless a new impulse from the first neuron releases more neurotransmitter.

Many synapses are termed excitatory, because the neurotransmitter causes the postsynaptic neuron to depolarize (become more negative outside as Na^+ ions enter the cell) and transmit an electrical impulse to another neuron, muscle cell, or gland. Some synapses, however, are inhibitory, meaning that the neurotransmitter causes the postsynaptic neuron to hyperpolarize (become even more positive outside as K^+ ions leave the cell or Cl^- ions enter the cell) and therefore *not* transmit an electrical impulse. Such inhibitory synapses are important, for example, for slowing the heart rate and for balancing the excitatory impulses transmitted to skeletal muscles. With respect to the skeletal muscles, this inhibition prevents excessive contraction and is necessary for coordination.

One important consequence of the presence of synapses is that they ensure one-way transmission of impulses in a living person. A nerve impulse cannot go backward across a synapse because no neurotransmitter is released by the dendrites or cell body. Neurotransmitters can be released only by a neuron's axon, which does not have receptor sites for it, as does the postsynaptic membrane. Keep this in mind when we discuss the types of neurons later in the chapter.

An example of a neurotransmitter is **acetylcholine**, which is found at neuromuscular junctions, in the CNS, and in much of the peripheral nervous system. Acetylcholine usually makes a postsynaptic membrane more permeable to Na^+ ions, which brings about depolarization of the postsynaptic neuron. **Cholinesterase** is the inactivator of acetylcholine. There are many other neurotransmitters, especially in the central nervous system. These include dopamine, GABA, norepinephrine, glutamate, and serotonin. Each of these neurotransmitters has its own chemical inactivator. Some neurotransmitters are reabsorbed into the neurons that secreted them; this process

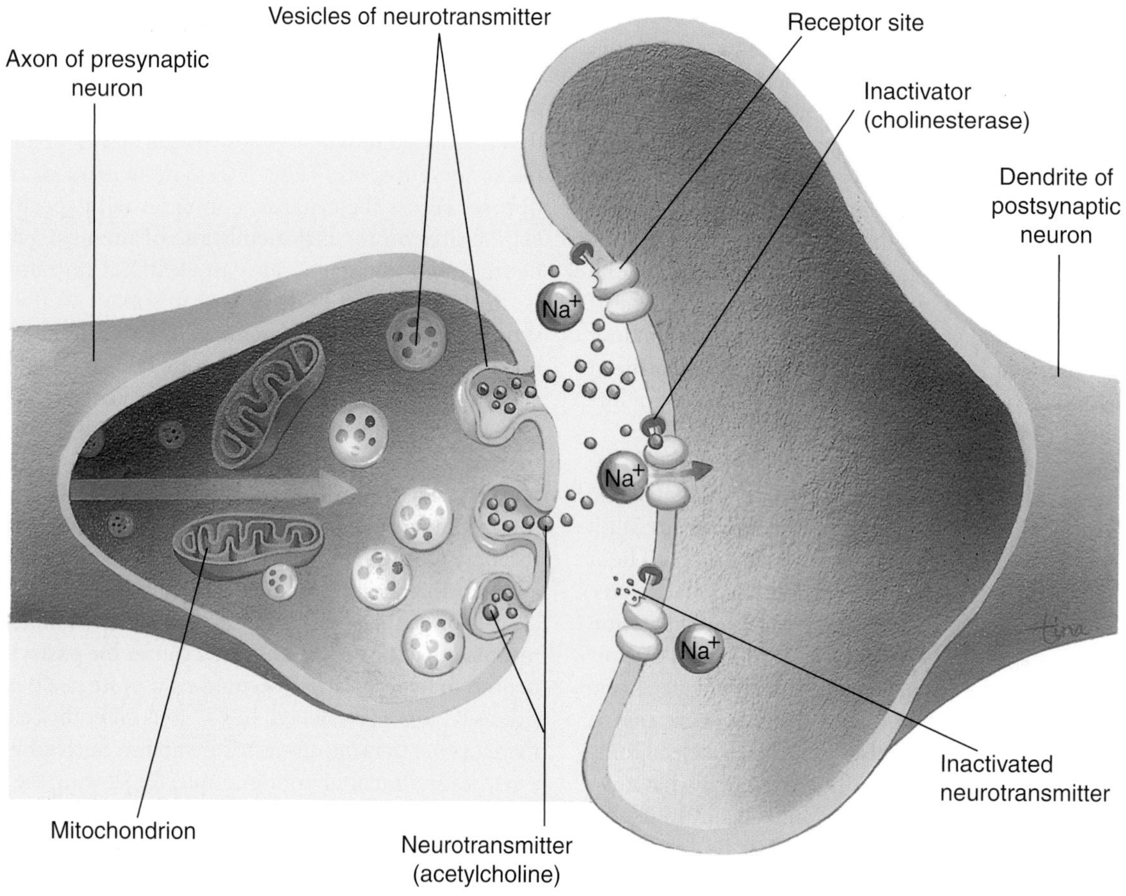

Figure 8–2 Impulse transmission at a synapse. The arrow indicates the direction of the electrical impulse.

QUESTION: Is this an excitatory synapse or an inhibitory synapse? Explain your answer.

is called **reuptake** and also terminates the effect of the transmitter.

The complexity and variety of synapses make them frequent targets of medications. For example, drugs that alter mood or behavior often act on specific neurotransmitters in the brain, and antihypertensive drugs affect synapse transmission at the smooth muscle of blood vessels.

TYPES OF NEURONS

Neurons may be classified into three groups: sensory neurons, motor neurons, and interneurons (Fig. 8–3). **Sensory neurons** (or **afferent neurons**) carry impulses from receptors to the central nervous system. **Receptors** detect external or internal changes and send the information to the CNS in the form of impulses by way of the afferent neurons. The central nervous system interprets these impulses as a sensation. Sensory neurons from receptors in skin, skeletal muscles, and joints are called **somatic**; those from receptors in internal organs are called **visceral** sensory neurons.

Motor neurons (or **efferent neurons**) carry impulses from the central nervous system to **effectors**. The two types of effectors are muscles and glands. In response to impulses, muscles contract or relax and glands secrete. Motor neurons linked to skeletal muscle are called somatic; those to smooth muscle, cardiac muscle, and glands are called visceral.

Sensory and motor neurons make up the peripheral nervous system. Visceral motor neurons form the autonomic nervous system, a specialized subdivision of the PNS that will be discussed later in this chapter.

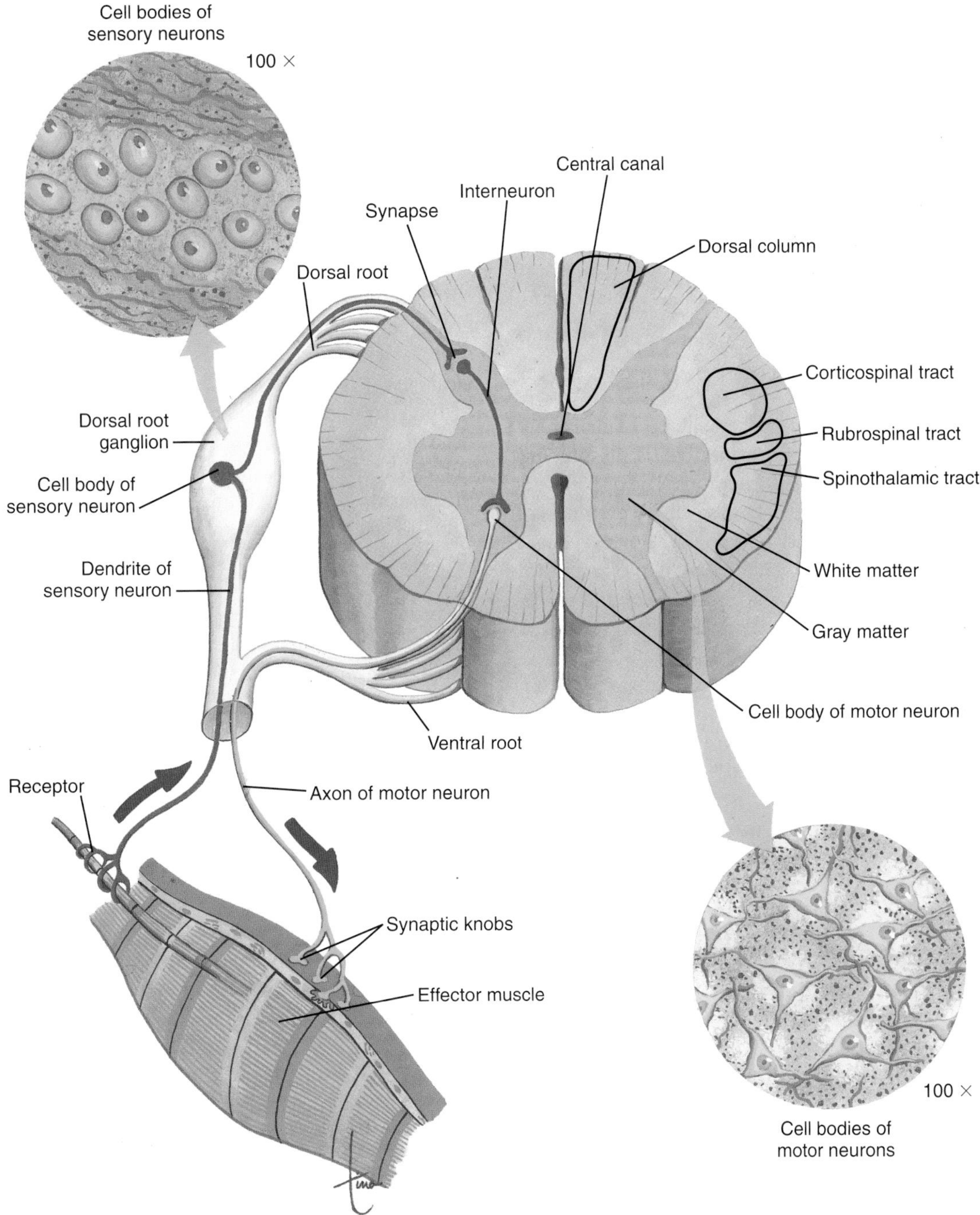

Figure 8–3 Cross-section of the spinal cord and the three types of neurons. Spinal nerve roots and their neurons are shown on the left side. Spinal nerve tracts are shown in the white matter on the right side. All tracts and nerves are bilateral (both sides). Cell bodies of sensory and somatic motor neurons are also shown.

QUESTION: The dorsal column is an ascending tract, and the corticospinal tract is descending. Explain what this means.

Interneurons are found entirely within the central nervous system. They are arranged so as to carry only sensory or motor impulses, or to integrate these functions. Some interneurons in the brain are concerned with thinking, learning, and memory.

A neuron carries impulses in only one direction. This is the result of the neuron's structure and location, as well as its physical arrangement with other neurons and the resulting pattern of synapses. The functioning nervous system, therefore, is an enormous network of "one-way streets," and there is no danger of impulses running into and canceling one another out.

NERVES AND NERVE TRACTS

A **nerve** is a group of axons and/or dendrites of many neurons, with blood vessels and connective tissue. **Sensory nerves** are made only of sensory neurons. The optic nerves for vision and olfactory nerves for smell are examples of nerves with a purely sensory function. **Motor nerves** are made only of motor neurons; autonomic nerves are motor nerves. A **mixed nerve** contains both sensory and motor neurons. Most of our peripheral nerves, such as the sciatic nerves in the legs, are mixed nerves.

The term **nerve tract** refers to groups of neurons within the central nervous system. All the neurons in a nerve tract are concerned with either sensory or motor activity. These tracts are often referred to as **white matter** because the myelin sheaths of the neurons give them a white color; this term is used for parts of both the brain and spinal cord.

THE SPINAL CORD

The **spinal cord** transmits impulses to and from the brain and is the integrating center for the spinal cord reflexes. Although this statement of functions is very brief and sounds very simple, the spinal cord is of great importance to the nervous system and to the body as a whole.

Enclosed within the vertebral canal and the meninges, the spinal cord is well protected from mechanical injury. In length, the spinal cord extends from the foramen magnum of the occipital bone to the disc between the first and second lumbar vertebrae.

A cross-section of the spinal cord is shown in Fig. 8–3; refer to it as you read the following. The internal **gray matter** is shaped like the letter H; gray matter consists of the cell bodies of motor neurons and interneurons. The external **white matter** is made of myelinated axons and dendrites of interneurons. These nerve fibers are grouped into nerve tracts on the basis of their functions. **Ascending tracts** (such as the dorsal columns and spinothalamic tracts) carry sensory impulses to the brain. **Descending tracts** (such as the corticospinal and rubrospinal tracts) carry motor impulses away from the brain. Lastly, find the **central canal**; this contains **cerebrospinal fluid** and is continuous with cavities in the brain called ventricles.

SPINAL NERVES

There are 31 pairs of **spinal nerves**, those that emerge from the spinal cord. The nerves are named according to their respective vertebrae: 8 cervical pairs, 12 thoracic pairs, 5 lumbar pairs, 5 sacral pairs, and 1 very small coccygeal pair. These are shown in Fig. 8–4; notice that each nerve is designated by a letter and a number. The 8th cervical nerve is C8, the 1st thoracic nerve is T1, and so on.

In general, the cervical nerves supply the back of the head, neck, shoulders, arms, and diaphragm (the phrenic nerves). The first thoracic nerve also contributes to nerves in the arms. The remaining thoracic nerves supply the trunk of the body. The lumbar and sacral nerves supply the hips, pelvic cavity, and legs. Notice that the lumbar and sacral nerves hang below the end of the spinal cord (in order to reach their proper openings to exit from the vertebral canal); this is called the **cauda equina**, literally, the "horse's tail." Some of the important peripheral nerves and their destinations are listed in Table 8–3.

Each spinal nerve has two roots, which are neurons entering or leaving the spinal cord (see Fig. 8–3). The **dorsal root** is made of sensory neurons that carry impulses into the spinal cord. The **dorsal root ganglion** is an enlarged part of the dorsal root that contains the cell bodies of the sensory neurons (see Fig. 8–3). The term **ganglion** means a group of cell bodies outside the CNS. These cell bodies are within the vertebral canal and are thereby protected from injury (see Box 8–2: Shingles).

The **ventral root** is the motor root; it is made of the axons of motor neurons carrying impulses from the spinal cord to muscles or glands. The cell bodies of these motor neurons, as mentioned previously, are in the gray matter of the spinal cord. When the two nerve roots merge, the spinal nerve thus formed is a mixed nerve.

SPINAL CORD REFLEXES

When you hear the term *reflex*, you may think of an action that "just happens," and in part this is so. A **reflex** is an involuntary response to a stimulus, that is, an automatic action stimulated by a specific change of some kind. **Spinal cord reflexes** are those that do not depend directly on the brain, although the brain may inhibit or enhance them. We do not have to think about these reflexes, which is very important, as you will see.

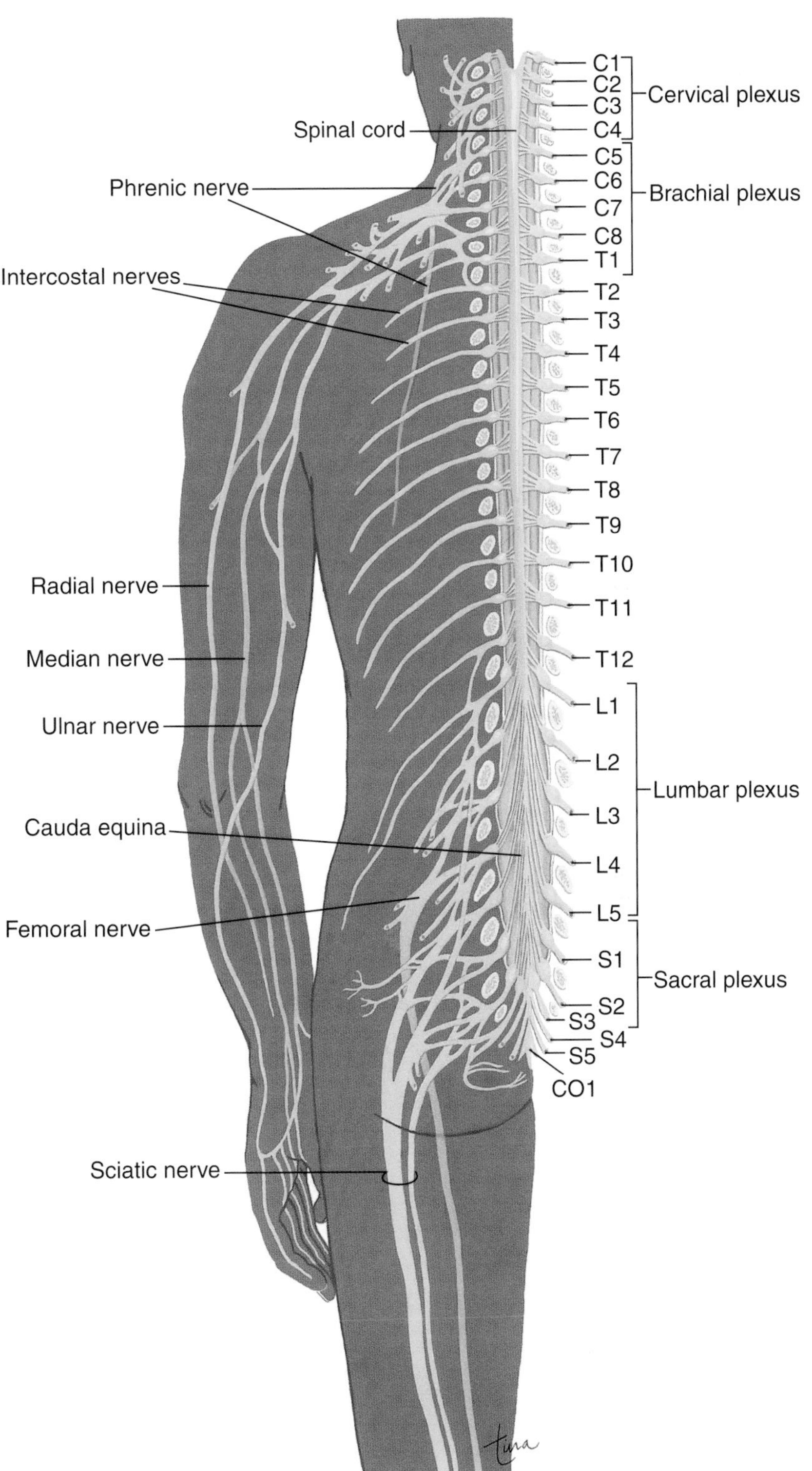

Figure 8–4 The spinal cord and spinal nerves. The distribution of spinal nerves is shown only on the left side. The nerve plexuses are labeled on the right side. A nerve plexus is a network of neurons from several segments of the spinal cord that combine to form nerves to specific parts of the body. For example, the radial and ulnar nerves to the arm emerge from the brachial plexus (see also Table 8–3).

QUESTION: Where does the spinal cord end? Why is this important clinically?

Table 8–3 | **MAJOR PERIPHERAL NERVES**

NERVE	SPINAL NERVES THAT CONTRIBUTE	DISTRIBUTION
Phrenic	C3–C5	Diaphragm
Radial	C5–C8, T1	Skin and muscles of posterior arm, forearm, and hand; thumb and first 2 fingers
Median	C5–C8, T1	Skin and muscles of anterior arm, forearm, and hand
Ulnar	C8, T1	Skin and muscles of medial arm, forearm, and hand; little finger and ring finger
Intercostal	T2–T12	Intercostal muscles, abdominal muscles; skin of trunk
Femoral	L2–L4	Skin and muscles of anterior thigh, medial leg, and foot
Sciatic	L4–S3	Skin and muscles of posterior thigh, leg, and foot

Box 8–2 | SHINGLES

Shingles is caused by the same virus that causes chickenpox: the herpes varicella-zoster virus. Varicella is chickenpox, which was once a common disease of children (there is now a vaccine). When a person recovers from chickenpox, the virus may survive in a dormant (inactive) state in the dorsal root ganglia of some spinal nerves. For most people, the immune system is able to prevent reactivation of the virus. With increasing age, however, the immune system is not as effective, and the virus may become active and cause zoster, or shingles.

The virus is present in sensory neurons, often those of the trunk, but the damage caused by the virus is seen in the skin over the affected nerve. The raised, red lesions of shingles are often very painful and follow the course of the nerve on the skin external to it. Pain may continue even after the rash heals; this is postherpetic neuralgia. Occasionally the virus may affect a cranial nerve and cause facial paralysis called Bell's palsy (7th cranial) or extensive facial lesions, or, rarely, blindness. Although not a cure, some antiviral medications lessen the duration of the illness. A vaccine is available for adults, especially those over 60 years of age, and though it may not completely prevent shingles, it may lessen the chance of postherpetic neuralgia.

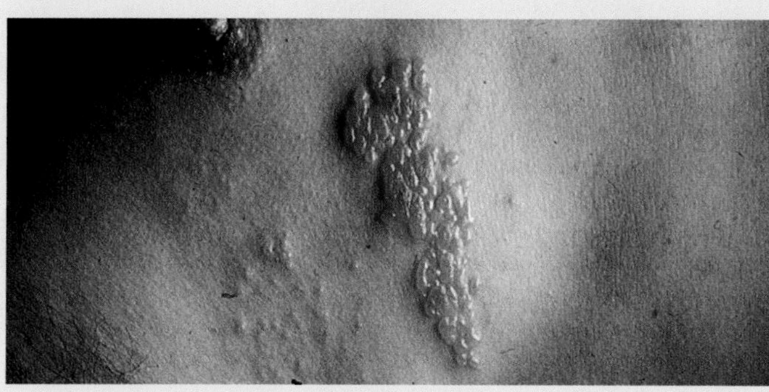

Box Figure 8–A Lesions of shingles on skin of trunk. (From Goldsmith, LA, Lazarus, GS, and Tharp, MD: Adult and Pediatric Dermatology: A Color Guide to Diagnosis and Treatment. FA Davis, Philadelphia, 1997, p 307, with permission.)

Reflex Arc

A reflex arc is the pathway that nerve impulses travel when a reflex is elicited, and there are five essential parts:

1. **Receptors**—detect a change (the stimulus) and generate impulses.
2. **Sensory neurons**—transmit impulses from receptors to the CNS.
3. **Central nervous system**—contains one or more synapses (interneurons may be part of the pathway).
4. **Motor neurons**—transmit impulses from the CNS to the effector.
5. **Effector**—performs its characteristic action.

Let us now look at the reflex arc of a specific reflex, the **patellar** (or knee-jerk) **reflex**, with which you are probably familiar. In this reflex, a tap on the patellar tendon just below the kneecap causes extension of the lower leg. This is a **stretch reflex**, which means that a muscle that is stretched will automatically contract. Refer now to Fig. 8–5 as you read the following:

In the quadriceps femoris muscle are (1) stretch receptors that detect the stretching produced by striking the patellar tendon. These receptors generate impulses that are carried along (2) sensory neurons in the femoral nerve to (3) the spinal cord. In the spinal cord, the sensory neurons synapse with (4) motor neurons (this is a two-neuron reflex). The motor neurons in the femoral nerve carry impulses back to (5) the quadriceps femoris, the effector, which contracts and extends the lower leg.

The patellar reflex is one of many used clinically to determine whether the nervous system is functioning properly. If the patellar reflex were absent in a patient, the problem could be in the thigh muscle, the femoral nerve, or the spinal cord. Further testing would be needed to determine the precise break in the reflex arc. If the reflex is normal, however, that means that all parts of the reflex arc are intact. So the testing of reflexes may be a first step in the clinical assessment of neurologic damage.

You may be wondering why we have such reflexes, these stretch reflexes. What is their importance in our everyday lives? Do they occur? If you have ever seen someone fall asleep while sitting, you may have seen one: the person's head droops and then suddenly snaps up. The posterior neck muscles were stretched by the droop and then contracted, abruptly pulling the head upright. Other stretch reflexes take place less dramatically. Imagine a person standing upright—is the body perfectly still? No, it isn't, because gravity exerts a downward pull. However, if the body tilts to the left, the right sides of the leg and trunk are stretched, and these stretched muscles automatically contract and pull the body upright again. This is the purpose of stretch reflexes; they help keep us upright without our having to think about doing so. If the brain had to

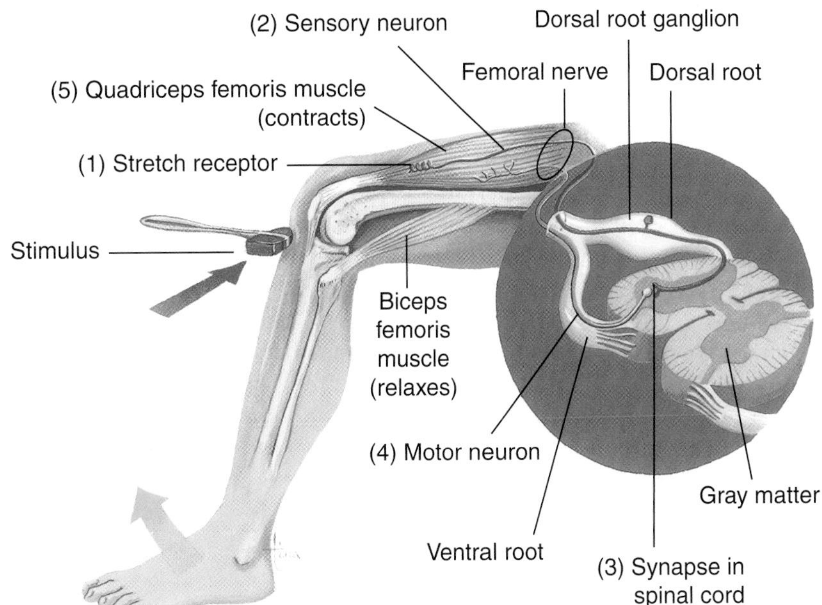

Figure 8–5 Patellar reflex. The reflex arc is shown. See text for description.

QUESTION: Why is this reflex called a stretch reflex?

make a decision every time we swayed a bit, all our concentration would be needed just to remain standing. Since these are spinal cord reflexes, the brain is not directly involved. The brain may become aware that a reflex has taken place, but that involves another set of neurons carrying impulses to the brain.

Flexor reflexes (or **withdrawal reflexes**) are another type of spinal cord reflex. The stimulus is something painful and potentially harmful, and the response is to pull away from it. If you inadvertently touch a hot stove, you automatically pull your hand away. Flexor reflexes are three-neuron reflexes because sensory neurons synapse with interneurons in the spinal cord, which in turn synapse with motor neurons. Again, however, the brain does not have to make a decision to protect the body; the flexor reflex does that automatically (see Box 8–3: Spinal Cord Injuries). The brain may know that the reflex has taken place, and may even learn from the experience, but that requires different neurons, not the reflex arc.

THE BRAIN

The **brain** is made of approximately 100 billion neurons and contains trillions of synapses, all of which function as an integrated whole. The major parts of the brain are the medulla, pons, and midbrain (collectively called the **brainstem**), the cerebellum, the hypothalamus, the thalamus, and the cerebrum. These parts are shown in Fig. 8–6. We will discuss each part separately, but keep in mind that they are all interconnected, by way of those trillions of synapses, and work together.

VENTRICLES

The **ventricles** are four cavities within the brain: two lateral ventricles, the third ventricle, and the fourth ventricle (Fig. 8–7). The ventricles are lined with ciliated ependymal cells (see Table Fig. 8–A in Table 8–1) and filled with **cerebrospinal fluid** (**CSF**). Each ventricle contains a capillary network called a **choroid plexus**, which forms the cerebrospinal fluid from blood plasma. Cerebrospinal fluid is the tissue fluid of the central nervous system; its circulation and functions will be discussed in the section on meninges.

MEDULLA

The **medulla** extends from the spinal cord to the pons and is anterior to the cerebellum. Its functions are those we think of as vital (as in "vital signs"). The medulla

Box 8–3 | SPINAL CORD INJURIES

Injuries to the spinal cord are most often caused by auto accidents, falls, and gunshot wounds. The most serious injury is transection, or severing, of the spinal cord. If, for example, the spinal cord is severed at the level of the 8th thoracic segment, there will be paralysis and loss of sensation below that level. Another consequence is spinal shock, the at-least-temporary loss of spinal cord reflexes. In this example, the spinal cord reflexes of the lower trunk and legs will not occur. The stretch reflexes and flexor reflexes of the legs will be at least temporarily abolished, as will the urination and defecation reflexes. Although these reflexes do not depend directly on the brain, spinal cord neurons depend upon impulses from the brain to enhance their own ability to generate impulses.

As spinal cord neurons below the injury recover their ability to generate impulses, these reflexes, such as the patellar reflex, often return. Urination and defecation reflexes may also be reestablished, but the person will not have an awareness of the need to urinate or defecate. Nor will voluntary control of these reflexes be possible, because inhibiting impulses from the brain can no longer reach the lower segments of the spinal cord.

Potentially less serious injuries are those in which the spinal cord is crushed rather than severed, and treatment is aimed at preserving whatever function remains. Minimizing inflammation and stimulating the production of nerve growth factors are aspects of such treatment.

Perhaps the most challenging research is the attempt to stimulate severed spinal cords to regenerate. Partial success has been achieved in rats and mice, with Schwann cells transplanted from their peripheral nerves and nerve growth factors produced by genetically engineered cells. The use of stem cells has also been successful in rats. The researchers caution, however, that it will take some time before their procedures will be tested on people.

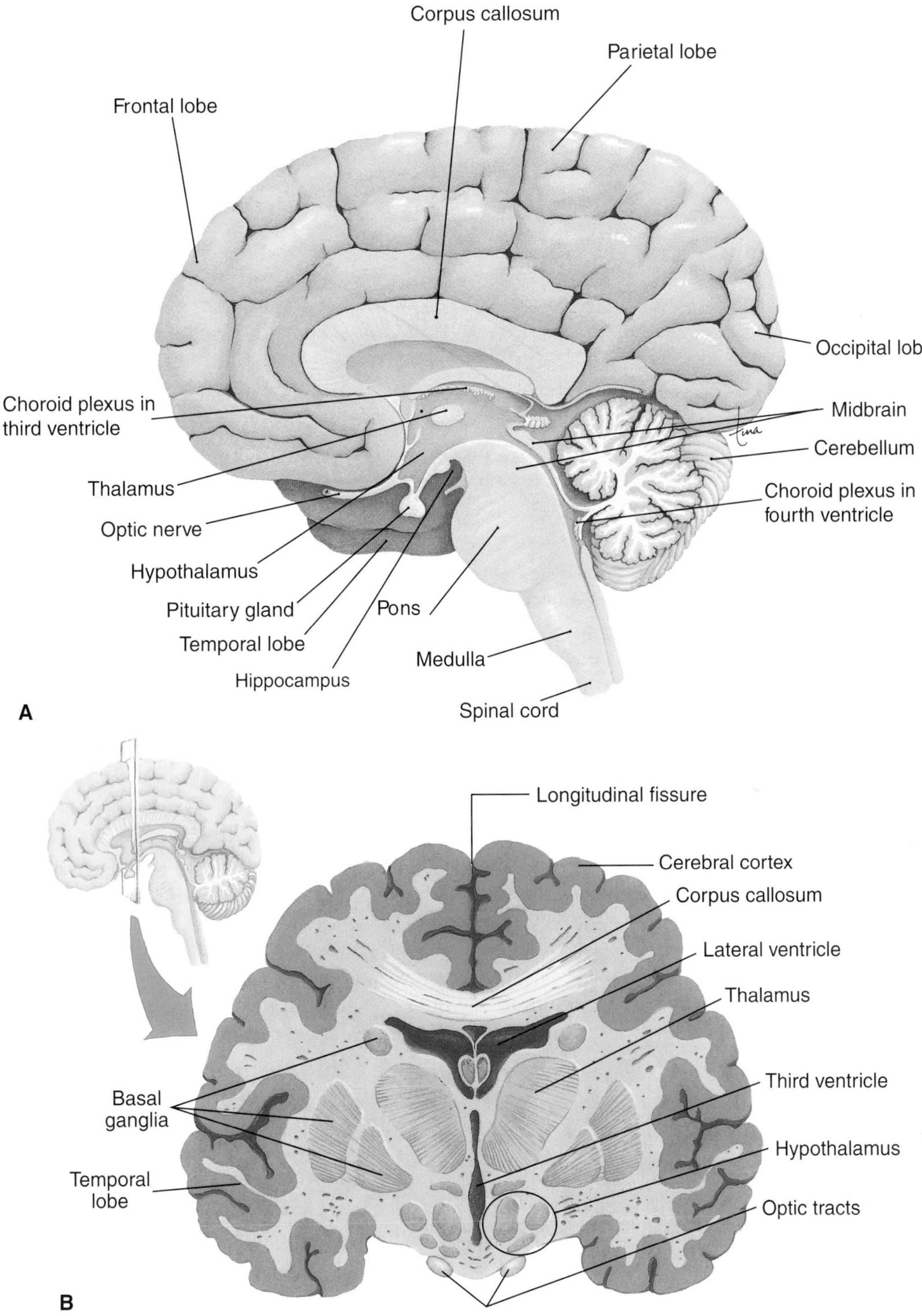

Figure 8–6 (**A**) Midsagittal section of the brain as seen from the left side. This medial plane shows internal anatomy and the lobes of the cerebrum. (**B**) Frontal section of the brain in anterior view.

QUESTION: Find the corpus callosum in parts A and B, and describe its shape. What is its function?

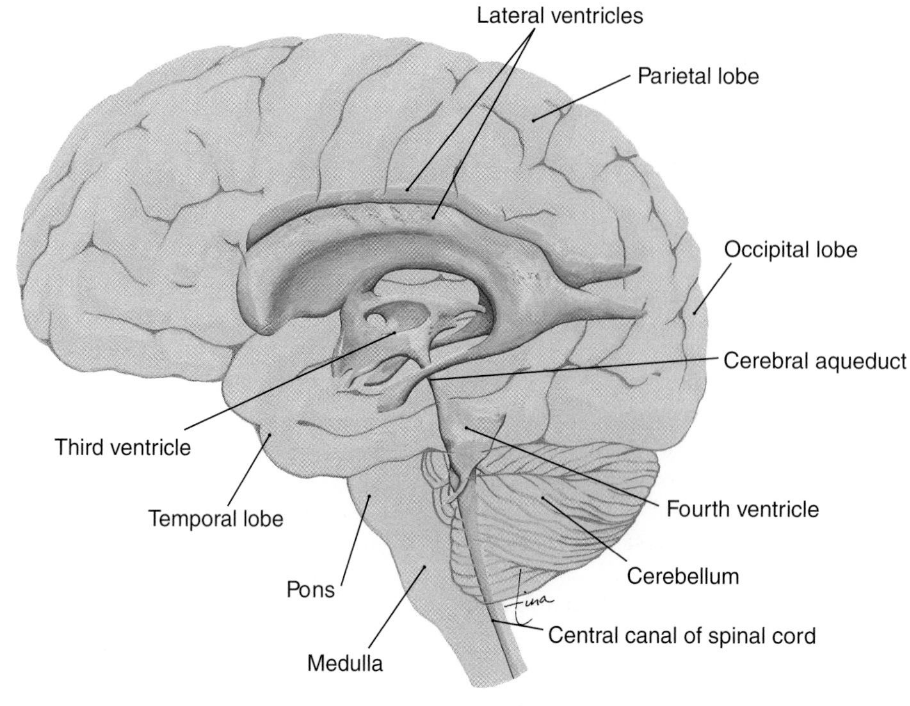

Figure 8–7 Ventricles of the brain as projected into the interior of the brain, which is seen from the left side.

QUESTION: Describe the extent of each lateral ventricle.

contains cardiac centers that regulate heart rate, vasomotor centers that regulate the diameter of blood vessels and, thereby, blood pressure, and respiratory centers that regulate breathing. You can see why a crushing injury to the occipital bone may be rapidly fatal—we cannot survive without the medulla. Also in the medulla are reflex centers for coughing, sneezing, swallowing, and vomiting.

PONS

The **pons** bulges anteriorly from the upper part of the medulla. Within the pons are two respiratory centers that work with those in the medulla to produce a normal breathing rhythm. (The function of all the respiratory centers is discussed in Chapter 15.) The many other neurons in the pons (*pons* is from the Latin for "bridge") connect the medulla with other parts of the brain.

MIDBRAIN

The **midbrain** extends from the pons to the hypothalamus and encloses the **cerebral aqueduct**, a tunnel that connects the third and fourth ventricles. Several different kinds of reflexes are integrated in the midbrain, including visual and auditory reflexes. If you see a wasp flying toward you, you automatically duck or twist away; this is a visual reflex. Keeping an eye on that wasp (actually both eyes) until it flies away is called tracking; the coordinated eye movements that make this possible are also a reflex. Other examples are following the flight of a home run ball or a long touchdown pass. The ability to read depends in part on the coordinated movement of the eyeballs from word to word; this is scanning and is another reflex mediated by the midbrain. Turning your head (ear) to a sound is an example of an auditory reflex, as is the "startle" reflex, a jump or cringe upon hearing a sudden loud sound such as thunder. The midbrain is also concerned with what are called righting reflexes, those that keep the head upright and maintain balance or equilibrium. When a cat falls from a tree and lands on its feet (if it was not too high up), its midbrain helped get its head upright, and other parts of the brain then swung the trunk and legs into position for a landing. Human midbrains are not nearly that efficient.

CEREBELLUM

The **cerebellum** is separated from the medulla and pons by the fourth ventricle and is inferior to the occipital lobes of the cerebrum. As you already know, many of the functions of the cerebellum are concerned with movement. These include coordination, regulation of muscle tone, the appropriate trajectory and end point of movements, and the maintenance of posture and equilibrium. Notice that these are all involuntary; that is, the cerebellum functions below the level of conscious thought. This is important to permit the conscious brain to work without being overburdened. If you decide to pick up a pencil, for example, the impulses for arm movement come from the cerebrum. The cerebellum then modifies these impulses so that your arm and finger movements are coordinated, and you don't reach past the pencil.

The cerebellum seems also to be involved in certain sensory functions. For example, if you close your eyes and someone places a tennis ball in one hand and a baseball in the other, could you tell which was which? Certainly you could, by the "feel" of each: the texture and the weight or heft. If you pick up a plastic container of coffee (with a lid on it) could you tell if the cup is full, half-full, or empty? Again, you certainly could. Do you have to think about it? No. The cerebellum is, in part, responsible for this ability.

To regulate equilibrium, the cerebellum (and midbrain) uses information about gravity and movement provided by receptors in the inner ears. These receptors are discussed further in Chapter 9.

HYPOTHALAMUS

Located superior to the pituitary gland and inferior to the thalamus, the **hypothalamus** is a small area of the brain with many diverse functions:

1. Production of **antidiuretic hormone** (ADH) and **oxytocin**; these hormones are then stored in the posterior pituitary gland. ADH enables the kidneys to reabsorb water back into the blood and thus helps maintain blood volume. Oxytocin causes contractions of the uterus to bring about labor and delivery.
2. Production of releasing hormones (also called releasing factors) that stimulate the secretion of hormones by the anterior pituitary gland. Because these hormones are covered in Chapter 10, a single example will be given here: The hypothalamus produces **growth hormone–releasing hormone** (GHRH), which stimulates the anterior pituitary gland to secrete growth hormone (GH).
3. Regulation of body temperature by promoting responses such as sweating in a warm environment or shivering in a cold environment (see Chapter 17).
4. Regulation of food intake; the hypothalamus is believed to respond to changes in blood nutrient levels, to chemicals secreted by fat cells, and to hormones secreted by the gastrointestinal tract. For example, during a meal, after a certain duration of digestion, the small intestine produces a hormone that circulates to the hypothalamus and brings about a sensation of satiety, or fullness, and we tend to stop eating.
5. Integration of the functioning of the autonomic nervous system, which in turn regulates the activity of organs such as the heart, blood vessels, and intestines. This will be discussed in more detail later in this chapter.
6. Stimulation of visceral responses during emotional situations. When we are angry, heart rate usually increases. Most of us, when embarrassed, will blush, which is vasodilation in the skin of the face. These responses are brought about by the autonomic nervous system when the hypothalamus perceives a change in emotional state. The neurologic basis of our emotions is not well understood, and the visceral responses to emotions are not something most of us can control.
7. Regulation of body rhythms such as secretion of hormones, sleep cycles, changes in mood, or mental alertness. This is often referred to as our biological clock, the rhythms as circadian rhythms, meaning "about a day." If you have ever had to stay awake for 24 hours, you know how disorienting it can be, until the hypothalamic biological clock has been reset.

THALAMUS

The **thalamus** is superior to the hypothalamus and inferior to the cerebrum. The third ventricle is a narrow cavity that passes through both the thalamus and hypothalamus. Many of the functions of the thalamus are concerned with sensation. Sensory impulses to the brain (except those for the sense of smell) follow neuron pathways that first enter the thalamus, which groups the impulses before relaying them to the cerebrum, where sensations are felt. For example, holding a cup of hot coffee generates impulses for heat, touch and texture, and the shape of the cup (muscle sense), but we do not experience these as separate sensations. The thalamus integrates the impulses from the cutaneous receptors and from the cerebellum; that is, it puts them together in a sort of electrochemical package and directs them to the sensory area in the parietal lobe of the cerebrum so that the neurons there feel the whole and are able to interpret the sensation quickly.

Some sensations, especially unpleasant ones such as pain, are believed to be felt by the thalamus. However, the thalamus cannot localize the sensation; that is, it does not know where the painful sensation is coming from. The sensory areas of the cerebrum are required for localization and precise awareness.

The thalamus may also suppress unimportant sensations. If you are reading an enjoyable book, you may not notice someone coming into the room. By temporarily blocking minor sensations, the thalamus permits the cerebrum to concentrate on important tasks.

Parts of the thalamus are also involved in alertness and awareness (being awake and knowing we are), and others contribute to memory. For these functions, as for others, the thalamus works very closely with the cerebrum.

CEREBRUM

The largest part of the human brain is the **cerebrum**, which consists of two hemispheres separated by the longitudinal fissure. At the base of this deep groove is the **corpus callosum**, a band of 200 million neurons that connects the right and left hemispheres. Within each hemisphere is a lateral ventricle.

The surface of the cerebrum is gray matter called the **cerebral cortex**. Gray matter consists of cell bodies of neurons, which carry out the many functions of the cerebrum. Internal to the gray matter is white matter, made of myelinated axons and dendrites that connect the lobes of the cerebrum to one another and to all other parts of the brain.

In the human brain the cerebral cortex is folded extensively. The folds are called **convolutions** or **gyri**, and the grooves between them are **fissures** or **sulci** (you can see the folding of the cortex in the frontal section of the brain in Fig. 8–6). This folding permits the presence of millions more neurons in the cerebral cortex. The cerebral cortex of an animal such as a dog or cat does not have this extensive folding. This difference enables us to read, speak, do long division, write poetry and songs, and do so many other "human" things that dogs and cats cannot do.

The cerebral cortex is divided into lobes that have the same names as the cranial bones external to them. Therefore, each hemisphere has a frontal lobe, parietal lobe, temporal lobe, and occipital lobe (Fig. 8–8). These lobes have been mapped; that is, certain areas are known to be associated with specific functions. We will discuss

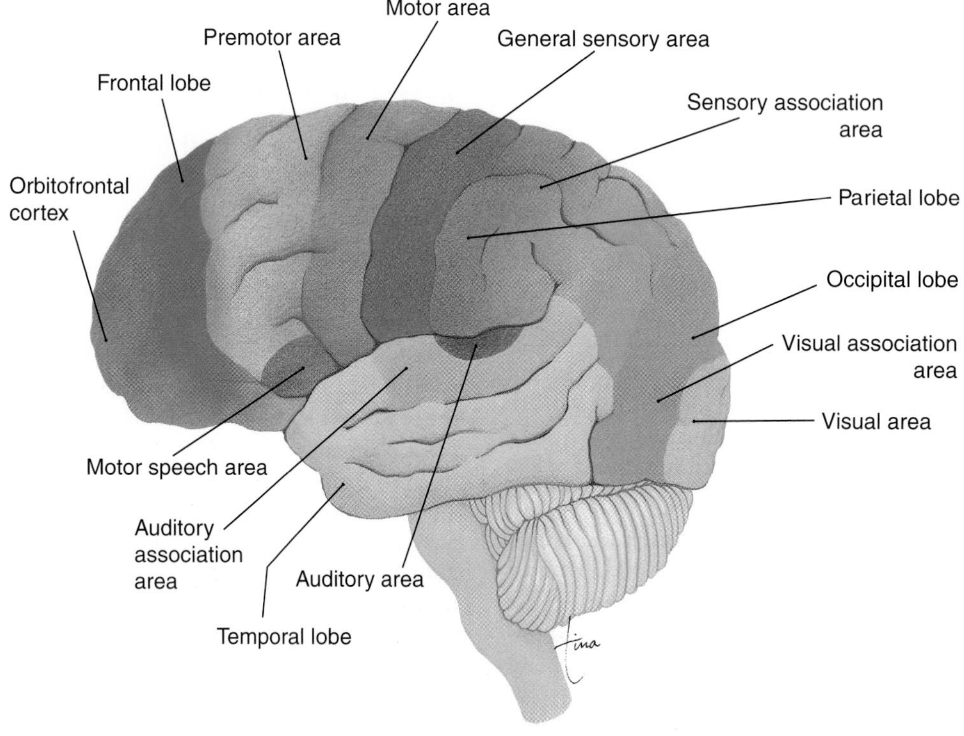

Figure 8–8 Left cerebral hemisphere showing some of the functional areas that have been mapped.

QUESTION: What sensations are felt in the general sensory area?

the functions of the cerebrum according to these mapped areas.

Frontal Lobes

Within the **frontal lobes** are the **motor areas** that generate the impulses for voluntary movement. The largest portions are for movement of the hands and face, those areas with many muscles capable of very fine or precise movements. It is the large size of the motor area devoted to them that gives these muscles their precision. The left motor area controls movement on the right side of the body, and the right motor area controls the left side of the body. This is why a patient who has had a cerebrovascular accident, or stroke, in the right frontal lobe will have paralysis of muscles on the left side (see Box 8–4: Cerebrovascular Accidents).

Anterior to the motor areas are the **premotor areas**, which are concerned with learned motor skills that require a sequence of movements. Tying shoelaces, for example, seems almost automatic to us; we forget having learned it. It is not a reflex, however; rather, the premotor cortex has learned the sequence so well that we are able to repeat it without consciously thinking about it.

The parts of the frontal lobes just behind the eyes are the **prefrontal** or **orbitofrontal cortex**. This area is concerned with things such as keeping emotional responses appropriate to the situation, realizing that there are standards of behavior (laws or rules of a game or simple courtesy) and following them, and anticipating and planning for the future. An example may be helpful to put all this together: Someone with damage to the prefrontal area might become enraged if a pen ran out of ink during class, might throw the pen at someone, and might not think that a pen will be needed tomorrow and that it is time to go buy one. As you can see, the prefrontal cortex is very important for social behavior. This is the part of the brain that enables us to realize that other people might not always think the way we do. This is the part that thinks "Ooops" and allows us to apologize for words or actions that were perhaps poorly considered. The prefrontal cortex greatly contributes to what makes us human and able to enjoy the humanity of others.

Also in the frontal lobe, usually only the left lobe for most right-handed people, is **Broca's motor speech** area, which controls the movements of the mouth involved in speaking.

Box 8–4 | CEREBROVASCULAR ACCIDENTS

A **cerebrovascular accident (CVA)**, or **stroke**, is damage to a blood vessel in the brain, resulting in lack of oxygen to that part of the brain. Possible types of vessel damage are thrombosis or hemorrhage.

A **thrombus** is a blood clot, which most often is a consequence of atherosclerosis, abnormal lipid deposits in cerebral arteries. The rough surface stimulates clot formation, which obstructs the blood flow to the part of the brain supplied by the artery. The symptoms depend upon the part of the brain affected and may be gradual in onset if clot formation is slow. Approximately 80% of CVAs are of this type.

A hemorrhage, the result of arteriosclerosis or **aneurysm** of a cerebral artery, allows blood out into brain tissue, which destroys brain neurons by putting excessive pressure on them, as well as depriving them of oxygen. Onset of symptoms in this type of CVA is usually rapid.

If, for example, the CVA is in the left frontal lobe, paralysis of the right side of the body will occur. Speech may also be affected if the speech areas are involved. Some CVAs are fatal because the damage they cause is very widespread or affects vital centers in the medulla or pons.

For CVAs of the thrombus type, a clot-dissolving drug may help reestablish blood flow. To be effective, however, the drug must be administered within 3 hours of symptom onset (see also Box 11–7 in Chapter 11).

Recovery from a CVA depends on its location and the extent of damage, as well as other factors. Two of these are the redundancy of the brain and its plasticity. Redundancy means repetition or exceeding what is necessary; the cerebral cortex has many more neurons than we actually use in daily activities. Plasticity means that these neurons are available for use, especially in younger people (younger than 50 years of age, but even in people much older). When a patient recovers from a disabling stroke, what has often happened is that the brain has established new pathways, with previously little-used neurons now carrying impulses "full time." Such recovery is highly individual and may take months. Yet another important factor is that CVA patients be encouraged and started on rehabilitation therapy as soon as their condition permits.

Parietal Lobes

The **general sensory areas** in the **parietal lobes** receive impulses from receptors in the skin and feel and interpret the cutaneous sensations. The left area is for the right side of the body and vice versa. These areas also receive impulses from stretch receptors in muscles for conscious muscle sense. The largest portions of these areas are for sensation in the hands and face, those parts of the body with the most cutaneous receptors and the most muscle receptors. The **taste areas**, which overlap the parietal and temporal lobes, receive impulses from taste buds on the tongue and elsewhere in the oral cavity.

Temporal Lobes

The **olfactory areas** in the **temporal lobes** receive impulses from receptors in the nasal cavities for the sense of smell. The olfactory association area learns the meaning of odors such as the smell of sour milk, or fire, or brownies baking in the oven, and enables the thinking cerebrum to use that information effectively.

The **auditory areas**, as their name suggests, receive impulses from receptors in the inner ear for hearing. The auditory association area is quite large. Part of it is concerned with the meanings of words we hear, that is, with speech. Other parts are for the interpretation of sounds such as thunder during a storm, an ambulance siren, or a baby crying. Without proper interpretation, we would hear the sound but would not know what it meant or be able to integrate it with other senses and could not respond appropriately.

Also in the temporal and parietal lobes in the left hemisphere (for most of us) are other speech areas concerned with the thought that precedes speech. Each of us can probably recall (and regret) times when we have "spoken without thinking," but in actuality that is not possible. The thinking takes place very rapidly and is essential in order to be able to speak (see Box 8–5: Aphasia).

Occipital Lobes

Impulses from the retinas of the eyes travel along the optic nerves to the **visual areas** in the **occipital lobes**. These areas "see." The visual association areas interpret what is seen and enable the thinking cerebrum to use the information. Imagine looking at a clock. Seeing the clock is far different from being able to interpret it. At one time we learned to interpret the clock face and hands, and now we do not have to consciously decide what time the clock is showing. We can simply use that information, such as hurrying a bit so as not to be late to class. Other parts of the occipital lobes are concerned with spatial relationships; that is, things such as judging distance and seeing in three dimensions or the ability to read a map and relate it to the physical world.

The cerebral cortex has the characteristic of **neural plasticity**, the ability to adapt to changing needs, to recruit different neurons for certain functions, as may occur during childhood or recovery from a stroke. Another example is the visual cortex of a person who is born blind. The neurons in the occipital lobes that would have been used for vision will often be used for another function; some may become

Box 8–5 | APHASIA

Our use of language sets us apart from other animals and involves speech, reading, and writing. Language is the use of symbols (words) to designate objects and to express ideas. Damage to the speech areas or interpretation areas of the cerebrum may impair one or more aspects of a person's ability to use language; this is called **aphasia**.

Aphasia may be a consequence of a cerebrovascular accident or physical trauma to the skull and brain such as a head injury sustained in an automobile accident. If the motor speech (Broca's) area is damaged, the person is still able to understand written and spoken words and knows what he wants to say, but he cannot say it. Without coordination and impulses from the motor speech area, the muscles used for speech cannot contract to form words properly.

Auditory aphasia is "**word deafness**," caused by damage to an interpretation area. The person can still hear but cannot comprehend what the words mean. Visual aphasia is "**word blindness**"; the person can still see perfectly well but cannot make sense of written words (the person retains the ability to understand spoken words). Imagine how you would feel if wms qsbbcljw jmqr rfc yzgjgrw rm pcyb. Frustrating isn't it? You know that those symbols are letters, but you cannot "decode" them right away. Those "words" were formed by shifting the alphabet two letters (A = C, B = D, C = E, etc.), and would normally be read as: "you suddenly lost the ability to read." That may give you a small idea of what word blindness is like.

part of an auditory area that is used to localize sounds and estimate their distance. Those of us who can see may not rely on hearing for localization; we simply look at where we think the sound came from. A blind person cannot do this, and may have an extensive mental catalogue of sounds, meanings of sounds, distances of sounds, and so on, some of these in the part of the cortex that normally is for vision.

The younger the person, the more plastic the brain. The brains of children are extraordinarily adaptable. As we get older, plasticity diminishes somewhat, but is still present.

Association Areas

As you can see in Fig. 8–8, many parts of the cerebral cortex are not concerned with movement or a particular sensation. These may be called **association areas** and perhaps are what truly make us individuals. It is probably these areas that give each of us a personality, a sense of humor, and the ability to reason and use logic. Learning and memory are also functions of these areas.

Although much has been learned about the formation of memories, the processes are still incompletely understood and mostly beyond the scope of this book. Briefly, however, we can say that memories of things such as people or books or what you did last summer involve the **hippocampus** (from the Greek for "seahorse," because of its shape), part of the temporal lobe on the floor of the lateral ventricle. The two hippocampi seem to collect information from many areas of the cerebral cortex. When you meet a friend, for example, the memory emerges as a whole: "Here's Fred," not in pieces. People whose hippocampi are damaged cannot form new memories that last more than a few seconds and have difficulty recalling old memories.

The right hippocampus is also believed to be involved in spatial cognition (literally: "space thinking"). For example, if you are in school and a friend asks you the shortest way to your home, you will probably quickly form a mental map. You can see how much memory that involves (streets, landmarks, and so on), but the hippocampus can take it a step further and make your memories three-dimensional and mentally visible. You can see your way home. That is spatial cognition.

It is believed that most, if not all, of what we have experienced or learned is stored somewhere in the brain. This is long-term memory, whether conscious or subconscious, and probably involves the creation of new connections in the brain. Sometimes a trigger may bring back memories from years or even decades ago; a certain scent or a song can act as possible triggers. Then we find ourselves recalling something from the past and wondering where it came from.

The loss of personality due to destruction of brain neurons is perhaps most dramatically seen in Alzheimer's disease (see Box 8–6: Alzheimer's Disease).

Box 8–6 | ALZHEIMER'S DISEASE

In the United States, **Alzheimer's disease**, a progressive, incurable form of mental deterioration, affects approximately 5 million people and is the cause of 100,000 deaths each year. The first symptoms, which usually begin after age 65, are memory lapses and slight personality changes. As the disease progresses, there is total loss of memory, reasoning ability, and personality, and those with advanced disease are unable to perform even the simplest tasks or self-care.

Structural changes in the brains of Alzheimer's patients may be seen at autopsy. Neurofibrillary tangles are made of abnormal fibrous proteins called tau and are found in cells of the cerebral cortex in areas important for memory and reasoning. Also present are plaques made of another protein called beta-amyloid (or amyloid-beta, an alternate name) that are damaging to neurons and impair the functioning of synapses. The cells' usual mechanisms (involving ubiquitin and proteasomes) for clearing old or misfolded proteins may be malfunctioning; the reason is not yet known.

A defective gene has been found in some patients who have late-onset Alzheimer's disease, the most common type. Yet another gene seems to trigger increased synthesis of amyloid-beta. Research is focused on the interaction of these genes and on inflammation as a contributing factor to this type of brain damage.

The diagnosis of Alzheimer's disease has been difficult, for in early stages the cognitive impairment resembles that of many other types of dementia. Timely diagnosis is important because it is likely that the treatment of Alzheimer's disease will one day mean delaying its severe manifestations with a variety of medications, each targeted at a different aspect of this complex disease.

Basal Ganglia

The **basal ganglia** are paired masses of gray matter within the white matter of the cerebral hemispheres (see Fig. 8–6). Their functions are certain subconscious aspects of voluntary movement, and they work with the cerebellum. The basal ganglia help regulate muscle tone, and they coordinate accessory movements such as swinging the arms when walking or gesturing while speaking. Gestures and facial expressions can be as eloquent as words and often accompany and complement our conversation. The most common disorder of the basal ganglia is Parkinson's disease (see Box 8–7: Parkinson's Disease).

Corpus Callosum

As mentioned previously, the **corpus callosum** is a band of nerve fibers that connects the left and right cerebral hemispheres. This enables each hemisphere to know what the other is doing. A person with musical training has a thicker corpus callosum (more neurons) than someone without. Music apparently makes demands on the cerebrum that nonmusical study does not, and the cerebrum responds with more neurons and synapses. For all people, even those who are not musicians, the corpus callosum is important because for most of us the left hemisphere contains speech areas and the right hemisphere does not. The corpus callosum, therefore, lets the left hemisphere know what the right hemisphere is thinking about, and the right hemisphere know what the left hemisphere is thinking and talking about. A brief example may be helpful. If you put your left hand behind your back and someone places a pencil in your hand (you are not looking at it) and asks you what it is, would you be able to say? Yes, you would. You would feel the shape and weight of the pencil, find the point and the eraser. The sensory impulses from your left hand are interpreted as "pencil" by the general sensory area in your right parietal lobe. Your right hemisphere probably cannot speak, but its thoughts can be conveyed by way of the corpus callosum to the left hemisphere, which does have speech areas. Your left hemisphere can say that you are holding a pencil. Other aspects of the "division of labor" of our cerebral hemispheres are beyond the scope of this book, but it is a fascinating subject that you may wish to explore further.

MENINGES AND CEREBROSPINAL FLUID

The connective tissue membranes that cover the brain and spinal cord are called **meninges**; the three layers are illustrated in Fig. 8–9. The thick outermost layer, made of fibrous connective tissue, is the **dura mater** (Latin for "tough mother"), which lines the skull and vertebral canal. The middle **arachnoid membrane** (arachnids are spiders) is made of web-like strands of connective tissue. The innermost **pia mater** (Latin for "gentle mother") is a very thin membrane on the surface of the spinal cord and brain. Between the arachnoid and the pia mater is the **subarachnoid space**, which contains cerebrospinal fluid (CSF), the tissue fluid of the central nervous system.

Recall the ventricles (cavities) of the brain: two lateral ventricles, the third ventricle, and the fourth ventricle. Each contains a choroid plexus, a capillary network that forms cerebrospinal fluid from blood plasma. This is a continuous process, and the cerebrospinal fluid then circulates in and around the central nervous system (Fig. 8–10).

Box 8–7 | PARKINSON'S DISEASE

Parkinson's disease is a disorder of the basal ganglia whose cause is unknown, and although there is a genetic component in some families, it is probably not the only factor. The disease usually begins after the age of 60. Neurons in the basal ganglia that produce the neurotransmitter dopamine begin to degenerate and die, and the deficiency of dopamine causes specific kinds of muscular symptoms. Tremor, or involuntary shaking, of the hands is probably the most common symptom. The accessory movements regulated by the basal ganglia gradually diminish, and the affected person walks slowly without swinging the arms. A mask-like face is characteristic of this disease, as the facial muscles become rigid. Eventually all voluntary movements become slower and much more difficult, and balance is seriously impaired.

Dopamine itself cannot be used to treat Parkinson's disease because it does not cross the blood–brain barrier. A related chemical called L-dopa does cross and can be converted to dopamine by brain neurons. Unfortunately, L-dopa begins to lose its therapeutic effectiveness within a few years.

Other medications in use may ameliorate symptoms but do not provide a cure. Current research is focusing on gene therapy and stem cell therapy.

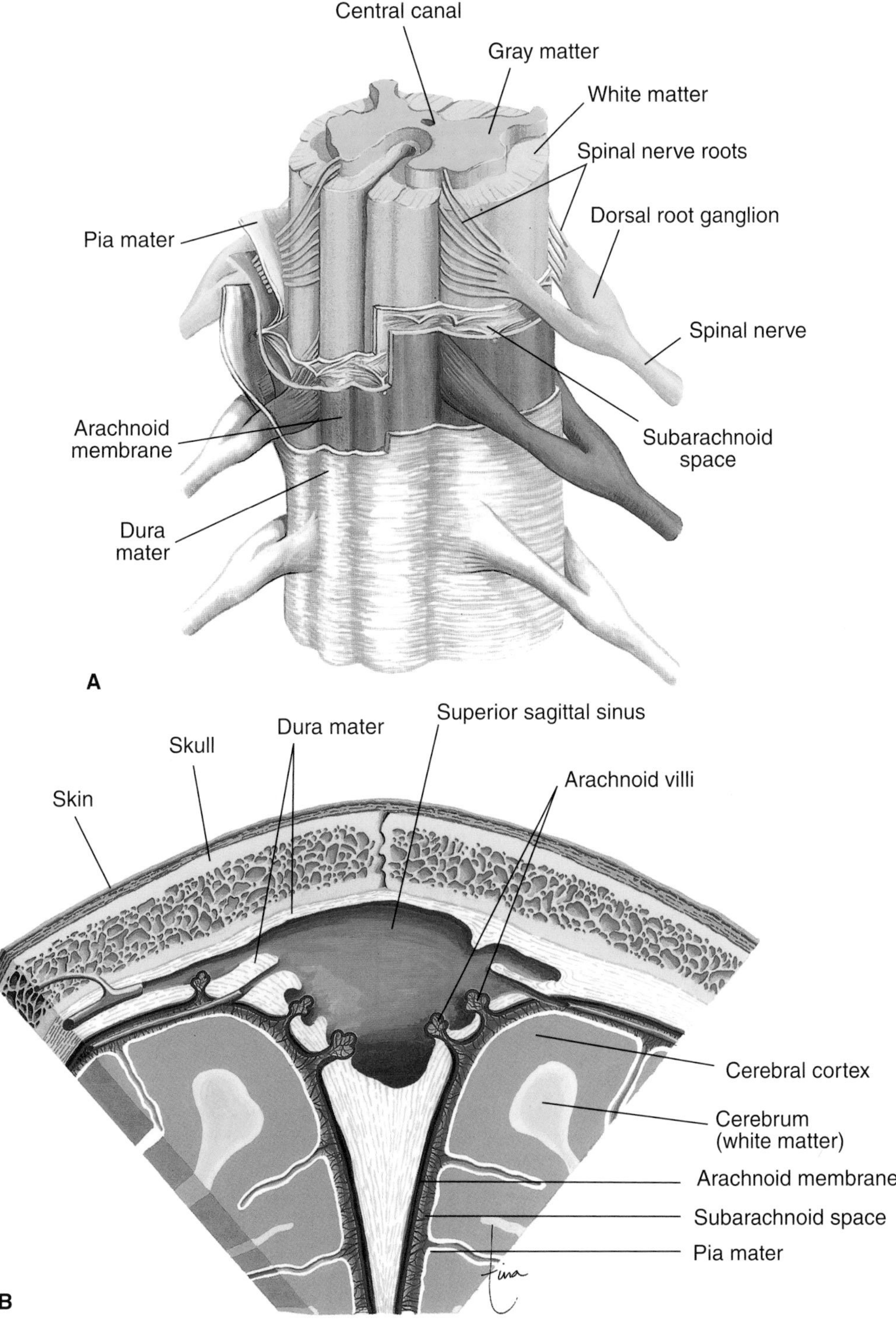

Figure 8–9 Structure of the meninges. (**A**) Meninges of the spinal cord. (**B**) Frontal section through the top of the skull showing the double-layered cranial dura mater and one of the cranial venous sinuses.

QUESTION: Describe the structural difference between the spinal dura mater and the cranial dura mater.

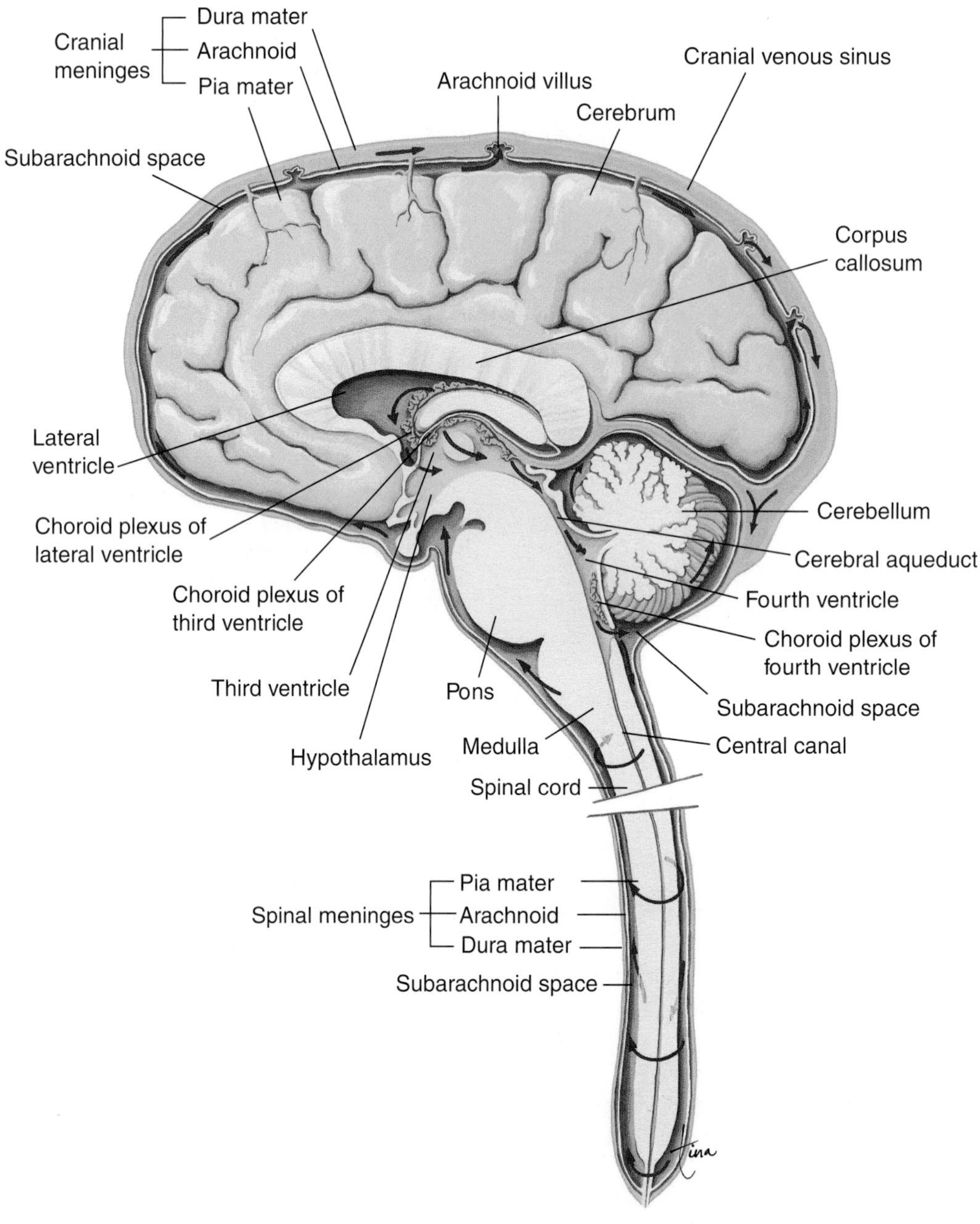

Figure 8–10 Formation, circulation, and reabsorption of cerebrospinal fluid. See text for description.

QUESTION: In this pathway, where is the CSF reabsorbed, and into what?

From the lateral and third ventricles, cerebrospinal fluid flows through the fourth ventricle, then to the central canal of the spinal cord, and to the cranial and spinal subarachnoid spaces. As more cerebrospinal fluid is formed, you might expect that some must be reabsorbed, and that is just what happens. From the cranial subarachnoid space, cerebrospinal fluid is reabsorbed through **arachnoid villi** into the blood in **cranial venous sinuses** (large veins within the double-layered cranial dura mater). The cerebrospinal fluid becomes blood plasma again, and the rate of reabsorption normally equals the rate of production.

Because cerebrospinal fluid is tissue fluid, one of its functions is to bring nutrients to CNS neurons and to remove waste products to the blood as the fluid is reabsorbed. The other function of cerebrospinal fluid is to act as a cushion for the central nervous system. The brain and spinal cord are enclosed in fluid-filled membranes that absorb shock. You can, for example, shake your head vigorously without harming your brain. Naturally, this protection has limits; very sharp or heavy blows to the skull will indeed cause damage to the brain.

Examination of cerebrospinal fluid may be used in the diagnosis of certain diseases (see Box 8–8: Lumbar Puncture).

CRANIAL NERVES

The 12 pairs of **cranial nerves** emerge from the brainstem or other parts of the brain—they are shown in Fig. 8–11. The name *cranial* indicates their origin, and many of them do carry impulses for functions involving the head. Some, however, have more far-reaching destinations.

The impulses for the senses of smell, taste, sight, hearing, and equilibrium are all carried by cranial nerves to their respective sensory areas in the brain. Some cranial nerves carry motor impulses to muscles of the face and eyes or to the salivary glands. The vagus nerves (*vagus* means "wanderer") branch extensively to the larynx, heart, stomach and intestines, and bronchial tubes.

The functions of the cranial nerves are summarized in Table 8–4.

THE AUTONOMIC NERVOUS SYSTEM

The **autonomic nervous system** (**ANS**) is actually part of the peripheral nervous system in that it consists of motor portions of some cranial and spinal nerves. Because its functioning is so specialized, however, the autonomic nervous system is usually discussed as a separate entity, as we will do here.

Box 8–8 | LUMBAR PUNCTURE

A **lumbar puncture** (spinal tap) is a diagnostic procedure that involves the removal of cerebrospinal fluid to determine its pressure and constituents. As the name tells us, the removal, using a syringe, is made in the lumbar area. Because the spinal cord ends between the 1st and 2nd lumbar vertebrae, the needle is usually inserted between the 4th and 5th lumbar vertebrae. The meningeal sac containing cerebrospinal fluid extends to the end of the lumbar vertebrae, permitting access to the cerebrospinal fluid with little chance of damaging the spinal cord.

Cerebrospinal fluid is a circulating fluid and has a normal pressure of 70 to 200 mm H_2O. An abnormal pressure usually indicates an obstruction in circulation, which may be caused by infection, a tumor, or mechanical injury. Other diagnostic tests would be needed to determine the precise cause.

Perhaps the most common reason for a lumbar puncture is suspected **meningitis**, which may be caused by several kinds of bacteria. If the patient does have meningitis, the cerebrospinal fluid will be cloudy rather than clear and will be examined for the presence of bacteria and many white blood cells. A few WBCs in CSF is normal because WBCs are found in all tissue fluid.

Another abnormal constituent of cerebrospinal fluid is red blood cells. Their presence indicates bleeding somewhere in the central nervous system. There may be many causes, and again, further testing would be necessary.

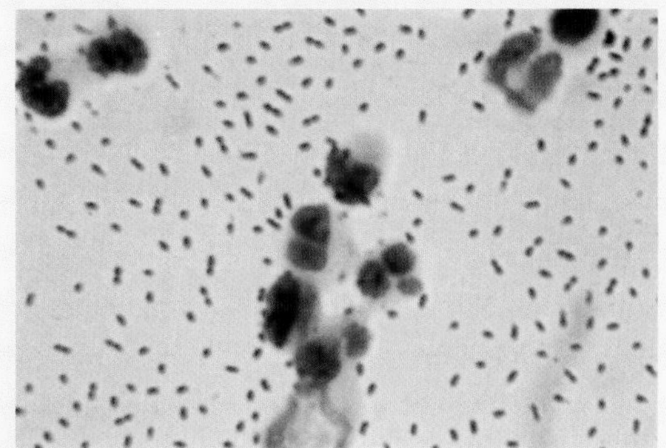

Box Figure 8–B Cerebrospinal fluid from a patient with meningitis. The bacteria are streptococci, seen here in pairs. The large cells are WBCs. (×500) (From Sacher, RA, and McPherson, RA: Widmann's Clinical Interpretation of Laboratory Tests, ed. 11. FA Davis, Philadelphia, 2000, Plate 52, with permission.)

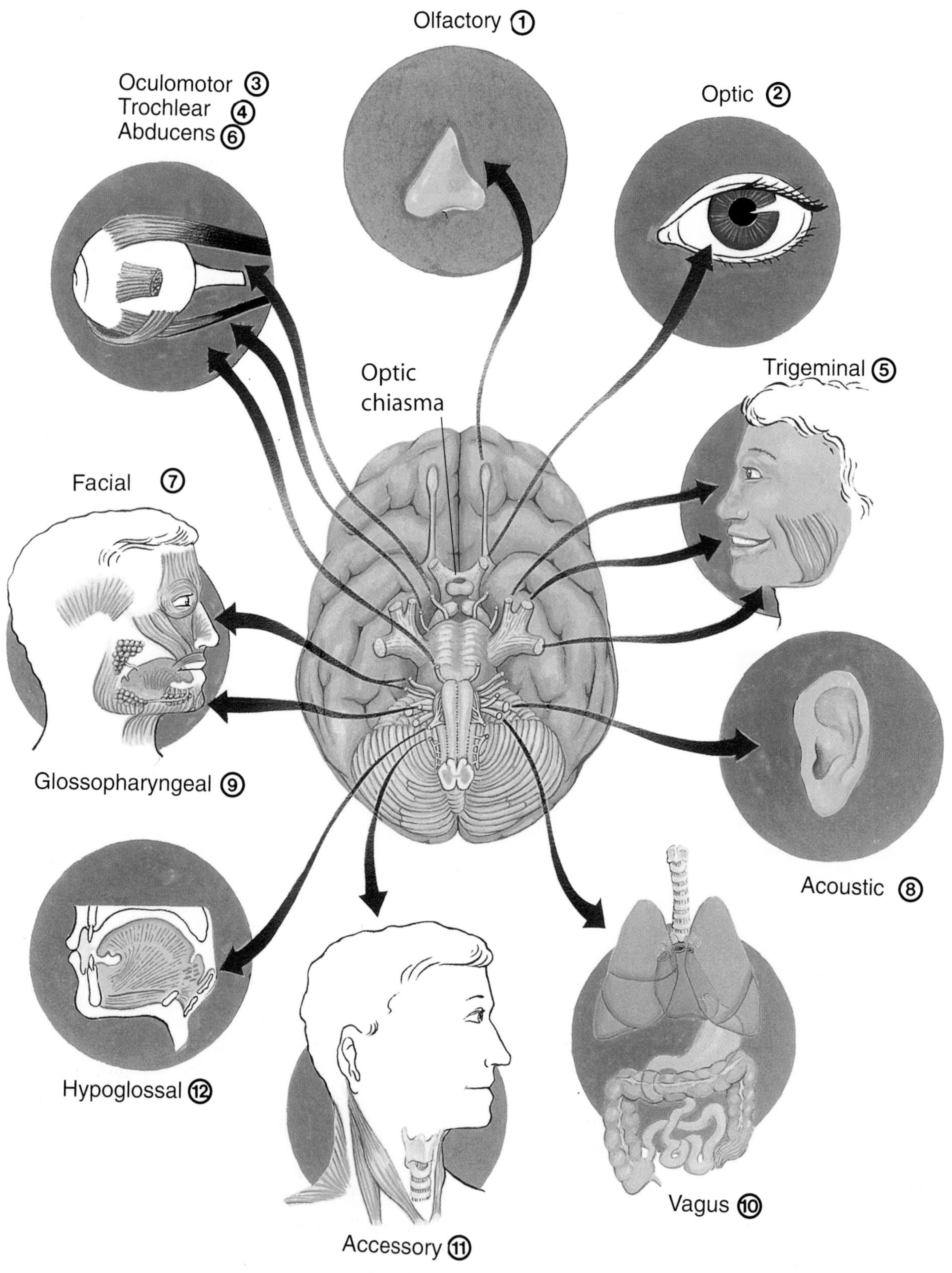

Figure 8–11 Cranial nerves and their distributions. The brain is shown in an inferior view. See Table 8–4 for descriptions.

QUESTION: Which cranial nerves bring about secretion of saliva? Which nerve brings about gastric and intestinal secretion?

Table 8–4 | CRANIAL NERVES

NUMBER AND NAME	FUNCTION(S)
I Olfactory	Sense of smell
II Optic	Sense of sight
III Oculomotor	Movement of the eyeball; constriction of pupil in bright light or for near vision
IV Trochlear	Movement of eyeball
V Trigeminal	Sensation in face, scalp, and teeth; contraction of chewing muscles
VI Abducens	Movement of the eyeball
VII Facial	Sense of taste; contraction of facial muscles; secretion of saliva
VIII Acoustic (vestibulocochlear)	Sense of hearing; sense of equilibrium
IX Glossopharyngeal	Sense of taste; sensory for cardiac, respiratory, and blood pressure reflexes; contraction of pharynx; secretion of saliva
X Vagus	Sensory in cardiac, respiratory, and blood pressure reflexes; sensory and motor to larynx (speaking); decreases heart rate; contraction of alimentary tube (peristalsis); increases digestive secretions
XI Accessory	Contraction of neck and shoulder muscles; motor to larynx (speaking)
XII Hypoglossal	Movement of the tongue

Making up the autonomic nervous system are **visceral motor neurons** to smooth muscle, cardiac muscle, and glands. These are the **visceral effectors**; muscle will either contract or relax, and glands will either increase or decrease their secretions.

The ANS has two divisions: **sympathetic** and **parasympathetic**. Often, they function in opposition to each other, as you will see. The activity of both divisions is integrated by the hypothalamus, which ensures that the visceral effectors will respond appropriately to the situation.

AUTONOMIC PATHWAYS

Autonomic nerve pathways going from the central nervous system to visceral effectors differ anatomically from somatic pathways that lead to skeletal muscle effectors. Turn back to Fig. 8–3 and find the motor neuron. This is a somatic motor neuron; its cell body is in the spinal cord and its axon extends all the way to the skeletal muscle, where it synapses with muscle cells. A somatic motor pathway, therefore, is a one-neuron pathway. An autonomic pathway, however, is a two-neuron pathway. It consists of two motor neurons that synapse in a ganglion outside the CNS. The first neuron is called the **preganglionic neuron**, from the CNS to the ganglion. The second neuron is called the **postganglionic neuron**, from the ganglion to the visceral effector. The ganglia are actually the cell bodies of the postganglionic neurons. Look at Fig. 8–12 as you read the next sections.

SYMPATHETIC DIVISION

Another name for the sympathetic division is thoracolumbar division, which tells us where the sympathetic preganglionic neurons originate. Their cell bodies are in the thoracic segments and some of the lumbar segments of the spinal cord. Their axons extend to the sympathetic ganglia, most of which are located in two chains just outside the spinal column (see Fig. 8–12). Within the ganglia are the synapses between preganglionic and postganglionic neurons; the postganglionic axons then go to the visceral effectors. One preganglionic neuron often synapses with many postganglionic neurons to many effectors. This anatomic arrangement has physiological importance: The sympathetic division brings about rapid and widespread responses in many organs. Aspects of the anatomy of both

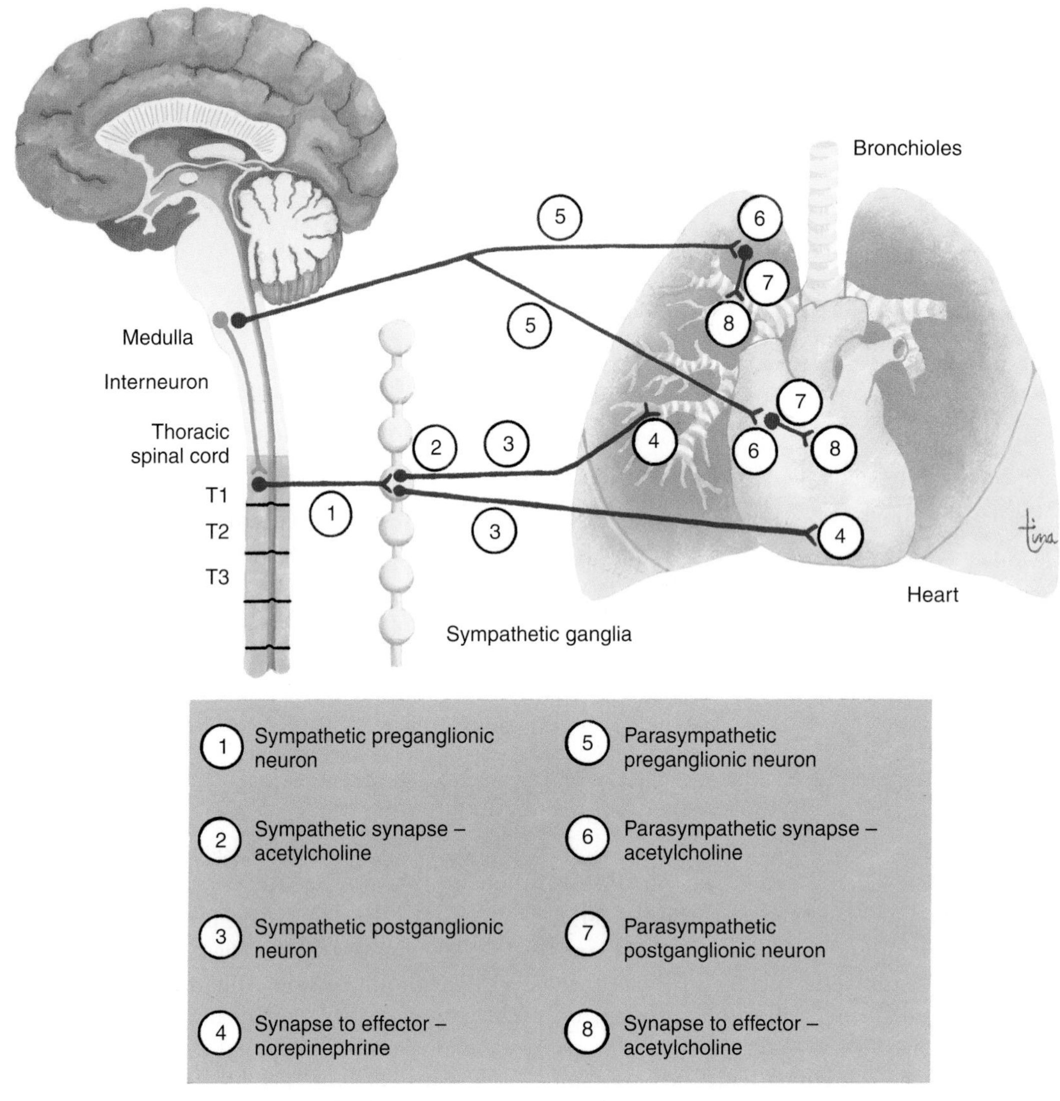

Figure 8–12 Neurons of the autonomic nervous system. A schematic of sympathetic (blue) and parasympathetic (red) neurons. See text and Table 8–5 for further description.

QUESTION: The parasympathetic neuron to the heart emerges from what part of the brain? Can you name this nerve?

ANS divisions as shown in Fig. 8–12 are summarized in Table 8–5.

The sympathetic division is dominant in stressful situations, which include anger, fear, or anxiety, as well as exercise. For our prehistoric ancestors, stressful situations often involved the need for intense physical activity—the "fight-or-flight response." Our nervous systems haven't changed very much in 50,000 years, and if you look at Table 8–6, you will see the kinds of responses the sympathetic division stimulates. The heart rate increases, vasodilation in skeletal muscles supplies them with more oxygen, the bronchioles dilate to take in more air, and the liver changes glycogen to glucose to supply energy. At the same time, digestive secretions decrease and peristalsis slows; these are not important in a stress situation. Vasoconstriction in the skin and viscera shunts blood to more

Table 8–5 | ANATOMY OF THE AUTONOMIC NERVOUS SYSTEM

CHARACTERISTIC	SYMPATHETIC	PARASYMPATHETIC
CNS location of preganglionic neuron cell bodies	Thoracic and lumbar spinal cord	Brainstem and sacral spinal cord
Location of ganglia	Most are in two chains beside the vertebral column	Near or in the visceral effectors
Preganglionic neurons	Relatively short Release acetylcholine at the synapse in the ganglion	Relatively long Release acetylcholine at the synapse in the ganglion
Postganglionic neurons	Relatively long Most release norepinephrine at the visceral effector	Relatively short All release acetylcholine at the visceral effector
Extent of neuron pathways	Widespread effect: One preganglionic neuron synapses with many postganglionic neurons to many effectors	Localized effect: One preganglionic neuron synapses with few postganglionic neurons to one effector

vital organs such as the heart, muscles, and brain. All of these responses enabled our ancestors to stay and fight or to get away from potential danger. Even though we may not always be in life-threatening situations during stress (such as figuring out our income taxes), our bodies are prepared for just that. Figure 8–13 depicts all of the organs innervated by the sympathetic division; the nerve pathways are in blue.

PARASYMPATHETIC DIVISION

The other name for the parasympathetic division is the craniosacral division. The cell bodies of parasympathetic preganglionic neurons are in the brainstem and the sacral segments of the spinal cord. Their axons are in cranial nerve pairs 3, 7, 9, and 10 (oculomotor, facial, glossopharyngeal, and vagus nerves) and in some sacral nerves and extend to the parasympathetic ganglia. These ganglia are very close to or actually in the visceral effector (see Figs. 8–12 and 8–13; nerve pathways are shown in red), and contain the postganglionic cell bodies, with very short axons to the cells of the effector.

In the parasympathetic division, one preganglionic neuron synapses with just a few postganglionic neurons to only one effector. With this anatomic arrangement, very localized (one organ) responses are possible.

The parasympathetic division dominates in relaxed (non-stress) situations to promote normal functioning of several organ systems. Digestion will be efficient, with increased secretions and peristalsis; defecation and urination may occur; and the heart will beat at a normal resting rate. Other functions of this division are listed in Table 8–6.

Notice that when an organ receives both sympathetic and parasympathetic impulses, the responses are opposites. Such an arrangement makes maintaining an appropriate level of activity quite simple, as in changing the heart rate to meet the needs of a situation. Notice also that some visceral effectors receive only sympathetic impulses. In such cases, the opposite response is brought about by a decrease in sympathetic impulses. Secretion by the sweat glands is an example.

NEUROTRANSMITTERS

Recall that neurotransmitters enable nerve impulses to cross synapses. In autonomic pathways there are two synapses: one between preganglionic and postganglionic neurons (within the autonomic ganglia) and the second between postganglionic neurons and the cells of the visceral effectors.

Look again at Fig. 8–12 and find the synapses for each division. **Acetylcholine** is the transmitter released by all preganglionic neurons, both sympathetic and parasympathetic; it is inactivated by **cholinesterase** in postganglionic neurons. Parasympathetic postganglionic neurons all release acetylcholine at the synapses with their visceral effectors. Most sympathetic postganglionic neurons

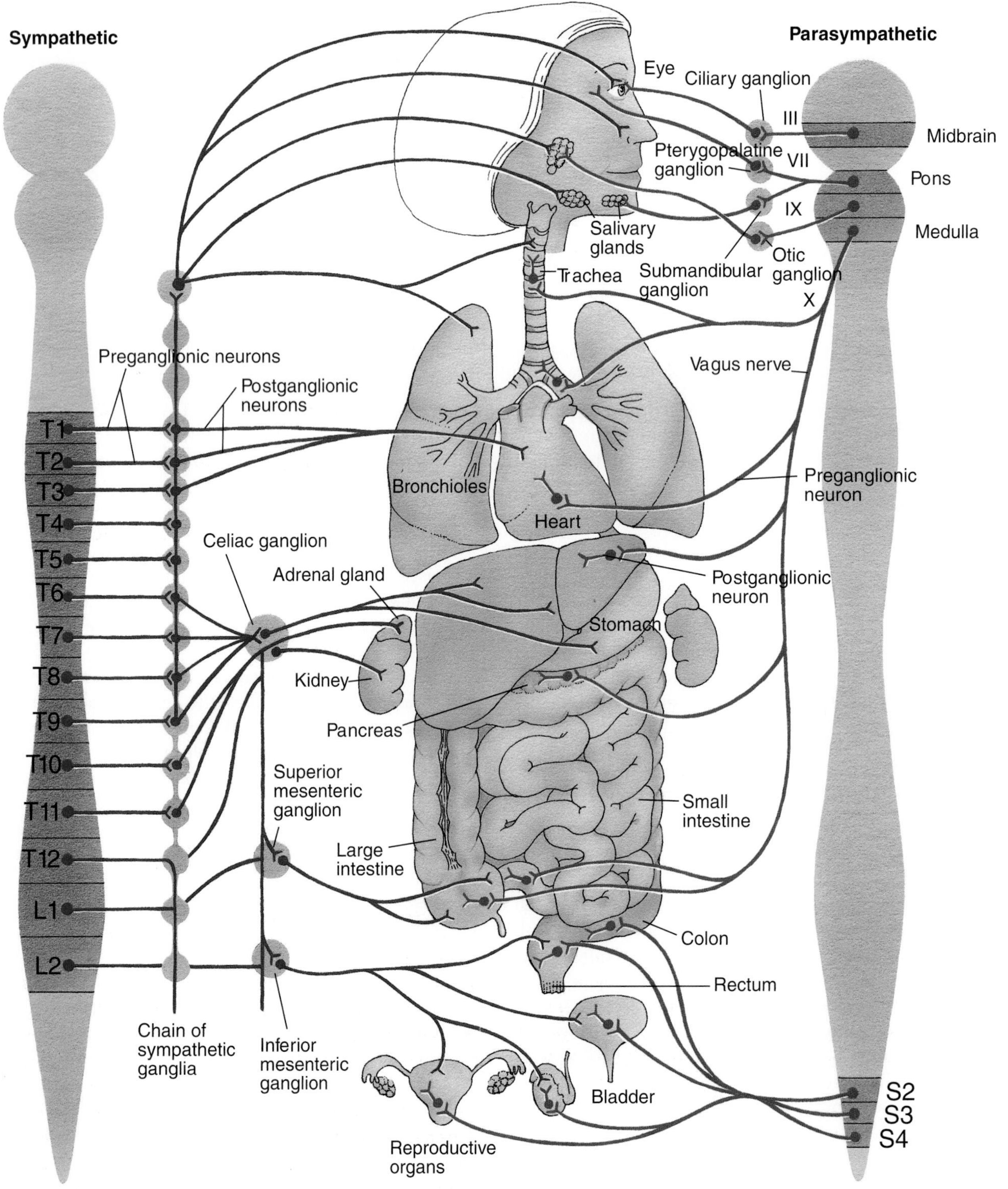

Figure 8–13 The autonomic nervous system. The sympathetic division is shown on the left, and the parasympathetic division is shown on the right (both divisions are bilateral).

QUESTION: Do both or just one division of the ANS supply the heart? What is the purpose of this arrangement?

Table 8–6 | FUNCTIONS OF THE AUTONOMIC NERVOUS SYSTEM

ORGAN	SYMPATHETIC RESPONSE	PARASYMPATHETIC RESPONSE
Heart (cardiac muscle)	Increase rate	Decrease rate (to resting normal)
Bronchioles (smooth muscle)	Dilate	Constrict (to normal)
Iris (smooth muscle)	Pupil dilates	Pupil constricts (to normal)
Salivary glands	Decrease secretion	Increase secretion (to normal)
Stomach and intestines (smooth muscle)	Decrease peristalsis	Increase peristalsis for normal digestion
Stomach and intestines (glands)	Decrease secretion	Increase secretion for normal digestion
Internal anal sphincter	Contracts to prevent defecation	Relaxes to permit defecation
Urinary bladder (smooth muscle)	Relaxes to prevent urination	Contracts for normal urination
Internal urethral sphincter	Contracts to prevent urination	Relaxes to permit urination
Liver	Changes glycogen to glucose	None
Pancreas	Secretes glucagon	Secretes insulin and digestive enzymes
Sweat glands	Increase secretion	None
Blood vessels (their smooth muscle) in skin and viscera	Constrict	None
Blood vessels (their smooth muscle) in skeletal muscle	Dilate (acetylcholine) Constrict (norepinephrine)	None
Adrenal glands	Increase secretion of epinephrine and norepinephrine	None

release the transmitter **norepinephrine** at the synapses with the effector cells. Norepinephrine is inactivated by either catechol-*O*-methyl transferase (COMT) or monoamine oxidase (MAO), or it may be removed from the synapse by reuptake. The sympathetic postganglionic neurons that release acetylcholine are the neurons to sweat glands and some of those to the smooth muscle in the walls of the blood vessels in skeletal muscle (to bring about vasodilation).

AGING AND THE NERVOUS SYSTEM

The aging brain does lose neurons, but the loss is only a small percentage of the total neurons. The formation of synaptic connections is believed to slow considerably as we get older, but this is not the usual cause of mental impairment in elderly people. (Far more common causes are depression, malnutrition, hypotension, and the side effects of medications.) Some forgetfulness is to be expected, however, as is a decreased ability for *rapid* problem solving, but most memory should remain intact. Voluntary movements become slower, as do reflexes and reaction time. Think of driving a car, an ability we sometimes take for granted. For elderly people, with their slower perceptions and reaction times, greater *consciousness* of driving is necessary.

As the autonomic nervous system ages, dry eyes and constipation may become problems. Transient hypotension may be the result of decreased sympathetic stimulation of vasoconstriction. In most cases, however, elderly people who are aware of these aspects of aging will be able to work with their physicians or nurses to adapt to them.

SUMMARY

The nervous system regulates many of our simplest and most complex activities. The impulses generated and carried by the nervous system are an example of the chemical level of organization of the body. These nerve impulses then regulate the functioning of tissues, organs, and organ systems, which permits us to perceive and respond to the world around us and the changes within us. The detection of such changes is the function of the sense organs, and they are the subject of our next chapter.

STUDY OUTLINE

Functions of the Nervous System

1. Detect changes and feel sensations.
2. Initiate responses to changes.
3. Organize and store information.

Nervous System Divisions

1. Central nervous system (CNS)—brain and spinal cord.
2. Peripheral nervous system (PNS)—cranial nerves and spinal nerves, including the autonomic nervous system (ANS) and the enteric nervous system in the alimentary tube.

Nerve Tissue—neurons (nerve fibers) and specialized cells (Schwann, neuroglia)

1. Neuron cell body contains the nucleus; cell bodies are in the CNS or in the trunk and are protected by bone.
2. An axon carries electrical impulses away from the cell body; dendrites carry impulses toward the cell body.
3. Schwann cells in PNS: Layers of cell membrane form the myelin sheath to electrically insulate neurons; nodes of Ranvier are spaces between adjacent Schwann cells. Nuclei and cytoplasm of Schwann cells form the neurolemma, which is essential for regeneration of damaged axons or dendrites.
4. Oligodendrocytes in CNS form the myelin sheaths; microglia phagocytize pathogens and damaged cells; astrocytes contribute to the blood–brain barrier and regulate localized blood flow (see Table 8–1).

The Nerve Impulse—see Table 8–2

1. Polarization—neuron membrane has a positive (+) charge outside and a negative (−) charge inside; many Na^+ ions outside and many K^+ ions inside.
2. Depolarization—entry of Na^+ ions and reversal of charges on either side of the membrane; the outside becomes negative relative to the inside.
3. An action potential, the impulse itself, is depolarization followed by repolarization. Repolarization is the exit of K^+ ions and return to a (+) charge outside.
4. Impulse transmission is rapid, often several meters per second.
   a. Saltatory conduction—in a myelinated neuron only the nodes of Ranvier depolarize; increases speed of impulses.
5. Electrical nerve impulses are all exactly alike; their different effects depend on their various destinations (muscles, glands, or other neurons).

6. Synapse—the space between the axon of one neuron and the dendrites or cell body of the next neuron. A neurotransmitter carries the impulse across a synapse and is then destroyed by a chemical inactivator or absorbed (reuptake). Synapses make impulse transmission one way in the living person.

Types of Neurons—nerve fibers

1. Sensory—carry impulses from receptors to the CNS; may be somatic (from skin, skeletal muscles, joints) or visceral (from internal organs).
2. Motor—carry impulses from the CNS to effectors; may be somatic (to skeletal muscle) or visceral (to smooth muscle, cardiac muscle, or glands). Visceral motor neurons make up the autonomic nervous system.
3. Interneurons—entirely within the CNS.

Nerves and Nerve Tracts

1. Sensory nerve—made only of sensory neurons.
2. Motor nerve—made only of motor neurons.
3. Mixed nerve—made of both sensory and motor neurons.
4. Nerve tract—a nerve within the CNS; also called white matter.

The Spinal Cord

1. Functions: transmits impulses to and from the brain, and integrates the spinal cord reflexes.
2. Location: within the vertebral canal; extends from the foramen magnum to the disc between the 1st and 2nd lumbar vertebrae.
3. Cross-section: internal H-shaped gray matter contains cell bodies of motor neurons and interneurons; external white matter is the myelinated axons and dendrites of interneurons.
4. Ascending tracts carry sensory impulses to the brain; descending tracts carry motor impulses away from the brain.
5. Central canal contains cerebrospinal fluid and is continuous with the ventricles of the brain.

Spinal Nerves—see Table 8–3 for major peripheral nerves

1. Eight cervical pairs to head, neck, shoulder, arm, and diaphragm; 12 thoracic pairs to trunk; 5 lumbar pairs and 5 sacral pairs to hip, pelvic cavity, and leg; 1 very small coccygeal pair.
2. Cauda equina—the lumbar and sacral nerves that extend below the end of the spinal cord.
3. Each spinal nerve has two roots: dorsal or sensory root; dorsal root ganglion contains cell bodies of sensory neurons; ventral or motor root; the two roots unite to form a mixed spinal nerve.

Spinal Cord Reflexes—do not depend directly on the brain

1. A reflex is an involuntary response to a stimulus.
2. Reflex arc—the pathway of nerve impulses during a reflex: (1) receptors, (2) sensory neurons, (3) CNS with one or more synapses, (4) motor neurons, (5) effector that responds.
3. Stretch reflex—a muscle that is stretched will contract; these reflexes help keep us upright against gravity. The patellar reflex is also used clinically to assess neurologic functioning, as are many other reflexes (Fig. 8–5).
4. Flexor reflex—a painful stimulus will cause withdrawal of the body part; these reflexes are protective.

The Brain—many parts that function as an integrated whole; see Figs. 8–6 and 8–8 for locations

1. Ventricles—four cavities: two lateral, 3rd, 4th; each contains a choroid plexus that forms cerebrospinal fluid (Figs. 8–6 and 8–7).
2. Medulla—regulates the vital functions of heart rate, breathing, and blood pressure; regulates reflexes of coughing, sneezing, swallowing, and vomiting.
3. Pons—contains respiratory centers that work with those in the medulla.
4. Midbrain—contains centers for visual reflexes, auditory reflexes, and righting (equilibrium) reflexes.
5. Cerebellum—regulates coordination of voluntary movement, muscle tone, stopping movements, and equilibrium; contributes to sensations involving texture and weight.
6. Hypothalamus
   a. Produces antidiuretic hormone (ADH), which increases water reabsorption by the kidneys
   b. Produces oxytocin, which promotes uterine contractions for labor and delivery
   c. Produces releasing hormones that regulate the secretions of the anterior pituitary gland
   d. Regulates body temperature
   e. Regulates food intake
   f. Integrates the functioning of the autonomic nervous system (ANS), and promotes visceral responses to emotional situations
   g. Acts as a biological clock that regulates body rhythms.
7. Thalamus—groups sensory impulses as to body part before relaying them to the cerebrum; awareness of pain but inability to localize; suppresses unimportant sensations to permit concentration; contributes to alertness and awareness, and to memory.
8. Cerebrum—two hemispheres connected by the corpus callosum, which permits communication between the hemispheres. The cerebral cortex is the surface gray matter, which consists of cell bodies of neurons and is folded extensively into convolutions. The internal white matter consists of nerve tracts that connect the lobes of the cerebrum to one another and to other parts of the brain.
   a. Frontal lobes—motor areas initiate voluntary movement; premotor area regulates sequences of movements for learned skills; prefrontal area for aspects of social behavior; Broca's motor speech area (left hemisphere) regulates the movements involved in speech.
   b. Parietal lobes—general sensory area feels and interprets the cutaneous senses and conscious muscle sense; taste area extends into temporal lobe, for sense of taste; speech areas (left hemisphere) for thought before speech.
   c. Temporal lobes—auditory areas for hearing and interpretation; olfactory areas for sense of smell and interpretation; speech areas for thought before speech.
   d. Occipital lobes—visual areas for vision; interpretation areas for spatial relationships.
   e. Association areas—in all lobes, for abstract thinking, reasoning, learning, memory, and personality. The hippocampi are essential for the formation of memories. Neural plasticity is the ability of the brain to adapt to changing needs.
   f. Basal ganglia—small masses of gray matter within the cerebral hemispheres; regulate accessory movements such as gestures and facial expressions, as well as muscle tone.

Meninges and Cerebrospinal Fluid (CSF) (see Figs. 8–9 and 8–10)

1. Three meningeal layers made of connective tissue: outer—dura mater; middle—arachnoid membrane; inner—pia mater; all three enclose the brain and spinal cord.
2. Subarachnoid space contains CSF, the tissue fluid of the CNS.
3. CSF is formed continuously in the ventricles of the brain by choroid plexuses, from blood plasma.
4. CSF circulates from the ventricles to the central canal of the spinal cord and to the cranial and spinal subarachnoid spaces.
5. CSF is reabsorbed from the cranial subarachnoid space through arachnoid villi into the blood in the cranial venous sinuses. The rate of reabsorption equals the rate of production.
6. As tissue fluid, CSF brings nutrients to CNS neurons and removes waste products. CSF also acts as a shock absorber to cushion the CNS.

Cranial Nerves—12 pairs of nerves that emerge from the brain (see Fig. 8–11)

1. Concerned with vision, hearing and equilibrium, taste and smell, and many other functions within the head and viscera.
2. See Table 8–4 for the functions of each pair.

The Autonomic Nervous System (ANS) (see Figs. 8–12 and 8–13 and Tables 8–5 and 8–6)

1. Has two divisions: sympathetic and parasympathetic; their functioning is integrated by the hypothalamus.
2. Consists of motor neurons to visceral effectors: smooth muscle, cardiac muscle, and glands.
3. An ANS pathway consists of two neurons that synapse in a ganglion:
   a. Preganglionic neurons—from the CNS to the ganglia
   b. Postganglionic neurons—from the ganglia to the effectors
   c. Most sympathetic ganglia are in two chains just outside the vertebral column; parasympathetic ganglia are very near or in the visceral effectors.
4. Neurotransmitters: acetylcholine is released by all preganglionic neurons and by parasympathetic postganglionic neurons; the inactivator is cholinesterase. Norepinephrine is released by most sympathetic postganglionic neurons; the inactivator is COMT or MAO.
5. Sympathetic division—dominates during stress situations; responses prepare the body to meet physical demands.
6. Parasympathetic division—dominates in relaxed situations to permit normal functioning.

REVIEW QUESTIONS

1. Name the divisions of the nervous system and state the parts of each. (p. 186)
2. State the function of the following parts of nerve tissue: (pp. 187–189)
   a. Axon
   b. Dendrites
   c. Myelin sheath
   d. Neurolemma
   e. Microglia
   f. Astrocytes
3. Explain the difference between: (pp. 192–194)
   a. Sensory neurons and motor neurons
   b. Interneurons and nerve tracts
4. Describe an electrical nerve impulse in terms of charges on either side of the neuron membrane. Describe how a nerve impulse crosses a synapse. (pp. 190–191)
5. With respect to the spinal cord: (p. 194)
   a. Describe its location
   b. State what gray matter and white matter are made of
   c. State the function of the dorsal root, ventral root, and dorsal root ganglion
6. State the names and number of pairs of spinal nerves. State the part of the body supplied by the phrenic nerves, radial nerves, and sciatic nerves. (pp. 194,196)
7. Define reflex, and name the five parts of a reflex arc. (pp. 194,197)
8. Define stretch reflexes, and explain their practical importance. Define flexor reflexes, and explain their practical importance. (pp. 197–198)
9. Name the part of the brain concerned with each of the following: (pp. 198–202)
   a. Regulates body temperature
   b. Regulates heart rate
   c. Suppresses unimportant sensations
   d. Regulates respiration (two parts)
   e. Regulates food intake
   f. Regulates coordination of voluntary movement
   g. Regulates secretions of the anterior pituitary gland
   h. Regulates coughing and sneezing
   i. Regulates muscle tone
   j. Regulates visual and auditory reflexes
   k. Regulates blood pressure
10. Name the part of the cerebrum concerned with each of the following: (pp. 203–206)
    a. Feels the cutaneous sensations
    b. Contains the auditory areas
    c. Contains the visual areas
    d. Connects the cerebral hemispheres
    e. Regulates accessory movements
    f. Contains the olfactory areas
    g. Initiates voluntary movement
    h. Contains the speech areas (for most people)
11. Name the three layers of the meninges, beginning with the outermost. (p. 206)
12. State all the locations of cerebrospinal fluid. What is CSF made from? Into what is CSF reabsorbed? State the functions of CSF. (pp. 206–209)
13. State a function of each of the following cranial nerves: (p. 211)
    a. Glossopharyngeal
    b. Olfactory
    c. Trigeminal
    d. Facial
    e. Vagus (three functions)
14. Explain how the sympathetic division of the ANS helps the body adapt to a stress situation; give three specific examples. (pp. 211–213)
15. Explain how the parasympathetic division of the ANS promotes normal body functioning; give three specific examples. (p. 213)

FOR FURTHER THOUGHT

1. Your friend Fred was telling a story, with eloquent gestures, while making a salad. He missed the tomato with the knife, cut his hand badly, and needed quite a few stitches. A local anesthetic was used. How might a local anesthetic stop nerve impulses? (Remember that a nerve impulse is very simple.) What part of Fred's brain got him into trouble?
2. Some pesticides kill insects by interfering with cholinesterase. We have cholinesterase too, and may be adversely affected. What would be the symptoms of such pesticide poisoning?
3. We cannot live without a central nervous system. Describe all the ways in which the central nervous system is protected.
4. Older drivers are sometimes said to have "lost their reflexes." Is this really true? Explain.
5. Look at Question Figure 8–A. Starting at the top of column A, read the words down as fast as you can. For column B, start at the top and name the colors as fast as you can. Did you have any trouble? Now column C: Start at the top and name the colors—do not read the words—as fast as you can. Was there any difference? Explain why.

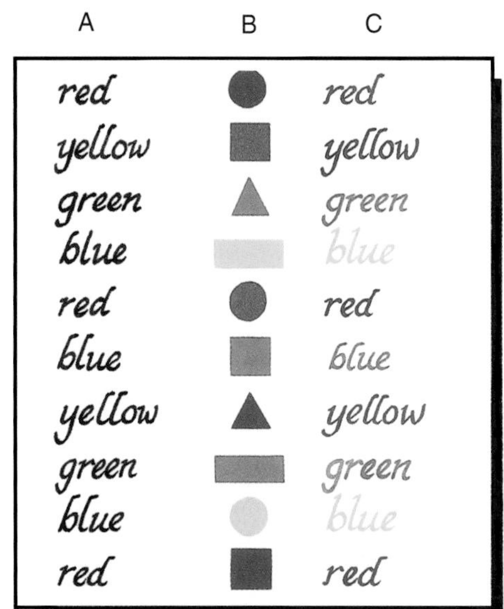

QUESTION FIGURE 8–A

6. Look at Question Figure 8–B: Nerve pathway. You have seen a similar picture in this chapter, with five numbered parts. Can you identify the numbered parts of this pathway? Can you give this pathway a name?

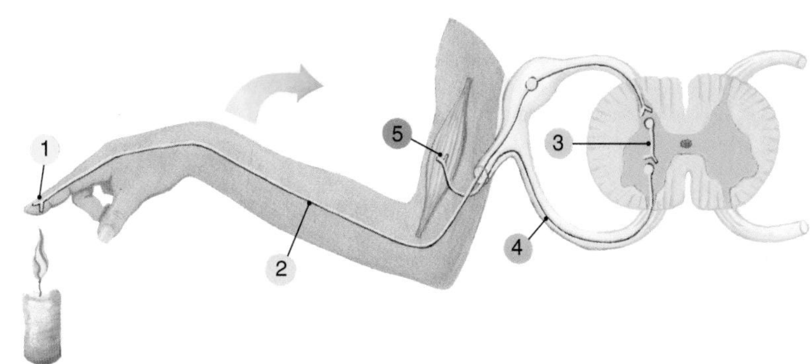

QUESTION FIGURE 8–B

CHAPTER

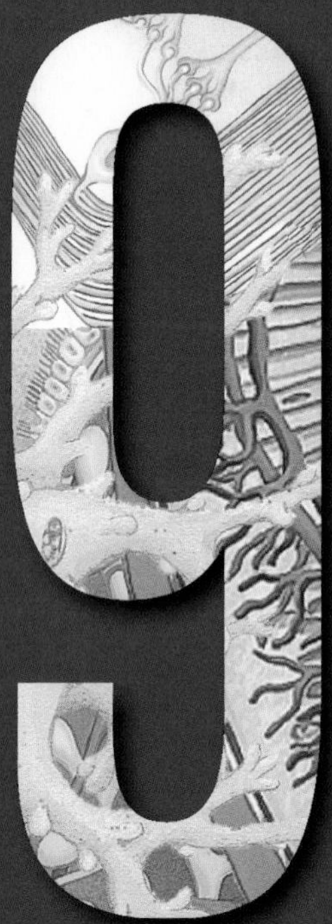

The Senses

STUDENT OBJECTIVES

- Explain the general purpose of sensations.
- Name the parts of a sensory pathway, and state the function of each.
- Describe the characteristics of sensations.
- Name the cutaneous senses, and explain their purpose.
- Explain referred pain and its importance.
- Explain the importance of muscle sense.
- Describe the pathways for the senses of taste and smell, and explain how these senses are interrelated.
- Name the parts of the eye and their functions.
- Describe the physiology of vision.
- Name the parts of the ear and their functions.
- Describe the physiology of hearing.
- Describe the physiology of equilibrium.
- Explain the importance of the arterial pressoreceptors and chemoreceptors.

NEW TERMINOLOGY

Adaptation *(A-dap-**TAY**-shun)*
After-image *(**AFF**-ter-im-ije)*
Aqueous humor *(**AY**-kwee-us **HYOO**-mer)*
Cochlea *(**KOK**-lee-uh)*
Cones *(KOHNES)*
Conjunctiva *(KON-junk-**TIGH**-vah)*
Contrast *(**KON**-trast)*
Cornea *(**KOR**-nee-ah)*
Eustachian tube *(yoo-**STAY**-shun TOOB)*
Iris *(**EYE**-ris)*
Lacrimal glands *(**LAK**-ri-muhl)*
Olfactory receptors *(ohl-**FAK**-toh-ree)*
Organ of Corti *(**KOR**-tee)*
Projection *(proh-**JEK**-shun)*
Referred pain *(ree-**FURRD** PAIN)*
Retina *(**RET**-i-nah)*
Rhodopsin *(roh-**DOP**-sin)*
Rods *(RAHDS)*
Sclera *(**SKLER**-ah)*
Semicircular canals *(SEM-ee-**SIR**-kyoo-lur)*
Tympanic membrane *(tim-**PAN**-ik)*
Vitreous humor *(**VIT**-ree-us **HYOO**-mer)*

*Terms that appear in **bold type** in the chapter text are defined in the glossary, which begins on page 603.*

CHAPTER OUTLINE

RELATED CLINICAL TERMINOLOGY

Age-related macular degeneration *(**MAK**-yoo-lar de-gen-er-**AY**-shun)*
Amblyopia *(am-blee-**OH**-pee-uh)*
Astigmatism *(uh-**STIG**-mah-TIZM)*
Cataract *(**KAT**-uh-rakt)*
Color blindness *(**KUHL**-or **BLIND**-ness)*
Conjunctivitis *(kon-JUNK-ti-**VIGH**-tis)*
Deafness *(**DEFF**-ness)*
Detached retina *(dee-**TACHD**)*
Glaucoma *(glaw-**KOH**-mah)*
Hyperopia *(HIGH-per-**OH**-pee-ah)*
Motion sickness *(**MOH**-shun)*
Myopia *(my-**OH**-pee-ah)*
Night blindness *(NIGHT **BLIND**-ness)*
Otitis media *(oh-**TIGH**-tis **MEE**-dee-ah)*
Phantom pain *(**FAN**-tum)*
Presbyopia *(PREZ-bee-**OH**-pee-ah)*
Strabismus *(strah-**BIZ**-miss)*

Have you ever been to a fireworks show? Bright bursts of lights in various colors, booms and crackles of explosions, and the scent of gunpowder are all part of the experience, which we can enjoy because of our senses. Even when our surroundings are not quite so dramatic, our senses constantly provide us with information. We see a friend waving, hear our names called, and then shake hands or give a hug because touch is important to us. The senses of taste and smell enable us to enjoy the flavor of our food or warn us that food has spoiled and may be dangerous to eat. Our sense of equilibrium keeps us upright. We also get information from our senses about what is happening inside the body. The pain of a headache, for example, prompts us to do something about it, such as take aspirin. In general, this is the purpose of sensations: to enable the body to respond appropriately to ever-changing situations and maintain homeostasis.

SENSORY PATHWAY

The impulses involved in sensations follow very precise pathways, which all have the following parts:

1. **Receptors**—detect changes (**stimuli**) and generate impulses. Receptors are usually very specific with respect to the kinds of changes they respond to. Those in the retina detect light rays, those in the nasal cavities detect vapors, and so on. Once a specific stimulus has affected receptors, however, they all respond in the same way by generating electrical nerve impulses. All receptors change the energy of a stimulus to the electrical energy of a nerve impulse.
2. **Sensory neurons**—transmit impulses from receptors to the central nervous system. These sensory neurons are found in both spinal nerves and cranial nerves, but each carries impulses from only one type of receptor.
3. **Sensory tracts**—white matter in the spinal cord or brain that transmits the impulses to a specific part of the brain.
4. **Sensory areas**—most are in the cerebral cortex (recall Fig. 8–8 in the last chapter). These areas feel and interpret the sensations. Learning to interpret nerve impulses as sensations begins in infancy (if not before birth), without our awareness of it, and continues throughout life.

CHARACTERISTICS OF SENSATIONS

Certain characteristics of sensations will help you understand how the sensory areas work with impulses from the receptors to produce useful information about the external and internal environments:

1. **Projection**—the sensation seems to come from the area where the receptors were stimulated. If you touch this book, the sensation of touch seems to be in your hand but is actually being felt by your cerebral cortex. That it is indeed the brain that feels sensations is demonstrated by patients who feel **phantom pain** after amputation of a limb. After loss of a hand, for example, the person may still feel that the hand is really there. Why does this happen? The receptors in the hand are no longer present, but the severed nerve endings continue to generate impulses. These impulses travel along the usual nerves to the spinal cord, arrive in the parietal lobe area for the hand, and the brain does what it has

always done with impulses from these pathways and creates the projection, the feeling that the hand is still there. For most amputees, phantom pain diminishes as the severed nerves heal, but the person often experiences a phantom "presence" of the missing part. This may be helpful when learning to use an artificial limb.

A slightly different situation, with the same outcome, occurs for some people who have become partially deaf and experience **tinnitus**, a buzzing, crackling, or ringing in the ears. Some of the receptors for hearing have been damaged and are not generating impulses, so the brain is no longer receiving impulses. The brain is so used to such impulses (rarely are we in complete silence for long) that the auditory areas try to "fill in" what they perceive they are missing. The abnormal hissing or buzzing is a creation of the brain, and projected to the ears.

2. **Intensity**—some sensations are felt more distinctly and to a greater degree than are others. A weak stimulus such as dim light will affect a small number of receptors, but a stronger stimulus, such as bright sunlight, will stimulate many more receptors. When more receptors are stimulated, more impulses will arrive in the sensory area of the brain. The brain "counts" the impulses and projects a more intense sensation.
3. **Contrast**—the effect of a previous or simultaneous sensation on a current sensation, which may then be exaggerated or diminished. Again, this is a function of the brain, which constantly compares sensations. If, on a very hot day, you jump into a swimming pool, the water may feel quite cold at first. The brain compares the new sensation with the previous one, and since there is a significant difference between the two, the water will seem colder than it actually is.
4. **Adaptation**—becoming unaware of a continuing stimulus. Receptors detect changes, but if the stimulus continues, it may not be much of a change, and the receptors will generate fewer impulses. The water in the swimming pool that seemed cold at first seems to "warm up" after a few minutes. The water has not changed temperature, and the receptors for cold have no changes to detect, therefore they generate fewer impulses. The sensation of cold lessens, and we interpret or feel that as increasing warmth. For another example, look at your left wrist (or perhaps the right one). Many of us wear a watch and are probably unaware of its presence on the arm most of the time. The cutaneous receptors for touch or pressure adapt very quickly to a continuing stimulus, and if there is no change, there is nothing for the receptors to detect.
5. **After-image**—the sensation remains in the consciousness even after the stimulus has stopped. A familiar example is the bright after-image seen after watching a flashbulb go off. The very bright light strongly stimulates receptors in the retina, which generate many impulses that are perceived as an intense sensation that lasts longer than the actual stimulus. And if you have ever thought "my ears are ringing" after hearing a sudden, loud sound, you have experienced an auditory after-image.

CUTANEOUS SENSES

As you know, the skin is a large organ that forms the outer boundary of the body, and because of its placement it contains thousands of receptors. The dermis of the skin and the subcutaneous tissue contain receptors for the sensations of touch, pressure, heat, cold, itch, and pain. The receptors for heat, cold, itch, and pain are **free nerve endings**, which also respond to any intense stimulus. Intense pressure or cold, for example, may be felt as pain. The receptors for touch and pressure are **encapsulated nerve endings**, meaning that there is a cellular structure around the nerve ending (Fig. 9–1).

The **cutaneous senses** provide us with information about the external environment and also about the skin itself. Much of the information about the environment is not of great importance and is processed at a subconscious level (suppressed by the thalamus), though we can choose to be aware of it. For example, could you distinguish a cotton T-shirt from denim jeans by touch alone? Probably, but you might not realize that you can do that until you try it by, say, sorting laundry in the dark. If you were walking barefoot, could you tell if you were walking on a carpet, a wood floor, concrete, or beach sand? Yes, you could. But are we usually aware of the sensation from the soles of our feet? If all is going well, probably not, because there is nothing unexpected for us to deal with. Some people with diabetes, however, develop diabetic **neuropathy**, damage to nerves that impairs sensation, and they may say that walking on a wood floor feels like walking on cotton balls or that the buttons of a shirt feel too large or too small. They are aware of such odd sensations simply because the feelings are odd. For most of us, the touch of the wood floor is not brought to awareness because it is what the brain expects from past experience, but if the floor has splinters or if the beach sand is hot, we are certainly aware. This is information we can bring to our conscious minds if necessary, but usually do not.

As for the skin itself, if you have ever had poison ivy, you may remember the itchiness of the rash. Itch has been

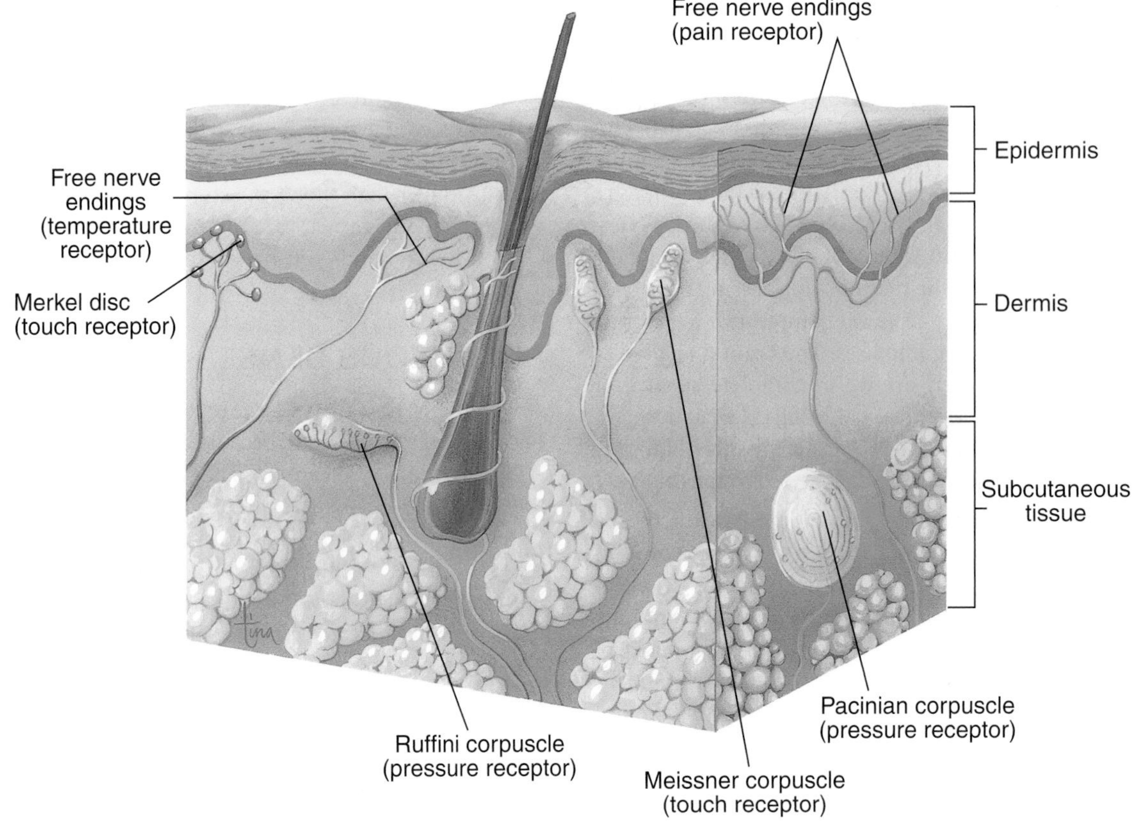

Figure 9–1 Cutaneous receptors in a section of the skin. Free nerve endings and encapsulated nerve endings are shown.

QUESTION: In which layers are most of the cutaneous receptors located?

found to be a rather complicated sensation, and there are at least two kinds of itch. One may be considered chemical itch and a second may be considered mechanical itch. Chemical itching is the result of an irritant such as poison ivy sap or mosquito saliva stimulating the release of histamine in the skin. This is part of the inflammatory response, and the histamine causes itching.

Mechanical itching may be caused by a coarse fabric against the skin or by the slight movement of something such as a flea. This type of itch may be a mild pain sensation, which may become more painful if not scratched.

Why does scratching help relieve mechanical itches, besides by removing an external irritant? One proposed mechanism is that scratching is a bit more painful than the itch, and the impulses it generates can distract the brain from the impulses generated by the itch. Another proposal is that the impulses generated by scratching inhibit the neurons in the spinal cord that are part of the itch pathway (a dog using its hind leg to scratch an itch is actually using a spinal cord reflex that does not require the brain). Scratching will not help relieve the itch of poison ivy, chickenpox, or a mosquito bite, however, because the irritating chemicals are in the skin, not on it. An antihistamine medication may help, and in such cases, scratching may do more damage and worsen inflammation at the site.

Clinicians have proposed a third type of itch, which they call "pathological." People with some types of liver or kidney disease, with certain cancers, or with HIV/AIDS may develop an unrelenting itchiness that disrupts sleep and even normal activities. The cause is not known, and no satisfactory treatment has yet been found for this type of painful and debilitating itching.

The sensory areas for the skin are in the parietal lobes. You may recall from Chapter 5 that the sensitivity of an area of skin is determined by the number of receptors present. Now we'll go a step further. The number of receptors corresponds to the size of the sensory area in the cerebral cortex. The greater the number of cutaneous receptors, the greater the number of cortex neurons devoted to receiving and interpreting their impulses. The largest parts of this sensory cortex are for the parts of the skin with the most receptors, that is, the hands and face.

As mentioned previously, sensory areas are not merely passive recipients of impulses. Consider the sensation of wetness. It is a distinct sensation, but there are no receptors for "wet" in the skin. Where does the sensation come from? Where all sensation comes from: the brain. The parietal lobes have learned to associate the simultaneous reception of temperature and pressure impulses with "wet." You can demonstrate this for yourself by putting on a plastic glove and dunking your fingers in a cup of water. Your fingers will feel wet, though they are perfectly dry inside the glove. Wetness is a learned sensation, created by the brain.

REFERRED PAIN

Free nerve endings are also found in internal organs. The smooth muscle of the small intestine, for example, has free nerve endings that are stimulated by excessive stretching or contraction; the resulting pain is called visceral pain. Sometimes pain that originates in an internal organ may be felt in a cutaneous area; this is called **referred pain**. The pain of a heart attack (myocardial infarction) may be felt in the left arm and shoulder, or the pain of gallstones may be felt in the right shoulder. These and other sites of referred pain are shown in Fig. 9–2.

Referred pain is actually a creation of the brain. Within the spinal cord are sensory tracts that are shared by cutaneous impulses and visceral impulses. Cutaneous impulses are much more frequent, and the brain correctly

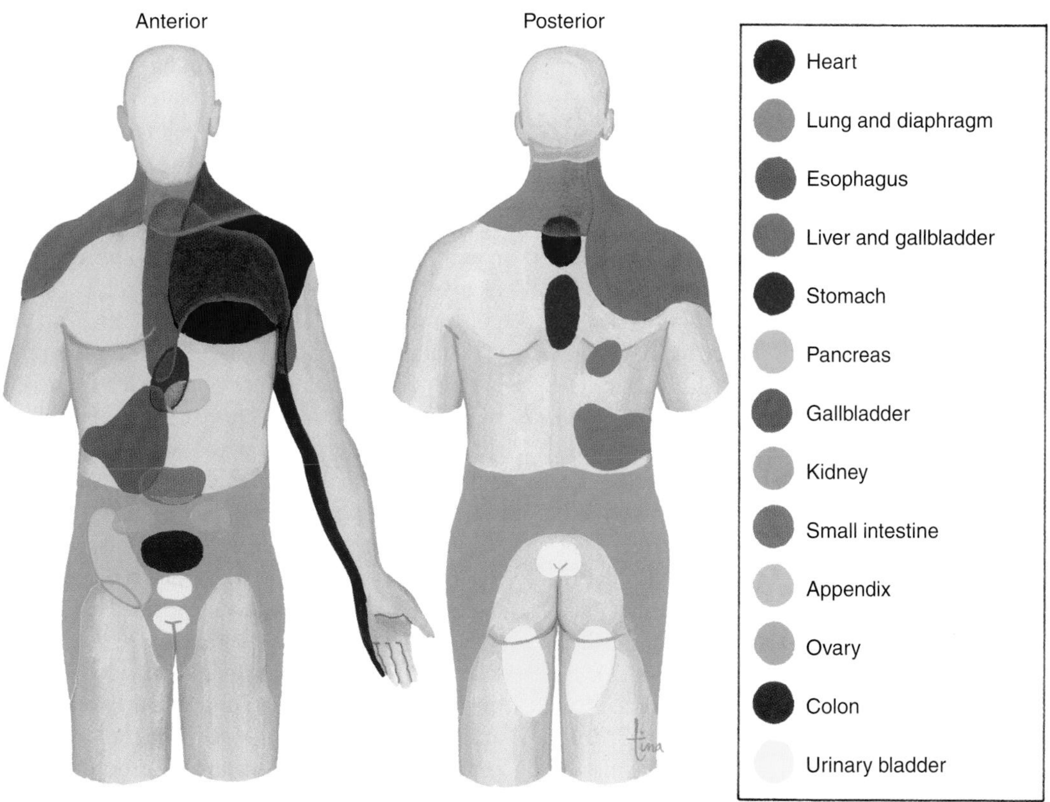

Figure 9–2 Referred pain. The sites for referred pain from various organs are shown.

QUESTION: From which visceral organs might pain be referred to a limb?

projects the sensation to the skin. When the impulses come from an organ such as the heart, however, the brain may still project the sensation to the "usual" cutaneous area, the left shoulder and left arm, and the left side of the neck. The brain projects sensation on the basis of past experience, and cutaneous pain is far more common than visceral pain. Knowledge of referred pain, as in the examples mentioned earlier, may often be helpful to clinicians but cannot be used in isolation. Notice in Fig. 9–2 that some referred pain areas are quite small but others are rather large, that some areas seem very logical and other areas (or parts of them) not as logical, and finally that some areas overlap. Nonetheless, referred pain can be a useful aspect of diagnosis.

MUSCLE SENSE

Muscle sense (also called proprioception or kinesthetic sense) was discussed in Chapter 7 and will be reviewed only briefly here. Stretch receptors (also called proprioceptors or muscle spindles) detect stretching of muscles and generate impulses, which enable the brain to create a mental picture to know where the muscles are and how they are positioned. Conscious muscle sense is felt by the parietal lobes. Unconscious muscle sense is used by the cerebellum to coordinate voluntary movements. We do not have to see our muscles to be sure that they are performing their intended actions. Muscle sense also contributes to our ability to distinguish the shape of objects.

SENSE OF TASTE

The receptors for taste are found in **taste buds**, most of which are in papillae on the tongue (Fig. 9–3). These **chemoreceptors** detect chemicals in solution in the mouth. The chemicals are foods and the solvent is saliva (if the mouth is very dry, taste is very indistinct). There are five (perhaps more) general types of taste receptors: sweet, sour, salty, bitter, and savory. Savory (also called umami or glutamate) is a taste like grilled meat. The tongue also has receptors for pain (as you know if you have ever accidentally bitten your tongue while chewing), and some of these receptors contain a molecular receptor that detects the "heat" of spicy foods such as "hot" peppers. We experience many more than five or six different tastes, however, because foods are often complex chemicals that stimulate different combinations of receptors, and the sense of smell also contributes to our perception of food.

Some taste preferences have been found to be genetic. People with more than the average number of taste buds find broccoli very bitter, whereas people with fewer taste buds may like the taste. Does adaptation occur with the sense of taste? With a moment's thought you know the answer. The first mouthful of a favorite food often tastes the best, but the rest also tastes pretty good. So yes, there is some adaptation.

The impulses from taste buds are transmitted by the facial and glossopharyngeal (7th and 9th cranial) nerves to the taste areas in the parietal-temporal cortex. The sense of taste is important because it makes eating enjoyable. Some medications may interfere with the sense of taste, and this sense becomes less acute as we get older. These may be contributing factors to poor nutrition in certain patients and in the elderly.

SENSE OF SMELL

As is true of the other senses, the sense of smell gives us a great deal of pleasure and practical information. The receptors for smell (**olfaction**) are **chemoreceptors** that detect vaporized chemicals that have been sniffed into the upper nasal cavities (see Fig. 9–3). Just as there are specific taste receptors, there are also specific scent receptors, and research indicates that humans have several hundred different receptors. When stimulated by vapor molecules, **olfactory receptors** generate impulses carried by the olfactory nerves (1st cranial) through the ethmoid bone to the olfactory bulbs. The pathway for these impulses ends in the olfactory areas of the temporal lobes. Vapors may stimulate many combinations of receptors, and it has been estimated that the human brain is capable of distinguishing among 10,000 different scents.

That may seem impressive, but the human sense of smell is very poorly developed compared with those of other animals. Dogs, for example, have a sense of smell about 2000 times more acute than that of people, with more receptors, but especially because the canine olfactory cortex is comparatively much larger than that of humans. (It has been said that most people live in a world of sights, whereas dogs live in a world of smells.) As mentioned earlier, however, much of what we call taste is actually the smell of food. If you have a cold and your nasal cavities are stuffed up, food just doesn't taste as good as it usually does. Adaptation occurs relatively quickly with odors. Pleasant scents may be sharply distinct at first but rapidly seem to dissipate or fade, and even unpleasant scents may fade with long exposure.

Loss of the sense of smell (gradual loss may be part of aging) not only deprives a person of much of the pleasure of food, but also can lead to harm. We tend to become aware of gas leaks, something burning, or the spoilage of food not by way of sight or hearing or touch, but by the sense of smell.

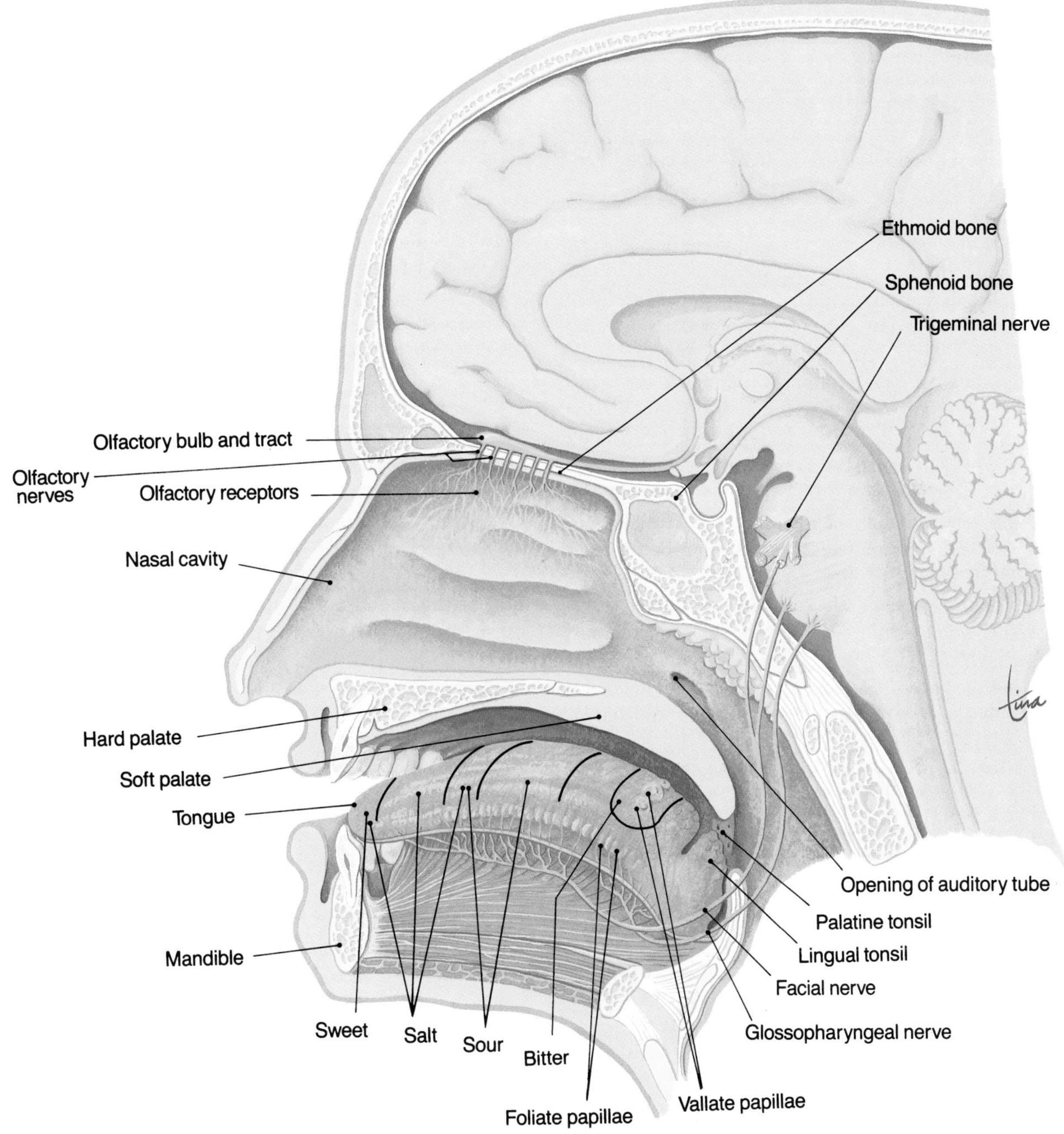

Figure 9–3 Structures concerned with the senses of smell and taste, shown in a midsagittal section of the head.

QUESTION: If we sniff something pungent, why can we often taste it as well? (Follow the inhaled air.)

HUNGER AND THIRST

Hunger and thirst may be called **visceral sensations**, in that they are triggered by internal changes. Hunger is a sensation that seems to be far more complex than was first thought, but thirst seems to be somewhat simpler. The receptors for both senses are specialized cells in the hypothalamus. Receptors for hunger are believed to detect changes in blood nutrient levels, the blood levels of hormones from the stomach and small intestine, and the hormone leptin released by adipose tissue; all of these chemical signals are collected by the hypothalamus. The receptors for thirst detect changes in the body water content, which is actually the water-to-salt proportion.

Naturally we do not feel these sensations in the hypothalamus: They are projected. Hunger is projected to the stomach, which contracts. Thirst is projected to the mouth and pharynx, and less saliva is produced.

If not satisfied by eating, the sensation of hunger gradually diminishes, that is, adaptation occurs. The reason is that after blood nutrient levels decrease, they become stable as fat in adipose tissue is used for energy. With little or no digestive activity in the gastrointestinal tract, secretion of hormones diminishes. With no sharp fluctuations of the chemical signals, the receptors in the hypothalamus have few changes to detect and hunger becomes much less intense. This adaptation has limits, however, and starvation can be very painful.

In contrast, the sensation of thirst, if not satisfied by drinking, is uncomfortable from the first and continues to worsen. There is no adaptation. As body water is lost, the amount keeps decreasing and does not stabilize. Therefore, there are constant changes for the receptors to detect, and prolonged thirst may be excruciatingly painful.

THE EYE

The eye contains the receptors for vision and a refracting system that focuses light rays on the receptors in the retina. We will begin our discussion, however, with the accessory structures of the eye, then later return to the eye itself and the physiology of vision.

EYELIDS AND THE LACRIMAL APPARATUS

The eyelids contain skeletal muscle that enables the eyelids to close and cover the front of the eyeball. Eyelashes along the border of each eyelid help keep dust out of the eyes. The eyelids are lined with a thin membrane called the **conjunctiva**, which is also folded over the white of the eye and merges with the corneal epithelium. Inflammation of this membrane, called **conjunctivitis**, may be caused by allergies or by certain bacteria or viruses and makes the eyes red, itchy, and watery.

Tears are produced by the **lacrimal glands**, located at the upper, outer corner of the eyeball, within the orbit (Fig. 9–4). Secretion of tears occurs constantly but is

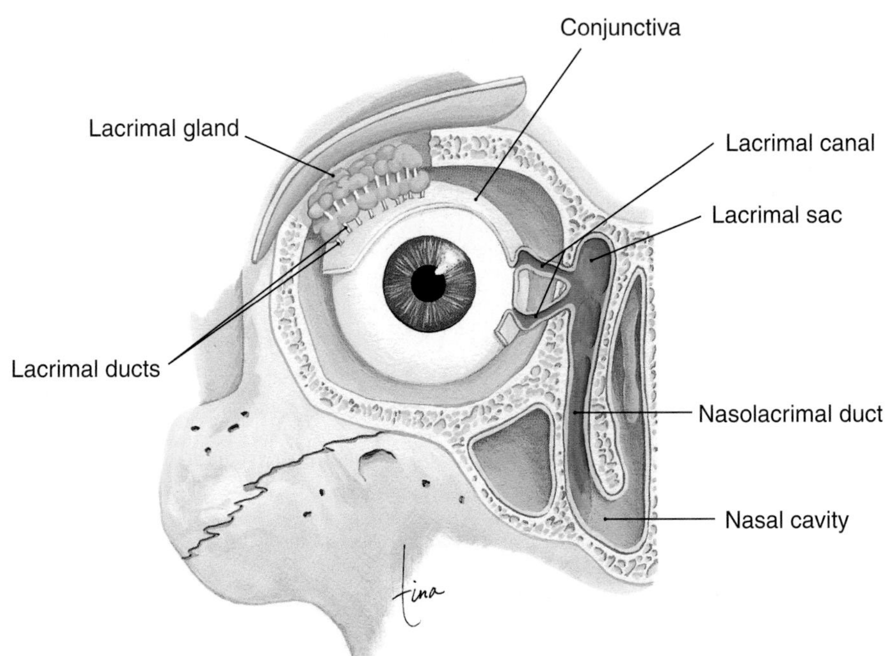

Figure 9–4 Lacrimal apparatus shown in an anterior view of the right eye.

QUESTION: Where do tears usually end up?

increased by the presence of irritating chemicals (onion vapors, for example) or dust, and in certain emotional situations (sad or happy). Small ducts take tears to the anterior of the eyeball, and blinking spreads the tears and washes the surface of the eye. Tears are mostly water, with about 1% sodium chloride, similar to other body fluids. Tears also contain **lysozyme**, an enzyme that inhibits the growth of most bacteria on the wet, warm surface of the eye. At the medial corner of the eyelids are two small openings into the superior and inferior lacrimal canals. These ducts take tears to the **lacrimal sac** (in the lacrimal bone), which leads to the **nasolacrimal duct**, which empties tears into the nasal cavity. This is why crying often makes the nose run and why cold or flu viruses transferred from a hand to an eye will end up in the nasal cavity, where they can infect cells of the lining.

EYEBALL

Most of the eyeball is within and protected by the **orbit**, formed by the lacrimal, maxilla, zygomatic, frontal, sphenoid, and ethmoid bones. The six **extrinsic muscles** of the eye (Fig. 9–5) are attached to this bony socket and to the surface of the eyeball. There are four rectus (straight) muscles that move the eyeball up and down or side to side; the name of the muscle tells you which direction.

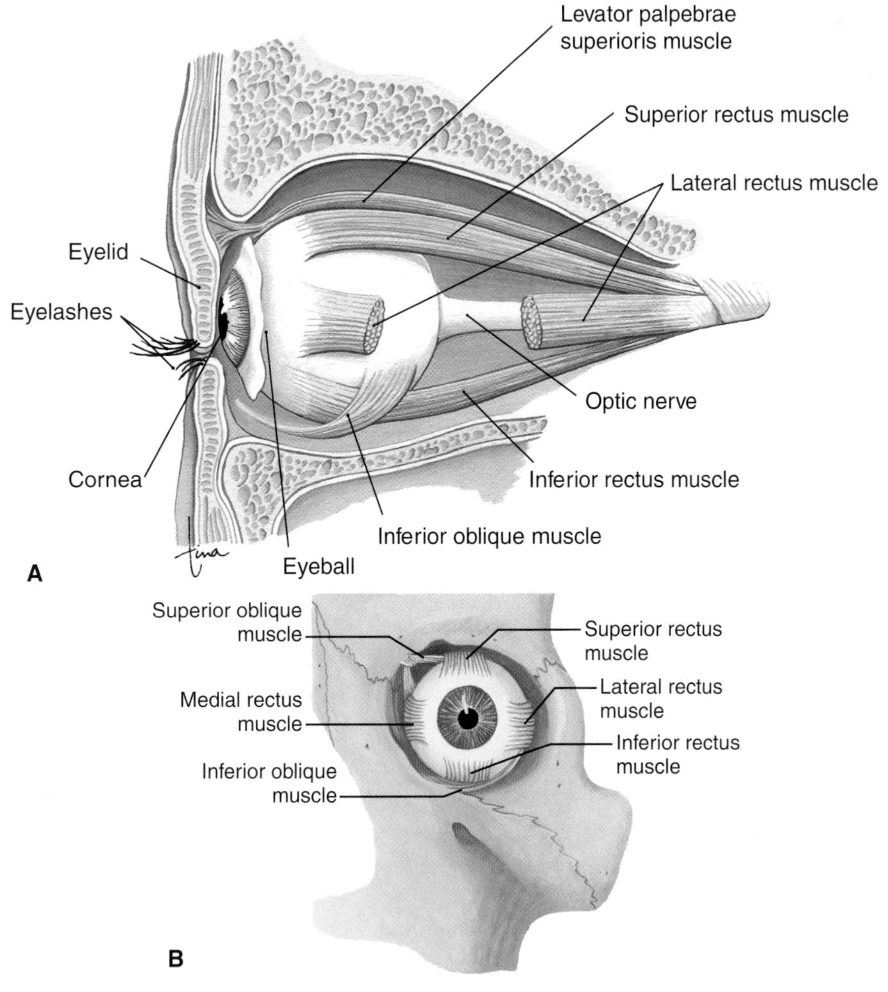

Figure 9–5 Extrinsic muscles of the eye. **(A)** Lateral view of left eye. **(B)** Frontal view of left eye.

QUESTION: Contraction of the inferior rectus muscle will have what effect on the eyeball?

The medial rectus muscle, for example, pulls the eyeball medially, as if to look at the nose. The two oblique (slanted) muscles rotate the eye. The cranial nerves that innervate these muscles are the oculomotor, trochlear, and abducens (3rd, 4th, and 6th cranial nerves, respectively). The very rapid and complex coordination of these muscles in both eyes is, fortunately, not something we have to think about. The convergence of both eyes on an object is very important to ensure a single image (that is, to prevent double vision) and to give us depth perception and a three-dimensional world.

Layers of the Eyeball

In its wall, the eyeball has three layers: the outer sclera, middle choroid layer, and inner retina (Fig. 9–6). The **sclera** is the thickest layer and is made of fibrous connective tissue that is visible as the white of the eye. The most anterior portion is the **cornea**, which differs from the rest

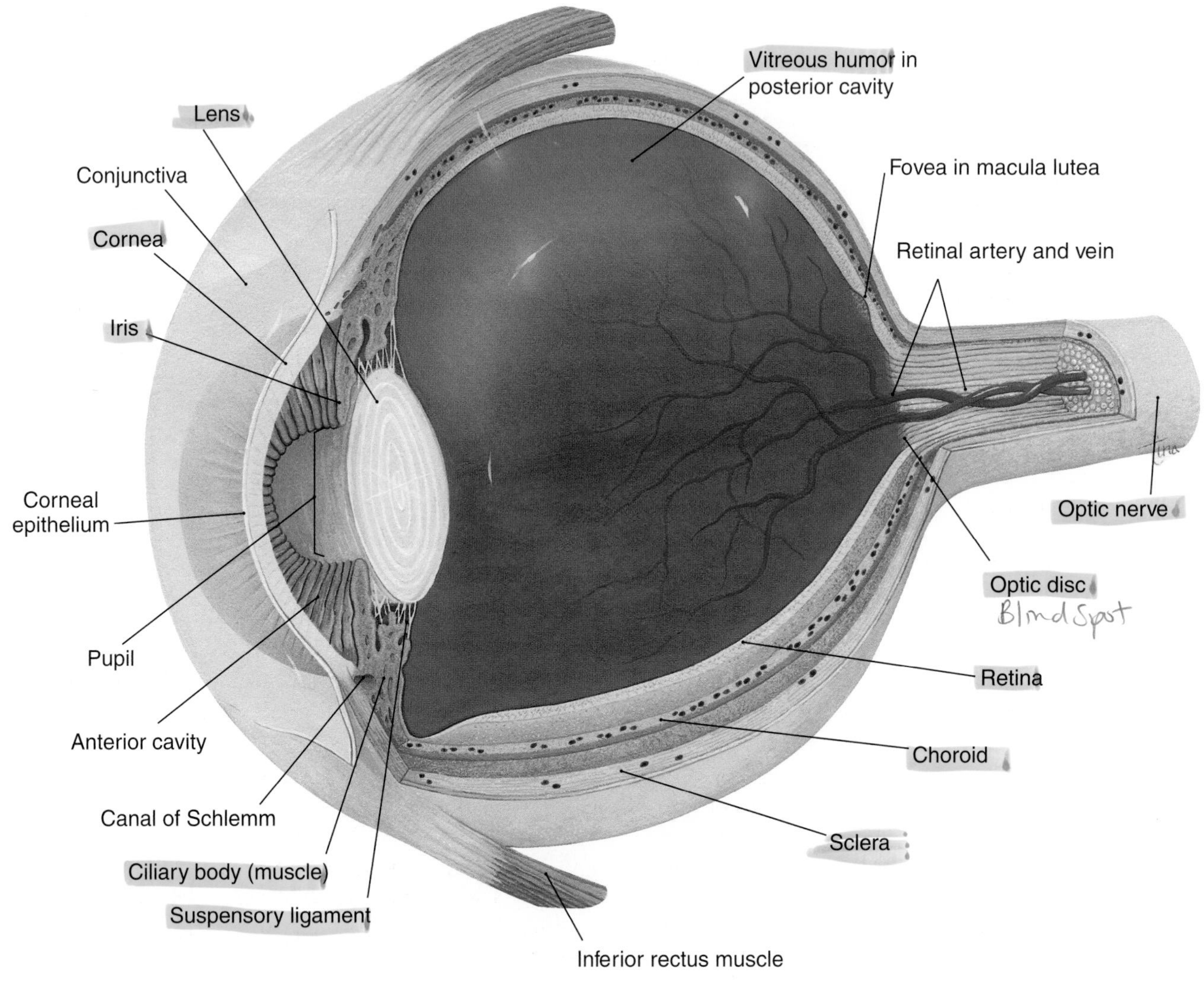

Figure 9–6 Internal anatomy of the eyeball.

QUESTION: What is the function of the iris?

of the sclera in that it is transparent. The cornea has no capillaries, covers the iris and pupil inside the eye, and is the first part of the eye that **refracts**, or bends, light rays.

The **choroid layer** contains blood vessels and a dark blue pigment (derived from melanin) that absorbs light within the eyeball and thereby prevents glare (just as does the black interior of a camera). The anterior portion of the choroid is modified into more specialized structures: the ciliary body and the iris. The **ciliary body** (muscle) is a circular smooth muscle that surrounds the edge of the lens and is connected to the lens by **suspensory ligaments**. The **lens** is made of a transparent, elastic protein, and, like the cornea, has no capillaries (see Box 9–1: Cataracts). The shape of the lens is changed by the ciliary muscle (contracting to form a smaller circle and a thick lens, or relaxing to form a larger circle with a thin lens), which enables the eye to focus light from objects at varying distances from the eye.

Just in front of the lens is the circular **iris**, the colored part of the eye; its pigment is a form of melanin. What we call "eye color" is the color of the iris and is a genetic characteristic, just as skin color is. Two sets of smooth muscle fibers in the iris change the diameter of the **pupil**, the central opening. Contraction of the radial fibers dilates the pupil and lets in more light; this is a sympathetic response. Contraction of the circular fibers constricts the pupil; this is a parasympathetic response (oculomotor nerves). Pupillary constriction is a reflex that protects the retina from intense light or that permits more acute near vision, as when reading.

The **retina** lines the posterior two-thirds of the eyeball and contains the visual receptors, the rods and cones (Fig. 9–7). **Rods** detect only the presence of light, whereas **cones** detect colors, which, as you may know from physics, are the different wavelengths of visible light. Rods are proportionally more abundant toward the periphery, or edge, of the retina. Our best vision in dim light or at night, for which we depend upon the rods, is at the sides of our visual fields. Cones are most abundant in the center of the retina, especially an area called the **macula lutea** directly behind the center of the lens on what is called the visual axis. The **fovea**, which contains only cones, is a small depression in the macula and is the area for best color vision.

An important cause of vision loss for people older than 65 years of age is **age-related macular degeneration** (**AMD**), that is, loss of central vision, and some cases seem to have a genetic component. In the dry form of AMD, small fatty deposits impair circulation to the macula and cells die from lack of oxygen. In the wet form of AMD, abnormal blood vessels begin leaking into the retina, and cells in the macula die from the damaging effects of blood outside its vessels. The macula, the center of the visual field, is the part of the retina we use most: for reading, for driving, for recognizing people, and for any kind of close work. People of all ages should be aware of this condition and that smoking and exposure to ultraviolet rays are risk factors.

When light strikes the retina, the rods and cones generate impulses. These impulses are carried by **ganglion neurons**, which all converge at the **optic disc** (see Figs. 9–6 and 9–7) and pass through the wall of the eyeball as the **optic nerve**. There are no rods or cones in the optic disc, so this part of the retina is sometimes called the "blind spot." We are not aware of a blind spot in our field of vision, however, in part because the eyes are constantly moving, and in part because the brain "fills in" the blank spot to create a "complete" picture.

Cavities of the Eyeball

There are two cavities within the eye: the posterior cavity and the anterior cavity (see Fig. 9–6). The larger, **posterior cavity** is found between the lens and retina and contains **vitreous humor** (or vitreous body). This semisolid substance keeps the retina in place. If the eyeball is punctured and vitreous humor is lost, the retina may fall away from the choroid; this is one possible cause of a **detached retina**.

Box 9–1 | CATARACTS

The lens of the eye is normally transparent but may become opaque; this cloudiness or opacity is called a **cataract**. Cataract formation is most common among elderly people. With age, the proteins of the lens break down and lose their transparency. Long-term exposure to ultraviolet light (sunlight) seems to be a contributing factor, as is smoking.

The cloudy lens does not refract light properly, and blurry vision throughout the visual field is the result. Small cataracts may be destroyed by laser surgery. Artificial lenses are available and may be surgically implanted to replace an extensively cloudy lens. The artificial lens is not adjustable, however, and the person may require glasses or contact lenses for vision at certain distances.

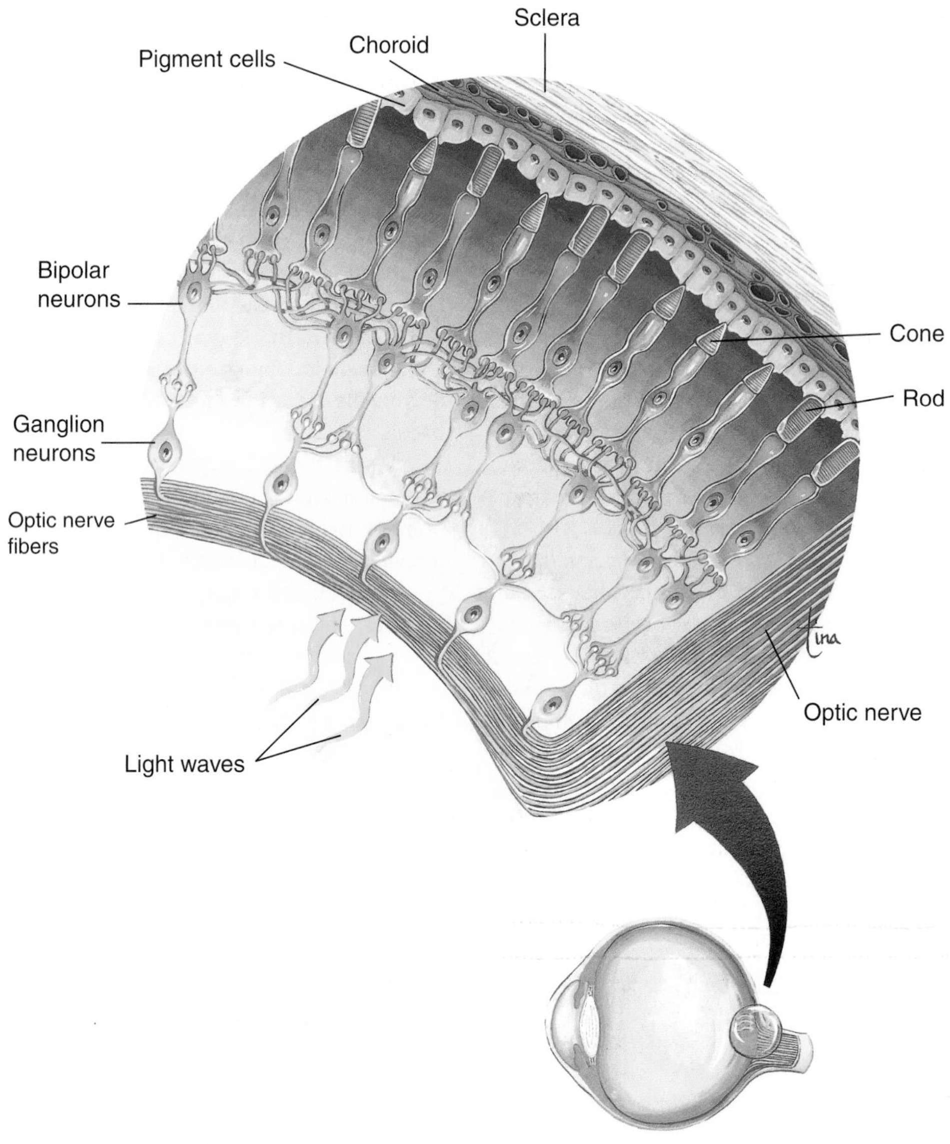

Figure 9–7 Microscopic structure of the retina in the area of the optic disc. See text for description.

QUESTION: Which type of neuron forms the optic nerve? Which cells are the photoreceptors?

The **anterior cavity** is found between the back of the cornea and the front of the lens and contains **aqueous humor**, the tissue fluid of the eyeball. Aqueous humor is formed by capillaries in the ciliary body, flows anteriorly through the pupil, and is reabsorbed by the **canal of Schlemm** (small veins also called the scleral venous sinus) at the junction of the iris and cornea. Because aqueous humor is tissue fluid, you would expect it to have a nourishing function, and it does. Recall that the lens and cornea have no capillaries; they are nourished by the continuous flow of aqueous humor (see Box 9–2: Glaucoma).

PHYSIOLOGY OF VISION

For us to see, light rays must be focused on the retina and the resulting nerve impulses must be transmitted to the visual areas of the cerebral cortex in the brain.

Box 9–2 | GLAUCOMA

The presence of aqueous humor in the anterior cavity of the eye creates a pressure called intraocular pressure. An increase in this pressure is an important risk factor for **glaucoma**, which is defined as a group of disorders that damage the optic nerve and cause loss of vision. Other risk factors include high blood pressure and diabetes. In the most common form of glaucoma, aqueous humor is not reabsorbed properly into the canal of Schlemm. Increased pressure in the anterior cavity is transmitted to the lens, the vitreous humor, and the retina and optic nerve. As pressure on the retina increases, halos may be seen around bright lights and peripheral vision is lost. Frequently, however, there are no symptoms. A person with glaucoma may not notice the shrinking visual field in one eye before vision loss is far advanced. This happens because the brain will suppress a faulty image from one eye that it cannot easily integrate with the normal image of the other eye. When both eyes are affected, the person may not become aware of the gradual loss of peripheral vision because close work such as reading does not require the edges of the visual fields.

Glaucoma may often be controlled with medications that constrict the pupil and flatten the iris, thus opening up access to the canal of Schlemm. If these or other medications are not effective, laser surgery may be used to create a larger drainage canal.

Anyone older than the age of 40 should have a test for glaucoma; anyone with a family history of glaucoma should have this test annually, as should those with diabetes or high blood pressure. If diagnosed early, glaucoma is treatable and blindness can usually be prevented.

Refraction of light rays is the deflection or bending of a ray of light as it passes through one object and into another object of greater or lesser density. The refraction of light within the eye takes place in the following pathway of structures: the cornea, aqueous humor, lens, and vitreous humor. The lens is the only adjustable part of the refraction system. When looking at distant objects, the ciliary muscle is relaxed (a larger circle) and the lens is stretched, becoming elongated and thin. When the eye is looking at near objects, the ciliary muscle contracts to form a smaller circle, the elastic lens recoils and bulges in the middle, and has greater refractive power (see Box 9–3: Errors of Refraction).

When light rays strike the retina, they stimulate chemical reactions in the rods and cones. In rods, the chemical **rhodopsin** breaks down to form scotopsin and retinal (a derivative of vitamin A). This chemical reaction generates an electrical impulse, and rhodopsin is then resynthesized in a slower reaction. Adaptation to darkness, such as going outside at night, takes a little while because being in a well-lit area has broken down most of the rhodopsin in the

Box 9–3 | ERRORS OF REFRACTION

Normal visual acuity is referred to as 20/20; that is, the eye should and does clearly see an object 20 feet away. **Nearsightedness** (**myopia**) means that the eye sees near objects well but not distant ones. If an eye has 20/80 vision, this means that what the normal eye can see at 80 feet, the nearsighted eye can see only if the object is brought to 20 feet away. The nearsighted eye focuses images from distant objects in front of the retina, because the eyeball is too long or the lens too thick. These structural characteristics of the eye are hereditary. Correction requires a concave lens to spread out light rays before they strike the eye.

Farsightedness (**hyperopia**) means that the eye sees distant objects well. Such an eye may have an acuity of 20/10, that is, it sees at 20 feet what the normal eye can see only at 10 feet. The farsighted eye focuses light from near objects "behind" the retina because the eyeball is too short or the lens too thin. Correction requires a convex lens to converge light rays before they strike the eye.

Continued

Box 9–3 | ERRORS OF REFRACTION *(Continued)*

As we get older, most of us will become more farsighted (**presbyopia**). As the aging lens loses its elasticity, it is not as able to recoil and thicken for near vision, and glasses for reading are often necessary.

Astigmatism is another error of refraction, caused by an irregular curvature of the cornea or lens that scatters light rays and blurs the image on the retina. Correction requires a lens ground specifically for the curvature of the individual eye.

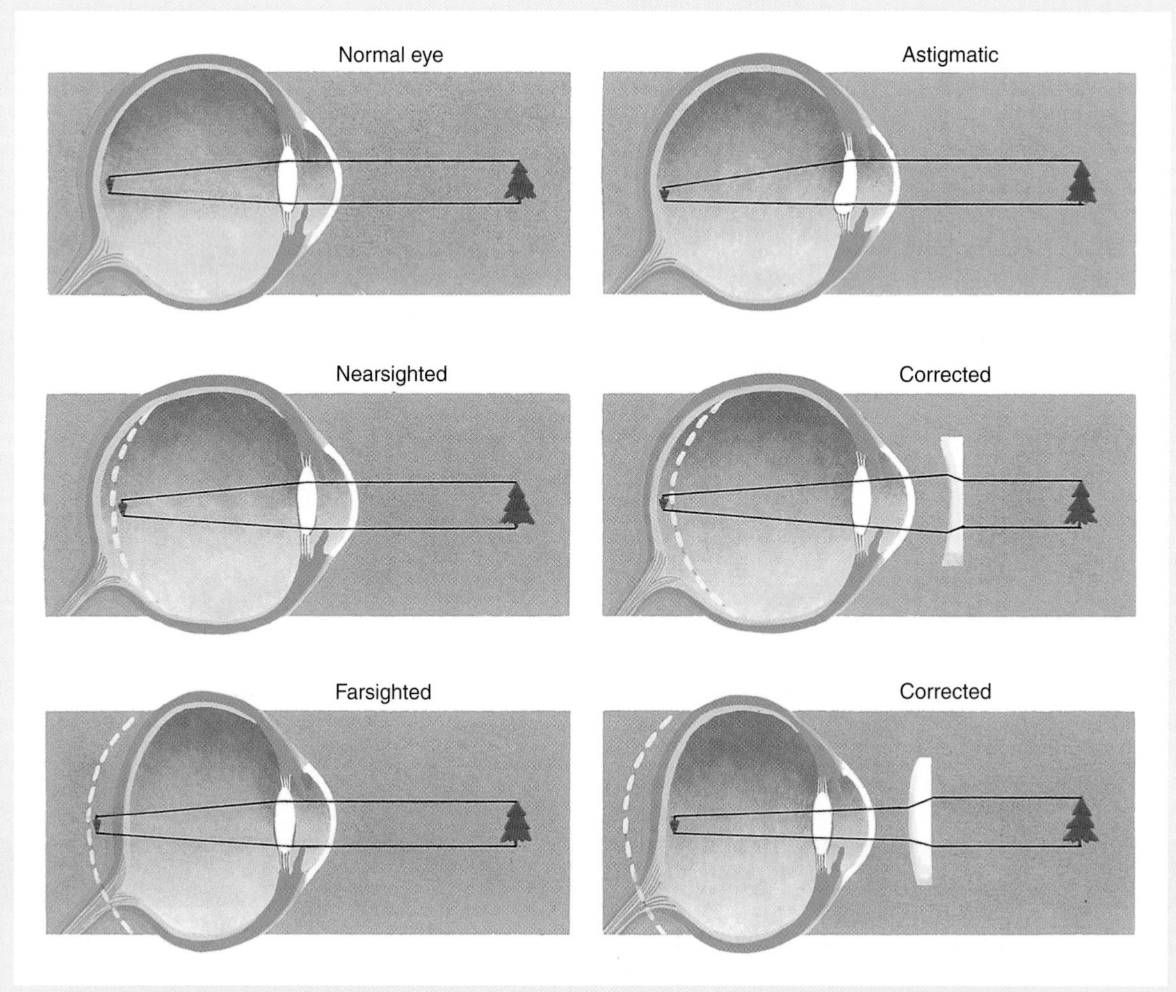

Box Figure 9–A Errors of refraction compared with refraction in normal eye. Corrective lenses are shown for nearsightedness and farsightedness.

rods, and resynthesis of rhodopsin is slow. The opposite situation, perhaps being suddenly awakened by a bright light, can seem almost painful. What happens is this: In darkness the rods have resynthesized a full supply of rhodopsin, and the sudden bright light breaks down all the rhodopsin at the same time. The barrage of impulses generated is very intense, and the brain may interpret any intense sensation as pain. A few minutes later the bright light seems fine because the rods are recycling their rhodopsin slowly, and it is not breaking down all at once.

Chemical reactions in the cones, also involving retinal, are brought about by different wavelengths of light. We have three types of cones: red-absorbing, blue-absorbing, and green-absorbing cones. Each type absorbs wavelengths over about a third of the visible light spectrum, so red cones, for example, absorb light of the red, orange, and yellow wavelengths. The chemical reactions in cones also generate electrical impulses (see Box 9–4: Night Blindness and Color Blindness).

The impulses from the rods and cones are transmitted to **ganglion neurons** (see Fig. 9–7); these converge at the optic disc and become the **optic nerve**, which passes posteriorly through the wall of the eyeball. Ganglion neurons also seem to have a photoreceptor chemical (called melanopsin) that may contribute to the daily resetting of our biological clocks.

The optic nerves from both eyes come together at the **optic chiasma** (or chiasm), just in front of the pituitary gland (see Fig. 9–8). Here, the medial fibers of each optic nerve cross to the other side. This crossing permits each visual area to receive impulses from both eyes, which is important for binocular vision.

The optic tracts continue from the optic chiasma to the occipital lobes. In Fig. 9–8, look first at the boxed image (lower left) to see the placement of the tracts from a familiar angle or perspective. Then look at the superior view and begin at the two retinas and optic nerves. Follow these to the optic chiasma and note the crossing of fibers. Follow the nerve tracts posteriorly and you will see branches to the midbrain. These branches provide the information for visual reflexes such as keeping both eyes on that wasp flying at you or the coordination of both eyeballs for reading; these are mediated by the midbrain. Continue farther posteriorly and you see that the nerve fibers converge at the thalamus. Recall that the thalamus is very important for the integration of sensory information. What do we use vision for? To see, yes, but also to respond to our surroundings. The thalamus integrates and disperses visual information; that is, it passes it on to other parts of the brain that will use it for judging distances or spatial relationships, or planning where and how a body part will be moved. What happens when you reach for a glass of

Box 9–4 | NIGHT BLINDNESS AND COLOR BLINDNESS

Night blindness, the inability to see well in dim light or at night, is usually caused by a deficiency of vitamin A, although some night blindness may occur with aging. Vitamin A is necessary for the synthesis of rhodopsin in the rods. Without sufficient vitamin A, there is not enough rhodopsin present to respond to low levels of light.

Color blindness is a genetic disorder in which one of the three sets of cones is lacking or nonfunctional. Total color blindness, the inability to see any colors at all, is very rare. The most common form is red-green color blindness, which is the inability to distinguish between these colors. If either the red cones or green cones are nonfunctional, the person will still see most colors but will not have the contrast that the nonworking set of cones would provide. So red and green shades will look somewhat similar, without the definite difference most of us see. This is a sex-linked trait; the recessive gene is on the X chromosome. A woman with one gene for color blindness and a gene for normal color vision on her other X chromosome will not be color blind but may pass the gene for color blindness to her children. A man with a gene for color blindness on his X chromosome has no gene at all for color vision on his Y chromosome and will be color blind.

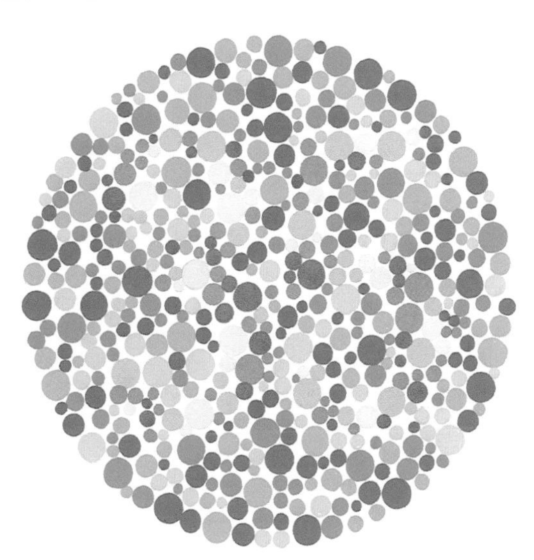

Box Figure 9–B Example of color patterns used to detect color blindness.

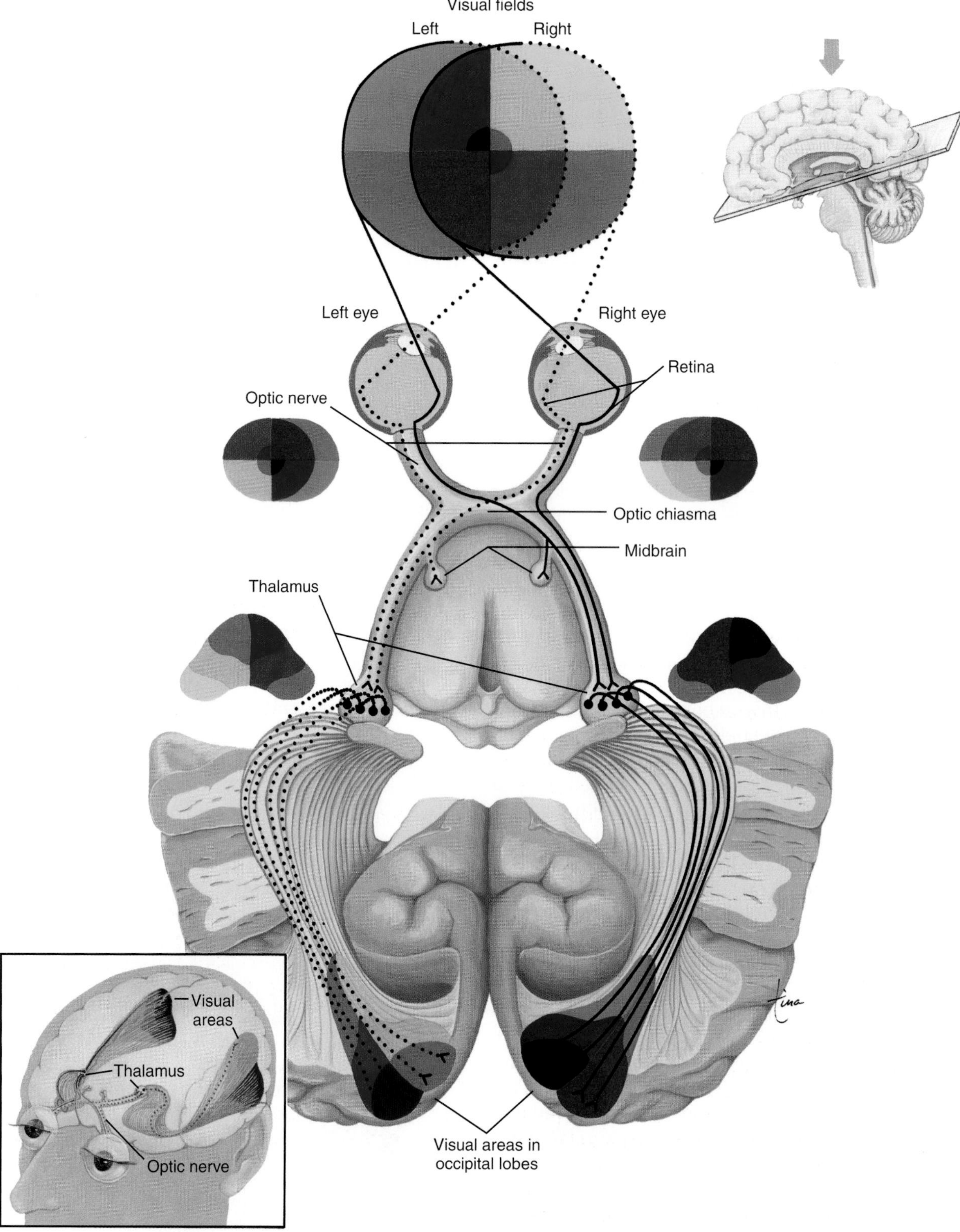

Figure 9–8 Optic tracts. The pathway of nerve impulses from the retinas to the visual areas is shown in a superior view. The insert box shows the tracts in a more familiar view. See text for further description.

QUESTION: If the right visual area were to become damaged and non-functional, what part of the visual field would be lost?

water? You see the glass, and because the thalamus has relayed that information to the cerebrum, the frontal lobe can generate the impulses for appropriate movements of the arm and hand. Finally, follow the optic tracts to the visual areas. This is where "seeing" takes place, where sensory impulses are interpreted as an image.

The visual areas are in the **occipital lobes** of the cerebral cortex. Notice in Fig. 9–8 that the left visual area gets information from the left half of each retina (the dotted lines) and "sees" the right half of the visual field of each eye. Similarly, the right visual area receives information from the right half of each retina (the solid lines) and "sees" the left half of the visual field of each eye. Although each eye transmits a slightly different picture (look straight ahead and close one eye at a time to see the difference between the two pictures), the visual areas put them together, or integrate them, to make a single image that has depth and three dimensions. This is **binocular vision**. The visual areas also turn the image upright because the image on the retina is upside down. The image on film in a camera is also upside down, but we don't even realize that because we look at the pictures right side up. The brain just as automatically ensures that we see our world right side up.

Also for near vision, such as reading, the pupils constrict to block out peripheral light rays that would otherwise blur the image, and the eyes converge even further to keep the images on the corresponding parts of both retinas. The importance of pupil constriction can be demonstrated by looking at this page through a pinhole in a piece of paper. You will be able to read with the page much closer to your eye because the paper blocks out light from the sides.

The importance of convergence can be demonstrated by looking at your finger placed on the tip of your nose. You can feel your eyes move medially ("cross") in maximum convergence. If the eyes don't converge, the result is double vision; the brain cannot make the very different images into one and settles for two. This is temporary, however, because the brain does not like seeing double and will eventually suppress one image.

You have probably heard of the condition called "lazy eye" (the formal name is **strabismus**), in which a person's eyes (the visual axis of each) cannot be directed at precisely the same point. True convergence is not possible and, if untreated, the brain simply will not use the image from the lazy eye. That eye may stop focusing and become functionally blind because the brain is ignoring the nerve impulses from it. Such loss of vision is called **amblyopia**. Correction of a lazy eye may involve eye exercises (to make the lazy eye straighten out), a patch over the good eye (to make the lazy eye straighten out and take over), or surgery to correct an imbalance of the extrinsic muscles. You can show yourself the benefits of converging eyes the next time you are a passenger in a car (*not* the driver). As the car is moving, close one eye. Does the oncoming landscape seem to flatten out, lose dimension? This is loss of depth perception and some of the three dimensionality that the brain provides when it has two images to work with.

THE EAR

The ear has three major areas: the outer ear, the middle ear, and the inner ear (Fig. 9–9). The ear contains the receptors for two senses: **hearing** and **equilibrium**. These receptors are all found in the inner ear.

OUTER EAR

The **outer ear** consists of the auricle and the ear canal. The **auricle**, or **pinna**, is made of cartilage covered with skin. For animals such as dogs, whose ears are movable, the auricle may act as a funnel for sound waves. For people, however, the flat and stationary auricle is not important. Hearing would not be negatively affected without it, although those of us who wear glasses would have our vision impaired without our auricles. The **ear canal** is lined with skin that contains ceruminous glands. It may also be called the **external auditory meatus** and is a tunnel into the temporal bone, curving slightly forward and down.

MIDDLE EAR

The **middle ear** is an air-filled cavity in the temporal bone. The **eardrum**, or **tympanic membrane**, is stretched across the end of the ear canal and vibrates when sound waves strike it. These vibrations are transmitted to the three auditory bones: the **malleus**, **incus**, and **stapes** (also called the hammer, anvil, and stirrup and shown in Fig. 9–9). The stapes then transmits vibrations to the fluid-filled inner ear at the **oval window**.

The **eustachian tube** (auditory tube) extends from the middle ear to the nasopharynx and permits air to enter or leave the middle ear cavity. The air pressure in the middle ear must be the same as the external atmospheric pressure in order for the eardrum to vibrate properly. You may have noticed your ears "popping" when in an airplane or when driving to a higher or lower altitude. Swallowing or yawning creates the "pop" by opening the eustachian tubes and equalizing the air pressures.

The eustachian tubes of children are short and nearly horizontal and may permit bacteria to spread from the pharynx to the middle ear. This is why **otitis media** may be a complication of strep throat.

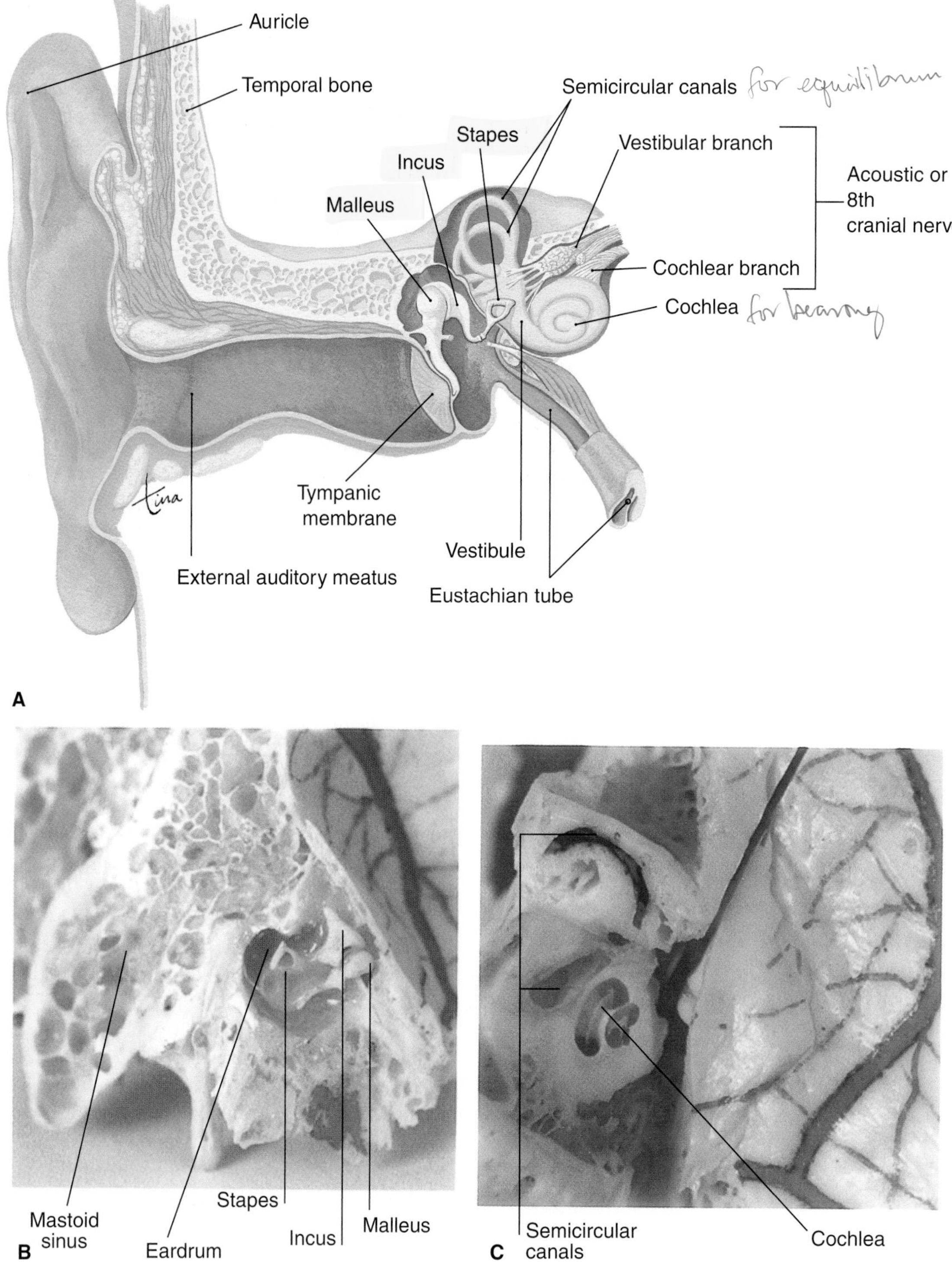

Figure 9–9 (**A**) Outer, middle, and inner ear structures as shown in a frontal section through the right temporal bone. (**B**) Section of temporal bone with the auditory bones. (**C**) Section of temporal bone showing bony labyrinth of inner ear. The colors on the bone are artificial. (Photographs by Dan Kaufman.)

QUESTION: What structure is first to vibrate when sound waves enter the ear canal? What is second?

INNER EAR

Within the temporal bone, the **inner ear** is a cavity called the **bony labyrinth** (a labyrinth is a series of interconnecting paths or tunnels, somewhat like a maze but without dead ends; see Fig. 9–9), which is lined with membrane called the **membranous labyrinth**. **Perilymph** is the fluid found between bone and membrane, and **endolymph** is the fluid within the membranous structures of the inner ear. These structures are the cochlea, concerned with hearing, and the utricle, saccule, and semicircular canals, all concerned with equilibrium (Fig. 9–10).

Cochlea

The **cochlea** is shaped like a snail shell with two-and-a-half structural turns. Internally, the cochlea is partitioned into three fluid-filled canals. The medial canal is the cochlear duct, the floor of which is the basilar membrane that supports the receptors for hearing in the **organ of Corti** (**spiral organ**). The receptors are called hair cells (their projections are not "hair," of course, but rather are specialized microvilli called stereocilia), which contain endings of the cochlear branch of the 8th cranial nerve. Overhanging the hair cells is the tectorial membrane (Fig. 9–11).

Very simply, the process of hearing involves the transmission of vibrations and the generation of nerve impulses. When sound waves enter the ear canal, vibrations are transmitted by the following sequence of structures: eardrum, malleus, incus, stapes, oval window of the inner ear, and perilymph and endolymph within the cochlea. Imagine the vibrations in the fluids as ripples or waves. The basilar membrane ripples and pushes the hair cells of the organ of Corti against the tectorial membrane. When the hair cells bend, they generate impulses that are carried by the 8th cranial nerve to the brain. Some of the fibers of each 8th cranial nerve cross to the other side, so the auditory areas in the **temporal lobes** of the cerebral cortex receive impulses from both ears. It is here that sounds are heard and interpreted (see Box 9–5: Deafness).

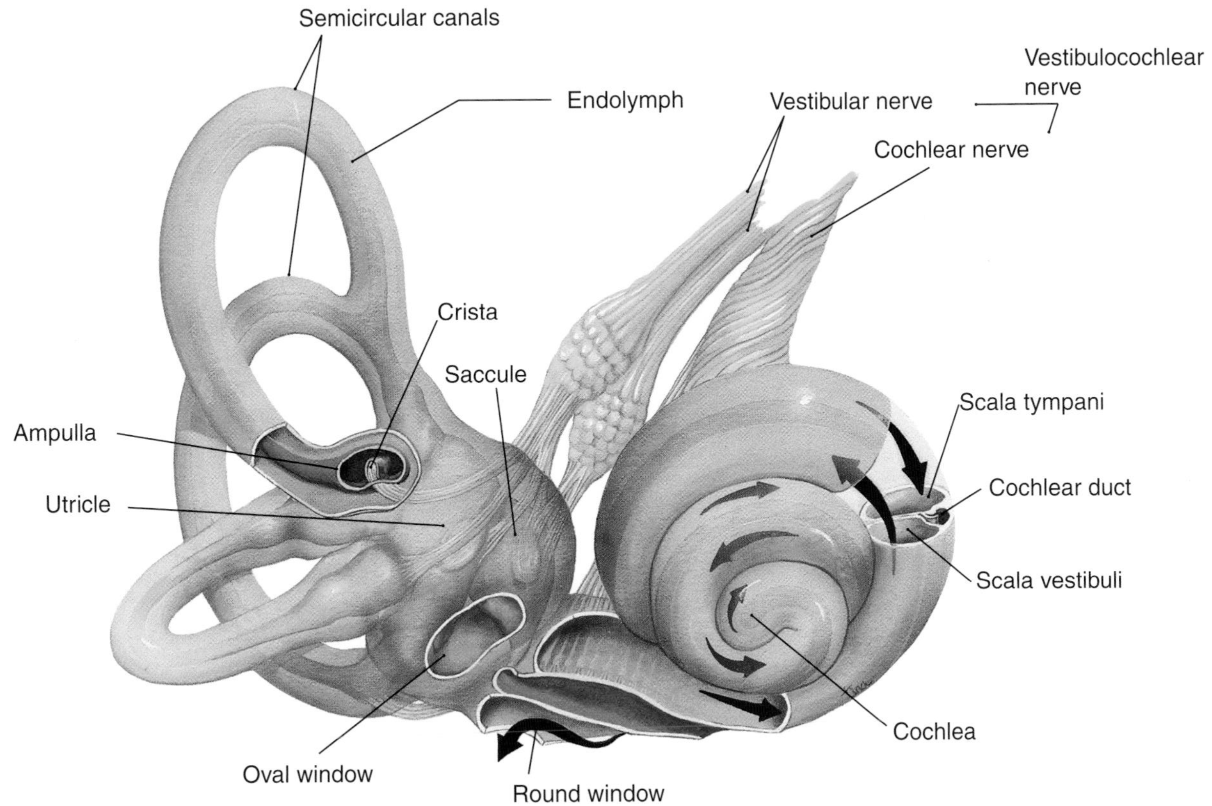

Figure 9–10 Inner ear structures. The arrows show the transmission of vibrations during hearing.

QUESTION: What is the function of the round window?

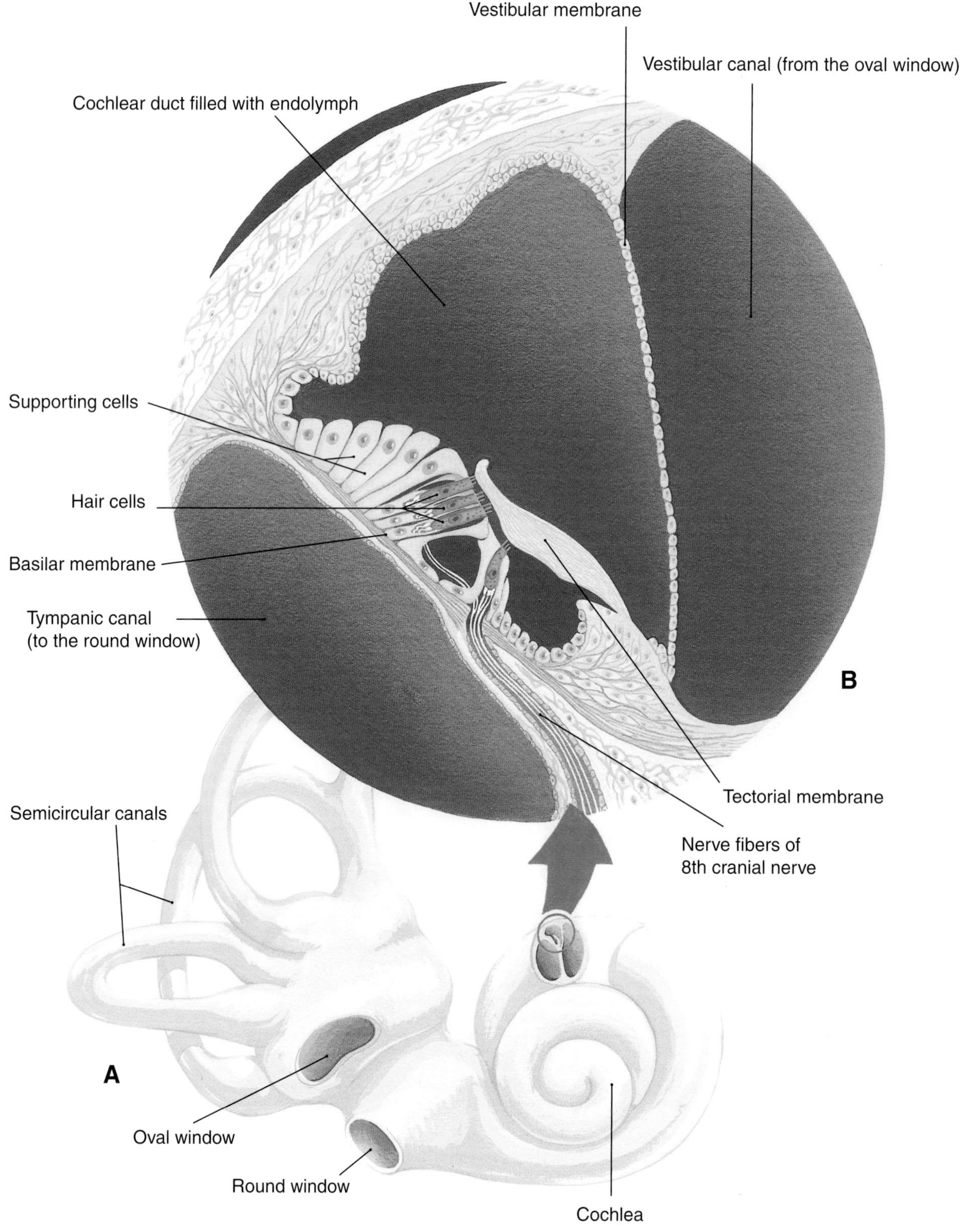

Figure 9–11 Organ of Corti. (**A**) Inner ear structures. (**B**) Magnification of organ of Corti within the cochlea.

QUESTION: What do the canals and cochlear duct contain (air or fluid)? What are the receptors for hearing?

Box 9–5 | DEAFNESS

Deafness is the inability to hear properly; the types are classified according to the part of the hearing process that is not functioning normally:

Conduction deafness—impairment of one of the structures that transmits vibrations. Examples of this type are a punctured eardrum, arthritis of the auditory bones, or a middle ear infection in which fluid fills the middle ear cavity.

Nerve deafness—impairment of the 8th cranial nerve or the receptors for hearing in the cochlea. The 8th cranial nerve may be damaged by some antibiotics used to treat bacterial infections. Nerve deafness is a rare complication of some viral infections such as mumps or congenital rubella (German measles). Deterioration of the hair cells in the cochlea is a natural consequence of aging, and the acuity of hearing diminishes as we get older. For example, it may be more difficult for an elderly person to distinguish conversation from background noise. Chronic exposure to loud noise accelerates degeneration of the hair cells and onset of this type of deafness. Listening to music by way of earphones is also believed to increase the risk of this type of damage.

Central deafness—damage to the auditory areas in the temporal lobes. This type of deafness is rare but may be caused by a brain tumor, meningitis, or a cerebrovascular accident in the temporal lobe.

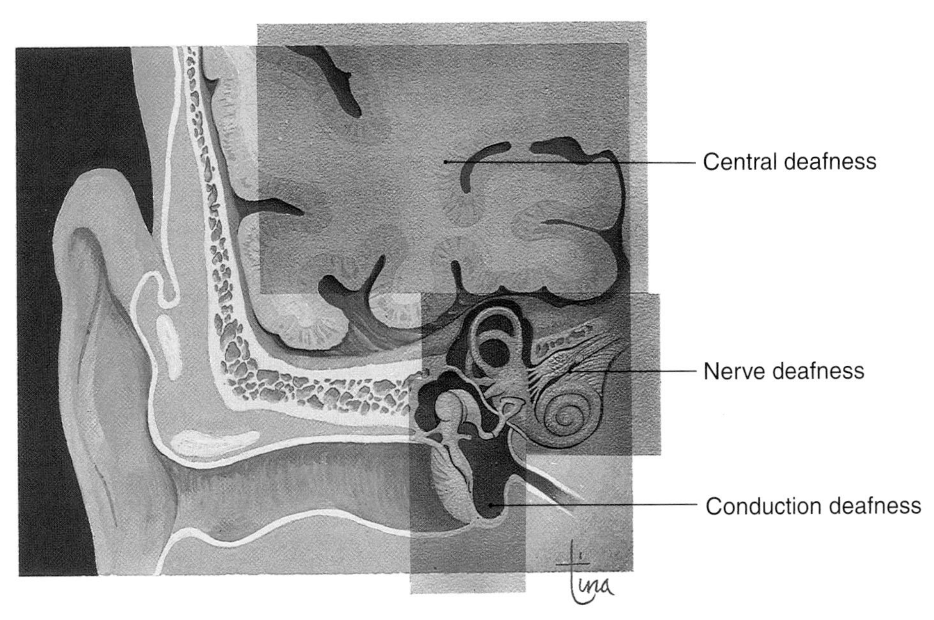

Box Figure 9–C Types of deafness.

The neurons of the auditory cortex are arranged in order of the pitch they "hear," from low to high, like a piano keyboard. Other aspects of sound "heard" by the brain are volume, rhythm and tempo (especially in music), and timbre, which is the quality of a tone (a piccolo compared with a tuba, for example, or a child's voice compared with an adult's voice). The auditory areas also enable us to determine from which direction a sound is coming. To do this, the auditory areas count and compare the number of impulses coming from each inner ear. For example, if more impulses arrive from the left cochlea than from the right one, the sound will be projected to the left and be perceived as coming from the left. If the source of a sound is directly above your head, the sound may seem to come from all directions, because each auditory area is receiving approximately the same number of impulses and cannot project the sensation to one side or the other.

Adaptation does occur in the sense of hearing. The hum of an air conditioner or a conversation in another room, for example, may be all but unnoticed after a while. Without such adaptation, what we call "background noise" would not exist. All sounds would be clamoring for our attention and concentration would not be possible. Adaptation does not occur with loud sounds, however, or frightening sounds, or grating sounds; we remain aware of those.

The final structure in the hearing pathway is the round window (see Fig. 9–10). The membrane-covered **round window**, just below the oval window, is important to relieve pressure within the cochlea. When the stapes pushes in the fluid at the oval window, the round window bulges out, which prevents damage to the hair cells.

Utricle and Saccule

The **utricle** and **saccule** are membranous sacs in an area called the **vestibule**, between the cochlea and semicircular canals. Within the utricle and saccule are hair cells embedded in a gelatinous membrane with tiny crystals of calcium carbonate called **otoliths**. Gravity pulls on the otoliths and bends the hair cells as the position of the head changes (Fig. 9–12). The impulses generated by these hair cells are carried by the vestibular portion of the 8th cranial nerve to the cerebellum, the midbrain, and the temporal lobes of the cerebrum.

The cerebellum and midbrain use this information to maintain equilibrium at a subconscious level. We can, of course, be aware of the position of the head, and it is the cerebrum that provides awareness.

Semicircular Canals

The three **semicircular canals** are fluid-filled membranous ovals oriented in three different planes. At the base of each is an enlarged portion called the ampulla (see Fig. 9–10), which contains hair cells (the crista) that are affected by movement. As the body moves forward, for example, the hair cells are bent backward at first and then straighten (see Fig. 9–12). The bending of the hair cells generates impulses carried by the vestibular branch of the 8th cranial nerve to the cerebellum, midbrain, and temporal lobes of the cerebrum. These impulses are interpreted as starting or stopping, and accelerating or decelerating, or changing direction, and this information is used to maintain equilibrium while we are moving (see Box 9–6: Motion Sickness).

In summary then, the utricle and saccule provide information about the position of the body at rest, while the semicircular canals provide information about the body in motion. Of course, there is some overlap, and the brain puts all the information together to create a single sense of body position.

ARTERIAL RECEPTORS

The aorta and carotid arteries contain receptors that detect changes in the blood. The **aortic arch**, which receives blood pumped by the left ventricle of the heart, curves over the top of the heart. The left and right **carotid arteries** are branches of the aortic arch that take blood through the neck on the way to the brain. In each of these vessels are pressoreceptors and chemoreceptors (see Fig. 12–8 in Chapter 12).

Pressoreceptors in the carotid sinuses and aortic sinus detect changes in blood pressure. **Chemoreceptors** in the carotid bodies and the aortic body detect changes in the oxygen and carbon dioxide content and the pH of blood. The impulses generated by these receptors are not interpreted as sensations that we feel, but rather as information used to make any necessary changes in respiration or circulation. We will return to this in later chapters, so one example will suffice for now.

If the blood level of oxygen decreases significantly, this change (hypoxemia) is detected by carotid and aortic chemoreceptors. The sensory impulses are carried by the glossopharyngeal (9th cranial) and vagus (10th cranial) nerves to the medulla. Centers in the medulla may then increase the respiratory rate and the heart rate to obtain and circulate more oxygen. These are the respiratory and cardiac reflexes that were mentioned in Chapter 8 as functions of the glossopharyngeal and vagus nerves. The importance of these reflexes is readily apparent: to maintain normal blood levels of oxygen and carbon dioxide and to maintain normal blood pressure.

AGING AND THE SENSES

All of the senses may be diminished in old age. In the eye, cataracts may make the lens cloudy or opaque. The lens also loses its elasticity and the eye becomes more farsighted, a condition called presbyopia. The risk of glaucoma increases, and elderly people should be tested for it. Macular degeneration, in which central vision becomes impaired, is a major cause of vision loss for people over 65. Reading and close work of any kind become difficult.

In the ear, cumulative damage to the hair cells in the organ of Corti usually becomes apparent some time after the age of 60. Hair cells that have been damaged in a lifetime of noise cannot be replaced (regrowth of cochlear hair cells has been stimulated in guinea pigs, and in gerbils with human stem cells, but not yet in people). The deafness of

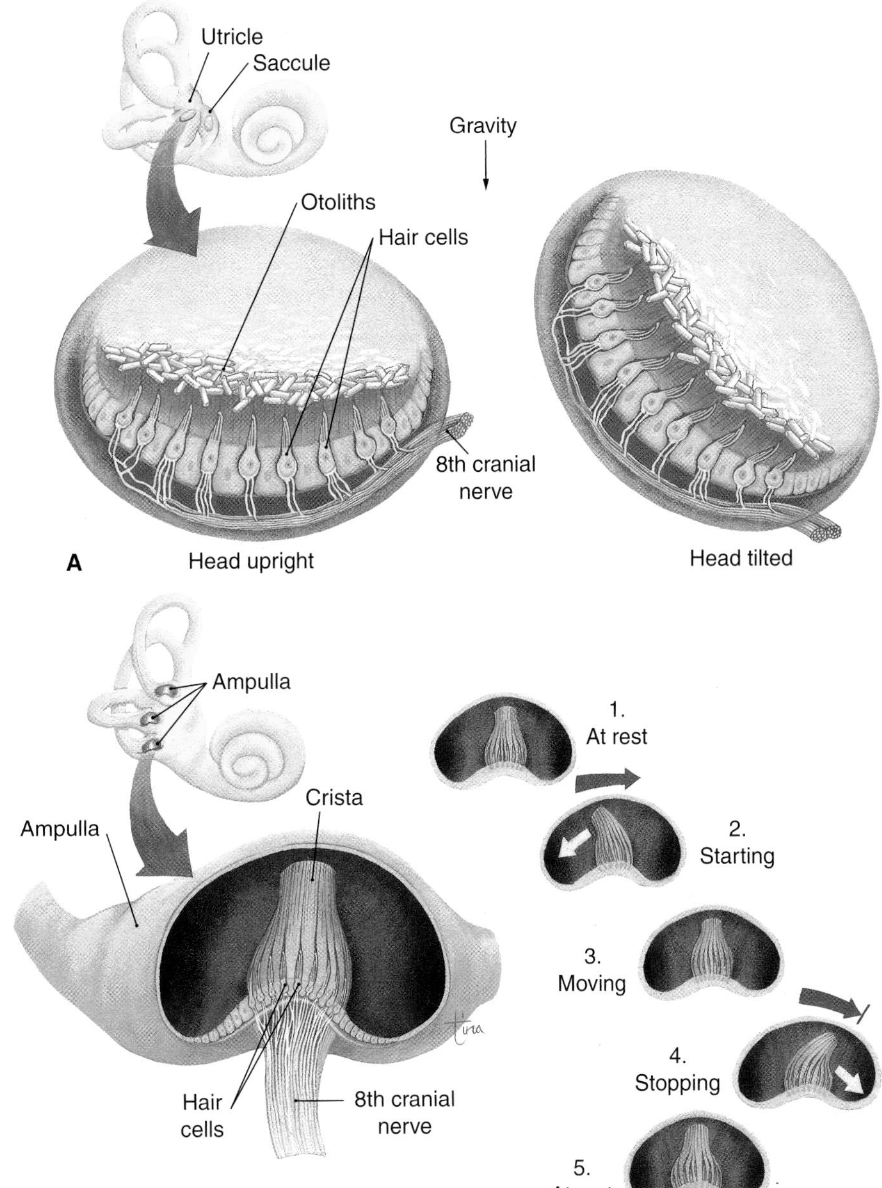

Figure 9–12 Physiology of equilibrium. (**A**) Utricle and saccule. (**B**) Semicircular canals. See text for description.

QUESTION: In part A, what causes the hair cells to bend? In part B, what causes the hair cells to sway?

Box 9–6 | MOTION SICKNESS

Motion sickness is characterized by cold sweats, hyperventilation, nausea, and vomiting when the person is exposed to repetitive motion that is unexpected or unfamiliar, or that cannot be controlled. Seasickness is a type of motion sickness, as is carsickness (why children are carsick more often than are adults is not known).

Some people are simply not affected by the rolling of a ship or train; for others, the constant stimulation of the receptors for position first becomes uncomfortable, then nauseating. For those who know they are susceptible to motion sickness, medications are available for use before traveling by plane, train, boat, or car.

old age ranges from slight to profound; very often high-pitched sounds are lost first, while hearing may still be adequate for low-pitched sounds. The sense of equilibrium may be diminished; the body is slower to react to tilting, and falls may become more frequent. Regular exercise, as simple as walking, and especially exercise to music, can minimize loss of the sense of balance.

Both taste and smell become less acute with age, which may contribute to poor nutrition in elderly people.

SUMMARY

Changes take place all around us, as well as within us. If the body could not respond appropriately to environmental and internal changes, homeostasis would soon be disrupted, resulting in injury, illness, or even death. To respond appropriately to changes, the brain must know what they are. Conveying this information to our brains is the function of our sensory pathways. Although we may sometimes take our senses for granted, we could not survive for very long without them.

You are familiar with the role of the nervous system in regulating the body's responses to the changes of sensations. In the next chapter we will discuss the other regulatory system, the endocrine system. The hormones of the endocrine glands are produced in response to changes, and their regulatory effects all contribute to homeostasis.

STUDY OUTLINE

Purpose of Sensations—to detect changes in the external or internal environment to enable the body to respond appropriately to maintain homeostasis

Sensory Pathway—pathway of impulses for a sensation

1. Receptors—detect a change (usually very specific) and generate electrical impulses.
2. Sensory neurons—transmit impulses from receptors to the CNS.
3. Sensory tracts—white matter in the CNS.
4. Sensory area—most are in the cerebral cortex; feels and interprets the sensation.

Characteristics of Sensations

1. Projection—the sensation seems to come from the area where the receptors were stimulated, even though it is the brain that truly feels the sensation.
2. Intensity—the degree to which a sensation is felt; a strong stimulus affects more receptors, more impulses are sent to the brain and are interpreted as a more intense sensation.
3. Contrast—the effect of a previous or simultaneous sensation on a current sensation as the brain compares them.
4. Adaptation—becoming unaware of a continuing stimulus; if the stimulus remains constant, there is no change for receptors to detect.
5. After-image—the sensation remains in the consciousness after the stimulus has stopped; often true for sensations of great intensity.

Cutaneous Senses—provide information about the external environment and the skin itself

1. The dermis has free nerve endings that are receptors for pain, itch, heat, and cold, as well as encapsulated nerve endings that are receptors for touch and pressure (see Fig. 9–1).
2. Sensory areas are in parietal lobes.
3. Referred pain is visceral pain that is felt as cutaneous pain (see Fig. 9–2). Common pathways in the CNS carry both cutaneous and visceral impulses; the brain usually projects sensation to the more frequent source of impulses, the cutaneous area.

Muscle Sense—knowing where our muscles are without looking at them

1. Stretch receptors in muscles detect stretching; brain creates a mental picture of the muscles.
2. Sensory areas for conscious muscle sense are in parietal lobes.
3. Cerebellum uses unconscious muscle sense to coordinate voluntary movement.

Sense of Taste (see Fig. 9–3)

1. Chemoreceptors are in taste buds on the tongue; detect chemicals (foods) in solution (saliva) in the mouth.

2. Five basic tastes: sweet, sour, salty, bitter, and savory; foods stimulate combinations of receptors; pain receptors for "hot" foods.
3. Pathway: facial and glossopharyngeal nerves to taste areas in parietal-temporal lobes.
4. Some adaptation does occur.

Sense of Smell (see Fig. 9–3)

1. Chemoreceptors are in upper nasal cavities; several hundred different ones; detect vaporized chemicals (many combinations possible).
2. Pathway: olfactory nerves to olfactory bulbs to olfactory areas in the temporal lobes.
3. Smell contributes greatly to what we call taste.
4. Adaptation occurs relatively quickly.

Hunger and Thirst—visceral (internal) sensations

1. Receptors for hunger: in hypothalamus, detect changes in GI hormones and nutrient levels in the blood; hunger is projected to the stomach; adaptation does occur at first.
2. Receptors for thirst: in hypothalamus, osmoreceptors detect changes in body water (water–salt proportions); thirst is projected to the mouth and pharynx; adaptation does not occur.

The Eye (see Figs. 9–4 through 9–8)

1. Eyelids and eyelashes spread tears and keep dust out of eyes; conjunctivae line the eyelids and cover white of eye.
2. Lacrimal glands produce tears, which flow across the eyeball to two lacrimal ducts, to lacrimal sac to nasolacrimal duct to nasal cavity. Tears wash the anterior eyeball and contain lysozyme to inhibit bacterial growth.
3. Most of the eyeball is protected by the bony orbit (socket).
4. The six extrinsic muscles move the eyeball; innervated by the 3rd, 4th, and 6th cranial nerves.
5. Sclera—outermost layer of the eyeball, made of fibrous connective tissue; anterior portion is the transparent cornea, the first light-refracting structure.
6. Choroid layer—middle layer of eyeball; dark blue pigment absorbs light to prevent glare within the eyeball.
7. Ciliary body (muscle) and suspensory ligaments—change shape of lens, which is made of a transparent, elastic protein and which refracts light.
8. Iris—two sets of smooth muscle fibers regulate diameter of pupil, that is, how much light strikes the retina.
   a. Radial fibers dilate pupil.
   b. Circular fibers constrict pupil.
9. Retina—innermost layer of eyeball; contains rods and cones.
   a. Rods—detect light; abundant toward periphery of retina.
   b. Cones—detect color; abundant in center of retina.
   c. Fovea—in the center of the macula lutea; contains only cones; area of best color vision.
   d. Optic disc—no rods or cones; optic nerve passes through eyeball.
10. Posterior cavity between lens and retina contains vitreous humor (semisolid) that keeps the retina in place.
11. Anterior cavity between cornea and lens contains aqueous humor that nourishes the lens and cornea; made by capillaries of the ciliary body, flows through pupil, is reabsorbed to blood at the canal of Schlemm.

Physiology of Vision

1. Refraction (bending and focusing) pathway of light: cornea, aqueous humor, lens, vitreous humor.
2. Lens is adjustable; ciliary muscle relaxes for distant vision, and lens is thin. Ciliary muscle contracts for near vision, and elastic lens thickens and has greater refractive power.
3. Light strikes retina and stimulates chemical reactions in the rods and cones.
4. In rods: rhodopsin breaks down to scotopsin and retinal (from vitamin A), and an electrical impulse is generated. In cones: specific wavelengths of light are absorbed (red, blue, green); chemical reactions generate nerve impulses.
5. Ganglion neurons from the rods and cones form the optic nerve, which passes through the eyeball at the optic disc.

6. Optic chiasma—site of the crossover of medial fibers of both optic nerves, permitting binocular vision.
7. Optic tracts—nerve pathways (see Fig. 9–8) from the optic chiasma to the brain; branches take impulses to the midbrain for visual reflexes; convergence at the thalamus for integration and dispersal; continuations to the occipital lobes for seeing and interpretation.
8. Visual areas in occipital lobes—each area receives impulses from both eyes; both areas create one image from the two slightly different images of each eye; both areas right the upside-down retinal image.

The Ear (see Figs. 9–9 through 9–12)

1. Outer ear—auricle or pinna has no real function for people; ear canal curves forward and down into temporal bone.
2. Middle ear—eardrum at end of ear canal vibrates when sound waves strike it. Auditory bones: malleus, incus, stapes; transmit vibrations to inner ear at oval window.
   a. Eustachian tube—extends from middle ear to nasopharynx; allows air in and out of middle ear to permit eardrum to vibrate; air pressure in middle ear should equal atmospheric pressure.
3. Inner ear—bony labyrinth in temporal bone, lined with membranous labyrinth. Perilymph is fluid between bone and membrane; endolymph is fluid within membrane. Membranous structures are the cochlea, utricle and saccule, and semicircular canals.
4. Cochlea—snail-shell shaped; three internal canals; cochlear duct contains receptors for hearing: hair cells in the organ of Corti; these cells contain endings of the cochlear branch of the 8th cranial nerve.
5. Physiology of hearing—sound waves stimulate vibration of eardrum, malleus, incus, stapes, oval window of inner ear, perilymph and endolymph of cochlea, and hair cells of organ of Corti. When hair cells bend, impulses are generated and carried by the 8th cranial nerve to the auditory areas in the temporal lobes. Round window prevents pressure damage to the hair cells.
6. Utricle and saccule—membranous sacs in the vestibule; each contains hair cells that are affected by gravity. When position of the head changes, otoliths bend the hair cells, which generate impulses along the vestibular branch of the 8th cranial nerve to the cerebellum, midbrain, and cerebrum. Impulses are interpreted as position of the head at rest.
7. Semicircular canals—three membranous ovals in three planes; enlarged base is the ampulla, which contains hair cells (crista) that are affected by movement. As body moves, hair cells bend in opposite direction, generate impulses along vestibular branch of 8th cranial nerve to cerebellum, midbrain, and cerebrum. Impulses are interpreted as movement of the body, changing speed, stopping or starting.

Arterial Receptors—in large arteries; detect changes in blood

1. Aortic arch—curves over top of heart. Aortic sinus contains pressoreceptors; aortic body contains chemoreceptors; sensory nerve is vagus (10th cranial).
2. Right and left carotid arteries in the neck; carotid sinus contains pressoreceptors; carotid body contains chemoreceptors; sensory nerve is the glossopharyngeal (9th cranial).
3. Pressoreceptors detect changes in blood pressure; chemoreceptors detect changes in pH or oxygen and CO_2 levels in the blood. This information is used by the vital centers in the medulla to change respiration or circulation to maintain normal blood oxygen and CO_2 and normal blood pressure.

REVIEW QUESTIONS

1. State the two general functions of receptors. Explain the purpose of sensory neurons and sensory tracts. (p. 224)
2. Name the receptors for the cutaneous senses, and explain the importance of this information. (pp. 225–227)
3. Name the receptors for muscle sense and the parts of the brain concerned with muscle sense. (p. 228)
4. State what the chemoreceptors for taste and smell detect. Name the cranial nerve(s) for each of these senses and the lobe of the cerebrum where each is felt. (p. 228)
5. Name the part of the eye with each of the following functions: (pp. 230–234)
   a. Change the shape of the lens
   b. Contains the rods and cones
   c. Forms the white of the eye
   d. Form the optic nerve
   e. Keep dust out of eye
   f. Changes the size of the pupil
   g. Produce tears
   h. Absorbs light within the eyeball to prevent glare
6. With respect to vision: (pp. 235–239)
   a. Name the structures and substances that refract light rays (in order)
   b. State what cones detect and what rods detect. What happens within these receptors when light strikes them?
   c. Name the cranial nerve for vision and the lobe of the cerebrum that contains the visual area
7. With respect to the ear: (pp. 239–244)
   a. Name the parts of the ear that transmit the vibrations of sound waves (in order)
   b. State the location of the receptors for hearing
   c. State the location of the receptors that respond to gravity
   d. State the location of the receptors that respond to motion
   e. State the two functions of the 8th cranial nerve
   f. Name the lobe of the cerebrum concerned with hearing
   g. Name the two parts of the brain concerned with maintaining balance and equilibrium
8. Name the following: (p. 244)
   a. The locations of arterial chemoreceptors, and state what they detect
   b. The locations of arterial pressoreceptors, and state what they detect
   c. The cranial nerves involved in respiratory and cardiac reflexes, and state the part of the brain that regulates these vital functions
9. Explain each of the following: adaptation, afterimage, projection, contrast. (pp. 224–225)

FOR FURTHER THOUGHT

1. Why are the inner ear labyrinths filled with fluid rather than air? One reason is directly concerned with hearing, the other with survival.
2. Michael's summer job in his town was collecting garbage. At first he thought the garbage and the truck smelled awful, but by the time he went home for lunch he decided that he didn't mind it at all. Explain what happened, and why his mother did mind.
3. When we are out in very cold weather, why don't our eyes freeze shut? Try to think of two reasons.
4. You probably have at one time hit your "funny bone," which is really the part of the ulnar nerve that crosses the elbow. Such a whack is very painful, and not just in the elbow but all the way down the forearm to the ring and little fingers of the hand. This is referred pain. Explain why it happens, and name the characteristic of sensations that it illustrates.
5. Albinism is a genetic characteristic in which melanin is not produced; it may occur in just about any type of animal. As you probably know, an albino person will have white skin and hair. Describe the consequences for the person's eyes.
6. We sometimes hear that blind people have a better sense of hearing than do sighted people. Do you think this is really true? Explain. Name two other senses a blind person may especially depend upon. Explain.
7. Look at Question Figure 9–A. In part A, which rectangle seems wider, the upper one or the lower one? Measure them, and explain your answer. Part B shows a Necker cube. Look at the cube and let your eyes relax. What seems to happen? Why do you think this happens? Part C has some lines and some shaded blocks. But what do we see? Explain.
8. Look at Question Figure 9–B. Part A shows a normal visual field. Parts B, C, and D are the visual fields of eye disorders you have read about in this chapter. Try to name each, with a reason for your answer.

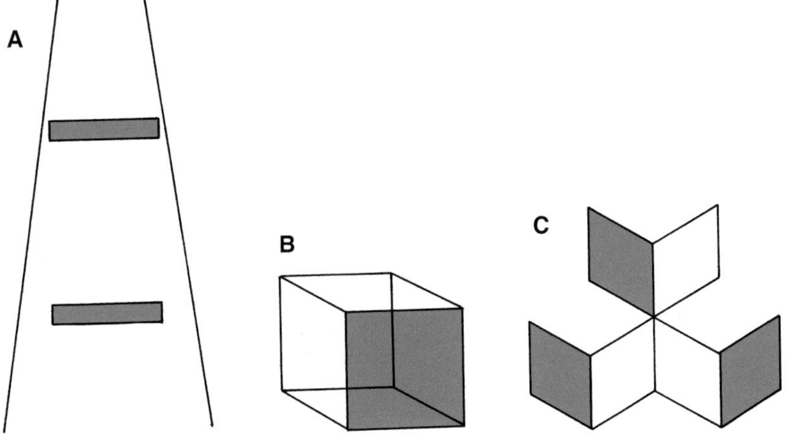

QUESTION FIGURE 9–A:

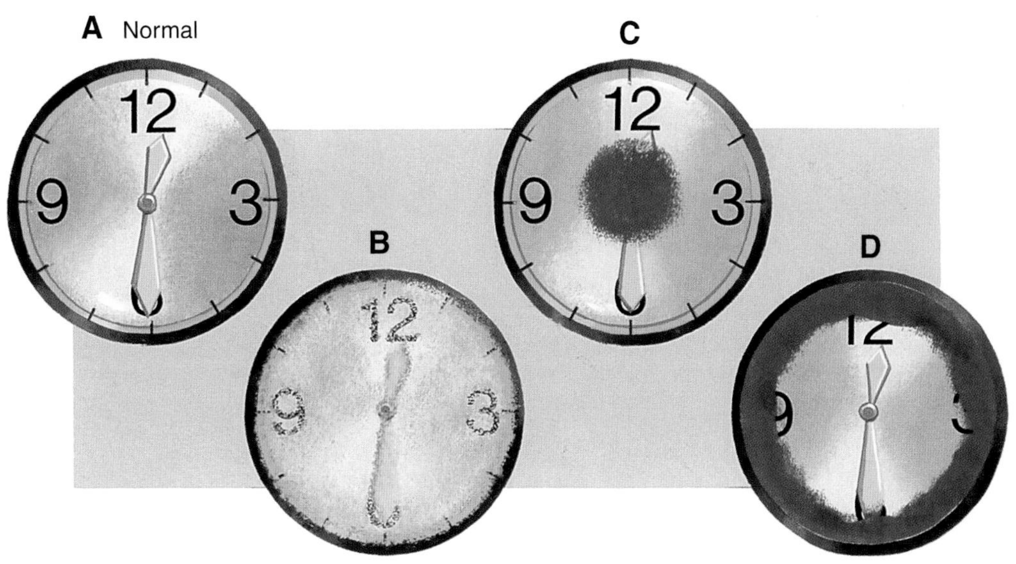

QUESTION FIGURE 9–B:

CHAPTER

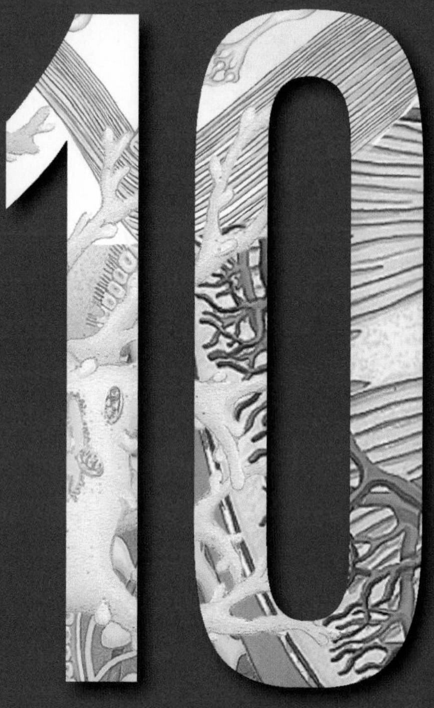

The Endocrine System

STUDENT OBJECTIVES

- Name the endocrine glands and the hormones secreted by each.
- Explain how a negative feedback mechanism works.
- Explain how the hypothalamus is involved in the secretion of hormones from the posterior pituitary gland and anterior pituitary gland.
- State the functions of oxytocin and antidiuretic hormone, and explain the stimulus for secretion of each.
- State the functions of the hormones of the anterior pituitary gland, and state the stimulus for secretion of each.
- State the functions of thyroxine and T_3, and describe the stimulus for their secretion.
- Explain how calcitonin and parathyroid hormone work as antagonists.
- Explain how glucagon and insulin work as antagonists.
- State the functions of epinephrine and norepinephrine, and explain their relationship to the sympathetic division of the autonomic nervous system.
- State the functions of aldosterone and cortisol, and describe the stimulus for secretion of each.
- State the functions of estrogen, progesterone, testosterone, and inhibin and state the stimulus for secretion of each.
- Explain what prostaglandins are made of, and state some of their functions.
- Explain how the protein hormones are believed to exert their effects.
- Explain how the steroid hormones are believed to exert their effects.

NEW TERMINOLOGY

Alpha cells *(**AL**-fah SELLS)*
Beta cells *(**BAY**-tah SELLS)*
Catecholamines *(**KAT**-e-kohl-ah-MEENZ)*
Corpus luteum *(**KOR**-pus **LOO**-tee-um)*
Gluconeogenesis *(GLOO-koh-nee-oh-**JEN**-i-sis)*
Glycogenesis *(GLIGH-koh-**JEN**-i-sis)*
Glycogenolysis *(GLIGH-ko-jen-**OL**-i-sis)*
Hypercalcemia *(HIGH-per-kal-**SEE**-mee-ah)*
Hyperglycemia *(HIGH-per-gligh-**SEE**-mee-ah)*
Hypocalcemia *(HIGH-poh-kal-**SEE**-mee-ah)*
Hypoglycemia *(HIGH-poh-gligh-**SEE**-mee-ah)*
Hypophysis *(high-**POFF**-e-sis)*
Islets of Langerhans *(**EYE**-lets of **LAHNG**-er-hanz)*
Prostaglandins *(PRAHS-tah-**GLAND**-ins)*
Renin-angiotensin mechanism *(**REE**-nin AN-jee-oh-**TEN**-sin)*
Sympathomimetic *(SIM-pah-tho-mi-**MET**-ik)*
Target organ *(**TAR**-get **OR**-gan)*

*Terms that appear in **bold type** in the chapter text are defined in the glossary, which begins on page 603.*

CHAPTER OUTLINE

RELATED CLINICAL TERMINOLOGY

Acromegaly *(AK-roh-**MEG**-ah-lee)*
Addison's disease *(**ADD**-i-sonz)*
Cretinism *(**KREE**-tin-izm)*
Cushing's syndrome *(**KOOSH**-ingz **SIN**-drohm)*
Diabetes mellitus *(DYE-ah-**BEE**-tis mel-**LYE**-tus)*
Giantism *(**JIGH**-an-tizm)*
Goiter *(**GOY**-ter)*
Graves' disease *(GRAYVES)*
Ketoacidosis *(KEY-toh-ass-i-**DOH**-sis)*
Myxedema *(MIK-suh-**DEE**-mah)*
Pituitary dwarfism *(pi-**TOO**-i-TER-ee **DWORF**-izm)*

We have already seen how the nervous system regulates body functions by means of nerve impulses and integration of information by the spinal cord and brain. The other regulating system of the body is the **endocrine system**, which consists of endocrine glands that secrete chemicals called **hormones**. These glands and the names of the hormones they secrete are shown in Fig. 10–1.

Endocrine glands are ductless; that is, they do not have ducts to take their secretions to specific sites. Instead, hormones are secreted directly into capillaries and circulate in the blood throughout the body. Each hormone then exerts very specific effects on certain organs, called **target organs** or **target tissues** (we will return to how this is accomplished, and just what makes an organ a "target," in a later section). Some hormones, such as insulin and thyroxine, have many target organs. Other hormones, such as calcitonin and some pituitary gland hormones, have only one or a few target organs.

In general, the endocrine system and its hormones help regulate growth, the use of foods to produce energy, resistance to stress, the pH of body fluids and fluid balance, and reproduction. In this chapter we will discuss the specific functions of the hormones and how each contributes to homeostasis.

CHEMISTRY OF HORMONES

With respect to their chemical structure, hormones may be classified into three groups: amines, proteins, and steroids.

1. **Amines**—these simple hormones are structural variations of the amino acid tyrosine. This group includes thyroxine from the thyroid gland and epinephrine and norepinephrine from the adrenal medulla.

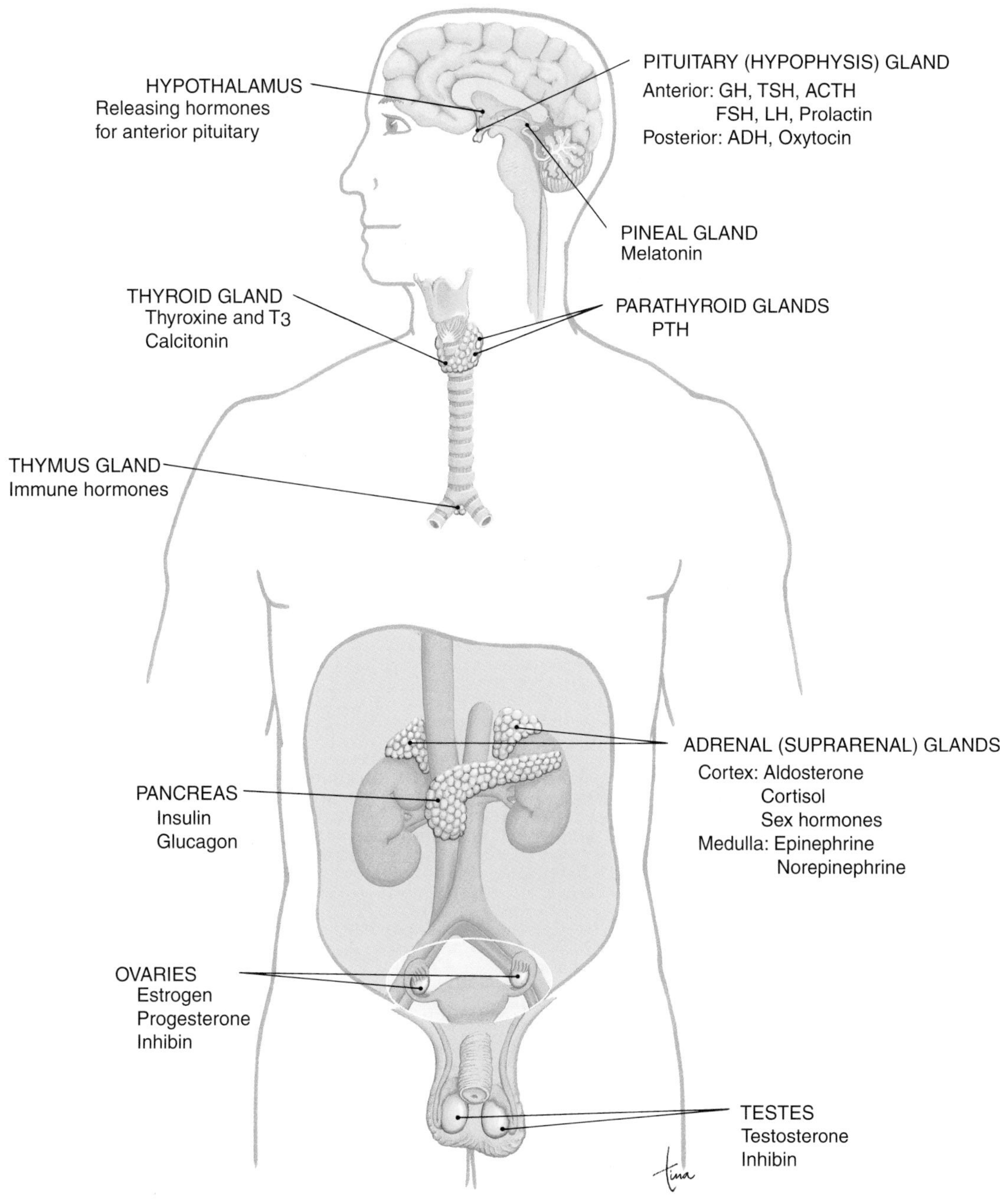

Figure 10–1 The endocrine system. Locations of many endocrine glands. Both male and female gonads (testes and ovaries) are shown.

QUESTION: Why is the location of the thyroid gland not really important for its function?

2. **Proteins**—these hormones are chains of from 50 to 200 amino acids. Insulin from the pancreas, growth hormone from the anterior pituitary gland, and calcitonin from the thyroid gland are all proteins. Short chains of amino acids may be called **peptides**. Antidiuretic hormone and oxytocin, synthesized by the hypothalamus, are peptide hormones of nine amino acids each.
3. **Steroids**—cholesterol is the precursor for the steroid hormones (the four carbon-ring structure of cholesterol is shown in Chapter 2), which include cortisol and aldosterone from the adrenal cortex, estrogen and progesterone from the ovaries, and testosterone from the testes.

REGULATION OF HORMONE SECRETION

Hormones are secreted by endocrine glands when there is a need for them, that is, for their effects on their target organs. The cells of endocrine glands respond to changes in the blood or perhaps to other hormones in the blood. These stimuli are the information the cells use to increase or decrease secretion of their own hormones. When a hormone brings about its effects, the stimulus is often reversed, and secretion of the hormone decreases until the stimulus reoccurs. You may recall from Chapter 1 that this is a negative feedback mechanism, and the mechanism for secretion of thyroxine was depicted in Fig. 1–3. Let us use insulin as a different example here.

Insulin is secreted by the pancreas when the blood glucose level is high; that is, hyperglycemia (such as after a meal) is the stimulus for secretion of insulin. Once circulating in the blood, insulin enables cells to remove glucose from the blood so that it can be used for energy production and enables the liver to store glucose as glycogen. As a result of these actions of insulin, the blood glucose level decreases, reversing the stimulus for secretion of insulin. Insulin secretion then decreases until the blood glucose level increases again. The blood glucose level rises, falls, rises, and falls within the range that is considered normal. The rises stimulate insulin secretion and the falls shut off the secretion of insulin.

In any hormonal **negative feedback mechanism**, information about the effects of the hormone is "fed back" to the gland, which then decreases its secretion of the hormone. This is why the mechanism is called "negative": The effects of the hormone reverse the stimulus and decrease the secretion of the hormone. Another way to put this is that the mechanism has its own brake; it turns itself off until the stimulus reoccurs. The secretion of many other hormones is regulated in a similar way. If we were to visualize such hormone secretion during the span of a day or two, it would look very much like the changes in blood sugar level just described. Secretion of insulin or thyroxine would rise and fall, rise and fall within a normal range. Picture ocean waves with crests and troughs much the same height and depth; this is what blood levels of the hormone would look like.

The hormones of the anterior pituitary gland are secreted in response to **releasing hormones** (also called releasing factors) secreted by the hypothalamus. You may recall this from Chapter 8. Growth hormone, for example, is secreted in response to growth hormone–releasing hormone (GHRH) from the hypothalamus. As growth hormone exerts its effects, the secretion of GHRH decreases, which in turn decreases the secretion of growth hormone. This is another type of negative feedback mechanism.

For each of the hormones to be discussed in this chapter, the stimulus for its secretion will also be mentioned. Some hormones function as an **antagonistic pair** to regulate a particular aspect of blood chemistry; these mechanisms will also be covered.

THE PITUITARY GLAND

The **pituitary gland** (or **hypophysis**) hangs by a short stalk (infundibulum) from the hypothalamus and is enclosed by the sella turcica of the sphenoid bone. Despite its small size, the pituitary gland regulates many body functions. Its two major portions are the posterior pituitary gland (**neurohypophysis**), which is an extension of the nerve tissue of the hypothalamus, and the anterior pituitary gland (**adenohypophysis**), which is separate glandular tissue. All of the hormones of the pituitary gland and their target organs are shown in Fig. 10–2. It may be helpful for you to look at this summary picture before you begin reading the following sections.

POSTERIOR PITUITARY GLAND

The two hormones of the **posterior pituitary gland**, antidiuretic hormone and oxytocin, are actually produced by the hypothalamus and simply stored in the posterior pituitary until needed. Their release is stimulated by nerve impulses from the hypothalamus (Fig. 10–3).

Antidiuretic Hormone

Antidiuretic hormone (ADH, also called **vasopressin**) increases the reabsorption of water by kidney tubules, which decreases the amount of urine formed. The water is reabsorbed into the blood, so as urinary output is decreased, blood volume is increased, which helps maintain

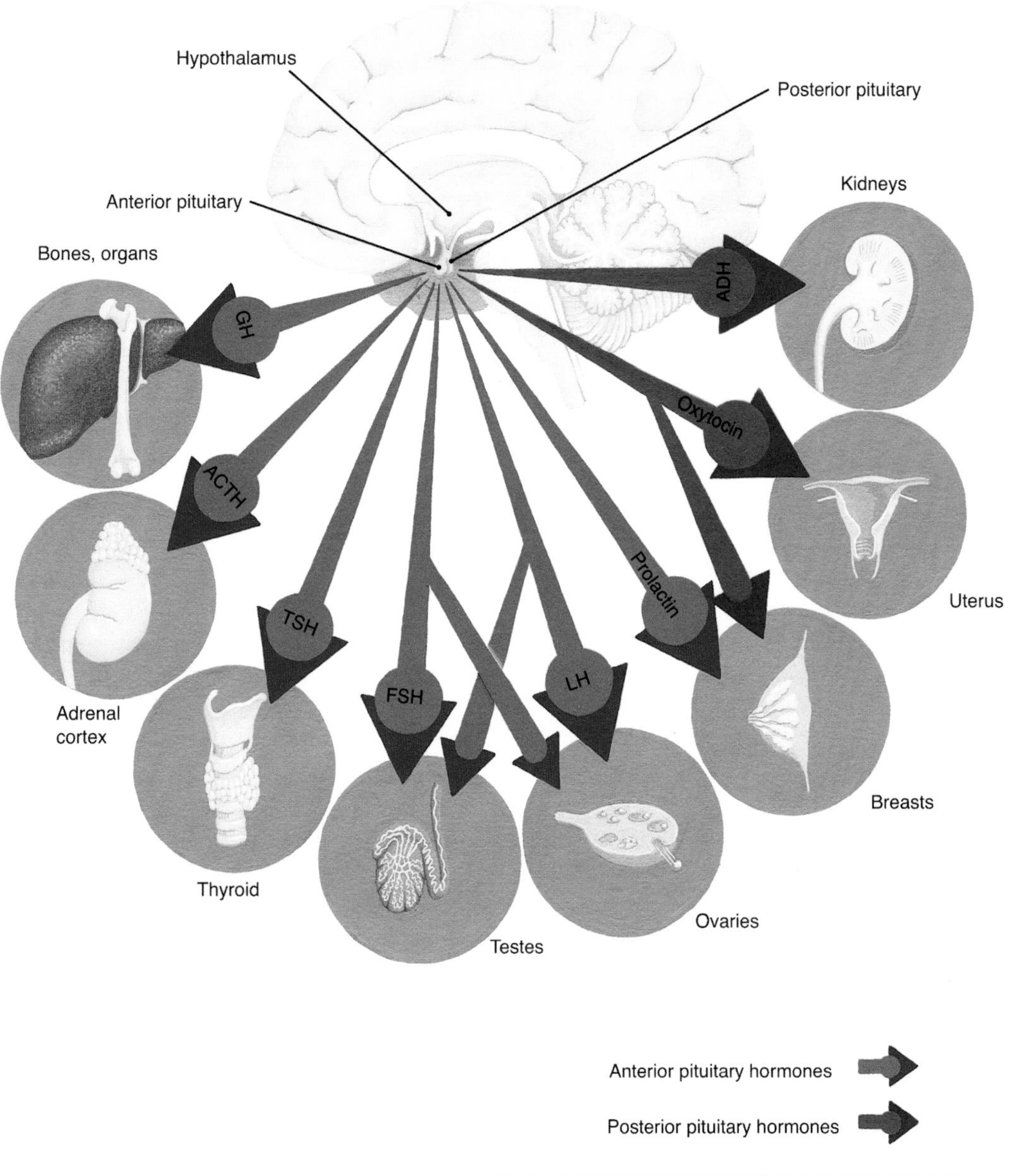

Figure 10–2 Hormones of the pituitary gland and their target organs.

QUESTION: Which pituitary hormones have other endocrine glands as their target organs?

normal blood pressure. ADH also decreases sweating, but the amount of water conserved is much less than that conserved by the kidneys.

The stimulus for secretion of ADH is decreased water content of the body. If too much water is lost through sweating or diarrhea, for example, **osmoreceptors** in the hypothalamus detect the increased "saltiness" of body fluids. The hypothalamus then transmits impulses to the posterior pituitary to increase the secretion of ADH and decrease the loss of more water in urine.

Any type of dehydration stimulates the secretion of ADH to conserve body water. In the case of severe hemorrhage, ADH is released in large amounts and will also cause vasoconstriction, especially in arterioles, which will help to raise or at least maintain blood pressure. This function gives ADH its other name, **vasopressin**.

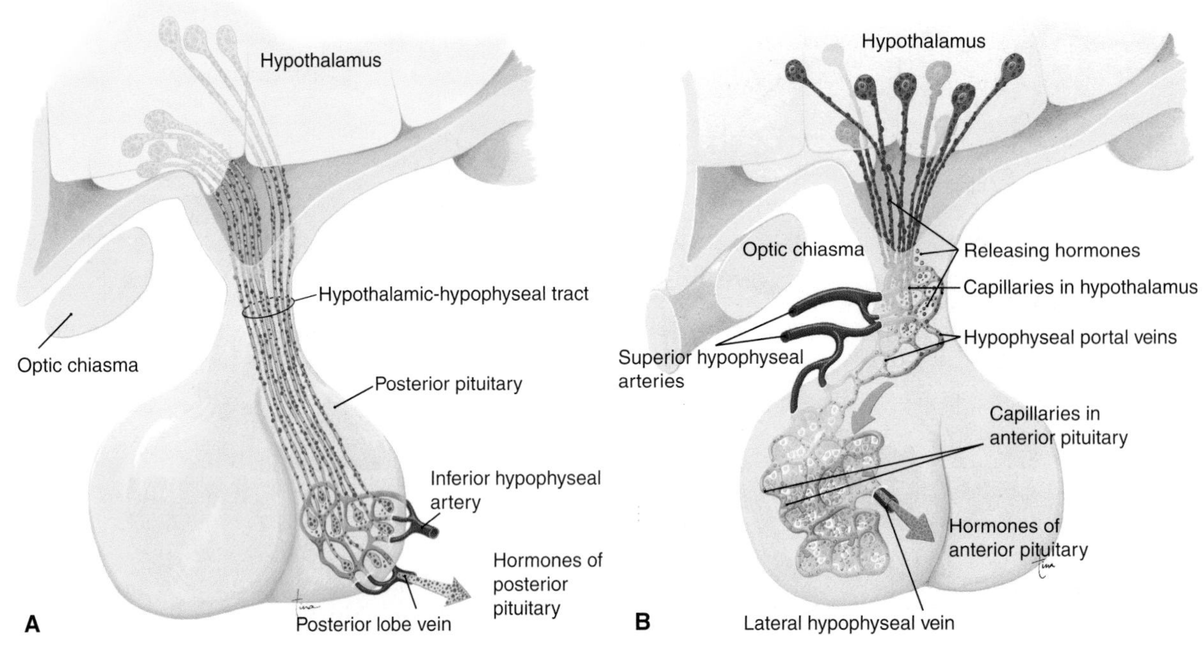

Figure 10–3 Structural relationships of hypothalamus and pituitary gland. (**A**) Posterior pituitary stores hormones produced in the hypothalamus. (**B**) Releasing hormones of the hypothalamus circulate directly to the anterior pituitary and influence its secretions. Notice the two networks of capillaries.

QUESTION: In part A, name the hormones of the posterior pituitary. In part B, what stimulates secretion of anterior pituitary hormones?

Ingestion of alcohol inhibits the secretion of ADH and increases urinary output. If alcohol intake is excessive and fluid is not replaced, a person will feel thirsty and dizzy the next morning. The thirst is due to the loss of body water, and the dizziness is the result of low blood pressure.

Oxytocin

Oxytocin stimulates contraction of the uterus at the end of pregnancy and stimulates release of milk from the mammary glands when the baby is nursing.

As labor begins, the cervix of the uterus is stretched, which generates sensory impulses to the hypothalamus, which in turn stimulates the posterior pituitary to release oxytocin. This cycle continues as the baby's head and body pass through the cervix. Oxytocin causes stronger and stronger contractions of the smooth muscle (myometrium) of the uterus to bring about delivery of the baby and the placenta. The secretion of oxytocin is one of the few positive feedback mechanisms within the body, and the external brake or shutoff of the feedback cycle is delivery of the baby and the placenta. With delivery, the distention of the cervix ends and there is no longer any stimulus for secretion of oxytocin. If we were to visualize this type of mechanism (say, from the beginning of labor for oxytocin), we would see that secretion of the hormone would rise, then rise some more, then rise some more. The stimulus keeps "bumping up" the secretion; this would look much like a stairway. Eventually the external brake, the birth of the baby in the case of oxytocin, shuts off secretion (a big step down to the starting level).

It has been discovered that the placenta itself secretes oxytocin at the end of gestation and in an amount far higher than that from the posterior pituitary gland. Research is continuing to determine the exact mechanism and precise role of the placenta in labor.

When a baby is breast-fed, the sucking of the baby stimulates sensory impulses from the mother's nipple to the hypothalamus. Nerve impulses from the hypothalamus to the posterior pituitary cause the release of oxytocin, which stimulates contraction of the smooth muscle cells around the mammary ducts. This release of milk is sometimes called the "milk let-down" reflex. The hormones of the posterior pituitary are summarized in Table 10–1.

Both ADH and oxytocin are peptide hormones with similar structure, having nine amino acids each. And both have been found to influence aspects of behavior such as nurturing and trustfulness. Certain brain cells have receptors for oxytocin and vasopressin, and they are involved in creating the bonds that sustain family life. Trust is part of many social encounters such as friendship, school, sports and games, and buying and selling, as well as family life (however, oxytocin does not make someone who is naturally mistrustful into a trusting person; it does not change a person's basic nature). The success of "pet therapy" (for some people, not everyone) is believed to result from the secretion of oxytocin in both the people and the animals that take part. These two small hormones have influences on us mentally and physically.

ANTERIOR PITUITARY GLAND

The hormones of the **anterior pituitary gland** regulate many body functions. They are in turn regulated by **releasing hormones** from the hypothalamus. These releasing hormones are secreted into capillaries in the hypothalamus and pass through the **hypophyseal portal** veins to another capillary network in the anterior pituitary gland. Here, the releasing hormones are absorbed and stimulate secretion of the anterior pituitary hormones. This small but specialized pathway of circulation is shown in Fig. 10–3. This pathway permits the releasing hormones to rapidly stimulate the anterior pituitary, without having to pass through general circulation.

Growth Hormone

Growth hormone (**GH**) is also called **somatotropin**, and it does indeed promote growth, though it does so indirectly. GH stimulates cells to produce chemicals called insulin-like growth factors (IGFs), intermediary molecules that bring about what we will consider the functions of GH in its target cells and organs (see Fig. 10–4). Growth hormone increases the transport of amino acids into cells and increases the rate of protein synthesis. Amino acids cannot be stored in the body, so when they are available, they must be used in the protein synthesis that is needed in a particular organ at that time. Excess amino acids, if any, are changed to carbohydrates or fat, to be used for energy right away, if needed, or for energy storage. Growth hormone ensures that amino acids will be used for whatever protein synthesis is necessary, before the amino acids can be changed to carbohydrates. Growth hormone also stimulates cell division in those tissues capable of mitosis. These functions contribute to the growth of the body during childhood, especially growth of bones and muscles.

You may now be wondering if GH is secreted in adults, and the answer is yes. The use of amino acids for the synthesis of proteins is still necessary. Even if the body is not growing in height, some tissues will require new proteins for repair or replacement. GH also stimulates the release of fat from adipose tissue and the use of fats for energy production. This is important any time we go for extended periods without eating, no matter what our ages.

Table 10–1 | HORMONES OF THE POSTERIOR PITUITARY GLAND

HORMONE	FUNCTION(S)	REGULATION OF SECRETION
Antidiuretic hormone (ADH or vasopressin)	■ Increases water reabsorption by the kidney tubules (water returns to the blood) ■ Decreases sweating ■ Causes vasoconstriction (in large amounts)	Decreased water content in the body (alcohol inhibits secretion)
Oxytocin	■ Promotes contraction of myometrium of uterus (labor) ■ Promotes release of milk from mammary glands	Nerve impulses from hypothalamus, the result of stretching of cervix or stimulation of nipple Secretion from placenta at end of gestation—stimulus unknown

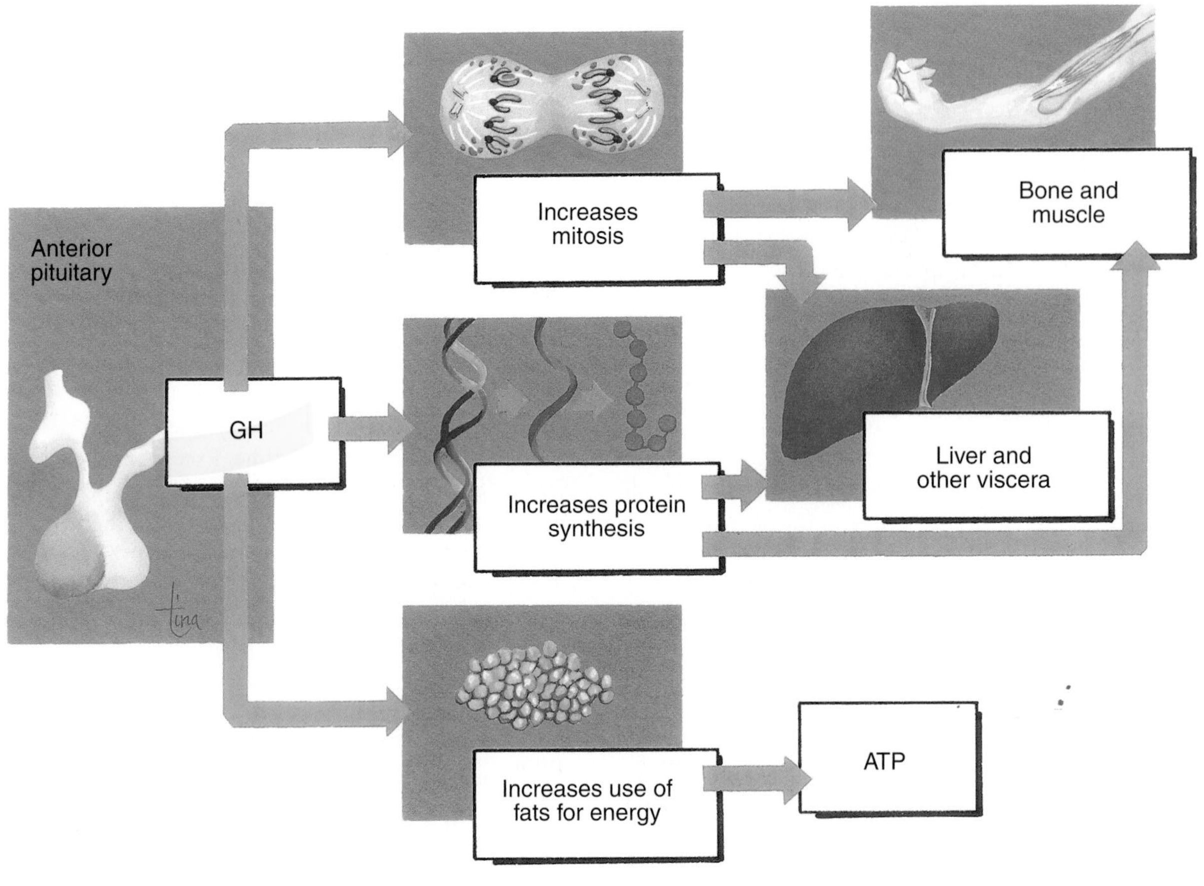

Figure 10–4 Functions of growth hormone.

QUESTION: Which functions of growth hormone directly help bones and muscles to grow?

The secretion of GH is regulated by two releasing hormones from the hypothalamus. Growth hormone–releasing hormone (GHRH), which increases the secretion of GH, is produced during hypoglycemia and during exercise. Another stimulus for GHRH is a high blood level of amino acids; the GH then secreted will ensure the conversion of these amino acids into protein. Growth hormone–inhibiting hormone (GHIH) may also be called **somatostatin** and, as its name tells us, it decreases the secretion of GH. Somatostatin is produced during hyperglycemia. Disorders of GH secretion are discussed in Box 10–1.

Thyroid-Stimulating Hormone

Thyroid-stimulating hormone (**TSH**) is also called thyrotropin, and its target organ is the thyroid gland. TSH stimulates the normal growth of the thyroid and the secretion of thyroxine (T_4) and triiodothyronine (T_3). The functions of these thyroid hormones will be covered later in this chapter.

The secretion of TSH is stimulated by thyrotropin-releasing hormone (TRH) from the hypothalamus. When metabolic rate (energy production) decreases, TRH is produced so that TSH is produced so that thyroxine is produced to increase energy production and raise the metabolic rate.

Adrenocorticotropic Hormone

Adrenocorticotropic hormone (**ACTH**) stimulates the secretion of cortisol and other hormones by the adrenal cortex. Secretion of ACTH is increased by corticotropin-releasing hormone (CRH) from the hypothalamus. CRH is produced in any type of physiological stress situation such as injury, disease, exercise, or hypoglycemia (being hungry is stressful).

Box 10–1 | DISORDERS OF GROWTH HORMONE

A deficiency or excess of growth hormone (GH) during childhood will have marked effects on the growth of a child. Hyposecretion of GH results in **pituitary dwarfism**, in which the person may attain a final height of only 3 to 4 feet but will have normal body proportions. GH can now be produced using genetic engineering and may be used to stimulate growth in children with this disorder. GH will not increase growth of children with the genetic potential for short stature. Reports that GH will reverse the effects of aging are simply not true.

Hypersecretion of GH results in **giantism** (or gigantism), in which the long bones grow excessively and the person may attain a height of 8 feet. Most very tall people, such as basketball players, do *not* have this condition; they are tall as a result of their genetic makeup and good nutrition.

In an adult, hypersecretion of GH is caused by a pituitary tumor and results in **acromegaly**. The long bones cannot grow because the epiphyseal discs are closed, but the growth of other bones is stimulated. The jaw and other facial bones become disproportionately large, as do the bones of the hands and feet. The skin becomes thicker, and the tongue also grows and may protrude. Other consequences include compression of nerves by abnormally growing bones and growth of the articular cartilages, which then erode and bring on arthritis. Treatment of acromegaly requires surgical removal of the tumor or its destruction by radiation.

Prolactin (PRL)

Prolactin, as its name suggests, is responsible for lactation. More precisely, prolactin initiates and maintains milk production by the mammary glands. The regulation of secretion of prolactin is complex, involving both prolactin-releasing hormone (PRH) and prolactin-inhibiting hormone (PIH) from the hypothalamus. The mammary glands must first be acted on by other hormones such as estrogen and progesterone, which are secreted in large amounts by the placenta during pregnancy. Then, after delivery of the baby, prolactin secretion increases and milk is produced. If the mother continues to breast-feed, prolactin levels remain high.

Follicle-Stimulating Hormone

Follicle-stimulating hormone (FSH) is one of the **gonadotropic hormones**; that is, it has its effects on the gonads: the ovaries or testes. FSH is named for one of its functions in women. Within the ovaries are ovarian follicles that contain potential ova (egg cells). FSH stimulates the growth of ovarian follicles; that is, it initiates egg development in cycles of approximately 28 days. FSH also stimulates secretion of estrogen by the follicle cells. In men, FSH initiates sperm production within the testes.

The secretion of FSH is stimulated by the hypothalamus, which produces **gonadotropin-releasing hormone (GnRH)**. FSH secretion is decreased by inhibin, a hormone produced by the ovaries or testes.

Luteinizing Hormone

Luteinizing hormone (LH) is another gonadotropic hormone. In women, LH is responsible for ovulation, the release of a mature ovum from an ovarian follicle. LH then stimulates that follicle to develop into the corpus luteum, which secretes progesterone, also under the influence of LH. In men, LH stimulates the interstitial cells of the testes to secrete testosterone. (LH is also called ICSH, interstitial cell stimulating hormone.)

Secretion of LH is also regulated by GnRH from the hypothalamus. We will return to FSH and LH, as well as a discussion of the sex hormones, in Chapter 20.

The hormones of the anterior pituitary are summarized in Table 10–2.

THYROID GLAND

The **thyroid gland** is located on the front and sides of the trachea just below the larynx and is shaped somewhat like a butterfly. Its two lobes (the "wings") are connected by a middle piece called the isthmus. The structural units of the thyroid gland are thyroid follicles (see Fig. 4–3, part A, in Chapter 4 for cross-sections of follicles) made of cuboidal epithelium. The follicles produce **thyroxine (T_4)** and **triiodothyronine (T_3)**. Iodine is necessary for the synthesis of these hormones; thyroxine contains four atoms of iodine, and T_3 contains three atoms of iodine.

The third hormone produced by the thyroid gland is **calcitonin**, which is secreted by parafollicular cells. Its

Table 10–2 | HORMONES OF THE ANTERIOR PITUITARY GLAND

HORMONE	FUNCTION(S)	REGULATION OF SECRETION
Growth hormone (GH)	■ Increases rate of mitosis ■ Increases amino acid transport into cells ■ Increases rate of protein synthesis ■ Increases use of fats for energy	GHRH (hypothalamus) stimulates secretion GHIH—somatostatin (hypothalamus) inhibits secretion
Thyroid-stimulating hormone (TSH)	■ Increases secretion of thyroxine and T_3 by thyroid gland	TRH (hypothalamus)
Adrenocorticotropic hormone (ACTH)	■ Increases secretion of cortisol by the adrenal cortex	CRH (hypothalamus)
Prolactin	■ Stimulates milk production by the mammary glands	PRH (hypothalamus) stimulates secretion PIH (hypothalamus) inhibits secretion
Follicle-stimulating hormone (FSH)	*In women:* ■ Initiates growth of ova in ovarian follicles ■ Increases secretion of estrogen by follicle cells *In men:* ■ Initiates sperm production in the testes	GnRH (hypothalamus) stimulates secretion Inhibin (ovaries or testes) inhibits secretion
Luteinizing hormone (LH) (ICSH)	*In women:* ■ Causes ovulation ■ Causes the ruptured ovarian follicle to become the corpus luteum ■ Increases secretion of progesterone by the corpus luteum *In men:* ■ Increases secretion of testosterone by the interstitial cells of the testes	GnRH (hypothalamus)

function is very different from those of thyroxine and T_3, as you may recall from Chapter 6.

THYROXINE AND T_3

Thyroxine (T_4) and T_3 have the same functions: regulation of energy production and protein synthesis, which contribute to growth of the body and to normal body functioning throughout life (Fig. 10–5). Thyroxine and T_3 increase cell respiration of all food types (carbohydrates, fats, and excess amino acids) and thereby increase energy and heat production. They also increase the rate of protein synthesis within cells. Normal production of thyroxine and T_3 is essential for physical growth, normal mental development, and maturation of the reproductive system. These hormones are the most important day-to-day regulators of metabolic rate; their activity is reflected in the functioning of the brain, muscles, heart, and virtually all other organs. Although thyroxine and T_3 are not vital hormones, in that they are not crucial to survival, their absence greatly diminishes physical and mental growth and abilities (see Box 10–2: Disorders of Thyroxine).

Secretion of thyroxine and T_3 is stimulated by **thyroid-stimulating hormone (TSH)** from the anterior pituitary gland (see also Fig. 1–3 in Chapter 1). When the metabolic rate (energy production) decreases, this change is detected by the hypothalamus, which secretes thyrotropin-releasing hormone (TRH). TRH stimulates the anterior pituitary to secrete TSH, which stimulates the thyroid to release

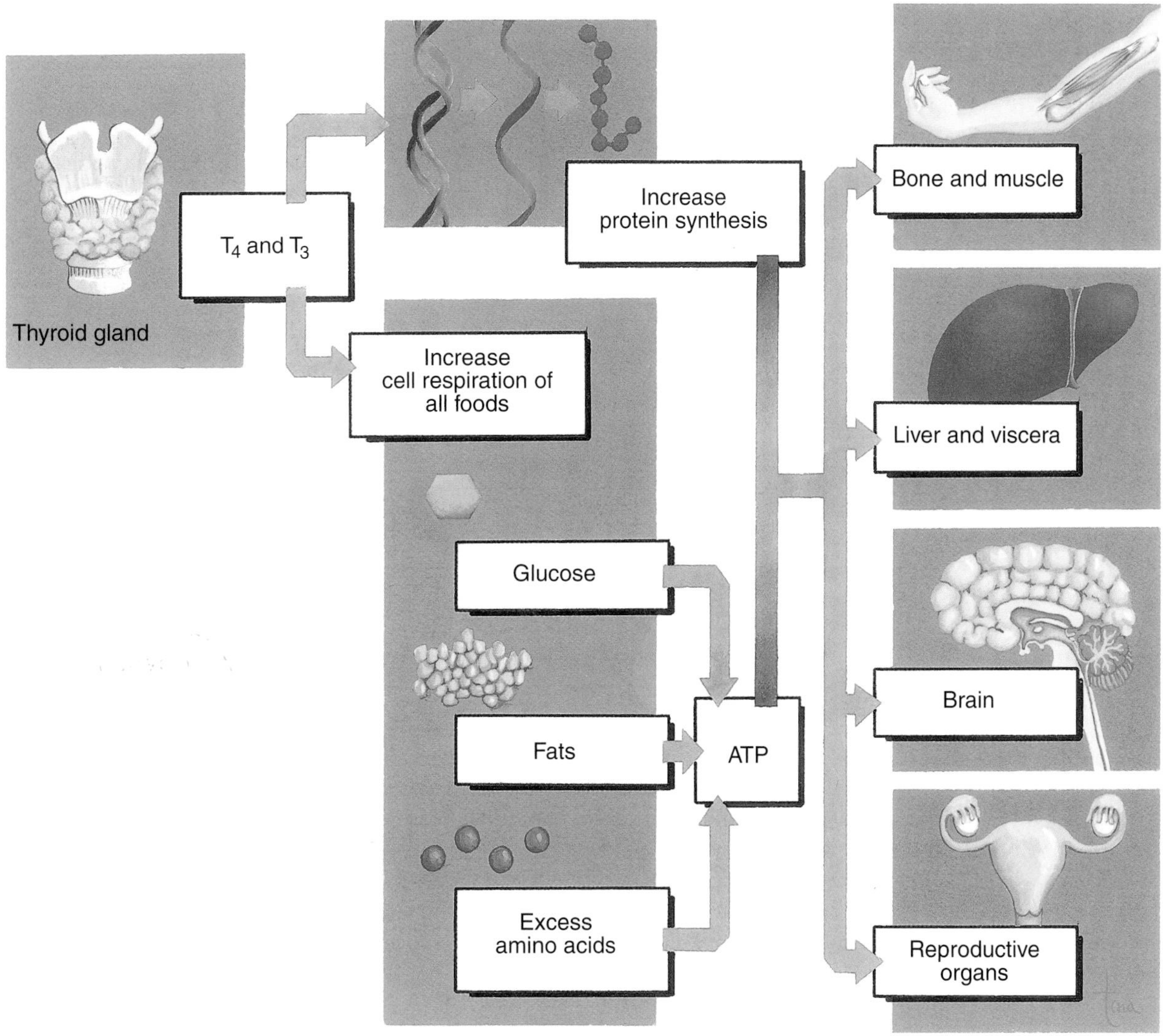

Figure 10–5 Functions of thyroxine and T_3.

QUESTION: Which functions of thyroxine help bones and muscles to grow and maintain their own functions?

Box 10–2 | DISORDERS OF THYROXINE

Iodine is an essential component of thyroxine (and T_3), and a dietary deficiency of iodine causes **goiter**. In an attempt to produce more thyroxine, the thyroid cells become enlarged, and hence the thyroid gland enlarges and becomes visible on the front of the neck. The use of iodized salt has made goiter a rare condition in many parts of the world.

Hyposecretion of thyroxine in a newborn has devastating effects on the growth of the child. Without thyroxine, physical growth is diminished, as is mental development. This condition is called **cretinism** and is characterized by severe mental and physical disabilities. If the thyroxine deficiency is detected shortly after birth, the child may

Continued

Box 10–2 | DISORDERS OF THYROXINE *(Continued)*

be treated with thyroid hormones to promote normal development.

Hyposecretion of thyroxine in an adult is called **myxedema**. Without thyroxine, the metabolic rate (energy production) decreases, resulting in lethargy, muscular weakness, slow heart rate, a feeling of cold, weight gain, and a characteristic puffiness of the face. The administration of thyroid hormones will return the metabolic rate to normal.

Graves' disease is an autoimmune disorder that causes hypersecretion of thyroxine. The autoantibodies seem to bind to TSH receptors on the thyroid cells and stimulate secretion of excess thyroxine. The symptoms are those that would be expected when the metabolic rate is abnormally elevated: weight loss accompanied by increased appetite, increased sweating, fast heart rate, feeling of warmth, and fatigue. Also present may be goiter and exophthalmos, which is protrusion of the eyes. Treatment is aimed at decreasing the secretion of thyroxine by the thyroid, and medications or radioactive iodine may be used to accomplish this.

thyroxine and T_3, which raise the metabolic rate by increasing energy production. This negative feedback mechanism then shuts off TRH from the hypothalamus until the metabolic rate decreases again.

CALCITONIN

Calcitonin decreases the reabsorption of calcium and phosphate from the bones to the blood, thereby lowering blood levels of these minerals. This function of calcitonin helps maintain normal blood levels of calcium and phosphate and also helps maintain a stable, strong bone matrix. It is believed that calcitonin exerts its most important effects during childhood, when bones are growing. A form of calcitonin obtained from salmon is used to help treat osteoporosis.

The stimulus for secretion of calcitonin is **hypercalcemia**, that is, a high blood calcium level. When blood calcium is high, calcitonin ensures that no more calcium will be removed from bones until there is a real need for more calcium in the blood (Fig. 10–6). The hormones of the thyroid gland are summarized in Table 10–3.

PARATHYROID GLANDS

There are four **parathyroid glands**: two on the back of each lobe of the thyroid gland (Fig. 10–7). The hormone they produce is called parathyroid hormone.

PARATHYROID HORMONE

Parathyroid hormone (**PTH**) is an antagonist to calcitonin and is important for the maintenance of normal blood levels of calcium and phosphate. The target organs of PTH are the bones, small intestine, and kidneys.

PTH increases the reabsorption of calcium and phosphate from bones to the blood, thereby raising their blood levels. Absorption of calcium and phosphate from food in the small intestine, which also requires vitamin D, is increased by PTH. This, too, raises the blood levels of these minerals. In the kidneys, PTH stimulates the activation of vitamin D and increases the reabsorption of calcium and the excretion of phosphate (more than is obtained from bones). Therefore, the overall effect of PTH is to raise the blood calcium level and lower the blood phosphate level. The functions of PTH are summarized in Table 10–4.

Secretion of PTH is stimulated by **hypocalcemia**, a low blood calcium level, and inhibited by hypercalcemia. The antagonistic effects of PTH and calcitonin are shown in Fig. 10–6. Together, these hormones maintain blood calcium within a normal range. Calcium in the blood is essential for the process of blood clotting and for normal activity of neurons and muscle cells.

As you might expect, a sustained hypersecretion of PTH, such as is caused by a parathyroid tumor, would remove calcium from bones and weaken them. It has been found, however, that an intermittent, brief excess of PTH, such as can occur by injection, will stimulate the formation of more bone matrix, rather than matrix reabsorption. This may seem very strange—the opposite of what we would expect—but it shows how much we have yet to learn about the body. PTH is used for some cases of osteoporosis, but this treatment is very expensive.

PANCREAS

The **pancreas** is located in the upper left quadrant of the abdominal cavity, extending from the curve of the duodenum to the spleen. Although the pancreas is both an exocrine gland (for digestion) and an endocrine gland, only

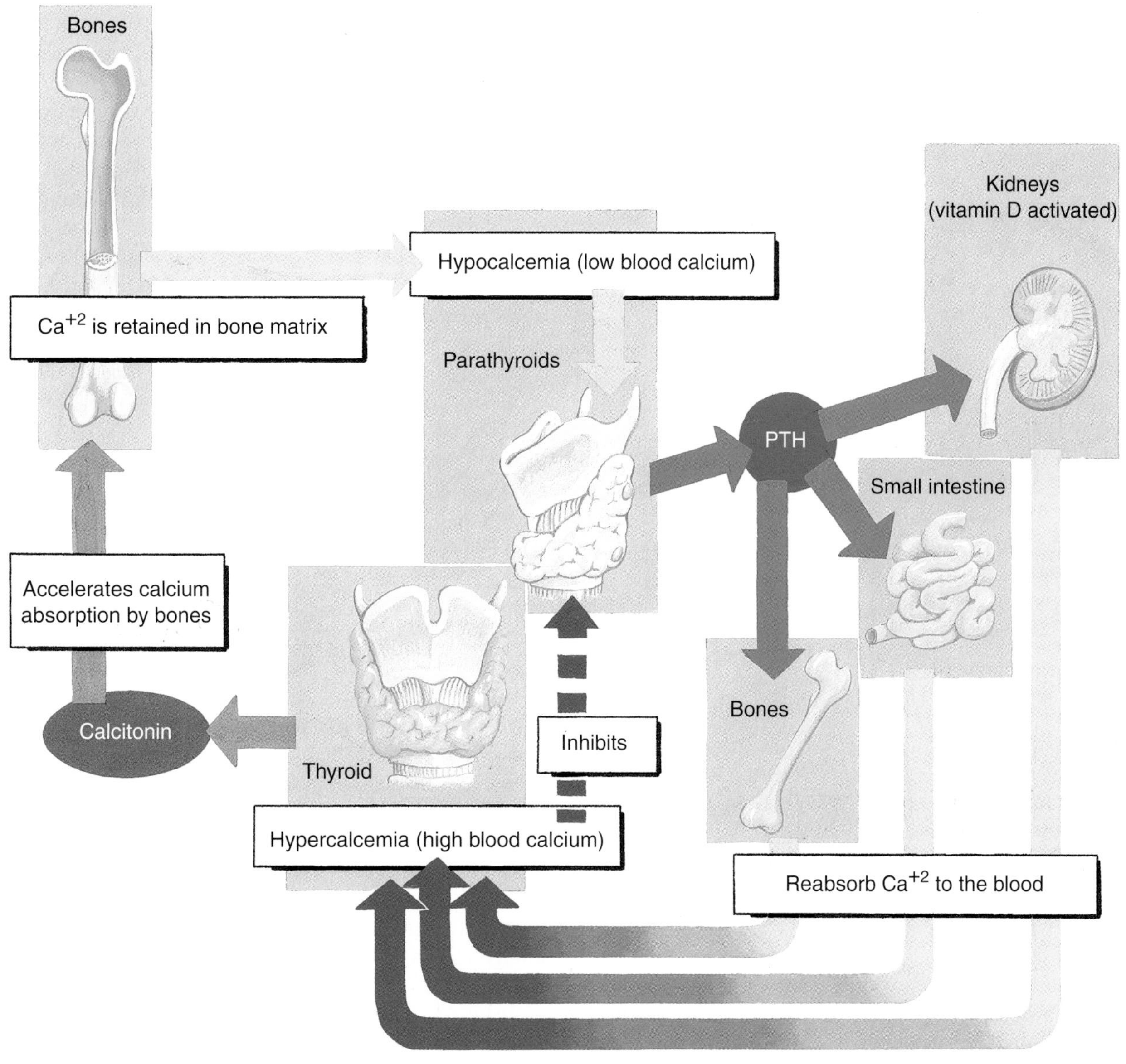

Figure 10–6 Calcitonin and parathyroid hormone (PTH) and their functions related to the maintenance of the blood calcium level.

QUESTION: Which hormone helps keep calcium in bones? What vitamin does PTH help activate, and where?

Table 10–3 | **HORMONES OF THE THYROID GLAND**

HORMONE	FUNCTION(S)	REGULATION OF SECRETION
Thyroxine (T_4) and triiodothyronine (T_3)	■ Increase energy production from all food types ■ Increase rate of protein synthesis	TSH (anterior pituitary)
Calcitonin	■ Decreases the reabsorption of calcium and phosphate from bones to blood	Hypercalcemia

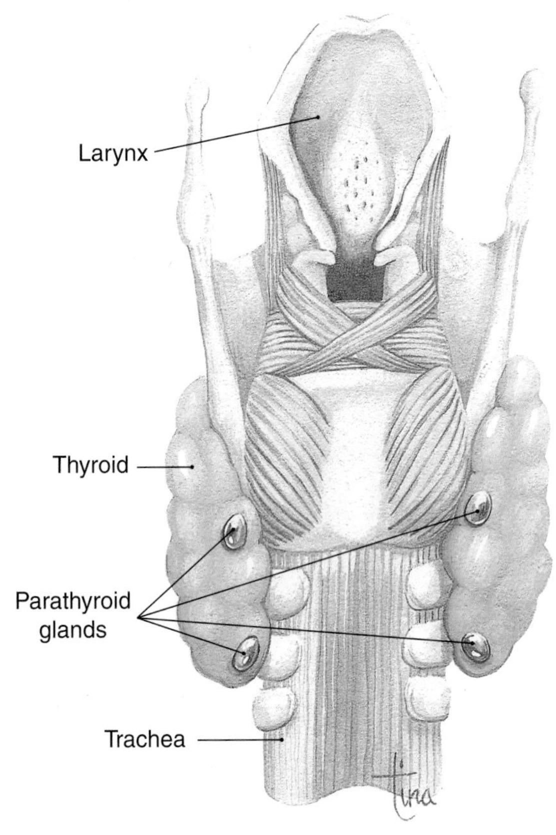

Figure 10–7 Parathyroid glands in posterior view, on lobes of the thyroid gland.

QUESTION: Which of the target organs of PTH may be called a reservoir, and what do they store?

its endocrine function will be discussed here. The hormone-producing cells of the pancreas are called **islets of Langerhans** (pancreatic islets; see Fig. 16–7 in Chapter 16); they contain **alpha cells** that produce glucagon and **beta cells** that produce insulin.

GLUCAGON

Glucagon stimulates the liver to change glycogen to glucose (this process is called **glycogenolysis**, which literally means "glycogen breakdown") and to increase the use of fats and excess amino acids for energy production. The process of **gluconeogenesis** (literally, "making new glucose") is the conversion of excess amino acids into simple carbohydrates that may enter the reactions of cell respiration. The overall effect of glucagon, therefore, is to raise the blood glucose level and to make all types of food available for energy production.

The secretion of glucagon is stimulated by **hypoglycemia**, a low blood glucose level. Such a state may occur between meals or during physiological stress situations such as exercise (Fig. 10–8).

INSULIN

Insulin increases the transport of glucose from the blood into cells by increasing the permeability of cell membranes to glucose. (Brain, liver, and kidney cells, however, are not dependent on insulin for glucose intake.) Once inside cells, glucose is used in cell respiration to produce energy. The liver and skeletal muscles also change glucose to glycogen (**glycogenesis**, which means "glycogen production") to be stored for later use. Insulin is also important in the metabolism of other food types; it enables cells to take in fatty acids and amino acids to use in the synthesis of lipids and proteins (*not* energy production). Without insulin, blood levels of lipids tend to rise and cells accumulate excess fatty acids. With respect to blood glucose, insulin decreases its level by promoting the use of glucose for energy production. The antagonistic functions of insulin and glucagon are shown in Fig. 10–8.

Insulin is a vital hormone; we cannot survive for very long without it. A deficiency of insulin or in its functioning is called **diabetes mellitus**, which is discussed in Box 10–3.

Table 10–4 | **HORMONE OF THE PARATHYROID GLANDS**

HORMONE	FUNCTIONS	REGULATION OF SECRETION
Parathyroid hormone (PTH)	■ Increases the reabsorption of calcium and phosphate from bone to blood ■ Increases absorption of calcium and phosphate by the small intestine ■ Increases the reabsorption of calcium and the excretion of phosphate by the kidneys; activates vitamin D	Hypocalcemia stimulates secretion. Hypercalcemia inhibits secretion.

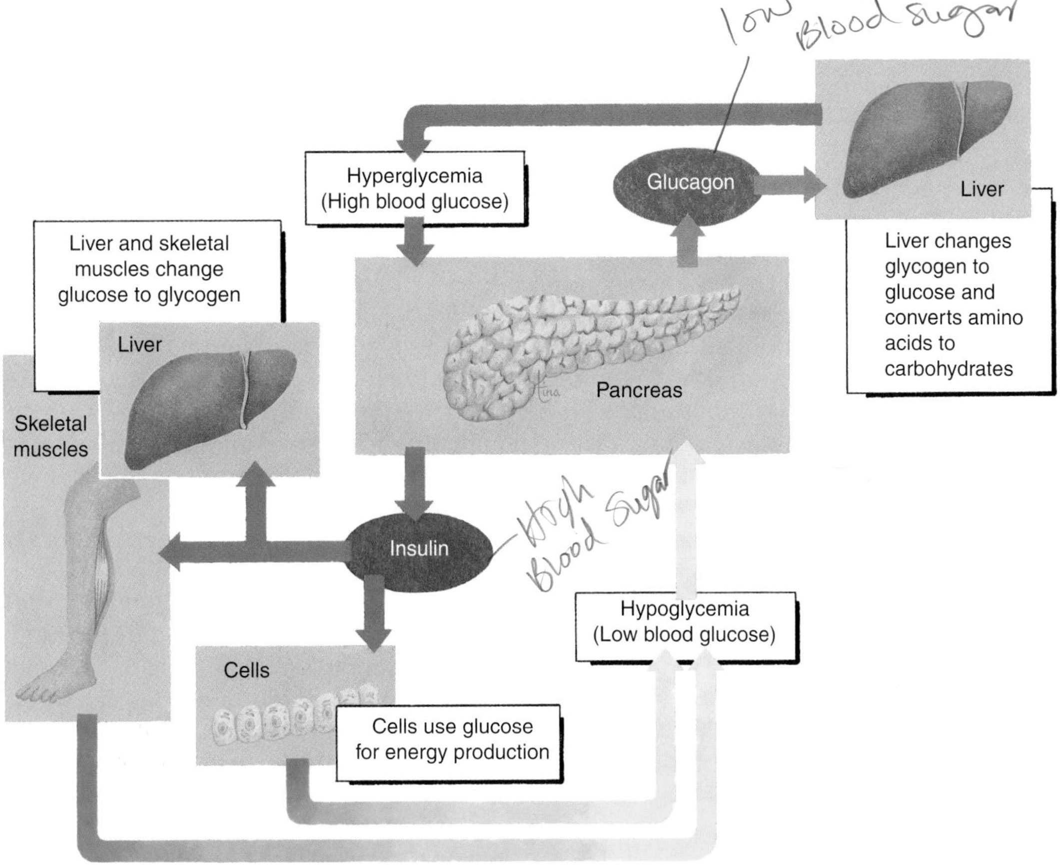

Figure 10–8 Insulin and glucagon and their functions related to the maintenance of the blood glucose level.

QUESTION: Which hormone enables cells to use glucose for energy production? What is the stimulus for secretion of this hormone?

Box 10–3 | DIABETES MELLITUS

There are two types of **diabetes mellitus**: Type 1 is called insulin-dependent diabetes and its onset is usually in childhood (juvenile onset). Type 2 is called non–insulin-dependent diabetes, and its onset is usually later in life (maturity onset).

Type 1 diabetes is characterized by destruction of the beta cells of the islets of Langerhans and a complete lack of insulin (see Box Figure 10–A); onset is usually abrupt. Destruction of the beta cells is an autoimmune response, perhaps triggered by a virus. There may be a genetic predisposition because certain HLA types are found more frequently in type 1 diabetics than in other children (see Box 11–5: White Blood Cell Types: HLA in Chapter 11). Insulin is essential to control type 1 diabetes. Research is continuing on the use of immunosuppressant medications to try to preserve some beta cells (if diagnosis is early), and also on the transplantation of stem cells to replace lost beta cells.

Continued

Box 10–3 | DIABETES MELLITUS *(Continued)*

In **type 2** diabetes, insulin is produced but cannot exert its effects on cells because of a loss of insulin receptors on cell membranes (see Box Figure 10–A). Onset of type 2 diabetes is usually gradual, and risk factors include a family history of diabetes and being overweight. Control may not require insulin, but rather medications that enable insulin to react with the remaining membrane receptors. For those with a family history of diabetes, a low-fat diet and regular exercise reduce the risk of developing the disease. The commitment to exercise must be lifelong but is well worth the effort, because diabetes is very destructive.

Without insulin (or its effects) blood glucose level remains high, and glucose is lost in urine. Because more water is lost as well, symptoms include greater urinary output (polyuria) and thirst (polydipsia).

The long-term effects of hyperglycemia produce distinctive vascular changes. The capillary walls thicken, and exchange of gases and nutrients diminishes. The most damaging effects are seen in the skin (especially of the feet), the retina (diabetic retinopathy), and the kidneys. Poorly controlled diabetes may lead to dry gangrene, blindness, and severe kidney damage. Atherosclerosis is common, because faulty triglyceride metabolism is linked to faulty glucose metabolism. Diabetics must control their blood pressure and cholesterol levels to prevent heart attacks. Neuropathy (damage to nerves) leads to impaired cutaneous sensation and difficulty with fine movements, such as buttoning a shirt. It is now possible for diabetics to prevent much of this tissue damage by precise monitoring of the blood glucose level and more frequent administration of insulin. Insulin pumps are able to more closely mimic the natural secretion of insulin.

A very serious potential problem for the type 1 diabetic is **ketoacidosis**. When glucose cannot be used for energy, the body turns to fats and proteins, which are converted by the liver to ketones. Ketones are organic acids (acetone, acetoacetic acid) that can be used in cell respiration, but cells are not able to utilize them rapidly so ketones accumulate in the blood. Ketones are acids, and lower the pH of the blood as they accumulate. The kidneys excrete excess ketones, but in doing so excrete more water as well, which leads to dehydration and worsens the acidosis. Without administration of insulin to permit the use of glucose, and IV fluids to restore blood volume to normal, ketoacidosis will progress to coma and death.

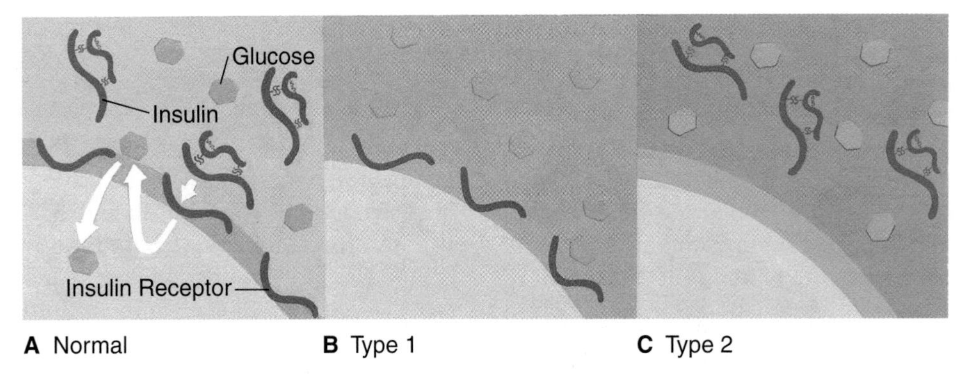

Box Figure 10–A (**A**) Cell membrane in normal state, with insulin receptors and insulin to regulate glucose intake. (**B**) Cell membrane in type 1 diabetes: insulin not present, glucose remains outside cell. (**C**) Cell membrane in type 2 diabetes: without insulin receptors, glucose remains outside cell.

Secretion of insulin is stimulated by **hyperglycemia**, a high blood glucose level. This state occurs after eating, especially of meals high in carbohydrates. As glucose is absorbed from the small intestine into the blood, insulin is secreted to enable cells to use the glucose for immediate energy. At the same time, any excess glucose will be stored in the liver and muscles as glycogen.

You will also notice in Fig. 16–7 the cells called delta cells. These produce the hormone somatostatin, which is identical to growth hormone–inhibiting hormone from the hypothalamus. Pancreatic somatostatin acts locally to inhibit the secretion of insulin and glucagon, and it seems to slow the absorption of the end products of digestion in the small intestine. The hormones of the pancreas are summarized in Table 10–5.

ADRENAL GLANDS

The two **adrenal glands** are each located on top of a kidney, which gives them their other name of **suprarenal glands**. Each adrenal gland consists of two parts: an inner adrenal medulla and an outer adrenal cortex. The hormones produced by each part have very different functions.

ADRENAL MEDULLA

The cells of the **adrenal medulla** secrete epinephrine and norepinephrine, which collectively are called **catecholamines** and are **sympathomimetic**. The secretion of both hormones is stimulated by sympathetic impulses from the hypothalamus, and their functions duplicate and prolong those of the sympathetic division of the autonomic nervous system (*mimetic* means "to mimic").

Epinephrine and Norepinephrine

Epinephrine (adrenalin) and norepinephrine (noradrenalin) are both secreted in stress situations and help prepare the body for "fight or flight." **Norepinephrine** is secreted in small amounts, and its most significant function is to cause vasoconstriction in the skin, viscera, and skeletal muscles (that is, throughout the body), which raises blood pressure.

Epinephrine, secreted in larger amounts, increases the heart rate and force of contraction and stimulates vasoconstriction in skin and viscera and vasodilation in skeletal muscles. It also dilates the bronchioles, decreases peristalsis, stimulates the liver to change glycogen to glucose, increases the use of fats for energy, and increases the rate of cell respiration. Many of these effects do indeed seem to be an echo of sympathetic responses, don't they? Responding to stress is so important that the body acts redundantly (that is, exceeds what is necessary, or repeats itself) and has both a nervous mechanism and a hormonal mechanism. Epinephrine is actually more effective than sympathetic stimulation, however, because the hormone increases energy production and cardiac output to a greater extent. The hormones of the adrenal medulla are summarized in Table 10–6, and their functions are shown in Fig. 10–9.

ADRENAL CORTEX

The **adrenal cortex** secretes three types of steroid hormones: mineralocorticoids, glucocorticoids, and sex hormones. The sex hormones, "female" estrogens and "male" androgens (similar to testosterone), are produced in very

Table 10–5 | HORMONES OF THE PANCREAS

HORMONE	FUNCTIONS	REGULATION OF SECRETION
Glucagon (alpha cells)	■ Increases conversion of glycogen to glucose in the liver ■ Increases the use of excess amino acids and of fats for energy	Hypoglycemia
Insulin (beta cells)	■ Increases glucose transport into cells and the use of glucose for energy production ■ Increases the conversion of excess glucose to glycogen in the liver and muscles ■ Increases amino acid and fatty acid transport into cells, and their use in synthesis reactions	Hyperglycemia
Somatostatin (delta cells)	■ Decreases secretion of insulin and glucagon ■ Slows absorption of nutrients	Rising levels of insulin and glucagon

Table 10–6 | HORMONES OF THE ADRENAL MEDULLA

HORMONE	FUNCTION(S)	REGULATION OF SECRETION
Norepinephrine	■ Causes vasoconstriction in skin, viscera, and skeletal muscles	Sympathetic impulses from the hypothalamus in stress situations
Epinephrine	■ Increases heart rate and force of contraction ■ Dilates bronchioles ■ Decreases peristalsis ■ Increases conversion of glycogen to glucose in the liver ■ Causes vasodilation in skeletal muscles ■ Causes vasoconstriction in skin and viscera ■ Increases use of fats for energy ■ Increases the rate of cell respiration	Sympathetic impulses from the hypothalamus in stress situations

small amounts, and their importance is not known with certainty. They may contribute to rapid body growth during early puberty. They may also be important in supplying estrogen to women after menopause and to men throughout life (see the "Estrogen" section later in this chapter).

The functions of the other adrenal cortical hormones are well known, however. Both kinds are secreted during stressful situations, and both are considered vital hormones.

Aldosterone

Aldosterone is the most abundant of the **mineralocorticoids**, and we will use it as a representative of this group of hormones. The target organs of aldosterone are the kidneys, but there are important secondary, or indirect, effects as well. Aldosterone increases the reabsorption of sodium and the excretion of potassium by the kidney tubules; this is its direct effect. Sodium ions (Na^+) are returned to the blood, and potassium ions (K^+) are excreted in urine. Look at Fig. 10–10 as you read the following.

As Na^+ ions are reabsorbed, hydrogen ions (H^+) may be excreted in exchange. This is one mechanism to prevent the accumulation of excess H^+ ions, which would cause acidosis of body fluids. Also, as Na^+ ions are reabsorbed, negative ions such as chloride (Cl^-) and bicarbonate (HCO_3^-) follow the Na^+ ions back to the blood, and water follows by osmosis. This indirect effect of aldosterone, the reabsorption of water by the kidneys, is very important to maintain normal blood volume and blood pressure. In summary, then, aldosterone directly maintains normal blood levels of sodium and potassium, and by doing so secondarily, or indirectly, contributes to the maintenance of normal blood pH, blood volume, and blood pressure.

A number of factors stimulate the secretion of aldosterone. These are a deficiency of sodium, loss of blood or dehydration that lowers blood pressure, or an elevated blood level of potassium. Low blood pressure or blood volume activates the **renin-angiotensin mechanism** of the kidneys. This mechanism is discussed in Chapters 13 and 18, so we will say for now that the process culminates in the formation of a chemical called **angiotensin II**. Angiotensin II causes vasoconstriction and stimulates the secretion of aldosterone by the adrenal cortex. Aldosterone then increases sodium and water retention by the kidneys to help restore blood volume and blood pressure to normal.

Cortisol

We will use **cortisol** as a representative of the group of hormones called **glucocorticoids** because it is responsible for most of the actions of this group (Fig. 10–11). Cortisol increases the use of fats and excess amino acids (gluconeogenesis) for energy and decreases the use of glucose. This is called the glucose-sparing effect, and it is important because it conserves glucose for use by the brain. Cortisol is secreted in any type of physiological stress situation: disease, physical injury, hemorrhage, fear or anger, exercise, and hunger. Although most body cells easily use fatty acids and excess amino acids in cell respiration, brain cells do not, so they must have glucose. By enabling other cells to use the alternative energy sources, cortisol ensures that whatever glucose is present will be available to the brain.

Cortisol also has an **anti-inflammatory effect**. During inflammation, **histamine** from damaged tissues and mast cells makes capillaries more permeable, and the

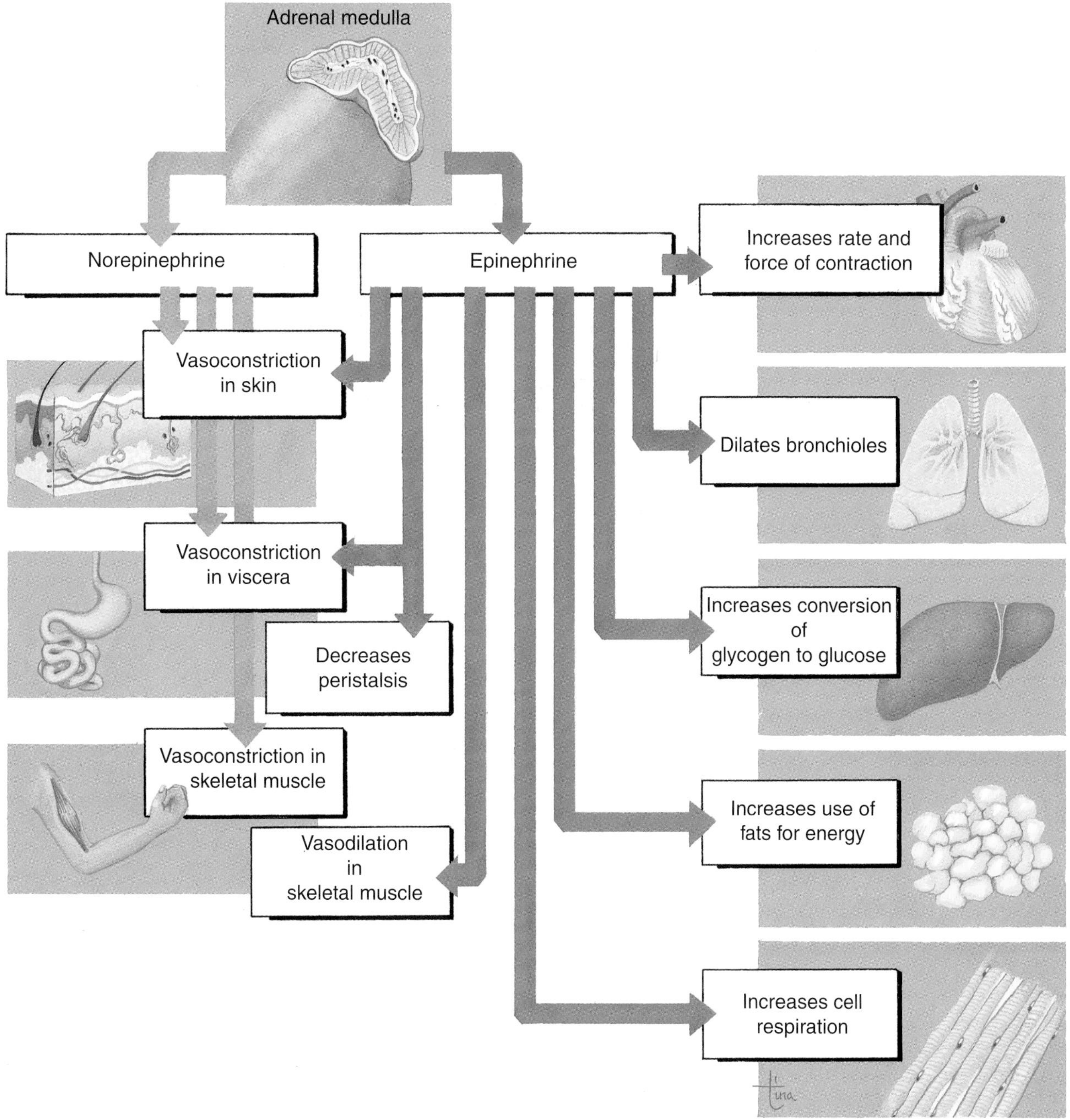

Figure 10–9 Functions of epinephrine and norepinephrine.

QUESTION: Do epinephrine and norepinephrine have the same effect on skeletal muscle? Explain your answer.

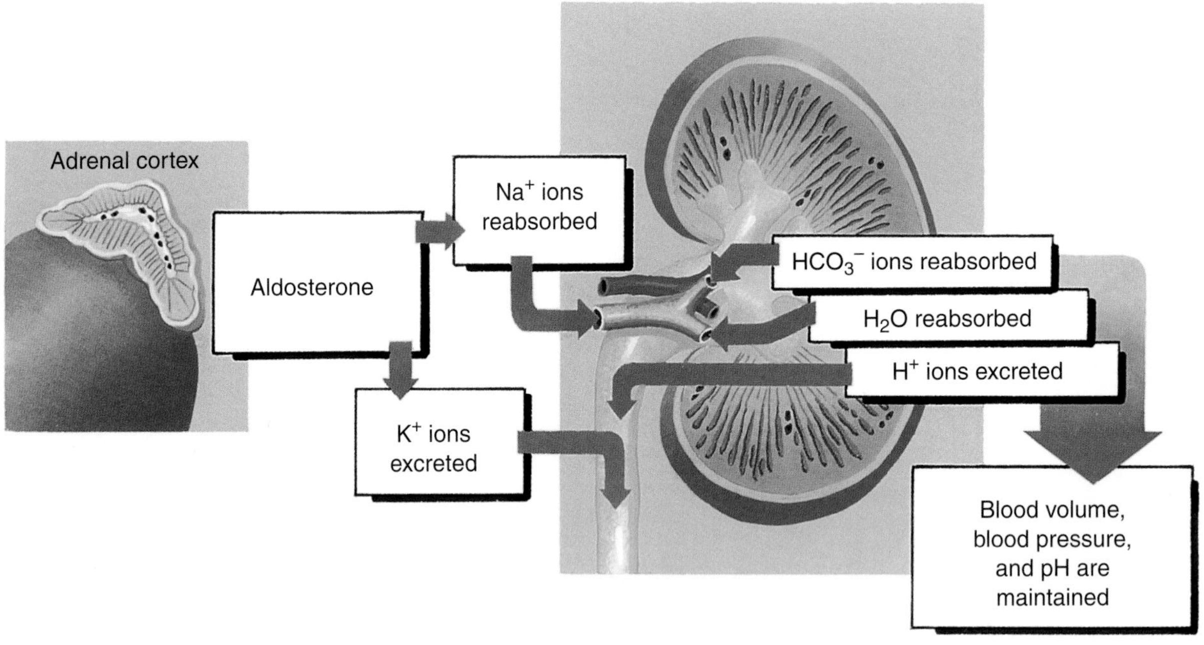

Figure 10–10 Functions of aldosterone. Direct and indirect functions are shown.

QUESTION: What ions does aldosterone have a direct effect on, and what is the effect?

lysosomes of damaged cells release their enzymes, which help break down damaged tissue for easier cleanup by macrophages but may also cause destruction of nearby healthy tissue. Cortisol blocks the effects of histamine and stabilizes lysosomal membranes, preventing excessive tissue destruction. Inflammation is a beneficial process up to a point and is an essential first step if tissue repair is to take place. It may, however, become a vicious cycle of damage, inflammation, more damage, more inflammation, and so on—a positive feedback mechanism. Recall that any positive feedback mechanism requires an external brake. Normal cortisol secretion seems to be the brake for this mechanism, to limit the inflammation process to what is useful for tissue repair, and to prevent excessive tissue destruction. Too much cortisol, however, decreases the immune response, leaving the body susceptible to infection and significantly slowing the healing of damaged tissue (see Box 10–4: Disorders of the Adrenal Cortex).

The direct stimulus for cortisol secretion is **ACTH** from the anterior pituitary gland, which in turn is stimulated by corticotropin-releasing hormone (CRH) from the hypothalamus. CRH is produced in the physiological stress situations mentioned earlier. Although we often think of epinephrine as a hormone important for coping with physiological stress, cortisol is also important. The hormones of the adrenal cortex are summarized in Table 10–7.

OVARIES

The **ovaries** are located in the pelvic cavity, one on each side of the uterus. The hormones produced by the ovaries are the steroids estrogen and progesterone, and the protein inhibin. Although their functions are an integral part of Chapters 20 and 21, we will briefly discuss some of them here.

ESTROGEN

Estrogen is secreted by the follicle cells of the ovary; secretion is stimulated by **FSH** from the anterior pituitary gland. Estrogen promotes the maturation of the ovum in the ovarian follicle and stimulates the growth of blood vessels in the endometrium (lining) of the uterus in preparation for a possible fertilized egg.

The **secondary sex characteristics** in women also develop in response to estrogen. These include growth of the duct system of the mammary glands, growth of the

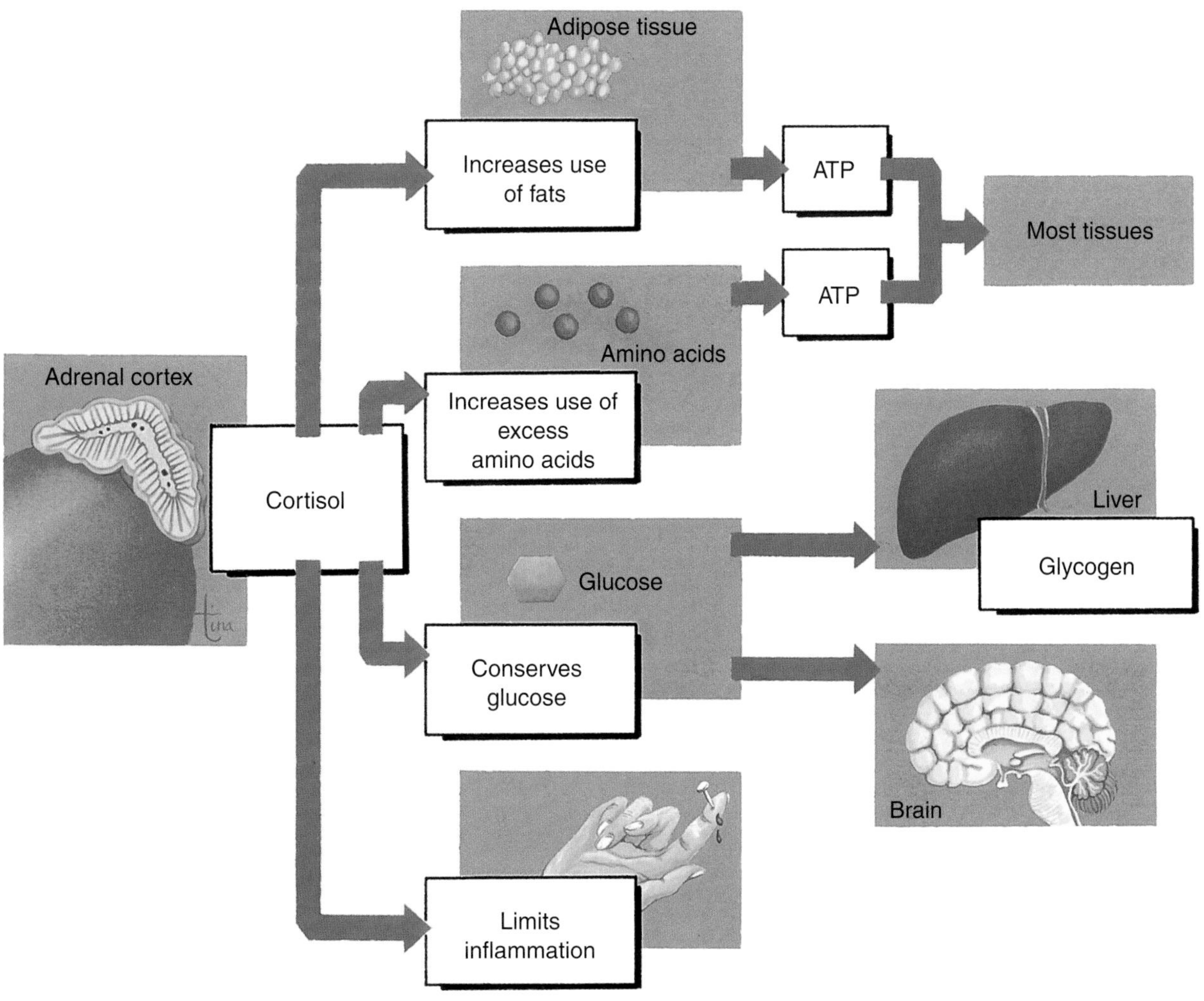

Figure 10–11 Functions of cortisol.

QUESTION: Which food types will be used for energy by most tissues? Which food type may be stored?

Box 10–4 | DISORDERS OF THE ADRENAL CORTEX

Addison's disease is the result of hyposecretion of the adrenal cortical hormones. Most cases are idiopathic, that is, of unknown cause; atrophy of the adrenal cortex decreases both cortisol and aldosterone secretion.

Deficiency of cortisol is characterized by hypoglycemia, decreased gluconeogenesis, and depletion of glycogen in the liver. Consequences are muscle weakness and the inability to resist physiological stress. Aldosterone deficiency leads to retention of potassium and excretion of sodium and water in urine. The result is severe dehydration, low blood volume, and low blood pressure. Without treatment, circulatory shock and death will follow. Treatment involves administration of hydrocortisone; in high doses this will also compensate for the aldosterone deficiency.

Continued

Box 10–4 | DISORDERS OF THE ADRENAL CORTEX *(Continued)*

Cushing's syndrome is the result of hypersecretion of the adrenal cortex, primarily cortisol. The cause may be a pituitary tumor that increases ACTH secretion or a tumor of the adrenal cortex itself.

Excessive cortisol promotes fat deposition in the trunk of the body, while the extremities remain thin. The skin becomes thin and fragile, and healing after injury is slow. The bones also become fragile because osteoporosis is accelerated. Also characteristic of this syndrome is the rounded appearance of the face. Treatment is aimed at removal of the cause of the hypersecretion, whether it be a pituitary or adrenal tumor.

Cushing's syndrome may also be seen in people who receive corticosteroids for medical reasons. Transplant recipients or people with rheumatoid arthritis or severe asthma who must take corticosteroids may exhibit any of the above symptoms. In such cases, the disadvantages of this medication must be weighed against the benefits provided.

Table 10–7 | HORMONES OF THE ADRENAL CORTEX

HORMONE	FUNCTION(S)	REGULATION OF SECRETION
Aldosterone	■ Increases reabsorption of Na^+ ions by the kidneys to the blood ■ Increases excretion of K^+ ions by the kidneys in urine	Low blood Na^+ level Low blood volume or blood pressure High blood K^+ level
Cortisol	■ Increases use of fats and excess amino acids for energy ■ Decreases use of glucose for energy (except for the brain) ■ Increases conversion of glucose to glycogen in the liver ■ Anti-inflammatory effect: stabilizes lysosomes and blocks the effects of histamine	ACTH (anterior pituitary) during physiological stress

uterus, and the deposition of fat subcutaneously in the hips and thighs. The closure of the epiphyseal discs in long bones is brought about by estrogen, and growth in height stops. Estrogen is also believed to lower blood levels of cholesterol and triglycerides. For women before the age of menopause this is beneficial in that it decreases the risk of atherosclerosis and coronary artery disease.

Research suggests that estrogen no longer be considered only a "female" hormone. Estrogen seems to have effects on many organs, including the brain, the heart, and blood vessels. In the brain, testosterone from the testes or the adrenal cortex can be converted to estrogen, which may be important for memory, especially for older people. Estrogen seems to have non-reproductive functions (such as influencing fat storage) in both men and women, although we cannot yet be as specific as we can be with the reproductive functions in women, mentioned previously.

PROGESTERONE

When a mature ovarian follicle releases an ovum, the follicle becomes the **corpus luteum** and begins to secrete **progesterone** in addition to estrogen. This is stimulated by **LH** from the anterior pituitary gland.

Progesterone seems to be necessary for the successful implantation of the very early embryo (5 to 8 days old) in the endometrium. It also promotes the storage of glycogen and the further growth of blood vessels in the endometrium, which thus becomes a potential placenta. The secretory cells of the mammary glands also develop under the influence of progesterone.

Both progesterone and estrogen are secreted by the placenta during pregnancy; these functions are covered in Chapter 21.

INHIBIN

The corpus luteum secretes another hormone, called inhibin. **Inhibin** helps decrease the secretion of FSH by the anterior pituitary gland, and GnRH by the hypothalamus.

TESTES

The **testes** are located in the scrotum, a sac of skin between the upper thighs. Two hormones, testosterone and inhibin, are secreted by the testes.

TESTOSTERONE

Testosterone is a steroid hormone secreted by the interstitial cells of the testes; the stimulus for secretion is LH from the anterior pituitary gland.

Testosterone promotes maturation of sperm in the seminiferous tubules of the testes; this process begins at puberty and continues throughout life. At puberty, testosterone stimulates development of the male **secondary sex characteristics**. These include growth of all the reproductive organs, growth of facial and body hair, growth of the larynx and deepening of the voice, and growth (protein synthesis) of the skeletal muscles. Testosterone also brings about closure of the epiphyses of the long bones.

INHIBIN

The hormone **inhibin** is secreted by the sustentacular cells of the testes; the stimulus for secretion is increased testosterone. The function of inhibin is to decrease the secretion of FSH by the anterior pituitary gland. The interaction of inhibin, testosterone, and the anterior pituitary hormones maintains spermatogenesis at a constant rate.

OTHER HORMONES

Melatonin is a hormone produced by the **pineal gland**, which is located at the back of the third ventricle of the brain. The secretion of melatonin is greatest during darkness and decreases when light enters the eye and the retina signals the hypothalamus. The retina also produces melatonin, which seems to indicate that the eyes and pineal gland work with the biological clock of the hypothalamus. In other mammals, melatonin helps regulate seasonal reproductive cycles. For people, melatonin definitely stimulates the onset of sleep and increases its duration. Other claims, such as that melatonin strengthens the immune system or prevents aging, are without evidence as yet.

Some organs produce hormones that have only one or a few target organs. For example, skeletal muscle produces irisin, which affects adipocytes, and adipose tissue produces the appetite-suppressing hormone leptin. The stomach and duodenum produce hormones that regulate aspects of digestion (pancreas and liver functioning) and appetite. The thymus gland produces hormones necessary for the normal functioning of the immune system, and the kidneys produce a hormone that stimulates red blood cell production in the red bone marrow. All of these will be discussed in later chapters.

PROSTAGLANDINS

Prostaglandins (PGs) are made by virtually all cells from the phospholipids of their cell membranes. They differ from other hormones in that they do not circulate in the blood to target organs, but rather exert their effects locally, where they are produced.

There are many types of prostaglandins, designated by the letters A through I, as in PGA, PGB, and so on. Prostaglandins have many functions, and we will list only a few of them here. Prostaglandins are known to be involved in inflammation, pain mechanisms, blood clotting, vasoconstriction and vasodilation, contraction of the uterus, reproduction, secretion of digestive glands, and nutrient metabolism. Current research is directed at determining the normal functioning of prostaglandins in the hope that many of them may eventually be used clinically.

One familiar example may illustrate the widespread activity of prostaglandins. For minor pain such as a headache, many people take aspirin. Aspirin inhibits the synthesis of prostaglandins involved in pain mechanisms and usually relieves the pain. Some people, however, such as those with rheumatoid arthritis, may take large amounts of aspirin to diminish pain and inflammation. These people may bruise easily because blood clotting has been impaired. This, too, is an effect of aspirin, which blocks the synthesis of prostaglandins necessary for blood clotting.

MECHANISMS OF HORMONE ACTION

Exactly how hormones exert their effects on their target organs involves a number of complex processes, which will be presented simply here.

All hormones are secreted into the blood and circulate throughout the body. What determines whether a hormone will affect a particular organ or tissue? That is, what makes a cell a target? A target is determined by the presence of receptors into which the hormone fits. A hormone must first bond to a **receptor** for it on or in the target cell. Cells respond to certain hormones and not to others; that is, they are targets or not because of the presence of specific receptors, which are proteins. These receptor proteins may be part of the cell membrane or within the cytoplasm or nucleus of the target cells. A hormone will affect only those cells that have its specific receptors. Liver cells, for example, have cell membrane receptors for insulin, glucagon, growth hormone, and epinephrine; bone cells have receptors for growth hormone, PTH, and calcitonin. Cells of the ovaries and testes do not have receptors for PTH and calcitonin but do have receptors for FSH and LH, which bone cells and liver cells do not have. Once a hormone has bonded to a receptor on or in its target cell, other reactions will take place (Fig. 10–12).

THE TWO-MESSENGER MECHANISM—PROTEIN HORMONES

The two-messenger mechanism of hormone action involves "messengers" that make something happen, that is, stimulate specific reactions. **Protein hormones** usually bond to receptors of the cell membrane, and the hormone is called the first messenger. The hormone–receptor bonding activates the enzyme adenyl cyclase on the inner surface of the cell membrane. Adenyl cyclase synthesizes a substance called cyclic adenosine monophosphate (**cyclic**

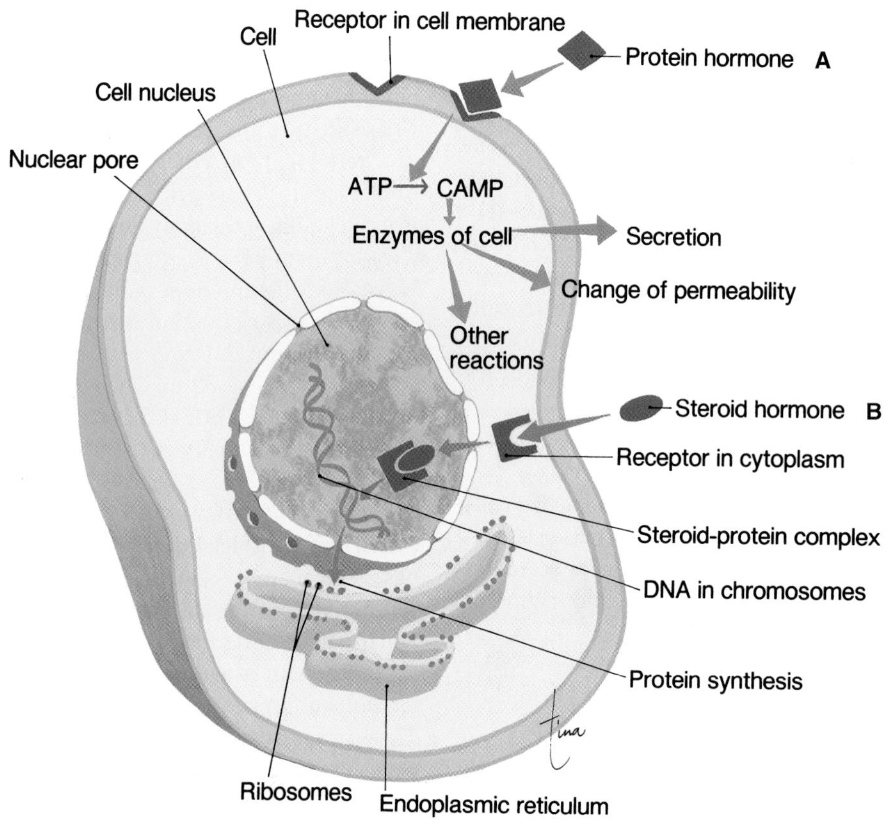

Figure 10–12 Mechanisms of hormone action. (**A**) Two-messenger mechanism of the action of protein hormones. (**B**) Action of steroid hormones. See text for description.

QUESTION: What must a cell have in order to be a target cell for a particular hormone?

AMP or **cAMP**) from ATP, and cyclic AMP is the second messenger.

Cyclic AMP activates specific enzymes within the cell, which bring about the cell's characteristic response to the hormone. These responses include a change in the permeability of the cell membrane to a specific substance, an increase in protein synthesis, activation of other enzymes, or the secretion of a cellular product.

In summary, a cell's response to a hormone is determined by the enzymes within the cell, that is, the reactions of which the cell is capable. These reactions are brought about by the first messenger, the hormone, which stimulates the formation of the second messenger, cyclic AMP. Cyclic AMP then activates the cell's enzymes to elicit a response to the hormone (see Fig. 10–12).

ACTION OF STEROID HORMONES

Steroid hormones are soluble in the lipids of the cell membrane and diffuse easily into a target cell. Once inside the cell, the steroid hormone combines with a protein receptor in the cytoplasm, and this steroid-protein complex enters the nucleus of the cell. Within the nucleus, the steroid-protein complex activates specific genes, which begin the process of **protein synthesis**. The enzymes produced bring about the cell's characteristic response to the hormone (see Fig. 10–12).

AGING AND THE ENDOCRINE SYSTEM

Most of the endocrine glands decrease their secretions with age, but normal aging usually does not lead to serious hormone deficiencies. There are decreases in adrenal cortical hormones, for example, but the levels are usually sufficient to maintain homeostasis of water, electrolytes, and nutrients. The decreased secretion of growth hormone leads to a decrease in muscle mass and an increase in fat storage. A lower basal metabolic rate is common in elderly people as the thyroid slows its secretion of thyroxine. Unless specific pathologies develop, however, the endocrine system usually continues to function adequately in old age.

SUMMARY

The hormones of endocrine glands are involved in virtually all aspects of normal body functioning. The growth and repair of tissues, the utilization of food to produce energy, responses to stress, the maintenance of the proper levels and pH of body fluids, and the continuance of the human species all depend on hormones. Some of these topics will be discussed in later chapters. As you might expect, you will be reading about the functions of many of these hormones again and reviewing their important contributions to the maintenance of homeostasis.

STUDY OUTLINE

Endocrine glands are ductless glands that secrete hormones into the blood. Hormones exert their effects on target organs or tissues.

Chemistry of Hormones

1. Amines—structural variations of the amino acid tyrosine; thyroxine, epinephrine.
2. Proteins—chains of amino acids; peptides are short chains. Insulin, GH, and glucagon are proteins; ADH and oxytocin are peptides.
3. Steroids—made from cholesterol; cortisol, aldosterone, estrogen, testosterone.

Regulation of Hormone Secretion

1. Hormones are secreted when there is a need for their effects. Each hormone has a specific stimulus for secretion.
2. The secretion of most hormones is regulated by negative feedback mechanisms: As the hormone exerts its effects, the stimulus for secretion is reversed, and secretion of the hormone decreases until the stimulus reoccurs.

Pituitary Gland (Hypophysis)—hangs from hypothalamus by the infundibulum; enclosed by sella turcica of sphenoid bone (see Figs. 10–1 and 10–2)

1. Posterior Pituitary (Neurohypophysis)—stores hormones produced by the hypothalamus (Figs. 10–2 and 10–3 and Table 10–1).
   - ADH—increases water reabsorption by the kidneys, decreases sweating, in large amounts causes vasoconstriction. Result: decreases urinary output and increases blood volume; increases BP. Stimulus: nerve impulses from hypothalamus when body water decreases for any reason.

- Oxytocin—stimulates contraction of myometrium of uterus during labor and release of milk from mammary glands. Stimulus: nerve impulses from hypothalamus as cervix is stretched or as infant sucks on nipple.

2. Anterior Pituitary (Adenohypophysis)—secretions are regulated by releasing hormones from the hypothalamus (Fig. 10–3 and Table 10–2).
   - GH—through intermediary molecules, IGFs, GH increases amino acid transport into cells and increases protein synthesis; increases rate of mitosis; increases use of fats for energy (Fig. 10–4). Stimulus: GHRH from the hypothalamus.
   - TSH—increases secretion of thyroxine and T_3 by the thyroid. Stimulus: TRH from the hypothalamus.
   - ACTH—increases secretion of cortisol by the adrenal cortex. Stimulus: CRH from the hypothalamus.
   - Prolactin—initiates and maintains milk production by the mammary glands. Stimulus: PRH from the hypothalamus.
   - FSH—*In women:* initiates development of ova in ovarian follicles and secretion of estrogen by follicle cells.

     In men: initiates sperm development in the testes. Stimulus: GnRH from the hypothalamus.
   - LH—*In women:* stimulates ovulation, transforms mature follicle into corpus luteum and stimulates secretion of progesterone.

     In men: stimulates secretion of testosterone by the testes. Stimulus: GnRH from the hypothalamus.

Thyroid Gland—on front and sides of trachea below the larynx (see Figs. 10–1 and 10–5 and Table 10–3)

- Thyroxine (T_4) and T_3—(Fig. 10–5) produced by thyroid follicles; both hormones contain iodine. Increase use of all food types for energy production and increase protein synthesis. Necessary for normal physical, mental, and sexual development. Stimulus: TSH from the anterior pituitary.
- Calcitonin—produced by parafollicular cells. Decreases reabsorption of calcium from bones and lowers blood calcium level. Stimulus: hypercalcemia.

Parathyroid Glands—four; two on posterior of each lobe of thyroid (see Figs. 10–6 and 10–7 and Table 10–4)

- PTH—increases reabsorption of calcium and phosphate from bones to the blood; increases absorption of calcium and phosphate by the small intestine; increases reabsorption of calcium and excretion of phosphate by the kidneys, and activates vitamin D. Result: raises blood calcium and lowers blood phosphate levels. Stimulus: hypocalcemia. Inhibitor: hypercalcemia.

Pancreas—extends from curve of duodenum to the spleen. Islets of Langerhans contain alpha cells and beta cells (see Figs. 10–1 and 10–8 and Table 10–5)

- Glucagon—secreted by alpha cells. Stimulates liver to change glycogen to glucose; increases use of fats and amino acids for energy. Result: raises blood glucose level. Stimulus: hypoglycemia.
- Insulin—secreted by beta cells. Increases use of glucose by cells to produce energy; stimulates liver and muscles to change glucose to glycogen; increases cellular intake of fatty acids and amino acids to use for synthesis of lipids and proteins. Result: lowers blood glucose level. Stimulus: hyperglycemia.
- Somatostatin—inhibits secretion of insulin and glucagon.

Adrenal Glands—one on top of each kidney; each has an inner adrenal medulla and an outer adrenal cortex (see Fig. 10–1)

1. Adrenal Medulla—produces catecholamines in stressful situations, preparing the body for "fight or flight" (Table 10–6 and Fig. 10–9).
   - Norepinephrine—stimulates vasoconstriction in skin, viscera, and skeletal muscles and thereby raises blood pressure.

- Epinephrine—increases heart rate and force of contraction, causes vasoconstriction in skin and viscera and vasodilation in skeletal muscles; dilates bronchioles; slows peristalsis; causes liver to change glycogen to glucose; increases use of fats for energy; increases rate of cell respiration. Stimulus: sympathetic impulses from the hypothalamus.

2. Adrenal Cortex—produces mineralocorticoids, glucocorticoids, and very small amounts of sex hormones (function not known with certainty) (Table 10–7).
   - Aldosterone—(Fig. 10–10) increases reabsorption of sodium and excretion of potassium by the kidneys. Results: hydrogen ions are excreted in exchange for sodium; chloride and bicarbonate ions and water follow sodium back to the blood; maintains normal blood pH, blood volume, and blood pressure. Stimulus: decreased blood sodium or elevated blood potassium; decreased blood volume or blood pressure (activates the renin-angiotensin mechanism of the kidneys).
   - Cortisol—(Fig. 10–11) increases use of fats and amino acids for energy; decreases use of glucose to conserve glucose for the brain; anti-inflammatory effect: blocks effects of histamine and stabilizes lysosomes to prevent excessive tissue damage. Stimulus: ACTH from the anterior pituitary during physiological stress.

Ovaries—in pelvic cavity on either side of uterus (see Fig. 10–1)

- Estrogen—produced by follicle cells. Promotes maturation of ovum; stimulates growth of blood vessels in endometrium; stimulates development of secondary sex characteristics: growth of duct system of mammary glands, growth of uterus, fat deposition. Promotes closure of epiphyses of long bones; lowers blood levels of cholesterol and triglycerides. Stimulus: FSH from anterior pituitary.
- Progesterone—produced by the corpus luteum. Promotes successful implantation of the very early embryo and storage of glycogen and further growth of blood vessels in the endometrium; promotes growth of secretory cells of mammary glands. Stimulus: LH from anterior pituitary.
- Inhibin—inhibits secretion of FSH.

Testes—in scrotum between the upper thighs (see Fig. 10–1)

- Testosterone—produced by interstitial cells. Promotes maturation of sperm in testes; stimulates development of secondary sex characteristics: growth of reproductive organs, facial and body hair, larynx, skeletal muscles; promotes closure of epiphyses of long bones. Stimulus: LH from anterior pituitary.
- Inhibin—produced by sustentacular cells. Inhibits secretion of FSH to maintain a constant rate of sperm production. Stimulus: increased testosterone.

Other Hormones

- Melatonin—secreted by the pineal gland during darkness; brings on sleep.
- Prostaglandins—synthesized by cells from the phospholipids of their cell membranes; exert their effects locally. Are involved in inflammation and pain, reproduction, nutrient metabolism, changes in blood vessels, blood clotting.

Mechanisms of Hormone Action (see Fig. 10–12)

1. The target cells for a hormone are those cells with receptors for it. Receptors are proteins with which hormones bond or fit; receptors may be part of the cell membrane, or within the cytoplasm or nucleus of the target cell.
   - The two-messenger mechanism: a protein hormone (1st messenger) bonds to a membrane receptor; this reaction stimulates formation of cyclic AMP (2nd messenger) inside the cell; cyclic AMP activates the cell's enzymes to bring about the cell's characteristic response to the hormone.
   - Steroid hormones diffuse easily through cell membranes and bond to cytoplasmic receptors. The steroid-protein complex enters the nucleus and activates certain genes, which initiate protein synthesis to bring about the cell's characteristic response to the hormone.

REVIEW QUESTIONS

1. Use the following to describe a negative feedback mechanism: TSH, TRH, decreased metabolic rate, thyroxine, and T_3. (pp. 262, 264)
2. Name the two hormones stored in the posterior pituitary gland. Where are these hormones produced? State the functions of each of these hormones. (pp. 256–258)
3. Name the two hormones of the anterior pituitary gland that affect the ovaries or testes, and state their functions. (p. 261)
4. Describe the antagonistic effects of PTH and calcitonin on bones and on blood calcium level. State the other functions of PTH. (p. 264)
5. Describe the antagonistic effects of insulin and glucagon on the liver and on blood glucose level. (pp. 266–267)
6. Describe how cortisol affects the use of foods for energy. Explain the anti-inflammatory effects of cortisol. (pp. 270, 272)
7. State the effect of aldosterone on the kidneys. Describe the results of this effect on the composition of the blood. (p. 270)
8. When are epinephrine and norepinephrine secreted? Describe the effects of these hormones. (p. 269)
9. Name the hormones necessary for development of egg cells in the ovaries. Name the hormones necessary for development of sperm in the testes. (pp. 272, 274–275)
10. State what prostaglandins are made from, and state three functions of prostaglandins. (p. 275)
11. Name the hormones that promote the growth of the endometrium of the uterus in preparation for a fertilized egg, and state precisely where each hormone is produced. (pp. 272, 274)
12. Explain the functions of growth hormone and thyroxine (also T_3) as they are related to normal growth. (pp. 259, 262)
13. State the direct stimulus for secretion of each of these hormones: (pp. 262, 269, 272, 264, 270, 264, 260, 266, 275, 257)
    a. Thyroxine
    b. Insulin
    c. Cortisol
    d. PTH
    e. Aldosterone
    f. Calcitonin
    g. GH
    h. Glucagon
    i. Progesterone
    j. ADH

FOR FURTHER THOUGHT

1. During a soccer game, 12-year-old Alicia got in a tangle with another player, fell hard on her hand, and fractured her radius. She is going to be fine, though she will be wearing a cast for a few weeks. What hormones will contribute to the repair of the fracture, and how?
2. Darren is 15 years old, tall for his age, but he wants to build more muscle. He decides that he will eat only protein foods, because, he says, "Muscle is protein, so protein will make protein, and the more protein, the more muscle." In part he is correct, and in part incorrect. Explain why, name the hormones involved in protein metabolism, and state how each affects protein metabolism.
3. Many people love pasta, others love potatoes, and still others love rice. Name the hormones involved in carbohydrate metabolism, and, for each, explain its specific function.
4. Unfortunately, more than 50% of the calories in many fast-food meals (such as a cheeseburger and fries) come from fat. Name the hormones involved in fat metabolism, and for each, explain its specific function.
5. You have read about the liver several times in this chapter and often seen its picture as a target organ. Many functions of the liver are stimulated by hormones. Name as many hormones as you can think of with effects on the liver, and state the function of each.

6. Look at Question Fig. 10–A, which depicts hormone feedback mechanisms for body processes. Each of these graph lines depicts the secretion of a hormone over time. One hormone is regulated by a positive feedback mechanism and the other by a negative feedback mechanism. Which is which? Give reasons for your answers.

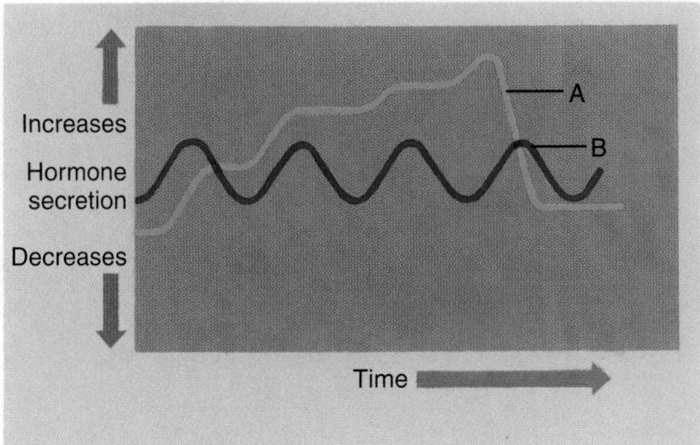

QUESTION FIGURE 10–A: Hormone feedback mechanisms for body processes.

7. Both parts of an adrenal gland contribute to our ability to respond to stressful situations. Look at Question Figure 10–B and label the parts indicated. The orange arrows represent hormones to target organs. To get you started, # 1 is the hypothalamus and corticotropin-releasing hormone to the anterior pituitary gland, and # 5 is an autonomic pathway. Once you have the hormones, describe a response of each target organ.

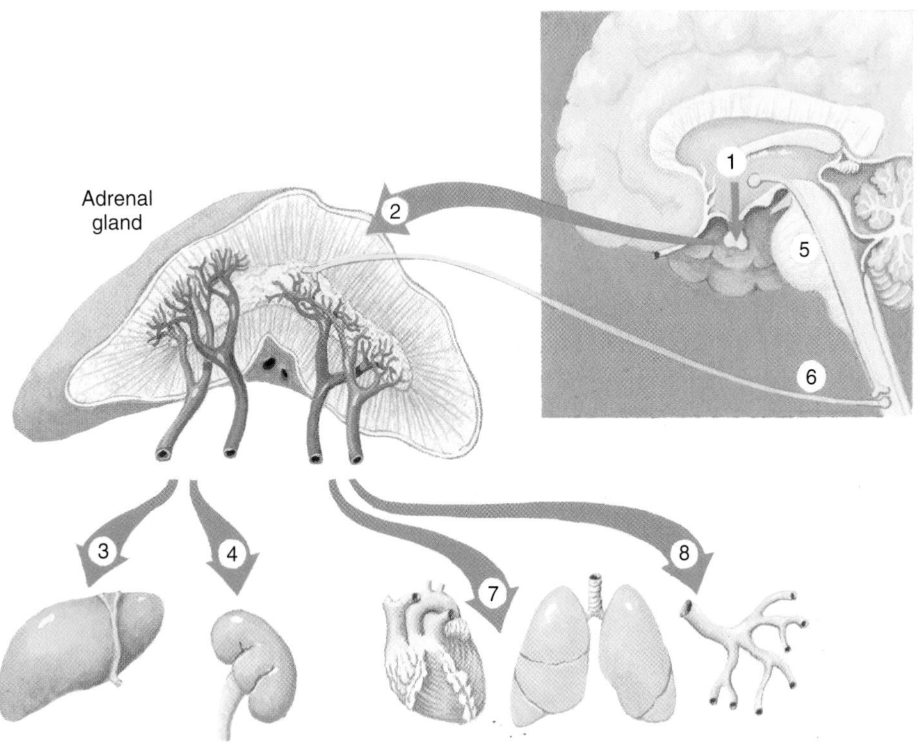

QUESTION FIGURE 10–B: Hormones secreted during stressful situations.

CHAPTER

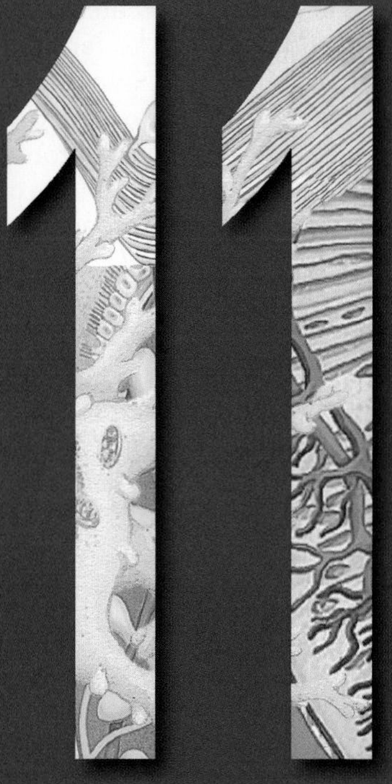

Blood

STUDENT OBJECTIVES

- Describe the composition and explain the functions of blood plasma.
- Name the primary hemopoietic tissue and the kinds of blood cells produced.
- State the function of red blood cells, including the protein and the mineral involved.
- Name the nutrients necessary for red blood cell production, and state the function of each.
- Explain how hypoxia may change the rate of red blood cell production.
- Describe what happens to red blood cells that have reached the end of their life span; what happens to the hemoglobin?
- Explain the ABO and Rh blood types.
- Name the five kinds of white blood cells and describe the function of each.
- State what platelets are, and explain how they are involved in hemostasis.
- Describe the three stages of chemical blood clotting.
- Explain how abnormal clotting is prevented in the vascular system.
- State the normal values in a complete blood count.

NEW TERMINOLOGY

ABO group *(A-B-O GROOP)*
Albumin *(al-**BYOO**-min)*
Bilirubin *(**BILL**-ee-roo-bin)*
Chemical clotting *(**KEM**-i-kuhl **KLAH**-ting)*
Embolism *(**EM**-boh-lizm)*
Erythrocyte *(e-**RITH**-roh-sight)*
Hemoglobin *(**HEE**-moh-GLOW-bin)*
Hemostasis *(HEE-moh-**STAY**-sis)*
Heparin *(**HEP**-ar-in)*
Immunity *(im-**MYOO**-ni-tee)*
Leukocyte *(**LOO**-koh-sight)*
Macrophage *(**MAK**-roh-fahj)*
Normoblast *(**NOR**-moh-blast)*
Reticulocyte *(re-**TIK**-yoo-loh-sight)*
Rh factor *(R-H **FAK**-ter)*
Thrombocyte *(**THROM**-boh-sight)*
Thrombus *(**THROM**-bus)*

RELATED CLINICAL TERMINOLOGY

Anemia *(uh-**NEE**-mee-yah)*
Differential count *(**DIFF**-er-EN-shul KOWNT)*
Erythroblastosis fetalis *(e-RITH-roh-blass-**TOH**-sis fee-**TAL**-is)*
Hematocrit *(hee-**MAT**-oh-krit)*
Hemophilia *(HEE-moh-**FILL**-ee-ah)*
Jaundice *(**JAWN**-diss)*
Leukemia *(loo-**KEE**-mee-ah)*
Leukocytosis *(LOO-koh-sigh-**TOH**-sis)*
RhoGAM *(**ROH**-gam)*
Tissue typing *(**TISH**-yoo-**TIGH**-ping)*
Typing and cross-matching *(**TIGH**-ping and **KROSS**-match-ing)*

*Terms that appear in **bold type** in the chapter text are defined in the glossary, which begins on page 603.*

CHAPTER OUTLINE

One of the simplest and most familiar life-saving medical procedures is a blood transfusion. As you know, however, the blood of one individual is not always compatible with that of another person. The ABO blood types were discovered in the early 1900s by Karl Landsteiner, an Austrian American. He also contributed to the discovery of the Rh factor in 1940. In the early 1940s, Charles Drew, an African American, developed techniques for processing and storing blood plasma, which could then be used in transfusions for people with any blood type. When we donate blood today, our blood may be given to a recipient as whole blood, or it may be separated into its component parts, and recipients will then receive only those parts they need, such as red cells, plasma, Factor 8, or platelets. Each of these parts has a specific function, and all of the functions of blood are essential to our survival.

The general functions of blood are transportation, regulation, and protection. Materials transported by the blood include nutrients, waste products, gases, and hormones. The blood contributes to the regulation of fluid–electrolyte balance, acid–base balance, and the body temperature. Protection against pathogens is provided by white blood cells, and the blood clotting mechanism prevents excessive loss of blood after injuries. Each of these functions is covered in more detail in this chapter.

CHARACTERISTICS OF BLOOD

Blood has distinctive physical characteristics:

Amount—a person has 4 to 6 liters of blood, depending on his or her size. Of the total blood volume in the human body, 38% to 48% is composed of the various blood cells, also called *formed elements*. The remaining 52% to 62% of the blood volume is plasma, the liquid portion of blood (Fig. 11–1).

Color—you're probably saying to yourself, "Of course, it's red!" Mention is made of this obvious fact, however, because the color does vary. Arterial blood is bright red because it contains high levels of oxygen. Venous blood has given up much of its oxygen in tissues, and has a darker, dull red color. This may be important in the assessment of the source of bleeding. If blood is bright red, it is probably from a severed artery, and dark red blood is probably venous blood.

pH—the normal pH range of blood is 7.35 to 7.45, which is slightly alkaline. Venous blood normally has a slightly lower pH than does arterial blood because of the presence of more carbon dioxide. Recall from Chapter 2 that blood contains buffer systems, pairs of chemicals (such as carbonic acid and sodium bicarbonate) that will react in less than a second to change a strong acid or base to molecules that will not bring about a drastic change in the pH of the blood.

Viscosity—this means thickness or resistance to flow. Blood is about three to five times thicker than water. Viscosity is increased by the presence of blood cells and the plasma proteins, and this thickness contributes to normal blood pressure.

PLASMA

Plasma is the liquid part of blood and is approximately 91% water. The solvent ability of water enables the plasma to transport many types of substances. Nutrients absorbed in the digestive tract, such as glucose, amino acids, vitamins, and minerals, are circulated to all body tissues. Waste products of the tissues, such as urea and creatinine, circulate through the kidneys and are excreted in urine. Hormones produced by endocrine glands are carried in the plasma to their target organs, and the antibodies produced by lymphocytes are also transported in plasma. Most of the carbon dioxide produced by cells is carried in the plasma in the form of bicarbonate ions (HCO_3^-). When the blood reaches the lungs, the CO_2 is re-formed, diffuses into the alveoli, and is exhaled.

Also in the plasma are the **plasma proteins**. The clotting factors **prothrombin**, **fibrinogen**, and others are synthesized by the liver and circulate until activated to form a clot in a ruptured or damaged blood vessel. **Albumin** is the most abundant plasma protein. It, too, is synthesized by the liver. Albumin contributes to the colloid osmotic pressure of blood, which pulls tissue fluid into capillaries. This is important to maintain normal blood volume and blood pressure. Other plasma proteins are called **globulins**. Alpha and beta globulins are synthesized by the liver and act as carriers for molecules such as fats. The gamma globulins (also called immunoglobulins) are the antibodies produced by lymphocytes. Antibodies are labels that initiate the destruction of pathogens and provide us with immunity.

Plasma also carries body heat. Heat is one of the byproducts of cell respiration (the production of ATP in cells). Blood becomes warmer as it flows through active organs such as the liver and muscles (blood flows slowly in capillaries, so there is time for warming). This heat is distributed to cooler parts of the body as blood continues to circulate.

BLOOD CELLS

There are three kinds of blood cells: red blood cells, white blood cells, and platelets. Blood cells are produced from stem cells in **hemopoietic tissue**. After birth this

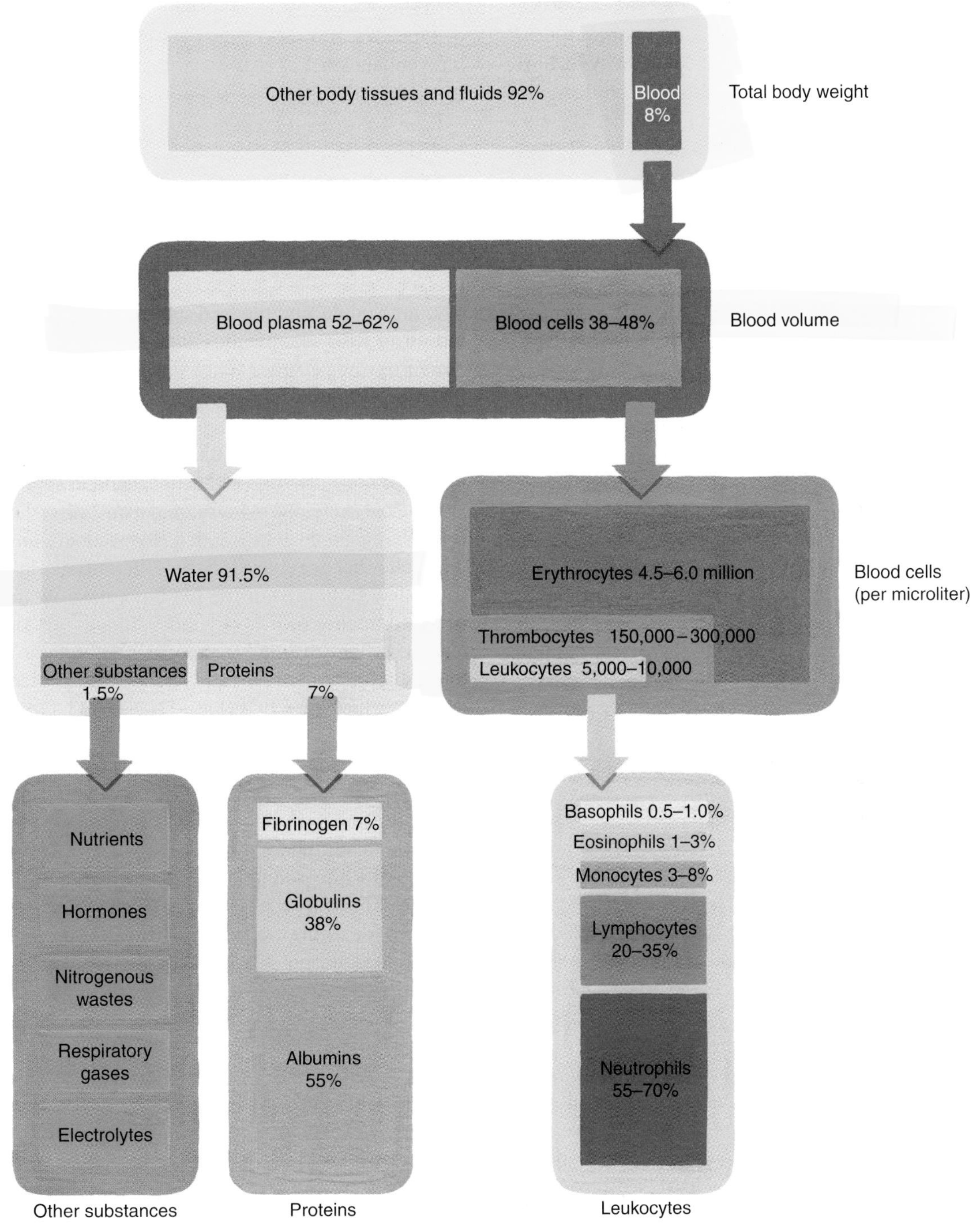

Figure 11–1 Components of blood and the relationship of blood to other body tissues.

QUESTION: Blood plasma is mostly what substance? Which blood cells are the most numerous?

is primarily the **red bone marrow**, found in flat and irregular bones such as the sternum, hip bone, and vertebrae. Lymphocytes mature and divide in **lymphatic tissue**, found in the spleen, lymph nodes, and thymus gland. The thymus contains stem cells that produce T lymphocytes, and the stem cells in other lymphatic tissue also produce lymphocytes.

RED BLOOD CELLS

Also called **erythrocytes**, red blood cells (RBCs) are biconcave discs, which means their centers are thinner than their edges. You may recall from Chapter 3 that red blood cells are the only human cells without nuclei. Their nuclei disintegrate as the red blood cells mature and are not needed for normal functioning.

A normal RBC count ranges from 4.5 to 6.0 million cells per microliter (μL) of blood (1 microliter = 1 mm^3 = one millionth of a liter, a very small volume). RBC counts for men are often toward the high end of this range; those for women are often toward the low end. Another way to measure the amount of RBCs is the **hematocrit**. This test involves drawing blood into a thin glass tube called a capillary tube and centrifuging the tube to force all the cells to one end. The percentages of cells and plasma can then be determined. Because RBCs are by far the most abundant of the blood cells, a normal hematocrit range is just like that of the total blood cells: 38% to 48%. Both RBC count and hematocrit (Hct) are part of a complete blood count (CBC).

Function

Red blood cells contain the protein **hemoglobin** (Hb), which gives them the ability to carry oxygen. Each red blood cell contains approximately 300 million hemoglobin molecules, each of which can bond to four oxygen molecules (see Box Fig. 3–B in Box 3–2 of Chapter 3 for the structure of hemoglobin). In the pulmonary capillaries, RBCs pick up oxygen and oxyhemoglobin is formed. This blood circulates from the lungs back to the heart and is then sent off to the body. In the systemic capillaries, hemoglobin gives up much of its oxygen and becomes reduced hemoglobin.

A determination of hemoglobin level is also part of a CBC; the normal range is 12 to 18 grams per 100 mL of blood. Essential to the formation of hemoglobin is the mineral iron; there are four atoms of iron in each molecule of hemoglobin. It is the iron that actually bonds to the oxygen and also makes RBCs red.

Hemoglobin is also able to bond to carbon dioxide (CO_2) and does transport some CO_2 from the tissues to the lungs. But hemoglobin accounts for only about 10% of total CO_2 transport (most is carried in the plasma as bicarbonate ions).

Production and Maturation

During embryonic and fetal development, the production of RBCs can be likened to a relay race, with the "baton" of production passed from one organ or tissue to another. In the embryo (the first 8 weeks after fertilization) RBCs are first produced by an external membrane called the yolk sac (see Fig. 21–3 in Chapter 21). The fetal liver then takes over for a while, and the fetal spleen also makes a contribution to RBC manufacture later in gestation. The red bone marrow becomes active during the fifth month of gestation, becomes ever more important, and shortly after birth is the only site of RBC formation.

In older children and adults, red blood cells are formed in the red bone marrow (RBM) in flat and irregular bones. Within red bone marrow are precursor cells called **stem cells**. Recall from Chapter 3 that stem cells are unspecialized cells that may develop, or differentiate, in several ways. The stem cells of the red bone marrow may also be called **hemocytoblasts** (hemo = "blood," cyto = "cell," blast = "producer"), and they constantly undergo mitosis to produce new stem cells and all the kinds of blood cells, many of which are RBCs (Figs. 11–2 and 11–3). The rate of production is very rapid (estimated at several million new RBCs every second), and a major regulating factor is oxygen. If the body is in a state of **hypoxia**, or lack of oxygen, the kidneys produce a hormone called **erythropoietin**, which stimulates the red bone marrow to increase the rate of RBC production (that is, the rate of stem cell mitosis). This will occur following hemorrhage or if a person stays for a time at a higher altitude. As a result of the action of erythropoietin, more RBCs will be available to carry oxygen and correct the hypoxic state.

The stem cells that will become RBCs go through a number of developmental stages, only the last two of which we will mention: normoblasts and reticulocytes (see Fig. 11–2). The **normoblast** is the last stage with a nucleus, which then disintegrates. Hemoglobin has been produced, and the chromosomes with the DNA code for hemoglobin are no longer needed. The **reticulocyte** has fragments of the endoplasmic reticulum (also no longer needed), which are visible as purple stippling when blood smears are stained for microscopic evaluation. These immature cells are usually found in the red bone marrow, although a small number of reticulocytes in the peripheral circulation is considered normal (up to 1.5% of the total RBCs). Large numbers of reticulocytes or normoblasts in the circulating blood mean that the number

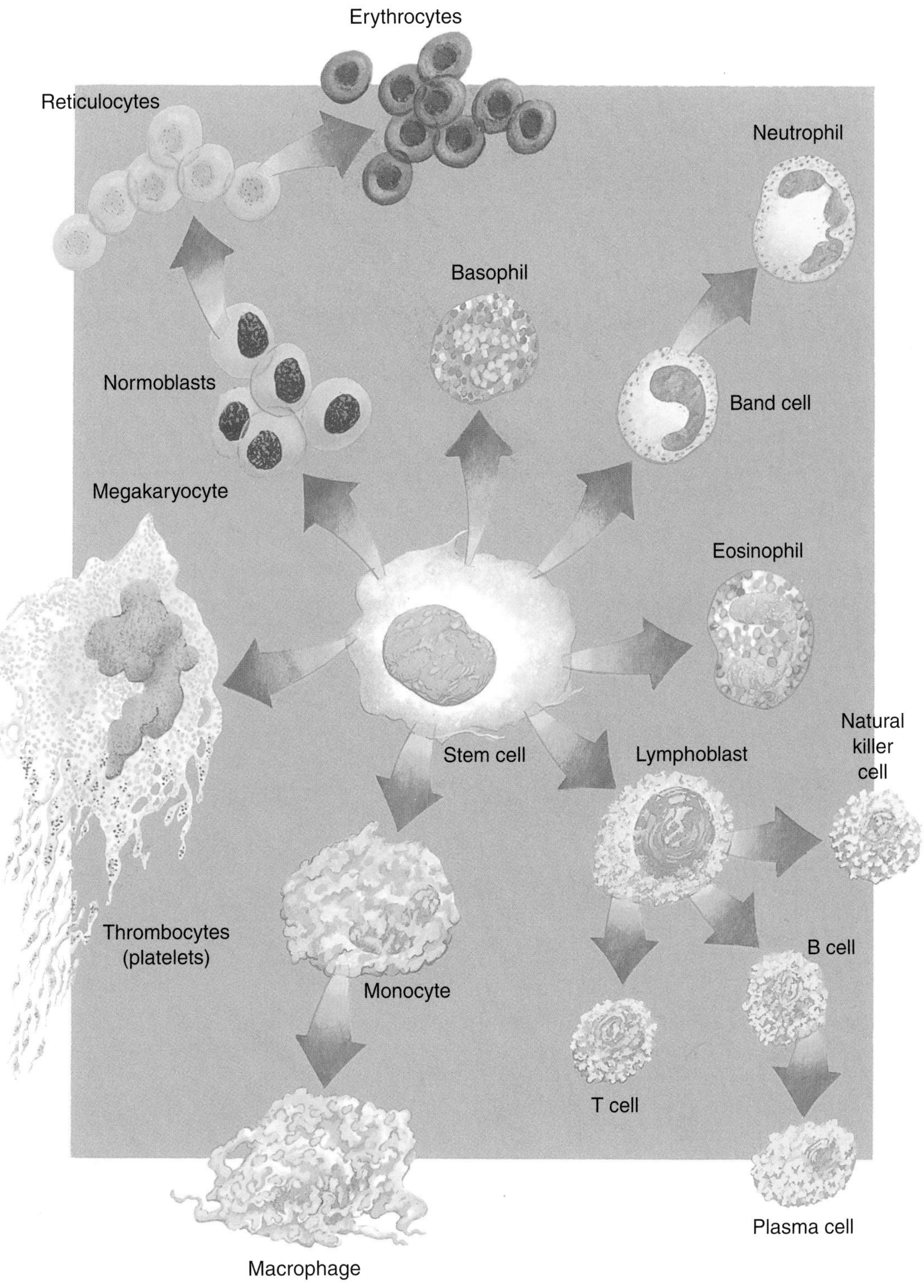

Figure 11–2 Production of blood cells. Stem cells are found primarily in red bone marrow and are the precursor cells for all the types of blood cells.

QUESTION: Where are normoblasts and reticulocytes usually found, and why?

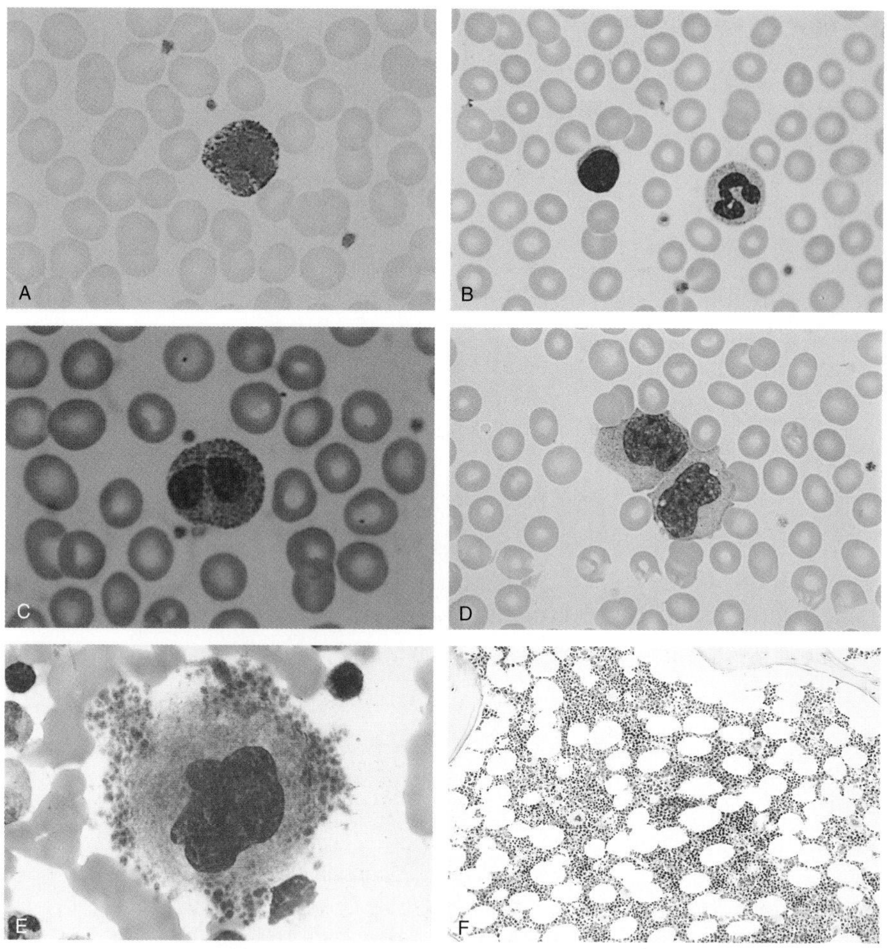

Figure 11–3 Blood cells. (**A**) Red blood cells, platelets, and a basophil. (**B**) Lymphocyte (left) and neutrophil (right). (**C**) Eosinophil. (**D**) Monocytes. (**E**) Megakaryocyte with platelets. (A–E ×600) (**F**) Normal bone marrow (×200). (From Harmening, DM: Clinical Hematology and Fundamentals of Hemostasis, ed. 3. FA Davis, Philadelphia, 1997, pp 14, 17, 19, 26, 48, with permission.)

QUESTION: Look at the RBCs in picture B. Why do they have pale centers?

of mature RBCs is not sufficient to carry the oxygen needed by the body. Such situations include hemorrhage, or when mature RBCs have been destroyed, as in Rh disease of the newborn, and malaria.

The maturation of red blood cells requires many nutrients. Protein and iron are necessary for the synthesis of hemoglobin and become part of hemoglobin molecules. Copper is part of some of the enzymes involved in hemoglobin synthesis, though it does *not* become part of hemoglobin itself (if it did, it would make our blood blue, like that of horseshoe crabs). The vitamins folic acid and B_{12} are required for DNA synthesis in the stem cells of the red bone marrow. As these cells undergo mitosis, they must continually produce new sets of chromosomes. Vitamin B_{12} contains the mineral cobalt and is also called the **extrinsic factor** because its source is external, our food. Parietal cells of the stomach lining produce the **intrinsic factor**, a chemical that combines with the vitamin B_{12} in food to prevent its digestion and promote its absorption in the small intestine. A deficiency of either vitamin B_{12} or the intrinsic factor results in **pernicious anemia** (see Box 11–1: Anemia).

Life Span

Red blood cells live for approximately 120 days. As they reach this age they become fragile; their membranes begin to disintegrate. These damaged cells are removed from circulation by cells of the **tissue macrophage system** (formerly called the reticuloendothelial or RE system). The organs that contain macrophages (literally, "big eaters") are the liver, spleen, and red bone marrow. Look at Fig. 11–4 as you read the following. The old RBCs are phagocytized and digested by macrophages, and the iron they contained is put into the blood to be returned to the red bone marrow to be used for the synthesis of new hemoglobin. If not needed immediately for this purpose, excess iron is stored in the liver. The iron of RBCs is actually recycled over and over again.

Box 11–1 | ANEMIA

Anemia is a deficiency of red blood cells, or insufficient hemoglobin within the red blood cells. There are many different types of anemia.

Iron-deficiency anemia is caused by a lack of dietary iron, when there is not enough of this mineral to form sufficient hemoglobin. A person with this type of anemia may have a normal RBC count and a normal hematocrit, but the hemoglobin level will always be below normal.

A deficiency of vitamin B_{12}, which is found only in animal foods, leads to **pernicious anemia**, in which the RBCs are large, misshapen, and fragile. Another cause of this form of anemia is lack of the intrinsic factor due to autoimmune destruction of the parietal cells of the stomach lining.

Sickle-cell anemia has already been discussed in Chapter 3. It is a genetic disorder of hemoglobin, which causes RBCs to sickle, clog capillaries, and rupture.

Aplastic anemia is suppression of the red bone marrow, with decreased production of RBCs, WBCs, and platelets. This is a very serious disorder that may be caused by exposure to radiation, certain chemicals such as benzene, or some medications. There are several antibiotics that must be used with caution because they may have this potentially fatal side effect.

Hemolytic anemia is any disorder that causes rupture of RBCs before the end of their normal life span. Sickle-cell anemia and Rh disease of the newborn are examples. Another example is malaria, in which a protozoan parasite reproduces in RBCs and destroys them. Hemolytic anemias are often characterized by jaundice because of the increased production of bilirubin.

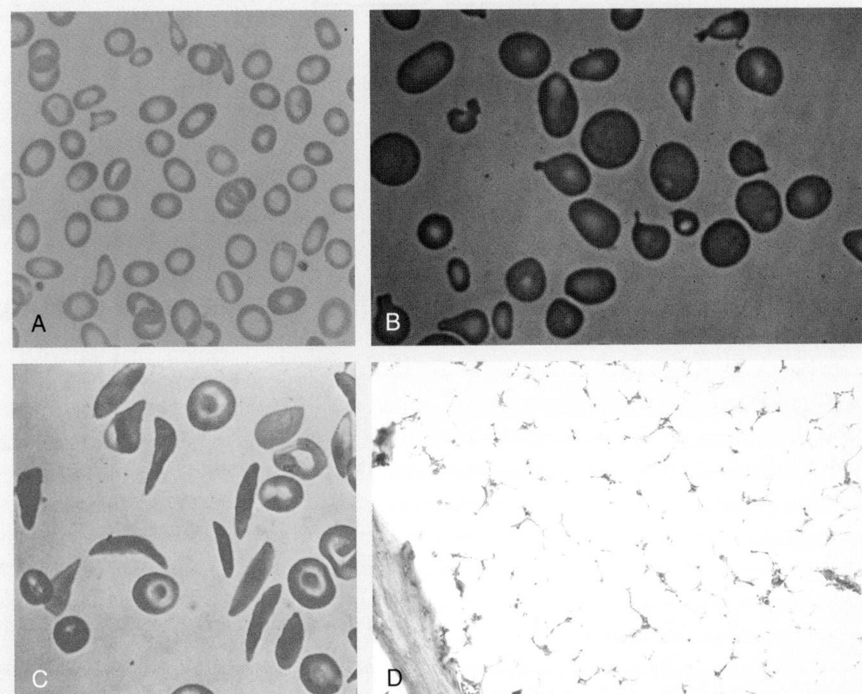

Box Figure 11–A Anemia. (**A**) Iron-deficiency anemia; notice the pale, oval RBCs (×400). (**B**) Pernicious anemia, with large, misshapen RBCs (×400). (**C**) Sickle-cell anemia (×400). (**D**) Aplastic anemia, bone marrow (×200). (**A**, **B**, and **C** from Listen, Look, and Learn, Vol 3; Coagulation, Hematology. The American Society of Clinical Pathologists Press, Chicago, 1973, with permission. **D** from Harmening, DM: Clinical Hematology and Fundamentals of Hemostasis, ed 3. FA Davis, Philadelphia, 1997, p 49, with permission.)

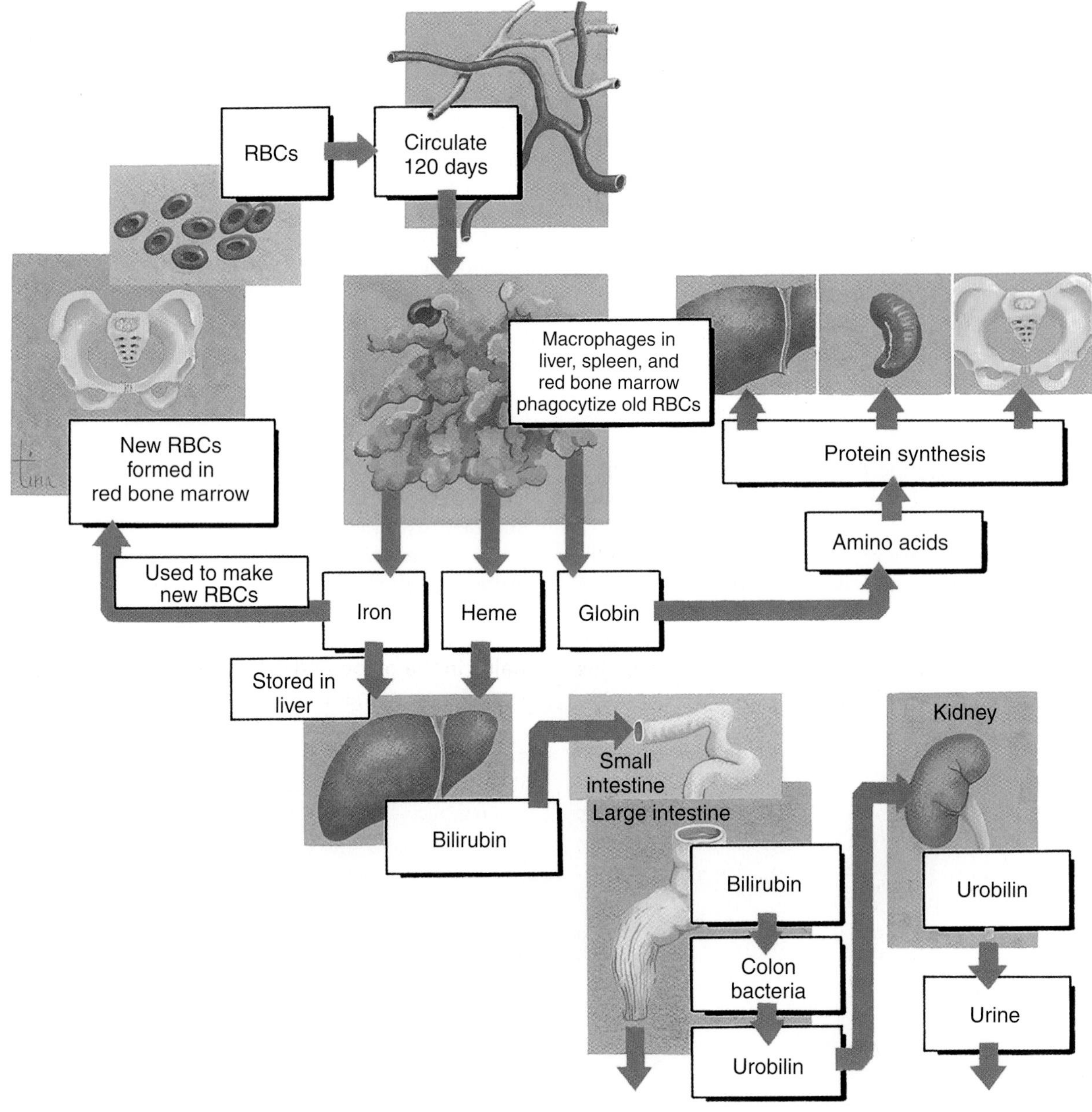

Figure 11–4 Life cycle of red blood cells. See text for description.

QUESTION: Which components of old RBCs are recycled? Which is excreted? (Go to the macrophage and follow the arrows.)

The globin or protein portion of the hemoglobin molecule is also recycled. It is digested to its amino acids, which may then be used for the synthesis of new proteins.

Another part of the hemoglobin molecule is the heme portion, which cannot be recycled and is a waste product. The heme is converted to **bilirubin** by macrophages. The liver removes bilirubin from circulation and excretes it into bile; bilirubin is a bile pigment. Bile is secreted by the liver into the duodenum and passes through the small intestine and colon, so bilirubin is eliminated in feces and gives feces their characteristic brown color. In the colon some bilirubin is changed to urobilinogen by the colon bacteria.

Some urobilinogen may be absorbed into the blood, but it is changed to urobilin and excreted by the kidneys in urine. If bilirubin is not excreted properly, perhaps because of liver disease such as hepatitis, it remains in the blood. This may cause **jaundice**, a condition in which the whites of the eyes appear yellow. This yellow color may also be seen in the skin of light-skinned people (see Box 11–2: Jaundice).

Blood Types

Our blood types are genetic; that is, we inherit genes from our parents that determine our own types. There are many red blood cell factors or types; we will discuss the two most important ones: the **ABO group** and the **Rh factor**. (The genetics of blood types is discussed in Chapter 21.)

The **ABO group** contains four blood types: A, B, AB, and O. The letters A and B represent antigens (protein-oligosaccharides) on the red blood cell membrane. A person with type A blood has the A antigen on the RBCs, and someone with type B blood has the B antigen. Type AB means that both A and B antigens are present, and type O means that neither the A nor the B antigen is present.

Circulating in the plasma of each person are natural antibodies for those antigens *not* present on the RBCs. Therefore, a type A person has anti-B antibodies in the plasma; a type B person has anti-A antibodies; a type AB person has neither anti-A nor anti-B antibodies; and a type O person has both anti-A and anti-B antibodies (see Table 11–1 and Fig. 11–5).

Box 11–2 | JAUNDICE

Jaundice is not a disease, but rather a sign caused by excessive accumulation of bilirubin in the blood. Because one of the liver's many functions is the excretion of bilirubin, jaundice may be a sign of liver disease such as hepatitis or cirrhosis. This may be called **hepatic jaundice** because the problem is with the liver.

Other types of jaundice are prehepatic jaundice and posthepatic jaundice: The name of each tells us where the problem is. Recall that bilirubin is the waste product formed from the heme portion of the hemoglobin of old RBCs. **Prehepatic jaundice** means that the problem is "before" the liver; that is, hemolysis of RBCs is taking place at a more rapid rate. Rapid hemolysis is characteristic of sickle-cell anemia, malaria, and Rh disease of the newborn; these are hemolytic anemias. As excessive numbers of RBCs are destroyed, bilirubin is formed at a faster rate than the liver can excrete it. The bilirubin that the liver cannot excrete remains in the blood and causes jaundice. Another name for this type is **hemolytic jaundice**.

Posthepatic jaundice means that the problem is "after" the liver. The liver excretes bilirubin into bile, which is stored in the gallbladder and then moved to the small intestine. If the bile ducts are obstructed, perhaps by gallstones or inflammation of the gallbladder, bile cannot pass to the small intestine and backs up in the liver. Bilirubin may then be reabsorbed back into the blood and cause jaundice. Another name for this type is **obstructive jaundice**.

Table 11–1 | ABO BLOOD TYPES

TYPE	ANTIGENS PRESENT ON RBCs	ANTIBODIES PRESENT IN PLASMA	PERCENTAGE IN U.S. POPULATION* WHITE	BLACK	ASIAN
A	A	anti-B	40	27	31
B	B	anti-A	11	20	26
AB	both A and B	neither anti-A nor anti-B	4	4	8
O	neither A nor B	both anti-A and anti-B	45	49	35

*Average.

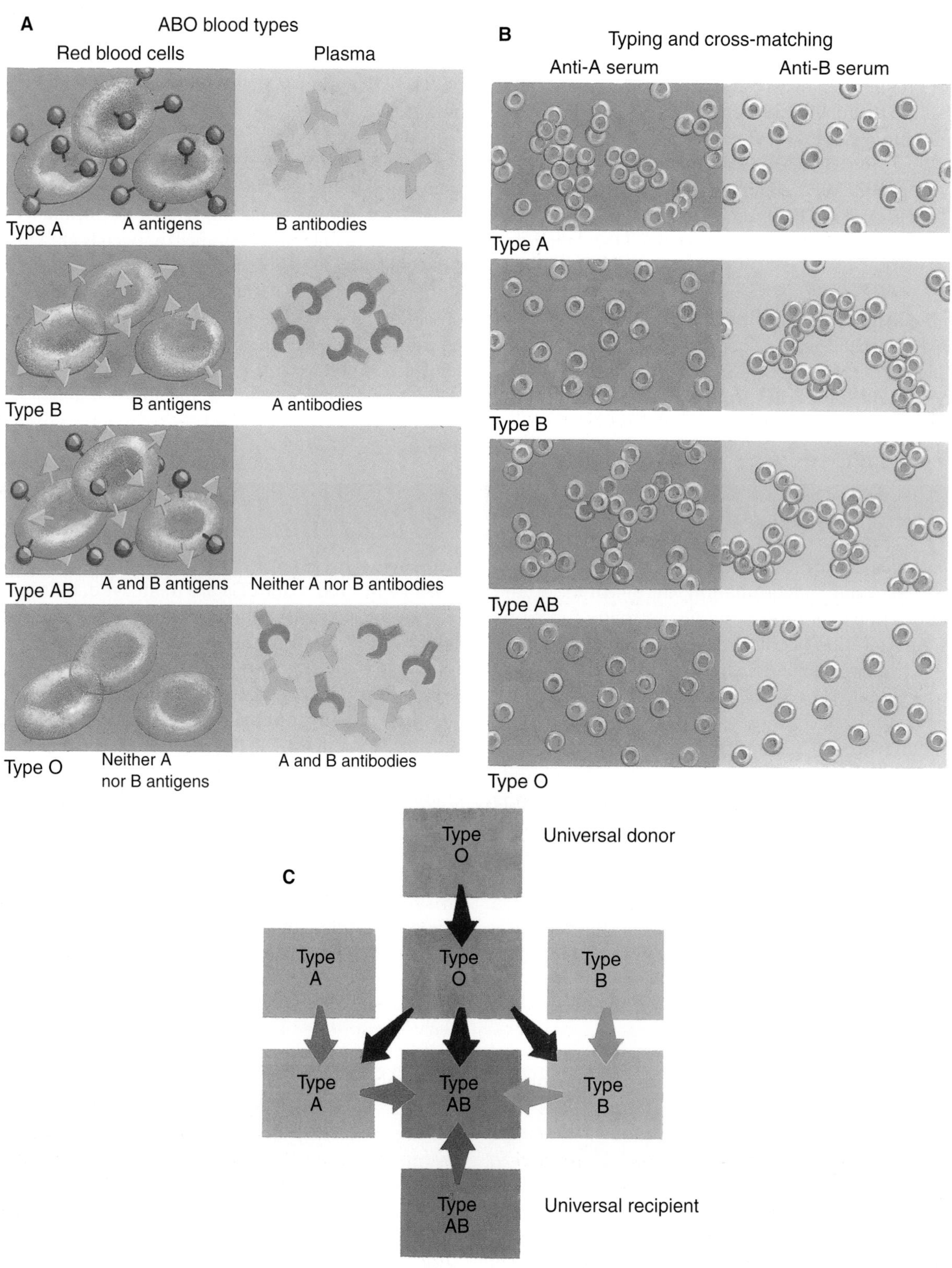

Figure 11–5 (**A**) The ABO blood types. Schematic representation of antigens on the RBCs and antibodies in the plasma. (**B**) Typing and cross-matching. The A or B antiserum causes agglutination of RBCs with the matching antigen. (**C**) Acceptable transfusions are diagrammed and presuppose compatible Rh factors.

QUESTION: In part C, find your blood type. To whom (that is, to which blood types) can you donate blood?

Why we have these natural antibodies is not known (they begin to be formed several months after birth), but we do know that they are of great importance for transfusions. If possible, a person should receive blood of his or her own type; only if this type is not available should type O negative blood be given. For example, let us say that a type A person needs a transfusion to replace blood lost in hemorrhage. If this person were to receive type B blood, what would happen? The type A recipient has anti-B antibodies that would bind to the type B antigens of the RBCs of the donated blood. The type B RBCs would first clump (**agglutination**) then rupture (**hemolysis**), thus defeating the purpose of the transfusion. An even more serious consequence is that the hemoglobin of the ruptured RBCs, now called free hemoglobin, may clog the capillaries of the kidneys and lead to renal damage or renal failure. You can see why **typing** and **cross-matching** of donor and recipient blood in the hospital laboratory is so important before any transfusion is given (see Fig. 11–5). This procedure helps ensure that donated blood will not bring about a hemolytic transfusion reaction in the recipient.

You may have heard of the concept that a person with type O blood is a "universal donor." Usually, a unit of type O negative blood may be given to people with any other blood type. This is so because type O RBCs have neither the A nor the B antigens and will not react with whatever antibodies the recipient may have. If only one unit (1 pint) of blood is given, the anti-A and anti-B antibodies in the type O blood plasma will be diluted in the recipient's blood plasma and will not have a harmful effect on the recipient's RBCs. The term *negative*, in O negative, the universal donor, refers to the Rh factor, which we will now consider.

The **Rh factor** is another antigen (often called D) that may be present on RBCs. People whose RBCs have the Rh antigen are Rh positive; those without the antigen are Rh negative. Rh-negative people do not have natural antibodies to the Rh antigen, and for them this antigen is foreign. If an Rh-negative person receives Rh-positive blood by mistake, antibodies will be formed just as they would be to bacteria or viruses. A first mistaken transfusion often does not cause problems because antibody production is slow upon the first exposure to Rh-positive RBCs, and those RBCs have a relatively short lifespan. A second transfusion, however, when anti-Rh antibodies are already present will bring about a transfusion reaction, with hemolysis and possible kidney damage (see also Box 11–3: Rh Disease of the Newborn).

WHITE BLOOD CELLS

White blood cells (WBCs) are also called **leukocytes**. There are five kinds of WBCs; all are larger than RBCs and have nuclei when mature. The nucleus may be in one piece

Box 11–3 | Rh DISEASE OF THE NEWBORN

Rh disease of the newborn may also be called **erythroblastosis fetalis** and is the result of an Rh incompatibility between mother and fetus. During a normal pregnancy, maternal blood and fetal blood do not mix in the placenta. However, during delivery of the placenta (the "afterbirth" that follows the birth of the baby), some fetal blood may enter maternal circulation.

If the woman is Rh negative and her baby is Rh positive, this exposes the woman to Rh-positive RBCs. In response, her immune system will now produce anti-Rh antibodies following this first delivery. In a subsequent pregnancy, these maternal antibodies will cross the placenta and enter fetal circulation. If this next fetus is also Rh positive, the maternal antibodies will cause destruction (hemolysis) of the fetal RBCs. In severe cases this may result in the death of the fetus. In less severe cases, the baby will be born anemic and jaundiced from the loss of RBCs. Such an infant may require a gradual exchange transfusion to remove the blood with the maternal antibodies and replace it with Rh-negative blood. The baby will continue to produce its own Rh-positive RBCs, which will not be destroyed once the maternal antibodies have been removed.

Much better than treatment, however, is prevention. If an Rh-negative woman delivers an Rh-positive baby, she should be given **RhoGAM** within 72 hours after delivery. RhoGAM is an anti-Rh antibody that will destroy any fetal RBCs that have entered the mother's circulation *before* her immune system can respond and produce antibodies. The RhoGAM antibodies themselves break down within a few months. The woman's next pregnancy will be like the first, as if she had never been exposed to Rh-positive RBCs.

or appear as several lobes or segments. Special staining for microscopic examination gives each kind of WBC a distinctive appearance (see Figs. 11–2 and 11–3).

A normal WBC count (part of a CBC) is 5,000 to 10,000 per µL. Notice that this number is quite small compared with a normal RBC count. Many of our WBCs are not circulating within blood vessels but are carrying out their functions in tissue fluid or in lymphatic tissue.

Classification

The five kinds of white blood cells, all produced in the red bone marrow (and some lymphocytes in lymphatic tissue), may be classified in two groups: granular and agranular. The granular leukocytes are the **neutrophils**, **eosinophils**, and **basophils**, which usually have nuclei in two or more lobes or segments and have distinctly colored granules when stained. Neutrophils have light blue granules, eosinophils have red granules, and basophils have dark blue granules. The agranular leukocytes are **lymphocytes** and **monocytes**, which have nuclei in one piece. Monocytes are usually quite a bit larger than lymphocytes. A **differential WBC count** (part of a CBC) is the percentage of each kind of leukocyte. Normal ranges are listed in Table 11–2, along with other normal values of a CBC.

Functions

White blood cells all contribute to the same general function, which is to protect the body from infectious disease and to provide **immunity** to certain diseases. Each kind

Table 11–2 | COMPLETE BLOOD COUNT

MEASUREMENT	NORMAL RANGE*	VARIATIONS
Red blood cells	4.5–6.0 million/µL	Decrease: anemia Increase: polycythemia
Hemoglobin	12–18 grams/100 mL	Decrease: iron deficiency, other anemias Increase: polycythemia
Hematocrit	38%–48%	Decrease: anemia Increase: polycythemia, heavy smoking
Reticulocytes	0%–1.5%	Decrease: RBM suppression Increase: insufficiency of mature RBCs
White blood cells (total)	5000–10,000/µL	Decrease: leucopenia Increase: leukocytosis
Neutrophils	55%–70%	Decrease: radiation, chemotherapy for cancer Increase: infection, inflammation
Eosinophils	1%–3%	Decrease: corticosteroid excess Increase: allergies, parasitic infections
Basophils	0.5%–1%	Decrease: cancer Increase: allergies
Lymphocytes	20%–35%	Decrease: HIV/AIDS, severe burns, cancer, radiation Increase: many viral diseases
Monocytes	3%–8%	Decrease: corticosteroid excess Increase: many viral diseases, chronic inflammation
Platelets	150,000–300,000/µL	Decrease: thrombocytopenia that may be idiopathic or accompany aplastic anemia Increase: not considered a clinical condition, but may follow removal of the spleen

*The values on hospital lab slips may vary somewhat but will be very similar to the normal ranges given here.

of leukocyte makes a contribution to this very important aspect of homeostasis.

Neutrophils and monocytes are capable of the **phagocytosis** of pathogens. Neutrophils are the more abundant phagocytes, but the monocytes are the more efficient phagocytes, because they differentiate into **macrophages**, which also phagocytize dead or damaged tissue at the site of any injury, helping to make tissue repair possible. Monocytes also contribute to tissue repair. During an infection, neutrophils are produced more rapidly, and the immature forms, called **band cells** (see Fig. 11–2), may appear in greater numbers in peripheral circulation (band cells are usually less than 10% of the total neutrophils). The term "band" refers to the nucleus that has not yet become segmented and may look somewhat like a dumbbell.

Eosinophils are believed to detoxify foreign proteins and will phagocytize anything labeled with antibodies. Eosinophils become more abundant during allergic reactions and parasitic infections such as trichinosis (caused by a worm parasite). Basophils contain granules of heparin and histamine. **Heparin** is an anticoagulant that helps prevent abnormal clotting within blood vessels. **Histamine**, you may recall, is released as part of the inflammation process, and it makes capillaries more permeable, allowing tissue fluid, proteins, and white blood cells to accumulate in the damaged area.

There are two major kinds of lymphocytes, T cells and B cells, and a less numerous third kind called natural killer cells. For now we will say that **T cells** (or T lymphocytes) help recognize foreign antigens and may directly destroy some foreign antigens. **B cells** (or B lymphocytes) become plasma cells that produce antibodies to foreign antigens. Both T cells and B cells provide memory for pathogens. The memory T cells and B cells are the reason vaccines or recovery from a disease can provide immunity to future cases of that disease. **Natural killer cells** (NK cells) destroy foreign cells by chemically rupturing their membranes. These functions of lymphocytes are discussed in the context of the mechanisms of immunity in Chapter 14.

As mentioned earlier, leukocytes function in tissue fluid and blood. Many WBCs are capable of self-locomotion (ameboid movement) and are able to squeeze between the cells of capillary walls and out into tissue spaces. Macrophages provide a good example of the dual locations of leukocytes. Some macrophages are "fixed," that is, stationary in organs such as the liver, spleen, and red bone marrow (part of the tissue macrophage or RE system—the same macrophages that phagocytize old RBCs) and in the lymph nodes. They phagocytize pathogens that circulate in blood or lymph through these organs. Other "wandering" macrophages move about in tissue fluid, especially in the areolar connective tissue of mucous membranes and below the skin. Pathogens that gain entry into the body through natural openings or through breaks in the skin are usually destroyed by the macrophages and other leukocytes in connective tissue before they can cause serious disease. The alveoli of the lungs, for example, have macrophages that very efficiently destroy pathogens that enter with inhaled air.

A high WBC count, called **leukocytosis**, is often an indication of infection. **Leukopenia** is a low WBC count, which may be present in the early stages of diseases such as tuberculosis. Exposure to radiation or to chemicals such as benzene may destroy WBCs and lower the total count. Such a person is then very susceptible to infection. **Leukemia**, or malignancy of leukocyte-forming tissues, is discussed in Box 11–4: Leukemia.

The white blood cell types (analogous to RBC types such as the ABO group) are called **human leukocyte antigens (HLAs)**. These cell types are created by cell membrane proteins that are a genetic characteristic. The genes for these self-antigens are collectively called the **major histocompatibility complex (MHC)** and are on chromosome number 6. The purpose of the antigens is discussed in Box 11–5: White Blood Cell Types: HLA.

PLATELETS

The more formal name for platelets is **thrombocytes**, which are not whole cells but rather fragments or pieces of cells. Some of the stem cells in the red bone marrow differentiate into large cells called **megakaryocytes** (see Figs. 11–2 and 11–3), which break up into small pieces that enter circulation. These small, oval, circulating pieces are platelets, which may last for 5 to 9 days, if not utilized before that. **Thrombopoietin** is a hormone produced by the liver that increases the rate of platelet production.

A normal platelet count (part of a CBC) is 150,000 to 300,000/μL (the high end of the range may be extended to 500,000). **Thrombocytopenia** is the term for a low platelet count.

Function

Platelets are necessary for **hemostasis**, which means prevention of blood loss. With respect to intact blood vessels, platelets help maintain the junctions between adjacent epithelial cells that form capillaries and line larger vessels (the endothelium). Without platelets, zipper-like

Box 11–4 | LEUKEMIA

Leukemia is the term for malignancy of a blood-forming tissue. There are many types of leukemia, which are classified as acute or chronic, by the types of abnormal cells produced, and by either childhood or adult onset.

In general, leukemia is characterized by an overproduction of immature white blood cells. These immature cells cannot perform their normal functions, and the person becomes very susceptible to infection. As a greater proportion of the body's nutrients are used by malignant cells, the production of other blood cells decreases. Severe anemia is a consequence of decreased red blood cell production, and the tendency to bruise easily, then hemorrhage, is the result of decreased platelets.

Chemotherapy may bring about cure or remission for some forms of leukemia, but other forms remain resistant to treatment and may be fatal within a few months of diagnosis. In such cases, the cause of death is often pneumonia or some other serious infection because the abnormal white blood cells cannot prevent the growth and spread of pathogens within the body.

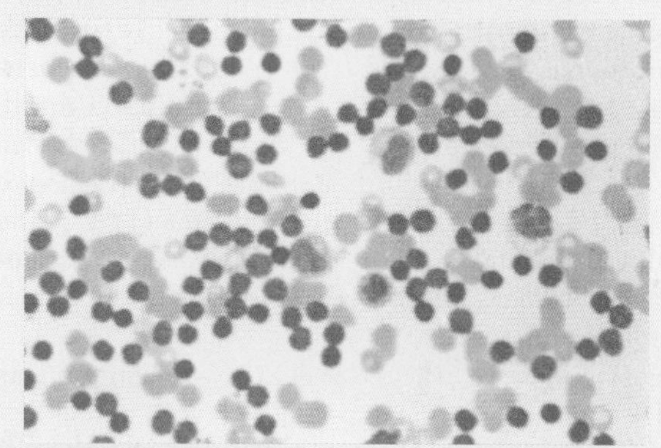

Box Figure 11–B Leukemia. Notice the many darkly staining WBCs (×300); compare with normal blood in Fig. 11–3 A and B. (From Sacher, RA, and McPherson, RA: Widmann's Clinical Interpretation of Laboratory Tests, ed 11. FA Davis, Philadelphia, 2000, with permission.)

Box 11–5 | WHITE BLOOD CELL TYPES: HLA

Human leukocyte antigens (HLAs) are antigens on WBCs that are representative of the antigens present on all the cells of an individual. These are our "self" antigens that identify cells that belong in the body.

Recall that in the ABO blood group of RBCs, there are only two antigens, A and B, and four possible types: A, B, AB, and O. HLA antigens are also given letter names. HLA A, B, and C are called class I proteins, with from 100 to more than 400 possibilities for the specific protein each can be. The several class II proteins are given various D designations and, again, there are many possibilities for each. Each person has two genes for each HLA type because these types are inherited, just as RBC types are inherited. Members of the same family may have some of the same HLA types, and identical twins have exactly the same HLA types.

The purpose of the HLA types is to provide a "self" comparison for the immune system to use when pathogens enter the body. The T lymphocytes compare the "self" antigens on macrophages to the antigens on bacteria and viruses. Because these antigens do not match ours, they are recognized as foreign; this is the first step in the destruction of a pathogen.

The surgical transplantation of organs has also focused on the HLA. The most serious problem for the recipient of a transplanted heart or kidney is rejection of the organ and its destruction by the immune system. You may be familiar with the term **tissue typing**. This process involves determining the HLA types of a donated organ to see if one or several will match the HLA types of the potential recipient. If even one HLA type matches, the chance of rejection is lessened. Although all transplant recipients (except corneal) must receive immunosuppressive medications to prevent rejection, such medications make them more susceptible to infection. The closer the HLA match of the donated organ, the lower the dosage of such medications,

Box 11–5 | WHITE BLOOD CELL TYPES: HLA *(Continued)*

and the less chance of serious infections. (The chance of finding a perfect HLA match in the general population is estimated at 1 in 20,000.)

There is yet another aspect of the importance of HLA: People with certain HLA types seem to be more likely to develop certain autoimmune diseases. For example, type 1 (insulin-dependent) diabetes mellitus is often found in people with HLA DR3 or DR4, and an arthritis of the spine called ankylosing spondylitis is often found in those with HLA B27. These are *not* genes for these diseases but may be predisposing factors. What may happen is this: A virus enters the body and stimulates the immune system to produce antibodies. The virus is destroyed, but one of the person's own antigens is so similar to the viral antigen that the immune system continues its activity and begins to destroy this similar part of the body. Another possibility is that a virus damages a self-antigen to the extent that it is now so different that it will be perceived as foreign. These are two theories of how autoimmune diseases are triggered, a topic that is the focus of much research in the field of immunology.

glycoproteins called **cadherins** tend to come apart, the epithelial cells separate, and RBCs and excess plasma leak out. Should a blood vessel rupture or be cut, three mechanisms help minimize blood loss, and platelets are involved in each. Two of these mechanisms are shown in Fig. 11–6.

1. **Vascular spasm**—when a large vessel such as an artery or vein is severed, the smooth muscle in its wall contracts in response to the damage (called the myogenic response). Platelets in the area of the rupture release serotonin, which also brings about vasoconstriction. The diameter of the vessel is thereby made smaller, and the smaller opening may then be blocked by a blood clot. If the vessel did not constrict first, the clot that formed would quickly be washed out by the force of the blood pressure.
2. **Platelet plugs**—when capillaries rupture, the damage is too slight to initiate the formation of a blood clot. The rough surface, however, causes platelets to change shape (become spiky) and become sticky. These activated platelets stick to the edges of the break and to each other. The platelets form a mechanical barrier or wall to close off the break in the capillary. Capillary ruptures are quite frequent, and platelet plugs, although small, are all that is needed to seal them.
   Would platelet plugs be effective for breaks in larger vessels? No, they are too small, and though they do form, they are washed away (until a clot begins to form that can contain them). Would vascular spasm be effective for capillaries? Again, the answer is no, because capillaries have no smooth muscle and cannot constrict at all.
3. **Chemical clotting**—The stimulus for clotting is a rough surface within a vessel, or a break in the vessel, which also creates a rough surface. The more damage there is, the faster clotting begins, usually within 15 to 120 seconds.

The clotting mechanism is a series of reactions involving chemicals that normally circulate in the blood and others that are released when a vessel is damaged.

The chemicals involved in clotting include platelet factors, chemicals released by damaged tissues, calcium ions, and the plasma proteins prothrombin, fibrinogen, Factor 8, and others synthesized by the liver. (These clotting factors are also designated by Roman numerals; Factor 8 would be Factor VIII.) Vitamin K is necessary for the liver to synthesize prothrombin and several other clotting factors (Factors 7, 9, and 10). Most of our vitamin K is produced by the intestinal microbiota, the bacteria that live in the colon; the vitamin is absorbed as the colon absorbs water and may be stored in the liver.

Chemical clotting is usually described in three stages, which are listed in Table 11–3 and illustrated in Fig. 11–7. Stage 1 begins when a vessel is cut or damaged internally and includes all of the factors shown. As you follow the pathway, notice that the product of stage 1 is prothrombin activator, which may also be called prothrombinase. Each name tells us something. The first name suggests that this chemical activates prothrombin, and that is true. The second name ends in "ase," which indicates that this is an enzyme. The traditional names for enzymes use the substrate of the enzyme as the first part of the name, and add "ase." So this chemical must be an enzyme whose substrate is prothrombin, and that is also true. The stages of clotting may be called a cascade, where one leads to the

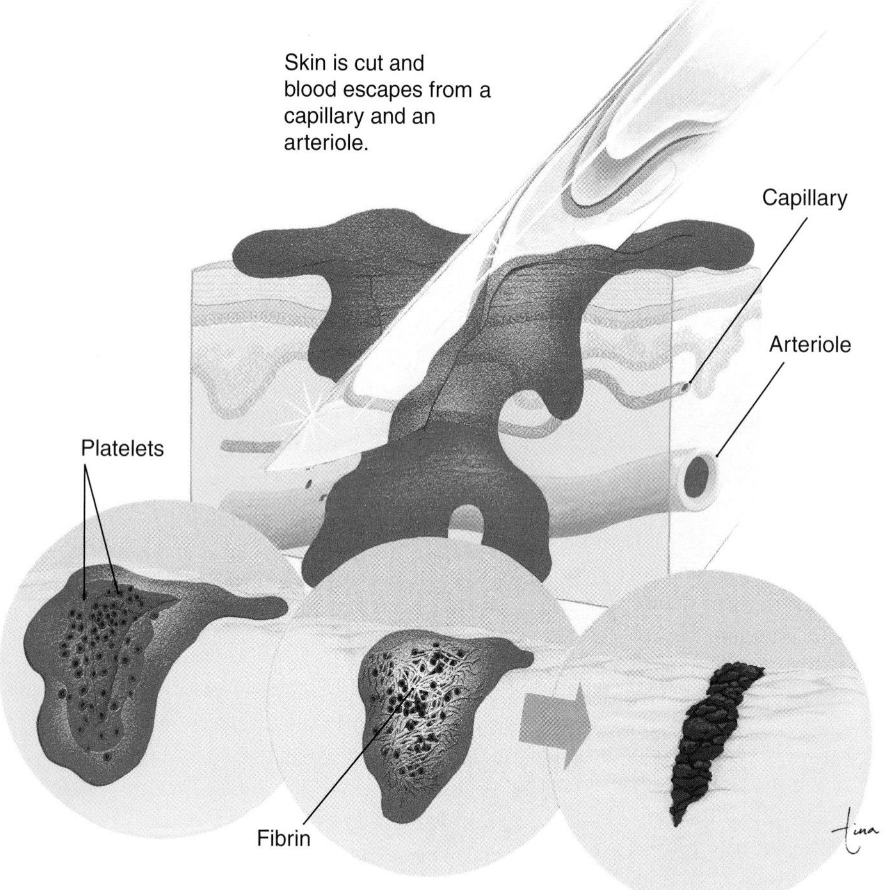

Figure 11–6 Hemostasis. Platelet plug formation in a capillary and chemical clotting and clot retraction in an arteriole.

QUESTION: Look at the diameter of the arteriole (compared with that of the capillary) and explain why platelet plugs would not be sufficient to stop the bleeding.

Table 11–3 | **CHEMICAL CLOTTING**

CLOTTING STAGE	FACTORS NEEDED	REACTION
Stage 1	■ Platelet factors ■ Chemicals from damaged tissue (tissue thromboplastin) ■ Factors 5, 7, 8, 9, 10, 11, 12 ■ Calcium ions	Platelet factors + tissue thromboplastin + other clotting factors + calcium ions form prothrombin activator (prothrombinase)
Stage 2	■ Prothrombin activator from stage 1 ■ Prothrombin ■ Calcium ions	Prothrombin activator converts prothrombin to thrombin
Stage 3	■ Thrombin from stage 2 ■ Fibrinogen ■ Calcium ions ■ Factor 13 (fibrin stabilizing factor)	Thrombin converts fibrinogen to fibrin

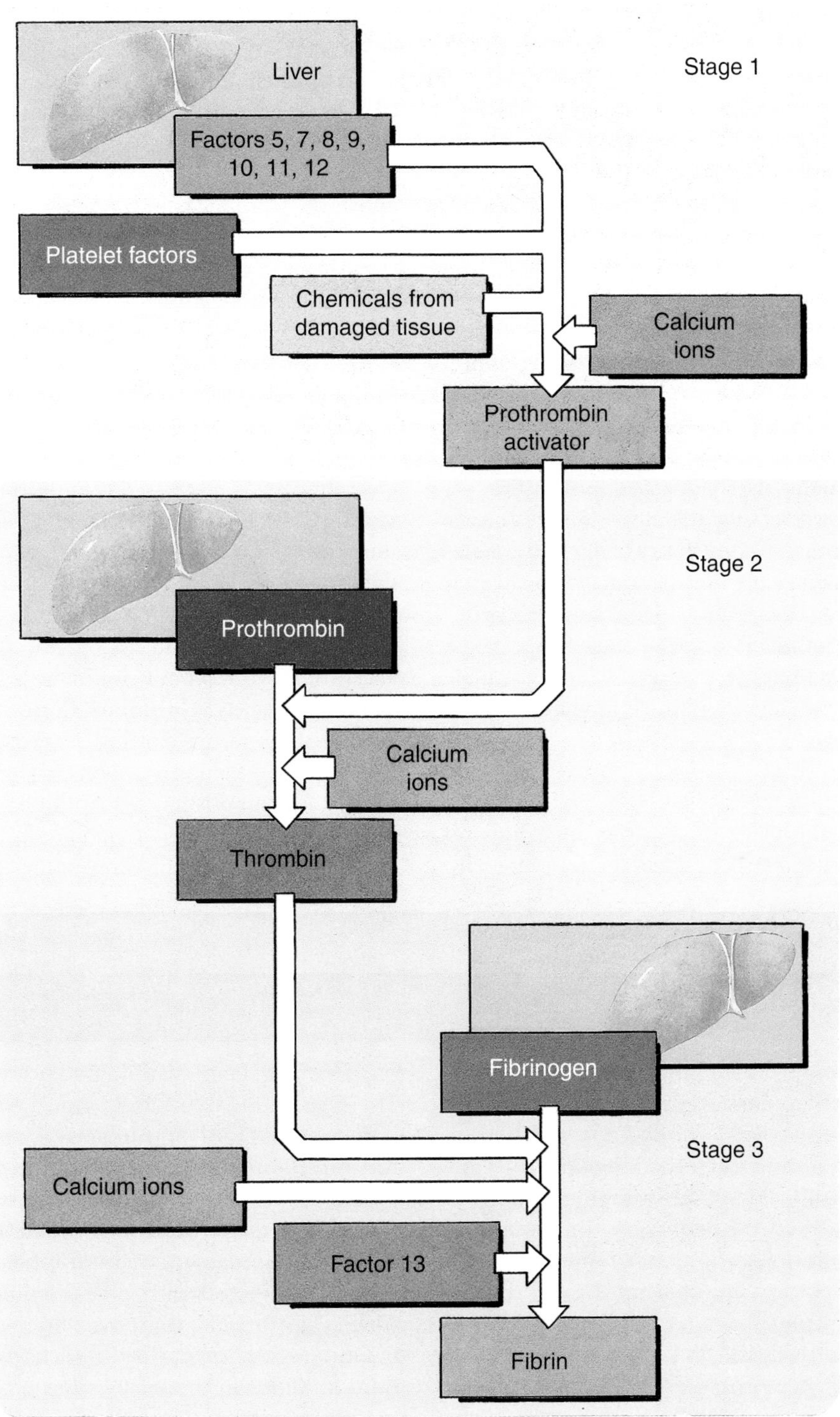

Figure 11–7 Stages of chemical blood clotting.

QUESTION: Based only on this picture, explain why the liver is a vital organ.

next, as inevitable as water flowing downhill. Prothrombin activator, the product of stage 1, brings about the stage 2 reaction: converting prothrombin to thrombin. The product of stage 2, thrombin, brings about the stage 3 reaction: converting fibrinogen to fibrin (see Box 11–6: Hemophilia).

The clot itself is made of **fibrin**, the product of stage 3. Fibrin is a threadlike protein. Many strands of fibrin form a mesh that traps RBCs and platelets and creates a wall across the break in the vessel.

Once the clot has formed and bleeding has stopped, **clot retraction** and **fibrinolysis** occur. Clot retraction requires platelets, ATP, and Factor 13 and involves folding of the fibrin threads to pull the edges of the rupture in the vessel wall closer together. This will make the area to be repaired smaller. The platelets contribute in yet another way because as they disintegrate they release platelet-derived growth factor (PDGF), which stimulates mitosis for the repair of blood vessels. As repair begins, the clot is dissolved, a process called fibrinolysis. It is important that the clot be dissolved because it is a rough surface, and if it were inside a vessel it would stimulate more and unnecessary clotting, which might eventually obstruct blood flow.

Prevention of Abnormal Clotting

Clotting should take place to stop bleeding, but too much clotting would obstruct vessels and interfere with normal circulation of blood. Clots do not usually form in intact vessels because the **endothelium** (simple squamous epithelial lining) is very smooth and repels the platelets and clotting factors. If the lining becomes roughened, as happens with the lipid deposits of atherosclerosis, a clot will form.

Heparin, produced by basophils, is a natural anticoagulant that inhibits the clotting process (although heparin is called a "blood thinner," it does not "thin" or dilute the blood in any way; rather it prevents a chemical reaction from taking place). The liver produces a globulin called **antithrombin**, which combines with and inactivates excess thrombin. Excess thrombin would exert a positive feedback effect on the clotting cascade and result in the splitting of more prothrombin to thrombin, more clotting, more thrombin formed, and so on. Antithrombin helps to prevent this, as does the fibrin of the clot, which adsorbs excess thrombin and renders it inactive. All of these factors are the external brake for this positive feedback mechanism. Together they usually limit the fibrin formed to what is needed to create a useful clot but not an obstructive one.

Thrombosis refers to clotting in an intact vessel; the clot itself is called a **thrombus**. Coronary thrombosis, for example, is abnormal clotting in a coronary artery, which will decrease the blood (oxygen) supply to part of the heart muscle. An **embolism** is a clot or other tissue transported from elsewhere that lodges in and obstructs a vessel (see Box 11–7: Dissolving and Preventing Clots).

Box 11–6 | HEMOPHILIA

There are several forms of **hemophilia**; all are genetic and are characterized by the inability of the blood to clot properly. Hemophilia A is the most common form and involves a deficiency of clotting Factor 8 (VIII). The gene for hemophilia A is located on the X chromosome, so this is a **sex-linked trait**, with the same pattern of inheritance as red-green color blindness and Duchenne's muscular dystrophy.

Without Factor 8, the first stage of chemical clotting cannot be completed, and prothrombin activator is not formed. Without treatment, a hemophiliac experiences prolonged bleeding after even minor injuries and extensive internal bleeding, especially in joints subjected to the stresses of weight bearing. Treatment, but not cure, is possible with Factor 8 obtained from blood donors. The Factor 8 is extracted from the plasma of donated blood and administered in concentrated form to hemophiliacs, enabling them to live normal lives.

In what is perhaps the most tragic irony of medical progress, many hemophiliacs were inadvertently infected with HIV, the virus that causes AIDS. Before 1985, there was no test to detect HIV in donated blood, and the virus was passed to hemophiliacs in the very blood product that was meant to control their disease and prolong their lives. Today, all donated blood and blood products are tested for HIV, and the risk of AIDS transmission to hemophiliacs, or anyone receiving donated blood, is now very small.

Box 11–7 | DISSOLVING AND PREVENTING CLOTS

Abnormal clots may cause serious problems in coronary arteries, pulmonary arteries, cerebral vessels, and even veins in the legs. However, if these clots can be dissolved before they cause death of tissue, normal circulation and tissue functioning may be restored.

One of the first substances used to dissolve clots in coronary arteries was **streptokinase**, which is actually a bacterial toxin produced by some members of the genus *Streptococcus*. Streptokinase did indeed dissolve clots, but its use created the possibility of clot destruction throughout the body, with serious hemorrhage a potential consequence.

Safer thrombolytic chemicals are now used (thrombo = "clot" and lytic = "to lyse" or "split"). In a case of a coronary thrombosis, if a thrombolytic can be directed into the affected vessel within a few hours, the clot may be dissolved and permanent heart damage prevented. The same procedure is also used to prevent permanent brain damage after strokes (CVAs) caused by blood clots.

Some people, such as those with atrial fibrillation or a tendency to form clots in veins of the legs, require clot prevention. You have probably heard of warfarin, which has been a standard clot-preventing drug for many years. Several new medications are available (and can be taken orally) that inhibit the action of thrombin or other clotting factors. Slower clotting and excessive bleeding are possible side effects, but episodes of major bleeding have been less likely with the newer medications than with warfarin.

SUMMARY

All of the functions of blood described in this chapter—transport, regulation, and protection—contribute to the homeostasis of the body as a whole. However, these functions could not be carried out if the blood did not circulate properly. The circulation of blood throughout the blood vessels depends on the proper functioning of the heart, the pump of the circulatory system, which is the subject of our next chapter.

STUDY OUTLINE

The general functions of blood are transportation, regulation, and protection.

Characteristics of Blood

1. Amount—4 to 6 liters; 38% to 48% is cells; 52% to 62% is plasma (Fig. 11–1).
2. Color—arterial blood has a high oxygen content and is bright red; venous blood has less oxygen and is dark red.
3. pH—7.35 to 7.45; venous blood has more CO_2 and a lower pH than arterial blood; buffer systems help maintain normal pH.
4. Viscosity—thickness or resistance to flow; due to the presence of cells and plasma proteins; contributes to normal blood pressure.

Plasma—the liquid portion of blood

1. 91% water.
2. Plasma transports nutrients, wastes, hormones, heat, antibodies, and CO_2 as HCO_3^-.
3. Plasma proteins: many are produced by the liver.
   a. Clotting factors (prothrombin, fibrinogen, and others) are synthesized by the liver.
   b. Albumin is synthesized by the liver and provides colloid osmotic pressure that pulls tissue fluid into capillaries to maintain normal blood volume and blood pressure.

c. Alpha and beta globulins are synthesized by the liver and are carriers for fats and other substances in the blood.

d. Gamma globulins (immunoglobulins) are antibodies produced by lymphocytes.

Blood Cells

1. Formed elements are RBCs, WBCs, and platelets (Figs. 11–2 and 11–3).
2. After birth the primary hemopoietic tissue is the red bone marrow, which contains stem cells. Lymphocytes mature and divide in the lymphatic tissue of the spleen, lymph nodes, and thymus, which also have stem cells for lymphocytes.

Red Blood Cells—erythrocytes (see Table 11–2 for normal values)

1. Biconcave discs; no nuclei when mature.
2. RBCs carry O_2 bonded to the iron in hemoglobin; oxyhemoglobin is formed in pulmonary capillaries; the oxygen is dropped off in systemic capillaries.
3. Before birth, RBCs are formed by the embryonic yolk sac and then by the fetal liver, spleen, and RBM.
4. After birth, RBCs are formed in the RBM from hemocytoblasts (stem cells, the precursor cells).
5. Hypoxia stimulates the kidneys to produce the hormone erythropoietin, which increases the rate of RBC production (mitosis of stem cells) in the RBM.
6. Immature RBCs: normoblasts (have nuclei) and reticulocytes; large numbers in peripheral circulation indicate a need for more RBCs to carry oxygen.
7. Vitamin B_{12} contains cobalt and is called the extrinsic factor, needed for DNA synthesis (mitosis) in stem cells in the RBM. Intrinsic factor is produced by the parietal cells of the stomach lining; it combines with B_{12} to prevent its digestion and promote its absorption in the small intestine.
8. RBCs live for 120 days and are then phagocytized by macrophages in the liver, spleen, and RBM (see Fig. 11–4).
   a. The iron is returned to the RBM or stored in the liver.
   b. The heme of the hemoglobin is converted to bilirubin, which the liver excretes into bile to be eliminated in feces.
   c. Colon bacteria change bilirubin to urobilinogen.
   d. Any urobilinogen absorbed is converted to urobilin and excreted by the kidneys in urine.
   e. Jaundice is the accumulation of bilirubin in the blood, perhaps the result of liver disease.
9. ABO blood types are hereditary.
   a. The type indicates the antigen(s) on the RBCs (see Table 11–1 and Fig. 11–5).
   b. Antibodies in plasma are for those antigens not present on the RBCs and are an important consideration for transfusions.
10. The Rh blood type (D antigen) is also hereditary.
   a. Rh positive means that the D antigen is present on the RBCs.
   b. Rh negative means that the D antigen is not present on the RBCs.
   c. Rh-negative people do not have natural antibodies but will produce them if given Rh-positive blood.

White Blood Cells—leukocytes (see Table 11–2 for normal values)

1. Larger than RBCs; have nuclei when mature; produced in the red bone marrow, except some lymphocytes produced in the thymus or other lymphatic tissue (Figs. 11–2 and 11–3).
2. Granular WBCs are the neutrophils, eosinophils, and basophils.
3. Agranular WBCs are the lymphocytes and monocytes.
4. Neutrophils and monocytes phagocytize pathogens; monocytes become macrophages, which also phagocytize dead tissue.
5. Eosinophils detoxify foreign proteins during allergic reactions and parasitic infections; they phagocytize anything labeled with antibodies.
6. Basophils contain the anticoagulant heparin and histamine, which makes capillaries more permeable during inflammation.
7. Lymphocytes: T cells, B cells, and natural killer cells.
   a. T cells recognize foreign antigens and destroy them and also provide memory for pathogens, in turn providing immunity.
   b. B cells become plasma cells, which produce antibodies to foreign antigens, and also provide memory.
   c. NK cells destroy the cell membranes of foreign cells.
8. WBCs carry out their functions in tissue fluid and lymphatic tissue, as well as in the blood.

Platelets—thrombocytes (see Table 11–2 for normal values)

1. Platelets are formed in the RBM and are fragments of megakaryocytes; the hormone thrombopoietin from the liver increases platelet production.
2. Platelets help maintain the endothelium of blood vessels and are involved in all mechanisms of hemostasis (prevention of blood loss) (Fig. 11–6).
3. Vascular spasm—large vessels constrict when damaged, the myogenic response. Platelets release serotonin, which also causes vasoconstriction. The break in the vessel is made smaller and may be closed with a blood clot.
4. Platelet plugs—rupture of a capillary creates a rough surface to which platelets stick and form a barrier over the break.
5. Chemical clotting involves platelet factors, chemicals from damaged tissue, prothrombin, fibrinogen and other clotting factors synthesized by the liver, and calcium ions. Vitamin K from the intestinal microbiota is required for synthesis of some clotting factors. See Table 11–3 and Fig. 11–7 for the three stages of chemical clotting.
   a. Stage 1: Prothrombin activator is formed.
   b. Stage 2: Prothrombin activator converts prothrombin to thrombin.
   c. Stage 3: Thrombin splits fibrinogen to fibrin. The clot is formed of fibrin threads that form a mesh over the break in the vessel.
6. Clot retraction is the folding of the fibrin threads to pull the cut edges of the vessel closer together to facilitate repair. Fibrinolysis is the dissolving of the clot once it has served its purpose.
7. Abnormal clotting (thrombosis) is prevented by the very smooth endothelium (simple squamous epithelium) that lines blood vessels; heparin, which inhibits the clotting process; and antithrombin (synthesized by the liver), which inactivates excess thrombin.

REVIEW QUESTIONS

1. Name four different kinds of substances transported in blood plasma. (p. 284)
2. Name the precursor cell of all blood cells. Name the primary hemopoietic tissue and state its locations. (p. 286)
3. State the normal values (CBC) for RBCs, WBCs, platelets, hemoglobin, and hematocrit. (p. 294)
4. State the function of RBCs; include the protein and mineral needed. (p. 286)
5. Explain why iron, protein, folic acid, vitamin B_{12}, and the intrinsic factor are needed for RBC production. (p. 288)
6. Explain how bilirubin is formed and excreted. (pp. 290–291)
7. Explain what will happen if a person with type O positive blood receives a transfusion of type A negative blood. (p. 293)
8. Name the WBC with each of the following functions: (p. 295)
   a. Become macrophages and phagocytize dead tissue
   b. Produce antibodies
   c. Detoxify foreign proteins
   d. Phagocytize pathogens
   e. Contain the anticoagulant heparin
   f. Recognize antigens as foreign
   g. Secrete histamine during inflammation
9. Explain how and why platelet plugs form in ruptured capillaries. (p. 297)
10. Describe what happens in vascular spasm, and explain how it prevents excessive blood loss when a large vessel is severed. (p. 297)
11. With respect to the chemical blood clotting mechanism: (pp. 297, 300)
    a. Name the mineral necessary
    b. Name the organ that produces many of the clotting factors
    c. Name the vitamin necessary for prothrombin synthesis
    d. State what the clot itself is made of
12. Explain what is meant by clot retraction and fibrinolysis and why they are important. (p. 300)
13. State two ways abnormal clotting is prevented in the vascular system. (p. 300)
14. Explain what is meant by blood viscosity, the factors that contribute, and why viscosity is important. (p. 284)
15. State the normal pH range of blood. What gas has an effect on blood pH? (p. 284)
16. Define anemia, leukocytosis, and thrombocytopenia. (pp. 289, 295)

FOR FURTHER THOUGHT

1. Explain why type AB+ blood may be called the "universal recipient" for blood transfusions. Explain why this would not be true if the transfusion required 6 units (about 3 liters) of blood.
2. The liver has many functions that are directly related to the composition and functions of blood. Name as many as you can.
3. Constructing a brick wall requires bricks *and* bricklayers. List all the nutrients that are needed for RBC production, and indicate which are bricks and which are bricklayers.
4. Anthony moved from New Jersey to a mountain cabin in Colorado, 8000 feet above sea level. When he first arrived, his hematocrit was 44%. After 6 months in his new home, what would you expect his hematocrit to be? Explain your answer and what brought about the change.
5. The lab results for a particular patient show these CBC values:
   RBCs—4.2 million/μL
   Hct—40%
   Hb—13 g/100 mL
   WBCs—8,500/μL
   Platelets—30,000/μL
   Is this patient healthy or would you expect any symptoms of a disorder? Explain your answer.
6. Using the model in Question 5, make a list of possible CBC values for a patient with iron-deficiency anemia. Then make a list of possible CBC values for a person with aplastic anemia.
7. An artificial blood may someday be available; many are being tested. What specific function of blood will it definitely have? Are there any advantages to an artificial blood compared with blood from a human donor?
8. Disseminated intravascular coagulation (DIC) is a serious condition that may follow certain kinds of infections or traumas. First, explain what the name means. This is best done one word at a time. In DIC, clotting becomes a vicious cycle, and the blood is depleted of clotting factors. What do you think will be the consequence for the affected person?
9. Look at Question Figure 11–A: Red blood cell production before birth. The graph shows the contributions made by the liver, spleen, yolk sac, and red bone marrow to RBC formation during the 9 months of gestation. Label each line with the proper organ or tissue.

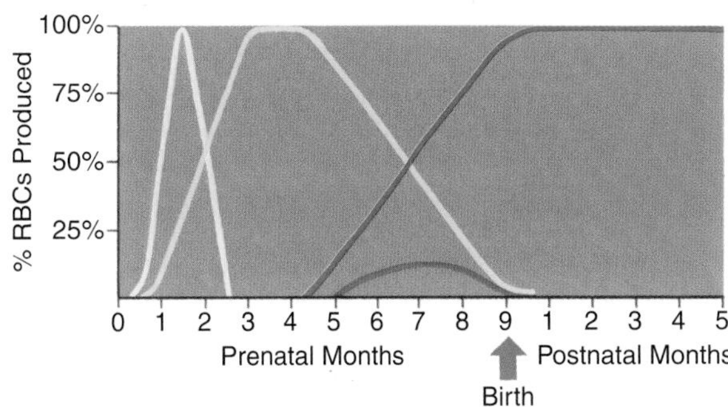

QUESTION FIGURE 11–A: Red blood cell production before birth.

CHAPTER

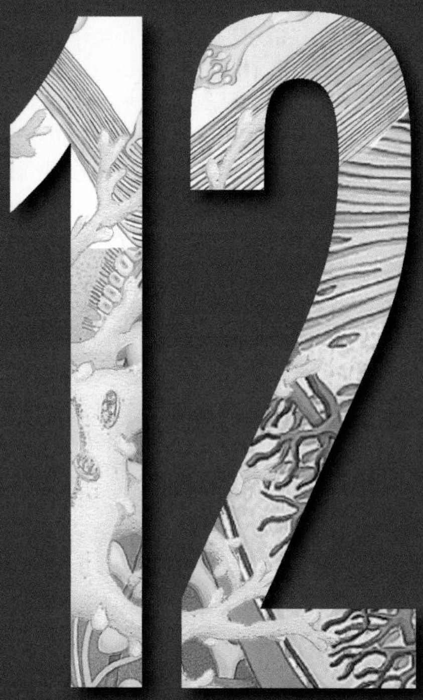

The Heart

STUDENT OBJECTIVES

- Describe the important characteristics of cardiac muscle tissue.
- Describe the location of the heart, the pericardial membranes, and the endocardium.
- Name the chambers of the heart and the vessels that enter or leave each.
- Name the valves of the heart, and explain their functions.
- Describe coronary circulation, and explain its purpose.
- Describe the cardiac cycle.
- Explain how heart sounds are created.
- Name the parts of the cardiac conduction pathway, and explain why it is the sinoatrial node that initiates each beat.
- Explain stroke volume, cardiac output, and Starling's law of the heart.
- Explain how the nervous system regulates heart rate and force of contraction.

NEW TERMINOLOGY

Aorta *(ay-**OR**-tah)*
Atrium *(**AY**-tree-um)*
Cardiac cycle *(**KAR**-dee-yak **SIGH**-kuhl)*
Cardiac output *(**KAR**-dee-yak **OUT**-put)*
Coronary arteries *(**KOR**-uh-na-ree **AR**-tuh-rees)*
Diastole *(dye-**AS**-tuh-lee)*
Endocardium *(EN-doh-**KAR**-dee-um)*
Epicardium *(EP-ee-**KAR**-dee-um)*
Mediastinum *(ME-dee-ah-**STYE**-num)*
Mitral valve *(**MY**-truhl VALV)*
Myocardium *(MY-oh-**KAR**-dee-um)*
Sinoatrial (SA) node *(**SIGH**-noh-AY-tree-al NOHD)*
Stroke volume *(STROHK **VAHL**-yoom)*
Systole *(**SIS**-tuh-lee)*
Tricuspid valve *(try-**KUSS**-pid VALV)*
Venous return *(**VEE**-nus ree-**TURN**)*
Ventricle *(**VEN**-tri-kuhl)*

RELATED CLINICAL TERMINOLOGY

Arrhythmia *(uh-**RITH**-me-yah)*
Ectopic focus *(ek-**TOP**-ik **FOH**-kus)*
Ejection fraction *(ee-**JEK**-shun **FRAK**-shun)*
Electrocardiogram (ECG) *(ee-LEK-troh-**KAR**-dee-oh-GRAM)*
Fibrillation *(fi-bri-**LAY**-shun)*
Heart murmur *(HART **MUR**-mur)*
Ischemic *(iss-**SKEE**-mik)*
Myocardial infarction *(MY-oh-**KAR**-dee-yuhl in-**FARK**-shun)*
Pulse *(PULS)*
Stenosis *(ste-**NOH**-sis)*

*Terms that appear in **bold type** in the chapter text are defined in the glossary, which begins on page 603.*

CHAPTER OUTLINE

In the embryo, the heart begins to beat at 4 weeks of age, even before its nerve supply has been established. If a person lives to be 80 years old, his or her heart continues to beat an average of 100,000 times a day, every day for each of those 80 years. Imagine trying to squeeze a tennis ball 70 times a minute. After a few minutes, your arm muscles would begin to tire. Then imagine increasing your squeezing rate to 120 times a minute. Most of us could not keep that up very long, but that is what the heart does during exercise. A healthy heart can increase its rate and force of contraction to meet the body's need for more oxygen, then return to its resting rate and keep on beating as if nothing very extraordinary had happened. In fact, it isn't extraordinary at all; this is the job the heart is meant to do.

The primary function of the heart is to pump blood through the arteries, capillaries, and veins. As you learned in the previous chapter, blood transports oxygen and nutrients and has other important functions as well. The heart is the pump that keeps blood circulating properly. Before we discuss the heart as a pump, however, let us look at the tissue that makes pumping possible: cardiac muscle.

CARDIAC MUSCLE TISSUE

Cardiac muscle cells (also called muscle fibers or myocytes) are branched, but in many other ways they are similar in structure to skeletal muscle cells (described in Chapter 7). As you would expect, many mitochondria are present. The cells are striated (see Fig. 12–1), which reflects the arrangement of the proteins myosin, actin, troponin, and others in the sarcomeres. Sarcomeres are the units of contraction. Contraction of cardiac muscle cells is also much the same as contraction of skeletal muscle fibers, and the action potential that is generated involves the same movements of sodium ions (entering the cell for depolarization) and potassium ions (leaving the cell for repolarization).

A significant difference is that cardiac myocytes generate their own action potentials; they do not require nerve impulses to contract. Another important difference is that the electrical activity of one cardiac muscle cell spreads quickly to adjacent muscle cells, by way of the **intercalated discs** that form end-to-end junctions. As you can see in Fig. 12–1, the cell membrane at the end of a cardiac muscle cell is folded extensively, and the folds fit into those of the next cell (like pudding in a mold or fingers in a glove). The folds create a great deal of surface area between cells for transmission of the action potential. When one cardiac muscle fiber depolarizes and contracts, the next one quickly does so as well, then the next one, and so on. The presence of intercalated discs enables the electrical impulse to travel so rapidly that in one heartbeat the two atria contract as a unit followed by the simultaneous contraction of the two ventricles.

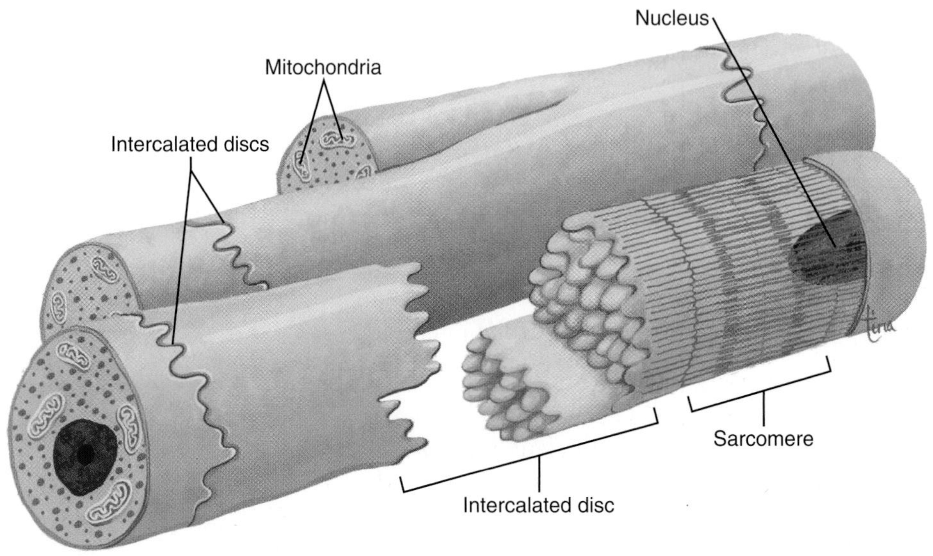

Figure 12–1 Cardiac muscle cells depicting sarcomeres and with intercalated discs at the ends of adjacent cells. The projections are folds of the cell membrane.

QUESTION: What cell membrane modification do intercalated discs resemble? Is the function the same?

Cardiac muscle is also an endocrine tissue, producing a group of hormones called the natriuretic peptides. We will use **atrial natriuretic peptide (ANP)**, also called **atrial natriuretic hormone (ANH),** as the representative of this group. ANP is produced when the walls of the atria are stretched by increased blood volume or blood pressure. ANP decreases the reabsorption of sodium ions by the kidneys, so that more sodium ions are excreted in urine, which in turn increases the elimination of water. The loss of water lowers blood volume and blood pressure and is protective for the heart, which can be damaged by chronic high blood pressure. (You may have noticed that ANP is an antagonist to the hormone aldosterone, which raises blood pressure.) Another target tissue for ANP is the smooth muscle layer of blood vessels; ANP stimulates vasodilation, which also contributes to lowering blood pressure.

Yet another target tissue for ANP is adipose tissue, and ANP promotes the conversion of white adipocytes to brown adipocytes. As you recall, white adipocytes store fat, but brown adipocytes metabolize fat in cell respiration, with the energy released as heat. Again, this is protective for the heart, in that excess fat is not stored, nor is it clogging arteries, but is broken down to CO_2 and H_2O. Additional stimuli for the secretion of ANP include exercise and exposure to cold. As you can see, by way of this chemical communication with kidney epithelium, vascular smooth muscle, and adipose tissue, the heart takes part in protecting itself.

LOCATION AND PERICARDIAL MEMBRANES

The heart is located in the thoracic cavity between the lungs. This area is called the **mediastinum**. The base of the cone-shaped heart is uppermost, behind the sternum, and the great vessels enter or leave here. The apex (tip) of the heart points downward and is just above the diaphragm to the left of the midline. This is why we may think of the heart as being on the left side, because the strongest beat can be heard or felt here.

The heart is enclosed in the **pericardial membranes**, of which there are three layers (Fig. 12–2). The outermost is the **fibrous pericardium**, a loose-fitting sac of strong fibrous connective tissue that extends inferiorly over the diaphragm and superiorly over the bases of the large vessels that enter and leave the heart. The serous pericardium is a folded membrane; the fold gives it two layers, parietal and visceral. Lining the fibrous pericardium is the **parietal pericardium**. On the surface of the heart muscle is the **visceral pericardium**, often called the **epicardium**. Between the parietal and visceral pericardial membranes is **serous fluid**, which prevents friction as the heart beats.

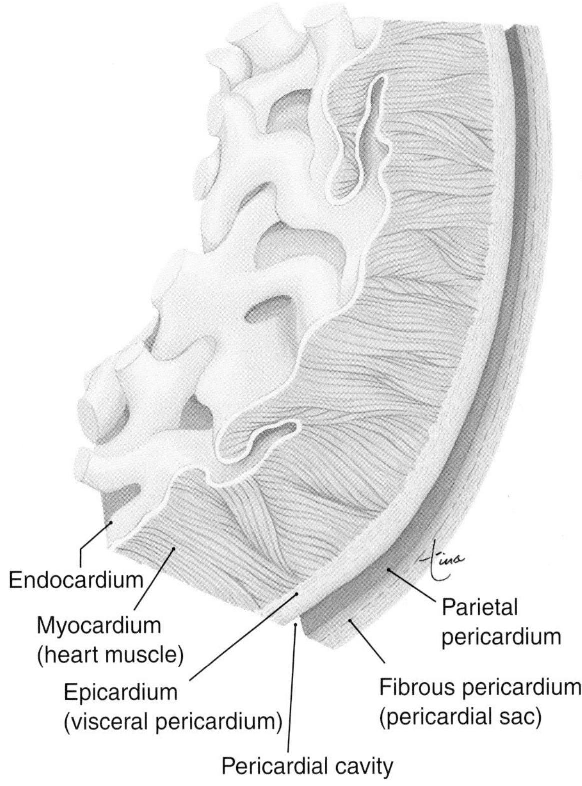

Figure 12–2 Layers of the wall of the heart and the pericardial membranes. The endocardium is the lining of the chambers of the heart. The fibrous pericardium is the outermost layer.

QUESTION: What is found between the parietal and visceral pericardial layers, and what is its function?

CHAMBERS—VESSELS AND VALVES

The thickest part of the walls of the four chambers of the heart is made of cardiac muscle. As a layer it is called the **myocardium**.

The chambers of the heart are lined with **endocardium**, simple squamous epithelium that also covers the valves of the heart and continues into the vessels as their lining (endothelium). The important physical characteristic of the endocardium is not its thinness, but rather its smoothness. This very smooth tissue prevents abnormal blood clotting, because clotting would be initiated by contact of blood with a rough surface.

The upper chambers of the heart are the right and left **atria** (singular: **atrium**), which have relatively thin walls and are separated by a common wall of myocardium called the **interatrial septum**. The lower chambers are the right and left **ventricles**, which have thicker walls and are separated by the **interventricular septum** (Fig. 12–3). As you will see, the atria receive blood, either from the body or the lungs, and the ventricles pump blood to either the lungs or the body.

RIGHT ATRIUM

The two large **caval veins** return blood from the body to the right atrium (see Fig. 12–3). The **superior vena cava** carries blood from the upper body, and the **inferior vena cava** carries blood from the lower body. From the right atrium, blood will flow through the **right atrioventricular (AV) valve**, or **tricuspid valve**, into the right ventricle.

The tricuspid valve is made of three flaps (or cusps) of endocardium reinforced with connective tissue. The general purpose of all valves in the circulatory system is to prevent backflow of blood. The specific purpose of the tricuspid valve is to prevent backflow of blood from the right ventricle to the right atrium when the right ventricle contracts. As the ventricle contracts, blood is forced behind the three valve flaps, forcing them upward and together to close the valve.

LEFT ATRIUM

The left atrium receives blood from the lungs, by way of four **pulmonary veins**. This blood will then flow into the left ventricle through the left atrioventricular (AV) valve, also called the **mitral valve** or **bicuspid** (two flaps) valve. The mitral valve prevents backflow of blood from the left ventricle to the left atrium when the left ventricle contracts.

RIGHT VENTRICLE

When the right ventricle contracts, the pressure closes the tricuspid valve and the blood is pumped to the lungs through the pulmonary artery (or trunk). At the junction of this large artery and the right ventricle is the **pulmonary semilunar valve** (or more simply, pulmonary valve). Its three flaps are forced open when the right ventricle contracts and pumps blood into the pulmonary artery. When the right ventricle relaxes, blood tends to come back, but this fills the valve flaps and closes the pulmonary valve to prevent backflow of blood into the right ventricle.

Projecting into the lower part of the right ventricle are columns of myocardium called **papillary muscles** (see Fig. 12–3). Strands of fibrous connective tissue, the **chordae tendineae**, extend from the papillary muscles to the flaps of the tricuspid valve. When the right ventricle contracts, the papillary muscles also contract and pull on the chordae tendineae to prevent inversion of the tricuspid valve. If you have ever had your umbrella blown inside out by a strong wind, you can imagine what would happen if the flaps of the tricuspid valve were not anchored by the chordae tendineae and papillary muscles.

LEFT VENTRICLE

The walls of the left ventricle are thicker than those of the right ventricle, which enables the left ventricle to contract more forcefully. The left ventricle pumps blood to the body through the **aorta**, the largest artery of the body. At the junction of the aorta and the left ventricle is the **aortic semilunar valve** (or aortic valve) (see Fig. 12–3). This valve is opened by the force of contraction of the left ventricle, which also closes the mitral valve. The aortic valve closes when the left ventricle relaxes, to prevent backflow of blood from the aorta to the left ventricle. When the mitral (left AV) valve closes, it prevents backflow of blood to the left atrium; the flaps of the mitral valve are also anchored by chordae tendineae and papillary muscles.

All of the valves are shown in Fig. 12–4, which also depicts the **fibrous skeleton of the heart**. This is fibrous connective tissue that anchors the outer edges of the valve flaps and keeps the valve openings from stretching. It also separates the myocardium of the atria and ventricles and prevents the contraction of the atria from reaching the ventricles except by way of the normal conduction pathway.

As you can see from this description of the chambers and their vessels, the heart is really a double, or two-sided, pump. The right side of the heart receives deoxygenated blood from the body and pumps it to the lungs to pick up oxygen and release carbon dioxide. The left side of the heart receives oxygenated blood from the lungs and pumps it to the body. Both pumps work simultaneously; that is, both atria contract together, followed by the contraction of both ventricles. Aspects of the anatomy of the heart are summarized in Table 12–1.

CORONARY VESSELS

The right and left **coronary arteries** are the first branches of the ascending aorta, just beyond the aortic semilunar valve (Fig. 12–5). The two arteries branch into smaller arteries and arterioles, then to capillaries. The coronary capillaries merge to form coronary veins, which empty

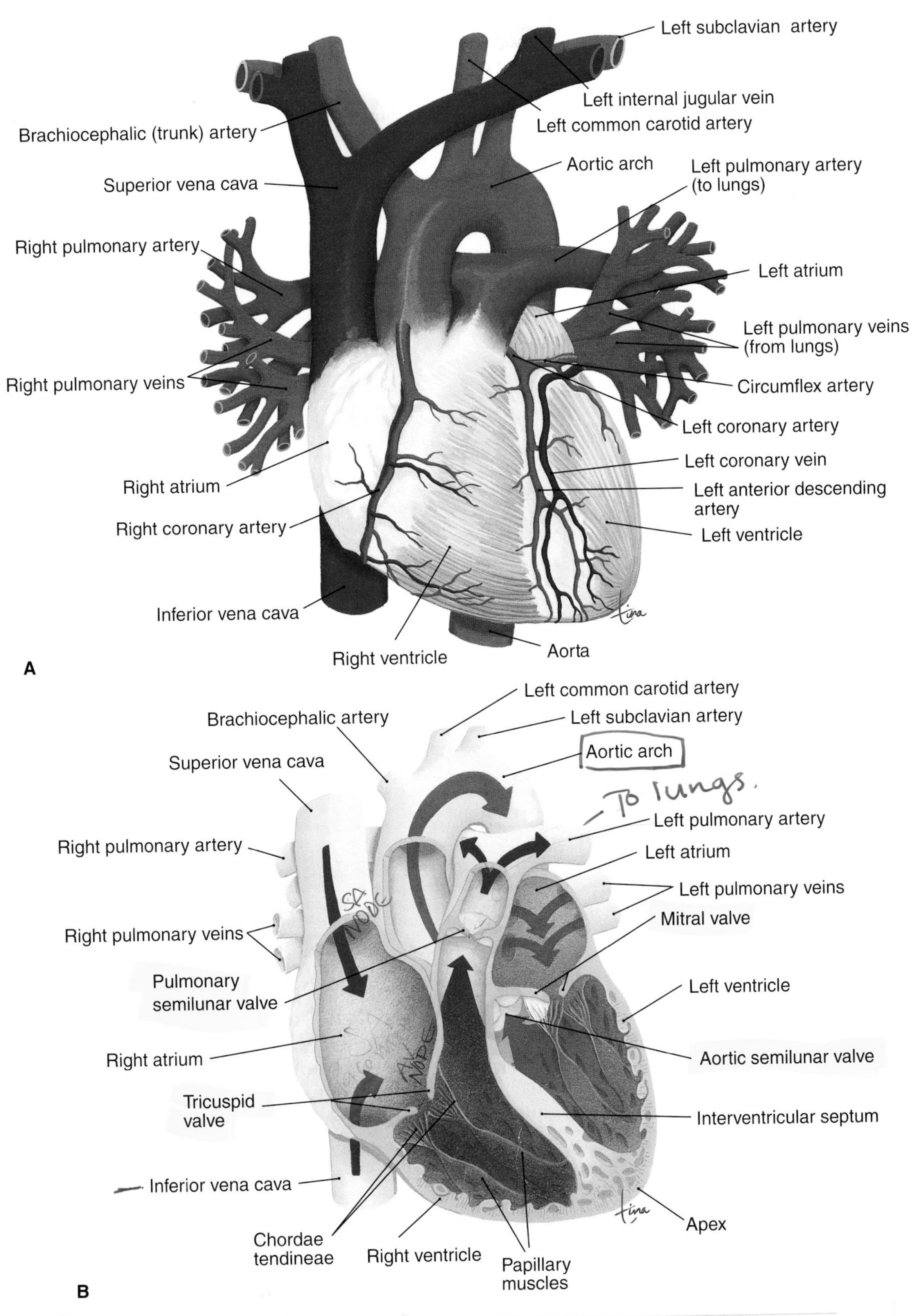

Figure 12–3 (**A**) Anterior view of the heart and major blood vessels. (**B**) Frontal section of the heart in anterior view, showing internal structures.

QUESTION: In part B, in the right atrium, what do the blue arrows represent?

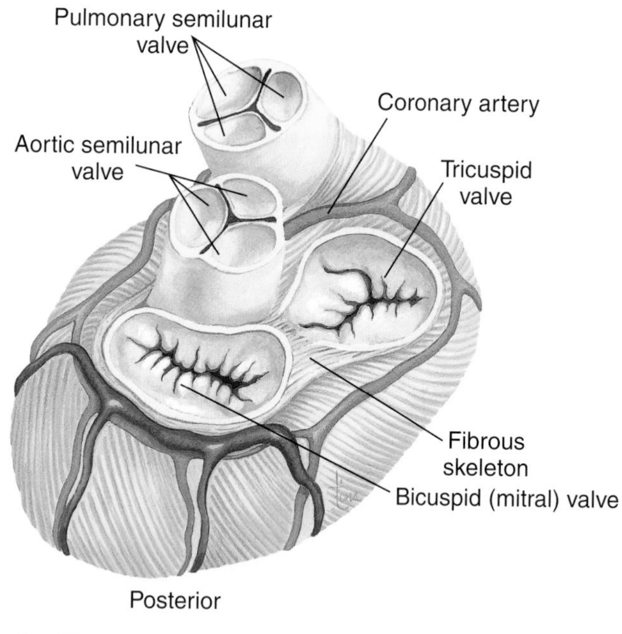

Figure 12–4 Heart valves in superior view. The atria have been removed. The fibrous skeleton of the heart is also shown.

QUESTION: When do the mitral and tricuspid valves close, and why is this important?

blood into a large coronary sinus that returns blood to the right atrium.

The purpose of the coronary vessels is to circulate oxygenated blood throughout the myocardium; oxygen is essential for normal myocardial contraction. If a coronary artery becomes obstructed, by a blood clot for example, part of the myocardium becomes **ischemic**, that is, deprived of its blood supply. Prolonged ischemia will create an **infarct**, an area of necrotic (dead) tissue. This is a **myocardial infarction**, commonly called a heart attack (see also Box 12–1: Coronary Artery Disease).

CARDIAC CYCLE AND HEART SOUNDS

The **cardiac cycle** is the sequence of events in one heartbeat. In its simplest form, the cardiac cycle is the simultaneous contraction of the two atria, followed a fraction of a second later by the simultaneous contraction of the two ventricles. **Systole** is another term for contraction. The term for relaxation is **diastole**. You are probably familiar with these terms as they apply to blood pressure readings. If we apply them to the cardiac cycle, we can say that atrial systole is followed by ventricular systole. There is, however, a significant difference between the movement of blood from the atria to the ventricles and the movement of blood from the ventricles to the arteries. The events of

Table 12–1 | **ANATOMY OF THE HEART**

STRUCTURE	DESCRIPTION
Epicardium	Serous membrane on the surface of the myocardium
Myocardium	Heart muscle; forms the walls of the four chambers
Endocardium	Endothelium that lines the chambers and covers the valves; smooth to prevent abnormal clotting
Right atrium (RA)	Receives deoxygenated blood from the body by way of the superior and inferior caval veins; the atria produce atrial natriuretic peptide (ANP), which increases urinary output and converts white adipocytes to brown fat cells
Tricuspid valve	Right AV valve; prevents backflow of blood from the RV to the RA when the RV contracts
Right ventricle (RV)	Pumps blood to the lungs by way of the pulmonary artery
Pulmonary semilunar valve	Prevents backflow of blood from the pulmonary artery to the RV when the RV relaxes
Left atrium (LA)	Receives oxygenated blood from the lungs by way of the four pulmonary veins; produces ANP

Table 12–1 | ANATOMY OF THE HEART—cont'd

STRUCTURE	DESCRIPTION
Mitral valve	Left AV valve; prevents backflow of blood from the LV to the LA when the LV contracts
Left ventricle (LV)	Pumps blood to the body by way of the aorta
Aortic semilunar valve	Prevents backflow of blood from the aorta to the LV when the LV relaxes
Papillary muscles and chordae tendineae	In both the RV and LV; prevent inversion of the AV valves when the ventricles contract
Fibrous skeleton of the heart	Fibrous connective tissue that anchors the four heart valves, prevents enlargement of the valve openings, and electrically insulates the ventricles from the atria

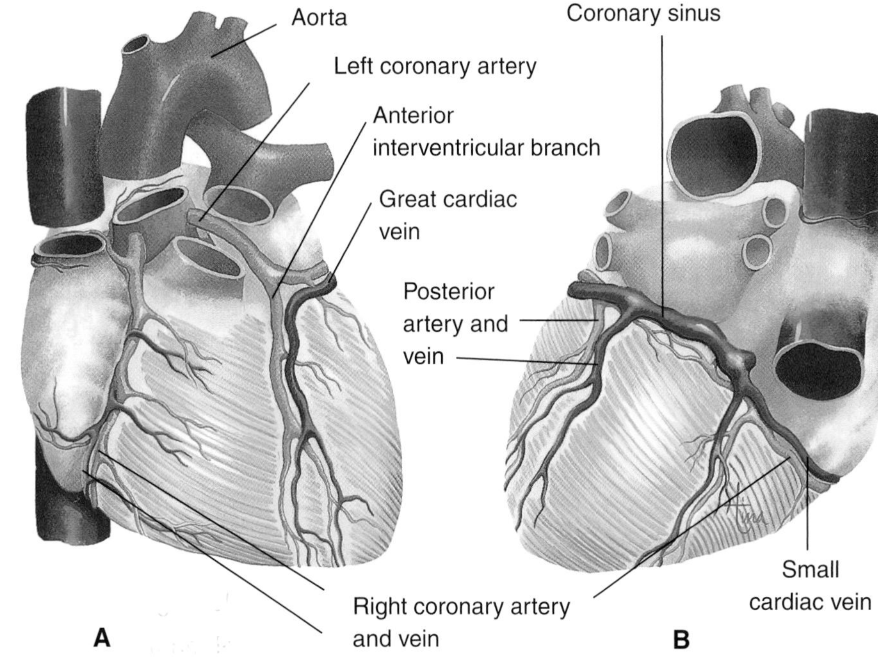

Figure 12–5 (**A**) Coronary vessels in anterior view. The pulmonary artery has been cut to show the left coronary artery emerging from the ascending aorta. (**B**) Coronary vessels in posterior view. The coronary sinus empties blood into the right atrium.

QUESTION: What is the function of the coronary vessels?

Box 12–1 | CORONARY ARTERY DISEASE

Coronary artery disease results in decreased blood flow to the myocardium. If blood flow is diminished but not completely obstructed, the person may experience difficulty breathing and angina, which is chest pain caused by lack of oxygen to part of the heart muscle. If blood flow is completely blocked, however, the result is a **myocardial infarction** (necrosis of cardiac muscle).

The most common cause of coronary artery disease is **atherosclerosis**. Plaques of cholesterol and inflammatory cells form in the walls of a coronary artery; this narrows the lumen (cavity) and

Continued

Box 12–1 | CORONARY ARTERY DISEASE *(Continued)*

creates a rough surface where a clot (thrombus) may form (see Box Fig. 12–A). A predisposing factor for such clot formation, one that cannot be changed, is a family history of coronary artery disease. There is no "gene for heart attacks," but we do have genes for the enzymes involved in cholesterol metabolism. Many of these are liver enzymes that regulate the transport of cholesterol in the blood in the form of lipoproteins and regulate the liver's excretion of excess cholesterol in bile. Some people, therefore, have a greater tendency than others to have higher blood levels of cholesterol and certain lipoproteins. In women before menopause, estrogen is believed to exert a protective effect by lowering blood lipid levels. This is why heart attacks in the 30- to 50-year-old age range are less frequent in women than in men.

Other predisposing factors for atherosclerosis include cigarette smoking, diabetes mellitus, and high blood pressure. Any one of these may cause damage to the lining of coronary arteries, which is the first step in the abnormal deposition of cholesterol. A diet high in cholesterol and saturated fats and high blood levels of these lipids will increase the rate of cholesterol deposition.

Chemical markers in the blood that signal the presence of inflammation include homocysteine and C-reactive protein (CRP). These markers do not cause heart attacks; they are instead indicators of increased inflammation, which may be a risk factor for a heart attack. There is still much to learn about the role of inflammation in atherosclerosis.

When coronary artery disease becomes life-threatening, coronary artery bypass surgery may be performed. In this procedure, a synthetic vessel or a vein (such as the saphenous vein of the leg) is grafted around the obstructed coronary vessel to restore blood flow to the myocardium. This is not a cure because atherosclerosis may occur in a grafted vein or at other sites in the coronary arteries.

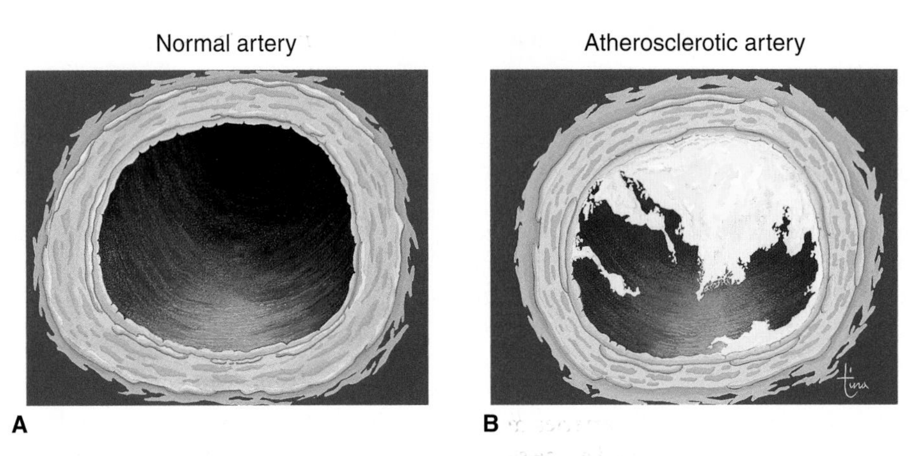

Box Figure 12–A (**A**) Cross-section of normal coronary artery. (**B**) Coronary artery with atherosclerosis narrowing the lumen.

the cardiac cycle are shown in Fig. 12–6. In this traditional representation, the cardiac cycle is depicted in a circle because one heartbeat follows another, and the beginning of atrial systole is at the top (12 o'clock). The size of the segment or arc of the circle indicates how long it takes. Find the segment for atrial systole and the one for ventricular systole, and notice how much larger (meaning "longer") ventricular systole is. Do you think this might mean that ventricular contraction is more important than atrial contraction? It does, as you will see. Refer to Fig. 12–5 as you read the following. We will begin at the bottom (6 o'clock) where the atria are in the midst of diastole and the ventricles have just completed their systole. The entire heart is relaxed and the atria are filling with blood.

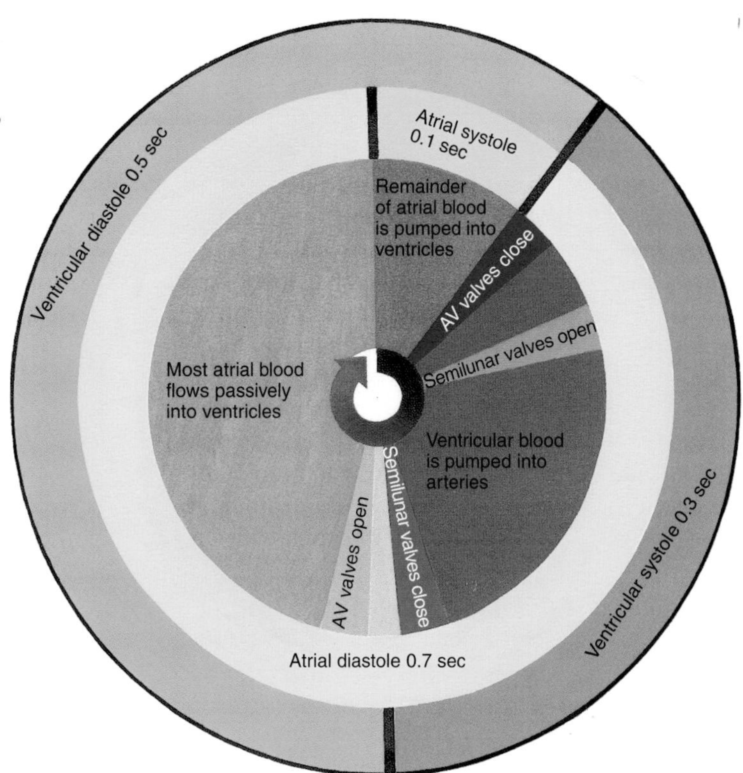

Figure 12–6 The cardiac cycle depicted in one heartbeat (pulse: 75). The outer circle represents the ventricles, the middle circle the atria, and the inner circle the movement of blood and its effect on the heart valves. See text for description.

QUESTION: What makes the AV valves close and the semilunar valves open?

Blood is constantly flowing from the veins into both atria. As more blood accumulates, its pressure forces open the right and left AV valves. Two-thirds of the atrial blood flows passively into the ventricles (which brings us to 12 o'clock); the atria then contract to pump the remaining blood into the ventricles.

Following their contraction, the atria relax and the ventricles begin to contract. Ventricular contraction forces blood against the flaps of the right and left AV valves and closes them; the force of blood also opens the aortic and pulmonary semilunar valves. As the ventricles continue to contract, they pump blood into the arteries. Notice that blood that enters the arteries must all be pumped. The ventricles then relax, and at the same time blood continues to flow into the atria, and the cycle begins again.

The important distinction here is that most blood flows passively from atria to ventricles, but *all* blood to the arteries is actively pumped by the ventricles. For this reason, the proper functioning of the ventricles is much more crucial to survival than is atrial functioning.

You may be asking: "All this in one heartbeat?" The answer is yes. The cardiac cycle is this precise sequence of events that keeps blood moving from the veins, through the heart, and into the arteries.

The cardiac cycle also creates the **heart sounds**: Each heartbeat produces two sounds, often called "lub-dup," that can be heard with a stethoscope. The first sound, the loudest and longest, is caused by ventricular systole closing the AV valves. The second sound is caused by the closure of the aortic and pulmonary semilunar valves. If any of the valves do not close properly, an extra sound called a **heart murmur** may be heard (see Box 12–2: Heart Murmur).

CARDIAC CONDUCTION PATHWAY

The cardiac cycle is a sequence of mechanical events that is regulated by the electrical activity of the myocardium. Cardiac muscle cells have the ability to contract spontaneously; that is, nerve impulses are not required to cause contraction, as they are to cause contraction of skeletal muscle cells. Cells of the myocardium generate their own electrical action potentials, which are similar to those brought about in skeletal muscle cells by nerve impulses (described in Chapter 7). Cardiac myocytes are branched and have intercalated discs; their electrical activity spreads quickly to adjacent muscle cells. The presence of intercalated discs enables the electrical impulse to travel so rapidly that the two atria contract as a unit in the cardiac cycle, followed by the simultaneous contraction of the two ventricles.

Box 12–2 | HEART MURMUR

A heart murmur is an abnormal or extra heart sound caused by a malfunctioning heart valve. The function of heart valves is to prevent backflow of blood, and when a valve does not close properly, blood will regurgitate (go backward), creating turbulence that may be heard with a stethoscope.

Rheumatic heart disease is a now uncommon complication of a streptococcal infection. In rheumatic fever, the heart valves are damaged by an abnormal response by the immune system. Erosion of the valves makes them "leaky" and inefficient, and a murmur of backflowing blood will be heard. Mitral valve regurgitation, for example, will be heard as a systolic murmur because this valve is meant to close and prevent backflow during ventricular systole.

Some valve defects involve a narrowing (**stenosis**) and are congenital; that is, the child is born with an abnormally narrow valve. In aortic stenosis, for example, blood cannot easily pass from the left ventricle to the aorta. The ventricle must then work harder to pump blood through the narrow valve to the arteries, and the turbulence created is also heard as a systolic murmur.

Children sometimes have heart murmurs that are called "functional" because no structural cause can be found. These murmurs usually disappear with no adverse effects on the child.

Each heartbeat is generated by the heart itself, and the electrical impulses follow a very specific route throughout the myocardium. You may find it helpful to refer to Fig. 12–7 as you read the following.

The natural pacemaker of the heart is the **sinoatrial (SA) node**, a specialized group of cardiac muscle cells located in the wall of the right atrium just below the opening of the superior vena cava. The SA node is considered specialized because it has the most rapid natural rate of contraction, that is, it depolarizes more rapidly than any other part of the myocardium (60 to 80 times per minute). Recall that depolarization is the rapid entry of Na^+ ions and the reversal of charges on either side of the cell membrane. The cells of the SA node are more permeable to Na^+ ions than are other cardiac muscle cells. Therefore, they depolarize more rapidly, then contract and initiate each heartbeat.

From the SA node, impulses for contraction travel to the **atrioventricular (AV) node**, located in the lower interatrial septum. The transmission of impulses from the SA node to the AV node and to the rest of the atrial myocardium brings about atrial systole.

Recall that the fibrous skeleton of the heart separates the atrial myocardium from the ventricular myocardium; the fibrous connective tissue acts as electrical insulation between the two sets of chambers. The only pathway for impulses from the atria to the ventricles, therefore, is the **atrioventricular bundle (AV bundle)**, also called the **bundle of His**. The AV bundle is within the upper interventricular septum; it receives impulses from the AV node and transmits them to the right and left **bundle branches**. From the bundle branches, impulses travel along **Purkinje fibers** to the rest of the ventricular myocardium and bring about ventricular systole. The electrical activity of the atria and ventricles is depicted by an electrocardiogram (ECG); this is discussed in Box 12–3: Electrocardiogram.

If the SA node does not function properly, the AV node will initiate the heartbeat, but at a slower rate (50 to 60 beats per minute). The AV bundle is also capable of generating the beat of the ventricles, but at a much slower rate (15 to 40 beats per minute). This may occur in certain kinds of heart disease in which transmission of impulses from the atria to the ventricles is blocked.

Arrhythmias are irregular heartbeats; their effects range from harmless to life-threatening. Nearly everyone experiences heart **palpitations** (becoming aware of an irregular beat) from time to time. These are usually not serious and may be the result of too much caffeine, nicotine, or alcohol. Much more serious is ventricular **fibrillation**, a very rapid and uncoordinated ventricular beat that is totally ineffective for pumping blood (see Box 12–4: Arrhythmias).

HEART RATE

A healthy adult has a resting heart rate (**pulse**) of 60 to 80 beats per minute, which is the rate of depolarization of the SA node. (The SA node actually has a slightly faster rate, closer to 100 beats per minute, but is slowed by parasympathetic nerve impulses to what we consider a normal resting rate.) A rate less than 60 (except for athletes) is called **bradycardia**; a prolonged or consistent rate greater than 100 beats per minute is called **tachycardia**.

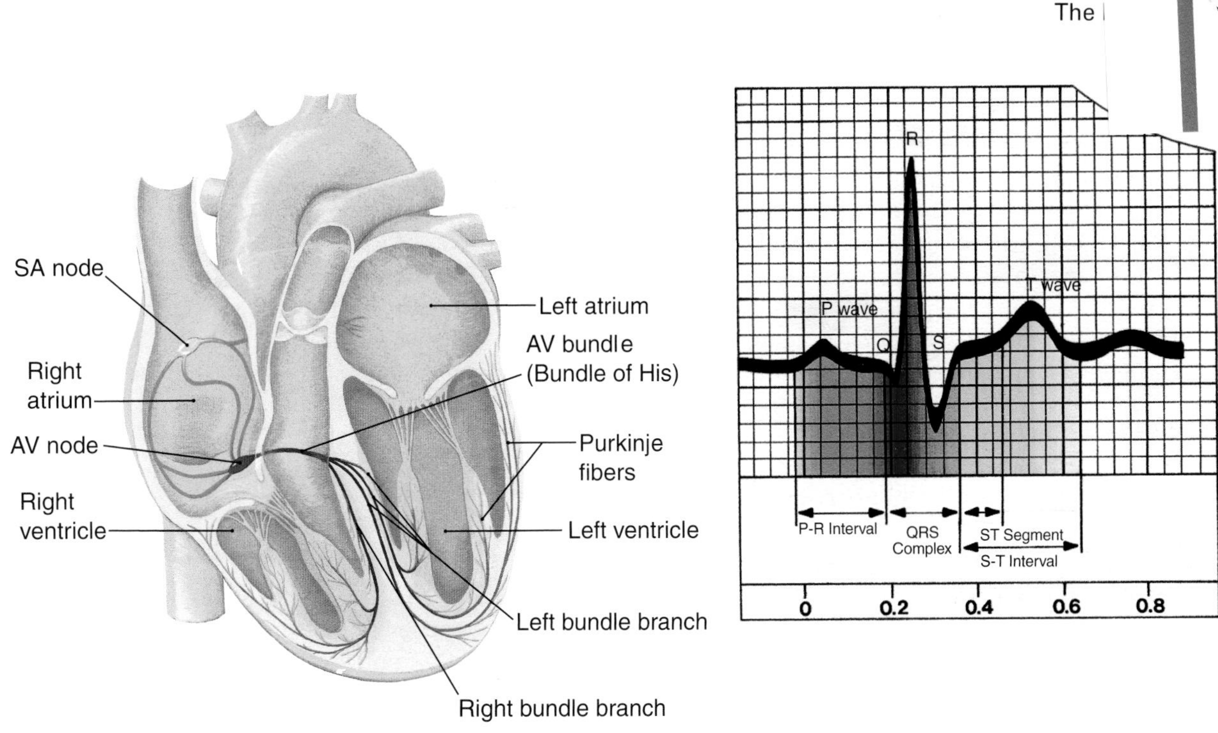

Figure 12–7 Conduction pathway of the heart. Anterior view of the interior of the heart. The electrocardiogram tracing is of one normal heartbeat. See text and Box 12–3 for description.

QUESTION: What structure is the pacemaker of the heart, and what is its usual rate of depolarization?

Box 12–3 | ELECTROCARDIOGRAM

A heartbeat is a series of electrical events, and the electrical changes generated by the myocardium can be recorded by placing electrodes on the body surface. Such a recording is called an **electrocardiogram (ECG)** (see Fig. 12–7).

A typical ECG consists of three distinguishable waves or deflections: the P wave, the QRS complex, and the T wave. Each represents a specific electrical event; all are shown in Fig. 12–7 in a normal ECG tracing.

The P wave represents depolarization of the atria, that is, the transmission of electrical impulses from the SA node throughout the atrial myocardium.

The QRS complex represents depolarization of the ventricles as the electrical impulses spread throughout the ventricular myocardium. The T wave represents repolarization of the ventricles (atrial repolarization does not appear as a separate wave because it is masked by the QRS complex).

Detailed interpretation of abnormal ECGs is beyond the scope of this book, but in general, the length of each wave and the time intervals between waves are noted. An ECG may be helpful in the diagnosis of coronary atherosclerosis, which deprives the myocardium of oxygen, or of rheumatic fever or other valve disorders that result in enlargement of a chamber of the heart and prolong a specific wave of an ECG. For example, the enlargement of the left ventricle that is often a consequence of hypertension may be indicated by an abnormal QRS complex.

Box 12–4 | ARRHYTHMIAS

Arrhythmias (also called dysrhythmias) are irregular heartbeats caused by damage to part of the conduction pathway, or by an **ectopic focus**, which is a beat generated in part of the myocardium other than the SA node.

Flutter is a very rapid but fairly regular heartbeat. In atrial flutter, the atria may contract up to 300 times per minute. Because atrial pumping is not crucial, however, blood flow to the ventricles may be maintained for a time, and flutter may not be immediately life-threatening. Ventricular flutter is usually only a brief transition between ventricular tachycardia and fibrillation.

Fibrillation is very rapid and uncoordinated contractions. Atrial fibrillation is usually not rapidly fatal, but pooling of blood in the atria increases the risk of clot formation and subsequent stroke. Ventricular fibrillation is a medical emergency that must be quickly corrected to prevent death. Normal contraction of the ventricles is necessary to pump blood into the arteries, but fibrillating ventricles are not pumping, and cardiac output decreases sharply.

Ventricular fibrillation may follow a non-fatal heart attack (myocardial infarction). Damaged cardiac muscle cells may not be able to maintain a normal state of polarization, and they depolarize spontaneously and rapidly. From this ectopic focus, impulses spread to other parts of the ventricular myocardium in a rapid and haphazard pattern, and the ventricles quiver rather than contract as a unit.

It is often possible to correct ventricular fibrillation with the use of an electrical defibrillator. This instrument delivers an electric shock to the heart, which causes the entire myocardium to depolarize and contract, then relax. If the first part of the heart to recover is the SA node (which usually has the most rapid rate of contraction), a normal heartbeat may be restored.

A child's normal heart rate may be as high as 100 beats per minute, that of an infant as high as 120, and that of a near-term fetus as high as 140 beats per minute. These higher rates are not related to age, but rather to size: the smaller the individual, the higher the metabolic rate and the faster the heart rate. Parallels may be found among animals of different sizes; the heart rate of a mouse is about 200 beats per minute and that of an elephant about 30 beats per minute.

Let us return to the adult heart rate and consider the person who is in excellent physical condition. As you may know, well-conditioned athletes have low resting pulse rates. Those of basketball players are often around 50 beats per minute, and the pulse of a marathon runner often ranges from 35 to 40 beats per minute. To understand why this is so, remember that the heart is a muscle. When our skeletal muscles are exercised, they become stronger and more efficient. The same is true for the heart; consistent exercise makes it a more efficient pump, as you will see in the next section.

CARDIAC OUTPUT

Cardiac output is the amount of blood pumped by a ventricle in 1 minute. A certain level of cardiac output is needed at all times to transport oxygen to tissues and to remove waste products. During exercise, cardiac output must increase to meet the body's need for more oxygen. We will return to exercise after first considering resting cardiac output.

To calculate cardiac output, we must know the **pulse** rate and how much blood is pumped per beat. **Stroke volume** is the term for the amount of blood pumped by a ventricle per beat; an average resting stroke volume is 60 to 80 mL per beat. A simple formula then enables us to determine cardiac output:

$$\text{Cardiac output} = \text{stroke volume} \times \text{pulse (heart rate)}$$

Let us put into this formula an average resting stroke volume, 70 mL, and an average resting pulse, 70 beats per minute (bpm):

$$\text{Cardiac output} = 70 \text{ mL} \times 70 \text{ bpm}$$
$$\text{Cardiac output} = 4900 \text{ mL per minute}$$
$$\text{(approximately 5 L)}$$

Naturally, cardiac output varies with the size of the person, but the average resting cardiac output is 5 to 6 L per minute. Notice that this amount is just about the same as a person's average volume of blood. At rest, the heart pumps all of the blood in the body within about a minute. Changes are possible, of course, depending on circumstances and extent of physical activity.

If we now reconsider the athlete, you will be able to see precisely why the athlete has a low resting pulse. In our formula, we will use an average resting cardiac output (5 L) and an athlete's pulse rate (50):

$$\text{Cardiac output} = \text{stroke volume} \times \text{pulse}$$
$$5000 \text{ mL} = \text{stroke volume} \times 50 \text{ bpm}$$
$$5000/50 = \text{stroke volume}$$
$$100 \text{ mL} = \text{stroke volume}$$

Notice that the athlete's resting stroke volume is significantly higher than the average. The athlete's more efficient heart pumps more blood with each beat and so can maintain a normal resting cardiac output with fewer beats.

Now let us see how the heart responds to exercise. Heart rate (pulse) increases during exercise, and so does stroke volume. The increase in stroke volume is the result of **Starling's law of the heart**, which states that the more the cardiac muscle fibers are stretched, the more forcefully they contract. During exercise, more blood returns to the heart; this is called **venous return**. Increased venous return stretches the myocardium of the ventricles, which contract more forcefully and pump more blood, thereby increasing stroke volume. Therefore, during exercise, our formula might have the following values:

$$\text{Cardiac output} = \text{stroke volume} \times \text{pulse}$$
$$\text{Cardiac output} = 100 \text{ mL} \times 100 \text{ bpm}$$
$$\text{Cardiac output} = 10{,}000 \text{ mL (10 liters)}$$

This exercise cardiac output is twice the resting cardiac output we first calculated, which should not be considered unusual. The cardiac output of a healthy young person may increase up to four times the resting level during strenuous exercise. This difference is the **cardiac reserve**, the extra volume the heart can pump when necessary. If resting cardiac output is 5 L and exercise cardiac output is 20 L, the cardiac reserve is 15 L. The marathon runner's cardiac output may increase six times or more compared to the resting level, and cardiac reserve is even greater than for the average young person; this is the result of the marathoner's extremely efficient heart. Because of Starling's law, it is almost impossible to overwork a healthy heart. No matter how much the volume of venous return increases, the ventricles simply pump more forcefully and increase the stroke volume and cardiac output.

Also related to cardiac output, and another measure of the health of the heart, is the **ejection fraction**. This is the percent of the blood in a ventricle that is pumped during systole. A ventricle does not empty completely when it contracts but should pump out 60% to 70% of the blood within it. A lower percentage would indicate that the ventricle is weakening. These aspects of physiology are summarized in Table 12–2.

REGULATION OF HEART RATE

Although the heart generates and maintains its own beat, the rate of contraction can be changed to adapt to different situations. The nervous system can and does bring about necessary changes in heart rate, as well as in force of contraction.

The **medulla** of the brain contains the two cardiac centers, the **accelerator center** and the **inhibitory center**. These centers send impulses to the heart along autonomic nerves. Recall from Chapter 8 that the autonomic nervous

Table 12–2 | PHYSIOLOGY OF THE HEART

ASPECT AND NORMAL RANGE	DESCRIPTION
Heart rate (pulse): 60–80 bpm	Generated by the SA node, propagated through the conduction pathway; parasympathetic impulses (vagus nerves) decrease the rate; sympathetic impulses increase the rate
Stroke volume: 60–80 mL/beat	The amount of blood pumped by a ventricle in 1 beat
Cardiac output: 5–6 L/min	The volume of blood pumped by a ventricle in 1 minute; stroke volume × pulse
Ejection fraction: 60%–70%	The percentage of blood within a ventricle that is pumped out per beat
Cardiac reserve: 15 L or more	The difference between resting cardiac output and maximum cardiac output during exercise

system has two divisions: sympathetic and parasympathetic. Sympathetic impulses from the accelerator center along sympathetic nerves increase heart rate and force of contraction during exercise and stressful situations (the neurotransmitter is norepinephrine). Parasympathetic impulses from the inhibitory center along the vagus nerves decrease the heart rate (the neurotransmitter is acetylcholine). At rest these impulses slow down the depolarization of the SA node to what we consider a normal resting rate, and they also slow the heart after exercise is over.

Our next question might be: What information is received by the medulla to initiate changes? Because the heart pumps blood, it is essential to maintain normal blood pressure. Blood contains oxygen, which all tissues must receive continuously. Therefore, changes in blood pressure and oxygen level of the blood are stimuli for changes in heart rate.

You may also recall from Chapter 9 that pressoreceptors and chemoreceptors are located in the carotid arteries and aortic arch. **Pressoreceptors** in the carotid sinuses and aortic sinus detect changes in blood pressure. **Chemoreceptors** in the carotid bodies and aortic body detect changes in the oxygen content of the blood. The sensory nerves for the carotid receptors are the glossopharyngeal (9th cranial) nerves; the sensory nerves for the aortic arch receptors are the vagus (10th cranial) nerves. If we now put all of these facts together in a specific example, you will see that the regulation of heart rate is a reflex, and the nerve impulses follow a reflex arc. Figure 12–8 depicts all of the structures just mentioned.

A person who stands up suddenly from a lying position may feel light-headed or dizzy for a few moments because blood pressure to the brain has decreased abruptly. The

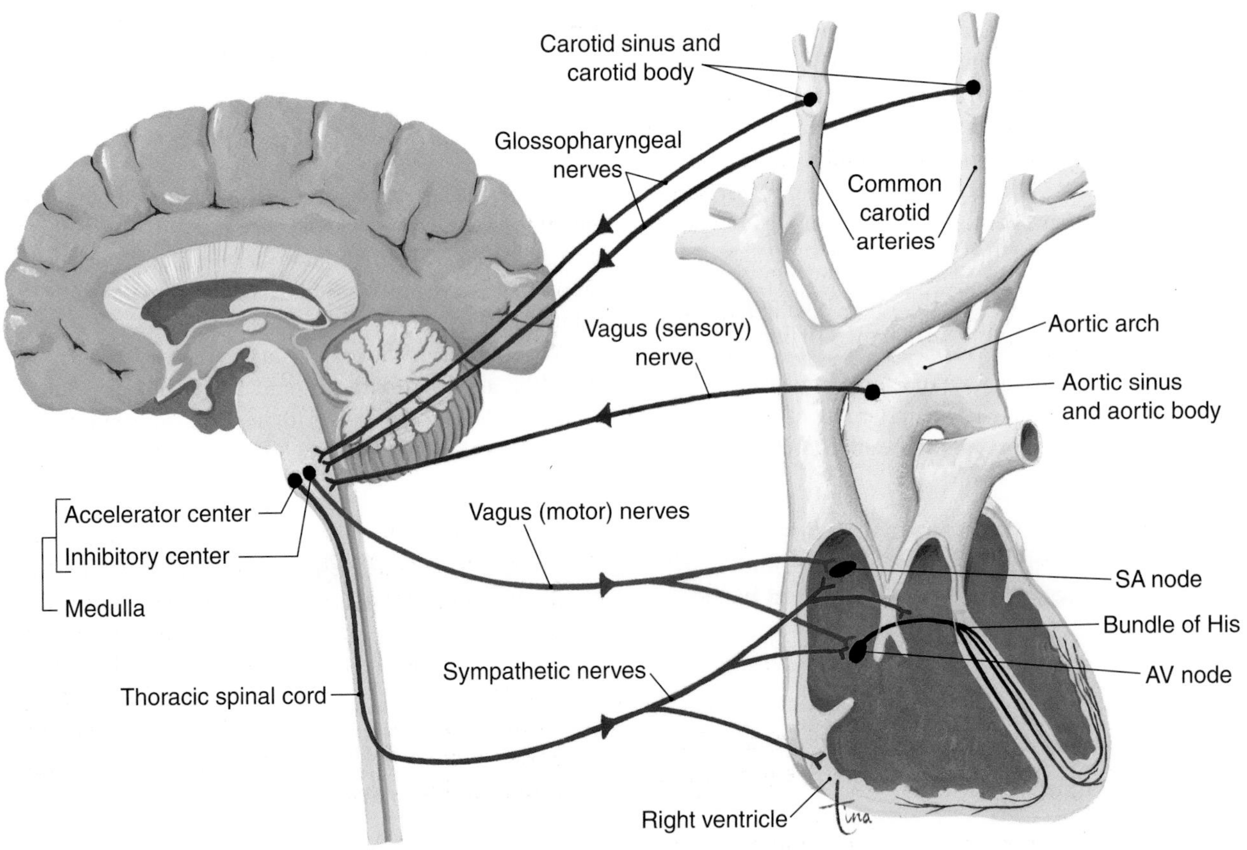

Figure 12–8 Nervous regulation of the heart. The brain and spinal cord are shown on the left. The heart and major blood vessels are shown on the right.

QUESTION: Sympathetic impulses to the ventricles will have what effect?

drop in blood pressure is detected by pressoreceptors in the carotid sinuses—notice that they are "on the way" to the brain, a very strategic location. The drop in blood pressure causes fewer impulses to be generated by the pressoreceptors. These impulses travel along the glossopharyngeal nerves to the medulla, and the decrease in the frequency of impulses stimulates the accelerator center. The accelerator center generates impulses that are carried by sympathetic nerves to the SA node, AV node, and ventricular myocardium. As heart rate and force increase, blood pressure to the brain is raised to normal, and the sensation of lightheadedness passes. When blood pressure to the brain is restored to normal, the heart receives more parasympathetic impulses from the inhibitory center along the vagus nerves to the SA node and AV node. These parasympathetic impulses slow the heart rate to a normal resting pace.

The heart will also be the effector in a reflex stimulated by a decrease in the oxygen content of the blood. The aortic receptors are strategically located so as to detect such an important change as soon as blood leaves the heart. The reflex arc in this situation would be (1) aortic chemoreceptors, (2) vagus nerves (sensory), (3) accelerator center in the medulla, (4) sympathetic nerves, and (5) the heart muscle, which will increase its rate and force of contraction to circulate more oxygen to correct the hypoxemia.

Recall also from Chapter 10 that the hormone epinephrine is secreted by the adrenal medulla in stressful situations. One of the many functions of epinephrine is to increase heart rate and force of contraction. This will help supply more blood to tissues in need of more oxygen to cope with the stressful situation.

AGING AND THE HEART

The heart muscle becomes less efficient with age, and there is a decrease in both maximum cardiac output and heart rate, although resting levels may be more than adequate. The health of the myocardium depends on its blood supply, and with age there is greater likelihood that atherosclerosis will narrow the coronary arteries. Atherosclerosis is the deposition of cholesterol on and in the walls of the arteries, which decreases blood flow and forms rough surfaces that may cause intravascular clot formation.

High blood pressure (hypertension) causes the left ventricle to work harder; it may enlarge and outgrow its blood supply, thus becoming weaker. A weak ventricle is not an efficient pump, and such weakness may progress to congestive heart failure; such a progression may be slow or rapid. The heart valves may become thickened by fibrosis, leading to heart murmurs and less efficient pumping. Arrhythmias are also more common with age, as the cells of the conduction pathway become less efficient.

SUMMARY

As you can see, the nervous system regulates the functioning of the heart on the basis of what the heart is supposed to do. The pumping of the heart maintains normal blood pressure and proper oxygenation of tissues, and the nervous system ensures that the heart will be able to meet these demands in different situations. Blood pressure and the blood vessels are the subjects of the next chapter.

STUDY OUTLINE

The heart pumps blood, which creates blood pressure, and circulates oxygen, nutrients, and other substances. The heart is located in the mediastinum, the area between the lungs in the thoracic cavity.

Cardiac muscle tissue (see Fig. 12–1)

1. Cardiac muscle fibers are branched and have many mitochondria; sarcomeres are the units of contraction.
2. Cardiac myocytes generate their own action potentials; the impulses spread rapidly from cell to cell by way of intercalated discs.
3. Cardiac muscle is an endocrine tissue; produces atrial natriuretic peptide (ANP) when the atria are stretched by increased blood volume or BP. ANP increases the loss of Na^+ ions and water in urine, which decreases blood volume and BP to normal. ANP is also stimulated by exercise and exposure to cold; promotes conversion of white adipocytes to thermogenic brown adipocytes.

Pericardial Membranes—three layers that enclose the heart (see Fig. 12–2)

1. The outer, fibrous pericardium, made of fibrous connective tissue, is a loose-fitting sac that surrounds the heart and extends over the diaphragm and the bases of the great vessels.
2. The parietal pericardium is a serous membrane that lines the fibrous pericardium.
3. The visceral pericardium, or epicardium, is a serous membrane on the surface of the myocardium.
4. Serous fluid between the parietal and visceral pericardial membranes prevents friction as the heart beats.

Chambers of the Heart: Vessels and Valves (see Figs. 12–3 and 12–4 and Table 12–1)

1. Cardiac muscle tissue, the myocardium, forms the walls of the four chambers of the heart.
2. Endocardium lines the chambers and covers the valves of the heart; is simple squamous epithelium that is very smooth and prevents abnormal clotting.
3. The right and left atria are the upper chambers, separated by the interatrial septum. The atria receive blood from veins.
4. The right and left ventricles are the lower chambers, separated by the interventricular septum. The ventricles pump blood into arteries.

Right Atrium

1. Receives blood from the upper body by way of the superior vena cava and receives blood from the lower body by way of the inferior vena cava.
2. The tricuspid (right AV) valve prevents backflow of blood from the right ventricle to the right atrium when the right ventricle contracts.

Left Atrium

1. Receives blood from the lungs by way of four pulmonary veins.
2. The mitral (left AV or bicuspid) valve prevents backflow of blood from the left ventricle to the left atrium when the left ventricle contracts.

Right Ventricle—has relatively thin walls

1. Pumps blood to the lungs through the pulmonary artery.
2. The pulmonary semilunar valve prevents backflow of blood from the pulmonary artery to the right ventricle when the right ventricle relaxes.
3. Papillary muscles and chordae tendineae prevent inversion of the right AV valve when the right ventricle contracts.

Left Ventricle—has thicker walls than does the right ventricle

1. Pumps blood to the body through the aorta.
2. The aortic semilunar valve prevents backflow of blood from the aorta to the left ventricle when the left ventricle relaxes.
3. Papillary muscles and chordae tendineae prevent inversion of the left AV valve when the left ventricle contracts.
4. The heart is a double pump: The right side of the heart receives deoxygenated blood from the body and pumps it to the lungs; the left side of the heart receives oxygenated blood from the lungs and pumps it to the body. Both sides of the heart work simultaneously.

Coronary Vessels (see Fig. 12–5)

1. Pathway: ascending aorta to right and left coronary arteries, to smaller arteries, to capillaries, to coronary veins, to the coronary sinus, to the right atrium.
2. Coronary vessels circulate oxygenated blood throughout the myocardium.
3. Obstruction of a coronary artery causes a myocardial infarction: death of an area of myocardium due to lack of oxygen.

Cardiac Cycle—the sequence of events in one heartbeat (see Fig. 12–6)

1. The atria continually receive blood from the veins; as pressure within the atria increases, the AV valves are opened.

2. Two-thirds of the atrial blood flows passively into the ventricles; atrial contraction pumps the remaining blood into the ventricles; the atria then relax.
3. The ventricles contract, which closes the AV valves and opens the aortic and pulmonary semilunar valves.
4. Ventricular contraction pumps all blood into the arteries. The ventricles then relax. Meanwhile, blood is filling the atria, and the cycle begins again.
5. Systole means contraction; diastole means relaxation. In the cardiac cycle, atrial systole is followed by ventricular systole. When the ventricles are in systole, the atria are in diastole.
6. The mechanical events of the cardiac cycle keep blood moving from the veins through the heart and into the arteries.

Heart Sounds—two sounds per heartbeat: lub-dup

1. The first sound is created by closure of the AV valves during ventricular systole.
2. The second sound is created by closure of the aortic and pulmonary semilunar valves.
3. Improper closing of a valve results in a heart murmur.

Cardiac Conduction Pathway—the pathway of impulses during the cardiac cycle (see Fig. 12–7)

1. The SA node in the wall of the right atrium initiates each heartbeat; the cells of the SA node are more permeable to Na^+ ions and depolarize more rapidly than any other part of the myocardium. The action potential spreads rapidly throughout the myocardium because of the intercalated discs at adjacent cells.
2. The AV node is in the lower interatrial septum. Depolarization of the SA node spreads to the AV node and to the atrial myocardium and brings about atrial systole.
3. The AV bundle (bundle of His) is in the upper interventricular septum; the first part of the ventricles to depolarize.
4. The right and left bundle branches in the interventricular septum transmit impulses to the Purkinje fibers in the ventricular myocardium, which complete ventricular systole.
5. An electrocardiogram (ECG) depicts the electrical activity of the heart (see Fig. 12–7).
6. If part of the conduction pathway does not function properly, the next part will initiate contraction, but at a slower rate.
7. Arrhythmias are irregular heartbeats; their effects range from harmless to life-threatening.

Heart Rate

1. Healthy adult: 60 to 80 beats per minute (heart rate equals pulse); children and infants have faster pulses because of their smaller size and higher metabolic rate.
2. A person in excellent physical condition has a slow resting pulse because the heart is a more efficient pump and pumps more blood per beat.

Cardiac Output (see Table 12–2)

1. Cardiac output is the amount of blood pumped by a ventricle in 1 minute.
2. Stroke volume is the amount of blood pumped by a ventricle in one beat; average is 60 to 80 mL.
3. Cardiac output equals stroke volume × pulse; average resting cardiac output is 5 to 6 L.
4. Starling's law of the heart—the more that cardiac muscle fibers are stretched, the more forcefully they contract.
5. During exercise, stroke volume increases as venous return increases and stretches the myocardium of the ventricles (Starling's law).
6. During exercise, the increase in stroke volume and the increase in pulse result in an increase in cardiac output: two to four times the resting level.
7. Cardiac reserve is the difference between resting cardiac output and the maximum cardiac output; may be 15 L or more.
8. The ejection fraction is the percent of its total blood that a ventricle pumps per beat; average is 60% to 70%.

Regulation of Heart Rate (see Fig. 12–8)

1. The heart generates its own beat, but the nervous system brings about changes to adapt to different situations.

2. The medulla contains the cardiac centers: the accelerator center and the inhibitory center. These are part of the reflex arc for changes in heart rate.
3. Sympathetic impulses to the heart increase rate and force of contraction; parasympathetic impulses (vagus nerves) to the heart decrease heart rate.
4. Pressoreceptors in the carotid and aortic sinuses detect changes in blood pressure.
5. Chemoreceptors in the carotid and aortic bodies detect changes in the oxygen content of the blood.
6. The glossopharyngeal nerves are sensory for the carotid receptors. The vagus nerves are sensory for the aortic receptors.
7. If blood pressure to the brain decreases, pressoreceptors in the carotid sinuses detect this decrease and send fewer sensory impulses along the glossopharyngeal nerves to the medulla. The accelerator center dominates and sends motor impulses along sympathetic nerves to increase heart rate and force of contraction to restore blood pressure to normal.
8. A similar reflex is activated by hypoxemia.
9. Epinephrine from the adrenal medulla increases heart rate and force of contraction during stressful situations.

REVIEW QUESTIONS

1. Describe the location of the heart with respect to the lungs and to the diaphragm. (p. 309)
2. Name the three pericardial membranes. Where is serous fluid found and what is its function? (p. 309)
3. Describe the location and explain the function of endocardium. (p. 309)
4. Name the veins that enter the right atrium; name those that enter the left atrium. For each, where does the blood come from? (p. 310)
5. Name the artery that leaves the right ventricle; name the artery that leaves the left ventricle. For each, where is the blood going? (p. 310)
6. Explain the purpose of the right and left AV valves and the purpose of the aortic and pulmonary semilunar valves. (p. 310)
7. Describe the coronary system of vessels and explain the purpose of coronary circulation. (pp. 310, 312)
8. Define systole, diastole, and cardiac cycle. (p. 312)
9. Explain how movement of blood from atria to ventricles differs from movement of blood from ventricles to arteries. (p. 315)
10. Explain why the heart is considered a double pump. Trace the path of blood from the right atrium back to the right atrium, naming the chambers of the heart and their vessels through which the blood passes. (p. 310)
11. Name the parts, in order, of the cardiac conduction pathway. Explain why it is the SA node that generates each heartbeat. State a normal range of heart rate for a healthy adult. (p. 316)
12. Calculate cardiac output if stroke volume is 75 mL and pulse is 75 bpm. Using the cardiac output you just calculated as a resting normal, what is the stroke volume of a marathoner whose resting pulse is 40 bpm? (p. 318)
13. Name the two cardiac centers and state their location. Sympathetic impulses to the heart have what effect? Parasympathetic impulses to the heart have what effect? Name the parasympathetic nerves to the heart. (pp. 319–320)
14. State the locations of arterial pressoreceptors and chemoreceptors, what they detect, and their sensory nerves. (p. 320)
15. Describe the reflex arc to increase heart rate and force when blood pressure to the brain decreases. (pp. 320–321)

FOR FURTHER THOUGHT

1. Endocarditis may be caused by bacteria or fungi that erode, or wear away, the heart valves, or in some cases make the valves bumpy (these bumps are called *vegetations*—think cauliflower). Explain the possible consequences of this.
2. Bob, a college freshman, is telling his new friends that he has been running seriously for 6 years and can run a marathon in a little over 3 hours. His friends aren't sure they should believe him but don't want to spend 3 hours waiting while Bob runs 26 miles. Bob says that he can prove he is telling the truth in 1 minute. Can he? Explain why or why not.
3. A neighbor, Mrs. G., age 62, tells you that she "doesn't feel right" and is suddenly tired for no apparent reason. She denies having chest pain, though she admits to a "full" feeling she calls indigestion. You suspect that she may be having a heart attack. What question can you ask to help you be more sure? Explain the physiological basis for your question.
4. Several types of artificial hearts are being developed and tested. What are the three essential characteristics a truly useful artificial heart must have? One is obvious, the others, perhaps not as much so.
5. Look at Question Fig. 12–A; this is a transverse section of the ventricles of the heart as seen from above. What parts of the heart are labeled A, B, and C? Give a reason for your answer. Label the anterior and posterior sides.

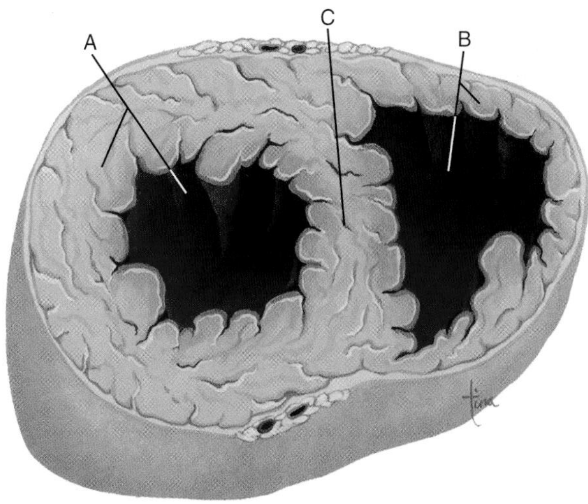

QUESTION FIGURE 12–A: Transverse section of the ventricles of the heart seen from above.

CHAPTER

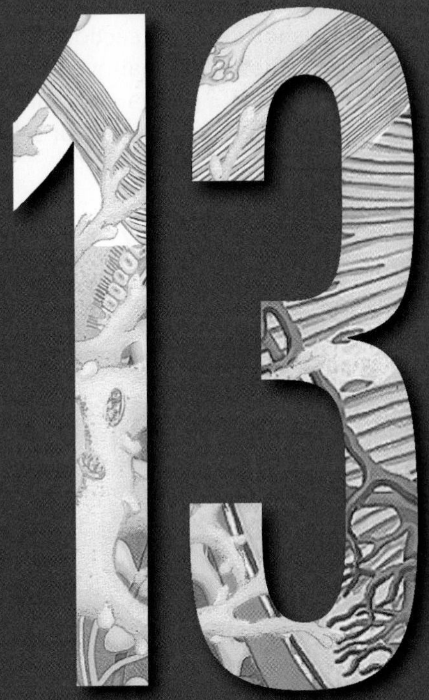

The Vascular System

STUDENT OBJECTIVES

- Describe the structure of arteries and veins, and relate their structure to function.
- Explain the purpose of arterial and venous anastomoses.
- Describe the structure of capillaries, and explain the exchange processes that take place in capillaries.
- Describe the pathway and purpose of pulmonary circulation.
- Name the branches of the aorta and their distributions.
- Name the major systemic veins and the parts of the body they drain of blood.
- Describe the pathway and purpose of hepatic portal circulation.
- Describe the modifications of fetal circulation, and explain the purpose of each.
- Explain the importance of slow blood flow in capillaries.
- Define blood pressure, and state the normal ranges for systemic and pulmonary blood pressure.
- Explain the factors that maintain systemic blood pressure.
- Explain how the heart and kidneys are involved in the regulation of blood pressure.
- Explain how the medulla and the autonomic nervous system regulate the diameter of blood vessels.

NEW TERMINOLOGY

Anastomosis *(a-NAS-ti-**MOH**-sis)*
Circle of Willis *(**SIR**-kuhl of **WILL**-iss)*
Ductus arteriosus *(**DUK**-tus ar-TIR-ee-**OH**-sis)*
Foramen ovale *(for-**RAY**-men oh-**VAHL**-ee)*
Hepatic portal *(hep-**PAT**-ik **POOR**-tuhl)*
Perfusion *(purr-**FEW**-zhun)*
Peripheral resistance *(puh-**RIFF**-uh-ruhl ree-**ZIS**-tense)*
Placenta *(pluh-**SEN**-tah)*
Precapillary sphincter *(pre-**KAP**-i-lar-ee **SFINK**-ter)*
Sinusoid *(**SIGH**-nuh-soyd)*
Umbilical arteries *(uhm-**BILL**-i-kull **AR**-tuh-rees)*
Umbilical vein *(uhm-**BILL**-i-kull VAIN)*
Venule *(**VEN**-yool)*

RELATED CLINICAL TERMINOLOGY

Anaphylactic *(AN-uh-fi-**LAK**-tik)*
Aneurysm *(**AN**-yur-izm)*
Arteriosclerosis *(ar-TIR-ee-oh-skle-**ROH**-sis)*
Hypertension *(HIGH-per-**TEN**-shun)*
Hypovolemic *(HIGH-poh-voh-**LEEM**-ik)*
Phlebitis *(fle-**BY**-tis)*
Pulse deficit *(PULS **DEF**-i-sit)*
Septic shock *(**SEP**-tik SHAHK)*
Varicose veins *(**VAR**-i-kohs VAINS).*

CHAPTER OUTLINE

*Terms that appear in **bold type** in the chapter text are defined in the glossary, which begins on page 603.*

The role of blood vessels in the circulation of blood has been known since 1628, when William Harvey, an English anatomist, demonstrated that blood in veins always flowed toward the heart. Before that time, it was believed that blood was static or stationary, some of it within the vessels but the rest sort of in puddles throughout the body. Harvey showed that blood indeed does move, and only in the blood vessels (though he did not know of the existence of capillaries). In the centuries that followed, the active (rather than merely passive) roles of the vascular system were discovered, and all contribute to homeostasis.

The vascular system consists of the arteries, capillaries, and veins through which the heart pumps blood throughout the body. As you will see, the major "business" of the vascular system, which is the exchange of materials between the blood and tissues, takes place in the capillaries. The arteries and veins, however, are just as important, transporting blood between the capillaries and the heart.

Another important topic of this chapter will be blood pressure (BP), which is the force the blood exerts against the walls of the vessels. Normal blood pressure is essential for circulation and for some of the material exchanges that take place in capillaries.

ARTERIES

Arteries carry blood from the heart to capillaries; smaller arteries are called **arterioles**. If we look at an artery in cross-section, we find three layers (or tunics) of tissues, each with different functions (Fig. 13–1).

The innermost layer, the **tunica intima** (or tunica interna), is the only part of a vessel that is in contact with blood. It is made of simple squamous epithelium called the **endothelium**. This lining is the same type of tissue that forms the endocardium, the lining of the chambers of the heart. As you might guess, its function is also the same: Its extreme smoothness and normal chemical composition prevent abnormal blood clotting by preventing the adhesion of platelets. The endothelium of blood vessels, however, also produces chemicals that affect blood pressure. Nitric oxide (NO) is a vasodilator; it stimulates relaxation of the smooth muscle of the middle layer of a vessel. The peptide **endothelin** stimulates contraction of this smooth muscle and is therefore a vasoconstrictor. Normal blood pressure depends in part upon a balance in the secretion of these opposing chemicals and others.

The **tunica media**, or middle layer, is made of smooth muscle and elastic connective tissue. Both of these tissues are involved in the maintenance of normal blood pressure, especially diastolic blood pressure when the heart is relaxed. The smooth muscle is the tissue affected by the chemicals produced by the endothelium. Relaxation of this smooth muscle brings about dilation of the vessel and a lower pressure. Contraction of the muscle layer brings about constriction and a higher blood pressure. Smooth muscle also has a nerve supply; increased sympathetic nerve impulses bring about vasoconstriction, and a decrease in impulses contributes to vasodilation. Fibrous connective tissue forms the outer layer, the **tunica externa**. This tissue is very strong, which is important to prevent the rupture or bursting of the larger arteries that carry blood under high pressure (see Box 13–1: Disorders of Arteries).

The outer and middle layers of large arteries are quite thick. In the smallest arterioles, however, only individual smooth muscle cells encircle the tunica intima. As mentioned, the smooth muscle layer enables arteries to constrict or dilate. Such changes in diameter are regulated in part by the endothelium and in part by the medulla and autonomic nervous system. For the terminal arterioles, those just before capillary networks, the level of oxygen in the surrounding tissue is a regulating factor. Hypoxia in tissues causes systemic arterioles to dilate, which will increase blood flow, called **perfusion**, to correct the hypoxia. In contrast, pulmonary terminal arterioles constrict in response to hypoxia; this is discussed in Chapter 15. Nervous regulation will be discussed in a later section on blood pressure.

VEINS

Veins carry blood from capillaries back to the heart; the smaller veins are called **venules**. The same three tissue layers are present in veins as in the walls of arteries, but they do have some differences when compared with the arterial layers. The inner layer of veins is smooth endothelium, but at intervals this lining is folded to form **valves** (see Fig. 13–1). Valves prevent backflow of blood and are most numerous in veins of the legs, where blood must often return to the heart against the force of gravity.

The middle layer of veins is a thin layer of smooth muscle. It is thin because veins do not regulate blood pressure and blood flow into capillaries as arteries do. Veins can constrict extensively, however, and this function becomes very important in certain situations such as severe hemorrhage. The outer layer of veins is also thin; not as much fibrous connective tissue as in arteries is necessary because blood pressure in veins is very low.

Veins have a greater capacity than arteries do; that is, their total volume is greater. The femoral vein, for

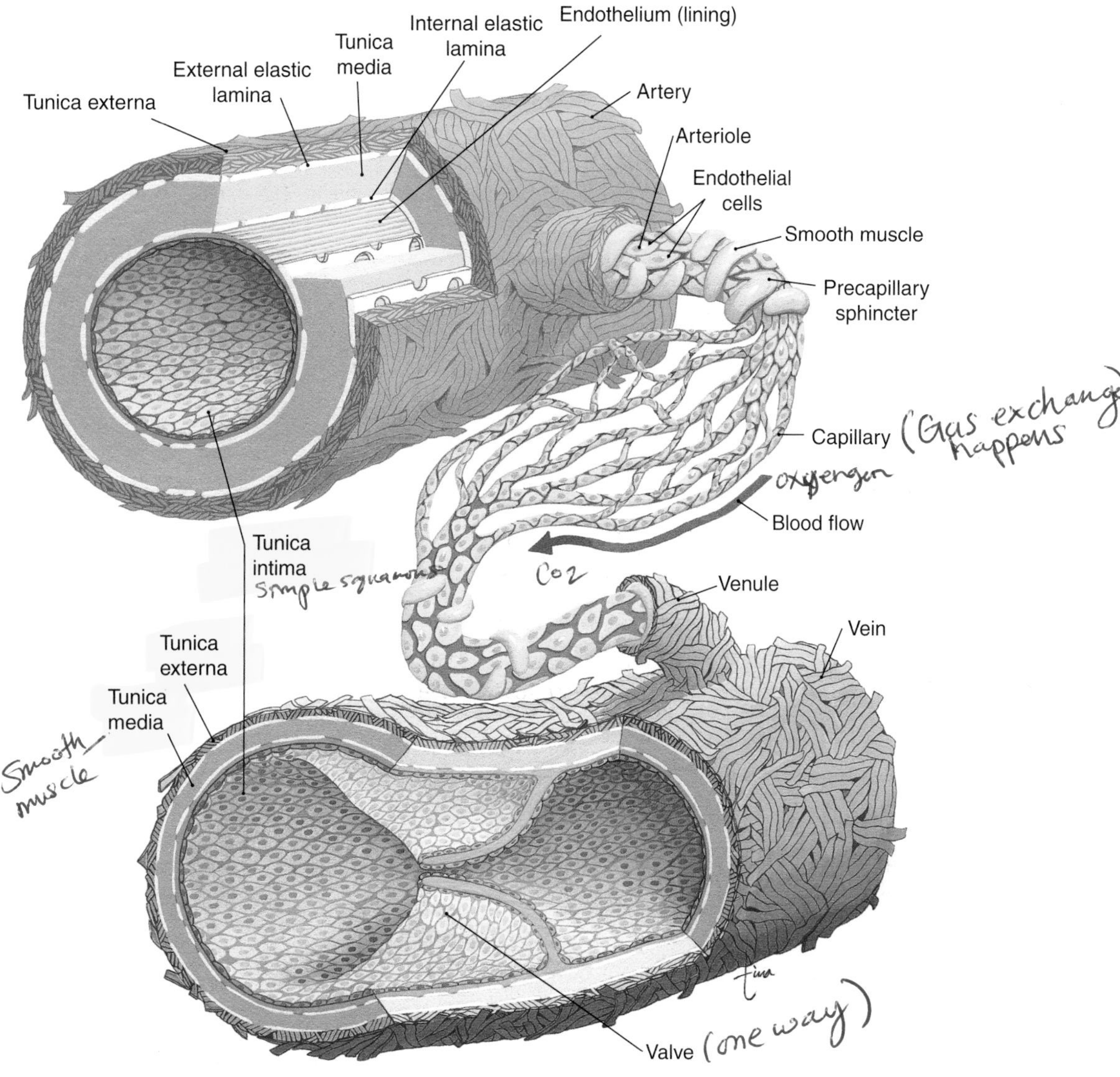

Figure 13–1 Structure of an artery, arteriole, capillary network, venule, and vein. See text for description.

QUESTION: What tissue is the tunica media made of, and how is this layer different in an artery and in a vein?

Box 13–1 | DISORDERS OF ARTERIES

Arteriosclerosis—although commonly called "hardening of the arteries," arteriosclerosis really means that the arteries lose their elasticity, and their walls become weakened. Arteries carry blood under high pressure, so deterioration of their walls is part of the aging process.

Aneurysm—a weak portion of an arterial wall may bulge out, forming a sac or bubble called an aneurysm. Arteriosclerosis is a possible cause, but some aneurysms are congenital. An aneurysm may be present for many years without any symptoms and may be discovered

Continued

Box 13–1 | DISORDERS OF ARTERIES *(Continued)*

only during diagnostic procedures for some other purpose.

The most common sites for aneurysm formation are the cerebral arteries and the aorta, especially the abdominal aorta. Rupture of a cerebral aneurysm is a possible cause of a cerebrovascular accident (CVA). Rupture of an aortic aneurysm is life-threatening and requires immediate corrective surgery. The damaged portion of the artery is removed and replaced with a graft. Such surgery may also be performed when an aneurysm is found before it ruptures.

Atherosclerosis—this condition has been mentioned previously; see Chapters 2 and 12.

example, has a larger lumen, or cavity, than does its counterpart, the femoral artery. When the body is at rest, approximately 63% to 65% of the blood is flowing through the systemic veins, compared with 12% to 15% flowing in the systemic arteries (the pulmonary vessels have 9% to 10%, and the heart and systemic capillaries have 7% to 8% each).

ANASTOMOSES

An **anastomosis** is a connection, or joining, of vessels, that is, artery to artery or vein to vein. The general purpose of these connections is to provide alternate pathways for the flow of blood if one vessel becomes obstructed.

An arterial anastomosis helps ensure that blood will get to the capillaries of an organ to deliver oxygen and nutrients and to remove waste products. There are arterial anastomoses, for example, between some of the coronary arteries that supply blood to the myocardium.

A venous anastomosis helps ensure that blood will be able to return to the heart in order to be pumped again. Venous anastomoses are most numerous among the veins of the legs, where the possibility of obstruction increases as a person gets older (see Box 13–2: Disorders of Veins).

Box 13–2 | DISORDERS OF VEINS

Phlebitis—inflammation of a vein. This condition is most common in the veins of the legs because they are subjected to great pressure as the blood is returned to the heart against the force of gravity. Often no specific cause can be determined, but advancing age, obesity, and blood disorders may be predisposing factors.

If a superficial vein is affected, the area may be tender or painful, but blood flow is usually maintained because there are so many anastomoses among these veins. Deep vein phlebitis is potentially more serious, with the possibility of clot formation (thrombophlebitis) and subsequent dislodging of the clot to form an embolism.

Varicose veins—swollen and distended veins that occur most often in the superficial veins of the legs. This condition may develop in people who must sit or stand in one place for long periods of time. Without contraction of the leg muscles, blood tends to pool in the leg veins, stretching their walls. If the veins become overly stretched, the valves within them no longer close properly. These incompetent valves no longer prevent backflow of blood, leading to further pooling and even further stretching of the walls of the veins. Varicose veins may cause discomfort and cramping in the legs, or become even more painful. Severe varicosities may be removed surgically.

This condition may also develop during pregnancy, when the enlarged uterus presses against the iliac veins and slows blood flow into the inferior vena cava. Varicose veins of the anal canal are called **hemorrhoids**, which may also be a result of pregnancy or of chronic constipation and straining to defecate. Hemorrhoids that cause discomfort or pain may also be removed surgically. Developments in laser surgery have made this a simpler procedure than it was in the past.

CAPILLARIES

Capillaries carry blood from arterioles to venules. Their walls are only one cell in thickness; capillaries are actually the extension of the endothelium, the simple squamous lining, of arteries and veins (see Fig. 13–1). Some tissues do not have capillaries; these are the epidermis, cartilage, and the lens and cornea of the eye.

Most tissues, however, have extensive capillary networks. The quantity or volume of capillary networks in an organ reflects the metabolic activity of the organ. The functioning of the kidneys, for example, depends upon a good blood supply. Figure 18–2 in Chapter 18 shows a vascular cast of a kidney; you can see how dense the vessels are, most of which are capillaries. In contrast, a tendon such as the Achilles tendon at the heel or the patellar tendon at the knee would have far fewer vessels because fibrous connective tissue is far less metabolically active.

Blood flow into capillary networks is regulated by smooth muscle cells called **precapillary sphincters**, found at the beginning of each network (see Fig. 13–1). Precapillary sphincters are not regulated by the nervous system but rather constrict or dilate depending on the needs of the tissues. Because there is not enough blood in the body to fill all of the capillaries at once, precapillary sphincters are usually slightly constricted. In an active tissue that requires more oxygen, such as exercising muscle, the precapillary sphincters dilate to increase blood flow. These automatic responses ensure that blood, the volume of which is constant, will circulate where it is needed most.

Some organs have another type of capillary called **sinusoids**, which are larger and more permeable than are other capillaries. The permeability of sinusoids permits large substances such as proteins and blood cells to enter or leave the blood. Sinusoids are found in the red bone marrow and spleen, where blood cells enter or leave the blood, and in organs such as the liver and pituitary gland, which produce and secrete proteins into the blood.

EXCHANGES IN CAPILLARIES

Capillaries are the sites of exchanges of materials between the blood and the tissue fluid surrounding cells. Some of these substances move from the blood to tissue fluid, and others move from tissue fluid to the blood. The processes by which these substances are exchanged are illustrated in Fig. 13–2.

Gases move by **diffusion**, that is, from their area of greater concentration to their area of lesser concentration. Oxygen, therefore, diffuses from the blood in systemic capillaries to the tissue fluid, and carbon dioxide diffuses from tissue fluid to the blood to be brought to the lungs and exhaled.

Let us now look at the blood pressure as blood enters capillaries from the arterioles. Blood pressure here is about 30 to 35 mm Hg, and the pressure of the surrounding tissue fluid is much lower, about 2 mm Hg. Because the capillary blood pressure is higher, the process of **filtration** occurs, which forces plasma and dissolved nutrients out of the capillaries and into tissue fluid. This is how nutrients such as glucose, amino acids, and vitamins are brought to cells.

Blood pressure decreases as blood reaches the venous end of capillaries, but notice that proteins such as albumin have remained in the blood. Albumin contributes to the **colloid osmotic pressure** (COP) of blood; this is an "attracting" pressure, a "pulling" rather than a "pushing" pressure. At the venous end of capillaries, the presence of albumin in the blood pulls tissue fluid into the capillaries, which also brings into the blood the waste products produced by cells. The tissue fluid that returns to the blood also helps maintain normal blood volume and blood pressure.

The amount of tissue fluid formed is slightly greater than the amount returned to the capillaries. If this were to continue, blood volume would be gradually depleted. The excess tissue fluid, however, enters lymph capillaries. Now called lymph, it will be returned to the blood to be recycled again as plasma, thus maintaining blood volume. This is discussed further in Chapter 14.

PATHWAYS OF CIRCULATION

The two major pathways of circulation are pulmonary and systemic. Pulmonary circulation begins at the right ventricle, and systemic circulation begins at the left ventricle. Hepatic portal circulation is a special segment of systemic circulation that will be covered separately. Fetal circulation involves pathways that are present only before birth and will also be discussed separately.

PULMONARY CIRCULATION

The right ventricle pumps blood into the pulmonary artery (or trunk), which divides into the right and left pulmonary arteries, one going to each lung. Within the lungs each artery branches extensively into smaller arteries and arterioles, then to capillaries. The pulmonary capillaries surround the alveoli of the lungs; it is here that exchanges of oxygen and carbon dioxide take place. The capillaries unite to form venules, which merge into veins, and finally into the two pulmonary veins from each lung that return blood to the left atrium.

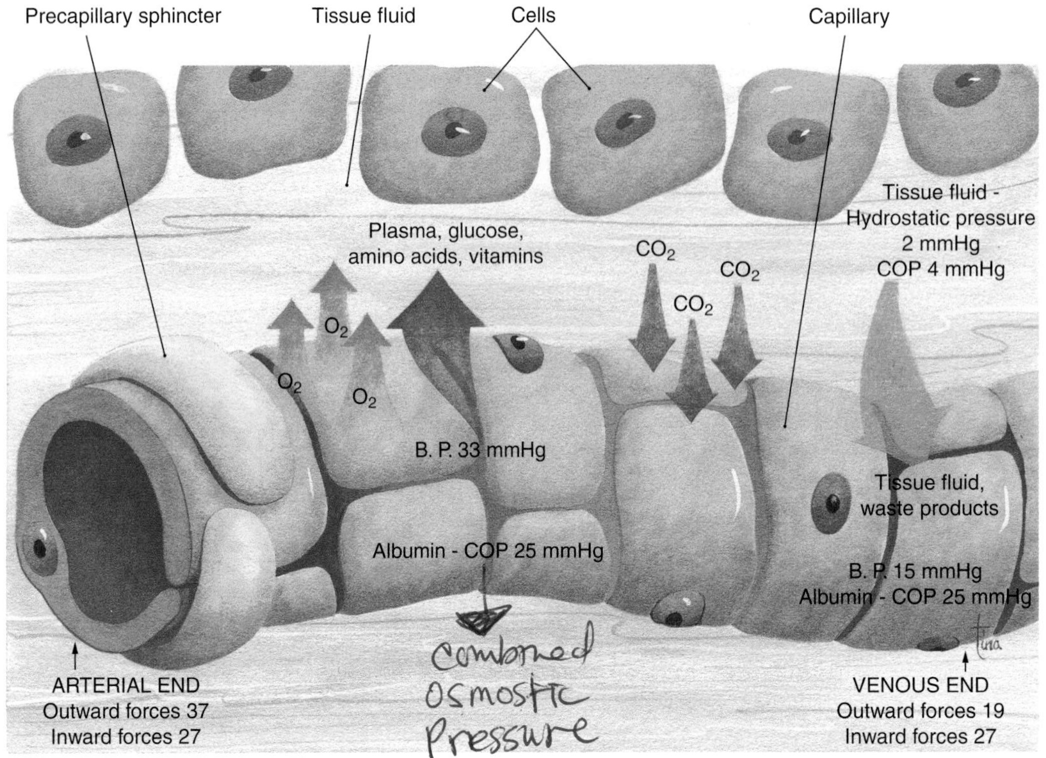

Figure 13–2 Exchanges between blood in a systemic capillary and the surrounding tissue fluid. Arrows depict the direction of movement. Filtration takes place at the arterial end of the capillary. Osmosis takes place at the venous end. Gases are exchanged by diffusion.

QUESTION: Of all the pressures shown here, which one is the highest, and what process does it bring about?

This oxygenated blood will then travel through the systemic circulation. (Notice that the pulmonary veins contain oxygenated blood; these are the only veins that carry blood with a high oxygen content. The blood in systemic veins has a low oxygen content; it is systemic arteries that carry oxygenated blood.)

SYSTEMIC CIRCULATION

The left ventricle pumps blood into the aorta, the largest artery of the body. We will return to the aorta and its branches in a moment, but first we will summarize the rest of systemic circulation. The branches of the aorta take blood into arterioles and capillary networks throughout the body. Capillaries merge to form venules and veins. The veins from the lower body take blood to the inferior vena cava; veins from the upper body take blood to the superior vena cava. These two caval veins return blood to the right atrium. The major arteries and veins are shown in Figs. 13–3 to 13–5, and their functions are listed in Tables 13–1 and 13–2.

The aorta is a continuous vessel, but for the sake of precise description it is divided into sections that are named anatomically: ascending aorta, aortic arch, thoracic aorta, and abdominal aorta. The ascending aorta is the first inch that emerges from the top of the left ventricle. The arch of the aorta curves posteriorly over the heart and turns downward. The thoracic aorta continues down through the chest cavity and through the diaphragm. Below the level of the diaphragm, the abdominal aorta continues to the level of the 4th lumbar vertebra, where it divides into the two common iliac arteries. Along its course, the aorta has many branches through which blood travels to specific organs and parts of the body.

The ascending aorta has only two branches: the right and left coronary arteries, which supply blood to the

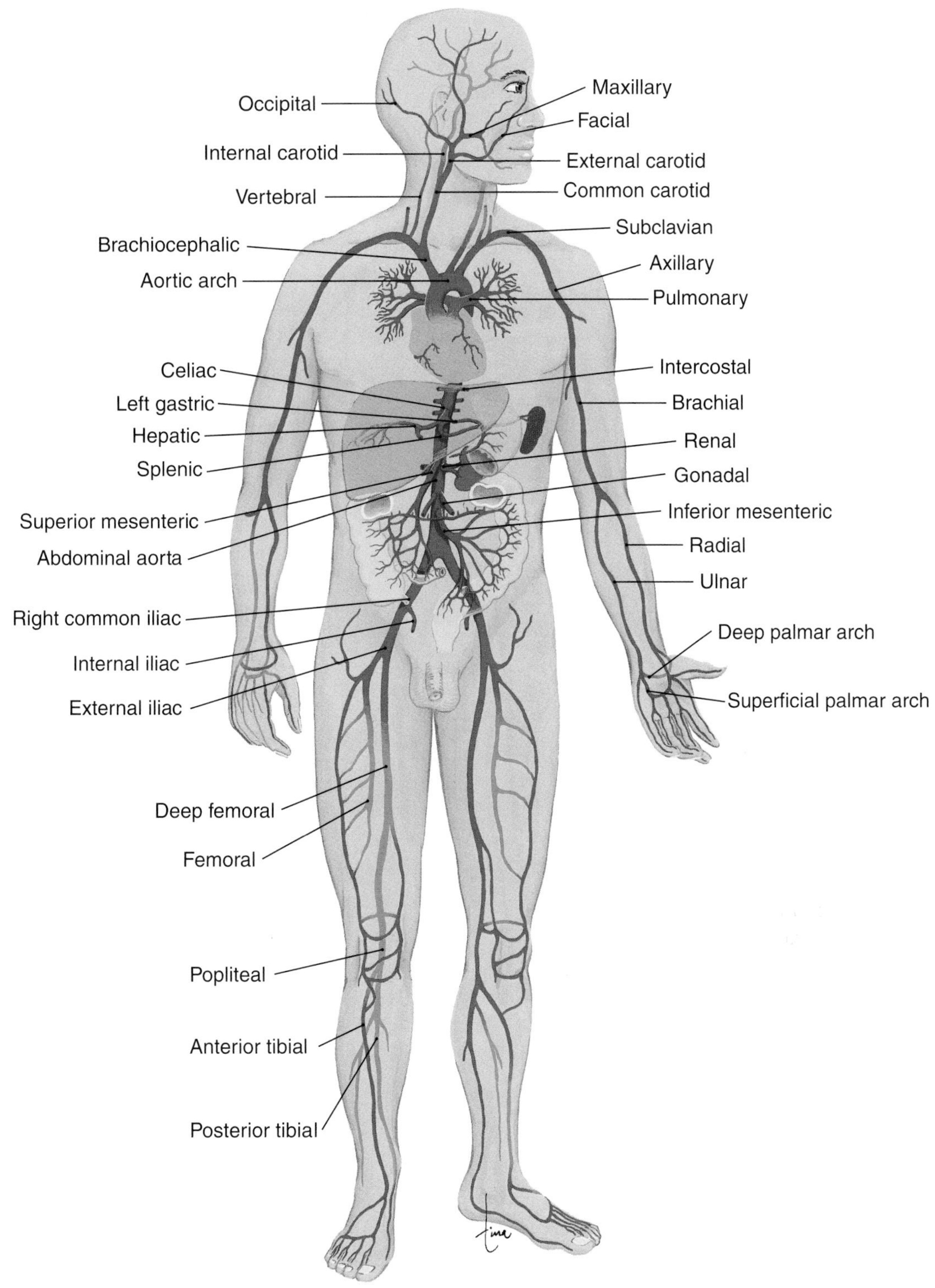

Figure 13–3 Systemic arteries. The aorta and its major branches are shown in anterior view.

QUESTION: Can you find three arteries named after bones? After organs?

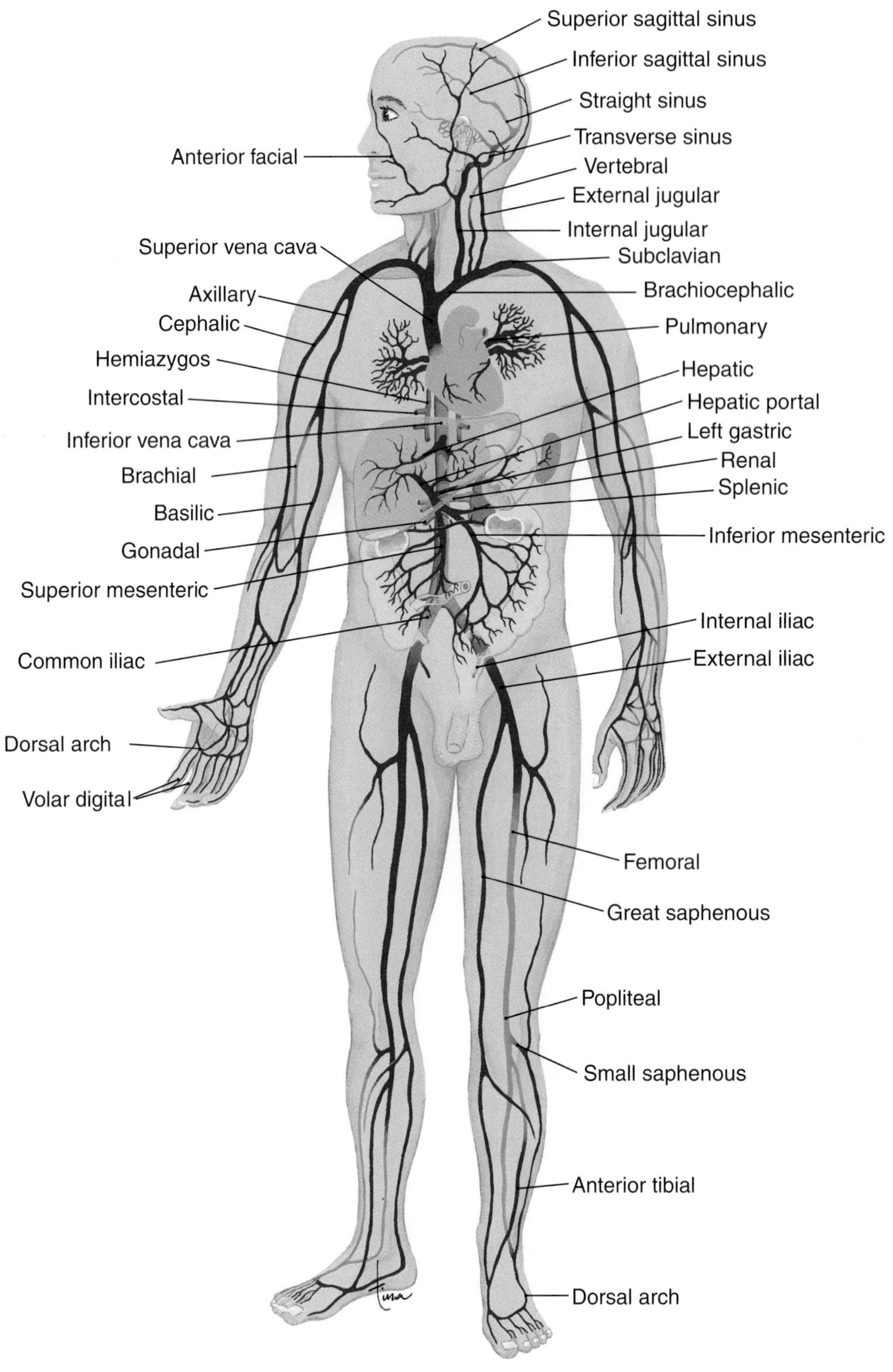

Figure 13–4 Systemic veins shown in anterior view.

QUESTION: Can you find three veins with the same name as the accompanying artery?

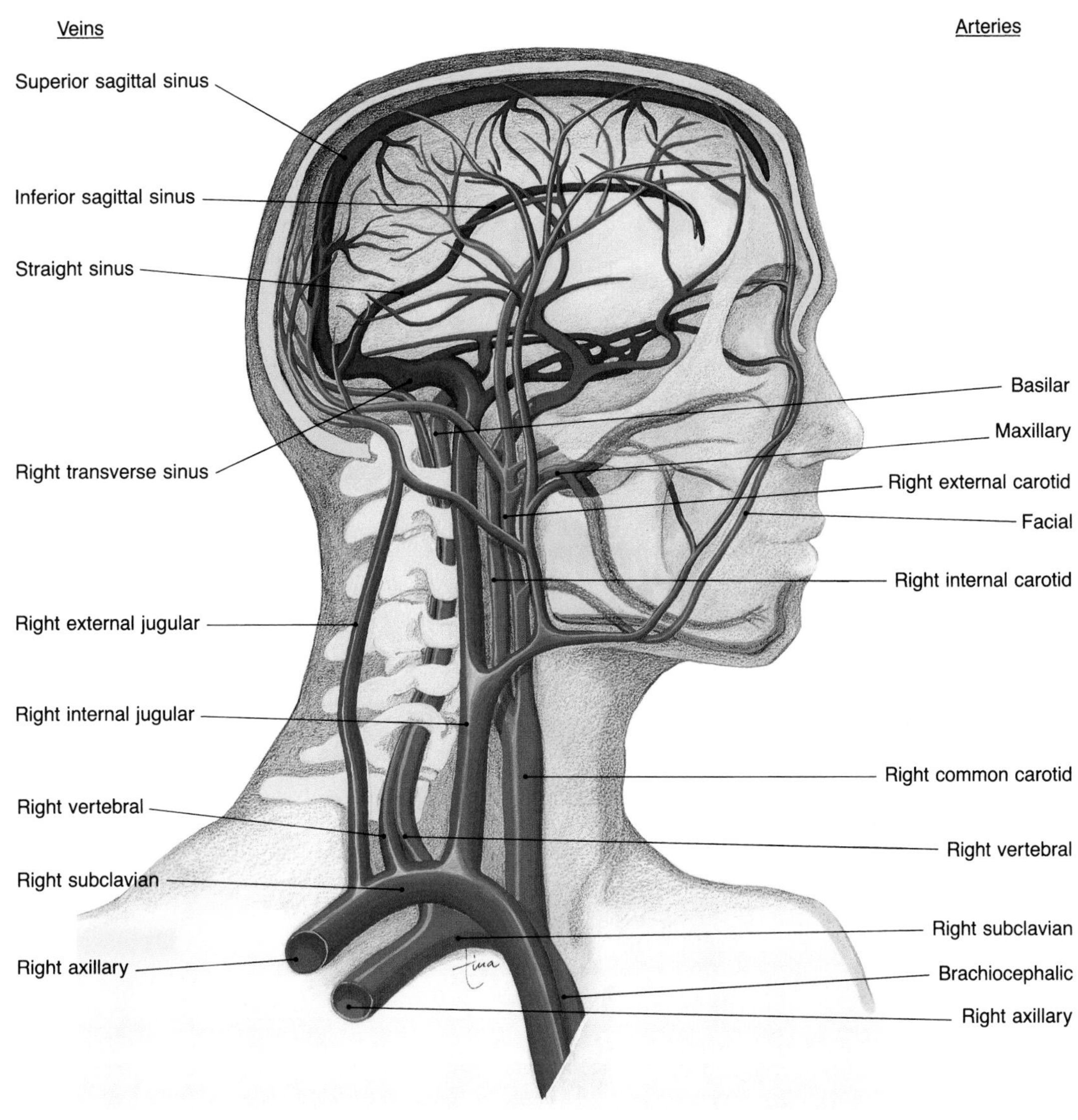

Figure 13–5 Arteries and veins of the head and neck shown in right lateral view. Veins are labeled on the left. Arteries are labeled on the right.

QUESTION: Which vein is the counterpart of the common carotid artery?

myocardium. This pathway of circulation was described previously in Chapter 12.

The aortic arch has three branches that supply blood to the head and arms: the brachiocephalic artery, left common carotid artery, and left subclavian artery. The brachiocephalic (literally, "arm-head") artery is very short and divides into the right common carotid artery and right subclavian artery. The right and left common carotid arteries extend into the neck, where each divides into an internal carotid artery and external carotid artery, which supply the head. The right and left subclavian arteries are in the shoulders behind the clavicles and continue into the arms. As the artery enters another body area (it may not "branch," simply continue), its name

Table 13–1 | **MAJOR SYSTEMIC ARTERIES**

BRANCHES OF THE ASCENDING AORTA AND AORTIC ARCH

ARTERY	BRANCH OF	REGION SUPPLIED
Coronary a.	Ascending aorta	■ Myocardium
Brachiocephalic a.	Aortic arch	■ Right arm and head
Right common carotid a.	Brachiocephalic a.	■ Right side of head
Right subclavian a.	Brachiocephalic a.	■ Right shoulder and arm
Left common carotid a.	Aortic arch	■ Left side of head
Left subclavian a.	Aortic arch	■ Left shoulder and arm
External carotid a.	Common carotid a.	■ Superficial head
Superficial temporal a.	External carotid a.	■ Scalp
Internal carotid a.	Common carotid a.	■ Brain (circle of Willis)
Ophthalmic a.	Internal carotid a.	■ Eye
Vertebral a.	Subclavian a.	■ Cervical vertebrae and circle of Willis
Axillary a.	Subclavian a.	■ Armpit
Brachial a.	Axillary a.	■ Upper arm
Radial a.	Brachial a.	■ Forearm
Ulnar a.	Brachial a.	■ Forearm
Volar arch	Radial and ulnar a.	■ Hand

BRANCHES OF THE THORACIC AORTA

ARTERY	REGION SUPPLIED
Intercostal a. (9 pairs)	■ Skin, muscles, bones of trunk
Superior phrenic a.	■ Diaphragm
Pericardial a.	■ Pericardium
Esophageal a.	■ Esophagus
Bronchial a.	■ Bronchioles and connective tissue of the lungs

BRANCHES OF THE ABDOMINAL AORTA

ARTERY	REGION SUPPLIED
Inferior phrenic a.	■ Diaphragm
Lumbar a.	■ Lumbar area of back
Middle sacral a.	■ Sacrum, coccyx, buttocks
Celiac a.	■ (see branches)
Hepatic a.	■ Liver
Left gastric a.	■ Stomach
Splenic a.	■ Spleen, pancreas
Superior mesenteric a.	■ Small intestine, part of colon
Suprarenal a.	■ Adrenal glands
Renal a.	■ Kidneys
Inferior mesenteric a.	■ Most of colon and rectum
Testicular or ovarian a.	■ Testes or ovaries

Table 13–1 | **MAJOR SYSTEMIC ARTERIES—cont'd**

BRANCHES OF THE ABDOMINAL AORTA

ARTERY	REGION SUPPLIED
Common iliac a.	■ The two large vessels that receive blood from the abdominal aorta; each branches as follows:
Internal iliac a.	■ Bladder, rectum, reproductive organs
External iliac a.	■ Lower pelvis to leg
Femoral a.	■ Thigh
Popliteal a.	■ Back of knee
Anterior tibial a.	■ Front of lower leg
Dorsalis pedis	■ Top of ankle and foot
Plantar arches	■ Foot
Posterior tibial a.	■ Back of lower leg
Peroneal a.	■ Medial lower leg
Plantar arches	■ Foot

Table 13–2 | **MAJOR SYSTEMIC VEINS**

VEIN	VEIN JOINED	REGION DRAINED
HEAD AND NECK		
Cranial venous sinuses	Internal jugular v.	■ Brain, including reabsorbed CSF
Internal jugular v.	Brachiocephalic v.	■ Face and neck
External jugular v.	Subclavian v.	■ Superficial face and neck
Subclavian v.	Brachiocephalic v.	■ Shoulder
Brachiocephalic v.	Superior vena cava	■ Upper body
Superior vena cava	Right atrium	■ Upper body
ARM AND SHOULDER		
Radial v.	Brachial v.	■ Forearm and hand
Ulnar v.	Brachial v.	■ Forearm and hand
Cephalic v.	Axillary v.	■ Superficial arm and forearm
Basilic v.	Axillary v.	■ Superficial upper arm
Brachial v.	Axillary v.	■ Upper arm
Axillary v.	Subclavian v.	■ Armpit
Subclavian v.	Brachiocephalic v.	■ Shoulder
TRUNK		
Brachiocephalic v.	Superior vena cava	■ Upper body
Azygos v.	Superior vena cava	■ Deep structures of chest and abdomen; links inferior vena cava to superior vena cava
Hepatic v.	Inferior vena cava	■ Liver
Renal v.	Inferior vena cava	■ Kidney

Continued

Table 13–2 | **MAJOR SYSTEMIC VEINS—cont'd**

VEIN	VEIN JOINED	REGION DRAINED
TRUNK		
Testicular or ovarian v.	Inferior vena cava and left renal v.	■ Testes or ovaries
Internal iliac v.	Common iliac v.	■ Rectum, bladder, reproductive organs
External iliac v.	Common iliac v.	■ Leg and abdominal wall
Common iliac v.	Inferior vena cava	■ Leg and lower abdomen
LEG AND HIP		
Anterior and posterior tibial v.	Popliteal v.	■ Lower leg and foot
Popliteal v.	Femoral v.	■ Knee
Small saphenous v.	Popliteal v.	■ Superficial leg and foot
Great saphenous v.	Femoral v.	■ Superficial foot, leg, and thigh
Femoral v.	External iliac v.	■ Thigh
External iliac v.	Common iliac v.	■ Leg and abdominal wall
Common iliac v.	Inferior vena cava	■ Leg and lower abdomen
Inferior vena cava	Right atrium	■ Lower body

changes: The subclavian artery becomes the axillary artery, which becomes the brachial artery. The branches of the carotid and subclavian arteries are diagrammed in Figs. 13–3 and 13–5. As you look at these diagrams, keep in mind that the name of the vessel often tells us where it is. The facial artery, for example, is found in the face.

Some of the arteries in the head contribute to an important arterial anastomosis, the **circle of Willis** (or cerebral arterial circle), which is a "circle" of arteries around the pituitary gland (Fig. 13–6). The circle of Willis is formed by the right and left internal carotid arteries and the basilar artery, which is the union of the right and left vertebral arteries (branches of the subclavian arteries). The brain is always active, even during sleep, and must have a constant flow of blood to supply oxygen and remove waste products. For this reason there are four vessels that bring blood to the circle of Willis. From this anastomosis, several paired arteries (the cerebral arteries) extend into the brain itself.

The thoracic aorta and its branches supply the chest wall and the organs within the thoracic cavity. These vessels are listed in Table 13–1.

The abdominal aorta gives rise to arteries that supply the abdominal wall and organs and to the common iliac arteries, which continue into the legs. Notice in Fig. 13–3 that the common iliac artery becomes the external iliac artery, which becomes the femoral artery, which becomes the popliteal artery; the same vessel has different names based on location. These vessels are also listed in Table 13–1 (see Box 13–3: Pulse Sites).

The systemic veins drain blood from organs or parts of the body and often parallel their corresponding arteries. The most important veins are diagrammed in Fig. 13–4 and listed in Table 13–2.

HEPATIC PORTAL CIRCULATION

Hepatic portal circulation is a subdivision of systemic circulation in which blood from the abdominal digestive organs and spleen circulates through the liver before returning to the heart.

Blood from the capillaries of the stomach, small intestine, colon, pancreas, and spleen flows into two large veins, the superior mesenteric vein and the splenic vein, which unite to form the portal vein (Fig. 13–7). The portal vein takes blood into the liver, where it branches extensively and empties blood into the sinusoids, the capillaries of the liver (see also Fig. 16–6 in Chapter 16). From the sinusoids, blood flows into hepatic veins, to the inferior vena cava and back to the right atrium. Notice that this pathway has two sets of capillaries, and keep in mind that it is in capillaries that exchanges take place. Let us use some specific examples to show the purpose and importance of portal circulation.

Glucose from carbohydrate digestion is absorbed into the capillaries of the small intestine; after a big meal this

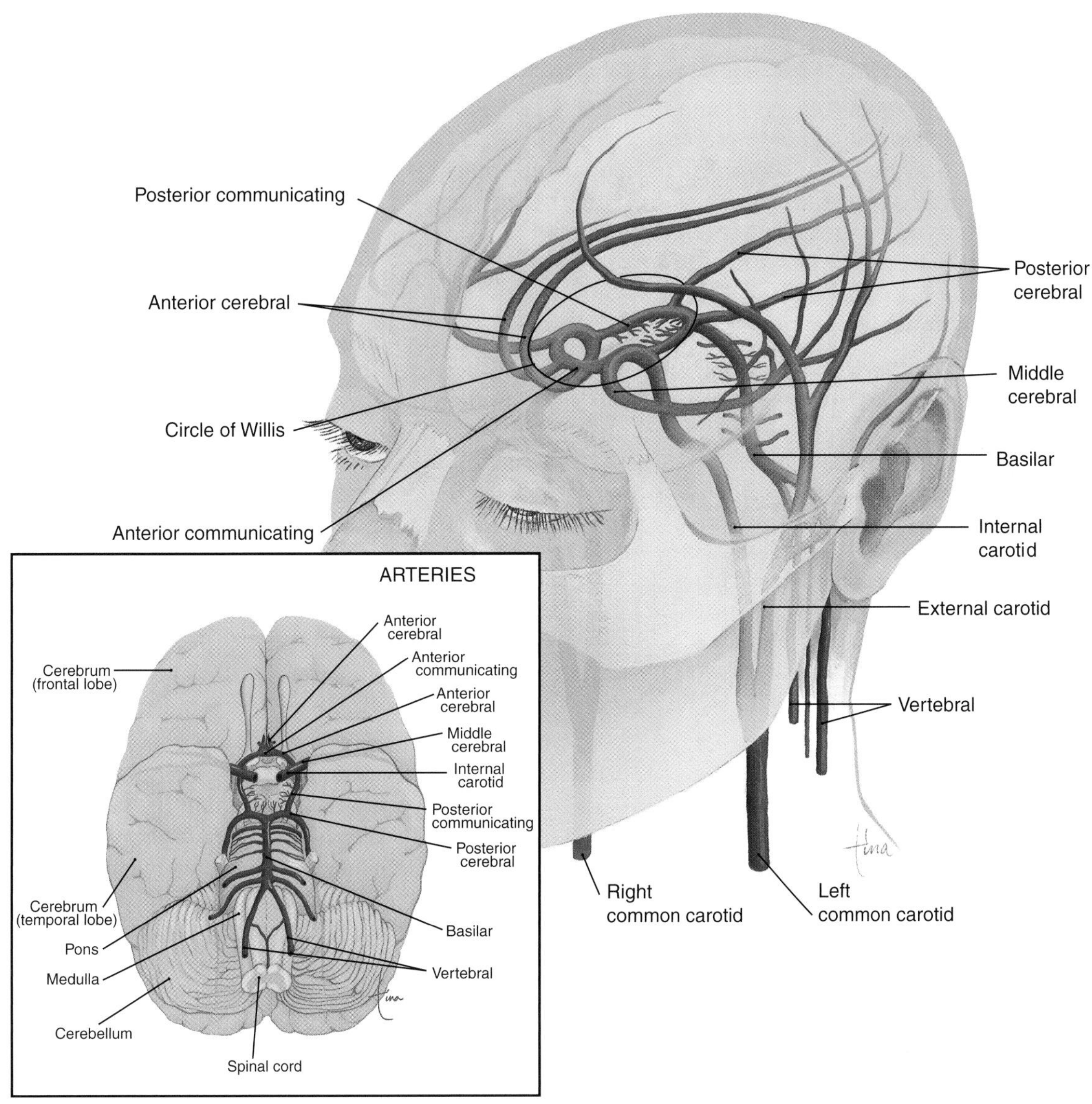

Figure 13–6 Circle of Willis. This anastomosis is formed by the following arteries: internal carotid, anterior communicating, posterior communicating, and basilar. The cerebral arteries extend from the circle of Willis into the brain. The insert box shows these vessels in an inferior view of the brain.

QUESTION: Why do so many vessels contribute to the circle of Willis?

may greatly increase the blood glucose level. If this blood were to go directly back to the heart and then circulate through the kidneys, some of the glucose might be lost in urine. However, blood from the small intestine passes first through the liver sinusoids, and the liver cells remove the excess glucose and store it as glycogen. The blood that returns to the heart will then have a blood glucose level in the normal range.

Another example: Alcohol is absorbed into the capillaries of the stomach and small intestine. If it were to circulate directly throughout the body, the alcohol would rapidly impair the functioning of the brain. Portal circulation,

Box 13–3 | PULSE SITES

A pulse is the heartbeat that is felt at an arterial site. What is felt is not actually the force exerted by the blood, but the force of ventricular contraction transmitted through the walls of the arteries. This is why pulses are not felt in veins; they are too far from the heart for the force to be detectable.

The most commonly used pulse sites are:

Radial—the radial artery on the thumb side of the wrist.

Carotid—the carotid artery lateral to the larynx in the neck.

Temporal—the temporal artery just in front of the ear.

Femoral—the femoral artery at the top of the thigh.

Popliteal—the popliteal artery at the back of the knee.

Dorsalis pedis—the dorsalis pedis artery on the top of the foot (commonly called the pedal pulse).

Pulse rate is, of course, the heart rate. However, if the heart is beating weakly, a radial pulse may be lower than an **apical pulse** (listening to the heart itself with a stethoscope). This is called a **pulse deficit** and indicates heart disease of some kind.

When taking a pulse, the careful observer also notes the rhythm and force of the pulse. Abnormal rhythms may reflect cardiac arrhythmias, and the force of the pulse (strong or weak) is helpful in assessing the general condition of the heart and arteries.

however, takes blood from the stomach and intestine to the liver, the organ that can detoxify the alcohol and prevent its detrimental effects on the brain. Of course, if alcohol consumption continues, the blood alcohol level rises faster than the liver's capacity to detoxify, and the well-known signs of alcohol intoxication appear.

As you can see, this portal circulation pathway enables the liver to modify the blood from the digestive organs and spleen. Some nutrients may be stored or changed, bilirubin from the spleen is excreted into bile, and potential poisons are detoxified before the blood returns to the heart and the rest of the body.

FETAL CIRCULATION

The fetus depends upon the mother for oxygen and nutrients and for the removal of carbon dioxide and other waste products. The site of exchange between fetus and mother is the **placenta**, which contains fetal and maternal blood vessels that are very close to one another (see Fig. 13–8 and also Fig. 21–5 in Chapter 21). The blood of the fetus does not mix with the blood of the mother; substances are exchanged by diffusion and active transport mechanisms.

The fetus is connected to the placenta by the umbilical cord, which contains two umbilical arteries and one umbilical vein (see Fig. 13–8). The **umbilical arteries** are branches of the fetal internal iliac arteries; they carry blood from the fetus to the placenta. In the placenta, carbon dioxide and waste products in the fetal blood enter maternal circulation, and oxygen and nutrients from the mother's blood enter fetal circulation.

The **umbilical vein** carries this oxygenated blood from the placenta to the fetus. Within the body of the fetus, the umbilical vein branches: One branch takes some blood to the fetal liver, but most of the blood passes through the **ductus venosus** to the inferior vena cava, to the right atrium. After birth, when the umbilical cord is cut, the remnants of these fetal vessels constrict and become nonfunctional.

The other modifications of fetal circulation concern the fetal heart and large arteries (also shown in Fig. 13–8). Because the fetal lungs are deflated and do not provide for gas exchange, blood is shunted away from the lungs and to the body. The **foramen ovale** is an opening in the interatrial septum that permits some blood to flow from the right atrium to the left atrium, not, as usual, to the right ventricle. The blood that does enter the right ventricle is pumped into the pulmonary artery. The **ductus arteriosus** is a short vessel that diverts most of the blood in the pulmonary artery to the aorta, to the body. Both the foramen ovale and the ductus arteriosus permit blood to bypass the fetal lungs.

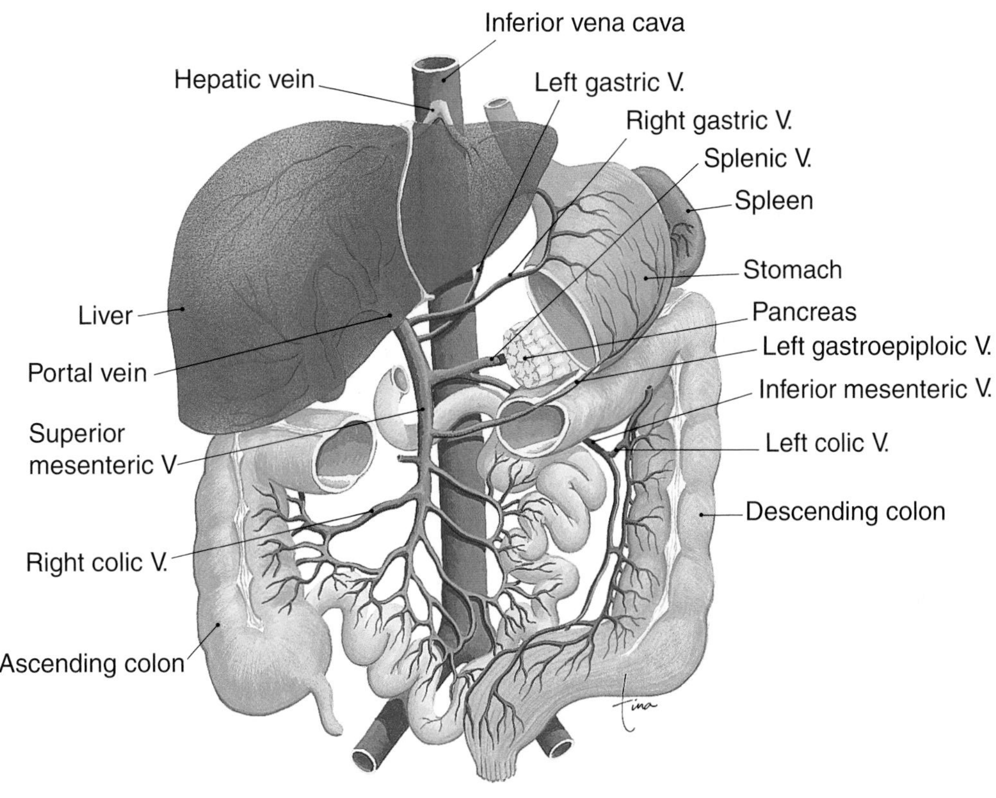

Figure 13–7 Hepatic portal circulation. Portions of some of the digestive organs have been removed to show the veins that unite to form the portal vein. See text for description.

QUESTION: The blood in the portal vein is going to what organ? Where is the blood coming from?

Just after birth, the baby breathes and expands its lungs, which pulls more blood into the pulmonary circulation. More blood then returns to the left atrium, and a flap on the left side of the foramen ovale is closed. The ductus arteriosus constricts, probably in response to the higher oxygen content of the blood, and pulmonary circulation becomes fully functional within a few days.

VELOCITY OF BLOOD FLOW

The velocity, or speed, with which blood flows differs in the various parts of the vascular system. Velocity is inversely related (meaning as one value goes up, the other goes down) to the cross-sectional area of the particular segment of the vascular system. Refer to Fig. 13–9 as you read the following. The aorta receives all the blood from the left ventricle, its cross-sectional area is small, about 3 cm^2 (0.5 sq. inch), and the blood moves very rapidly, at least 30 cm (about 12 inches) per second. Each time the aorta or any artery branches, the total cross-sectional area becomes larger, and the speed of blood flow decreases. Think of a river that begins in a narrow bed and is flowing rapidly. If the river bed widens, the water spreads out to fill it and flows more slowly. If the river were to narrow again, the water would flow faster. This is just what happens in the vascular system.

The capillaries in total have the greatest cross-sectional area, and blood velocity there is slowest, less than 0.1 cm per second. When capillaries unite to form venules, and then veins, the cross-sectional area decreases and blood flow speeds up.

Recall that it is in capillary networks that exchanges of nutrients, wastes, and gases take place between the blood and tissue fluid. The slow rate of blood flow in capillaries permits sufficient time for these essential exchanges. Think of a train slowing down (not actually stopping) at

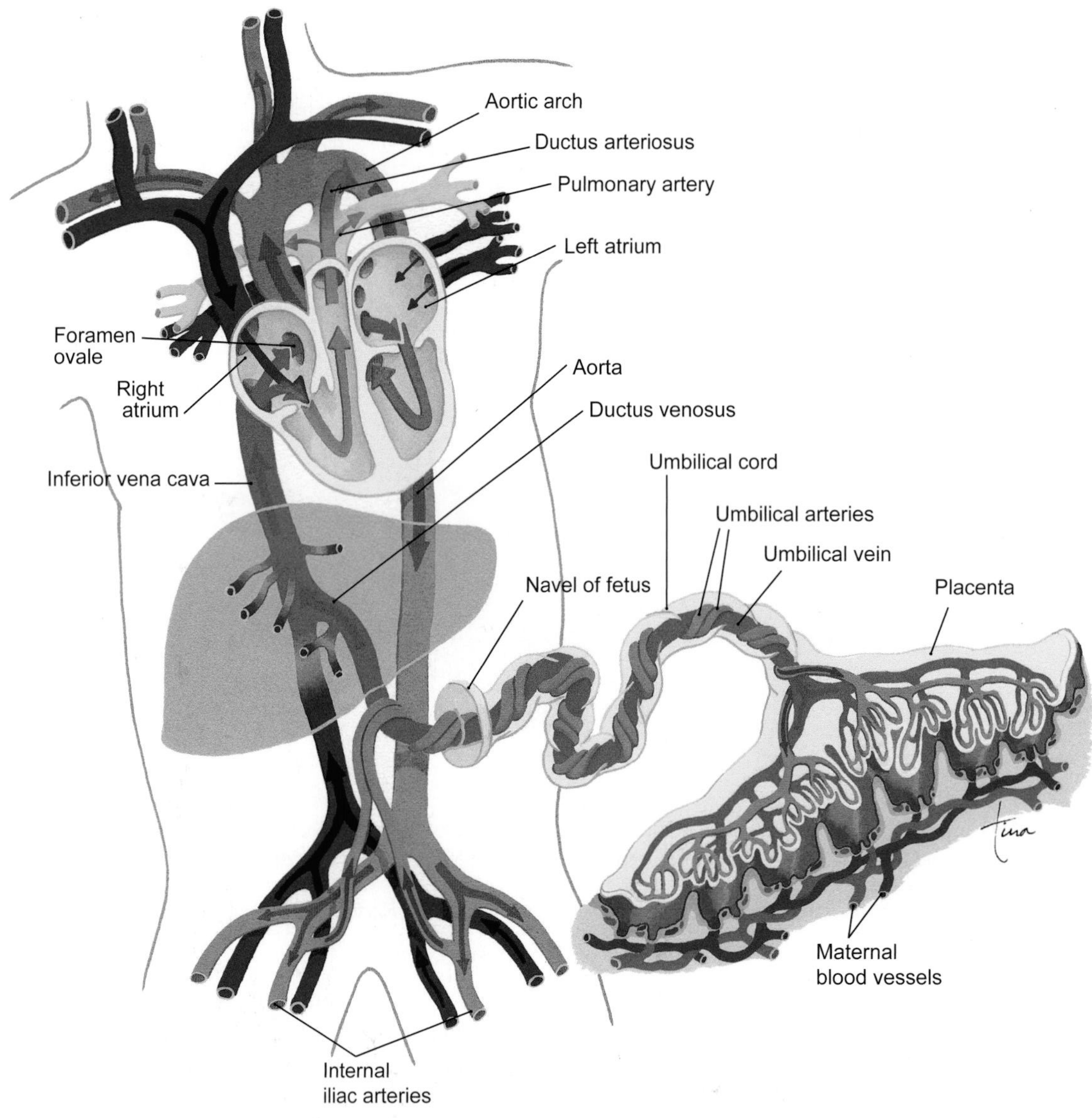

Figure 13–8 Fetal circulation. Fetal heart and blood vessels are shown on the left. Arrows depict the direction of blood flow. The placenta and umbilical blood vessels are shown on the right. See text for description.

QUESTION: Find the foramen ovale in the fetal heart. Which way does blood flow through it, and why?

stations to allow people to jump on and off, then speeding up again to get to the next station. The capillaries are the "stations" of the vascular system.

The more rapid blood velocity in other vessels makes circulation time quite short. This is the time it takes for blood to go from the right ventricle to the lungs, back to the heart to be pumped by the left ventricle to the body, and return to the heart again. Circulation time is about 1 minute or less and ensures an adequate exchange of gases.

BLOOD PRESSURE

Blood pressure is the force the blood exerts against the walls of the blood vessels. Filtration in capillaries depends

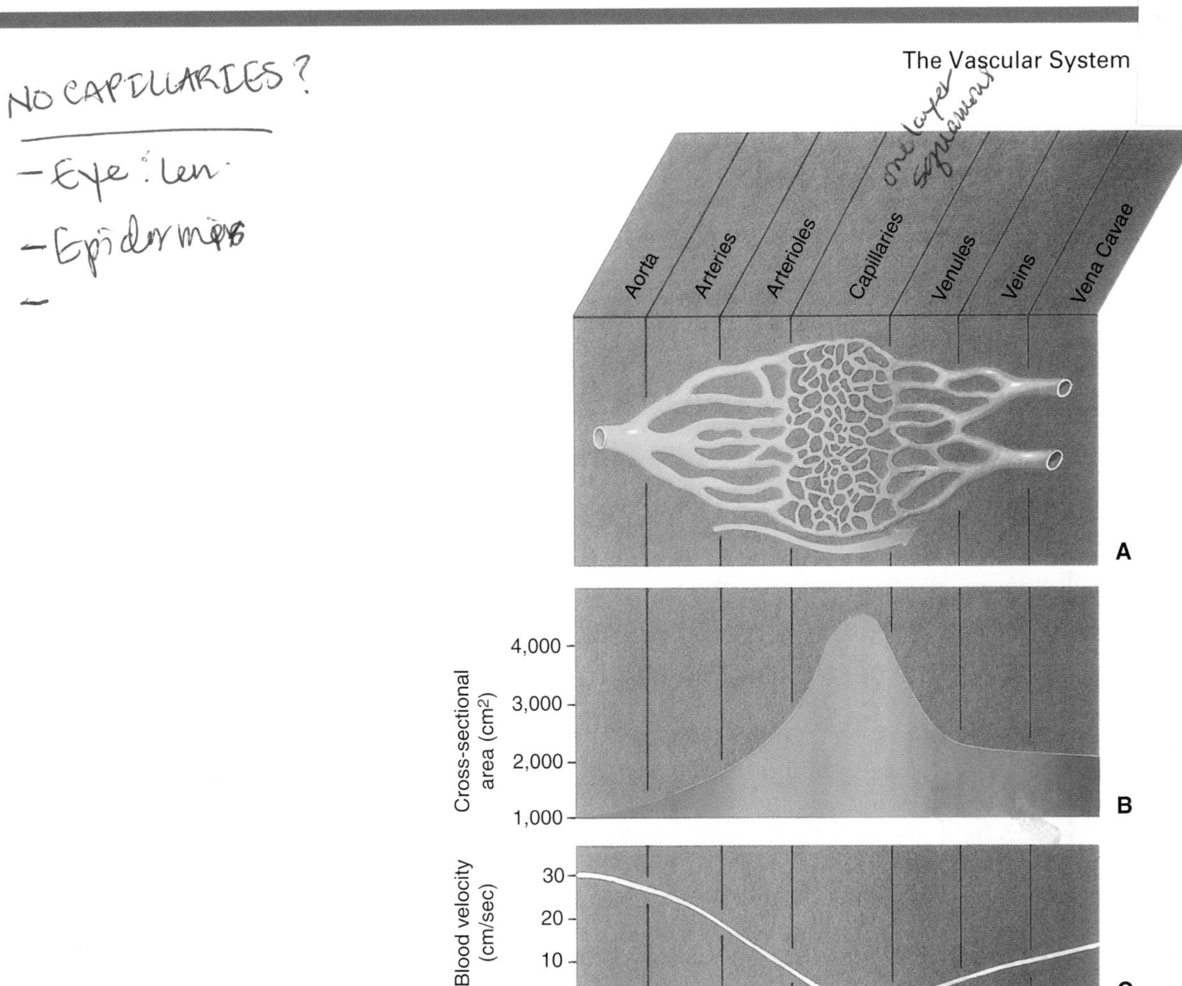

Figure 13–9 Characteristics of the vascular system. (**A**) Schematic of the branching of vessels. (**B**) Cross-sectional area in square centimeters. (**C**) Blood velocity in centimeters per second. (**D**) Systemic blood pressure changes. Notice that systolic and diastolic pressures become one pressure in the capillaries.

QUESTION: Look at the cross-sectional area and blood velocity. As area increases, what happens to velocity? Where is velocity slowest?

upon blood pressure; filtration brings nutrients to tissues, and as you will see in Chapter 18, is the first step in the formation of urine. Blood pressure is one of the "vital signs" often measured, and indeed a normal blood pressure is essential to life.

The pumping of the ventricles creates blood pressure, which is measured in mm Hg (millimeters of mercury). When a systemic blood pressure reading is taken, two numbers are obtained: systolic and diastolic, as in 110/70 mm Hg. **Systolic** pressure is always the higher of the two and represents the blood pressure when the left ventricle is contracting. The lower number is the **diastolic** pressure, when the left ventricle is relaxed and does not exert force. Diastolic pressure is maintained by the arteries and arterioles and is discussed in a later section.

Systemic blood pressure is highest in the aorta, which receives all of the blood pumped by the left ventricle. As blood travels farther away from the heart, blood pressure decreases (see Fig. 13–9). The brachial artery is most often used to take a blood pressure reading; here a normal systolic range is 90 to 120 mm Hg, and a normal diastolic range is 60 to 80 mm Hg. In the arterioles, blood pressure decreases further, and systolic and diastolic pressures merge into one pressure. At the arterial end of capillary networks, blood pressure is about 30 to 35 mm Hg, decreasing to 12 to 15 mm Hg at the venous end of capillaries. This is high enough to permit filtration but low enough to prevent rupture of the capillaries. As blood flows through veins, the pressure decreases further, and in the caval veins, blood pressure approaches zero as blood enters the right atrium.

The upper limit of the normal blood pressure range is now 120/80 mm Hg. The levels of 125 to 139/85 to 89 mm Hg, once considered high-normal, are now called "prehypertension," that is, with the potential to become even higher. A systemic blood pressure consistently higher than the normal range is called **hypertension** (see also Box 13–4: Hypertension). A lower than normal blood pressure is called **hypotension**. The

Box 13–4 | HYPERTENSION

Hypertension is high blood pressure, that is, a resting systemic pressure consistently above the normal range (90 to 120/60 to 80 mm Hg). Clinicians now consider 125 to 139/85 to 89 mm Hg to be prehypertension. A systolic reading of 140 to 159 mm Hg or a diastolic reading of 90 to 99 mm Hg may be called stage 1 hypertension, and a systolic reading above 160 mm Hg or a diastolic reading above 100 mm Hg may be called stage 2 hypertension.

The term "essential" or "primary hypertension" means that no specific cause can be determined; most cases are in this category. For some people, however, an overproduction of renin by the kidneys is the cause of their hypertension. Excess renin increases the production of angiotensin II, which raises blood pressure. Although hypertension often produces no symptoms, the long-term consequences may be very serious. Chronic hypertension has its greatest effects on the arteries and on the heart.

Although the walls of arteries are strong, hypertension weakens them and contributes to arteriosclerosis. Such weakened arteries may rupture or develop aneurysms, which may in turn lead to a CVA or kidney damage.

Hypertension affects the heart because the left ventricle must now pump blood against the higher arterial pressure. The left ventricle works harder and, like any other muscle, enlarges as more work is demanded; this is called **left ventricular hypertrophy**. This abnormal growth of the myocardium, however, is not accompanied by a corresponding growth in coronary capillaries, and the blood supply of the left ventricle may not be adequate for all situations. Exercise, for example, puts further demands on the heart, and the person may experience angina due to a lack of oxygen or a myocardial infarction if the oxygen deficiency is severe.

Although several different kinds of medications (diuretics, vasodilators) are used to treat hypertension, people with moderate hypertension may limit their dependence on medications by following certain guidelines:

1. Don't smoke because nicotine stimulates vasoconstriction, which raises BP. Smoking also damages arteries, contributing to arteriosclerosis.
2. Lose weight if overweight. A weight loss of as little as 10 pounds can lower BP. A diet high in fruits and vegetables may, for some people, contribute to lower BP.
3. Cut salt intake. Although salt consumption may not be the *cause* of hypertension, reducing salt intake may help lower blood pressure by decreasing blood volume.
4. Exercise on a regular basis. A moderate amount of aerobic exercise (such as a half hour walk every day) is beneficial for the entire cardiovascular system and may also contribute to weight loss.

regulation of systemic blood pressure is discussed in a later section.

Pulmonary blood pressure is created by the right ventricle, which has relatively thin walls and thus exerts about one-sixth the force of the left ventricle. The result is that pulmonary arterial pressure is always low: 20 to 25/8 to 10 mm Hg, and in pulmonary capillaries is lower still. This is important to *prevent* filtration in pulmonary capillaries, which in turn prevents tissue fluid from accumulating in the alveoli of the lungs.

MAINTENANCE OF SYSTEMIC BLOOD PRESSURE

Because blood pressure is so important, many physiological factors and processes interact to keep blood pressure within normal limits:

1. **Venous return**—the amount of blood that returns to the heart by way of the veins. Venous return is important because the heart can pump only the blood it receives. If venous return decreases, the cardiac muscle fibers will not be stretched, the force of ventricular systole will decrease (Starling's law), and blood pressure will decrease. This is what might happen following a severe hemorrhage.

   When the body is horizontal, venous return can be maintained fairly easily, but when the body is vertical, gravity must be overcome to return blood from the lower body to the heart. Three mechanisms help promote venous return: constriction of veins, the skeletal muscle pump, and the respiratory pump.

   Veins contain smooth muscle, which enables them to constrict and force blood toward the heart; the valves prevent backflow of blood. The second mechanism is the **skeletal muscle pump**, which is especially effective for the deep veins of the legs. These veins are surrounded by skeletal muscles that contract and relax during normal activities such as walking. Contractions of the leg muscles squeeze the veins to force blood toward the heart. The third mechanism is the **respiratory pump**, which affects veins that pass through the chest cavity. The pressure changes of inhalation and exhalation alternately expand and compress the veins, and blood is returned to the heart.

2. **Heart rate and force**—in general, if heart rate and force increase, blood pressure increases; this is what happens during exercise. However, if the heart is beating extremely rapidly, the ventricles may not fill completely between beats, and cardiac output and blood pressure will decrease.

3. **Peripheral resistance**—this term refers to the resistance the vessels offer to the flow of blood. The arteries and veins are usually slightly constricted, which maintains normal diastolic blood pressure. It may be helpful to think of the vessels as the "container" for the blood. If a person's body has 5 liters of blood, the "container" must be smaller in order for the blood to exert a pressure against its walls. This is what normal vasoconstriction does: It makes the container (the vessels) smaller than the volume of blood so that the blood will exert pressure even when the left ventricle is relaxed.

   If more vasoconstriction occurs, blood pressure will increase (the container has become even smaller). This is what happens in a stress situation, when greater vasoconstriction is brought about by sympathetic impulses. If vasodilation occurs, blood pressure will decrease (the container is larger). After eating a large meal, for example, there is extensive vasodilation in the digestive tract to supply more oxygenated blood for digestive activities. To keep blood pressure within the normal range, vasoconstriction must, and does, occur elsewhere in the body. This is why strenuous exercise should be avoided right after eating; there is not enough blood to completely supply oxygen to exercising muscles and an active digestive tract at the same time.

4. **Elasticity of the large arteries**—when the left ventricle contracts, the blood that enters the large arteries stretches the arteries' walls. The arterial walls are elastic and absorb some of the force. When the left ventricle relaxes, the arterial walls recoil or snap back, which helps keep diastolic pressure within the normal range. Normal elasticity, therefore, lowers systolic pressure, raises diastolic pressure, and maintains a normal pulse pressure. (Pulse pressure is the difference between systolic and diastolic pressure. The usual ratio of systolic to diastolic to pulse pressure is approximately 3:2:1. For example, with a blood pressure of 120/80 mm Hg, the pulse pressure is 40 and the ratio is 120:80:40, or 3:2:1.)

5. **Viscosity of the blood**—normal blood viscosity depends upon the presence of red blood cells and plasma proteins, especially albumin. Having too many red blood cells is rare but does occur in the disorder called polycythemia vera and in people who are heavy smokers. This will increase blood viscosity and blood pressure.

   A decreased number of red blood cells, as is seen with severe anemia, or decreased albumin, as may occur in liver disease or kidney disease, will decrease blood viscosity and blood pressure. In these situations, other mechanisms such as vasoconstriction will maintain blood pressure as close to normal as is possible.

6. **Loss of blood**—a small loss of blood, as when donating a pint of blood, will cause a temporary drop in blood pressure followed by rapid compensation in the form of a more rapid heart rate and greater vasoconstriction. After a severe hemorrhage, however, these compensating mechanisms may not be sufficient to maintain normal blood pressure and blood flow to the brain. Although a person may survive loss of 50% of the body's total blood, the possibility of brain damage increases as more blood is lost and not rapidly replaced.
7. **Hormones**—several hormones have effects on blood pressure. You may recall them from Chapters 10 and 12, but we will summarize them here and in Fig. 13–10. The adrenal medulla secretes norepinephrine and epinephrine in stressful situations. Norepinephrine stimulates vasoconstriction, which raises blood pressure. Epinephrine also causes vasoconstriction and increases heart rate and force of contraction, both of which increase blood pressure.

   Antidiuretic hormone (ADH) is secreted by the posterior pituitary gland when the water content of the body decreases. ADH increases the reabsorption of water by the kidneys to prevent further loss of water in urine and a further decrease in blood pressure.

   Aldosterone, a hormone from the adrenal cortex, has a similar effect on blood volume. When blood pressure decreases, secretion of aldosterone stimulates the reabsorption of Na^+ ions by the kidneys. Water follows sodium back to the blood, which

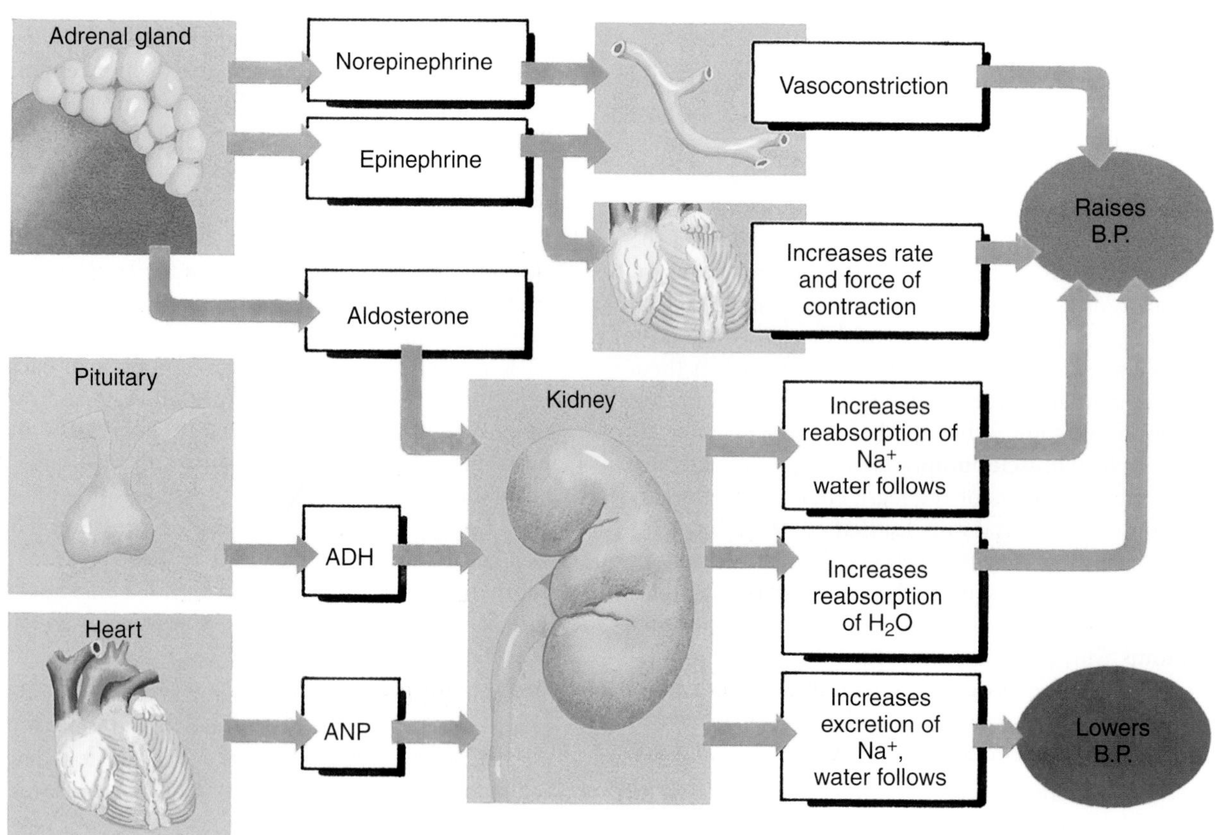

Figure 13–10 Hormones that affect blood pressure. See text for further description.

QUESTION: Which two hormones have opposite functions, and what are these functions?

maintains blood volume to prevent a further drop in blood pressure.

Atrial natriuretic peptide (ANP), secreted by the atria of the heart, functions in opposition to aldosterone. ANP increases the excretion of Na^+ ions and water by the kidneys, which decreases blood volume and lowers blood pressure.

DISTRIBUTION OF BLOOD FLOW

An individual's blood volume remains relatively constant within the normal range appropriate to the size of the person. Active tissues, however, require more blood, that is, more oxygen, than do less active tissues. As active tissues and organs receive a greater proportion of the total blood flow, less active organs must receive less, or blood pressure will decrease markedly.

As mentioned previously, precapillary sphincters dilate in active tissues and constrict in less active ones. The arterioles also constrict to reduce blood flow to less active organs (where the oxygen level remains relatively high because the cells are not using it quickly to produce ATP). This ensures that metabolically active organs will receive enough oxygen to function properly and that blood pressure for the body as a whole will be maintained within normal limits.

An example will be helpful here; let us use the body at rest and the body during exercise. Consult Fig. 13–11 as you read the following. Resting cardiac output is approximately 5000 mL per minute. Exercise cardiac output is three times

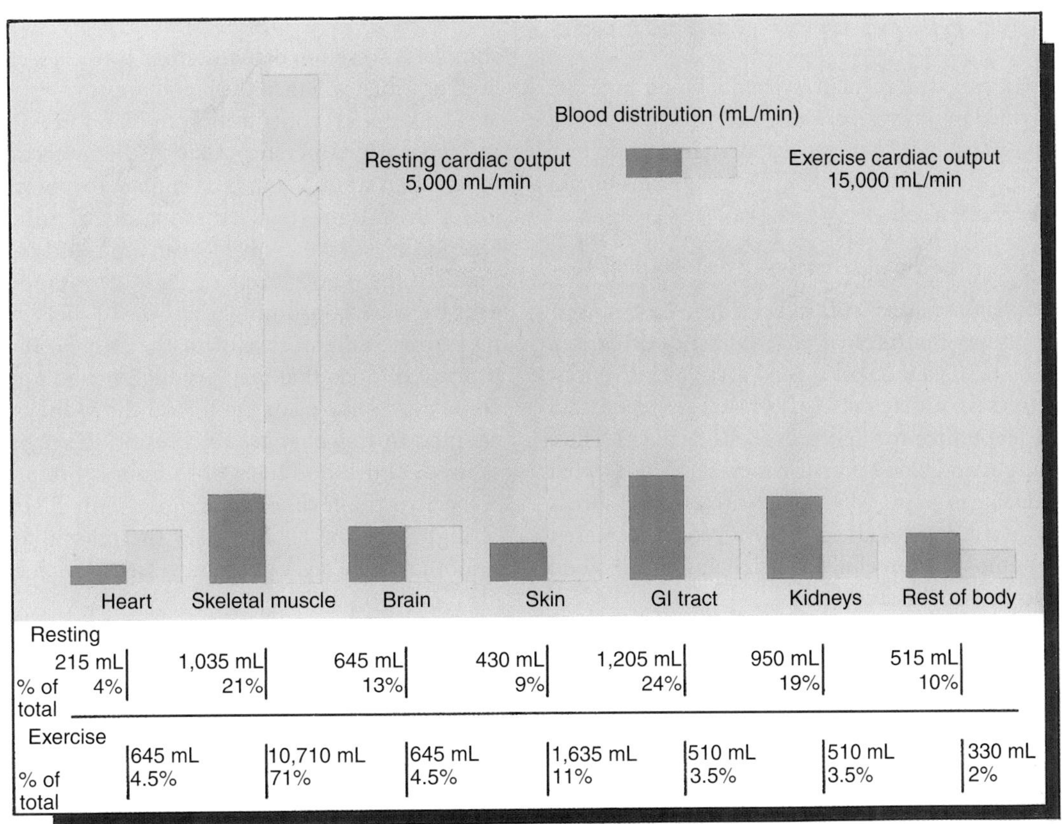

Figure 13–11 Blood flow through various organs when the body is at rest and during exercise. For each organ, the percentage of the total blood flow is given.

QUESTION: During exercise, which organs have the greatest increase in blood flow? Which organs have the greatest decrease?

that, about 15,000 mL per minute. Keep in mind that the volume of blood is the same in both cases, but that during exercise the blood is being circulated more rapidly.

Compare the amounts of blood flowing to various organs and tissues during exercise and at rest. During exercise, the heart receives about three times as much blood as it does when the body is at rest. The very active skeletal muscles receive about 10 times as much blood. The skin, as an organ of heat loss, receives about four times as much blood. Other organs, however, can function adequately with less blood. Blood flow is reduced to the digestive tract, to the kidneys, and to other parts of the body such as bones.

When the exercise ceases, cardiac output will gradually return to the resting level, as will blood flow to the various organs. These changes in the distribution of blood ensure sufficient oxygen for active tissues and an appropriate blood pressure for the body as a whole.

REGULATION OF BLOOD PRESSURE

The mechanisms that regulate systemic blood pressure may be divided into two types: intrinsic mechanisms and nervous mechanisms. The nervous mechanisms involve the nervous system, and the intrinsic mechanisms do not require nerve impulses.

INTRINSIC MECHANISMS

The term *intrinsic* means "within." Intrinsic mechanisms work because of the internal characteristics of certain organs. The first such organ is the heart. When venous return increases, cardiac muscle fibers are stretched, and the ventricles pump more forcefully (Starling's law). Thus, cardiac output and blood pressure increase. This is what happens during exercise, when a higher blood pressure is needed. When exercise ends and venous return decreases, the heart pumps less forcefully, which helps return blood pressure to a normal resting level.

The second intrinsic mechanism involves the kidneys. When blood flow through the kidneys decreases, the process of filtration decreases and less urine is formed. This decrease in urinary output preserves blood volume so that it does not decrease further. Following severe hemorrhage or any other type of dehydration, this is very important to maintain blood pressure.

The kidneys are also involved in the **renin-angiotensin mechanism**. When blood pressure decreases, the kidneys secrete the enzyme **renin**, which initiates a series of reactions that result in the formation of **angiotensin II**. These reactions are described in Table 13–3 and depicted in Fig. 13–12. Angiotensin II causes vasoconstriction and stimulates secretion of aldosterone by the adrenal cortex, both of which will increase blood pressure.

Table 13–3 | **THE RENIN-ANGIOTENSIN MECHANISM**

1. Decreased blood pressure stimulates the kidneys to secrete renin.
2. Renin splits the plasma protein angiotensinogen (synthesized by the liver) to angiotensin I.
3. Angiotensin I is converted to angiotensin II by an enzyme (called converting enzyme) secreted by lung tissue and vascular endothelium.
4. Angiotensin II:
   - causes vasoconstriction
   - stimulates the adrenal cortex to secrete aldosterone

The kidneys' contribution to blood pressure is also influenced by a person's diet. A diet with more plant foods than animal foods is higher in potassium and lower in sodium than a diet mainly of animal foods. Our kidneys have evolved over thousands of years to regulate the blood levels of these two important ions as if we were consuming plant-based diets, as did our prehistoric ancestors. But in the past 50 to 60 years, processed foods that are very high in sodium have become much more common, and the kidneys have not adapted to this change. As a result, the proportion is skewed: Our blood level of sodium is often high with respect to the level of potassium. This disproportion of high Na^+/low K^+ increases the muscle tone of the smooth muscle layer of blood vessels, which raises resting blood pressure.

NERVOUS MECHANISMS

The medulla and the autonomic nervous system are directly involved in the regulation of blood pressure. The first of these nervous mechanisms concerns the heart; this was described previously, so we will not review it here but refer you to Chapter 12 and Fig. 12–8, as well as Fig. 13–13.

The second nervous mechanism involves peripheral resistance, that is, the degree of constriction of the arteries and arterioles and, to a lesser extent, the veins (see Fig. 13–13). The medulla contains the **vasomotor center**, which consists of a vasoconstrictor area and

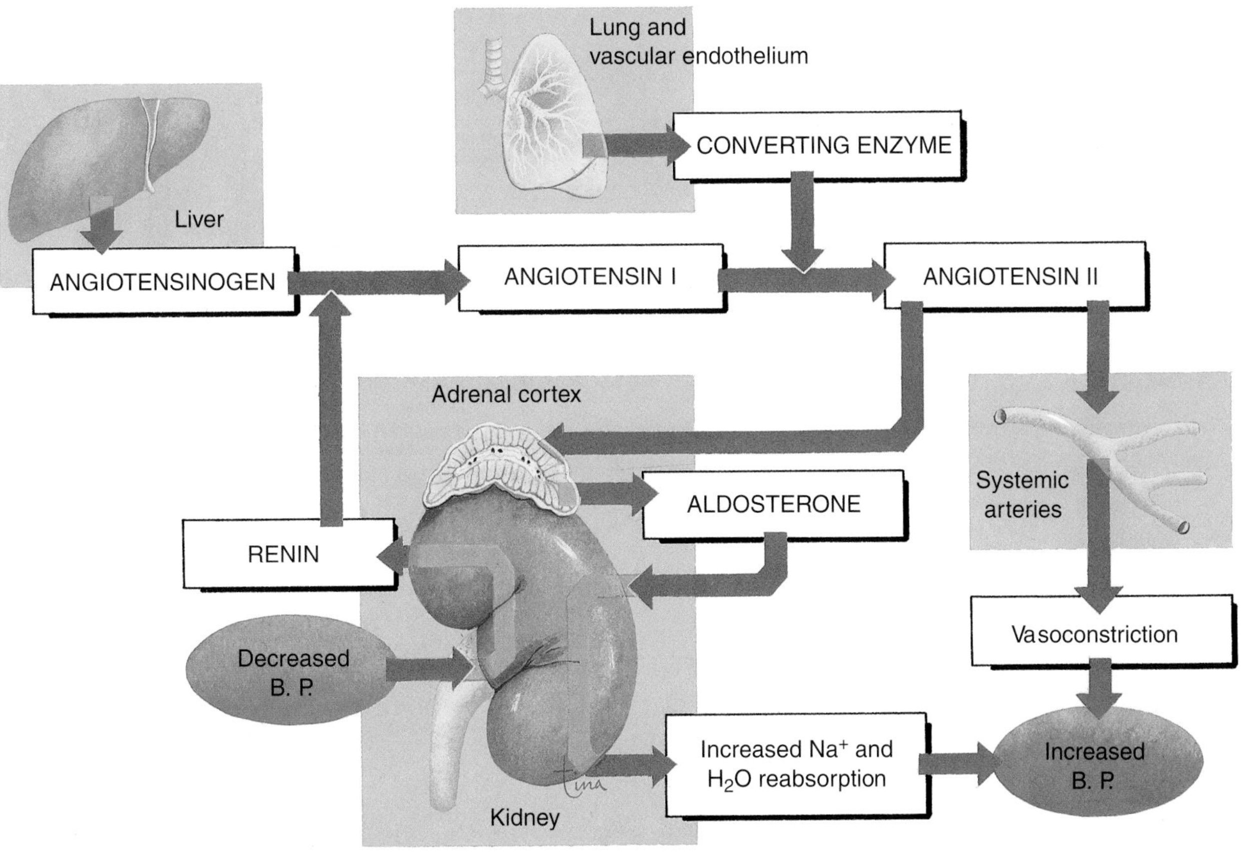

Figure 13–12 The renin-angiotensin mechanism. Begin at "Decreased B. P." and see Table 13–3 for numbered steps.

QUESTION: Where is renin produced? What are the functions of angiotensin II?

a vasodilator area. The vasodilator area may depress the vasoconstrictor area to bring about vasodilation, which will decrease blood pressure. The vasoconstrictor area may bring about more vasoconstriction by way of the sympathetic division of the autonomic nervous system.

Sympathetic vasoconstrictor fibers innervate the smooth muscle of all arteries and veins, and several impulses per second along these fibers maintain normal vasoconstriction. More impulses per second bring about greater vasoconstriction, and fewer impulses per second cause vasodilation. The medulla receives the information to make such changes from the pressoreceptors in the carotid sinuses and the aortic sinus. The inability to maintain normal blood pressure is one aspect of circulatory shock (see Box 13–5: Circulatory Shock).

AGING AND THE VASCULAR SYSTEM

It is believed that the aging of blood vessels, especially arteries, begins in childhood, although the effects are not apparent for decades. The cholesterol deposits of atherosclerosis are to be expected with advancing age, with the most serious consequences in the coronary arteries. A certain degree of arteriosclerosis is to be expected, and average resting blood pressure may increase, which further damages arterial walls. Consequences include

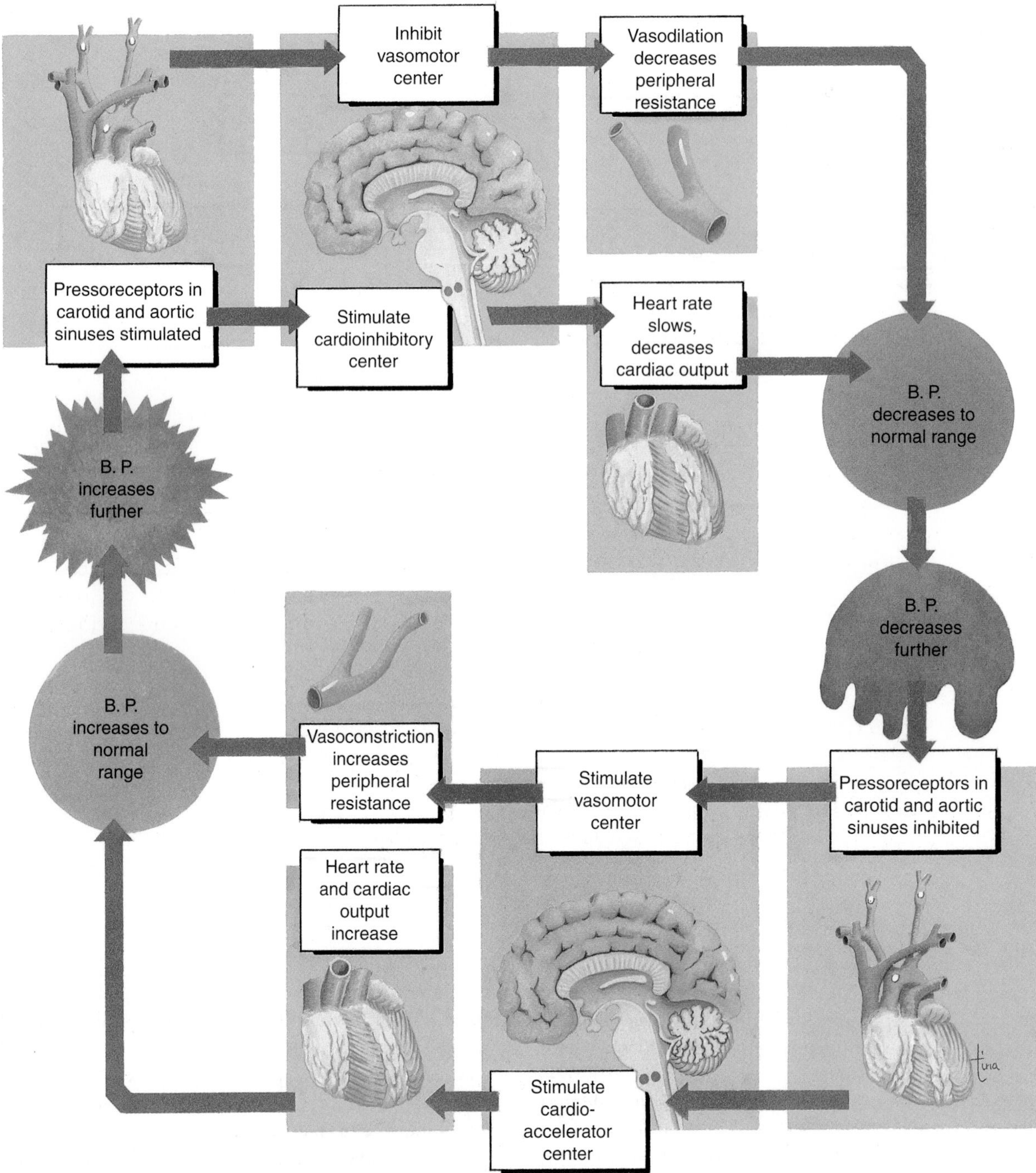

Figure 13–13 Nervous mechanisms that regulate blood pressure. See text for description.

QUESTION: What kind of sensory information is used to make changes in BP, and where are the receptors located?

Box 13–5 | CIRCULATORY SHOCK

Circulatory shock is any condition in which cardiac output decreases to the extent that tissues are deprived of oxygen and waste products accumulate.

CAUSES OF SHOCK

Cardiogenic shock occurs most often after a severe myocardial infarction but may also be the result of ventricular fibrillation. In either case, the heart is no longer an efficient pump, and cardiac output decreases.

Hypovolemic shock is the result of decreased blood volume, often due to severe hemorrhage. Other possible causes are extreme sweating (heat stroke) or extreme loss of water through the kidneys (diuresis) or intestines (diarrhea). In these situations, the heart simply does not have enough blood to pump, and cardiac output decreases. **Anaphylactic** shock, also in this category, is a massive allergic reaction in which great amounts of histamine increase capillary permeability and vasodilation throughout the body. Much plasma is then lost to tissue spaces, which decreases blood volume, blood pressure, and cardiac output.

Septic shock is the result of septicemia, the presence of bacteria in the blood. The bacteria and damaged tissues release inflammatory chemicals that cause vasodilation and extensive loss of plasma into tissue spaces.

STAGES OF SHOCK

Compensated shock—the responses by the body maintain cardiac output. Following a small hemorrhage, for example, the heart rate increases, the blood vessels constrict, and the kidneys decrease urinary output to conserve water. These responses help preserve blood volume and maintain blood pressure, cardiac output, and blood flow to tissues.

Progressive shock—the state of shock leads to more shock. Following a severe hemorrhage, cardiac output decreases and the myocardium itself is deprived of blood. The heart weakens, which further decreases cardiac output. Arteries that are deprived of their blood supply cannot remain constricted. As the arteries dilate, venous return decreases, which in turn decreases cardiac output. Progressive shock is a series of such vicious cycles, and medical intervention is required to restore cardiac output to normal.

Irreversible shock—no amount of medical assistance can restore cardiac output to normal. The usual cause of death is that the heart has been damaged too much to recover. A severe myocardial infarction, massive hemorrhage, or septicemia may all be fatal despite medical treatment.

left-sided heart failure, and stroke if cerebral vessels are damaged.

The veins also deteriorate with age; their thin walls weaken and stretch, making their valves incompetent. This is most likely to occur in the veins of the legs; their walls are subject to great pressure as blood is returned to the heart against the force of gravity. Varicose veins and phlebitis are more likely to occur among elderly people.

SUMMARY

Although the vascular system does form passageways for the blood, you can readily see that the blood vessels are not simply pipes through which the blood flows. The vessels are not passive tubes, but rather active contributors to homeostasis. The arteries and veins help maintain blood pressure, and the capillaries provide sites for the exchanges of materials between the blood and the tissues. Some very important sites of exchange are discussed in later chapters: the lungs, the digestive tract, and the kidneys.

STUDY OUTLINE

The vascular system consists of the arteries, capillaries, and veins through which blood travels.

Arteries (and arterioles) (see Fig. 13–1)

1. Carry blood from the heart to capillaries; three layers in their walls.
2. Inner layer (tunica intima): simple squamous epithelial tissue (endothelium), very smooth to prevent adhesion of platelets and abnormal blood clotting; secretes the vasodilator nitric oxide and the vasoconstrictor endothelin.
3. Middle layer (tunica media): smooth muscle and elastic connective tissue; contributes to maintenance of diastolic blood pressure (BP).
4. Outer layer (tunica externa): fibrous connective tissue to prevent rupture.
5. Constriction or dilation is regulated by chemicals of the endothelium and by the autonomic nervous system.

Veins (and venules) (see Fig. 13–1)

1. Carry blood from capillaries to the heart; three layers in walls.
2. Inner layer: endothelium folded into valves to prevent the backflow of blood.
3. Middle layer: thin smooth muscle; thin because veins are not as important in the maintenance of BP.
4. Outer layer: thin fibrous connective tissue; thin because veins do not carry blood under high pressure.

Anastomoses—connections between vessels of the same type

1. Provide alternate pathways for blood flow if one vessel is blocked.
2. Arterial anastomoses provide for blood flow to the capillaries of an organ (e.g., circle of Willis to the brain).
3. Venous anastomoses provide for return of blood to the heart and are most numerous in veins of the legs.

Capillaries (see Figs. 13–1 and 13–2)

1. Carry blood from arterioles to venules.
2. Walls are one cell thick (simple squamous epithelial tissue) to permit exchanges between blood and tissue fluid.
3. Oxygen and carbon dioxide are exchanged by diffusion.
4. BP in capillaries brings nutrients to tissues and forms tissue fluid in the process of filtration.
5. Albumin in the blood provides colloid osmotic pressure, which pulls waste products and tissue fluid into capillaries. The return of tissue fluid maintains blood volume and BP.
6. Precapillary sphincters regulate blood flow into capillary networks on the basis of tissue needs; in active tissues they dilate; in less active tissues they constrict.
7. Sinusoids are very permeable capillaries found in the liver, spleen, pituitary gland, and red bone marrow to permit proteins and blood cells to enter or leave the blood.

Pathways of Circulation

1. Pulmonary: Right ventricle → pulmonary artery → pulmonary capillaries (exchange of gases) → pulmonary veins → left atrium.
2. Systemic: left ventricle → aorta → capillaries in body tissues → superior and inferior caval veins → right atrium (see Table 13–1 and Fig. 13–3 for systemic arteries and Table 13–2 and Fig. 13–4 for systemic veins).
3. Hepatic portal circulation: blood from the digestive organs and spleen flows through the portal vein to the liver before returning to the heart. Purpose: the liver stores some nutrients or regulates their blood levels and detoxifies potential poisons before blood enters the rest of peripheral circulation (see Fig. 13–7).

Fetal Circulation—the fetus depends on the mother for oxygen and nutrients and for the removal of waste products (see Fig. 13–8)

1. The placenta is the site of exchange between fetal blood and maternal blood.
2. Umbilical arteries (two) carry blood from the fetus to the placenta, where CO_2 and waste products enter maternal circulation.
3. The umbilical vein carries blood with O_2 and nutrients from the placenta to the fetus.
4. The umbilical vein branches; some blood flows through the fetal liver; most blood flows through the ductus venosus to the fetal inferior vena cava.

5. The foramen ovale permits blood to flow from the right atrium to the left atrium to bypass the fetal lungs.
6. The ductus arteriosus permits blood to flow from the pulmonary artery to the aorta to bypass the fetal lungs.
7. These fetal structures become nonfunctional after birth, when the umbilical cord is cut and breathing takes place.

Velocity of Blood Flow (see Fig. 13–9)

1. Velocity is inversely related to the cross-sectional area of a segment of the vascular system.
2. The total capillaries have the greatest cross-sectional area and slowest blood flow.
3. Slow flow in the capillaries is important to permit sufficient time for exchange of gases, nutrients, and wastes.

Blood Pressure (BP)—the force exerted by the blood against the walls of the blood vessels (Fig. 13–9)

1. BP is measured in mm Hg: systolic/diastolic. Systolic pressure occurs during ventricular contraction; diastolic pressure occurs during ventricular relaxation.
2. Normal range of systemic arterial BP: 90 to 120/60 to 80 mm Hg.
3. BP in capillaries is 30 to 35 mm Hg at the arterial end and 12 to 15 mm Hg at the venous end—high enough to permit filtration but low enough to prevent rupture of the capillaries.
4. BP decreases in the veins and approaches zero in the caval veins.
5. Pulmonary BP is always low (the right ventricle pumps with less force): 20 to 25/8 to 10 mm Hg. This low BP prevents filtration and accumulation of tissue fluid in the alveoli.

Maintenance of Systemic BP

1. Venous return—the amount of blood that returns to the heart. If venous return decreases, the heart contracts less forcefully (Starling's law) and BP decreases. The mechanisms that maintain venous return when the body is vertical are:
   a. Constriction of veins with the valves preventing backflow of blood
   b. Skeletal muscle pump—contraction of skeletal muscles, especially in the legs, squeezes the deep veins
   c. Respiratory pump—the pressure changes of inhalation and exhalation expand and compress the veins in the chest cavity
2. Heart rate and force—if heart rate and force increase, BP increases.
3. Peripheral resistance—the resistance of the arteries and arterioles to the flow of blood. These vessels are usually slightly constricted to maintain normal diastolic BP. Greater vasoconstriction will increase BP; vasodilation will decrease BP. In the body, vasodilation in one area requires vasoconstriction in another area to maintain normal BP.
4. Elasticity of the large arteries—ventricular systole stretches the walls of large arteries, which recoil during ventricular diastole. Normal elasticity lowers systolic BP, raises diastolic BP, and maintains normal pulse pressure.
5. Viscosity of blood—depends on RBCs and plasma proteins, especially albumin. Severe anemia tends to decrease BP. Deficiency of albumin as in liver or kidney disease tends to decrease BP. In these cases, compensation such as greater vasoconstriction will keep BP close to normal.
6. Loss of blood—a small loss will be rapidly compensated for by a faster heart rate and greater vasoconstriction. After severe hemorrhage, these mechanisms may not be sufficient to maintain normal BP.
7. Hormones—(see Fig. 13–10)
   a. Norepinephrine stimulates vasoconstriction, which raises BP.
   b. Epinephrine increases cardiac output and raises BP.
   c. ADH increases water reabsorption by the kidneys, which increases blood volume and BP.
   d. Aldosterone increases reabsorption of Na^+ ions by the kidneys; water follows Na^+ and increases blood volume and BP.
   e. ANP increases excretion of Na^+ ions and water by the kidneys, which decreases blood volume and BP.

Distribution of Blood Flow

1. Metabolically active tissues require more oxygen, and receive a greater proportion of the blood volume as it circulates (see Fig. 13–11).
2. Blood flow is increased by the dilation of arterioles and precapillary sphincters.

3. In less active tissues, arterioles and precapillary sphincters constrict.
4. Organs receive sufficient oxygen, and BP for the body is maintained within the normal range.

Regulation of Blood Pressure—intrinsic mechanisms and nervous mechanisms

Intrinsic Mechanisms

1. The heart—responds to increased venous return by pumping more forcefully (Starling's law), which increases cardiac output and BP.
2. The kidneys—decreased blood flow decreases filtration, which decreases urinary output to preserve blood volume. Decreased BP stimulates the kidneys to secrete renin, which initiates the renin-angiotensin mechanism (Table 13–3 and Fig. 13–12) that results in the formation of angiotensin II, which causes vasoconstriction and stimulates secretion of aldosterone.

Nervous Mechanisms (see Fig. 13–13)

1. Heart rate and force—see also Chapter 12.
2. Peripheral resistance—the medulla contains the vasomotor center, which consists of a vasoconstrictor area and a vasodilator area.
   a. The vasodilator area brings about vasodilation by suppressing the vasoconstrictor area.
   b. The vasoconstrictor area maintains normal vasoconstriction by generating several impulses per second along sympathetic vasoconstrictor fibers to all arteries and veins.
   c. More impulses per second increase vasoconstriction and raise BP.
   d. Fewer impulses per second bring about vasodilation and a drop in BP.
   e. The information to make changes in BP comes from the carotid and aortic pressoreceptors.

REVIEW QUESTIONS

1. Describe the structure of the three layers of the walls of arteries, and state the function of each layer. Describe the structural differences in these layers in veins, and explain the reason for each difference. (p. 328)
2. Describe the structure and purpose of anastomoses, and give a specific example. (p. 330)
3. Describe the structure of capillaries. State the process by which each of the following is exchanged between capillaries and tissue fluid: nutrients, oxygen, waste products, and carbon dioxide. (pp. 331–332)
4. State the part of the body supplied by each of the following arteries: (pp. 333, 336–337)
   a. Bronchial
   b. Femoral
   c. Hepatic
   d. Brachial
   e. Inferior mesenteric
   f. Internal carotid
   g. Subclavian
   h. Intercostal
5. Describe the pathway of blood flow in hepatic portal circulation. Use a specific example to explain the purpose of portal circulation. (pp. 338–340)
6. Begin at the right ventricle and describe the pathway of pulmonary circulation. Explain the purpose of this pathway. (pp. 331–332)
7. Name the fetal structure with each of the following functions: (p. 340)
   a. Permits blood to flow from the right atrium to the left atrium
   b. Carries blood from the placenta to the fetus
   c. Permits blood to flow from the pulmonary artery to the aorta
   d. Carry blood from the fetus to the placenta
   e. Carries blood from the umbilical vein to the inferior vena cava
8. Describe the three mechanisms that promote venous return when the body is vertical. (p. 345)
9. Explain how the normal elasticity of the large arteries affects both systolic and diastolic blood pressure. (p. 345)

10. Explain how Starling's law of the heart is involved in the maintenance of blood pressure. (p. 345)
11. Name two hormones involved in the maintenance of blood pressure, and state the function of each. (pp. 346–347)
12. Describe two different ways the kidneys respond to decreased blood flow and blood pressure. (p. 348)
13. State two compensations that will maintain blood pressure after a small loss of blood. (p. 346)
14. State the location of the vasomotor center and name its two parts. Name the division of the autonomic nervous system that carries impulses to blood vessels. Which blood vessels? Which tissue in these vessels? Explain why normal vasoconstriction is important. Explain how greater vasoconstriction is brought about. Explain how vasodilation is brought about. How will each of these changes affect blood pressure? (pp. 348–350)

FOR FURTHER THOUGHT

1. Some old textbooks used the term *descending aorta*. Explain what is meant by that, and why it is not a very good term. Explain why an aneurysm of the aorta is quite likely to rupture sooner or later.
2. Renee, a nurse, is first on the scene of a car accident. The driver has been thrown from the car, and even from 15 feet away, Renee knows that a large artery in the man's leg has been severed. How does she know this? What two things does she see? Renee stops the bleeding, but the ambulance has not arrived. She wants to assess the man's condition after he has lost so much blood. She cannot take a blood pressure, but what other vital sign can be helpful? Explain. If Renee could take a blood pressure reading, what might it be? Might it be within the normal range? Explain.
3. A friend tells you that her grandmother has a tendency to develop blood clots in the veins of her legs. Your friend fears that her grandmother will have a stroke as a result. How would you explain that a stroke from a clot there is not likely? Because you are a good friend, you want to explain the serious result that may occur. How would you do that?
4. Some people with hypertension take prescribed diuretics. Some call these "water pills." Is this an accurate name? How can a diuretic help lower blood pressure? What disadvantage does the use of diuretics have?
5. Sinusoids are found in the liver and pituitary gland. For each of these organs, name four specific large molecules that enter the blood by way of sinusoids.
6. Question Figure 13–A is a circle graph that depicts the distribution of blood within the compartments of the circulatory system. The segments for the heart and pulmonary vessels have been labeled. Can you name vessels for the remaining three segments?

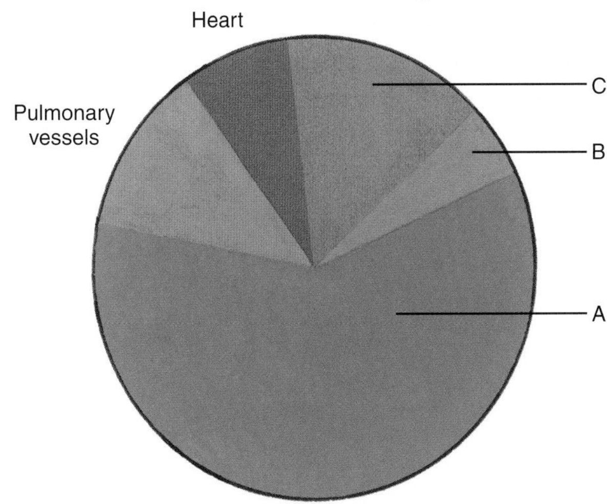

QUESTION FIGURE 13–A: Blood distribution in the compartments of the circulatory system.

CHAPTER

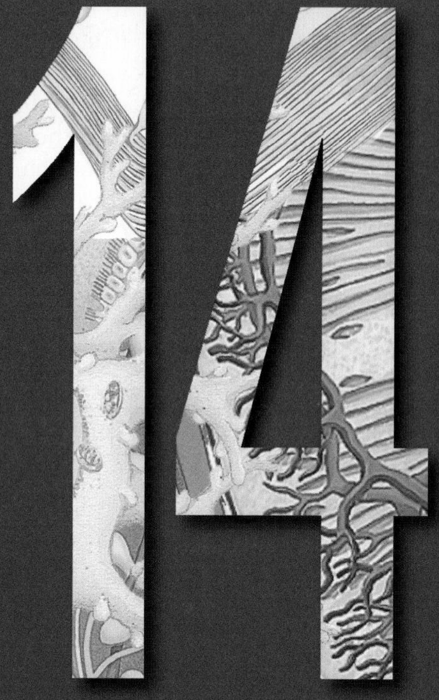

14

The Lymphatic System and Immunity

STUDENT OBJECTIVES

- Describe the functions of the lymphatic system.
- Describe how lymph is formed.
- Describe the system of lymph vessels, and explain how lymph is returned to the blood.
- State the locations and functions of the lymph nodes and nodules.
- State the location and functions of the spleen and thymus.
- Explain what is meant by immunity.
- Describe the aspects of innate immunity.
- Describe adaptive immunity: cell-mediated and antibody-mediated.
- Describe the responses to a first and second exposure to a pathogen.
- Explain the difference between genetic immunity and acquired immunity.
- Explain the difference between passive acquired immunity and active acquired immunity.
- Explain how vaccines work.

NEW TERMINOLOGY

Acquired immunity *(uh-**KWHY**-erd)*
Active immunity *(**AK**-tiv)*
Antibody-mediated immunity *(**AN**-ti-BAH-dee **ME**-dee-ay-ted)*
Antigen *(**AN**-ti-jen)*
B cells *(B SELLS)*
Cell-mediated immunity *(SELL **ME**-dee-ay-ted)*
Complement *(**KOM**-ple-ment)*
Cytokines *(**SIGH**-toh-kines)*
Genetic immunity *(je-**NET**-ik)*
Humoral immunity *(**HYOO**-mohr-uhl)*
Interferon *(in-ter-**FEER**-on)*
Lymph *(LIMF)*
Lymph nodes *(LIMF NOHDS)*
Lymph nodules *(LIMF **NAHD**-yools)*
Opsonization *(OP-sah-ni-**ZAY**-shun)*
Passive immunity *(**PASS**-iv)*
Plasma cell *(**PLAZ**-mah SELL)*
Spleen *(SPLEEN)*
T cells *(T SELLS)*
Thymus *(**THIGH**-mus)*
Tonsils *(**TAHN**-sills)*

RELATED CLINICAL TERMINOLOGY

AIDS *(AYDS)*
Allergy *(**AL**-er-jee)*
Antibody titer *(**AN**-ti-BAH-dee **TIGH**-ter)*
Attenuated *(uh-**TEN**-yoo-AY-ted)*
Complement fixation test *(**KOM**-ple-ment fik-**SAY**-shun)*
Fluorescent antibody test *(floor-**ESS**-ent)*
Hodgkin's disease *(**HODJ**-kinz)*
Tonsillectomy *(TAHN-si-**LEK**-toh-mee)*
Toxoid *(**TOK**-soyd)*
Vaccine *(vak-**SEEN**)*

Terms that appear in **bold type** *in the chapter text are defined in the glossary, which begins on page 603.*

CHAPTER OUTLINE

A child falls and scrapes her knee. Is this likely to be a life-threatening injury? Probably not, even though the breaks in the skin have permitted the entry of thousands or even millions of bacteria. Those bacteria, however, will be quickly destroyed by the cells and organs of the lymphatic system.

Although the lymphatic system may be considered part of the circulatory system, we will consider it separately because its functions are so different from those of the heart and blood vessels. Keep in mind, however, that all of these functions are interdependent. The lymphatic system is responsible for returning tissue fluid to the blood and for protecting the body against foreign material. The parts of the lymphatic system are the lymph, the system of lymph vessels, and lymphatic tissue, which includes lymph nodes and nodules, the spleen, and the thymus gland.

LYMPH

Lymph is the name for tissue fluid that enters lymph capillaries. As you may recall from Chapter 13, filtration in capillaries creates tissue fluid from blood plasma, most of which returns almost immediately to the blood in the capillaries by osmosis. Some tissue fluid, however, remains in interstitial spaces and must be returned to the blood by way of the lymphatic vessels. Without this return, blood volume and blood pressure would very soon decrease. The relationship of the lymphatic vessels to the cardiovascular system is depicted in Fig. 14–1.

LYMPH VESSELS

The system of lymph vessels begins as dead-end **lymph capillaries** found in most tissue spaces (Fig. 14–2). Lymph capillaries are very permeable and collect tissue fluid and proteins. **Lacteals** are specialized lymph capillaries in the villi of the small intestine; they absorb the fat-soluble end products of digestion, such as fatty acids and vitamins A, D, E, and K.

Lymph capillaries unite to form larger lymph vessels, whose structure is very much like that of veins. There is no pump for lymph (as the heart is the pump for blood), but the lymph is kept moving within lymph vessels by the same mechanisms that promote venous return. The smooth muscle layer of the larger lymph vessels constricts, and the one-way valves (just like those of veins) prevent backflow of lymph. Lymph vessels in the extremities, especially the legs, are compressed by the skeletal muscles that surround them; this is the **skeletal muscle pump**. The **respiratory pump** alternately expands and compresses the lymph vessels in the chest cavity and keeps the lymph moving.

Where is the lymph going? Back to the blood to become plasma again. Refer to Fig. 14–3 as you read the following. The lymph vessels from the lower body unite in front of the lumbar vertebrae to form a vessel called the **cisterna chyli**, which continues upward in front of the backbone as the **thoracic duct**. Lymph vessels from the upper left quadrant of the body join the thoracic duct, which empties lymph into the left subclavian vein. Lymph vessels from the upper right quadrant of the body unite to form the right lymphatic duct, which empties lymph into the right subclavian vein. Flaps in both subclavian veins permit the entry of lymph but prevent blood from flowing into the lymph vessels.

LYMPHATIC TISSUE

Lymphatic tissue consists mainly of lymphocytes in a mesh-like framework of connective tissue; various numbers of stem cells are present. Recall that after birth, most lymphocytes are produced from stem cells in the red bone marrow, then migrate to the lymph nodes and nodules, to the spleen, and to the thymus. In these structures, lymphocytes become activated and proliferate in response to infection (this is a function of all lymphatic tissue). The thymus has stem cells that produce a significant portion of the T lymphocytes.

LYMPH NODES AND NODULES

Lymph nodes and nodules are masses of lymphatic tissue. Nodes and nodules differ with respect to size and location. Nodes are usually larger, 10 to 20 mm in length, and are encapsulated; nodules range from a fraction of a millimeter to several millimeters in length and do not have capsules.

Lymph nodes are found in groups along the pathways of lymph vessels, and lymph flows through these nodes on its way to the subclavian veins. Lymph enters a node through several afferent lymph vessels and leaves through one or two efferent vessels (Fig. 14–4). As lymph passes through a lymph node, bacteria and other foreign materials are phagocytized by fixed (stationary) **macrophages**. **Plasma cells** develop from B lymphocytes exposed to pathogens in the lymph and produce antibodies. These antibodies will eventually reach the blood and circulate throughout the body.

There are many groups of lymph nodes along all the lymph vessels throughout the body, but three paired groups deserve mention because of their strategic locations. These are the **cervical**, **axillary**, and **inguinal** lymph

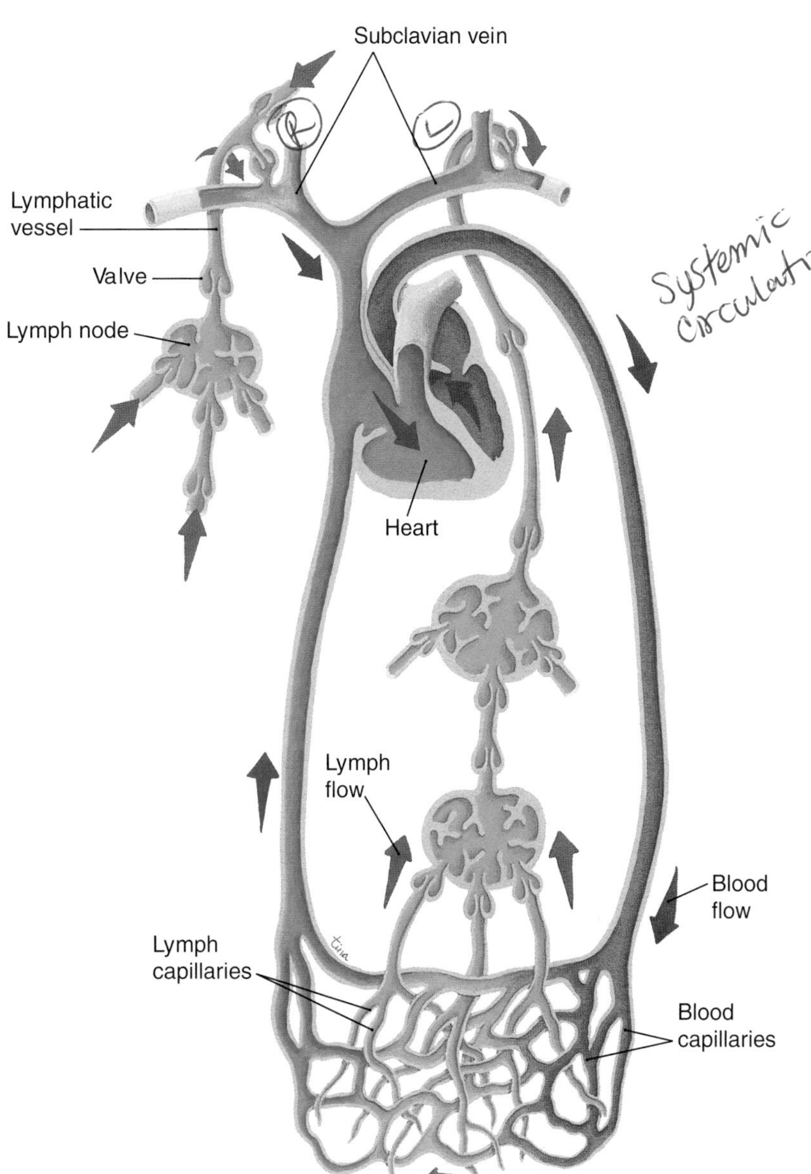

Figure 14–1 Relationship of lymphatic vessels to the cardiovascular system. Lymph capillaries collect tissue fluid, which is returned to the blood. The arrows indicate the direction of flow of the blood and lymph.

QUESTION: To which large veins is lymph returned, and why is this return important?

nodes (see Fig. 14–3). Notice that these are at the junctions of the head and extremities with the trunk of the body. Breaks in the skin, with entry of pathogens, are much more likely to occur in the arms or legs or head rather than in the trunk. If these pathogens get to the lymph, they will be destroyed by the lymph nodes before they get to the trunk and before the lymph is returned to the blood in the subclavian veins.

You may be familiar with the expression "swollen glands," as when a child has strep throat (an inflammation of the pharynx caused by *Streptococcus* bacteria). These "glands" are the cervical lymph nodes that have enlarged as their macrophages attempt to destroy the bacteria in the lymph from the pharynx (see Box 14–1: Hodgkin's Disease).

Lymph nodules are small masses of lymphatic tissue found just beneath the epithelium of all **mucous membranes**. The body systems lined with mucous membranes are those that have openings to the environment: the respiratory, digestive, urinary, and reproductive tracts. You can probably see that these are also strategic locations for lymph nodules, because any natural body opening is a

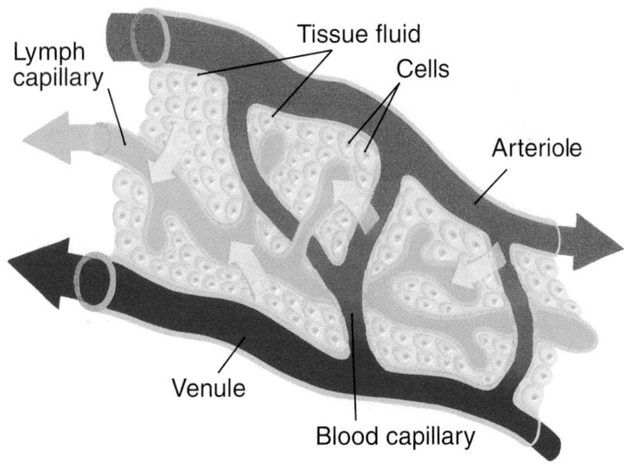

Figure 14–2 Dead-end lymph capillaries found in tissue spaces. Arrows indicate the movement of plasma, lymph, and tissue fluid.

QUESTION: Just before water enters lymph capillaries, what name does it have?

possible portal of entry for pathogens. For example, if bacteria in inhaled air get through the epithelium of the trachea, lymph nodules with their macrophages are in position to destroy these bacteria before they get to the blood.

Some of the lymph nodules have specific names. Those of the pharynx are called **tonsils**. The palatine tonsils are on the lateral walls of the pharynx, the adenoid (pharyngeal tonsil) is on the posterior wall, and the lingual tonsils are on the base of the tongue. The tonsils, therefore, form a ring of lymphatic tissue around the pharynx, which is a common pathway for food and air and for the pathogens they contain. A **tonsillectomy** is the surgical removal of the palatine tonsils and the adenoid and may be performed if the tonsils are chronically inflamed and swollen, as may happen in children. As mentioned earlier, the body has redundant structures to help ensure survival if one structure is lost or seriously impaired. Thus, there are many other lymph nodules in the pharynx to take over the function of the surgically removed tonsils.

The lymph nodules of the small intestine are called **Peyer's patches**, and despite their small size, they are extremely important. From the time we are born and every day thereafter, hundreds of foreign proteins enter the body by way of the mouth. Absorption of nutrients takes place in the small intestine. Foreign proteins and peptides in foods are absorbed as well, and they are picked up by the roaming dendritic cells and brought to lymphocytes in the nearest lymph nodule. In infancy the lymphocytes develop tolerance for proteins from food, while retaining their destructive potential for pathogens. Without such tolerance, allergies to common foods may develop. The lymphocytes of the Peyer's patches "learn" to distinguish friend (that is, food) from foe.

SPLEEN

The **spleen** is located in the upper left quadrant of the abdominal cavity, just below the diaphragm, behind the stomach. The lower rib cage protects the spleen from physical trauma (see Fig. 14–3).

In the fetus, the spleen produces red blood cells, a function assumed by the red bone marrow after birth. After birth the spleen is very much like a large lymph node, except that its functions affect the blood that flows through it rather than lymph.

The functions of the spleen after birth are:

1. Contains plasma cells that produce antibodies to foreign antigens.
2. Contains monocytes and fixed macrophages (RE cells) that phagocytize pathogens or other foreign material in the blood. The macrophages of the spleen also phagocytize old red blood cells and form bilirubin. By way of portal circulation, the bilirubin is sent to the liver for excretion in bile. The monocytes of the spleen may enter circulation when tissue is damaged and in need of cleanup and repair.
3. Stores platelets and destroys them when they are no longer useful.

The spleen is not considered a vital organ because other organs compensate for its functions if the spleen must be removed. The liver and red bone marrow will remove old red blood cells and platelets from circulation. The many lymph nodes and nodules will phagocytize pathogens (as will the liver) and have lymphocytes to be activated and plasma cells to produce antibodies. Despite this redundancy, a person without a spleen is somewhat more susceptible to certain bacterial infections such as pneumonia and meningitis.

THYMUS

The **thymus** is located inferior to the thyroid gland. In the fetus and infant, the thymus is large and extends beneath the sternum (Fig. 14–5). With increasing age, the thymus shrinks, and relatively little thymus tissue is found in adults, though it is still active.

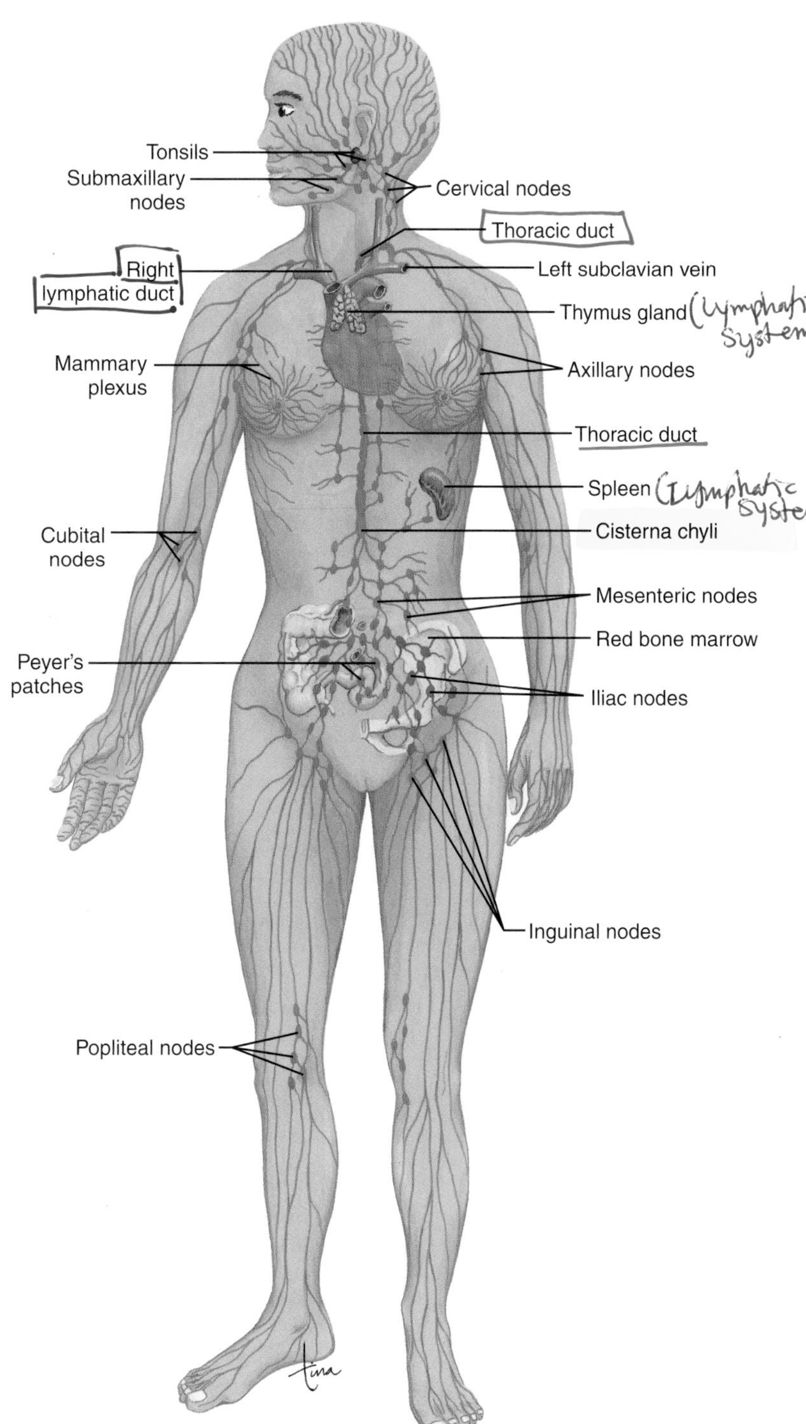

Figure 14–3 System of lymph vessels and the major groups of lymph nodes and nodules. Lymph is returned to the blood in the right and left subclavian veins.

QUESTION: Where are the major paired groups of lymph nodes located?

The stem cells of the thymus produce T lymphocytes or **T cells**; their specific functions are discussed in the next section. Thymic hormones are necessary for what may be called "immunological competence." To be competent means to be able to do something well. The thymic hormones and other cells of the thymus enable the T cells to participate in the recognition of foreign antigens and to provide immunity. This ability of T cells is established

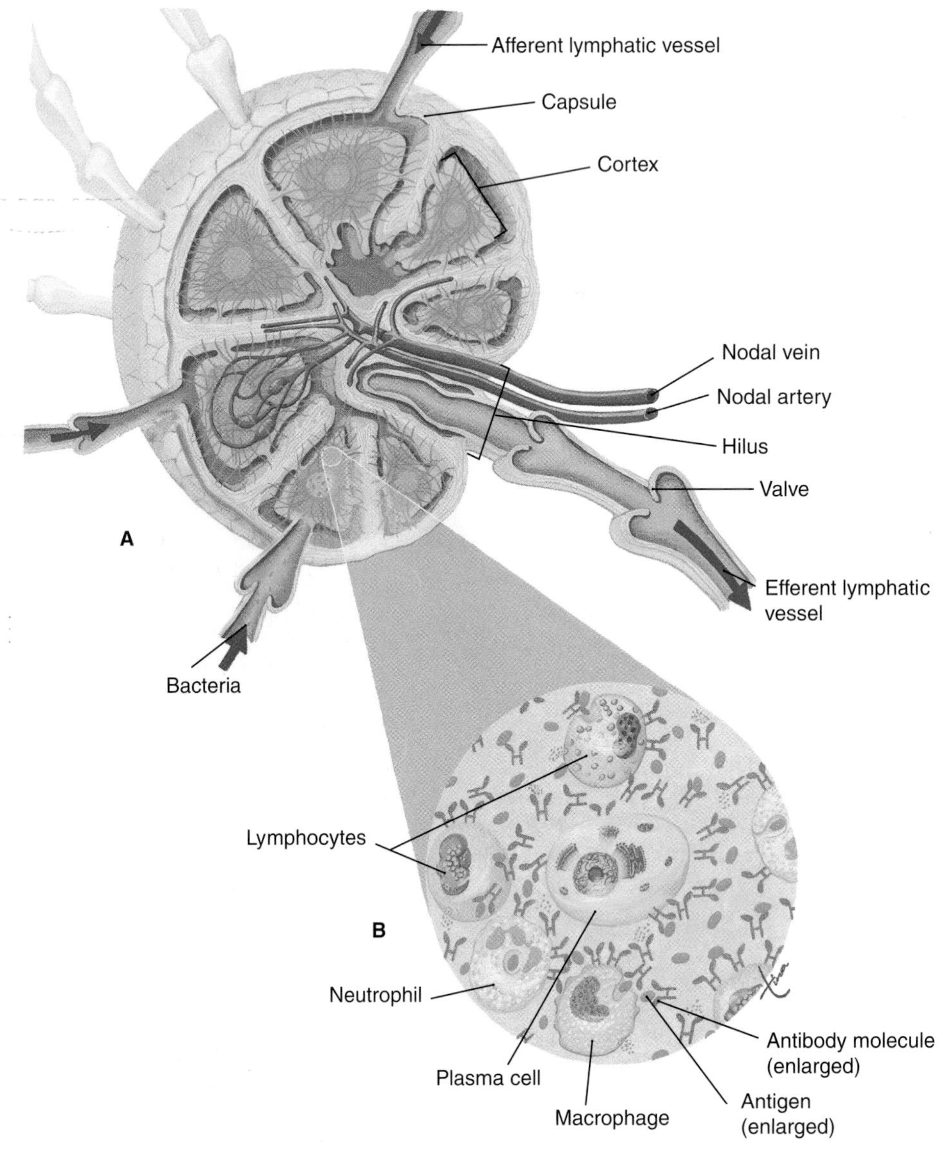

Figure 14–4 Lymph node. (**A**) Section through a lymph node, showing the flow of lymph. (**B**) Microscopic detail of bacteria being destroyed within the lymph node.

QUESTION: What is the function of the plasma cells in a lymph node?

Box 14–1 | HODGKIN'S DISEASE

Hodgkin's disease is a malignant disorder of the lymph nodes; the cause is not known. The first symptom is usually a swollen but painless lymph node, often in the cervical region. The individual is prompted to seek medical attention because of other symptoms: chronic fever, fatigue, and weight loss. The diagnosis involves biopsy of the lymph node and the finding of characteristic cells.

Treatment of Hodgkin's disease requires chemotherapy, radiation, or both. With early diagnosis and proper treatment, this malignancy is very often curable.

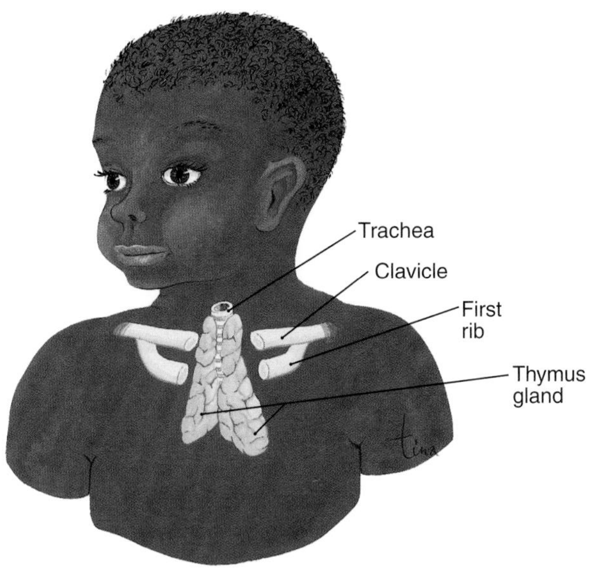

Figure 14–5 Location of the thymus in a young child.

QUESTION: Which blood cells mature in the thymus?

early in life and then is perpetuated by the lymphocytes themselves. But what exactly do the T cells learn that makes them competent? In the thymus, immature T cells are "introduced" to the cells and organic molecules of the body and develop two capabilities: self-recognition and self-tolerance.

Self-recognition is the ability to distinguish the cells that belong in the body from those that do not. Some of the immature T cells react with the cell membrane "self" proteins on the cells of the thymus and "learn" them. These are the antigens of the major histocompatibility complex (MHC; also called HLA on white blood cells). All of our cells have these proteins, so these T cells will accept all of a person's cells as belonging. T cells that do not do this will undergo apoptosis (programmed cell death).

Self-tolerance is the ability *not* to react to proteins and other organic molecules our cells produce. Immature T cells interact with dendritic cells of the thymus that have collected such "self" molecules. The T cells that do *not* react to these molecules, but rather accept or tolerate them, are the ones that will survive. Those T cells that do react will be inactivated or destroyed.

All of these "introductions" in the thymus begin taking place during fetal development. But the newborn's immune system is not yet fully mature, and infants are more susceptible to certain infections than are older children and adults. Usually by the age of 2 years, the immune system matures and becomes fully functional. This is why some vaccines, such as the measles vaccine, are not recommended for infants younger than 15 to 18 months of age. Their immune systems are not mature enough to respond strongly to the vaccine, and the protection provided by the vaccine may be incomplete.

IMMUNITY

Immunity may be defined as the ability to destroy pathogens or other foreign material and to prevent further cases of certain infectious diseases. This ability is of vital importance because the body is exposed to pathogens from the moment of birth.

Antigens are chemical markers that identify cells. Human cells have their own antigens that identify all the cells in an individual as "self," the HLA types. When antigens are foreign, or "non-self," they may be recognized as such and destroyed. Bacteria, viruses, fungi, and protozoa are all foreign antigens that activate immune responses, as are cell products such as bacterial toxins.

Malignant cells, which may be formed within the body as a result of mutations of normal cells, are also recognized as foreign and are usually destroyed before they can establish themselves and cause cancer. Unfortunately, transplanted organs are also foreign tissue, and the immune system may reject (destroy) a transplanted kidney or heart. Sometimes the immune system mistakenly reacts to part of the body itself and causes an autoimmune disease; several of these were mentioned in previous chapters. Most often, however, the immune mechanisms function to protect the body from the microorganisms around us and within us.

Immunity has two main components: innate immunity and adaptive immunity. Before we describe each component, a brief general comparison may be helpful. Innate immunity may be called nonspecific, it does not create memory, and its responses are always the same regardless of the target. Adaptive immunity is very specific as to its target, it may involve antibodies, it does create memory, and it may become more efficient. Both kinds of immunity work together to prevent damage and disease.

INNATE IMMUNITY

Innate immunity has several aspects: anatomic and physiological barriers, phagocytic and other defensive cells, and chemical secretions and reactions, including inflammation. Although we will describe each aspect separately, keep in mind that they all work together. There is also a great deal of overlap among the three aspects, as you will see. The innate immune responses are always the same, and their degree of efficiency does not increase with repeated exposure.

Barriers

The stratum corneum of the epidermis of the skin is non-living, and when unbroken is an excellent barrier to pathogens of all kinds. The microbiota (normal bacterial population) of the skin surface and the fatty acids in sebum help limit the growth of bacteria on the skin. The living cells of the epidermis produce defensins, which are antimicrobial chemicals.

The mucous membranes of the respiratory, digestive, urinary, and reproductive tracts are living tissue yet still a good barrier. The ciliated epithelium of the upper respiratory tract is an especially effective barrier. Dust and pathogens are trapped on the mucus, the cilia sweep the mucus to the pharynx, and it is swallowed. The hydrochloric acid of the gastric juice destroys most pathogens that enter the stomach, either in mucus or with food and drink. Lysozyme, an enzyme found in saliva and tears, inhibits the growth of bacteria in the oral cavity and on the warm, wet surface of the eye. The subcutaneous tissue contains many white blood cells (WBCs), as does the areolar connective tissue below the epithelium of mucous membranes (Fig. 14–6).

Defensive Cells

Recall from Chapter 11 that many of our defensive cells are white blood cells. Macrophages, both fixed and wandering, have receptors for the pathogens humans are likely to encounter (this probably reflects millions of years of coexistence) and are very efficient phagocytes. Other cells capable of phagocytosis of pathogens or other foreign antigens are the neutrophils and, to a lesser extent, the eosinophils. Phagocytic cells use intracellular enzymes and chemicals such as hydrogen peroxide (H_2O_2) to destroy ingested pathogens.

The Langerhans cells of the skin and the many other dendritic cells throughout the body also phagocytize foreign material, not merely to destroy it, but to take it to a lymph node or nodule where the lymphocytes of adaptive immune mechanisms are then activated. The macrophages are also involved in activating these lymphocytes. This is a very important link between the two components of immunity.

Natural killer cells (NK cells) circulate in the blood but are also found in the red bone marrow, spleen, and lymph nodes. They are a small portion (about 10%) of the total lymphocytes but are able to destroy many kinds of pathogens and tumor cells. NK cells make direct contact with foreign cells and kill them by rupturing their cell membranes (with chemicals called perforins) or by inflicting some other kind of chemical damage.

Basophils and mast cells (a type of connective tissue cell formed in the red bone marrow) are also defensive cells that are found throughout the areolar connective tissue of mucous membranes and the subcutaneous tissue. They produce histamine and leukotrienes. Histamine causes vasodilation and makes capillaries more permeable; these are aspects of inflammation. Leukotrienes also increase capillary permeability and attract phagocytic cells to the area.

Chemical Defenses

Chemicals that help the body resist infection include the interferons, the complement, and the chemicals involved in inflammation. The **interferons** (alpha-, beta-, and gamma-interferons) are proteins produced by cells infected with viruses and by T cells. Viruses must be inside a living cell to reproduce, and although interferon cannot prevent the entry of viruses into cells, it does block their reproduction. When viral reproduction is blocked, the viruses cannot infect new cells and cause disease. Interferon is probably a factor in the self-limiting nature of many viral diseases (and is used in the treatment of some diseases, such as hepatitis C).

Complement is a group of more than 20 plasma proteins that circulate in the blood until activated. They are involved in the lysis of cellular antigens and the labeling of noncellular antigens. Some stimulate the release of histamine in inflammation; others attract WBCs to the site.

Inflammation is a general response to damage of any kind: microbial, chemical, or physical. Basophils and mast cells release histamine and leukotrienes, which affect blood vessels as previously described. Vasodilation increases blood flow to the damaged area, and capillaries become more permeable; tissue fluid and WBCs collect at the site. The purpose of inflammation is to try to contain the damage, keep it from spreading, eliminate the cause, and permit repair of the tissue to begin. From even this brief description you can see why the four signs of inflammation are redness, heat, swelling, and pain: redness from greater blood flow, heat from the blood and greater metabolic activity, swelling from the accumulation of tissue fluid, and pain from the damage itself and perhaps the swelling.

As mentioned in Chapter 10, inflammation is a positive feedback mechanism that may become a vicious cycle of damage and more damage. The hormone cortisol is

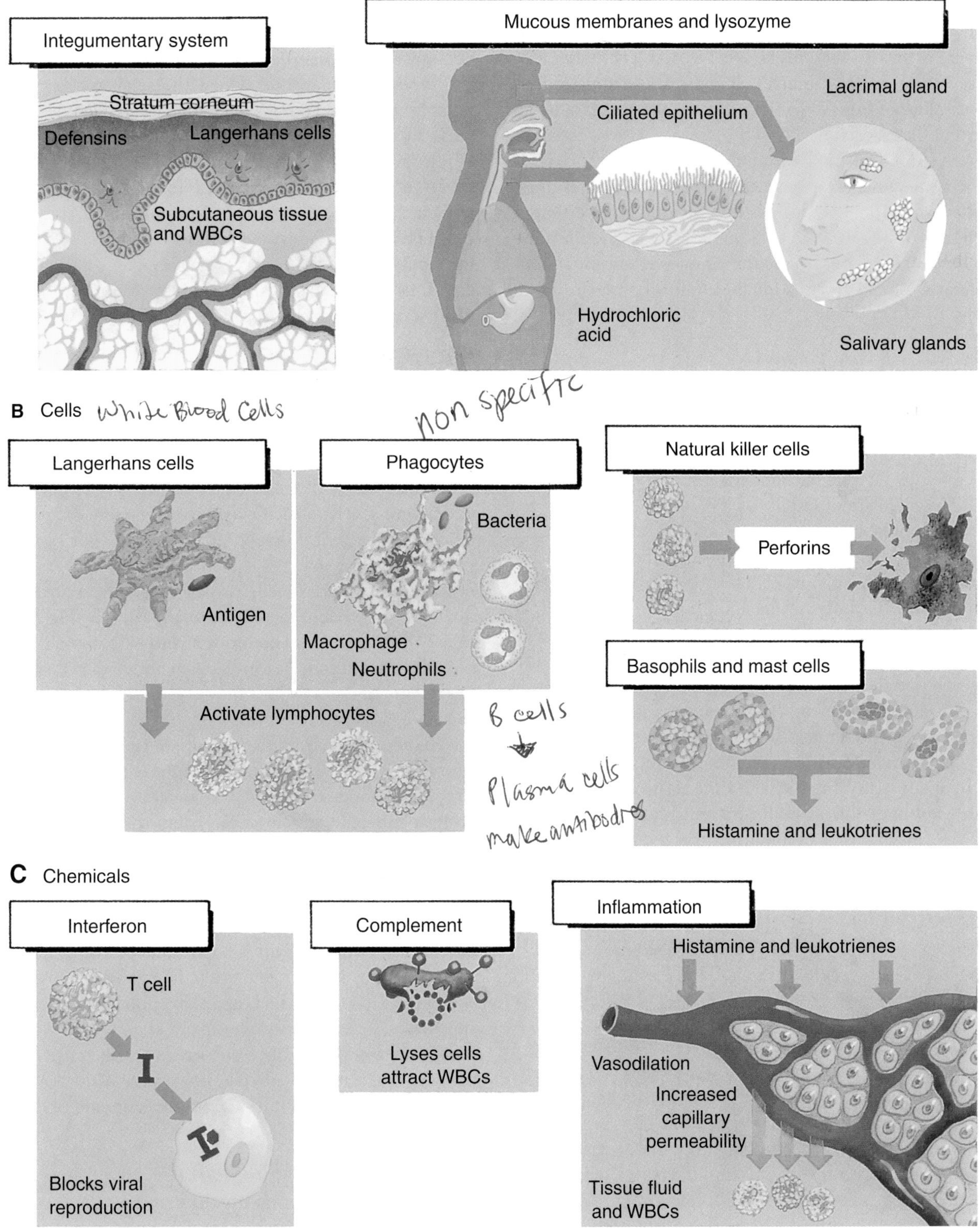

Figure 14–6 Innate immunity. (**A**) Barriers. (**B**) Defensive cells. (**C**) Chemical defenses. See text for description.

QUESTION: The three aspects of innate immunity are interconnected; describe two of these connections.

one brake that prevents this, and at least one of the complement proteins has this function as well. There are probably other chemical signals (in general called **cytokines** and **chemokines**) that help limit inflammation to an extent that is useful.

In summary, innate immunity is nonspecific, it is always the same, it does not create memory, and, though often very effective, it does not become more efficient upon repeated exposures. Some cells of innate immune mechanisms also activate the adaptive immune mechanisms. The aspects of innate immunity are shown in Fig. 14–6.

ADAPTIVE IMMUNITY

To adapt means to become suitable, and adaptive immunity can become "suitable" for and respond to almost any foreign antigen. Adaptive immunity is specific and is carried out by lymphocytes and macrophages.

The majority of lymphocytes are the T lymphocytes and B lymphocytes, or, more simply, **T cells** and **B cells**. In the embryo, T cells are produced in the bone marrow and thymus. They must pass through the thymus, where the thymic hormones bring about their maturation; that is, the ability to distinguish between "self" and "non-self." The T cells then migrate to the spleen, lymph nodes, and lymph nodules, where they are found after birth.

Produced in the embryonic bone marrow, B cells migrate directly to the spleen and lymph nodes and nodules. When activated during an immune response, some B cells will divide many times and become plasma cells that produce antibodies to a specific foreign antigen.

The mechanisms of immunity that involve T cells and B cells are specific, meaning that one foreign antigen is the target each time a mechanism is activated. A macrophage has receptor sites for foreign chemicals such as those of bacterial cell walls or flagella and may phagocytize just about any foreign material it comes across (as will the Langerhans or dendritic cells). T cells and B cells, however, become very specific, as you will see.

The first step in the destruction of a pathogen or foreign cell is the recognition of its antigens as foreign. Both T cells and B cells are capable of this, but the immune mechanisms are activated especially well when this recognition is accomplished by macrophages and a specialized group of T lymphocytes called **helper T cells** (also called CD4 T cells). The foreign antigen is first phagocytized by a macrophage, and parts of it are "presented" on the macrophage's cell membrane. Also on the macrophage membrane are "self" antigens that are representative of the antigens found on all of the cells of the individual. Therefore, the helper T cell that encounters this macrophage is presented not only with the foreign antigen but also with "self" antigens for comparison (Fig. 14–7). The helper T cell becomes sensitized to and specific for the foreign antigen, the one that does not belong in the body (see Box 14–2: AIDS).

The recognition of an antigen as foreign initiates one or both of the mechanisms of adaptive immunity. These are **cell-mediated immunity** (sometimes called simply cellular immunity), in which T cells and macrophages participate, and **antibody-mediated immunity** (or **humoral immunity**), which involves T cells, B cells, and macrophages.

Cell-Mediated Immunity

This mechanism of immunity does not result in the production of antibodies, but it is effective against intracellular pathogens (such as viruses), fungi, malignant cells, and grafts of foreign tissue. As mentioned earlier, the first step is the recognition of the foreign antigen by macrophages and helper T cells, which become activated and are specific. (You may find it helpful to refer to Fig. 14–7 as you read the following.)

These activated T cells, which are antigen specific, divide many times to form **cytotoxic** (**killer**) **T cells** (also called CD8 T cells) and **memory T cells**. Cytotoxic T cells are able to chemically destroy foreign antigens by disrupting cell membranes. This is how cytotoxic T cells destroy cancer cells, or cells infected with viruses to prevent the viruses from reproducing. These T cells also produce cytokines, which are chemicals that attract macrophages to the area and activate them to phagocytize the foreign antigen and cellular debris. The memory T cells will remember the specific foreign antigen and become active if it enters the body again.

Besides being activated or started appropriately, these immune responses must be stopped when their targets have been eliminated. This is important because an excessive immune response can be very damaging to tissues. A subset of CD4 T cells called **regulatory T cells** (once called suppressor T cells) produces feedback chemicals that limit the immune response once the foreign antigen has been destroyed. The memory T cells, however, will quickly initiate the cell-mediated immune response should there be a future exposure to the antigen.

Antibody-Mediated Immunity

This mechanism of immunity does involve the production of antibodies and is also diagrammed in Fig. 14–7. Again, the first step is the recognition of the foreign antigen, this time by B cells, as well as by macrophages and helper T cells. The sensitized helper T cell presents the

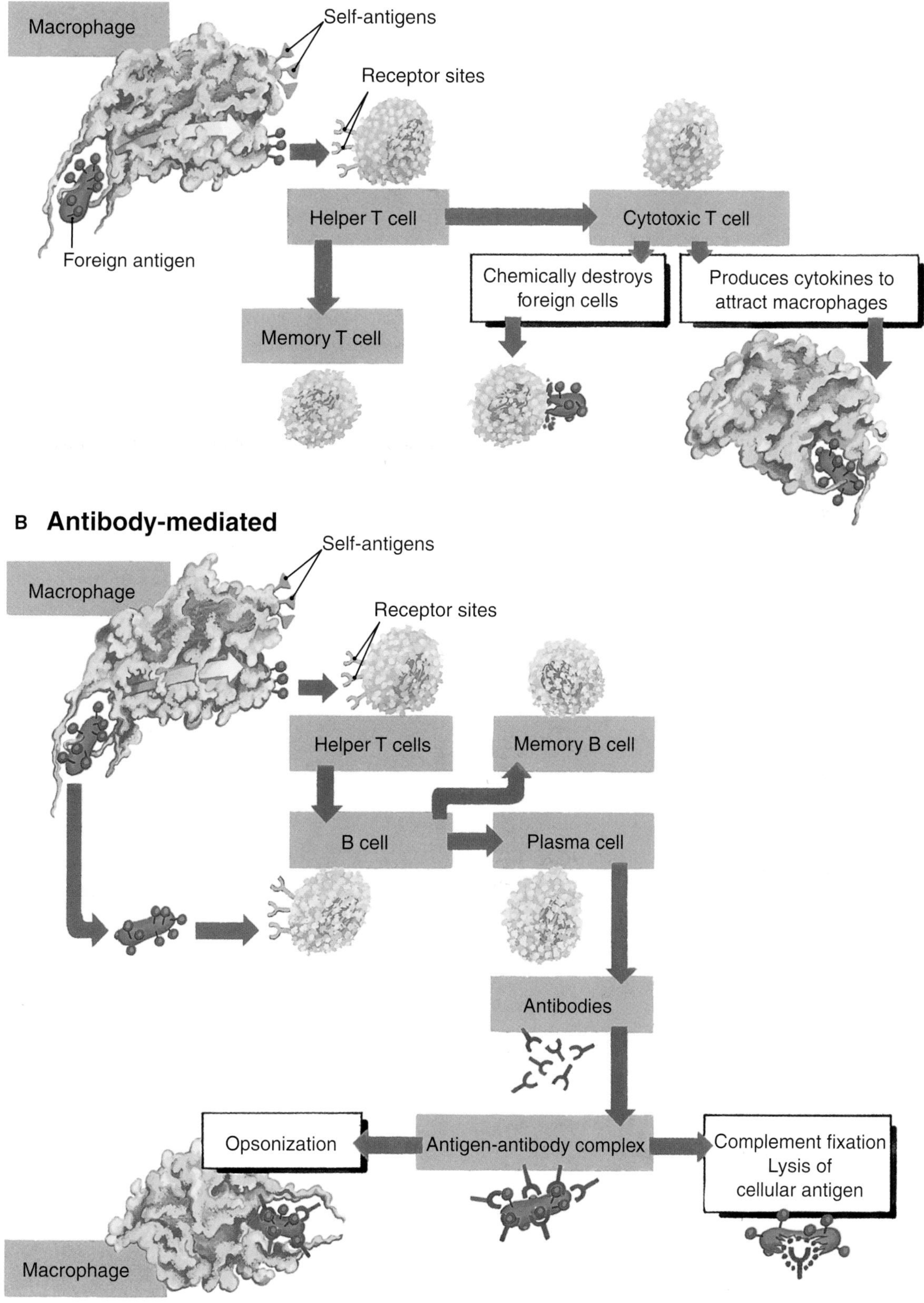

Figure 14–7 Adaptive immunity. (**A**) Cell-mediated immunity. (**B**) Antibody-mediated immunity. See text for description.

QUESTION: Adaptive immunity has memory; which cells provide this? What kind of memory is it?

Box 14–2 | AIDS

As of early 2014, more than 26 million people had died of acquired immunodeficiency syndrome (**AIDS**), which is caused by the human immunodeficiency virus (HIV). Worldwide, more than 34 million people are HIV positive or have AIDS. The disease was first described in 1981 among young homosexual men in New York and California. These men had opportunistic infections such as Kaposi's sarcoma and *Pneumocystis* pneumonia and would develop other fungal or protozoan infections that would not occur in those with healthy immune systems. Where did this virus come from? It is likely that HIV evolved from a chimpanzee virus in Africa sometime during the 1930s. Spread of the virus among people was very slow at first, and only when air travel became commonplace did the virus spread worldwide.

HIV is a retrovirus that infects helper T cells, macrophages, and many other human cells. Without sufficient helper T cells, the immune system is seriously impaired. Pathogens are not recognized as foreign, B cells are not activated, and killer T cells are not stimulated to proliferate. Although some opportunistic infections may be treated with medications and even temporarily cured, the immune system cannot prevent the next infection, or the next.

The incubation period of AIDS is highly variable, ranging from a few months to several years. An infected person may unknowingly spread HIV to others before any symptoms appear. It should be emphasized that AIDS, although communicable, is not a contagious disease. It is not spread by casual contact as is measles or the common cold. Transmission of AIDS occurs through sexual contact, by contact with infected blood, or by placental transmission of the virus from mother to fetus.

In the United States, most of the cases of AIDS during the 1980s were in homosexual men and IV drug users who shared syringes contaminated with their blood. By the 1990s, however, it was clear that AIDS was heterosexually transmitted as well. In much of the rest of the world, especially Africa and Asia, the transmission of AIDS has always been primarily by heterosexual contact, with equal numbers of women and men infected. In many of these countries AIDS remains an enormous public health problem.

As of this writing, AIDS is still an incurable disease. At present we have no medications that will eradicate HIV, although certain combinations of drugs effectively suppress the virus in some people. For these people, AIDS may become a chronic but not fatal disease. Unfortunately, the medications do not work for everyone, and they are very expensive, placing them beyond the means of most of the world's AIDS patients.

We have no vaccine for AIDS as yet, despite extensive ongoing work. HIV is a mutating virus; it constantly changes itself, making previously produced antibodies ineffective. Even a healthy immune system might find it difficult to keep up with such a rapidly mutating virus, and an impaired immune system simply cannot. A constant antigen, one that does not change and could be used in a vaccine, has not yet been discovered.

Behavioral prevention remains extremely important, and that requires education. Everyone should know how AIDS is spread and know the high-risk behaviors that make acquiring HIV more likely. Health care personnel have a special responsibility, not only to educate themselves, but to provide education about AIDS for their patients and the families of their patients and to encourage HIV testing when appropriate.

foreign antigen to B cells, which provides a strong stimulus for the activation of B cells specific for this antigen. The activated B cells begin to divide many times, and two subsets of cells are formed. Some of the new B cells produced are **plasma cells** that produce antibodies specific for this one foreign antigen. Other B cells become **memory B cells**, which will remember the specific antigen and initiate a rapid response upon a second exposure.

Antibodies, also called **immune globulins (Ig)**, **immunoglobulins**, or **gamma globulins**, are proteins shaped somewhat like the letter Y. Antibodies do not themselves destroy foreign antigens, but rather become attached to such antigens to "label" them for destruction. Each antibody produced is specific for only one antigen. Because there are so many different pathogens, you might think that the immune system would have to be capable of producing many different antibodies, and in fact this is so. It is estimated that millions of different antigen-specific antibodies can be produced, should there be a need for them. The structure of antibodies is shown in Fig. 14–8, and the five classes of antibodies are described in Table 14–1.

The antibodies produced will bond to the antigen, forming an antigen–antibody complex. This complex results in **opsonization**, which means that the antigen is now "labeled" for phagocytosis by macrophages or neutrophils. The antigen–antibody complex also stimulates the process of complement fixation (see Box 14–3: Diagnostic Tests).

Some of the circulating complement proteins are activated, or fixed, by an antigen–antibody complex. Complement fixation may be complete or partial. If the foreign antigen is cellular, the complement proteins bond to the antigen–antibody complex, then to one another, forming an enzymatic ring that punches a hole in the cell to bring about the death of the cell. This is complete (or entire) complement fixation and is what happens to bacterial cells (it is also the cause of hemolysis in a transfusion reaction).

If the foreign antigen is not a cell—let's say it's a virus, for example—partial complement fixation takes place, in which some of the complement proteins bond to the antigen–antibody complex. This is a chemotactic factor. *Chemotaxis* means "chemical movement" and is actually another label that attracts macrophages to engulf and destroy the foreign antigen.

In summary, adaptive immunity is very specific, does create memory, and, because it does, often becomes more efficient with repeated exposures.

Before we continue, let us consider one final comparison of our two major components of immunity. It may be

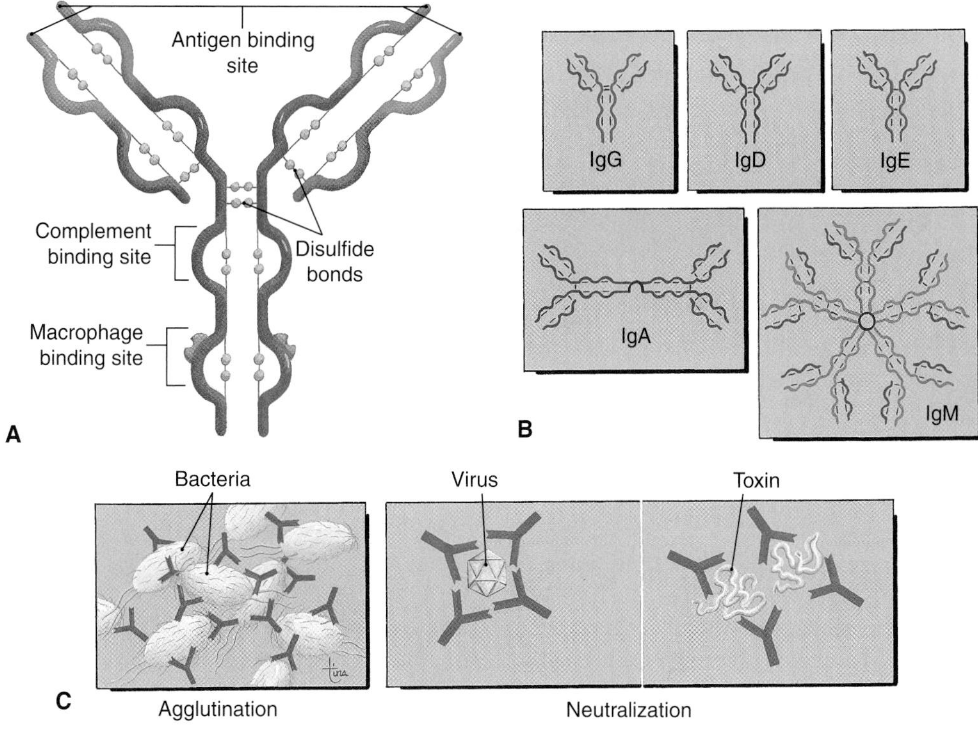

Figure 14–8 Antibodies. (**A**) Structure of one IgG molecule. Notice how the many disulfide bonds maintain the shape of the molecule. (**B**) Structure of the five classes of antibodies. (**C**) Antibody activity: Agglutination of bacteria and neutralization of viruses or toxins.

QUESTION: In part C, why does neutralization inactivate a bacterial toxin?

Table 14–1 | CLASSES OF ANTIBODIES

NAME	LOCATION	FUNCTIONS
IgG	Blood and extracellular fluid	A monomer; the most abundant immune globulin; crosses the placenta to provide passive immunity for newborns; provides long-term immunity to a disease following recovery or a vaccine
IgA	External and internal secretions (tears, saliva, intestinal, etc.)	A dimer; present in breast milk to provide passive immunity for breast-fed infants; found in secretions of all mucous membranes to provide local defense where pathogens enter
IgM	Blood	A pentamer; produced first by the maturing immune system of infants; produced first during an infection (IgG production follows); the antibodies of the ABO blood group
IgD	B lymphocytes	A monomer; forms receptors on B lymphocytes
IgE	Mast cells or basophils	A monomer; is important in allergic reactions (mast cells release histamine) and responses to parasites such as worms

Box 14–3 | DIAGNOSTIC TESTS

Several important laboratory tests involve antibodies and may be very useful to confirm a diagnosis.

Complement fixation test—determines the presence of a particular antibody in the patient's blood but does not indicate when the infection occurred.

Antibody titer—determines the level or amount of a specific antibody in the patient's blood. If another titer is done one to several weeks later, an increase in the antibody level shows the infection to be current.

Fluorescent antibody test—uses antibodies tagged with fluorescent dyes, which are added to a clinical specimen such as blood, sputum, or a biopsy of tissue. If the suspected pathogen is present, the fluorescent antibodies will bond to it and the antigen–antibody complex will "glow" when examined with a fluorescent microscope.

Tests such as these are used in conjunction with patient history and symptoms to arrive at a diagnosis.

helpful to think of innate and adaptive immunity as teams in a sport such as soccer, baseball, or basketball. If you have a favorite team sport, you know that any good team needs a good defense. The innate immunity team uses the same defense game after game, no matter who the opponent is. Why? Because it is the only strategy the innate immunity team knows, and because it often works. Although it cannot recognize the star player on an opposing team and adapt accordingly, innate immunity is often very effective, as a zone defense may be in basketball. Of great importance as well is that the cells of innate immunity activate lymphocytes of the adaptive immune response—as if players on the team were giving a scouting report to the team that will be playing this opponent next week. The adaptive immunity team *will* focus on and go after the opponent's star player (as with a man-to-man defense) and will remember and be prepared for that player should there ever be a rematch.

Antibody Responses

The first exposure to a foreign antigen does stimulate antibody production, but antibodies are produced slowly and in small amounts (see Fig. 14–9). Let us take as a specific example, the measles virus. On a person's first

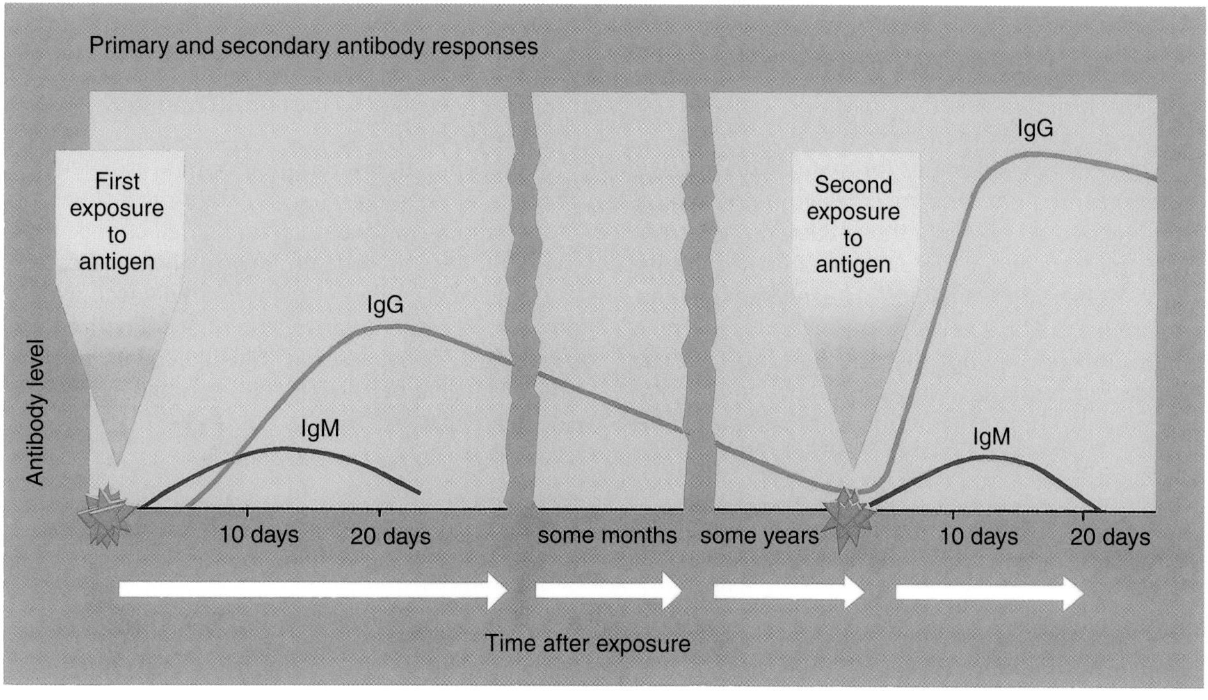

Figure 14–9 Antibody responses to first and subsequent exposures to a pathogen. See text for description.

QUESTION: State the two differences in IgG production after a first and a second exposure to the same antigen.

exposure to this virus, antibody production is usually too slow to prevent the disease itself, and the person will have clinical measles. Most people who get measles recover and, upon recovery, have antibodies and memory cells that are specific for the measles virus.

On a second exposure to this virus, the memory cells initiate rapid production of large amounts of antibodies, enough to prevent a second case of measles. This is the reason why we develop immunity to certain diseases, and this is also the basis for the protection given by **vaccines** (see Box 14–4: Vaccines).

As mentioned previously, antibodies label pathogens or other foreign antigens for phagocytosis or complement fixation. More specifically, antibodies cause agglutination or neutralization of pathogens before their eventual destruction. **Agglutination** means "clumping,"

Box 14–4 | VACCINES

The purpose of vaccines is to prevent disease. A vaccine contains an antigen that the immune system will respond to, just as it would to the actual pathogen. The types of vaccine antigens are a killed or weakened (**attenuated**) pathogen, part of a pathogen such as a bacterial capsule, or an inactivated bacterial toxin called a **toxoid**.

Because the vaccine itself does not cause disease (with very rare exceptions), the fact that antibody production to it is slow is not detrimental to the person. The vaccine takes the place of the first exposure to the pathogen and stimulates production of antibodies and memory cells. On exposure to the pathogen itself, the memory cells

Continued

Box 14–4 | VACCINES *(Continued)*

initiate rapid production of large amounts of antibody, enough to prevent disease.

We now have vaccines for many diseases. The tetanus and diphtheria vaccines contain toxoids, the inactivated toxins of these bacteria. Vaccines for pneumococcal pneumonia and meningitis contain bacterial capsules. These vaccines cannot cause disease because the capsules are non-toxic and non-living; there is nothing that can cause harm or reproduce. Influenza and rabies vaccines contain killed viruses. Measles and the oral polio vaccines contain attenuated (weakened) viruses.

Although attenuated pathogens are usually strongly antigenic and stimulate a protective immune response, there is a very small chance that the pathogen may regain its virulence and cause the disease. The live-virus oral polio vaccine (still being used in the quest to eliminate polio throughout the world) has a risk of 1 in 500,000 of causing polio. The killed-virus injectable polio vaccine has no such risk.

Box 14–5 | ALLERGIES

An **allergy** is a hypersensitivity to a particular foreign antigen, called an **allergen**. Allergens include plant pollens, foods, chemicals in cosmetics, antibiotics such as penicillin, and mold spores. Such allergens are not themselves harmful. Most people, for example, can inhale pollen, eat peanuts and shrimp, or take penicillin with no ill effects.

Hypersensitivity means that the immune system mistakenly responds—and overresponds—to the allergen and produces tissue damage by doing so. The development of a food allergy to shrimp is shown in Box Figure 14–A. On a first exposure to shrimp protein, the roaming dendritic cells pick up the protein in the mucosa of the small intestine and take it to the T cells in a Peyer's patch. For

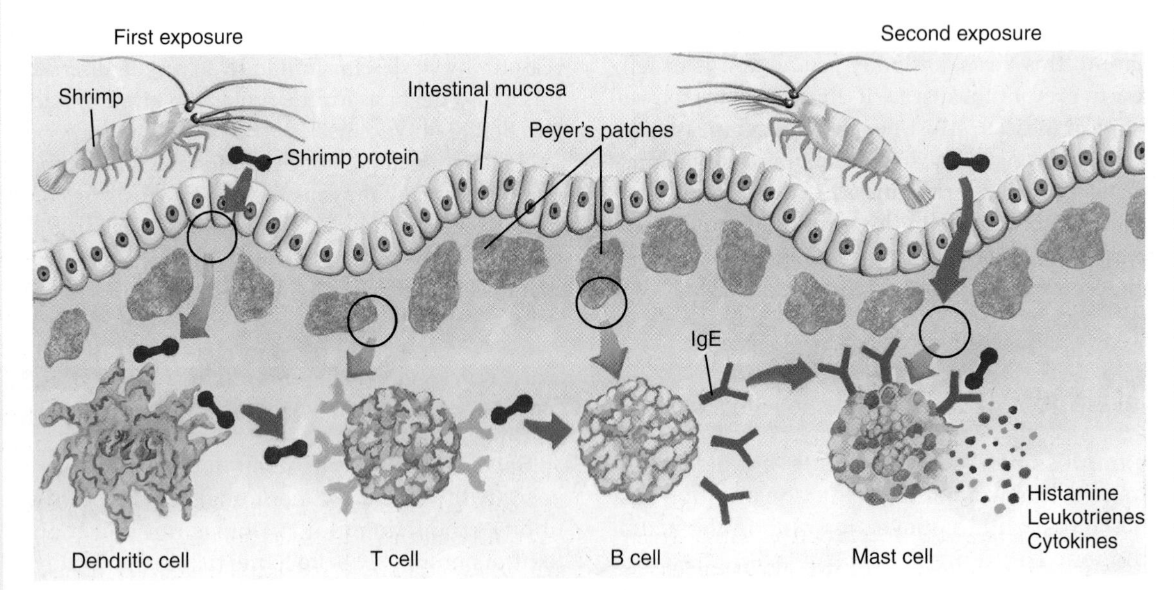

Box Figure 14–A Development of an allergy to shrimp protein.

Box 14–5 | ALLERGIES *(Continued)*

reasons we do not yet know, a person's T cells may not be able to "learn" the shrimp protein and tolerate it as food. If that happens, the T cells activate B cells, and they produce IgE antibodies to the shrimp protein. These antibodies then bond to mast cells, which contain histamine and leukotrienes. Then, on a second exposure to shrimp protein, the protein bonds to the IgE antibodies on the mast cells, which triggers the release of histamine and the other cytokines. These chemicals contribute to inflammation by increasing the permeability of capillaries and venules.

In an allergic reaction, however, inflammation serves no useful purpose—it is simply damaging and creates symptoms such as hives, or watery eyes and runny nose (hay fever), or the more serious wheezing and difficult breathing that characterize asthma (see Chapter 15). Several medications are available to counteract these effects.

Anaphylactic shock is an extreme allergic response that may be elicited by exposure to penicillin, insect venoms, or certain foods. On the first exposure, the person becomes highly sensitized to the foreign antigen. On the second exposure, histamine and other cytokines are released from mast cells throughout the body and cause a drastic decrease in blood volume. The resulting drop in blood pressure may be fatal in only a few minutes. People who know they are allergic to bee stings, for example, may obtain a syringe of epinephrine to carry with them. Epinephrine can delay the progression of anaphylactic shock long enough for the person to seek medical attention.

Clinical studies to help the immune system (the T cells) learn to tolerate allergens are ongoing. Children with severe (likely to be fatal) allergies to milk or peanuts are first given, in food, a minute amount of the problem protein. The following week they get a little more, then a little more, and so on. After months of these very gradual increases, some children could eat up to a dozen peanuts or drink 6 to 8 ounces of milk. Such studies must proceed slowly and under strict medical supervision.

and this is what happens when antibodies bind to bacterial cells. The bacteria that are clumped together by attached antibodies are more easily phagocytized by macrophages (see Fig. 14–8).

The activity of viruses may be neutralized by antibodies. A virus must get inside a living cell in order to reproduce itself. However, a virus with antibodies attached to it is unable to enter a cell, cannot reproduce, and will soon be phagocytized. Bacterial toxins may also be neutralized by attached antibodies. The antibodies change the shape of the toxin, prevent it from exerting its harmful effects, and promote its phagocytosis by macrophages.

Allergies are also the result of antibody activity (see Box 14–5: Allergies).

TYPES OF IMMUNITY

If we consider the source of immunity, that is, where it comes from, we can begin with two major categories: genetic immunity and acquired immunity. Genetic immunity is conferred by our DNA, and acquired immunity is developed or acquired by natural or artificial means.

Genetic immunity does not involve antibodies or the immune system; it is the result of our genetic makeup. What this means is that some pathogens cause disease in certain host species but not in others. Dogs and cats, for example, have genetic immunity to the measles virus, which is a pathogen only for people. Mouse leukemia viruses affect only mice, not people; we have genetic immunity to them. This is not because we have antibodies against these mouse viruses, but rather that we have genes that are the codes for proteins that make it impossible for such pathogens to reproduce in our cells and tissues. Monkeys have similar protective genes and proteins for the human AIDS virus; HIV does not cause disease in these monkeys. Because this is a genetic characteristic programmed in DNA, genetic immunity always lasts a lifetime.

Acquired immunity does involve antibodies. **Passive immunity** means that the antibodies are from another source, whereas **active immunity** means that the individual produces his or her own antibodies.

One type of naturally acquired passive immunity is the placental transmission of antibodies (IgG) from maternal blood to fetal circulation. The baby will then be born temporarily immune to the diseases the mother is immune to. Such passive immunity may be prolonged by breast-feeding because breast milk also contains maternal antibodies (IgA).

Artificially acquired passive immunity is obtained by the injection of immune globulins (gamma globulins or preformed antibodies) after presumed exposure to a particular pathogen. Such immune globulins are available for German measles, hepatitis A and B, tetanus and botulism (anti-toxins), and rabies. These are *not* vaccines; they do not stimulate immune mechanisms, but rather provide immediate antibody protection. Passive immunity is always temporary, lasting a few weeks to a few months, because antibodies from another source eventually break down.

Active immunity is the production of one's own antibodies and may be stimulated by natural or artificial means. Naturally acquired active immunity means that a person has recovered from a disease and now has antibodies and memory cells specific for that pathogen. Artificially acquired active immunity is the result of a vaccine that has stimulated production of antibodies and memory cells (see Box 14–6: Vaccines That Have Changed Our Lives). No general statement can be made about the duration of active immunity. Recovering from bubonic plague, for example, confers lifelong immunity, but the plague vaccine does not. Duration of active immunity, therefore, varies with the particular disease or vaccine.

The types of immunity are summarized in Table 14–2.

AGING AND THE LYMPHATIC SYSTEM

The aging of the lymphatic system is apparent in the decreased efficiency of immune responses. Elderly people are more likely than younger ones to develop shingles, when an aging immune system cannot keep the chickenpox virus dormant. They are also more susceptible to

Box 14–6 | VACCINES THAT HAVE CHANGED OUR LIVES

In England in 1797, Edward Jenner published his results on the use of the cowpox virus called vaccinia as the first vaccine for smallpox, a closely related virus. (He was unaware of the actual pathogens because viruses had not yet been discovered, but he had noticed that milkmaids who got cowpox rarely got smallpox.) In 1980, the World Health Organization declared that smallpox had been eradicated throughout the world. A disease that had killed or disfigured millions of people throughout recorded history is now considered part of history (except for the possible use of the virus as a biological weapon).

In the 19th century in the northern United States, thousands of children died of diphtheria every winter. Today there are fewer than 10 cases of diphtheria each year in the entire country. In the early 1950s, 50,000 cases of paralytic polio were reported in the United States each year. Today, wild-type polio virus is not found in North America.

Smallpox, diphtheria, and polio are no longer the terrible diseases they once were, and this is because of the development and widespread use of vaccines. When people are protected by a vaccine, they are no longer possible reservoirs or sources of the pathogen for others, and the spread of disease may be greatly limited.

Other diseases that have been controlled by the use of vaccines are tetanus, mumps, influenza, measles, and German measles. Whooping cough had been controlled until recently, when the vaccination rate decreased. With that decrease, the annual number of cases in the United States has increased markedly. The vaccine for hepatitis B has significantly decreased the number of cases of this disease among health-care workers, and the vaccine is recommended for all children. People who have been exposed to rabies, which otherwise is virtually always fatal, can be protected by a safe vaccine.

Without such vaccines our lives would be very different. Infant mortality or death in childhood would be much more frequent, and all of us would have to be much more aware of infectious diseases. In many parts of the world this is still true; many of the developing countries in Africa and Asia still cannot afford extensive vaccination programs for their children. Many of the diseases mentioned here, which we may rarely think of, are still a significant part of the lives of millions of people.

Table 14–2 | TYPES OF IMMUNITY

TYPE	DESCRIPTION
GENETIC	Does not involve antibodies; is programmed in DNA Some pathogens affect certain host species but not others
ACQUIRED	Does involve antibodies
PASSIVE	Antibodies from another source
Natural	Placental transmission of IgG antibodies from mother to fetus Transmission of IgA antibodies in breast milk
Artificial	Injection of preformed antibodies (gamma globulins or immune globulins) after presumed exposure
ACTIVE	Production of one's own antibodies
Natural	Recovery from a disease, with production of antibodies and memory cells
Aпcial	A vaccine stimulates production of antibodies and memory cells

infections such as influenza and to what are called secondary infections, such as pneumonia following a case of the flu. Vaccines for both of these are available, and elderly people should be encouraged to get them. Elderly people should also be sure to get a tetanus-diphtheria-pertussis booster every 10 years.

Autoimmune disorders are also more common among older people; the immune system mistakenly perceives a body tissue as foreign and initiates its destruction. Rheumatoid arthritis and myasthenia gravis are examples of autoimmune diseases. The incidence of cancer is also higher. Malignant cells that once might have been quickly destroyed remain alive and proliferate.

SUMMARY

The preceding discussions of immunity should give you a small idea of the complexity of the body's defense system. However, much more remains to be learned, especially about the effects of the nervous system and endocrine system on immunity. For example, it is known that people under great stress have immune systems that may not function as they did when stress was absent.

At present, much research is being done in this field. The goal is not to eliminate all disease because that would not be possible. Rather, the aim is to enable people to live healthier lives by preventing certain diseases.

STUDY OUTLINE

Functions of the Lymphatic System

1. To return tissue fluid to the blood to maintain blood volume (see Fig. 14–1).
2. To protect the body against pathogens and other foreign material.

Parts of the Lymphatic System

1. Lymph and lymph vessels.
2. Lymphatic tissue: lymph nodes and nodules, spleen, and thymus; lymphocytes mature and proliferate; stem cells are present.

Lymph—the tissue fluid that enters lymph capillaries

1. Similar to plasma, but more WBCs are present, and has less protein.
2. Must be returned to the blood to maintain blood volume and blood pressure.

Lymph Vessels

1. Dead-end lymph capillaries are found in most tissue spaces; collect tissue fluid and proteins (see Fig. 14–2).

2. The structure of larger lymph vessels is like that of veins; valves prevent the backflow of lymph.
3. Lymph is kept moving in lymph vessels by:
   a. Constriction of the lymph vessels
   b. The skeletal muscle pump
   c. The respiratory pump
4. Lymph from the lower body and upper left quadrant enters the thoracic duct and is returned to the blood in the left subclavian vein (see Fig. 14–3).
5. Lymph from the upper right quadrant enters the right lymphatic duct and is returned to the blood in the right subclavian vein.

Lymph Nodes—encapsulated masses of lymphatic tissue

1. Found in groups along the pathways of lymph vessels.
2. As lymph flows through the nodes:
   a. Foreign material is phagocytized by fixed macrophages
   b. Lymphocytes are activated and fixed plasma cells produce antibodies to foreign antigens (see Fig. 14–4)
3. The major paired groups of lymph nodes are the cervical, axillary, and inguinal groups. These are at the junctions of the head and extremities with the trunk; remove pathogens from the lymph from the extremities before the lymph is returned to the blood.

Lymph Nodules—small unencapsulated masses of lymphatic tissue

1. Found beneath the epithelium of all mucous membranes, that is, the tracts that have natural openings to the environment.
2. Destroy pathogens that penetrate the epithelium of the respiratory, digestive, urinary, or reproductive tracts.
3. Tonsils are the lymph nodules of the pharynx; Peyer's patches are those of the small intestine.

Spleen—located in the upper left abdominal quadrant behind the stomach

1. The fetal spleen produces RBCs.
2. Functions after birth:
   a. Contains lymphocytes to be activated and fixed plasma cells that produce antibodies
   b. Contains monocytes and fixed macrophages (RE cells) that phagocytize pathogens and old RBCs; bilirubin is formed and sent to the liver for excretion in bile
   c. Stores platelets and destroys damaged platelets

Thymus—inferior to the thyroid gland; in the fetus and infant the thymus is large (see Fig. 14–5); with age the thymus shrinks

1. Produces T lymphocytes (T cells).
2. Produces other cells and thymic hormones that enable T cells to become immunologically competent: able to recognize foreign antigens and provide immunity.
3. The two aspects of immunological competence are self-recognition (for cells) and self-tolerance (for proteins and other organic molecules that the body's cells produce).

Immunity—the ability to destroy foreign antigens and prevent future cases of certain infectious diseases

1. Antigens are chemical markers that identify cells. Human cells have "self" antigens—the HLA types.
2. Foreign antigens stimulate antibody production or other immune responses and include bacteria, viruses, fungi, protozoa, and malignant cells.

Innate Immunity (see Fig. 14–6)

1. Is nonspecific, responses are always the same, does not create memory, and does not become more efficient. Consists of barriers, defensive cells, and chemical defenses.

2. Barriers
   a. Unbroken stratum corneum an excellent barrier; microbiota and sebum limit other bacterial growth; living epidermal cells secrete defensins
   b. Subcutaneous tissue with WBCs
   c. Mucous membranes and areolar CT with WBCs; upper respiratory epithelium is ciliated
   d. HCl in gastric juice
   e. Lysozyme in saliva and tears
3. Defensive cells
   a. Phagocytes—macrophages, neutrophils, eosinophils; macrophages also activate the lymphocytes of adaptive immunity
   b. Langerhans cells and other dendritic cells—activate lymphocytes
   c. Natural killer cells—destroy foreign cells by rupturing their cell membranes
   d. Basophils and mast cells—produce histamine and leukotrienes (inflammation)
4. Chemical defenses
   a. Interferon blocks viral reproduction
   b. Complement proteins lyse foreign cells, attract WBCs, and contribute to inflammation
   c. Inflammation—the response to any kind of damage; vasodilation and increased capillary permeability bring tissue fluid and WBCs to the area. Purpose: to contain the damage, eliminate the cause, and make tissue repair possible. Signs: redness, heat, swelling, and pain.

Adaptive Immunity (see Fig. 14–7)

1. Is very specific, may involve antibodies, does create memory, and responses become more efficient. Consists of cell-mediated and antibody-mediated immunity; is carried out by T cells, B cells, and macrophages.
2. T lymphocytes (T cells)—in the embryo are produced in the thymus and RBM; they require the hormones of the thymus for maturation; migrate to the spleen, lymph nodes, and nodules.
3. B lymphocytes (B cells)—in the embryo are produced in the RBM; migrate to the spleen, lymph nodes, and nodules.
4. The antigen must first be recognized as foreign; this is accomplished by B cells or by helper T cells that compare the foreign antigen with "self" antigens present on macrophages.
5. Helper T cells strongly initiate one or both of the immune mechanisms: cell-mediated immunity and antibody-mediated immunity.

Cell-Mediated (cellular) Immunity (see Fig. 14–7)

1. Does not involve antibodies; is effective against intracellular pathogens, malignant cells, and grafts of foreign tissue.
2. Macrophages and helper T cells recognize the foreign antigen; helper T cells are antigen specific and begin to divide to form different subsets of T cells.
3. Memory T cells will remember the specific foreign antigen.
4. Cytotoxic (killer) T cells chemically destroy foreign cells and produce cytokines to attract macrophages.
5. Regulatory T cells stop the immune response when the pathogen has been eliminated.

Antibody-Mediated (Humoral) Immunity (see Fig. 14–7)

1. Does involve antibody production; is effective against pathogens and foreign cells.
2. B cells, macrophages, and helper T cells recognize the foreign antigen; the B cells are antigen specific and begin to divide.
3. Memory B cells will remember the specific foreign antigen.
4. Other B cells become plasma cells that produce antigen-specific antibodies.
5. An antigen–antibody complex is formed, which attracts macrophages (opsonization).
6. Complement fixation is stimulated by antigen–antibody complexes. The complement proteins bind to the antigen–antibody complex and lyse cellular antigens or enhance the phagocytosis of noncellular antigens.

Antibodies—immune globulins (Ig) or gamma globulins (see Table 14–1 and Fig. 14–8)

1. Proteins produced by plasma cells in response to foreign antigens.
2. Each antibody is specific for only one foreign antigen.
3. Bond to the foreign antigen to label it for phagocytosis (opsonization).

Antibody Responses and Functions (see Fig. 14–9)

1. On the first exposure to a foreign antigen, antibodies are produced slowly and in small amounts, and the person may develop clinical disease.
2. On the second exposure, the memory cells initiate rapid production of large amounts of antibodies, and a second case of the disease may be prevented. This is the basis for the protection given by vaccines, which take the place of the first exposure.
3. Antibodies cause agglutination (clumping) of bacterial cells; clumped cells are easier for macrophages to phagocytize (see Fig. 14–8).
4. Antibodies neutralize viruses by bonding to them and preventing their entry into cells.
5. Antibodies neutralize bacterial toxins by bonding to them and changing their shape.

Types of Immunity (see Table 14–2)

REVIEW QUESTIONS

1. Explain the relationships among plasma, tissue fluid, and lymph, in terms of movement of water throughout the body. (p. 358)
2. Describe the system of lymph vessels. Explain how lymph is kept moving in these vessels. Into which veins is lymph emptied? (p. 358)
3. State the locations of the major groups of lymph nodes, and explain their functions. (pp. 358–359)
4. State the locations of lymph nodules, and explain their functions. (pp. 359–360)
5. Describe the location of the spleen and explain its functions. If the spleen is removed, what organs will compensate for its functions? (p. 360)
6. Explain the function of the thymus, and state when (age) this function is most important. (pp. 360–361, 363)
7. Name the different kinds of foreign antigens to which the immune system responds, and state three general differences between innate immunity and adaptive immunity. (p. 363)
8. Innate immunity includes barriers, defensive cells, and chemicals; give two examples of each. (p. 364)
9. Explain how a foreign antigen is recognized as foreign. Which mechanism of adaptive immunity involves antibody production? Explain what opsonization means. (pp. 366, 368–369)
10. State the functions of helper T cells, cytotoxic T cells, regulatory T cells, and memory T cells. Plasma cells differentiate from which type of lymphocyte? State the function of plasma cells. What other type of cell comes from B lymphocytes? (pp. 366, 368)
11. What is the stimulus for complement fixation? How does this process destroy cellular antigens and non-cellular antigens? (p. 369)
12. Explain the antibody reactions of agglutination and neutralization. (pp. 371, 373)
13. Explain how a vaccine provides protective immunity in terms of first and second exposures to a pathogen. (pp. 370–371)
14. Explain the difference between the following: (pp. 373–375)
    a. Genetic immunity and acquired immunity
    b. Passive acquired immunity and active acquired immunity
    c. Natural and artificial passive acquired immunity
    d. Natural and artificial active acquired immunity

FOR FURTHER THOUGHT

1. Bubonic plague, also called black plague, is a serious disease caused by a bacterium and spread by fleas from rats or other rodents to people. It got its "black" name from "buboes," dark swellings found in the groin or armpit of people with plague. Explain what buboes are and why they were usually found in the groin and armpit.
2. In Rh disease of the newborn, maternal antibodies enter fetal circulation and destroy the red blood cells of the fetus. A mother with type O blood has anti-A and anti-B antibodies but may have a dozen type A children without any problem at all. Explain why. (Look at Table 14–1 and Fig. 14–8.)
3. Most vaccines are given by injection. The oral polio vaccine (OPV), however, is not; it is given by mouth. Remembering that the purpose of a vaccine is to expose the individual to the pathogen, what does this tell you about the polio viruses (there are three) and their usual site of infection?
4. Everyone should have a tetanus booster shot every 10 years. That is what we often call a "tetanus shot." Someone who sustains a soil-contaminated injury should also receive a tetanus booster (if none in the past 10 years). But someone who has symptoms of tetanus should get TIG, tetanus immune globulin. Explain the difference, and why TIG is so important.
5. People with AIDS are susceptible to many other diseases. Which of these would be least likely: pneumonia, rheumatoid arthritis, yeast infection of the mouth, or protozoan infection of the intestines? Explain your answer.
6. A cut in the skin has permitted bacteria to enter the epidermis and dermis. Both innate and adaptive immune mechanisms will respond. The graph in Question Figure 14–A is a time line that depicts the sequence of responses. Try to match each immune cell and antibody production with its proper place in the sequence. To get started, for the red line, # 1: what kind of cell is present in the epidermis to pick up incoming pathogens?

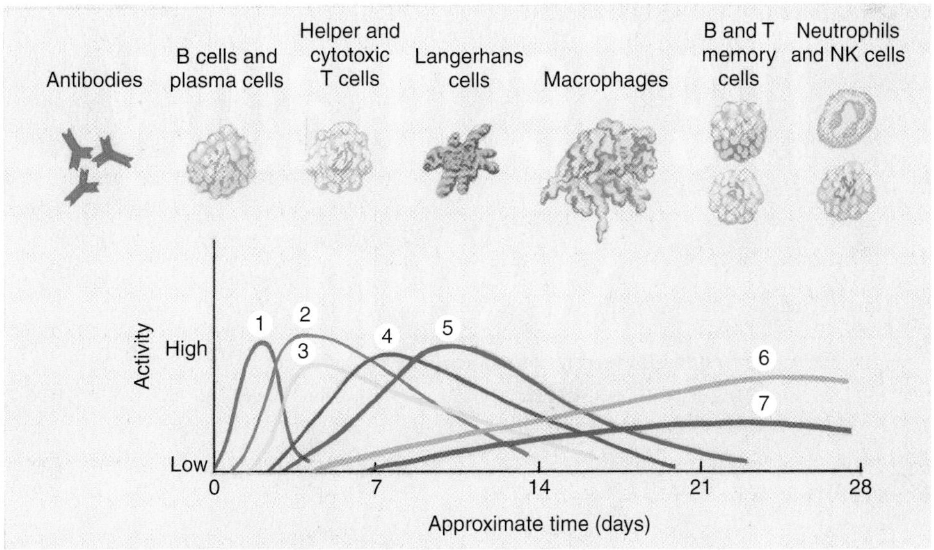

QUESTION FIGURE 14–A: Time line of responses to a pathogen.

CHAPTER

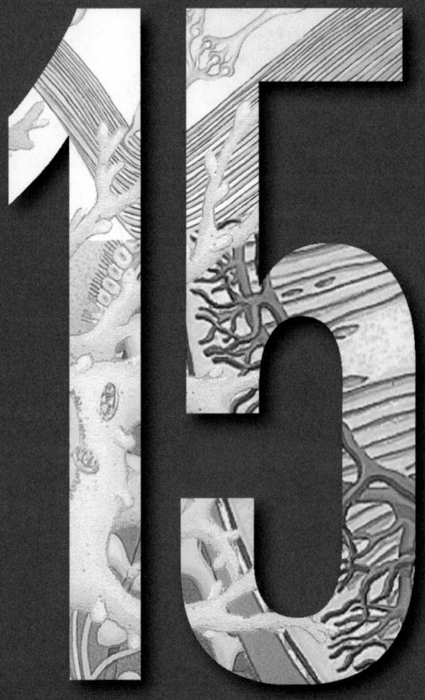

15 The Respiratory System

STUDENT OBJECTIVES

- State the general function of the respiratory system.
- Describe the structure and functions of the nasal cavities and pharynx.
- Describe the structure of the larynx, and explain the speaking mechanism.
- Describe the structure and functions of the trachea and bronchial tree.
- State the locations of the pleural membranes, and explain the functions of serous fluid.
- Describe the structure of the alveoli and pulmonary capillaries, and explain the importance of pulmonary surfactant.
- Name and describe the important air pressures involved in breathing.
- Describe normal inhalation and exhalation and forced exhalation.
- Name the pulmonary volumes and define each.
- Explain the diffusion of gases in external respiration and internal respiration.
- Describe how oxygen and carbon dioxide are transported in the blood.
- Explain the nervous and chemical mechanisms that regulate respiration.
- Explain how respiration affects the pH of body fluids.

NEW TERMINOLOGY

Alveoli *(al-**VEE**-oh-lye)*

Bronchial tree *(**BRONG**-kee-uhl TREE)*

Epiglottis *(ep-i-**GLAH**-tis)*

Glottis *(**GLAH**-tis)*

Intrapleural pressure *(IN-trah-**PLOOR**-uhl **PRES**-shur)*

Intrapulmonic pressure *(IN-trah-pull-**MAHN**-ik **PRES**-shur)*

Larynx *(**LA**-rinks)*

Partial pressure *(**PAR**-shul **PRES**-shur)*

Phrenic nerves *(**FREN**-ik NURVZ)*

Pulmonary surfactant *(**PULL**-muh-ner-ee sir-**FAK**-tent)*

Residual air *(ree-**ZID**-yoo-al AIR)*

Respiratory acidosis *(RES-pi-rah-**TOR**-ee ass-i-**DOH**-sis)*

Respiratory alkalosis *(RES-pi-rah-**TOR**-ee al-kah-**LOH**-sis)*

Soft palate *(SAWFT **PAL**-uht)*

Tidal volume *(**TIGH**-duhl **VAHL**-yoom)*

Ventilation *(VEN-ti-**LAY**-shun)*

Vital capacity *(**VY**-tuhl kuh-**PASS**-i-tee)*

*Terms that appear in **bold type** in the chapter text are defined in the glossary, which begins on page 603.*

CHAPTER OUTLINE

RELATED CLINICAL TERMINOLOGY

Cyanosis (*SIGH-uh-**NOH**-sis*)
Dyspnea (***DISP**-nee-ah or disp-**NEE**-ah*)
Emphysema (*EM-fi-**SEE**-mah*)
Heimlich maneuver (***HIGHM**-lik ma-**NEW**-ver*)
Hyaline membrane disease (***HIGH**-e-lin **MEM**-brain di-**ZEEZ***)
Pneumonia (*new-**MOH**-nee-ah*)
Pneumothorax (*NEW-moh-**THAW**-raks*)
Pulmonary edema (***PULL**-muh-ner-ee uh-**DEE**-muh*)

Sometimes a person will describe a habit as being "as natural as breathing." Indeed, what could be more natural? We rarely think about breathing, and it isn't something we look forward to, as we might look forward to a good dinner. We just breathe, usually at the rate of 12 to 20 times per minute, and faster when necessary (such as during exercise). You may have heard of trained singers "learning how to breathe," but they are really learning how to make their breathing more efficient.

Most of the **respiratory system** is concerned with what we think of as breathing: moving air into and out of the lungs. The lungs are the site of the exchanges of oxygen and carbon dioxide between the air and the blood. Both of these exchanges are important. All of our cells must obtain oxygen to carry out cell respiration to produce ATP. Just as crucial is the elimination of the CO_2 produced as a waste product of cell respiration, and, as you already know, the proper functioning of the circulatory system is essential for the transport of these gases in the blood.

DIVISIONS OF THE RESPIRATORY SYSTEM

The respiratory system may be divided into the upper respiratory tract and the lower respiratory tract. The **upper respiratory tract** consists of the parts outside the chest cavity: the air passages of the nose, nasal cavities, pharynx, larynx, and upper trachea. The **lower respiratory tract** consists of the parts found within the chest cavity: the lower trachea and the lungs themselves, which include the bronchial tubes and alveoli. Also part of the respiratory system are the pleural membranes and the respiratory muscles that form the chest cavity: the diaphragm and intercostal muscles.

Have you recognized some familiar organs and structures thus far? There will be more because this chapter includes material from all of the previous chapters. Even though we are discussing the body system by system, the respiratory system is an excellent example of the interdependent functioning of all the body systems.

NOSE AND NASAL CAVITIES

Air usually enters and leaves the respiratory system through the **nose**, which is made of bone and cartilage covered with skin. Just inside the nostrils are hairs, which help block the entry of dust.

The two **nasal cavities** are within the skull, separated by the **nasal septum**, which is a bony plate made of the ethmoid bone and vomer. The **nasal mucosa** (lining) is ciliated epithelium, with goblet cells that produce mucus. Three shelf-like or scroll-like bones called **conchae** project from the lateral wall of each nasal cavity (Fig. 15–1; see also Fig. 6–6 in Chapter 6). Just as shelves in a cabinet provide more flat space for storage, the conchae increase the surface area of the nasal mucosa. As air passes through the nasal cavities, it picks up heat and moisture from the nasal mucosa. The air that reaches the lungs is warmed almost to body temperature and has a humidity of 100%; this is important to prevent drying of the cells of the alveoli. Bacteria and particles of air pollution that enter with inhaled air are trapped on the mucus; the cilia continuously sweep the mucus toward the pharynx. Most of this mucus is eventually swallowed, and most bacteria present will be destroyed by the hydrochloric acid in the gastric juice.

In the upper nasal cavities are the **olfactory receptors**, which detect vaporized chemicals that have been inhaled. The olfactory nerves pass through the ethmoid bone to the brain.

You may also recall our earlier discussion of the **paranasal sinuses**, air cavities in the maxillae, frontal, sphenoid, and ethmoid bones (see Fig. 15–1 and also Fig. 6–9 in Chapter 6). These sinuses are lined with ciliated epithelium, and the mucus produced drains into the nasal cavities. The functions of the paranasal sinuses are to lighten the skull and provide resonance (more vibrating air) for the voice.

PHARYNX

The **pharynx** is a muscular tube posterior to the nasal and oral cavities and anterior to the cervical vertebrae. For descriptive purposes, the pharynx may be divided into three parts: the nasopharynx, oropharynx, and laryngopharynx (see Fig. 15–1).

The uppermost portion is the **nasopharynx**, which is behind the nasal cavities. The **soft palate** is elevated during swallowing to block the nasopharynx and prevent food or saliva from going up rather than down. The uvula is the part of the soft palate you can see at the back of the throat. On the posterior wall of the nasopharynx is the adenoid or pharyngeal tonsil, a lymph nodule that contains macrophages. Opening into the nasopharynx are the two eustachian tubes, which extend to the middle ear cavities. The purpose of the eustachian tubes is to permit air to enter or leave the middle ears, allowing the eardrums to vibrate properly.

The nasopharynx is a passageway for air only, but the remainder of the pharynx serves as both an air and food passageway, although not for both at the same time. The **oropharynx** is behind the mouth; its mucosa is stratified squamous epithelium, continuous with that of the oral cavity. On its lateral walls are the palatine tonsils, also lymph nodules. Together with the adenoid and the lingual tonsils on the base of the tongue, they form a ring of lymphatic tissue around the pharynx to destroy pathogens that penetrate the mucosa.

The **laryngopharynx** is the most inferior portion of the pharynx. It opens anteriorly into the larynx and posteriorly into the esophagus. Contraction of the muscular wall of the oropharynx and laryngopharynx is part of the swallowing reflex.

LARYNX

The **larynx** is often called the voice box, a name that indicates one of its functions, which is speaking. The other function of the larynx is to be an air passageway between the pharynx and the trachea. Air passages must be kept open at all times, so the larynx is made of nine pieces of cartilage connected by ligaments. Cartilage is a firm yet flexible tissue that prevents collapse of the larynx. In comparison, the esophagus (which is behind the larynx) is a collapsed tube except when food is passing through it.

The largest cartilage of the larynx is the **thyroid cartilage** (Fig. 15–2), which you can feel on the anterior surface of your neck. The **epiglottis** is the uppermost cartilage. During swallowing, the larynx is elevated and the epiglottis closes over the top, rather like a trap door or hinged lid, to prevent the entry of saliva or food into the larynx.

The mucosa of the larynx is ciliated epithelium, except for the vocal cords (stratified squamous epithelium). The cilia of the mucosa sweep upward to remove mucus and trapped dust and microorganisms.

The **vocal cords** (or vocal folds) are on either side of the **glottis**, the opening between them. During breathing, the vocal cords are held at the sides of the glottis, so that air passes freely into and out of the trachea (Fig. 15–3). During speaking, the intrinsic muscles of the larynx pull the vocal cords across the glottis, and exhaled air vibrates the vocal cords to produce sounds that can be turned into speech. It is also physically possible to speak

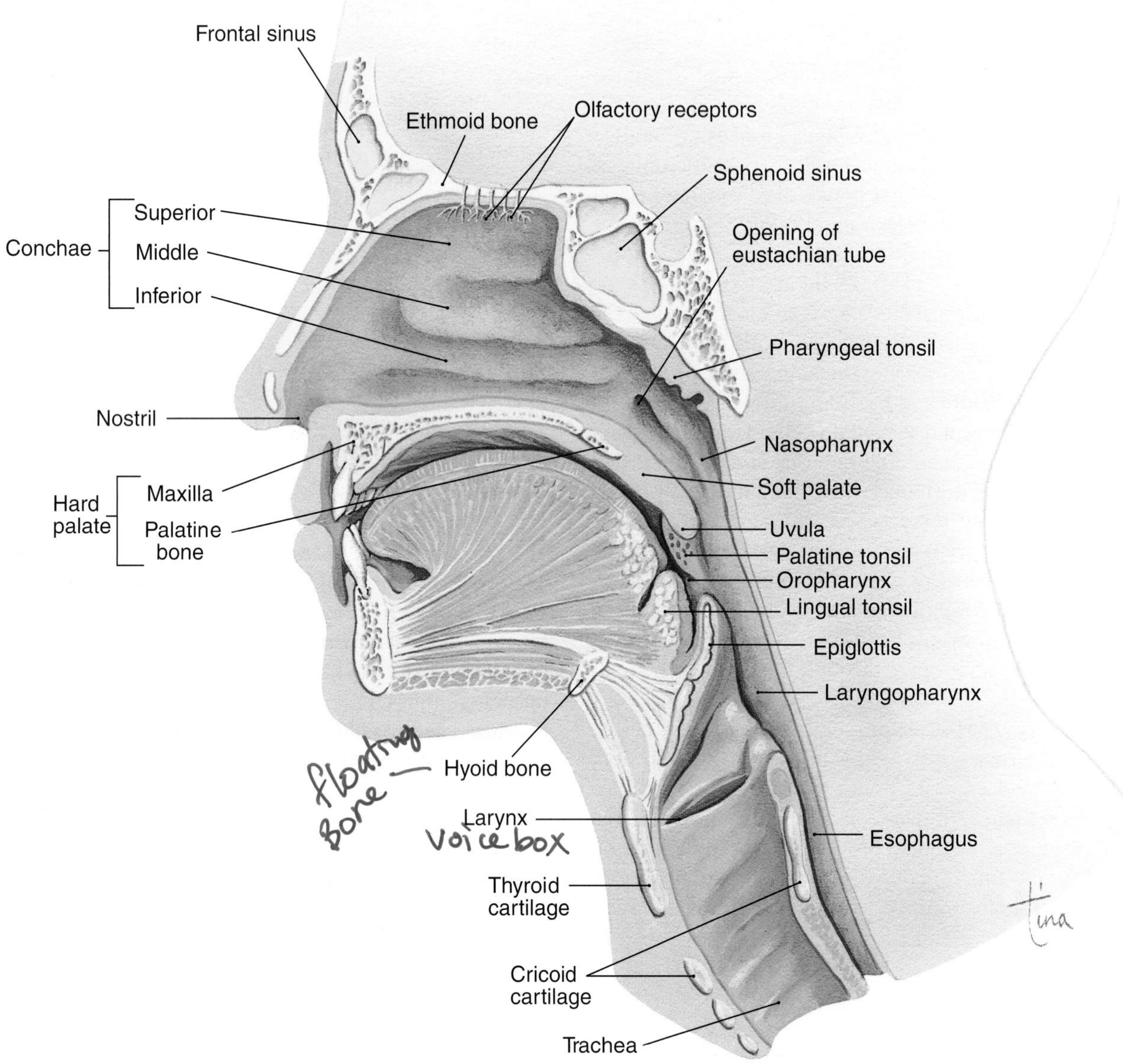

Figure 15–1 Midsagittal section of the head and neck showing the structures of the upper respiratory tract.

QUESTION: Describe the shape of the conchae by using a familiar object. What is the function of the conchae?

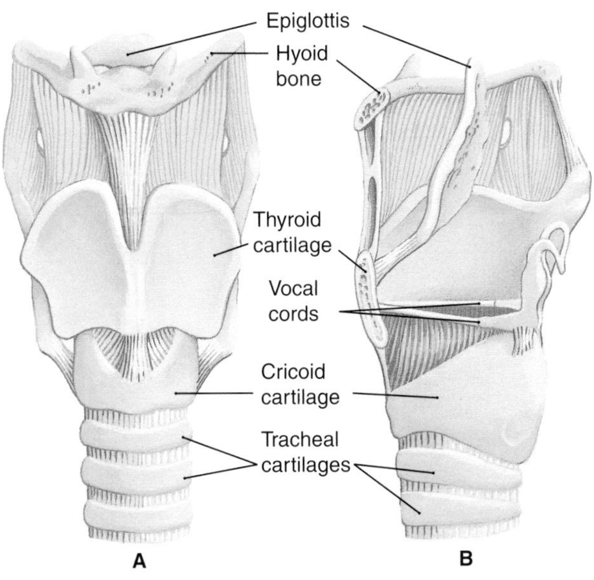

Figure 15–2 Larynx. (**A**) Anterior view. (**B**) Midsagittal section through the larynx, viewed from the left side.

QUESTION: What is the function of the epiglottis?

while inhaling, but this is not what we are used to. The cranial nerves that are motor nerves to the larynx for speaking are the vagus and accessory nerves. You may also recall that for most people, the speech areas are in the left cerebral hemisphere.

TRACHEA AND BRONCHIAL TREE

The **trachea** is about 4 to 5 inches (10 to 13 cm) long and extends from the larynx to the primary bronchi; it is anterior to the esophagus. If you place your fingertips at the base of your neck just above your sternum, you can feel the firmness of the trachea. The wall of the trachea contains 16 to 20 C-shaped pieces of cartilage, which keep the trachea open (see Figs. 15–2 and 15–4). The gaps in these incomplete cartilage rings are posterior, to permit the expansion of the esophagus when food is swallowed. The mucosa of the trachea is ciliated epithelium with goblet cells (see Fig. 4–3, part C, in Chapter 4). As in the larynx, the cilia sweep upward toward the pharynx.

The right and left **primary bronchi** (Fig. 15–4) are the branches of the trachea that enter the lungs. Their structure is just like that of the trachea, with C-shaped cartilages and ciliated epithelium. Within the lungs, each primary bronchus branches into secondary bronchi leading to the lobes of each lung (three right, two left). The further branching of the bronchial tubes is often called the **bronchial tree**. Imagine the trachea as the trunk of an upside-down tree with extensive branches that become smaller and smaller; these smaller branches are the **bronchioles**. No cartilage is present in the walls of the bronchioles; this becomes clinically important in asthma (see Box 15–1: Asthma). The smallest bronchioles terminate in clusters of alveoli, the air sacs of the lungs.

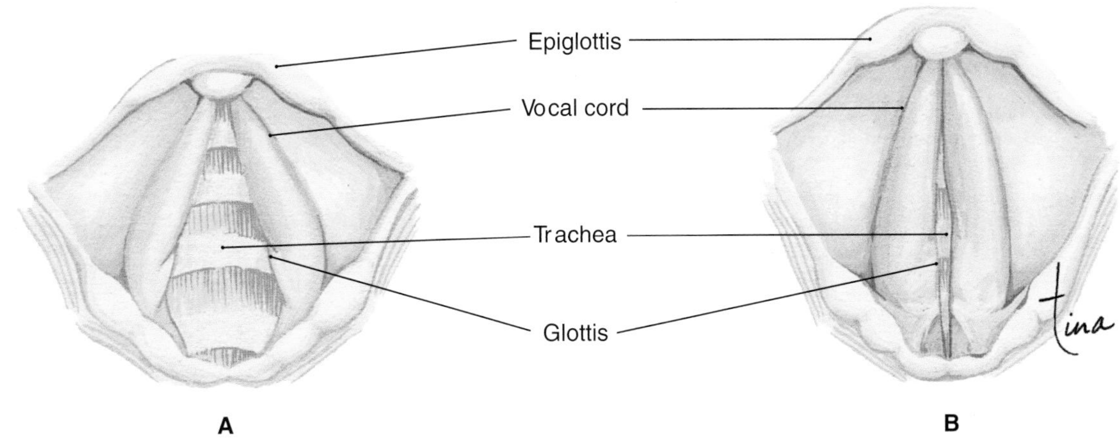

Figure 15–3 Vocal cords and glottis, superior view. (**A**) Position of the vocal cords during breathing. (**B**) Position of the vocal cords during speaking.

QUESTION: What makes the vocal cords vibrate?

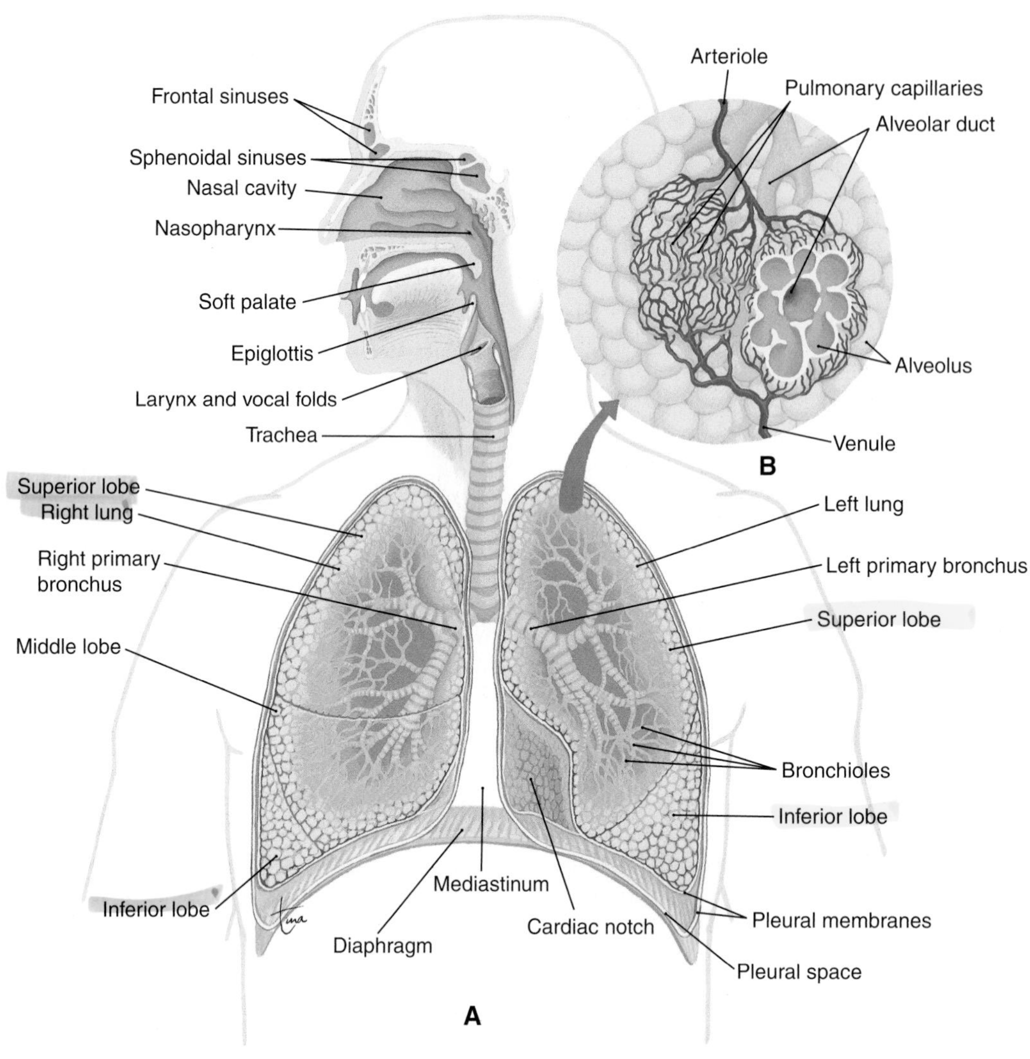

Figure 15–4 Respiratory system. (**A**) Anterior view of the upper and lower respiratory tracts. (**B**) Microscopic view of alveoli and pulmonary capillaries. (The colors represent the vessels, not the oxygen content of the blood within the vessels.)

QUESTION: What are the first branches of the trachea, and how do they resemble the trachea in structure?

LUNGS AND PLEURAL MEMBRANES

The **lungs** are located on either side of the heart in the chest cavity and are encircled and protected by the rib cage. The base of each lung rests on the diaphragm below; the apex (superior tip) is at the level of the clavicle. On the medial surface of each lung is an indentation called the **hilus**, where the primary bronchus and the pulmonary artery and veins enter the lung.

The pleural membranes are the serous membranes of the thoracic cavity. The **parietal pleura** lines the chest wall, and the **visceral pleura** is on the surface of the lungs. Between the pleural membranes is serous fluid, which prevents friction and keeps the two membranes together during breathing.

Box 15–1 | ASTHMA

Asthma is an inflammation of the bronchial tree and is usually triggered by an infection or allergic reaction that affects the smooth muscle and glands of the bronchioles. Allergens include foods and inhaled substances such as dust, pollen, pet dander, and chitin from the exoskeletons of insects or the cell walls of fungi. Wheezing and dyspnea (difficult breathing) characterize an asthma attack, which may range from mild to fatal.

As part of the allergic response, the smooth muscle of the bronchioles constricts (see Box Fig. 15–A). Because there is no cartilage present in their walls, the bronchioles may close completely. As part of inflammation, the lining of the bronchioles swells and the secretion of mucus increases, perhaps markedly, so the already constricted bronchioles may become clogged or completely obstructed with mucus.

Chronic asthma is a predisposing factor for emphysema. When obstructed bronchioles prevent ventilation of alveoli, the walls of the alveoli begin to deteriorate and break down, leaving large cavities that do not provide much surface area for gas exchange.

One possible way to prevent serious lung damage is to prevent asthma attacks with a medication that blocks the release of IgE antibodies. An allergy is an immune overreaction, and blocking it would prevent the damaging effects of inflammation. Correcting a deficiency of vitamin D (if present) lessens the severity of asthma attacks for some children. Some asthma medications block the actions of leukotrienes or other inflammatory cytokines. In the United States the incidence of asthma is increasing among children who grow up in cities (children who grow up on farms have far lower rates of asthma); this may be a result of exposure to air pollution, or the lack of exposure to a variety of plant and animal antigens when the immune system is maturing.

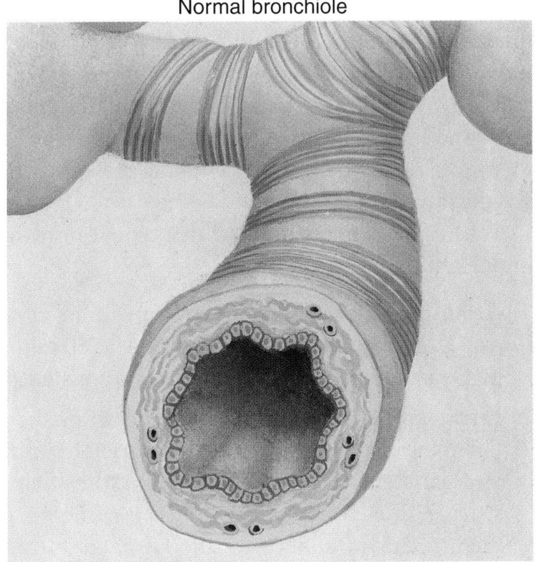

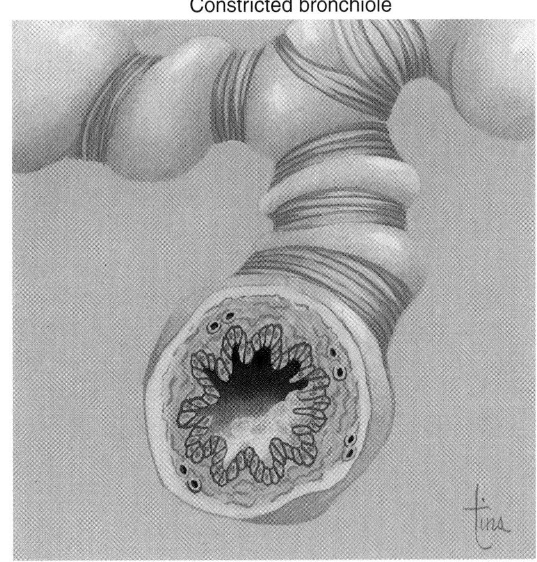

Box Figure 15–A (**A**) Cross-section of normal bronchiole. (**B**) Bronchiole with asthmatic inflammation narrowing the airway.

Alveoli

The functional units of the lungs are the air sacs called **alveoli**. There are millions of alveoli in each lung, and their total surface area is estimated to be 700 to 800 square feet (picture a sidewalk 2 ½ feet wide that is as long as an American football field [300 feet], or a rectangle measuring 25 feet by 30 feet); this is the surface area available for exchange of oxygen and carbon dioxide. The flat alveolar type I cells that form most of the alveolar walls are simple squamous epithelium. But before we go inside the alveoli, let us take a look at their surroundings.

In the spaces between clusters of alveoli is elastic connective tissue; the elastin fibers contribute to exhalation. Each alveolus is surrounded by a network of pulmonary capillaries (see Fig. 15–4). Recall that capillaries are also made of simple squamous epithelium, so there are only two cells between the air in the alveoli and the blood in the pulmonary capillaries, which permits efficient diffusion of gases (Fig. 15–5). The pulmonary arterioles that bring blood to these capillary networks differ from systemic arterioles in their response to varying levels of oxygen in the lung tissue. In response to hypoxia, pulmonary arterioles constrict (rather than dilate), reducing blood flow in their capillary networks. What purpose might this have? Let us use as an example bacterial pneumonia, a disease in which alveoli become filled with fluid. These alveoli are poorly ventilated, little new air gets in, and blood that is circulating through the surrounding pulmonary capillaries has little or no oxygen to pick up. This blood would leave the lungs without oxygen to deliver to body tissues. Under these conditions, however, the pulmonary arterioles will constrict, decreasing the blood flow around these poorly ventilated alveoli. As a result, greater blood flow will occur around better-ventilated clusters of alveoli, where oxygen pick-up is much more likely.

We now return to the interior of the alveoli, where we find much more than air. Within the alveoli are wandering macrophages (Fig. 15–5) that phagocytize pathogens or other foreign material that may not have been swept out by the ciliated epithelium of the bronchial tree. Each alveolus is lined with a thin layer of tissue fluid, which is essential for the diffusion of gases, because a gas must dissolve in a liquid in order to enter or leave a cell (the earthworm principle—an earthworm breathes through its moist skin and will suffocate if its skin dries out). Although this tissue fluid is necessary, it creates a potential problem in that, by itself, would make the walls of an alveolus stick together internally. Imagine a plastic bag that is wet inside; its walls would stick together because of the surface tension of the water. The cohesion of water molecules and adhesion to the plastic would keep the walls together. This is just what would happen in alveoli, with the tissue fluid and alveolar cells, and inflation of these air sacs would be very difficult.

This problem is overcome by **pulmonary surfactant**, a lipoprotein secreted by alveolar type II cells, also called septal cells. Surfactant mixes with the tissue fluid within the alveoli and decreases its surface tension, permitting inflation of the alveoli (see Box 15–2: Hyaline Membrane Disease). Normal inflation of the alveoli in turn permits the exchange of gases, but before we discuss this process, we will first see how air gets into and out of the lungs.

MECHANISM OF BREATHING

Ventilation is the term for the movement of air to and from the alveoli. The two aspects of ventilation are inhalation and exhalation, which are brought about by the nervous system and the respiratory muscles. The respiratory centers are located in the medulla and pons. Their specific functions will be covered in a later section, but it is the medulla that generates impulses to the respiratory muscles.

These muscles are the diaphragm and the external and internal intercostal muscles (Fig. 15–6). The **diaphragm** is a dome-shaped muscle below the lungs; when it contracts, the diaphragm flattens and moves downward. The intercostal muscles are found between the ribs. The **external intercostal muscles** pull the ribs upward and outward, and the **internal intercostal muscles** pull the ribs downward and inward. Ventilation is the result of the respiratory muscles producing changes in the pressure within the alveoli and bronchial tree.

With respect to breathing, three types of pressure are important:

1. **Atmospheric pressure**—the pressure of the air around us. At sea level, atmospheric pressure is 760 mm Hg. At higher altitudes, of course, atmospheric pressure is lower.
2. **Intrapleural pressure**—the pressure within the potential pleural space between the parietal pleura and visceral pleura. This is a potential rather than a real space. A thin layer of serous fluid causes the two pleural membranes to adhere to one another. Intrapleural pressure is always slightly below atmospheric pressure (about 756 mm Hg) and is called a *negative* pressure. The elastic lungs are always tending to collapse and pull the visceral pleura away from the parietal pleura. The serous fluid, however, prevents actual separation of the pleural membranes (see Box 15–3: Pneumothorax).
3. **Intrapulmonic pressure**—the pressure within the bronchial tree and alveoli. This pressure fluctuates

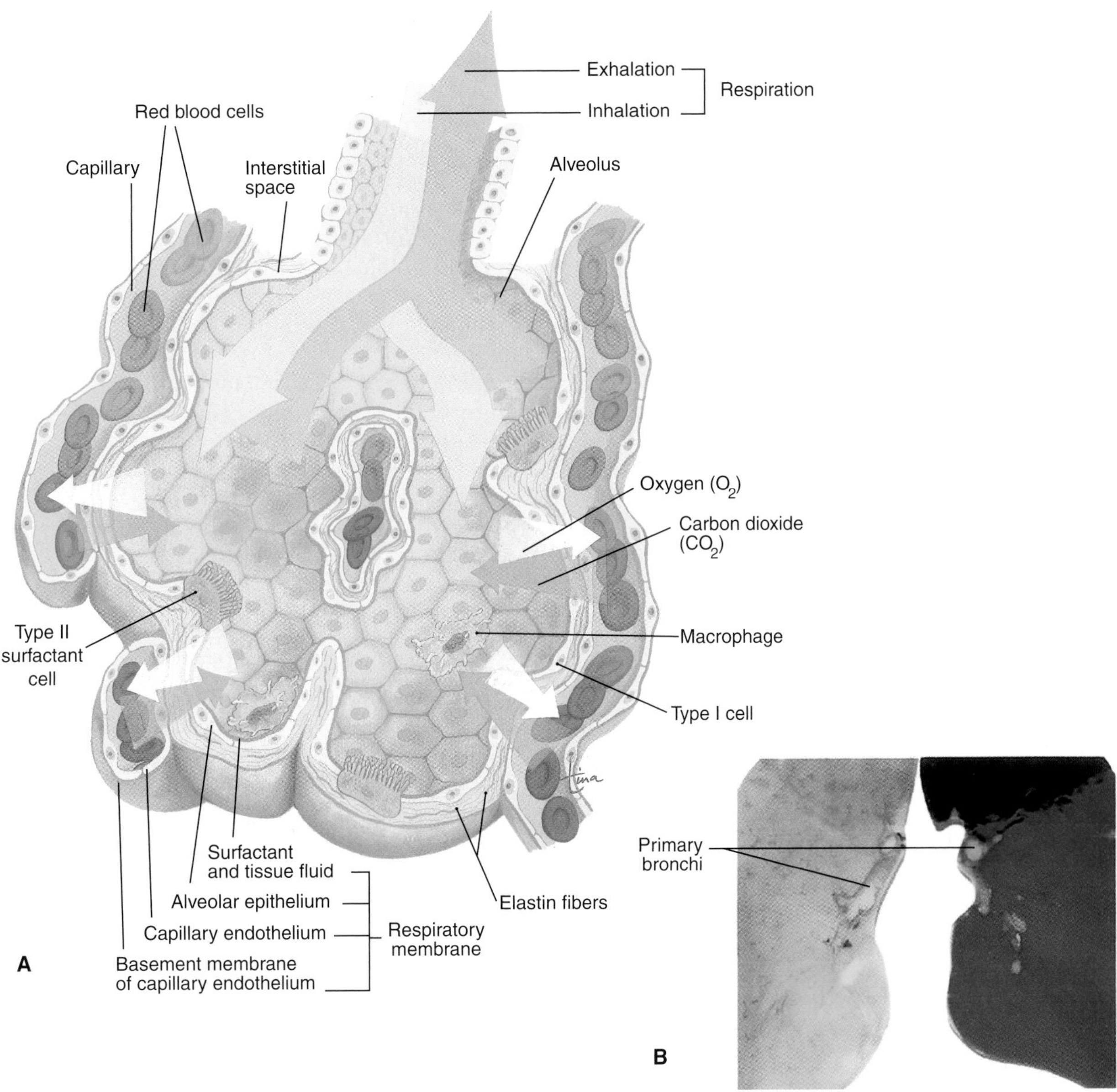

Figure 15–5 (**A**) Alveolar structure showing type I and type II cells, as well as alveolar macrophages. The respiratory membrane: the structures and substances through which gases must pass as they diffuse from air to blood (oxygen) or from blood to air (CO_2). (**B**) Sections of human lungs embedded in plastic. On the left is a normal adult lung; on the right is a smoker's lung. (Photograph by Dan Kaufman.)

QUESTION: Which cells shown here are part of the respiratory membrane? Which cells are not, and what are their functions?

Box 15–2 | HYALINE MEMBRANE DISEASE

Hyaline membrane disease is also called respiratory distress syndrome (RDS) of the newborn and most often affects premature infants whose lungs have not yet produced sufficient quantities of pulmonary surfactant.

The first few breaths of a newborn inflate most of the previously collapsed lungs, and the presence of surfactant permits the alveoli to remain open. The following breaths become much easier, and normal breathing is established.

Without surfactant, the surface tension of the tissue fluid lining the alveoli causes the air sacs to collapse after each breath rather than remain inflated. Each breath, therefore, is difficult, and the newborn must expend a great deal of energy just to breathe.

Premature infants may require respiratory assistance until their lungs are mature enough to produce surfactant. Use of a synthetic surfactant has significantly helped some infants, and because they can breathe more normally, their dependence on respirators is minimized. Still undergoing evaluation are the effects of the long-term use of this surfactant in the most premature babies, who may require it for much longer periods of time.

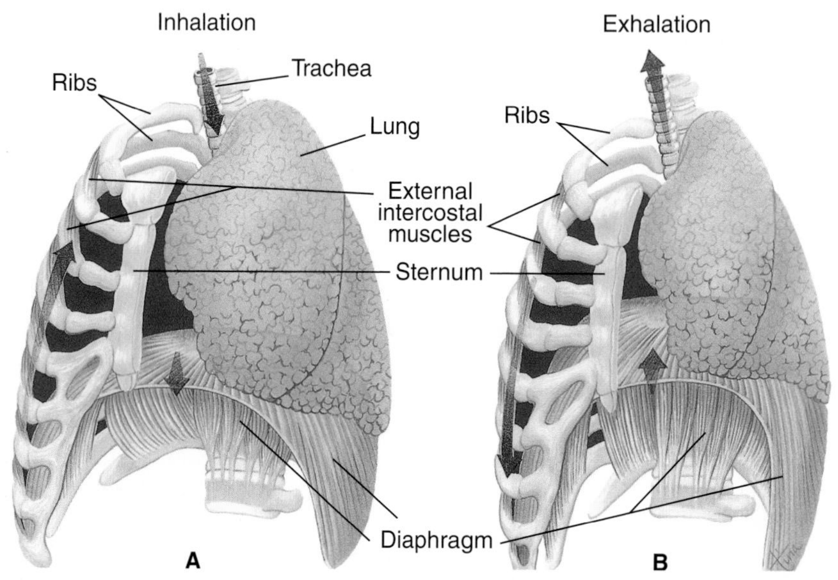

Figure 15–6 Actions of the respiratory muscles. (**A**) Inhalation: diaphragm contracts downward; external intercostal muscles pull rib cage upward and outward; lungs are expanded. (**B**) Normal exhalation: diaphragm relaxes upward; rib cage falls down and in as external intercostal muscles relax; lungs are compressed.

QUESTION: Why is a normal exhalation a passive process?

below and above atmospheric pressure during each cycle of breathing.

INHALATION

Inhalation, also called **inspiration**, is a precise sequence of events that may be described as follows: Motor impulses from the medulla travel along the **phrenic nerves** to the diaphragm and along the **intercostal nerves** to the external intercostal muscles. The diaphragm contracts, moves downward, and expands the chest cavity from top to bottom. The external intercostal muscles pull the ribs up and out, which expands the chest cavity from side to side and front to back.

Box 15–3 | PNEUMOTHORAX

Pneumothorax is the presence of air in the pleural space, which causes collapse of the lung on that side. Recall that the pleural space is only a potential space because the serous fluid keeps the pleural membranes adhering to one another, and the intrapleural pressure is always slightly below atmospheric pressure. Should air at atmospheric pressure enter the pleural cavity, the suddenly higher pressure outside the lung will contribute to its collapse (the other factor is the normal elasticity of the lungs).

A spontaneous pneumothorax, without apparent trauma, may result from rupture of weakened alveoli on the lung surface. Pulmonary diseases such as emphysema may weaken alveoli.

Puncture wounds of the chest wall also allow air into the pleural space, with resulting collapse of a lung. In severe cases, large amounts of air push the heart, great vessels, trachea, and esophagus toward the opposite side (mediastinal shift), putting pressure on the other lung and making breathing difficult. This is called tension pneumothorax and requires rapid medical intervention to remove the trapped air.

As the chest cavity is expanded, the parietal pleura expands with it. Intrapleural pressure becomes even more negative as a sort of suction is created between the pleural membranes. The adhesion created by the serous fluid, however, permits the visceral pleura to be expanded, too, and this expands the lungs as well.

As the lungs expand, intrapulmonic pressure falls below atmospheric pressure, and air enters the nose and travels through the respiratory passages to the alveoli. Entry of air continues until intrapulmonic pressure is equal to atmospheric pressure; this is a normal inhalation. Of course, inhalation can be continued beyond normal, that is, a deep breath. This requires a more forceful contraction of the respiratory muscles to further expand the lungs, permitting the entry of more air.

EXHALATION

Exhalation may also be called **expiration** and begins when motor impulses from the medulla decrease and the diaphragm and external intercostal muscles relax. As the chest cavity becomes smaller, the lungs are compressed, and their elastic connective tissue, which was stretched during inhalation, recoils and also compresses the alveoli. As intrapulmonic pressure rises above atmospheric pressure, air is forced out of the lungs until the two pressures are again equal.

Notice that inhalation is an active process that requires muscle contraction, but normal exhalation is a passive process, with relaxation of muscles, and depending to a great extent on the normal elasticity of healthy lungs. In other words, under normal circumstances we must expend energy to inhale but not to exhale (see Box 15–4: Emphysema).

We can, however, go beyond a normal exhalation and expel more air, such as when talking, singing, or blowing up a balloon. Such a forced exhalation is an active process that requires contraction of other muscles. Contraction of the internal intercostal muscles pulls the ribs down and in and squeezes even more air out of the lungs. Contraction of abdominal muscles, such as the rectus abdominis, compresses the abdominal organs and pushes the diaphragm upward, which also forces more air out of the lungs (see Box 15–5: The Heimlich Maneuver).

PULMONARY VOLUMES

The capacity of the lungs varies with the size and age of the person. Taller people have larger lungs than do shorter people. Also, as we get older our lung capacity diminishes as lungs lose their elasticity and the respiratory muscles become less efficient. For the following pulmonary volumes, the values given are those for healthy young adults. These are also shown in Fig. 15–7.

1. **Tidal volume**—the amount of air involved in one normal inhalation and exhalation. The average tidal volume is 500 mL, but many people often have lower tidal volumes because of shallow breathing.
2. **Minute respiratory volume** (MRV)—the amount of air inhaled and exhaled in 1 minute. MRV is calculated by multiplying tidal volume by the number of respirations per minute (average range: 12 to 20 per minute). If tidal volume is 500 mL and the respiratory rate is 12 breaths per minute, the MRV is 6000 mL, or 6 liters of air per minute, which is average. Shallow breathing usually indicates a smaller than average tidal volume

Box 15–4 | EMPHYSEMA

Emphysema, a form of chronic obstructive pulmonary disease (COPD), is a degenerative disease in which the alveoli lose their elasticity and cannot recoil. Perhaps the most common (and avoidable) cause is cigarette smoking; other causes are long-term exposure to severe air pollution or industrial dusts, chronic asthma, or chronic bronchitis. Inhaled irritants damage the alveolar walls and cause deterioration of the elastic connective tissue surrounding the alveoli. Macrophages migrate to the damaged areas and seem to produce an enzyme that contributes to the destruction of the protein elastin. This is an instance of a useful body response (for cleaning up damaged tissue) becoming damaging when it is excessive. As the alveoli break down, larger air cavities are created that are not efficient in gas exchange (see Box Fig. 15–B).

In progressive emphysema, damaged lung tissue is replaced by fibrous connective tissue (scar tissue), which further limits the diffusion of gases. Blood oxygen level decreases, and blood carbon dioxide level increases. Accumulating carbon dioxide decreases the pH of body fluids; this is a respiratory acidosis.

For some people who develop COPD, the damage to lung tissue caused by tobacco smoke triggers autoimmune mechanisms. The mistaken activity of immune system cells causes additional damage, even if the person has stopped smoking.

One of the most characteristic signs of emphysema is that the affected person must make an effort to exhale. The loss of lung elasticity makes normal exhalation an active process, rather than the passive process it usually is. The person must expend energy to exhale in order to make room in the lungs for inhaled air. This extra "work" required for exhalation may be exhausting for the person and contributes to the debilitating nature of emphysema.

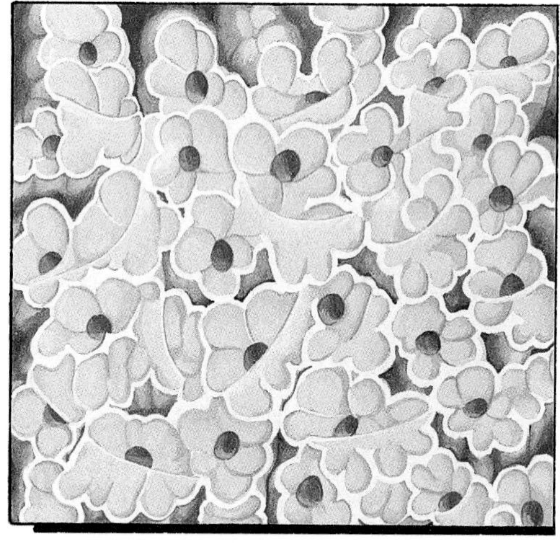

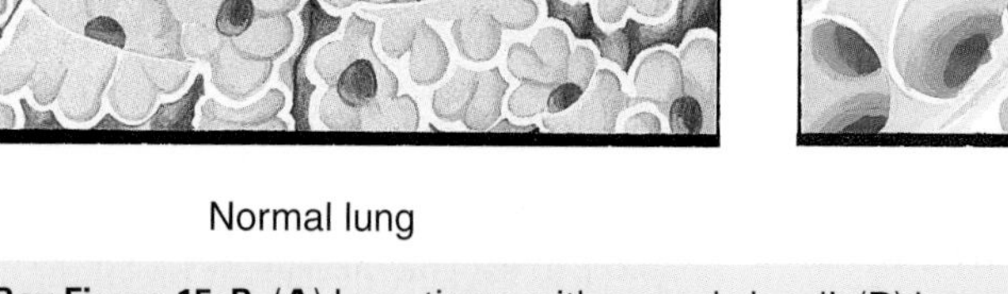

Normal lung

Emphysema

Box Figure 15–B (**A**) Lung tissue with normal alveoli. (**B**) Lung tissue in emphysema.

and would thus require more respirations per minute to obtain the necessary MRV.

3. **Inspiratory reserve**—the amount of air, beyond tidal volume, that can be taken in with the deepest possible inhalation. Normal inspiratory reserve ranges from 2000 to 3000 mL.
4. **Expiratory reserve**—the amount of air, beyond tidal volume, that can be expelled with the most forceful exhalation. Normal expiratory reserve ranges from 1000 to 1500 mL.
5. **Vital capacity**—the sum of tidal volume, inspiratory reserve, and expiratory reserve. Stated another way,

Box 15–5 | THE HEIMLICH MANEUVER

The **Heimlich maneuver** has received much well-deserved publicity, and indeed it is a life-saving technique.

If a person is choking on a foreign object (such as food) lodged in the pharynx or larynx, the air in the lungs may be utilized to remove the object. The physiology of this technique is illustrated in Box Fig. 15–C.

The person performing the maneuver stands behind the choking victim and puts both arms around the victim's waist. One hand forms a fist that is placed between the victim's navel and rib cage (below the diaphragm), and the other hand covers the fist. It is important to place hands correctly, in order to avoid breaking the victim's ribs. With both hands, a quick, forceful upward thrust is made and repeated if necessary. This forces the diaphragm upward to compress the lungs and force air out. The forcefully expelled air is often sufficient to dislodge the foreign object.

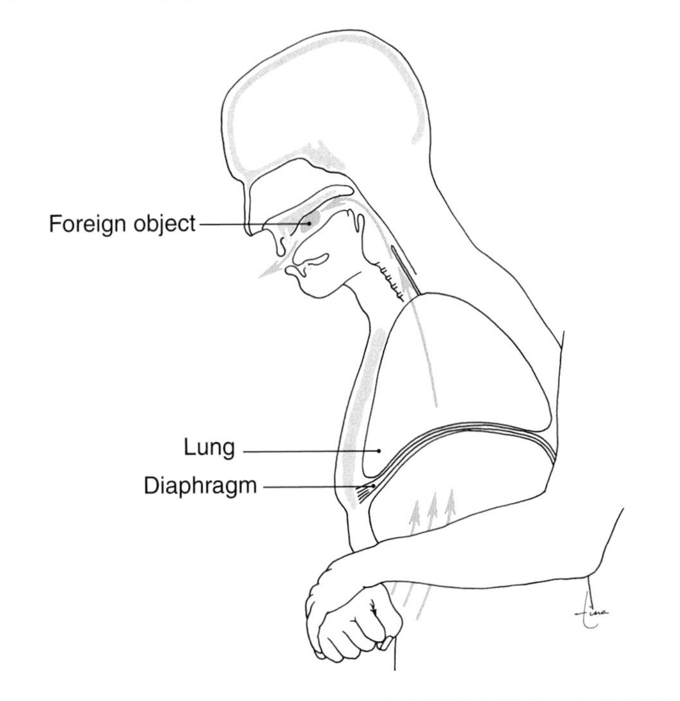

Box Figure 15–C The Heimlich maneuver.

vital capacity is the amount of air involved in the deepest inhalation followed by the most forceful exhalation. Average range of vital capacity is 3500 to 5000 mL.

6. **Residual air (volume)**—the amount of air that remains in the lungs after the most forceful exhalation; the average range is 1000 to 1500 mL. Residual air is important to ensure that there is some air in the lungs at all times, so that exchange of gases is a continuous process, even between breaths.

Some of the volumes just described can be determined with instruments called spirometers, which measure movement of air. Trained singers and musicians who play wind instruments often have vital capacities much larger than would be expected for their height and age because their respiratory muscles have become more efficient with "practice." The same is true for athletes who exercise regularly. A person with emphysema, however, must "work" to exhale, and vital capacity and expiratory reserve volume are often much lower than average.

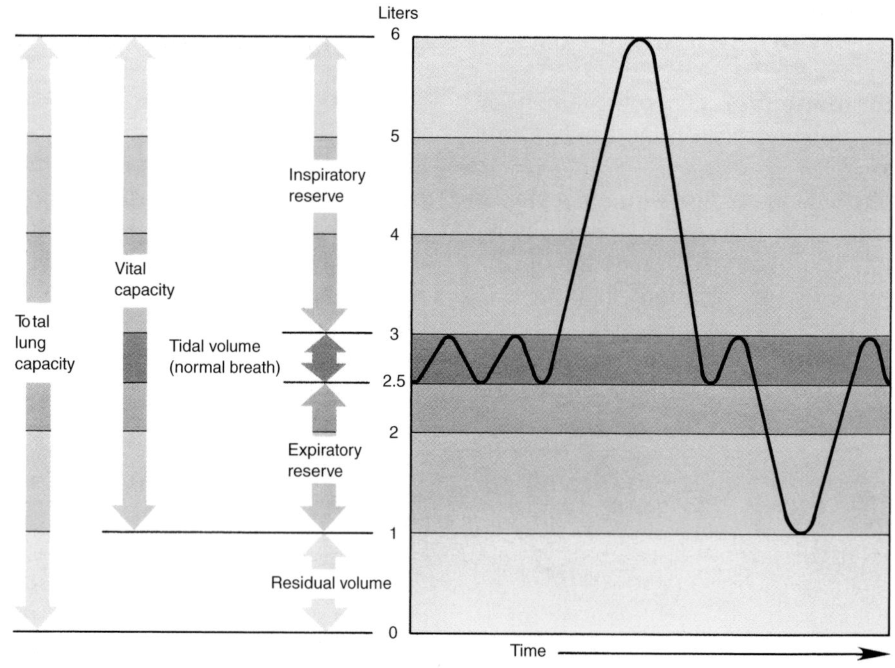

Figure 15–7 Pulmonary volumes. See text for description.

QUESTION: Which volumes make up vital capacity? Which volume cannot be measured with a spirometer?

A related volume, and one that may be measured as part of a diagnosis for emphysema, is **forced expiratory volume** (FEV). The name tells us how FEV is measured: After a deep inhalation, the person exhales as rapidly and forcefully as possible and the volume is determined at 1, 2, and 3 seconds (FEV_1 or FEV_2, for example). Any widespread damage to alveoli will decrease the FEV.

A different kind of pulmonary volume is **alveolar ventilation**, which is the amount of air that actually reaches the alveoli and participates in gas exchange. An average tidal volume is 500 mL, of which 350 to 400 mL is in the alveoli at the end of an inhalation. The remaining 100 to 150 mL of air is **anatomic dead space**, the air still within the respiratory passages. Despite its rather grim name, anatomic dead space is normal; everyone has it.

Physiological dead space is not normal and is the volume of non-functioning alveoli that decrease gas exchange. Causes of increased physiological dead space include bronchitis, pneumonia, tuberculosis, emphysema, asthma, pulmonary edema, and a collapsed lung.

The **compliance** of the thoracic wall and the lungs, that is, their normal expansibility, is necessary for sufficient alveolar ventilation. Thoracic compliance (expansion of the thoracic cavity) may be decreased by pleurisy or fractured ribs, which make inhalation painful, or by scoliosis or ascites, which obstruct the normal contraction of the respiratory muscles. Lung compliance, the natural expansibility of healthy air-filled lungs, will be decreased by any condition that increases physiological dead space. Normal compliance thus ensures that the expansion of the lungs will be sufficient to promote the necessary gas exchange in the alveoli.

EXCHANGE OF GASES

There are two sites of exchange of oxygen and carbon dioxide: the lungs and the tissues of the body. The exchange of gases between the air in the alveoli and the blood in the pulmonary capillaries is called **external respiration**. This term may be a bit confusing at first because we often think of "external" as being outside the body. In this case, however, "external" means the exchange that involves air from the external environment, though the exchange takes place within the lungs. **Internal respiration** is the exchange of gases between the blood in the systemic capillaries and the tissue fluid (cells) of the body.

The air we inhale (the earth's atmosphere) is approximately 21% oxygen and 0.04% carbon dioxide. Although most (78%) of the atmosphere is nitrogen, this gas is not physiologically available to us, and we simply exhale it. This exhaled air also contains about 16% oxygen and 4.5% carbon dioxide, so it is apparent that some oxygen is retained within the body and the carbon dioxide produced by cells is exhaled.

DIFFUSION OF GASES—PARTIAL PRESSURES

Within the body, a gas will diffuse from an area of greater concentration to an area of lesser concentration. The concentration of each gas in a particular site (alveolar air, pulmonary blood, and so on) is expressed in a value called **partial pressure**. The partial pressure of a gas, measured in mm Hg, is the pressure it exerts within a mixture of gases, whether the mixture is actually in a gaseous state or is in a liquid such as blood. The partial pressures of oxygen and carbon dioxide in the atmosphere and in the sites of exchange in the body are listed in Table 15–1. The abbreviation for partial pressure is "P," which is used, for example, on hospital lab slips for blood gases and will be used here.

The partial pressures of oxygen and carbon dioxide at the sites of external respiration (lungs) and internal respiration (body) are shown in Fig. 15–8. Because partial pressure reflects concentration, a gas will diffuse from an area of higher partial pressure to an area of lower partial pressure.

The air in the alveoli has a high PO_2 and a low PCO_2. The blood in the pulmonary capillaries, which has just come from the body, has a low PO_2 and a high PCO_2. Therefore, in external respiration, oxygen diffuses from the air in the alveoli to the blood, and carbon dioxide diffuses from the blood to the air in the alveoli. The blood that returns to the heart now has a high PO_2 and a low PCO_2 and is pumped by the left ventricle into systemic circulation.

The arterial blood that reaches systemic capillaries has a high PO_2 and a low PCO_2. The body cells and tissue fluid have a low PO_2 and a high PCO_2 because cells continuously use oxygen in cell respiration (energy production) and produce carbon dioxide in this process. Therefore, in internal respiration, oxygen diffuses from the blood to tissue fluid (cells), and carbon dioxide diffuses from tissue fluid to the blood. The blood that enters systemic veins to return to the heart now has a low PO_2 and a high PCO_2 and is pumped by the right ventricle to the lungs to participate in external respiration.

Disorders of gas exchange often involve the lungs, that is, external respiration (see Box 15–6: Pulmonary Edema and Box 15–7: Pneumonia).

Table 15–1 | PARTIAL PRESSURES AND OXYGEN SATURATION

SITE	PO_2 (mm Hg)	PCO_2 (mm Hg)	HEMOGLOBIN SATURATION (SaO_2)
Atmosphere	160	0.15	—
Alveolar air	104	40	—
Systemic venous blood (to pulmonary arteries)	40	45	70–75%
Systemic arterial blood (from pulmonary veins)	100	40	95–100%
Tissue fluid	40	50	—

Partial pressure is calculated as follows:
% of the gas in the mixture × total pressure = P_{GAS}
Example: **O_2 in the atmosphere**
21% × 760 mm Hg = 160 mm Hg (PO_2)
Example: **CO_2 in the atmosphere**
0.04% × 760 mm Hg = 0.15 mm Hg (PCO_2)
Notice that alveolar partial pressures are not exactly those of the atmosphere. Alveolar air contains significant amounts of water vapor and the CO_2 diffusing in from the blood. Oxygen also diffuses readily from the alveoli into the pulmonary capillaries. Therefore, alveolar PO_2 is lower than atmospheric PO_2, and alveolar PCO_2 is significantly higher than atmospheric PCO_2.

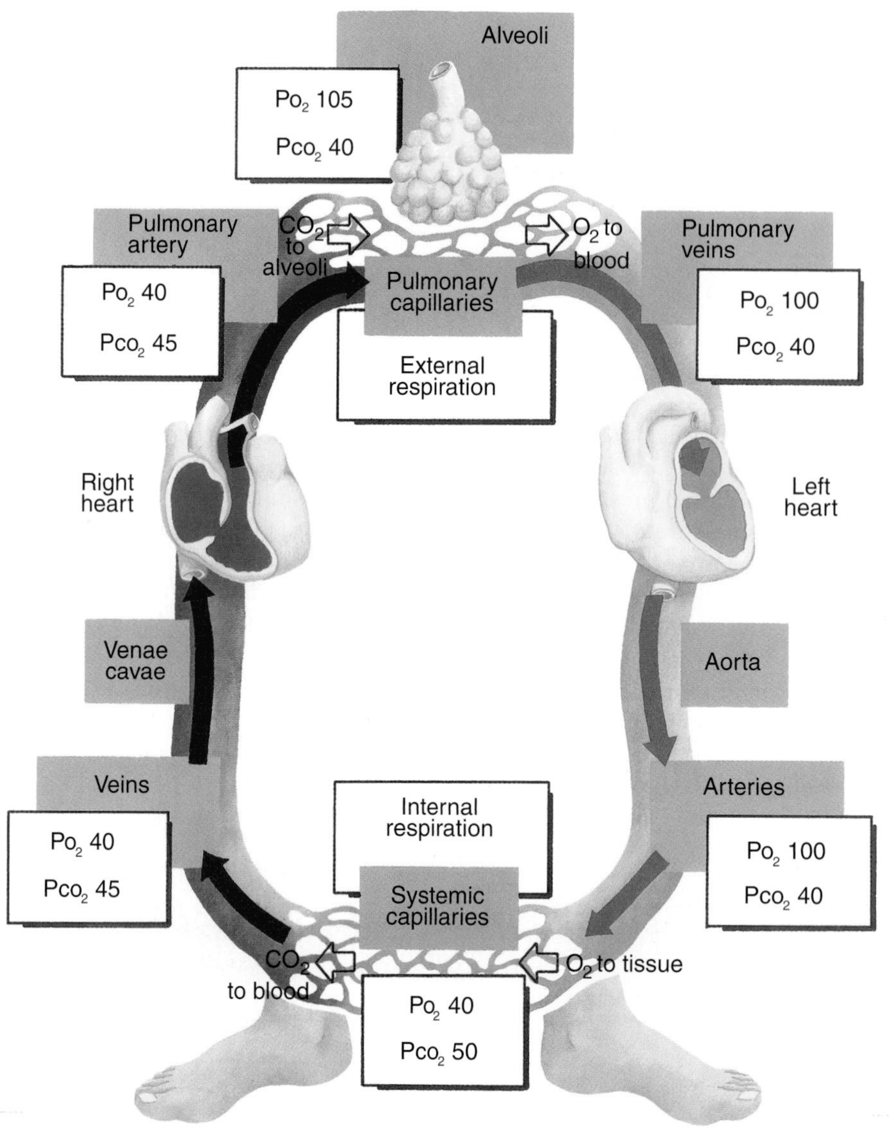

Figure 15–8 External respiration in the lungs and internal respiration in the body. The partial pressures of oxygen and carbon dioxide are shown at each site.

QUESTION: In external respiration, describe the movement of oxygen. In internal respiration, describe the movement of carbon dioxide.

TRANSPORT OF GASES IN THE BLOOD

Although some oxygen is dissolved in blood plasma and does create the Po_2 values, it is only about 1.5% of the total oxygen transported, not enough to sustain life. As you already know, most oxygen is carried in the blood bonded to the **hemoglobin** in red blood cells (RBCs). The mineral iron is part of hemoglobin and gives this protein its oxygen-carrying ability.

The oxygen–hemoglobin bond is formed in the lungs where Po_2 is high. This bond, however, is relatively unstable, and when blood passes through tissues with a low Po_2, the bond breaks and oxygen is released to the tissues. The lower the oxygen concentration in a tissue, the more oxygen

Box 15–6 | PULMONARY EDEMA

Pulmonary edema is the accumulation of fluid in the alveoli. This is often a consequence of congestive heart failure in which the left side of the heart (or the entire heart) is not pumping efficiently. If the left ventricle does not pump strongly, the chamber does not empty as it should and cannot receive all the blood flowing in from the left atrium. Blood flow, therefore, is "congested," and blood backs up in the pulmonary veins and then in the pulmonary capillaries. As blood pressure increases in the pulmonary capillaries, filtration creates tissue fluid that collects in the alveoli.

Fluid-filled alveoli are no longer sites of efficient gas exchange, and the resulting hypoxia leads to the symptoms of **dyspnea** and increased respiratory rate. The most effective treatment is that which restores the pumping ability of the heart to normal.

Box 15–7 | PNEUMONIA

Pneumonia is a bacterial infection of the lungs. Although many bacteria can cause pneumonia, the most common one is probably *Streptococcus pneumoniae*. This species is estimated to cause at least 500,000 cases of pneumonia every year in the United States, with 50,000 deaths.

S. pneumoniae is a transient inhabitant of the upper respiratory tract; it is not considered part of our beneficial microbiota, but for most of us, it is not a virulent pathogen. In otherwise healthy people, the ciliated epithelium and the immune system prevent infection. Most cases of pneumonia occur in elderly people following a primary infection such as influenza, or in the very young.

When the bacteria are able to establish themselves in the alveoli, the alveolar cells secrete fluid that accumulates in the air sacs. Many neutrophils migrate to the site of infection and attempt to phagocytize the bacteria. The alveoli become filled with fluid, bacteria, and neutrophils (this is called consolidation); this decreases the exchange of gases.

Pneumovax is a vaccine for this type of pneumonia. It contains only the capsules of the most common types of *S. pneumoniae* and cannot cause the disease (the bacterial capsules are nontoxic, but antigenic, meaning they stimulate antibody production). The vaccine is recommended for people older than the age of 60 years and for those with chronic pulmonary disorders or any debilitating disease. It is also recommended for infants.

the hemoglobin will release. This ensures that active tissues, such as exercising muscles, receive as much oxygen as possible to continue cell respiration. Other factors that increase the release of oxygen from hemoglobin are a high Pco_2 (actually a lower pH) and a high temperature, both of which are also characteristic of active tissues.

Another measure of blood oxygen is the percent of oxygen saturation of hemoglobin (Sao_2). The higher the Po_2, the higher the Sao_2, and as Po_2 decreases, so does Sao_2, though not as rapidly. A Po_2 of 100 is an Sao_2 of about 97%, as is found in systemic arteries. A Po_2 of 40, as is found in systemic veins, is an Sao_2 of about 75%. Notice that venous blood still has quite a bit of oxygen. Had this blood flowed through a very active tissue, more of its oxygen would have been released from hemoglobin. This venous reserve of oxygen provides active tissues with the oxygen they need (see also Box 15–8: Carbon Monoxide).

Carbon dioxide transport is a little more complicated. Some carbon dioxide is dissolved in the plasma, and some is carried by hemoglobin (**carbaminohemoglobin**), but these account for only about 20% of total CO_2 transport. Most carbon dioxide is carried in the plasma in the form of bicarbonate ions (HCO_3^-). Let us look at the reactions that transform CO_2 into a bicarbonate ion.

When carbon dioxide enters the blood, most diffuses into red blood cells, which contain the enzyme **carbonic anhydrase**. This enzyme (which contains zinc) catalyzes

Box 15–8 | CARBON MONOXIDE

Carbon monoxide (CO) is a colorless, odorless gas that is produced during the combustion of fuels such as gasoline, coal, oil, and wood. As you know, CO is a poison that may cause death if inhaled in more than very small quantities or for more than a short period of time.

The reason CO is so toxic is that it forms a very strong and stable bond with the hemoglobin in RBCs (**carboxyhemoglobin**). Hemoglobin with CO bonded to it cannot bond to and transport oxygen. The effect of CO, therefore, is to drastically decrease the amount of oxygen carried in the blood. As little as 0.1% CO in inhaled air can saturate half the total hemoglobin with CO.

Lack of oxygen is often apparent in people with light skin as **cyanosis**, a bluish cast to the skin, lips, and nail beds. This is because hemoglobin is dark red unless something (usually oxygen) is bonded to it. When hemoglobin bonds to CO, however, it becomes a bright, cherry red. This color may be seen in light skin and may be very misleading; the person with CO poisoning is in a severely hypoxic state. The most frequent symptoms of carbon monoxide poisoning are headache and dizziness. Shortness of breath, confusion, and nausea may also be present. The heart may be damaged because CO bonds to the myoglobin that stores oxygen in cardiac muscle cells and interferes with the functioning of mitochondria, diminishing ATP production.

Although CO is found in cigarette smoke, it is present in such minute quantities that it is not lethal. Heavy smokers, however, may be in a mild but chronic hypoxic state because much of their hemoglobin is firmly bonded to CO. As a compensation, RBC production may increase, and a heavy smoker may have a hematocrit over 50%.

Treatment of severe CO poisoning may require use of a hyperbaric chamber in which a person breathes oxygen under pressure. Other conditions for which hyperbaric therapy may be helpful include burns, bone infections, gangrene in any tissue, and severe anemia.

the reaction of carbon dioxide and water to form carbonic acid:

$$CO_2 + H_2O \rightarrow H_2CO_3$$

The carbonic acid then dissociates:

$$H_2CO_3 \rightarrow H^+ + HCO_3^-$$

The bicarbonate ions diffuse out of the red blood cells into the plasma, leaving the hydrogen ions (H^+) in the red blood cells. The many H^+ ions would tend to make the red blood cells too acidic, but hemoglobin acts as a buffer to prevent acidosis. To maintain an ionic equilibrium, chloride ions (Cl^-) from the plasma enter the red blood cells; this is called the chloride shift. Where is the CO_2? It is in the plasma as part of HCO_3^- ions. When the blood reaches the lungs, an area of lower P_{CO_2}, these reactions are reversed, and CO_2 is re-formed and diffuses into the alveoli to be exhaled.

REGULATION OF RESPIRATION

Two types of mechanisms regulate breathing: nervous mechanisms and chemical mechanisms. Because any changes in the rate or depth of breathing are ultimately brought about by nerve impulses, we will consider nervous mechanisms first.

NERVOUS REGULATION

The respiratory centers are located in the **medulla** and **pons**, which are parts of the brain stem (see Fig. 15–9). Within the medulla are the inspiration center and expiration center.

The **inspiration center** automatically generates impulses in rhythmic spurts. These impulses travel along nerves to the respiratory muscles to stimulate their contraction. The result is inhalation. As the lungs inflate, baroreceptors in lung tissue detect this stretching and generate sensory impulses to the medulla; these impulses begin to depress the inspiration center. This is called the Hering-Breuer inflation reflex, which also helps prevent overinflation of the lungs.

As the inspiration center is depressed, the result is a decrease in impulses to the respiratory muscles, which relax to bring about exhalation. Then the inspiration center becomes active again to begin another cycle of breathing. When there is a need for more forceful exhalations, such

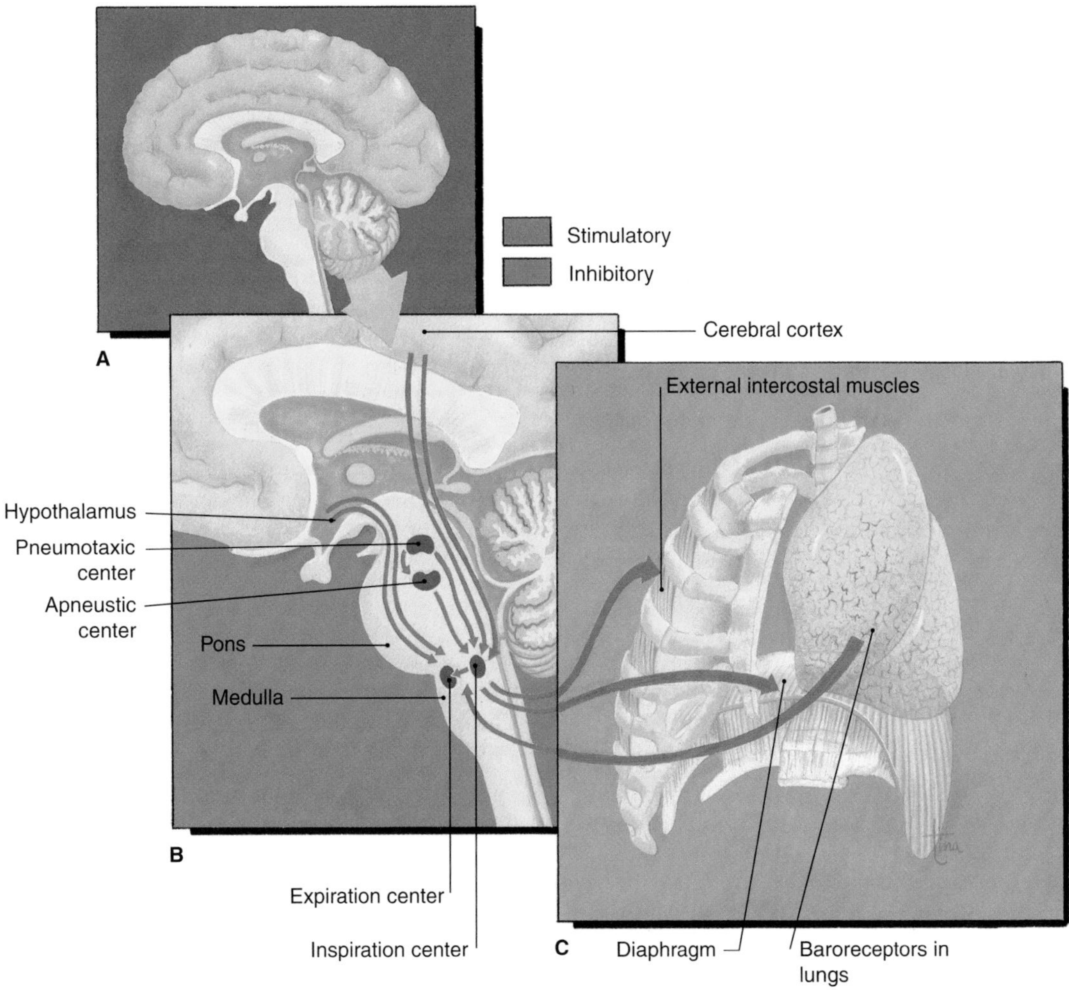

Figure 15–9 Nervous regulation of respiration. (**A**) Midsagittal section of brain. (**B**) Respiratory centers in medulla and pons. (**C**) Respiratory muscles. See text for description.

QUESTION: Which center directly stimulates inhalation? How can you tell from this picture?

as during exercise, the inspiration center activates the **expiration center**, which generates impulses to the internal intercostal and abdominal muscles.

The two respiratory centers in the pons work with the inspiration center to produce a normal rhythm of breathing. The **apneustic center** prolongs inhalation and is then interrupted by impulses from the **pneumotaxic center**, which contributes to exhalation. In normal breathing, inhalation lasts 1 to 2 seconds, followed by a slightly longer (2 to 3 seconds) exhalation, producing the normal respiratory rate range of 12 to 20 breaths per minute.

What has just been described is normal breathing, but variations are possible and quite common. Emotions often affect respiration; a sudden fright may bring about a gasp or a scream, and anger usually increases the respiratory rate. In these situations, impulses from the **hypothalamus** modify the output from the medulla. The **cerebral cortex** enables us to voluntarily change our breathing rate or rhythm to talk, sing, breathe faster or slower, or even to stop breathing for 1 or 2 minutes. Such changes cannot be continued indefinitely, however, and the medulla will eventually resume control.

Coughing and **sneezing** are reflexes that remove irritants from the respiratory passages; the medulla contains the centers for both of these reflexes. Sneezing is stimulated by an irritation of the nasal mucosa, and coughing is stimulated by irritation of the mucosa of the pharynx, larynx, or trachea. The reflex action is essentially the same for both: An inhalation is followed by exhalation beginning with the glottis closed to build up pressure. Then the glottis opens suddenly, and the exhalation is explosive. A cough directs the exhalation out the mouth, while a sneeze directs the exhalation out the nose. Some people sneeze upon exposure to bright light such as sunlight. This is called photic sneezing and is genetic. It is an autosomal dominant trait; expression of the trait requires only one gene, maternal or paternal (it is believed to be caused by misrouted sneeze-reflex neurons and light-detecting neurons and does not seem to have a useful purpose).

Hiccups, also a reflex, are spasms of the diaphragm. The result is a quick inhalation that is stopped when the glottis snaps shut, causing the "hic" sound. The stimulus may be irritation of the phrenic nerves or nerves of the stomach. Excessive alcohol is an irritant that can cause hiccups. Some causes are simply unknown.

Yet another respiratory reflex is yawning. Many of us yawn when we are tired, but the stimulus for and purpose of yawning are not known with certainty. One possible stimulus is an accumulation of carbon dioxide, such as may happen when we are bored or sleepy and breathing becomes shallow. But evidence now suggests that yawning helps keep the brain cool by shunting warm blood away from the brain and to the face, where the heat is closer to the body surface and can be lost. This would be advantageous because a cooler brain is a more alert brain. Research is continuing. Also not known at present is why yawning is contagious, but seeing someone yawn is almost sure to elicit a yawn of one's own. You may even have yawned while reading this paragraph about yawning.

CHEMICAL REGULATION

Chemical regulation refers to the effect on breathing of blood pH and blood levels of oxygen and carbon dioxide. This is shown in Fig. 15–10. **Chemoreceptors** that detect changes in blood gases and pH are located in the carotid and aortic bodies and in the medulla itself.

A decrease in the blood level of oxygen (hypoxemia) is detected by the chemoreceptors in the **carotid** and **aortic bodies**. The sensory impulses generated by these receptors travel along the glossopharyngeal and vagus nerves to the medulla, which responds by increasing respiratory rate or depth (or both). This response will bring more air into the lungs so that more oxygen can diffuse into the blood to correct the hypoxic state.

Carbon dioxide becomes a problem when it is present in excess in the blood, because excess CO_2 (**hypercapnia**) lowers the pH when it reacts with water to form carbonic acid (a source of H^+ ions). That is, excess CO_2 makes the blood or other body fluids less alkaline (or more acidic). The **medulla** contains **chemoreceptors** that are very sensitive to changes in pH, especially decreases. If accumulating CO_2 lowers blood pH, the medulla responds by increasing respiration. This is not for the purpose of inhaling, but rather to exhale more CO_2 to raise the pH back to normal.

Of the two respiratory gases, which is the more important as a regulator of respiration? Our guess might be oxygen, because it is essential for energy production in cell respiration. However, the respiratory system can maintain a normal blood level of oxygen even if breathing decreases

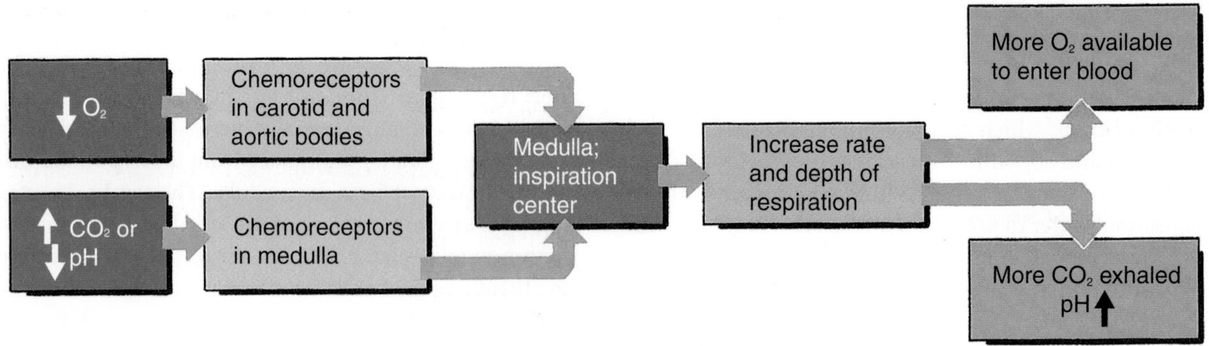

Figure 15–10 Chemical regulation of respiration. See text for description.

QUESTION: The body's response to two very different changes (less O_2 or more CO_2) is the same. Explain why.

to half the normal rate or stops for a few moments. Recall that exhaled air is 16% oxygen. This oxygen did not enter the blood but was available to do so if needed. Also, the residual air in the lungs supplies oxygen to the blood even if breathing rate slows.

Therefore, carbon dioxide must be the major regulator of respiration, and the reason is that carbon dioxide affects the pH of the blood. As was just mentioned, an excess of CO_2 causes the blood pH to decrease, a process that must not be allowed to continue. Therefore, any increase in the blood CO_2 level is quickly compensated for by increased breathing to exhale more CO_2. If, for example, you hold your breath, what is it that makes you breathe again? Have you run out of oxygen? Probably not, for the reasons mentioned. What has happened is that accumulating CO_2 has lowered blood pH enough to stimulate the medulla to start the breathing cycle again.

In some situations, oxygen does become the major regulator of respiration. People with severe, chronic pulmonary diseases such as emphysema have decreased exchange of both oxygen and carbon dioxide in the lungs. The decrease in pH caused by accumulating CO_2 is corrected by the kidneys, but the blood oxygen level keeps decreasing. Eventually, the oxygen level may fall so low that it does provide a very strong stimulus to increase the rate and depth of respiration.

RESPIRATION AND ACID–BASE BALANCE

As you have just seen, respiration affects the pH of body fluids because it regulates the amount of carbon dioxide in these fluids. Remember that CO_2 reacts with water to form carbonic acid (H_2CO_3), which ionizes into H^+ ions and HCO_3^- ions. The more hydrogen ions present in a body fluid, the lower the pH, and the fewer hydrogen ions present, the higher the pH.

The respiratory system may be the cause of a pH imbalance, or it may help correct a pH imbalance created by some other cause.

RESPIRATORY ACIDOSIS AND ALKALOSIS

Respiratory acidosis occurs when the rate or efficiency of respiration decreases, permitting carbon dioxide to accumulate in body fluids. The excess CO_2 results in the formation of more H^+ ions, which decrease the pH. Holding one's breath can bring about a mild respiratory acidosis, which will soon stimulate the medulla to initiate breathing again. More serious causes of respiratory acidosis are pulmonary diseases such as pneumonia and emphysema, or severe asthma. Each of these impairs gas exchange and allows excess CO_2 to remain in body fluids.

Respiratory alkalosis occurs when the rate of respiration increases, and CO_2 is very rapidly exhaled. Less CO_2 decreases H^+ ion formation, which increases the pH. Breathing faster for a few minutes can bring about a mild state of respiratory alkalosis. Babies who cry for extended periods (crying is a noisy exhalation) put themselves in this condition. In general, however, respiratory alkalosis is not a common occurrence. Severe physical trauma and shock, or certain states of mental or emotional anxiety, may be accompanied by hyperventilation and also result in respiratory alkalosis. In addition, traveling to a higher altitude (less oxygen in the atmosphere) may cause a temporary increase in breathing rate before compensation occurs (increased rate of RBC production—see Chapter 11).

RESPIRATORY COMPENSATION

If a pH imbalance is caused by something other than a change in respiration, it is called metabolic acidosis or alkalosis. In either case, the change in pH stimulates a change in respiration that may help restore the pH of body fluids to normal.

Metabolic acidosis may be caused by untreated diabetes mellitus (ketoacidosis), kidney disease, or severe diarrhea. In such situations, the H^+ ion concentration of body fluids is increased. Respiratory compensation involves an increase in the rate and depth of respiration to exhale more CO_2 to decrease H^+ ion formation, which will raise the pH toward the normal range.

Metabolic alkalosis is not a common occurrence but may be caused by ingestion of excessive amounts of alkaline medications such as those used to relieve gastric disturbances. Another possible cause is vomiting of stomach contents only. In such situations, the H^+ ion concentration of body fluids is decreased. Respiratory compensation involves a decrease in respiration to retain CO_2 in the body to increase H^+ ion formation, which will lower the pH toward the normal range.

Respiratory compensation for an ongoing metabolic pH imbalance cannot be complete, because there are limits to the amounts of CO_2 that may be exhaled or retained. At most, respiratory compensation is only about 75% effective. A complete discussion of acid–base balance is found in Chapter 19.

AGING AND THE RESPIRATORY SYSTEM

Perhaps the most important way to help your respiratory system age gracefully is not to smoke. In the absence of chemical assault, respiratory function does diminish but usually remains adequate. The respiratory muscles, like all skeletal muscles, weaken with age (exercise, even if only brisk walking, helps maintain the strength of the respiratory muscles). Lung tissue loses its elasticity and alveoli are lost as their walls deteriorate. All of this results in decreased ventilation and lung capacity, but the remaining capacity is usually sufficient for ordinary activities. The cilia of the respiratory mucosa deteriorate with age, and the alveolar macrophages are not as efficient, which make elderly people more prone to pneumonia, a serious pulmonary infection.

Chronic alveolar hypoxia from diseases such as emphysema or chronic bronchitis may lead to pulmonary hypertension, which in turn overworks the right ventricle of the heart. Systemic hypertension often weakens the left ventricle of the heart, leading to congestive heart failure and pulmonary edema, in which excess tissue fluid collects in the alveoli and decreases gas exchange. Though true at any age, the interdependence of the respiratory and circulatory systems is particularly apparent in elderly people.

SUMMARY

As you have learned, respiration is much more than the simple mechanical actions of breathing. Inhalation provides the body with the oxygen that is necessary for the production of ATP in the process of cell respiration. Exhalation removes the CO_2 that is a product of cell respiration. Breathing also regulates the level of CO_2 within the body, and this contributes to the maintenance of the acid–base balance of body fluids. Although the respiratory gases do not form structural components of the body, their contributions to the chemical level of organization are essential to the functioning of the body at every level.

STUDY OUTLINE

The respiratory system moves air into and out of the lungs, the site of exchange for O_2 and CO_2 between the air and the blood. The functioning of the respiratory system depends directly on the proper functioning of the circulatory system.

1. The upper respiratory tract consists of those parts outside the chest cavity.
2. The lower respiratory tract consists of those parts within the chest cavity.

Nose—made of bone and cartilage covered with skin

1. Hairs inside the nostrils block the entry of dust.

Nasal Cavities—within the skull; separated by the nasal septum (see Fig. 15–1)

1. Nasal mucosa is ciliated epithelium with goblet cells; surface area is increased by the conchae.
2. Nasal mucosa warms and moistens the incoming air; dust and microorganisms are trapped on mucus and swept by the cilia to the pharynx.
3. Olfactory receptors respond to vapors in inhaled air.
4. Paranasal sinuses in the maxillae, frontal, sphenoid, and ethmoid bones open into the nasal cavities: functions are to lighten the skull and provide resonance for the voice.

Pharynx—posterior to nasal and oral cavities (see Fig. 15–1)

1. Nasopharynx—above the level of the soft palate, which blocks it during swallowing; a passageway for air only. The eustachian tubes from the middle ears open into it. The adenoid is a lymph nodule on the posterior wall.
2. Oropharynx—behind the mouth; a passageway for both air and food. Palatine tonsils are on the lateral walls.
3. Laryngopharynx—a passageway for both air and food; opens anteriorly into the larynx and posteriorly into the esophagus.

Larynx—the voice box and the airway between the pharynx and trachea (see Fig. 15–2)

1. Made of nine cartilages; the thyroid cartilage is the largest and most anterior.
2. The epiglottis is the uppermost cartilage; covers the larynx during swallowing.
3. The vocal cords are lateral to the glottis, the opening for air (see Fig. 15–3).
4. During speaking, the vocal cords are pulled across the glottis and vibrated by exhaled air, producing sounds that may be turned into speech.
5. The cranial nerves for speaking are the vagus and accessory.

Trachea—extends from the larynx to the primary bronchi (see Fig. 15–4)

1. Sixteen to 20 C-shaped cartilages in the tracheal wall keep the trachea open.
2. Mucosa is ciliated epithelium with goblet cells; cilia sweep mucus, trapped dust, and microorganisms upward to the pharynx.

Bronchial Tree—extends from the trachea to the alveoli (see Fig. 15–4)

1. The right and left primary bronchi are branches of the trachea; one to each lung; same structure as the trachea.
2. Secondary bronchi: to the lobes of each lung (three right, two left)
3. Bronchioles—no cartilage in their walls.

Lungs—on either side of the heart in the chest cavity; extend from the diaphragm below up to the level of the clavicles

1. The rib cage protects the lungs from mechanical injury.
2. Hilus—indentation on the medial side: primary bronchus and pulmonary artery and veins enter (also bronchial vessels).

Pleural Membranes—serous membranes of the thoracic cavity

1. Parietal pleura lines the chest wall.
2. Visceral pleura covers the lungs.
3. Serous fluid between the two layers prevents friction and keeps the membranes together during breathing.

Alveoli—sites of gas exchange in the lungs

1. Made of alveolar type I cells, simple squamous epithelium; thin to permit diffusion of gases.
2. Surrounded by pulmonary capillaries, which are also made of simple squamous epithelium (see Fig. 15–4); pulmonary arterioles constrict in response to the hypoxia of poorly ventilated alveoli; blood is shunted to better-ventilated alveoli.
3. Elastic connective tissue between alveoli is important for normal exhalation.
4. A thin layer of tissue fluid lines each alveolus; essential to permit diffusion of gases (see Fig. 15–5).
5. Alveolar type II cells produce pulmonary surfactant that mixes with the tissue fluid lining to decrease surface tension to permit inflation of the alveoli.
6. Alveolar macrophages phagocytize foreign material.

Mechanism of Breathing

1. Ventilation is the movement of air into and out of the lungs: inhalation and exhalation.
2. Respiratory centers are in the medulla and pons.
3. Respiratory muscles are the diaphragm and external and internal intercostal muscles (see Fig. 15–6).
   a. Atmospheric pressure is air pressure: 760 mm Hg at sea level.
   b. Intrapleural pressure is within the potential pleural space; always slightly below atmospheric pressure ("negative").
   c. Intrapulmonic pressure is within the bronchial tree and alveoli; fluctuates during breathing.

Inhalation (inspiration)

1. Motor impulses from medulla travel along phrenic nerves to diaphragm, which contracts and moves down. Impulses are sent along intercostal nerves to external intercostal muscles, which pull ribs up and out.
2. The chest cavity is expanded and expands the parietal pleura.
3. The visceral pleura adheres to the parietal pleura and is also expanded and in turn expands the lungs.
4. Intrapulmonic pressure decreases, and air rushes into the lungs.

Exhalation (expiration)

1. Motor impulses from the medulla decrease, and the diaphragm and external intercostal muscles relax.
2. The chest cavity becomes smaller and compresses the lungs.

3. The elastic lungs recoil and further compress the alveoli.
4. Intrapulmonic pressure increases, and air is forced out of the lungs. Normal exhalation is passive.
5. Forced exhalation: contraction of the internal intercostal muscles pulls the ribs down and in; contraction of the abdominal muscles forces the diaphragm upward.

Pulmonary Volumes (see Fig. 15–7)

1. Tidal volume—the amount of air in one normal inhalation and exhalation.
2. Minute respiratory volume—the amount of air inhaled and exhaled in 1 minute.
3. Inspiratory reserve—the amount of air beyond tidal in a maximal inhalation.
4. Expiratory reserve—the amount of air beyond tidal in the most forceful exhalation.
5. Vital capacity—the sum of tidal volume, inspiratory and expiratory reserves.
6. Residual air—the amount of air that remains in the lungs after the most forceful exhalation; provides for continuous exchange of gases.
7. Forced expiratory volume—the maximum amount of air that can be exhaled in 1, 2, or 3 seconds.
8. Alveolar ventilation—air that reaches the alveoli for gas exchange; depends on normal thoracic and lung compliance.
   a. Anatomic dead space—air still in the respiratory passages at the end of inhalation (is normal).
   b. Physiological dead space—the volume of nonfunctional alveoli; decreases compliance (the expansibility of the lungs) and thus decreases gas exchange.

Exchange of Gases

1. External respiration is the exchange of gases between the air in the alveoli and the blood in the pulmonary capillaries.
2. Internal respiration is the exchange of gases between blood in the systemic capillaries and tissue fluid (cells).
3. Inhaled air (atmosphere) is 21% O_2 and 0.04% CO_2. Exhaled air is 16% O_2 and 4.5% CO_2.
4. Diffusion of O_2 and CO_2 in the body occurs because of pressure gradients (see Table 15–1). A gas will diffuse from an area of higher partial pressure to an area of lower partial pressure.
5. External respiration: in the lungs
   a. Po_2 in the alveoli is high, and Po_2 in the pulmonary capillaries is low, so O_2 diffuses from the air to the blood.
   b. Pco_2 in the alveoli is low, and Pco_2 in the pulmonary capillaries is high, so CO_2 diffuses from the blood to the air and is exhaled (see Fig. 15–8).
6. Internal respiration: in the tissues
   a. Po_2 in the systemic capillaries is high, and Po_2 in the tissue fluid is low, so O_2 diffuses from the blood to the tissue fluid and cells.
   b. Pco_2 in the systemic capillaries is low, and Pco_2 in the tissue fluid is high, so CO_2 diffuses from the tissue fluid to the blood (see Fig. 15–8).

Transport of Gases in the Blood

1. Oxygen is carried by the iron of hemoglobin (Hb) in the RBCs. The O_2–Hb bond is formed in the lungs where the Po_2 is high.
2. In tissues, Hb releases much of its O_2; the important factors are low Po_2 in tissues, high Pco_2 in tissues, and a high temperature in tissues.
3. Oxygen saturation of hemoglobin (Sao_2) is 95% to 97% in systemic arteries and averages 70% to 75% in systemic veins.
4. Most CO_2 is carried as HCO_3^- ions in blood plasma. CO_2 enters the RBCs and reacts with H_2O to form carbonic acid (H_2CO_3). Carbonic anhydrase is the enzyme that catalyzes this reaction. H_2CO_3 dissociates to H^+ ions and HCO_3^- ions. The HCO_3^- ions leave the RBCs and enter the plasma; Hb buffers the H^+ ions that remain in the RBCs. Cl^- ions from the plasma enter the RBCs to maintain ionic equilibrium (the chloride shift).
5. When blood reaches the lungs, CO_2 is re-formed, diffuses into the alveoli, and is exhaled.

Nervous Regulation of Respiration (see Fig. 15–9)

1. The medulla contains the inspiration center and expiration center.
2. Impulses from the inspiration center to the respiratory muscles cause their contraction; the chest cavity is expanded.
3. Baroreceptors in lung tissue detect stretching and send impulses to the medulla to depress the inspiration center. This is the Hering-Breuer inflation reflex, which also prevents overinflation of the lungs.
4. The expiration center is stimulated by the inspiration center when forceful exhalations are needed.
5. In the pons: the apneustic center prolongs inhalation, and the pneumotaxic center helps bring about exhalation. These centers work with the inspiration center in the medulla to produce a normal breathing rhythm.
6. The hypothalamus influences changes in breathing in emotional situations. The cerebral cortex permits voluntary changes in breathing.
7. Coughing and sneezing remove irritants from the upper respiratory tract; the centers for these reflexes are in the medulla.

Chemical Regulation of Respiration (see Fig. 15–10)

1. Decreased blood O_2 is detected by chemoreceptors in the carotid body and aortic body. Response: increased respiration to take more air into the lungs.
2. Increased blood CO_2 level is detected by chemoreceptors in the medulla. Response: increased respiration to exhale more CO_2.
3. CO_2 is the major regulator of respiration because excess CO_2 decreases the pH of body fluids ($CO_2 + H_2O \rightarrow H_2CO_3 \rightarrow H^+ + HCO_3^-$). Excess H^+ ions lower pH.
4. Oxygen becomes a major regulator of respiration when blood level is very low, as may occur with severe, chronic pulmonary disease.

Respiration and Acid–Base Balance

1. Respiratory acidosis: a decrease in the rate or efficiency of respiration permits excess CO_2 to accumulate in body fluids, resulting in the formation of excess H^+ ions, which lower pH. Occurs in severe pulmonary disease.
2. Respiratory alkalosis: an increase in the rate of respiration increases the CO_2 exhaled, which decreases the formation of H^+ ions and raises pH. Occurs during hyperventilation or when first at a high altitude.
3. Respiratory compensation for metabolic acidosis: increased respiration to exhale CO_2 to decrease H^+ ion formation to raise pH to normal.
4. Respiratory compensation for metabolic alkalosis: decreased respiration to retain CO_2 to increase H^+ ion formation to lower pH to normal.

REVIEW QUESTIONS

1. State the three functions of the nasal mucosa. (p. 383)
2. Name the three parts of the pharynx; state whether each is an air passage only or an air and food passage. (p. 383)
3. Name the tissue that lines the larynx and trachea, and describe its function. State the function of the cartilage of the larynx and trachea. (pp. 383, 385)
4. Name the pleural membranes, state the location of each, and describe the functions of serous fluid. (p. 386)
5. Name the tissue of which the alveoli and pulmonary capillaries are made, and explain the importance of this tissue in these locations. Explain the function of pulmonary surfactant. (p. 388)
6. Name the respiratory muscles, and describe how they are involved in normal inhalation and exhalation. Define these pressures and relate them to a cycle of breathing: atmospheric pressure, intrapulmonic pressure. (pp. 388, 390–391)
7. Describe external respiration in terms of partial pressures of oxygen and carbon dioxide. (p. 395)

8. Describe internal respiration in terms of partial pressures of oxygen and carbon dioxide. (p. 395)
9. Name the cell, protein, and mineral that transport oxygen in the blood. State the three factors that increase the release of oxygen in tissues. (pp. 396–397)
10. Most carbon dioxide is transported in what part of the blood, and in what form? Explain the function of hemoglobin with respect to carbon dioxide transport. (p.397)
11. Name the respiratory centers in the medulla and pons, and explain how each is involved in a breathing cycle. (pp. 398–399)
12. State the location of chemoreceptors affected by a low blood oxygen level; describe the body's response to hypoxia and its purpose. State the location of chemoreceptors affected by a high blood CO_2 level; describe the body's response and its purpose. (p. 400)
13. For respiratory acidosis and alkalosis: state a cause and explain what happens to the pH of body fluids. (p. 401)
14. Explain how the respiratory system may compensate for metabolic acidosis or alkalosis. For an ongoing pH imbalance, what is the limit of respiratory compensation? (p. 401)

FOR FURTHER THOUGHT

1. The success of an organ transplant depends on many factors. What unavoidable factor would diminish the chance of success of a lung transplant but is not a factor at all in a heart transplant?
2. As recently as 50 years ago (the early 1960s) it was believed that mouth-to-mouth resuscitation was not really helpful to another person. What mistaken belief about the air we exhale contributed to that thinking, and what are the facts?
3. You are making a list of vital organs, organs we cannot live without. Should you include the larynx on your list? Explain why or why not.
4. At a construction site, a hole caved in and buried a workman up to his shoulders in wet sand. The supervisor told the trapped man that a crane would be there in 20 minutes to pull him out, but another worker said they couldn't wait, and had to dig *now*. The other worker was right. Why was this a life-threatening emergency?
5. A patient's blood pH is 7.34, and his respirations are 32 per minute. What acid–base situation is this patient in? State your reasoning step-by-step.

6. Mrs. D is in the emergency department because of severe abdominal pain that may be appendicitis. Her blood pH is 7.47 and her respirations are 34 per minute. What acid–base situation is Mrs. D in? State your reasoning step-by-step.

7. Look at Question Fig. 15–A. This is a transverse section through the neck, with the anterior at the top of the picture. If you put your hand just above your interclavicular notch (where your two clavicles meet your sternum), that is the site of the section. Name the indicated structures, and give reasons for your answers.

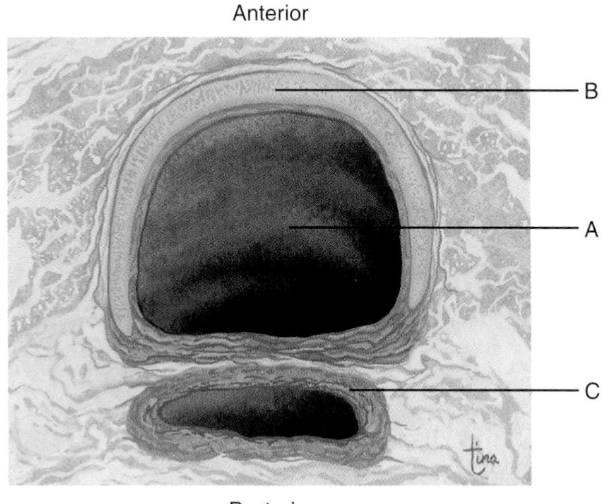

QUESTION FIGURE 15–A: A Transverse section of the base of the neck.

CHAPTER

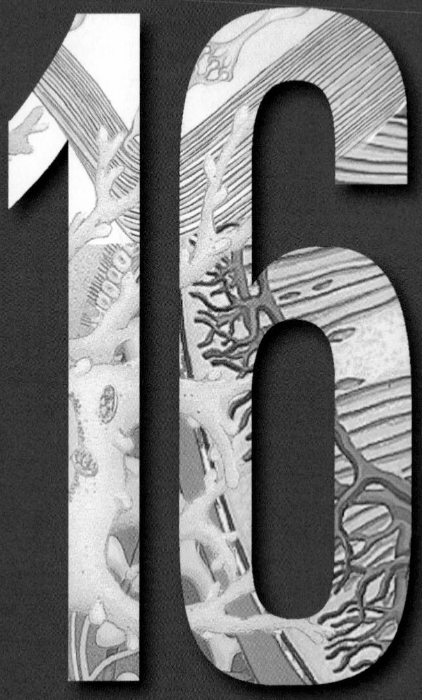

The Digestive System

STUDENT OBJECTIVES

- Describe the general functions of the digestive system, and name its major divisions.
- Explain the difference between mechanical and chemical digestion, and name the end products of digestion.
- Describe the structure and functions of the teeth and tongue.
- Explain the functions of saliva.
- Describe the location and functions of the pharynx and esophagus.
- Describe the structure and function of each of the four layers of the alimentary tube.
- Describe the location, structure, and function of the stomach, small intestine, liver, gallbladder, and pancreas.
- Describe absorption in the small intestine.
- Describe the location and functions of the large intestine.
- Explain the functions of the normal flora of the colon.
- Describe the functions of the liver.

NEW TERMINOLOGY

Alimentary tube *(AL-i-**MEN**-tah-ree TOOB)*
Chemical digestion *(**KEM**-i-kuhl dye-**JES**-chun)*
Common bile duct *(**KOM**-mon BYL DUKT)*
Defecation reflex *(DEF-e-**KAY**-shun)*
Duodenum *(dew-**AH**-den-um or DEW-oh-**DEE**-num)*
Emulsify *(e-**MULL**-si-fye)*
Enamel *(e-**NAM**-uhl)*
Essential amino acids *(e-**SEN**-shul ah-**ME**-noh **ASS**-ids)*
External anal sphincter *(eks-**TER**-nuhl **AY**-nuhl **SFINK**-ter)*
Ileocecal valve *(ILL-ee-oh-**SEE**-kuhl VALV)*
Internal anal sphincter *(in-**TER**-nuhl **AY**-nuhl **SFINK**-ter)*
Lower esophageal sphincter *(e-SOF-uh-**JEE**-uhl **SFINK**-ter)*
Mechanical digestion *(muh-**KAN**-i-kuhl dye-**JES**-chun)*
Non-essential amino acids *(NON-e-**SEN**-shul ah-**ME**-noh **ASS**-ids)*
Normal flora *(**NOR**-muhl **FLOOR**-ah)*
Periodontal membrane *(PER-ee-oh-**DON**-tal)*
Pyloric sphincter *(pye-**LOR**-ik **SFINK**-ter)*
Rugae *(**ROO**-gay)*
Villi *(**VILL**-eye)*

*Terms that appear in **bold type** in the chapter text are defined in the glossary, which begins on page 603.*

CHAPTER OUTLINE

RELATED CLINICAL TERMINOLOGY

Appendicitis *(uh-PEN-di-**SIGH**-tis)*
Dental caries *(**DEN**-tuhl **KAIR**-eez)*
Diverticulitis *(DYE-ver-TIK-yoo-**LYE**-tis)*
Gastric ulcer *(**GAS-trik UL**-ser)*
Hepatitis *(HEP-uh-**TIGH**-tis)*
Lactose intolerance *(**LAK**-tohs in-**TAHL**-er-ense)*
Lithotripsy *(LITH-oh-**TRIP**-see)*
Paralytic ileus *(**PAR**-uh-LIT-ik **ILL**-ee-us)*
Peritonitis *(per-i-toh-**NIGH**-tis)*
Pyloric stenosis *(pye-**LOR**-ik ste-**NOH**-sis)*

A hurried breakfast when you are late for work or school . . . Thanksgiving dinner . . . going on a diet to lose 5 pounds . . . what do these experiences all have in common? Food. We may take food for granted, celebrate with it, or wish we wouldn't eat quite so much of it. Although food is not as immediate a need for human beings as is oxygen, it is a very important part of our lives. Food provides the raw materials or nutrients that cells use to reproduce and to build new tissue. The energy needed for cell reproduction and tissue building is released from food in the process of cell respiration. In fact, a supply of nutrients from regular food intake is so important that the body can even store any excess for use later. Those "extra 5 pounds" are often stored fat in adipose tissue.

The food we eat, however, is not in a form that our body cells can use. A turkey sandwich, for example, consists of complex proteins, fats, and carbohydrates. The function of the **digestive system** is to change these complex organic nutrient molecules into simple organic and inorganic molecules that can then be absorbed into the blood or lymph to be transported to cells. In this chapter we will discuss the organs of digestion and the contribution each makes to digestion and absorption.

DIVISIONS OF THE DIGESTIVE SYSTEM

The two divisions of the digestive system are the alimentary tube and the accessory organs (Fig. 16–1). The **alimentary tube** extends from the mouth to the anus. It consists of the oral cavity, pharynx, esophagus, stomach, small intestine, and large intestine. Digestion takes place within the oral cavity, stomach, and small intestine; most absorption of nutrients takes place in the small intestine. Undigestible material, primarily cellulose, is eliminated by the large intestine (also called the colon).

The **accessory organs** of digestion are the teeth, tongue, salivary glands, liver, gallbladder, and pancreas. Digestion does not take place *within* these organs, but each contributes something *to* the digestive process.

TYPES OF DIGESTION

The food we eat is broken down in two complementary processes: mechanical digestion and chemical digestion. **Mechanical digestion** is the physical breaking up of food into smaller pieces. Chewing is an example of this. As food is broken up, more of its surface area is exposed for the action of digestive enzymes (enzymes

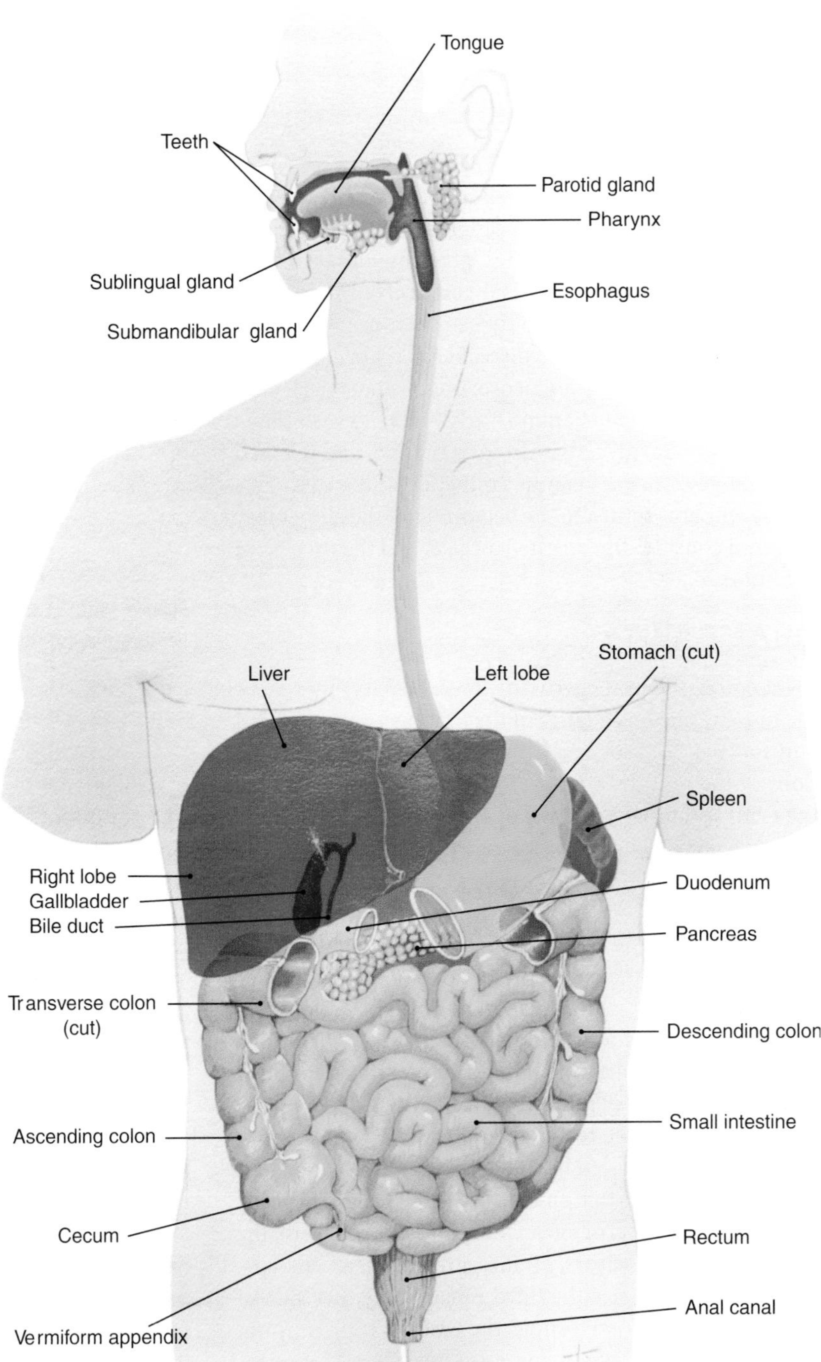

Figure 16–1 The digestive organs shown in anterior view of the trunk and left lateral view of the head. (The spleen is not a digestive organ but is included to show its location relative to the stomach, pancreas, and colon.)

QUESTION: In which parts of the digestive system does digestion actually take place?

are discussed in Chapter 2). The work of the digestive enzymes is the **chemical digestion** of broken-up food particles, in which complex chemical molecules are changed into much simpler chemicals that the body can utilize. Such enzymes are specific with respect to the fat, protein, or carbohydrate food molecules each can digest. For example, protein-digesting enzymes work only on proteins, not on carbohydrates or fats. Each enzyme is produced by a particular digestive organ and functions at a specific site. However, the enzyme's site of action may or may not be its site of production. These digestive enzymes and their functions are discussed in later sections.

END PRODUCTS OF DIGESTION

Before we describe the organs of digestion, let us see where the process of digestion will take us, or rather, will take our food. The three types of complex organic molecules found in food are carbohydrates, proteins, and fats. Each of these complex molecules is digested to a much more simple substance that the body can then use. Carbohydrates, such as starches and disaccharides, are digested to monosaccharides such as glucose, fructose, and galactose. Proteins are digested to amino acids, and fats are digested to fatty acids and glycerol. Also part of food, and released during digestion, are vitamins, minerals, and water.

We will now return to the beginning of the alimentary tube and consider the digestive organs and the process of digestion.

ORAL CAVITY

Food enters the **oral cavity** (or **buccal cavity**) by way of the mouth. The boundaries of the oral cavity are the hard and soft palates superiorly; the cheeks laterally; and the floor of the mouth inferiorly. Within the oral cavity are the teeth and tongue and the openings of the ducts of the salivary glands.

TEETH

The function of the **teeth** is, of course, chewing. This is the process that mechanically breaks food into smaller pieces and mixes it with saliva. An individual develops two sets of teeth: deciduous and permanent. The **deciduous teeth** begin to erupt through the gums at about 6 months of age, and the set of 20 teeth is usually complete by the age of 2 years. These teeth are gradually lost throughout childhood and replaced by the **permanent teeth**, the first of which are molars that emerge around the age of 6 years. A complete set of permanent teeth consists of 32 teeth; the types of teeth are incisors, canines, premolars, and molars. The wisdom teeth are the third molars on either side of each jawbone. In some people, the wisdom teeth may not emerge from the jawbone because there is no room for them along the gum line. These wisdom teeth are said to be impacted and may put pressure on the roots of the second molars. In such cases, extraction of a wisdom tooth may be necessary to prevent damage to other teeth.

The structure of a tooth is shown in Fig. 16–2. The crown is visible above the gum (**gingiva**). The root is enclosed in a socket in the mandible or maxillae; the portion of each bone that contains sockets is called the dental arch. The **periodontal membrane** lines the socket and produces a bone-like cement that anchors the tooth. The outermost layer of the crown is **enamel**, which is made by cells called ameloblasts. Enamel provides a hard chewing surface and is more resistant to decay than are other parts of the tooth. Within the enamel is **dentin**, which is very similar to bone and is produced by cells called odontoblasts. Dentin also forms the roots of a tooth. The innermost portion of a tooth is the **pulp cavity**, which contains blood vessels and nerve endings of the trigeminal nerve (5th cranial).

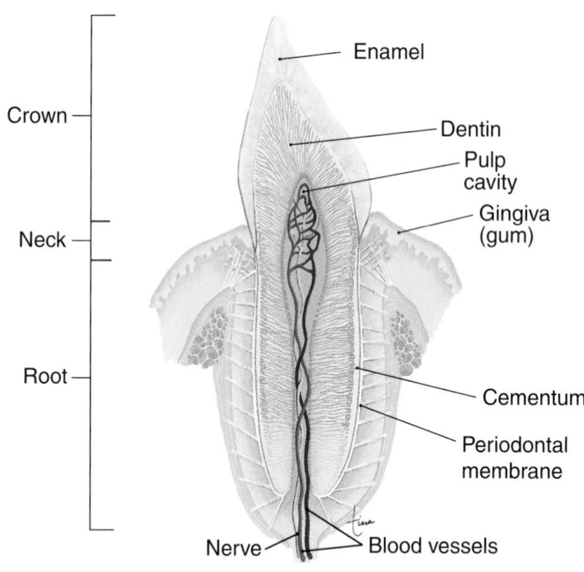

Figure 16–2 Tooth structure. Longitudinal section of a tooth showing internal structure.

QUESTION: Which parts of a tooth are living? How do you know?

As you know, the oral cavity is a microbiome, the home of one of our bacterial populations. The normal flora of the oral cavity includes small numbers of yeasts and protozoa as well as bacteria, and as usual, the "good" bacteria help to prevent the overgrowth of pathogens. Oral yeast infections usually occur only in people with compromised immune systems (as by HIV–AIDS) or who are taking antibiotics for a bacterial infection. Some common bacteria, however, can be detrimental when they metabolize sugars in our food as their food. Byproducts of this include acids that erode (decalcify) the enamel and dentin layers of teeth, leading to **dental caries** or cavities. In caries left untreated, bacteria may invade the pulp cavity, causing a very painful toothache, and possibly death of the tooth and infection of the bony socket.

TONGUE

The **tongue** is made of skeletal muscle that is innervated by the hypoglossal nerves (12th cranial). On the upper surface of the tongue are small projections called **papillae**, many of which contain taste buds (see also Chapter 9). The sensory nerves for taste are also cranial nerves: the facial (7th) and glossopharyngeal (9th). As you know, the sense of taste is important because it makes eating enjoyable, but the tongue has other functions as well.

Chewing is efficient because of the action of the tongue in keeping the food between the teeth and mixing it with saliva. These movements of the tongue are reflexive; if they were not, we would have to pay very close attention to chewing and might bite our tongues several times a day. Elevation of the tongue is the first step in swallowing. This is a voluntary action, in which the tongue contracts and meets the resistance of the hard palate. The mass of food, called a bolus, is thus pushed backward toward the pharynx. The remainder of swallowing is a reflex, which is described in the section on the pharynx.

SALIVARY GLANDS

The digestive secretion in the oral cavity is **saliva**, produced by three pairs of **salivary glands**, which are shown in Fig. 16–3. The **parotid glands** are just below and in front of the ears. The **submandibular** (also called submaxillary) glands are at the posterior corners of the mandible, and the **sublingual** glands are below the floor of the mouth. Each gland has at least one duct that takes saliva to the oral cavity.

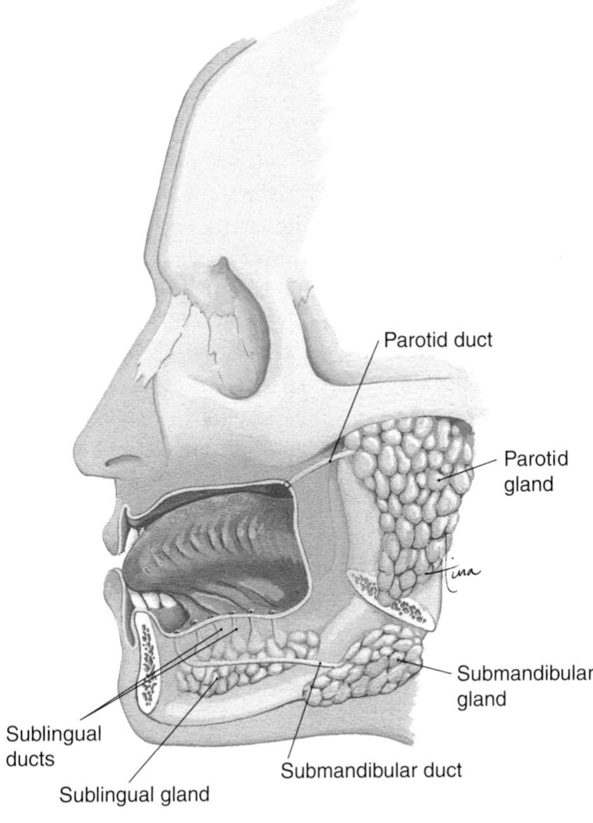

Figure 16–3 The salivary glands shown in left lateral view.

QUESTION: Why are these exocrine glands? What is saliva made from?

Secretion of saliva is continuous, but the amount varies in different situations. The presence of food (or anything else) in the mouth increases saliva secretion. This is a parasympathetic response mediated by the facial and glossopharyngeal nerves. The sight or smell of food also increases secretion of saliva. Sympathetic stimulation in stress situations decreases secretion, making the mouth dry and swallowing difficult. If you have ever been badly frightened suddenly (even by a scary movie) or been anxious for an extended period of time, you know what that dry mouth feels like.

Saliva is mostly water, which is important to dissolve food for tasting and to moisten food for swallowing. The enzyme **lysozyme** in saliva is similar to the one in tears and has the same function: to inhibit the growth of many kinds of bacteria. It does not outright kill them, as does HCl in gastric juice (or it might do the same to the living cells of the oral mucous membranes), but it does slow down bacterial reproduction. The digestive enzyme in saliva is salivary **amylase**, which breaks down starch molecules to shorter chains of glucose molecules, or to maltose, a disaccharide. Most of us, however, do not chew our food long enough for the action of salivary amylase to be truly effective. As you will see, another amylase from the pancreas is also available to digest starch. Table 16–1 summarizes the functions of digestive secretions.

Saliva is made from blood plasma and thus contains many of the chemicals that are found in plasma. Considerable research is focused on detecting in saliva chemical markers for diseases such as cancer, with the goal of using saliva rather than blood for diagnostic tests.

PHARYNX

As described in the preceding chapter, the oropharynx and laryngopharynx, besides being air passageways to the larynx, are food passageways connecting the oral cavity to the esophagus. No digestion takes place in the pharynx. Its only related function is swallowing, the mechanical movement of food. When the bolus of food is pushed backward by the tongue, the constrictor muscles of the pharynx contract as part of the swallowing reflex. The reflex center for swallowing is in the medulla, which coordinates the many actions that take place: constriction of the pharynx, cessation of breathing, elevation of the soft palate to block the nasopharynx, elevation of the larynx and closure of the epiglottis, and peristalsis of the esophagus.

As you can see, swallowing is rather complicated, but because it is a reflex we don't have to think about making it happen correctly. Talking or laughing while eating, however, may interfere with the reflex and cause food to go into the "wrong pipe," the larynx. When that happens, the cough reflex is usually effective in clearing the airway.

ESOPHAGUS

The **esophagus** is a muscular tube that takes food from the pharynx to the stomach; no digestion takes place here. Peristalsis of the esophagus propels food in one direction and ensures that food gets to the stomach even if the body is horizontal or upside down. At the junction with the stomach, the lumen (cavity) of the esophagus is surrounded by the **lower esophageal sphincter** (LES or cardiac sphincter), a circular smooth muscle. The LES relaxes to permit food to enter the stomach, then contracts to prevent the backup of stomach contents. If the LES does not close completely, gastric juice may splash up into the esophagus; this is a painful condition we call heartburn, or gastroesophageal reflux disease (GERD). Most people experience heartburn once in a while, and it is merely uncomfortable, but chronic GERD is more serious. The lining of the esophagus cannot withstand the corrosive action of gastric acid and will be damaged, perhaps resulting in bleeding or even perforation. Medications are available to treat this condition.

STRUCTURAL LAYERS OF THE ALIMENTARY TUBE

Before we continue with our discussion of the organs of digestion, we will first examine the typical structure of the alimentary tube. When viewed in cross-section, the alimentary tube has four layers (Fig. 16–4): the mucosa, submucosa, external muscle layer, and serosa. Each layer has a specific structure, and its functions contribute to the functioning of the organs of which it is a part.

Table 16–1 | THE PROCESS OF DIGESTION

ORGAN	ENZYME OR OTHER SECRETION	FUNCTION	SITE OF ACTION
Salivary glands	Amylase	Converts starch to maltose	Oral cavity
Stomach	Pepsin	Converts proteins to polypeptides	Stomach
	HCl	Changes pepsinogen to pepsin; maintains pH 1–2; destroys pathogens	Stomach
Liver	Bile salts	Emulsify fats	Small intestine
Pancreas	Amylase	Converts starch to maltose	Small intestine
	Trypsin	Converts polypeptides to peptides	Small intestine
	Lipase	Converts emulsified fats to fatty acids and glycerol	Small intestine
Small intestine	Peptidases	Convert peptides to amino acids	Small intestine
	Sucrase	Converts sucrose to glucose and fructose	Small intestine
	Maltase	Converts maltose to glucose (2)	Small intestine
	Lactase	Converts lactose to glucose and galactose	Small intestine

Table 16–1 | THE PROCESS OF DIGESTION—cont'd

ORGAN	ENZYME OR OTHER SECRETION	FUNCTION	SITE OF ACTION

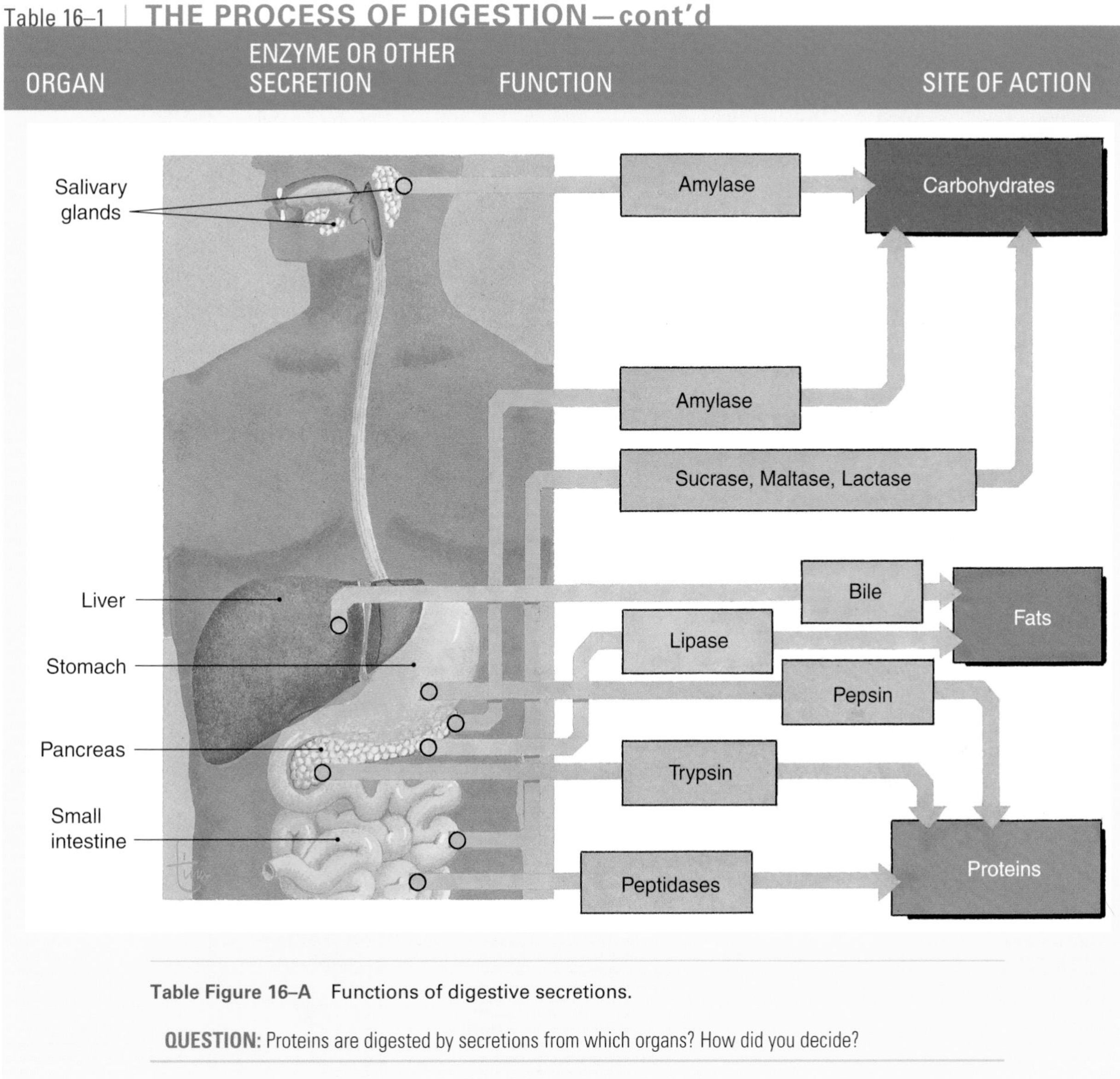

Table Figure 16–A Functions of digestive secretions.

QUESTION: Proteins are digested by secretions from which organs? How did you decide?

MUCOSA

The **mucosa**, or lining, of the alimentary tube is made of epithelial tissue, areolar connective tissue, and two thin layers of smooth muscle. In the esophagus the epithelium is stratified squamous epithelium; in the stomach and intestines it is simple columnar epithelium. The epithelium secretes mucus, which lubricates the passage of food, and also secretes the digestive enzymes of the stomach and small intestine. Just below the epithelium, within the areolar connective tissue, are lymph nodules that contain lymphocytes to produce antibodies and macrophages to phagocytize bacteria or other foreign material that get through the epithelium. The thin layers of smooth muscle create folds in the mucosa, and ripples, so that all of the epithelial cells are in touch with the contents of the organ. In the stomach and small intestine this is important for absorption.

SUBMUCOSA

The **submucosa** is made of areolar connective tissue with many blood vessels and lymphatic vessels. Many millions of nerve fibers are also present, part of what is called the

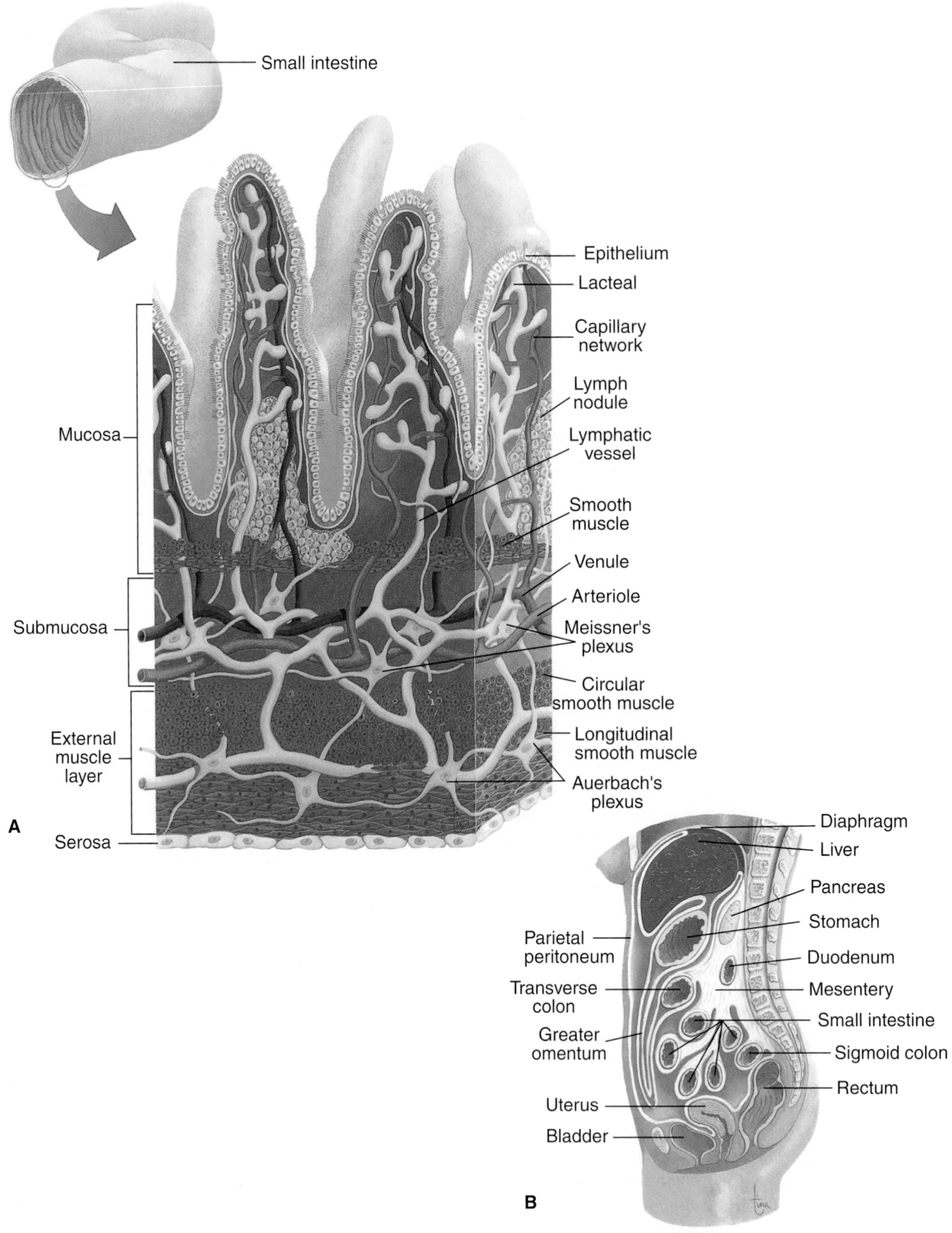

Figure 16–4 (**A**) The four layers of the wall of the alimentary tube. A small part of the wall of the small intestine has been magnified to show the four layers typical of the alimentary tube. (**B**) Sagittal section through the abdomen showing the relationship of the peritoneum and mesentery to the abdominal organs.

QUESTION: What is the function of the external muscle layer?

enteric nervous system, or the "brain of the gut," which extends the entire length of the alimentary tube. The enteric nervous system can function independently of the CNS but is also influenced by the autonomic nervous system. The nerve networks in the submucosa are called **Meissner's plexus** (or submucosal plexus), and they innervate the mucosa to regulate secretions. Parasympathetic impulses to enteric neurons increase secretions, whereas sympathetic impulses decrease secretions. Sensory neurons are also present to the smooth muscle (a stretched or cramping gut is painful), as are motor neurons to blood vessels, to regulate vessel diameter and blood flow.

EXTERNAL MUSCLE LAYER

The external muscle layer typically contains two layers of smooth muscle: an inner, circular layer and an outer, longitudinal layer. Variations from the typical do occur, however. In the esophagus, this layer is striated muscle in the upper third, which gradually changes to smooth muscle in the lower portions. The stomach has three layers of smooth muscle, rather than two.

Contractions of this muscle layer help break up food and mix it with digestive juices. The one-way contractions of **peristalsis** move the food toward the anus. **Auerbach's plexus** (or myenteric plexus) is the portion of the enteric nervous system in this layer, and some of its millions of neurons receive autonomic impulses. Sympathetic impulses decrease contractions and peristalsis, whereas parasympathetic impulses increase contractions and peristalsis, promoting normal digestion. The parasympathetic nerves are the vagus (10th cranial) nerves; they truly live up to the meaning of *vagus*, which is "wanderer."

SEROSA

Above the diaphragm, for the esophagus, the serosa, the outermost layer, is fibrous connective tissue. Below the diaphragm, the serosa is the **mesentery** or visceral peritoneum, a serous membrane. Lining the abdominal cavity is the parietal peritoneum, usually simply called the **peritoneum**. The peritoneum-mesentery is actually one continuous membrane (see Fig. 16–4). The serous fluid between the peritoneum and mesentery prevents friction when the alimentary tube contracts and the organs slide against one another.

The preceding descriptions are typical of the layers of the alimentary tube. As noted, variations are possible, and any important differences are mentioned in the sections that follow on specific organs.

STOMACH

The **stomach** is located in the upper left quadrant of the abdominal cavity, to the left of the liver and in front of the spleen. Although part of the alimentary tube, the stomach is not a tube, but rather a sac that extends from the esophagus to the small intestine. Because it is a sac, the stomach is a reservoir for food, so digestion proceeds gradually and we do not have to eat constantly. Both mechanical and chemical digestion take place in the stomach.

The parts of the stomach are shown in Fig. 16–5. The cardiac orifice is the opening of the esophagus, and the fundus is the portion above the level of this opening. The body of the stomach is the large central portion, bounded laterally by the greater curvature and medially by the lesser curvature. The pylorus is adjacent to the duodenum of the small intestine, and the **pyloric sphincter** surrounds the junction of the two organs. The fundus and body are mainly storage areas, whereas most digestion takes place in the pylorus.

When the stomach is empty, the mucosa appears wrinkled or folded. These folds are called **rugae**; they flatten out as the stomach is filled and permit expansion of the lining without tearing it. The **gastric pits** are the glands of the stomach and consist of several types of cells; their collective secretions are called gastric juice. **Mucous cells** secrete mucus, which coats the stomach lining and helps prevent erosion by the gastric juice. **Chief cells** secrete **pepsinogen**, an inactive form of the enzyme **pepsin**. **Parietal cells** produce hydrochloric acid (HCl); these cells have enzymes called **proton pumps**, which secrete H^+ ions into the stomach cavity. The H^+ ions unite with Cl^- ions that have diffused from the parietal cells to form HCl in the lumen of the stomach. HCl converts pepsinogen to pepsin, which then begins the digestion of proteins to polypeptides, and also gives gastric juice its pH of 1 to 2. This very acidic pH is necessary for pepsin to function and also kills most microorganisms that enter the stomach. The parietal cells also secrete intrinsic factor, which is necessary to prevent the digestion of vitamin B_{12}, and promote its absorption by the small intestine. Enteroendocrine cells called G cells secrete the hormone gastrin.

Gastric juice is secreted in small amounts at the sight or smell of food. This is a parasympathetic response that ensures that some gastric juice will be present in the stomach when food arrives. The presence of food in the stomach causes the G cells to secrete **gastrin**, a hormone that stimulates the secretion of greater amounts of gastric juice.

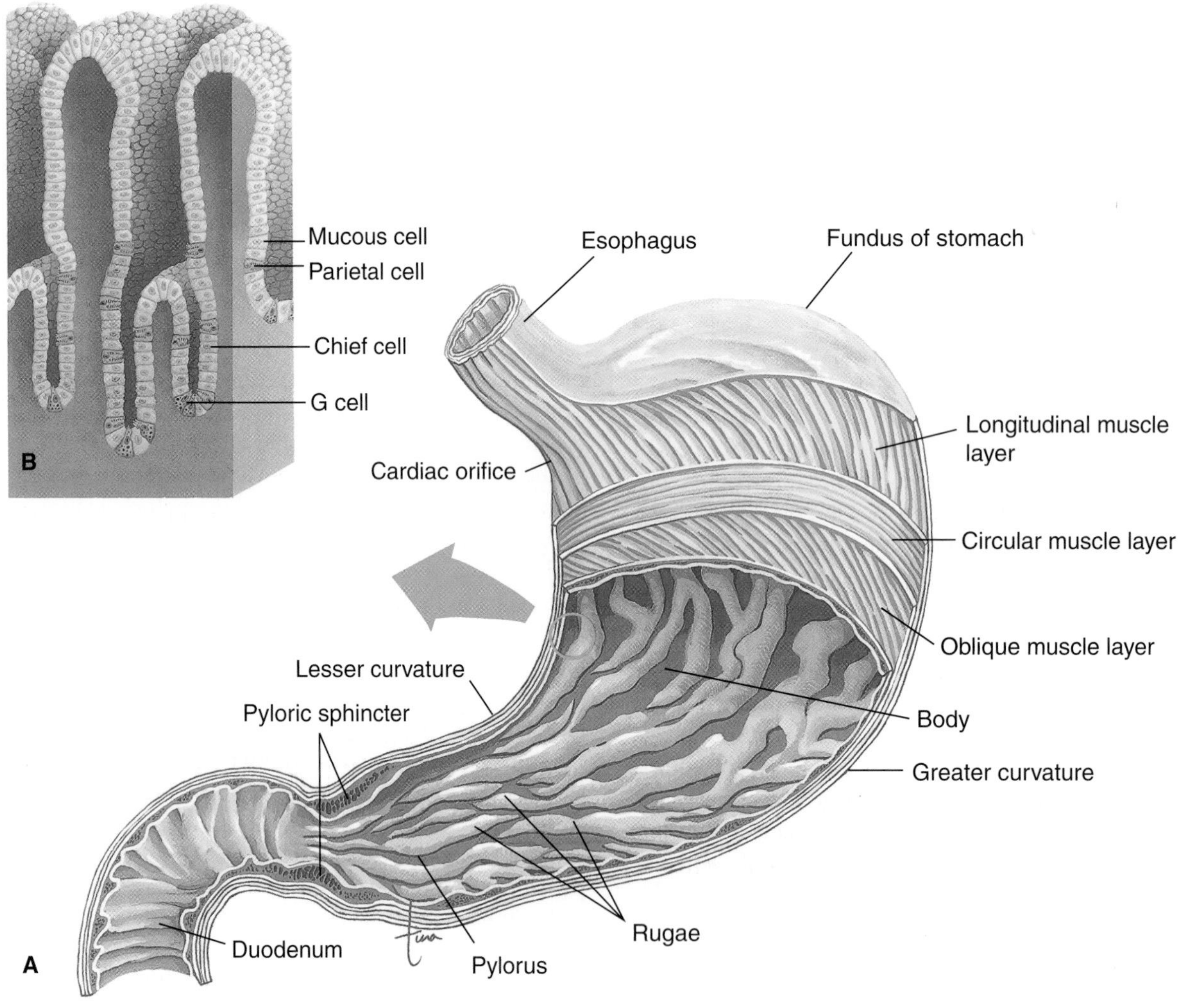

Figure 16–5 (**A**) The stomach in anterior view. The stomach wall has been sectioned to show the muscle layers and the rugae of the mucosa. (**B**) Gastric pits (glands) showing the types of cells present. See text for functions.

QUESTION: What is the function of the pyloric sphincter?

This is an instance of the source and the target organ of a hormone being the same organ (but different cells in that organ).

The external muscle layer of the stomach consists of three layers of smooth muscle: circular, longitudinal, and oblique layers. These three layers are innervated by the myenteric plexuses of the enteric nervous system. Stimulatory impulses are carried from the CNS by the vagus nerves (10th cranial) and provide for very efficient mechanical digestion to change food into a thick liquid called chyme. The pyloric sphincter is usually contracted when the stomach is churning food; it relaxes at intervals to permit small amounts of chyme to pass into the duodenum. This sphincter then contracts again to prevent the backup of intestinal contents into the stomach (see Box 16–1: Disorders of the Stomach).

SMALL INTESTINE

The **small intestine** is about 1 inch (2.5 cm) in diameter and approximately 20 feet (6 m) long and extends from the stomach to the cecum of the large intestine. Within

Box 16–1 | DISORDERS OF THE STOMACH

Vomiting is the expulsion of stomach and intestinal contents through the esophagus and mouth. Stimuli include irritation of the stomach, motion sickness, food poisoning, or diseases such as meningitis. The vomiting center is in the medulla, which coordinates the simultaneous contraction of the diaphragm and the abdominal muscles. This squeezes the stomach and upper intestine, expelling their contents. As part of the reflex, the lower esophageal sphincter relaxes, and the glottis closes. If the glottis fails to close, as may happen in alcohol or drug intoxication, aspiration of vomitus may occur and result in fatal obstruction of the respiratory passages.

Pyloric stenosis is a narrowing of the opening of the pyloric sphincter, which impairs emptying of the stomach. This is most often a congenital disorder caused by hypertrophy of the pyloric sphincter. For reasons unknown, this condition is more common in male infants than in female infants. When the stomach does not empty efficiently, its internal pressure increases. Vomiting relieves the pressure; this is a classic symptom of pyloric stenosis. Correcting this condition requires surgery to widen the opening in the sphincter.

A **gastric ulcer** is an erosion of the mucosa of the stomach. With a rapid rate of mitosis in the gastric pits and continuous secretion of mucus, the normal stomach lining is well adapted to resist the corrosive action of gastric juice, and ulcer formation is the result of oversecretion of HCl or undersecretion of mucus.

As erosion reaches the submucosa, small blood vessels are ruptured and bleed. If vomiting occurs, the vomitus has a "coffee-grounds" appearance because of the presence of blood acted on by gastric juice. A more serious complication is perforation of the stomach wall, with leakage of gastric contents into the abdominal cavity, and **peritonitis**.

The bacterium called *Helicobacter pylori* is the cause of most gastric ulcers. For many patients, a few weeks of antibiotic therapy to eradicate this bacterium has produced rapid healing of their ulcers. This bacterium also seems to be responsible for virtually all cases of stomach cancer.

The medications that decrease the secretion of HCl are useful for ulcer patients not helped by antibiotics.

the abdominal cavity, the large intestine encircles the coils of the small intestine (see Fig. 16–1).

The **duodenum** is the first 10 inches (25 cm) of the small intestine. The common bile duct enters the duodenum at the ampulla of Vater (or hepatopancreatic ampulla). The **jejunum** is about 8 feet long, and the **ileum** is about 11 feet in length. In a living person, however, the small intestine is always contracted and is therefore somewhat shorter.

Digestion is completed in the small intestine, and the end products of digestion are absorbed into the blood and lymph. The mucosa (see Fig. 16–4) has simple columnar epithelium that includes cells with microvilli and goblet cells that secrete mucus. Enteroendocrine cells secrete the hormones of the small intestine. Lymph nodules called Peyer's patches are abundant throughout the intestinal mucosa, and especially so in the ileum to destroy absorbed pathogens. The external muscle layer has the typical circular and longitudinal smooth muscle layers that mix the chyme with digestive secretions and propel the chyme toward the colon. Stimulatory impulses to the enteric nerves of these muscle layers are carried by the vagus nerves. The waves of peristalsis, however, can take place without stimulation by the central nervous system; the enteric nervous system can function entirely on its own and promote normal peristalsis.

There are three sources of digestive secretions that function within the small intestine: the liver, the pancreas, and the small intestine itself. We will return to the small intestine after considering these other organs.

LIVER

The **liver** (Fig. 16–6) consists of two large lobes, right and left, and fills the upper right and center of the abdominal cavity, just below the diaphragm. The structural unit of the liver is the **liver lobule**, a roughly hexagonal column of liver cells (hepatocytes). Between adjacent lobules are branches of the hepatic artery and portal vein. The capillaries of a lobule are sinusoids, large and very permeable vessels between the rows of liver cells. The sinusoids receive blood from both the hepatic artery and portal vein,

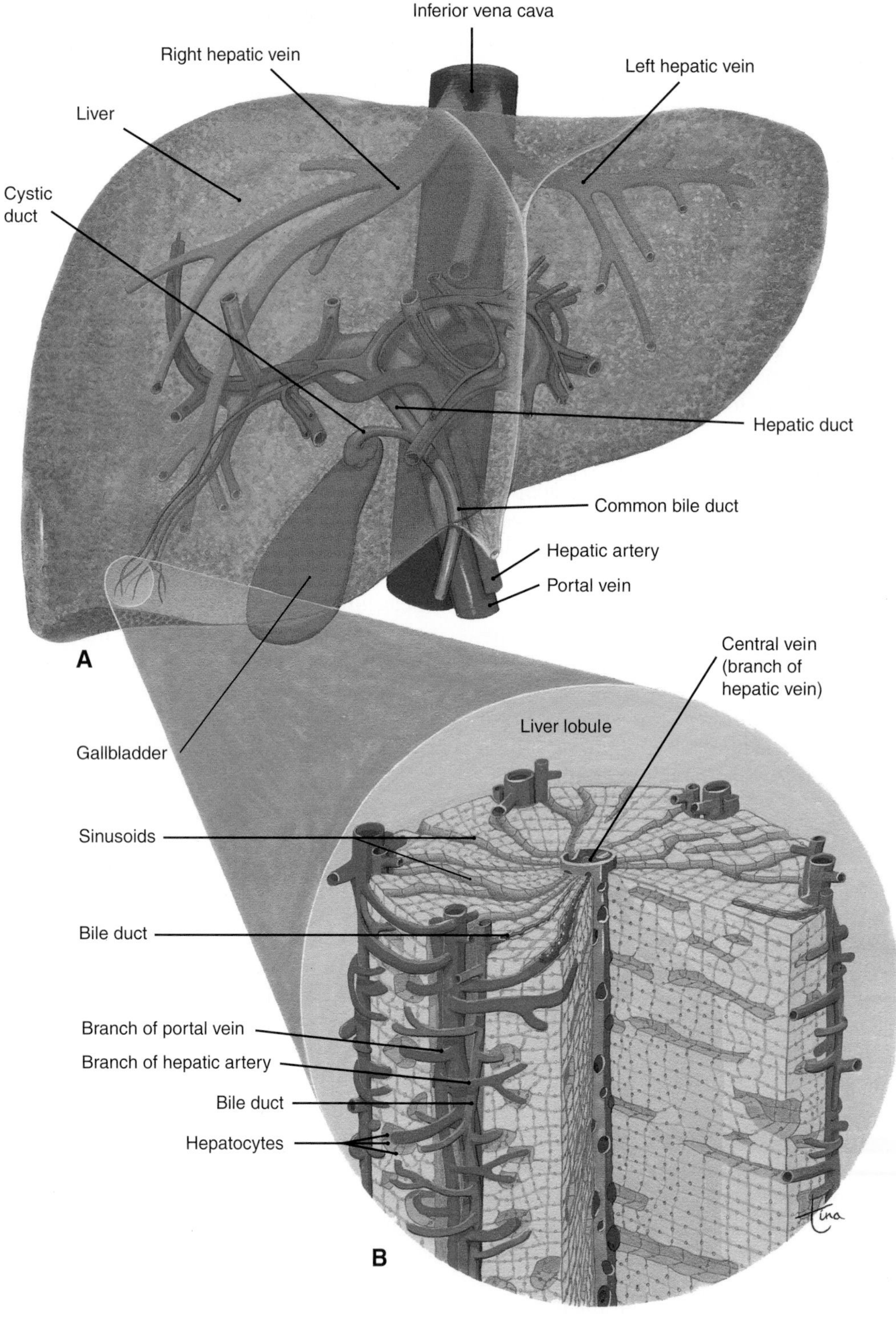

Figure 16–6 (**A**) The liver and gallbladder with blood vessels and bile ducts. (**B**) Magnified view of one liver lobule. See text for description.

QUESTION: In part B, trace the pathway of blood flow through a liver lobule.

and it is with this mixture of blood that the liver cells carry out their functions. The hepatic artery brings oxygenated blood, and the portal vein brings blood from the digestive organs and spleen (see Fig. 13–7 in Chapter 13). Each lobule has a central vein. The central veins of all the lobules unite to form the hepatic veins, which take blood out of the liver to the inferior vena cava.

The cells of the liver have many functions (which are discussed in a later section), but their only digestive function is the production of **bile**. Bile enters the small bile ducts, called bile canaliculi, on the liver cells, which unite to form larger ducts and finally merge to form the **hepatic duct**, which takes bile out of the liver (see Fig. 16–6). The hepatic duct unites with the cystic duct of the gallbladder to form the **common bile duct**, which takes bile to the duodenum.

Bile is mostly water and has an excretory function in that it carries bilirubin and excess cholesterol to the intestines for elimination in feces. The digestive function of bile is accomplished by **bile salts**, which **emulsify** fats in the small intestine. Emulsification means that large fat globules are broken into smaller globules. This is mechanical, not chemical, digestion; the fat is still fat but now has more surface area to facilitate chemical digestion.

Production of bile is stimulated by the hormone **secretin**, which is produced by the duodenum when food enters the small intestine. Table 16–2 summarizes the regulation of secretion of all digestive secretions.

GALLBLADDER

The **gallbladder** is a sac about 3 to 4 inches (7.5 to 10 cm) long located on the undersurface of the right lobe of the liver. Bile in the hepatic duct of the liver flows through the **cystic duct** into the gallbladder (see Fig. 16–6), which stores bile until it is needed in the small intestine. The gallbladder also concentrates bile by absorbing water (see Box 16–2: Gallstones).

Table 16–2 | REGULATION OF DIGESTIVE SECRETIONS

SECRETION	NERVOUS REGULATION	CHEMICAL REGULATION
Saliva	Presence of food in mouth or sight or smell of food; parasympathetic impulses along 7th and 9th cranial nerves	None
Gastric juice	Sight or smell of food; parasympathetic impulses along 10th cranial nerves	Gastrin—produced by the G cells of the gastric mucosa when food is present in the stomach
Bile		
Secretion by the liver	None	Secretin—produced by the enteroendocrine cells of the duodenum when chyme enters
Contraction of the gallbladder	None	Cholecystokinin—produced by the enteroendocrine cells of the duodenum when chyme enters
Enzyme pancreatic juice	None	Cholecystokinin—from the duodenum
Bicarbonate pancreatic juice	None	Secretin—from the duodenum
Intestinal juice	Presence of chyme in the duodenum; parasympathetic impulses along 10th cranial nerves	None

Box 16–2 | GALLSTONES

One of the functions of the gallbladder is to concentrate bile by absorbing water. If the bile contains a high concentration of cholesterol, absorption of water may lead to precipitation and the formation of cholesterol crystals. These crystals are **gallstones**.

If the gallstones are small, they will pass through the cystic duct and common bile duct to the duodenum without causing symptoms. If large, however, the gallstones cannot pass out of the gallbladder and may cause mild to severe pain that often radiates to the right shoulder. Obstructive jaundice may occur if bile backs up into the liver and bilirubin is reabsorbed into the blood.

Several treatments are available for gallstones. Medications that dissolve gallstones work slowly, over the course of several months, and are useful if biliary obstruction is not severe. An instrument that generates shock waves (called a lithotripter) may be used to pulverize the stones into smaller pieces that may easily pass into the duodenum; this procedure is called **lithotripsy**. Surgery to remove the gallbladder (cholecystectomy) is required in some cases. The hepatic duct is then connected directly to the common bile duct, and dilute bile flows into the duodenum. Following such surgery, the patient should avoid meals high in fats.

When fatty foods enter the duodenum, the enteroendocrine cells of the duodenal mucosa secrete the hormone **cholecystokinin**. This hormone stimulates contraction of the smooth muscle in the wall of the gallbladder, which forces bile into the cystic duct, then into the common bile duct, and on into the duodenum.

PANCREAS

The **pancreas** is located in the upper left abdominal quadrant between the curve of the duodenum and the spleen and is about 6 inches (15 cm) in length. The endocrine functions of the pancreas were discussed in Chapter 10, so only the exocrine functions will be considered here. The exocrine glands of the pancreas are called acini (singular: acinus) (Fig. 16–7). They produce enzymes that are involved in the digestion of all three types of complex food molecules.

The pancreatic enzyme **amylase** digests starch to maltose. You may recall that this is the "backup" enzyme for salivary amylase, though pancreatic amylase is responsible for most digestion of starch. **Lipase** converts emulsified fats to fatty acids and glycerol. The emulsifying or fat-separating action of bile salts increases the surface area of fats so that lipase works effectively. Trypsinogen is an inactive enzyme that is changed to active **trypsin** in the duodenum. Trypsin digests polypeptides to shorter chains of amino acids.

The pancreatic enzyme juice is carried by small ducts that unite to form larger ducts, then finally the main **pancreatic duct**. An accessory duct may also be present. The main pancreatic duct emerges from the medial side of the pancreas and joins the common bile duct to the duodenum (see Fig. 16–7).

The pancreas also produces a **bicarbonate juice** (containing sodium bicarbonate), which is alkaline. Because the gastric juice that enters the duodenum is very acidic, it must be neutralized to prevent damage to the duodenal mucosa. This neutralizing is accomplished by the sodium bicarbonate in pancreatic juice, and the pH of the duodenal chyme is raised to about 7.5.

Secretion of pancreatic juice is stimulated by the hormones secretin and cholecystokinin, which are produced by the duodenal mucosa when chyme enters the small intestine. **Secretin** stimulates the production of bicarbonate juice by the pancreas, and **cholecystokinin** stimulates the secretion of the pancreatic enzymes.

COMPLETION OF DIGESTION AND ABSORPTION

SMALL INTESTINE

The secretion of the epithelium of the intestinal glands (or crypts of Lieberkühn) is stimulated by the presence of food in the duodenum. The intestinal enzymes are the peptidases and sucrase, maltase, and lactase. **Peptidases** complete the digestion of protein by breaking down short polypeptide chains to amino acids. **Sucrase**, **maltase**, and **lactase**, respectively, digest the disaccharides sucrose, maltose, and lactose to monosaccharides.

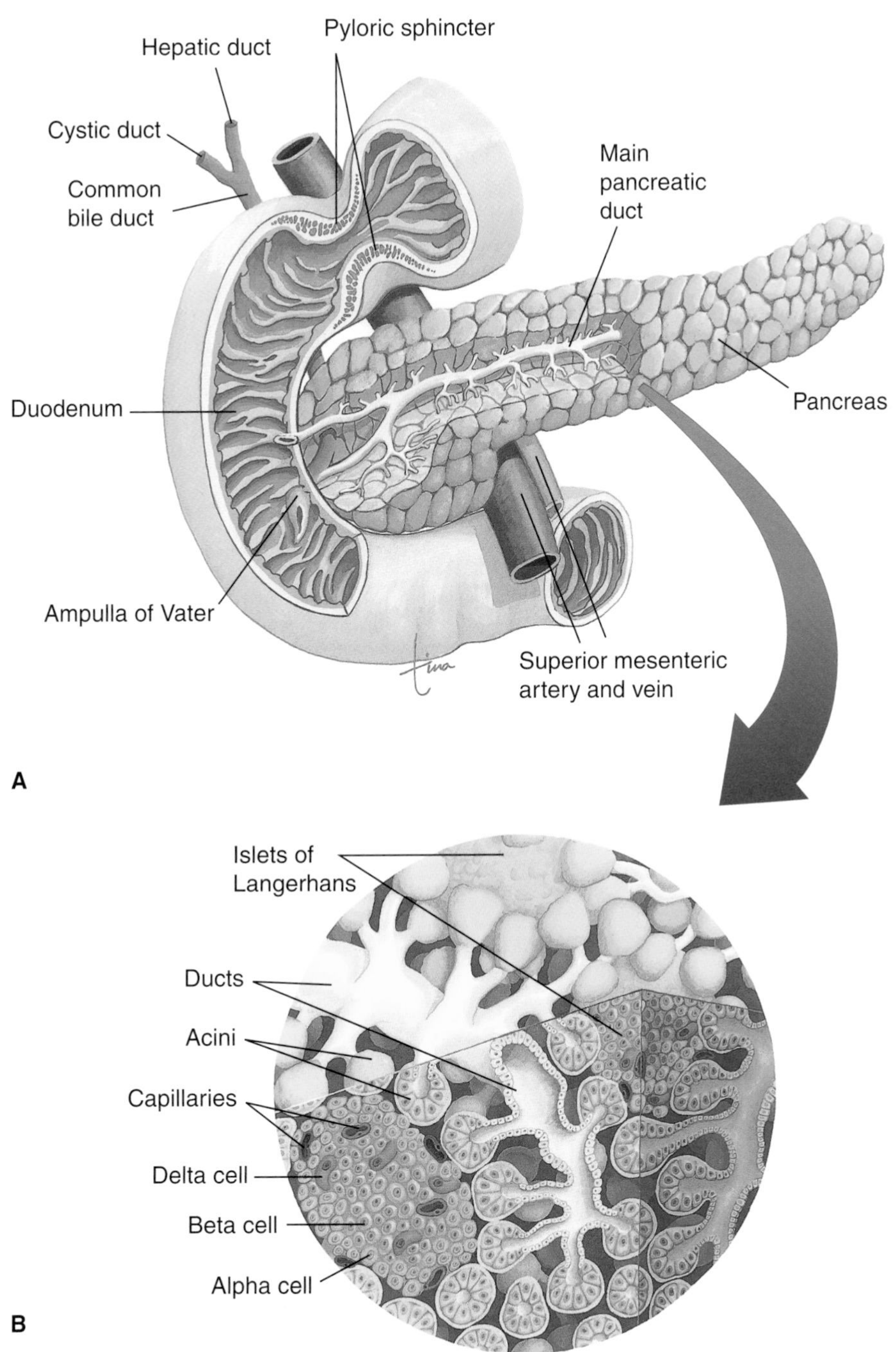

Figure 16–7 (**A**) The pancreas, sectioned to show the pancreatic ducts. The main pancreatic duct joins the common bile duct. (**B**) Microscopic section showing acini with their ducts and several islets of Langerhans.

QUESTION: In part B, what do the acini secrete?

The enteroendocrine cells of the intestinal glands secrete the hormones of the small intestine. Secretion is stimulated by food entering the duodenum.

A summary of the digestive secretions and their functions is found in Table 16–1. Regulation of these secretions is shown in Table 16–2.

ABSORPTION

Most absorption of the end products of digestion takes place in the small intestine (although the stomach does absorb water and alcohol). The process of absorption requires a large surface area, which is provided by several structural modifications of the small intestine; these are shown in Fig. 16–8. **Plica circulares**, or circular folds, are macroscopic folds of the mucosa and submucosa, somewhat like accordion pleats. The mucosa is further folded into projections called **villi**, which give the inner surface of the intestine a velvet-like appearance. Each columnar cell (except the mucus-secreting goblet cells) of the villi also has **microvilli** on its free surface.

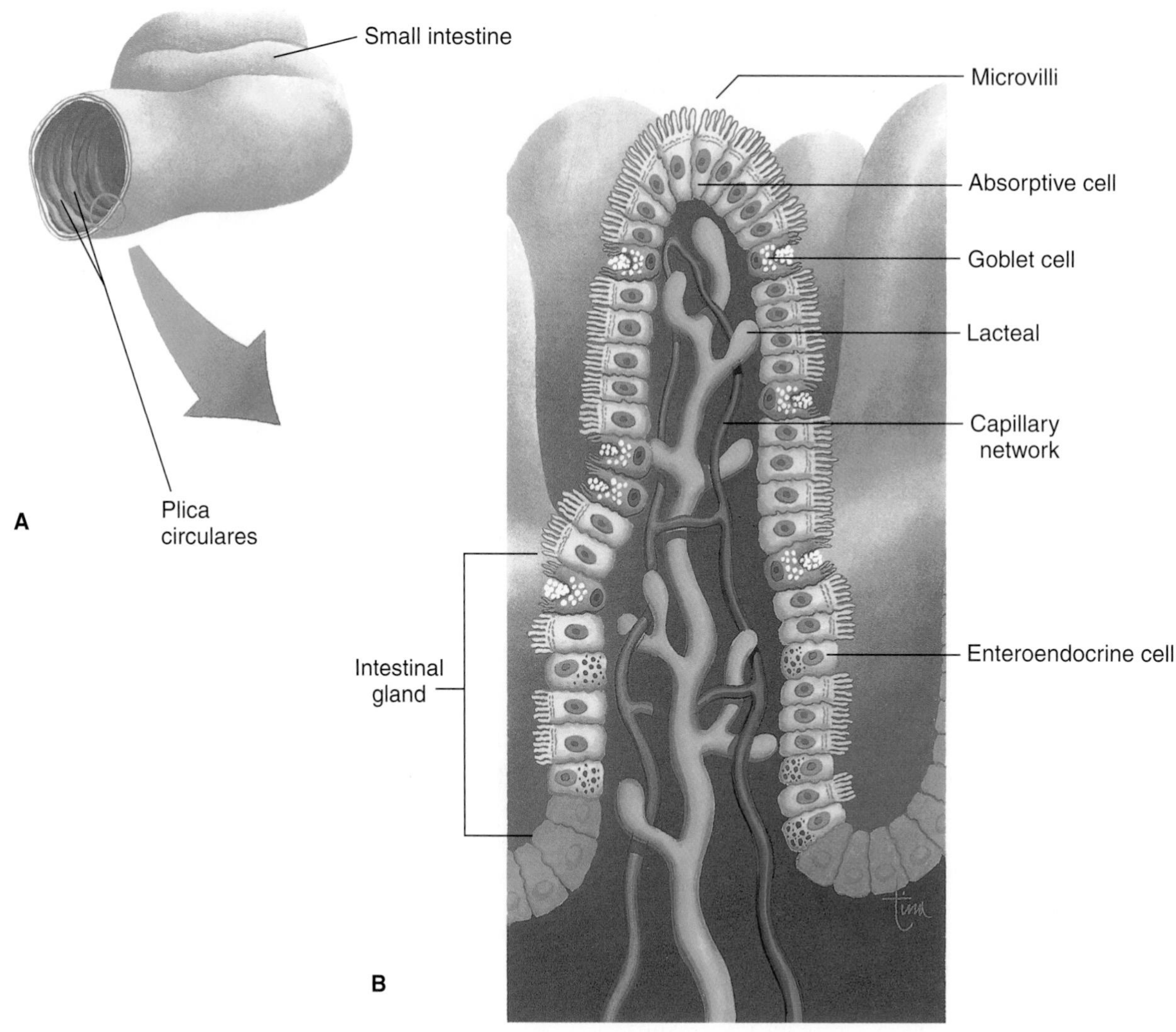

Figure 16–8 The small intestine. (**A**) Section through the small intestine showing plica circulares. (**B**) Microscopic view of a villus showing the internal structure. The enteroendocrine cells secrete the intestinal hormones.

QUESTION: What is the purpose of the villi? What other structures have the same purpose?

Microvilli are microscopic folds of the cell membrane and are collectively called the brush border. All of these folds greatly increase the surface area of the intestinal lining. It is estimated that if the intestinal mucosa could be flattened out, it would cover more than 2000 square feet (half a basketball court).

The absorption of nutrients takes place from the lumen of the intestine into the vessels within the villi. Refer to Fig. 16–8 and notice that within each villus is a **capillary network** and a **lacteal**, which is a dead-end lymph capillary. Water-soluble nutrients are absorbed into the blood in the capillary networks. Monosaccharides, amino acids, positive ions, and the water-soluble vitamins (vitamin C and the B vitamins) are absorbed by active transport. Negative ions may be absorbed by either passive or active transport mechanisms. Water is absorbed by osmosis following the absorption of minerals, especially sodium. Certain nutrients have additional special requirements for their absorption: For example, vitamin B_{12} requires the intrinsic factor produced by the parietal cells of the gastric mucosa, and the efficient absorption of calcium ions requires parathyroid hormone and vitamin D.

Fat-soluble nutrients are absorbed into the lymph in the lacteals of the villi. Bile salts are necessary for the efficient absorption of fatty acids and the fat-soluble vitamins (A, D, E, and K). Once absorbed, fatty acids are recombined with glycerol to form triglycerides. These triglycerides then form globules that include cholesterol and protein; these lipid–protein complexes are called **chylomicrons**. In the form of chylomicrons, most absorbed fat is transported by the lymph and eventually enters the blood in the left subclavian vein.

Blood from the capillary networks in the villi does not return directly to the heart but first travels through the portal vein to the liver. You may recall the importance of portal circulation, discussed in Chapter 13. This pathway enables the liver to regulate the blood levels of glucose and amino acids, store certain vitamins, and remove potential poisons from the blood (see Box 16–3: Disorders of the Intestines).

LARGE INTESTINE

The **large intestine**, also called the **colon**, is approximately 2.5 inches (6.3 cm) in diameter and 5 feet (1.5 m) in length. It extends from the ileum of the small intestine to the anus, the terminal opening. The parts of the colon are shown in Fig. 16–9. The **cecum** is the first portion, and at its junction with the ileum is the **ileocecal valve**, which is not a sphincter but serves the same purpose. The ileocecal valve is a fold of the intestinal mucosa that surrounds the opening from ileum to cecum. After undigested food (which is now mostly cellulose) and water pass into the cecum, this fold is pressed flat during peristalsis and effectively closed, which prevents the backflow of fecal material into the ileum.

Attached to the cecum is the **appendix**, a small, dead-end tube with abundant lymphatic tissue. The appendix seems to be a **vestigial organ**, that is, one whose size and function seem to be reduced. Although there is abundant lymphatic tissue in the wall of the appendix, the possibility that the appendix has special functions concerned with immunity is not known with certainty. **Appendicitis** is inflammation of the appendix, which may occur if fecal material becomes impacted within it. This usually necessitates an **appendectomy**, the surgical removal of the appendix.

The remainder of the colon consists of the ascending, transverse, and descending colon, which encircle the small intestine; the sigmoid colon, which turns medially and downward; the rectum; and the anal canal. The rectum is about 6 inches long, and the anal canal is the last inch of the colon that surrounds the anus. Clinically, however, the terminal end of the colon is usually referred to as the rectum.

No digestion takes place in the colon. The only secretion of the colonic mucosa is mucus, which lubricates the passage of fecal material. The longitudinal smooth muscle layer of the colon is in three bands called **taeniae coli**. The rest of the colon is "gathered" to fit these bands. This gives the colon a puckered appearance; the puckers or pockets are called **haustra**, which provide for more surface area within the colon.

The functions of the colon are the absorption of water, minerals, and vitamins and the elimination of undigestible material. Everything absorbed by the colon circulates first to the liver by way of portal circulation. About 80% of the water that enters the colon is absorbed (400 to 800 mL per day). Positive and negative ions are also absorbed. The vitamins absorbed are those produced by the **normal flora** (our **microbiota**, first mentioned in Chapter 1), the trillions of bacteria that live in the colon.

A person and his or her colon bacteria (or any of our normal flora) is an example of **symbiosis**, or "life together." We give the bacteria a home (and not just any home, rather one with a splendid climate-control system to keep it warm) and we supply food. The colon bacteria digest or ferment our undigested food and produce their own metabolic products, useful to them. Some of these

Box 16–3 | DISORDERS OF THE INTESTINES

Duodenal ulcers are erosions of the duodenal wall caused by the gastric juice that enters from the stomach. The most serious consequences are bleeding and perforation.

Paralytic ileus is the cessation of contraction of the smooth muscle layer of the intestine. This is a possible complication of abdominal surgery, but it may also be the result of peritonitis or inflammation elsewhere in the abdominal cavity. In the absence of peristalsis, intestinal obstruction may occur. Bowel movements cease, and vomiting occurs to relieve the pressure within the alimentary tube. Treatment involves suctioning the intestinal contents to eliminate any obstruction and to allow the intestine to regain its normal motility.

Lactose intolerance is the inability to digest lactose because of deficiency of the enzyme lactase. Lactase deficiency may be congenital, a consequence of prematurity, or acquired later in life. The delayed form is quite common among people of African or Asian ancestry, and in part is genetic. When lactose, or milk sugar, is not digested, it undergoes fermentation by the bacteria residing in the intestine. Symptoms include diarrhea, abdominal pain, bloating, and flatulence (gas formation).

Celiac disease is an autoimmune disorder that involves a destructive reaction to the protein gluten, found in wheat, oats, rye, and other grains. The immunological reaction (as if gluten were a pathogen) and subsequent inflammation damage the lining of the small intestine, resulting in poor absorption of nutrients. Symptoms include abdominal pain and bloating; controlling the inflammation requires a gluten-free diet. As with other autoimmune disorders, the trigger is not yet known.

Diverticula are small outpouchings through weakened areas of the intestinal wall. They are more likely to occur in the colon than in the small intestine and may exist for years without causing any symptoms. The presence of diverticula is called **diverticulosis**. Inflammation of diverticula is called **diverticulitis**, which is usually the result of entrapment of feces and bacteria. Symptoms include abdominal pain and tenderness and fever. If uncomplicated, diverticulitis may be treated with antibiotics and modifications in diet. The most serious complication is perforation of diverticula, allowing fecal material into the abdominal cavity, causing peritonitis. A diet high in fiber is believed to be an important aspect of prevention, to provide bulk in the colon and prevent weakening of its wall.

are beneficial to us as well. Vitamin K is produced and absorbed in amounts usually sufficient to meet a person's daily need for synthesis of the clotting factors by the liver. Other vitamins produced in smaller amounts include riboflavin, thiamin, biotin, and folic acid. Bacteria also contribute to the development of the immune system. Some bacterial products, however, may not be helpful to us and may influence weight gain, inflammation, or atherosclerosis. Yet another function of the normal colon flora is to inhibit the growth of pathogens. They do this either simply by their presence taking up space and food or by producing antibiotic chemicals. Our normal colon microbiota are not a perfect defense against pathogens, in that they do not inhibit viruses and may be overwhelmed by an onslaught of a bacterium such as *Salmonella* (food poisoning, from undercooked eggs or chicken, for example) but for an ongoing success for adults, see Box 16–4: Infant Botulism. Keep in mind as well that we still have much more to learn about our relationship with our microbiota.

ELIMINATION OF FECES

Feces consist of cellulose and other undigestible material, dead and living bacteria, and water. The colon moves feces along by contracting in waves of peristalsis, which become more numerous after eating. The gastrocolic reflex and duodenocolic reflex are named appropriately: The presence of food and subsequent peristalsis in the stomach or in the duodenum cause reflex contractions of the colon. These reflexes are brought about by the enteric nervous system; the intestines do have a mind of their own. Elimination of feces is accomplished by the **defecation reflex**, a spinal cord reflex that may be controlled voluntarily. The rectum is usually empty until

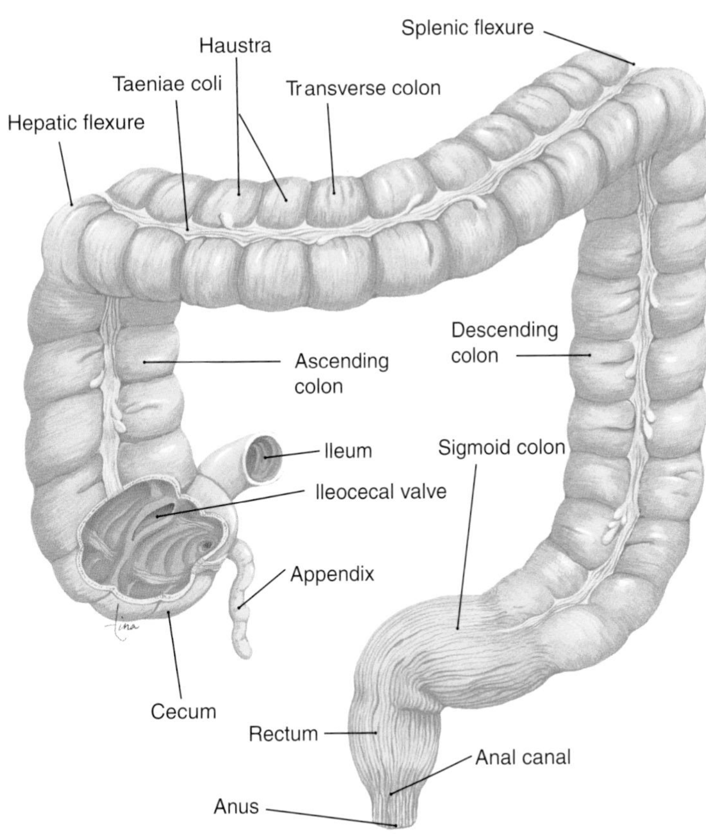

Figure 16–9 The large intestine shown in anterior view. The term *flexure* means a turn or bend.

QUESTION: What is the function of the ileocecal valve?

Box 16–4 | INFANT BOTULISM

Botulism is most often acquired from food. When the spores of the botulism bacteria (ubiquitous in soil) are in an anaerobic (without oxygen) environment such as a can of food, they germinate into active bacteria that produce a neurotoxin. If people ingest food containing this toxin, they will develop the paralysis that is characteristic of botulism.

For infants younger than 1 year of age, however, and especially those 6 months or younger, ingestion of just the bacterial spores may be harmful. The infant's stomach does not produce much HCl, so ingested botulism spores may not be destroyed. Of equal importance, the infant's normal colon flora is not yet established. Without the normal population of colon bacteria to provide competition, spores of the botulism bacteria may germinate and produce their toxin.

An affected infant becomes lethargic and weak (when first recognized in 1976, the condition was called "floppy-baby syndrome"); paralysis may progress slowly or rapidly. Treatment (antitoxin) is available, but may be delayed if botulism is not suspected. Many cases of infant botulism have been traced to honey that was found to contain botulism spores. Such spores are not harmful to older children and adults, who have a normal colon flora that prevents the botulism bacteria from becoming established.

peristalsis of the colon pushes feces into it. The wall of the rectum is stretched by the entry of feces, and this is the stimulus for the defecation reflex.

Stretch receptors in the smooth muscle layer of the rectum generate sensory impulses that travel to the sacral spinal cord. The returning motor impulses cause the smooth muscle of the rectum to contract. Surrounding the anus is the **internal anal sphincter**, which is made of smooth muscle. As part of the reflex, this sphincter relaxes, permitting defecation to take place.

The **external anal sphincter** is made of skeletal muscle and surrounds the internal anal sphincter (Fig. 16–10). If defecation must be delayed, the external sphincter may be voluntarily contracted to close the anus. The awareness of the need to defecate passes as the stretch receptors of the rectum adapt. These receptors will be stimulated again when the next wave of peristalsis reaches the rectum (see Box 16–5: Fiber).

OTHER FUNCTIONS OF THE LIVER

The **liver** is a remarkable organ, and only the brain is capable of a greater variety of functions. The liver cells (hepatocytes) produce many enzymes that catalyze many different chemical reactions. These reactions are the functions of the liver. As blood flows through the sinusoids (capillaries) of the liver (see Fig. 16–6), materials are removed by the liver cells, and the products of the liver cells are secreted into the blood. Some of the liver functions will already be familiar to you. Others are mentioned again and discussed in more detail in the next chapter. Because the liver has such varied effects on so many body systems, we will use the categories below to summarize the liver functions.

1. **Carbohydrate metabolism**—As you know, the liver regulates the blood glucose level. Excess glucose is converted to glycogen (glycogenesis) when blood glucose is high; the hormones insulin and cortisol facilitate this

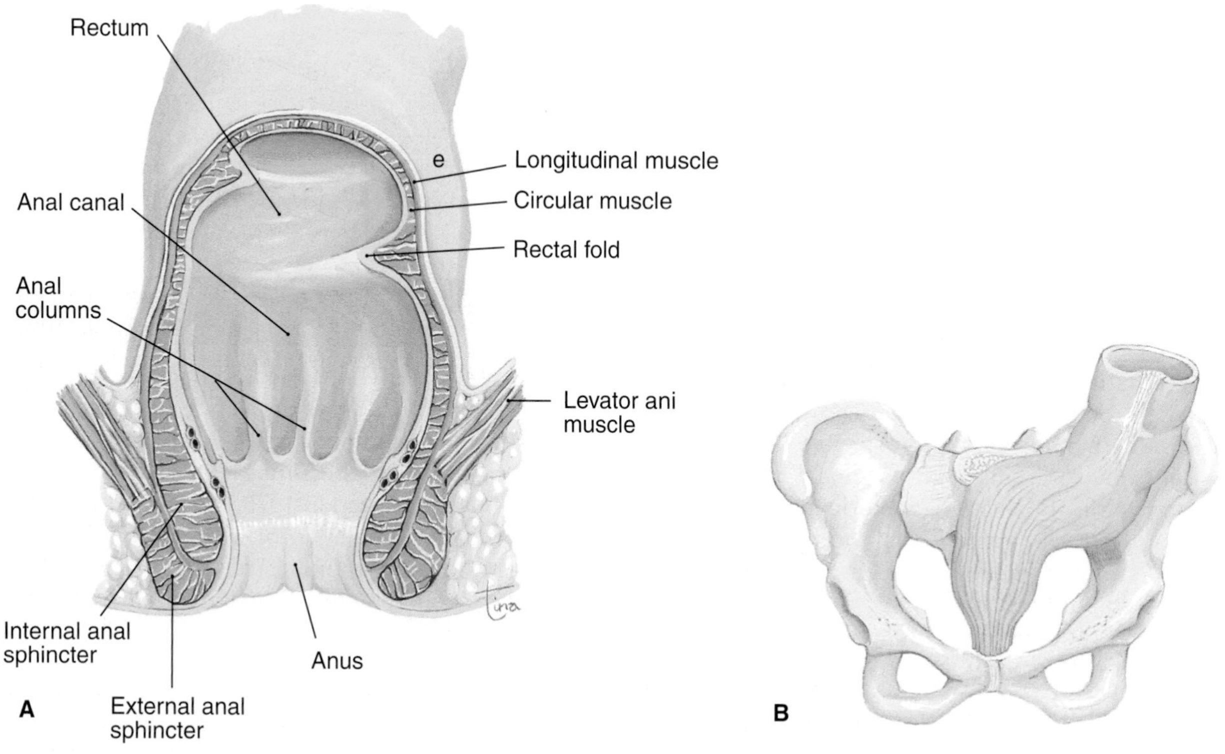

Figure 16–10 (**A**) Internal and external anal sphincters shown in a frontal section through the lower rectum and anal canal. (**B**) Position of rectum and anal canal relative to pelvic bone.

QUESTION: The internal anal sphincter is a continuation of which part of the rectum?

Box 16–5 | FIBER

Fiber is a term we use to refer to the organic materials in the cell walls of plants. These are mainly cellulose, pectins, and other complex carbohydrates. The role of dietary fiber and the possible benefits that a high-fiber diet may provide are currently the focus of a great deal of research, especially because fiber is the food of much of our intestinal microbiota, our bacterial flora. It is important to differentiate what is known from what is, at present, merely speculation.

Many studies have shown that populations (large groups of people, especially those of different cultures) who consume high-fiber diets tend to have a lower frequency of certain diseases. These include diverticulitis, colon cancer, coronary artery disease, diabetes, and hypertension. Such diseases are much more common in populations whose diets are low in vegetables, fruits, and whole grains, and high in meat and processed foods. In contrast, other studies have shown no protective effect of fiber against colon cancer. What we can say for sure is that fiber is not the only factor involved.

Claims that high-fiber diets directly lower blood levels of cholesterol and fats are not supported by clinical or experimental studies. One possible explanation may be that a person whose diet consists largely of high-fiber foods simply eats less of the foods high in fat, and this is the reason for that person's lower blood levels of fats and cholesterol. However, in addition to the possible benefits of fiber (including keeping our microbiota well fed), a diet that includes significant quantities of vegetables and fruits provides the body with important amounts of vitamins and minerals.

process. During hypoglycemia or stress situations, glycogen is converted back to glucose (glycogenolysis) to raise the blood glucose level. Epinephrine and glucagon are the hormones that facilitate this process.

The liver also changes other monosaccharides to glucose. Fructose and galactose, for example, are end products of the digestion of sucrose and lactose. Because most cells, however, cannot readily use fructose and galactose as energy sources, they are converted by the liver to glucose, which is easily used by cells.

2. **Amino acid metabolism**—The liver regulates blood levels of amino acids on the basis of tissue needs for protein synthesis. Of the 20 different amino acids needed for the production of human proteins, the liver is able to synthesize 12, called the **non-essential amino acids**. The chemical process by which this is done is called **transamination**, the transfer of an amino group (NH_2) from an amino acid present in excess to a free carbon chain that forms a complete, new amino acid molecule. The other 8 amino acids, which the liver cannot synthesize, are called the **essential amino acids**. In this case, "essential" means that the amino acids must be supplied by our food, because the liver cannot manufacture them. Similarly, "non-essential" means that the amino acids do not have to be supplied in our food because the liver *can* make them. All 20 amino acids are required in order to make our body proteins.

   Excess amino acids, those not needed right away for protein synthesis, cannot be stored. However, they do serve another useful purpose. By the process of **deamination**, which also occurs in the liver, the NH_2 group is removed from an amino acid and the remaining carbon chain may be converted to a simple carbohydrate molecule or to fat. Thus, excess amino acids are utilized for energy production: either for immediate energy or for the potential energy stored as fat in adipose tissue. The NH_2 groups that were detached from the original amino acids are combined to form urea, a waste product that will be removed from the blood by the kidneys and excreted in urine.

3. **Lipid metabolism**—The liver forms lipoproteins, which as their name tells us, are molecules of lipids and proteins, for the transport of fats in the blood to other tissues. The liver also synthesizes cholesterol and excretes excess cholesterol into bile to be eliminated in feces.

   Fatty acids are a potential source of energy, but in order to be used in cell respiration they must be broken down to smaller molecules. In the process of **beta-oxidation**, the long carbon chains of fatty acids are split into two-carbon molecules called acetyl groups, which are simple carbohydrates. These acetyl groups may be used by the liver cells to produce ATP or may be combined to form ketones to be transported in the blood to other cells. These other cells then use the ketones to produce ATP in cell respiration.

4. **Synthesis of plasma proteins**—This is a liver function that you will probably remember from Chapter 11. The liver synthesizes many of the proteins that circulate in the blood. **Albumin**, the most abundant plasma protein, helps maintain blood volume by pulling tissue fluid into capillaries.

   The **clotting factors** are also produced by the liver. These, as you recall, include prothrombin, fibrinogen, and Factor 8, which circulate in the blood until needed in the chemical clotting mechanism. The liver also synthesizes alpha and beta **globulins**, which are proteins that serve as carriers for other molecules, such as fats, in the blood.

5. **Formation of bilirubin**—This is another familiar function: The liver contains fixed macrophages that phagocytize old red blood cells (RBCs). Bilirubin is then formed from the heme portion of the hemoglobin. The liver also removes from the blood the bilirubin formed in the spleen and red bone marrow and excretes it into bile to be eliminated in feces.

6. **Phagocytosis by Kupffer cells**—The fixed macrophages of the liver are called **Kupffer cells** (or stellate reticuloendothelial cells). Besides destroying old RBCs, Kupffer cells phagocytize pathogens or other foreign material that circulate through the liver. Many of the bacteria that get to the liver come from the colon. These bacteria are normal residents of the colon but would be very harmful elsewhere in the body. The bacteria that enter the blood with the water absorbed by the colon are carried to the liver by way of portal circulation. The Kupffer cells in the liver phagocytize and destroy these bacteria, removing them from the blood before the blood returns to the heart and is pumped to the lungs.

7. **Storage**—The liver stores the fat-soluble vitamins A, D, E, and K, as well as the water-soluble vitamin B_{12}. Up to a 6- to 12-month supply of vitamins A and D may be stored, and beef or chicken liver is an excellent dietary source of these vitamins.

   Also stored by the liver are the minerals iron and copper. You already know that iron is needed for hemoglobin and myoglobin and enables these proteins to bond to oxygen. Copper (as well as iron) is part of some of the proteins needed for cell respiration and is part of some of the enzymes necessary for hemoglobin synthesis.

8. **Detoxification**—The liver is capable of synthesizing enzymes that will detoxify harmful substances, that is, change them to less harmful ones. Alcohol, for example, is changed to acetate, which is a two-carbon molecule (an acetyl group) that can be used in cell respiration.

   Medications are all potentially toxic, but the liver produces enzymes that break them down or change them. When given in a proper dosage, a medication exerts its therapeutic effect but is then changed to less active substances that are usually excreted by the kidneys. An overdose of a drug means that there is too much of it for the liver to detoxify in a given time, and the drug will remain in the body with possibly harmful effects. This is why alcohol should never be consumed when taking medication. Such a combination may cause the liver's detoxification ability to be overworked and ineffective, with the result that both the alcohol and the medication will remain toxic for a longer time. Barbiturates taken as sleeping pills after consumption of alcohol have too often proved fatal for just this reason.

   Ammonia is a toxic substance produced by the bacteria in the colon. Because it is soluble in water, some ammonia is absorbed into the blood, but it is carried first to the liver by portal circulation. The liver converts ammonia to urea, a less toxic substance, before the ammonia can circulate and damage other organs, especially the brain. The urea formed is excreted by the kidneys (see Box 16–6: Hepatitis).

AGING AND THE DIGESTIVE SYSTEM

Many changes can be expected in the aging digestive system. The sense of taste becomes less acute, less saliva is produced, and there is greater likelihood of periodontal disease and loss of teeth. Secretions are reduced throughout the digestive system, and the effectiveness of peristalsis diminishes. Indigestion may become more frequent, especially if the LES loses its tone, and there is a greater chance of esophageal damage. In the colon, diverticula may form; these bubble-like outpouchings of the weakened wall of the colon may be asymptomatic or become infected. Intestinal obstruction, of the large or small bowel, occurs with greater frequency among the elderly. Sluggish peristalsis contributes to constipation, which in turn may contribute to the formation of hemorrhoids. The risk of oral cancer or colon cancer also increases with age.

The liver usually continues to function adequately even well into old age, unless damaged by pathogens such as the hepatitis viruses or by toxins such as alcohol. There is a greater tendency for gallstones to form, perhaps necessitating removal of the gallbladder. Inflammation of the

Box 16–6 | HEPATITIS

Hepatitis is inflammation of the liver caused by any of several viruses. The most common of these hepatitis viruses have been designated A, B, and C, although there are others. Symptoms of hepatitis include anorexia, nausea, fatigue, and possibly jaundice. Severity of disease ranges from very mild (even asymptomatic) to fatal. Thousands of cases of hepatitis occur in the United States every year, and although liver inflammation is common to all of them, the three hepatitis viruses have different modes of transmission and different consequences for affected people.

Hepatitis A is an intestinal virus that is spread by the fecal–oral route. Food contaminated by the hands of people with mild cases is the usual vehicle of transmission, although shellfish harvested from water contaminated with human sewage are another possible source of this virus. Hepatitis A is most often mild, recovery provides lifelong immunity, and the carrier state is not known to occur. A vaccine is available, but people who have been exposed to hepatitis A may receive gamma globulin by injection; that is, antibodies to provide immediate protection and prevent the disease.

Hepatitis B is contracted by exposure to the body fluids of an infected person; these fluids include blood and semen. Hepatitis B may be severe or even fatal, and approximately 10% of those who recover become carriers of the virus. Possible consequences of the carrier state are chronic hepatitis progressing to cirrhosis or primary liver cancer. Of equal importance, carriers are sources of the virus for others, especially their sexual partners.

A vaccine is available for hepatitis B; it is one of the standard ones for infants, and for health-care workers who have contact with blood, even only occasional contact. Other potential recipients of the vaccine are the sexual partners of carriers.

The **hepatitis C** virus is also present in body fluids and is spread by blood or mucous membrane contact. Most people develop chronic disease, but many may remain asymptomatic for years after being infected. With active disease the virus may cause liver failure. The only therapy then is a liver transplant.

It is important for health-care personnel and their patients to know that these types of hepatitis are not spread by blood transfusions. Donated blood is tested for all three viruses.

gallbladder (cholecystitis) is also more frequent in older adults. In the absence of specific diseases, the pancreas usually functions well, although acute pancreatitis of unknown cause is somewhat more likely in elderly people.

SUMMARY

The processes of the digestion of food and the absorption of nutrients enable the body to use complex food molecules for many purposes. Much of the food we eat literally becomes part of us. The body synthesizes proteins and lipids for the growth and repair of tissues and produces enzymes to catalyze all of the reactions that contribute to homeostasis. Some of our food provides the energy required for growth, repair, movement, sensation, and thinking. In the next chapter we will discuss the chemical basis of energy production from food and consider the relationship of energy production to the maintenance of body temperature.

STUDY OUTLINE

Function of the Digestive System—to break down food into simple chemicals that can be absorbed into the blood and lymph and utilized by cells

Divisions of the Digestive System

1. Alimentary tube—oral cavity, pharynx, esophagus, stomach, small intestine, large intestine. Digestion takes place in the oral cavity, stomach, and small intestine.

2. Accessory organs—salivary glands, teeth, tongue, liver, gallbladder, and pancreas. Each contributes to digestion.

Types of Digestion

1. Mechanical—breaks food into smaller pieces to increase the surface area for the action of enzymes.
2. Chemical—enzymes break down complex organics into simpler organics and inorganics; each enzyme is specific for the food it will digest.

End Products of Digestion

1. Carbohydrates are digested to monosaccharides.
2. Proteins are digested to amino acids.
3. Fats are digested to fatty acids and glycerol.
4. Other end products are vitamins, minerals, and water.

Oral Cavity—food enters by way of the mouth

1. Teeth and tongue break up food and mix it with saliva.
2. Tooth structure (see Fig. 16–2)
   a. Enamel covers the crown and provides a hard chewing surface.
   b. Dentin is within the enamel and forms the roots.
   c. The pulp cavity contains blood vessels and endings of the trigeminal nerve.
   d. The periodontal membrane produces cement to anchor the tooth in the jawbone.
3. The tongue is skeletal muscle innervated by the hypoglossal nerves. Papillae on the upper surface contain taste buds (facial and glossopharyngeal nerves). Functions: taste, keeps food between the teeth when chewing, elevates to push food backward for swallowing.
4. Salivary glands—parotid, submandibular, and sublingual (see Fig. 16–3); ducts take saliva to the oral cavity; cranial nerves are the facial and glossopharyngeal; parasympathetic impulses increase secretion.
5. Saliva—(see Tables 16–1 and 16–2).
   a. Amylase digests starch to maltose.
   b. Water dissolves food for tasting and moistens food for swallowing
   c. Lysozyme inhibits the growth of bacteria.

Pharynx—food passageway from the oral cavity to the esophagus

1. No digestion takes place.
2. Contraction of pharyngeal muscles is part of swallowing reflex, regulated by the medulla.

Esophagus—food passageway from pharynx to stomach

1. No digestion takes place.
2. Lower esophageal sphincter (LES) at junction with stomach prevents backup of stomach contents.

Structural Layers of the Alimentary Tube (see Fig. 16–4)

1. Mucosa (lining)—made of epithelial tissue that produces the digestive secretions; lymph nodules contain macrophages to phagocytize pathogens that penetrate the mucosa; thin layer of smooth muscle to ripple the epithelium.
2. Submucosa—areolar connective tissue with blood vessels and lymphatic vessels; Meissner's plexus is a nerve network that innervates the mucosa, part of the enteric nervous system that extends the entire length of the alimentary tube.
3. External muscle layer—typically an inner circular layer and an outer longitudinal layer of smooth muscle; function is mechanical digestion and peristalsis; innervated by Auerbach's plexus, part of the enteric nervous system; sympathetic impulses decrease motility; parasympathetic impulses increase motility.
4. Serosa—outermost layer; above the diaphragm is fibrous connective tissue; below the diaphragm is the mesentery (serous). The peritoneum (serous) lines the abdominal cavity; serous fluid prevents friction between the serous layers.

Stomach—in upper left abdominal quadrant; a muscular sac that extends from the esophagus to the small intestine (see Fig. 16–5)

1. Reservoir for food; churns it to chyme; begins the digestion of protein.
2. Gastric juice is secreted by gastric pits (see Tables 16–1 and 16–2).
   a. Pepsin converts proteins to polypeptides; secreted by chief cells.

b. HCl (pH 1–2) activates pepsin, destroys pathogens; secreted by parietal cells.
c. Mucus coats the lining, prevents erosion; secreted by mucous cells.
d. The hormone gastrin increases secretion of gastric juice; secreted by G cells.

3. The pyloric sphincter at the junction with the duodenum prevents backup of intestinal contents.

Liver—consists of two lobes in the upper right and center of the abdominal cavity (see Figs. 16–1 and 16–6)

1. Functional unit is the hexagonal liver lobule: liver cells, sinusoids, branches of the hepatic artery and portal vein, and bile ducts.
2. The only digestive secretion is bile; the hepatic duct takes bile out of the liver and unites with the cystic duct of the gallbladder to form the common bile duct to the duodenum.
3. Bile salts emulsify fats, a type of mechanical digestion (see Table 16–1).
4. Excess cholesterol and bilirubin are excreted by the liver into bile.

Gallbladder—on undersurface of right lobe of liver (see Fig. 16–6)

1. Stores and concentrates bile until needed in the duodenum (see Table 16–2).
2. The cystic duct joins the hepatic duct to form the common bile duct.

Pancreas—in upper left abdominal quadrant between the duodenum and the spleen (see Fig. 16–1, Tables 16–1 and 16–2).

1. Pancreatic juice is secreted by acini, carried by pancreatic duct to the common bile duct to the duodenum (see Fig. 16–7).
2. Enzyme pancreatic juice contains enzymes for the digestion of all three food types.
   a. Amylase digests starch to maltose.
   b. Trypsin digests polypeptides to peptides.
   c. Lipase digests emulsified fats to fatty acids and glycerol.
3. Bicarbonate pancreatic juice neutralizes HCl from the stomach in the duodenum.

Small Intestine—coiled within the center of the abdominal cavity (see Fig. 16–1); extends from stomach to colon

1. Duodenum—first 10 inches; the common bile duct brings in bile and pancreatic juice. Jejunum (8 feet) and ileum (11 feet).
2. Enzymes secreted by the intestinal glands complete digestion (see Tables 16–1 and 16–2).
   a. Peptidases digest peptides to amino acids.
   b. Sucrase, maltase, and lactase digest disaccharides to monosaccharides.
3. The hormones cholecystokinin and secretin are produced by enteroendocrine cells; these hormones influence the liver, gall bladder, and secretion of the pancreas.
4. Surface area for absorption is increased by plica circulares, villi, and microvilli (see Fig. 16–8); microvilli are the brush border.
5. The villi contain capillary networks for the absorption of water-soluble nutrients: monosaccharides, amino acids, vitamin C and the B vitamins, minerals, and water. Blood from the small intestine goes to the liver first by way of portal circulation.
6. The villi contain lacteals (lymph capillaries) for the absorption of fat-soluble nutrients: vitamins A, D, E, and K, fatty acids, and glycerol, which are combined to form chylomicrons. Lymph from the small intestine is carried back to the blood in the left subclavian vein.

Large Intestine (colon)—extends from the small intestine to the anus

1. Colon—parts (see Fig. 16–9): cecum, ascending colon, transverse colon, descending colon, sigmoid colon, rectum, anal canal.
2. Ileocecal valve—at the junction of the cecum and ileum; prevents backup of fecal material into the small intestine.
3. Colon—functions: absorption of water, minerals, vitamins; elimination of undigestible material.
4. Normal flora—the microbiota of the colon, the bacteria that produce vitamins, especially vitamin K, inhibit the growth of pathogens, and have other beneficial functions.

5. Defecation reflex—stimulus: stretching of the rectum when peristalsis propels feces into it. Sensory impulses go to the sacral spinal cord, and motor impulses return to the smooth muscle of the rectum, which contracts. The internal anal sphincter relaxes to permit defecation. Voluntary control is provided by the external anal sphincter, made of skeletal muscle (see Fig. 16–10).

Liver—other functions

1. Carbohydrate metabolism—excess glucose is stored in the form of glycogen and converted back to glucose during hypoglycemia; fructose and galactose are changed to glucose.
2. Amino acid metabolism—the non-essential amino acids are synthesized by transamination; excess amino acids are changed to carbohydrates or fats by deamination; the amino groups are converted to urea and excreted by the kidneys.
3. Lipid metabolism—formation of lipoproteins for transport of fats in the blood; synthesis of cholesterol; excretion of excess cholesterol into bile; beta-oxidation of fatty acids to form two-carbon acetyl groups for energy use.
4. Synthesis of plasma proteins—albumin to help maintain blood volume; clotting factors for blood clotting; alpha and beta globulins as carrier molecules.
5. Formation of bilirubin—old RBCs are phagocytized, and bilirubin is formed from the heme and put into bile to be eliminated in feces.
6. Phagocytosis by Kupffer cells—fixed macrophages; phagocytize old RBCs and bacteria, especially bacteria absorbed by the colon.
7. Storage—vitamins: B_{12}, A, D, E, and K, and the minerals iron and copper.
8. Detoxification—liver enzymes change potential poisons to less harmful substances; examples of toxic substances are alcohol, medications, and ammonia absorbed by the colon.

REVIEW QUESTIONS

1. Name the organs of the alimentary tube, and describe the location of each. Name the accessory digestive organs, and describe the location of each. (pp. 412–414, 417–422, 425)
2. Explain the purpose of mechanical digestion, and give two examples. Explain the purpose of chemical digestion, and give two examples. (pp. 410–412)
3. Name the end products of digestion, and explain how each is absorbed in the small intestine. (pp. 412, 425)
4. Explain the function of teeth and tongue, salivary amylase, enamel of teeth, lysozyme, and water of saliva. (pp. 412–413)
5. Describe the function of the pharynx, esophagus, and lower esophageal sphincter. (pp. 413–414)
6. Name and describe the four layers of the alimentary tube. (pp. 414–415, 417)
7. State the two general functions of the stomach and the function of the pyloric sphincter. Explain the function of pepsin, HCl, and mucus. (pp. 417–418)
8. Describe the general functions of the small intestine, and name the three parts. Describe the structures that increase the surface area of the small intestine. (pp. 419, 424)
9. Explain how the liver, gallbladder, and pancreas contribute to digestion. (pp. 419, 421–422)
10. Describe the internal structure of a villus, and explain how its structure is related to absorption. (p. 425)
11. Name the parts of the large intestine, and describe the function of the ileocecal valve. (p. 425)
12. Describe the functions of the colon and of the microbiota of the colon. (pp. 425–426)
13. With respect to the defecation reflex, explain the stimulus, the part of the CNS directly involved, the effector muscle, the function of the internal anal sphincter, and the voluntary control possible. (pp. 426, 428)
14. Name the vitamins and minerals stored in the liver and the substances excreted by the liver into bile. Name the fixed macrophages of the liver, and explain their function. (p. 430)
15. Describe how the liver regulates blood glucose level. Explain the purpose of the processes of deamination and transamination. (pp. 428–429)
16. Name the plasma proteins produced by the liver, and state the function of each. (p. 430)

FOR FURTHER THOUGHT

1. Many people with GERD take proton-pump inhibitors, medications that reduce stomach acid. Why should these people be especially careful about what they eat or drink?
2. The colon does not have villi as part of its mucosa. Explain why villi are not necessary.
3. Food remains in the stomach for several hours. Passage of food through the small intestine also requires several hours. These two organs have very different shapes. Explain why they are able to retain food for so long, for efficient digestion and absorption.
4. Diarrhea can be unpleasant, but does have a purpose. Explain, and state the disadvantages as well.
5. Explain how a spinal cord transection at the level of T10 will affect the defecation reflex.
6. Look at Question Figure 16–A: Hormones of the duodenum. The passage of food from the stomach into the duodenum (white arrows) stimulates the secretion of two hormones into the capillaries of the duodenum (gray arrows to capillary network). The target organs of these two hormones are indicated by orange arrows from the duodenum. Name each hormone (a letter) and its effects on its target organs (the numbers).

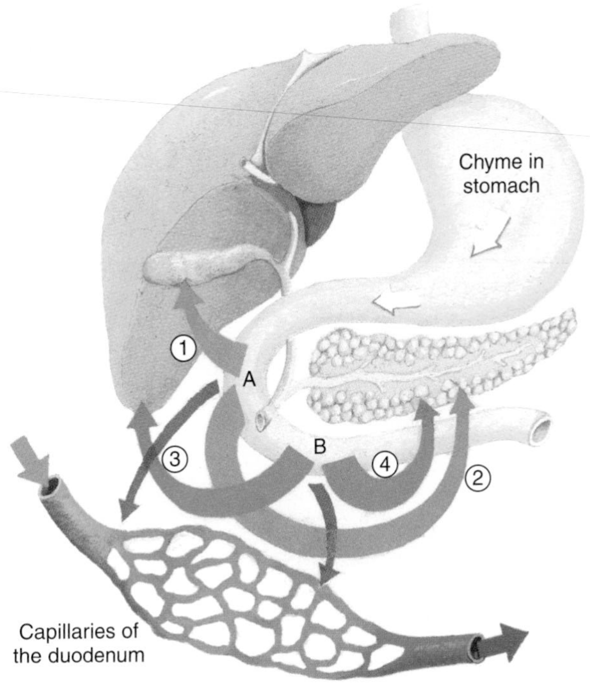

QUESTION FIGURE 16–A: Hormones of the duodenum

CHAPTER

Body Temperature and Metabolism

STUDENT OBJECTIVES

- State the normal range of human body temperature.
- Explain how cell respiration produces heat and the factors that affect heat production.
- Describe the pathways of heat loss through the skin and respiratory tract.
- Explain why the hypothalamus is called the "thermostat" of the body.
- Describe the mechanisms to increase heat loss.
- Describe the mechanisms to conserve heat.
- Explain the cause of a fever and the advantages and disadvantages of a fever.
- Define metabolism, anabolism, and catabolism.
- Describe what happens to a glucose molecule during the three stages of cell respiration.
- State what happens to each of the products of cell respiration.
- Explain how amino acids and fats may be used for energy production.
- Describe the synthesis uses for glucose, amino acids, and fats.
- Explain what is meant by metabolic rate and kilocalories.
- Describe the factors that affect a person's metabolic rate.

NEW TERMINOLOGY

Anabolism *(an-**NAB**-uh-lizm)*
Catabolism *(kuh-**TAB**-uh-lizm)*
Coenzyme *(koh-**EN**-zime)*
Conduction *(kon-**DUK**-shun)*
Convection *(kon-**VEK**-shun)*
Cytochromes *(**SIGH**-toh-krohms)*
Endogenous pyrogen *(en-**DOJ**-en-us **PYE**-roh-jen)*
Fever *(**FEE**-ver)*
Glycolysis *(gly-**KAHL**-ah-sis)*
Kilocalorie *(KILL-oh-**KAL**-oh-ree)*
Krebs cycle *(KREBS **SIGH**-kuhl)*
Pyrogen *(**PYE**-roh-jen)*
Radiation *(RAY-dee-**AY**-shun)*
Vitamins *(**VY**-tah-mins)*

RELATED CLINICAL TERMINOLOGY

Antipyretic *(AN-tigh-pye-**RET**-ik)*
Basal metabolic rate *(**BAY**-zuhl met-ah-**BAHL**-ik RAYT)*
Frostbite *(**FRAWST**-bite)*
Heat exhaustion *(HEET ig-**ZAWS**-chun)*
Heat stroke *(HEET STROHK)*
Hypothermia *(HIGH-poh-**THER**-mee-ah)*

*Terms that appear in **bold type** in the chapter text are defined in the glossary, which begins on page 603.*

CHAPTER OUTLINE

During every moment of our lives, our cells are breaking down food molecules to obtain ATP (adenosine triphosphate) for energy-requiring cellular processes. Naturally, we are not aware of the process of cell respiration, but we may be aware of one of the products—energy in the form of heat. The human body is indeed warm, and its temperature is regulated very precisely. Though we cannot stand barefoot on the ice of Antarctica for months in winter, as penguins do, we can adapt to and survive a wide range of environmental temperatures.

This chapter discusses the regulation of body temperature and also discusses **metabolism**, which is the total of all reactions that take place within the body. These reactions include the energy-releasing ones of cell respiration and energy-requiring ones such as protein synthesis or DNA synthesis for mitosis. As you will see, body temperature and metabolism are inseparable.

BODY TEMPERATURE

The normal range of human body temperature is 96.5° to 99.5°F (36° to 38°C), with an average oral temperature of 98.6°F (37°C). (A 1992 study suggested a slightly lower average oral temperature: 98.2° or 36.8°. But everyone seems to prefer the "traditional" average temperature.) Within a 24-hour period, an individual's temperature fluctuates 1° to 2°, with the lowest temperatures occurring during sleep.

At either end of the age spectrum, however, temperature regulation may not be as precise as it is in older children or younger adults. Infants have more surface area (skin) relative to volume and are likely to lose heat more rapidly. In the elderly, the mechanisms that maintain body temperature may not function as efficiently as they once did, and changes in environmental temperature may not be compensated for as quickly or effectively. This is especially important to remember when caring for patients who are very young or very old.

HEAT PRODUCTION

Cell respiration, the process that releases energy from food to produce ATP, also produces heat as one of its energy products. Although cell respiration takes place constantly, many factors influence the rate of this process:

1. The hormone **thyroxine** (and T_3), produced by the thyroid gland, increases the rate of cell respiration and heat production in all of the body tissues. The secretion of thyroxine is regulated by the body's rate of energy production, the metabolic rate itself. (See Chapter 10 for a discussion of the feedback mechanism involving the hypothalamus and anterior pituitary gland and Chapter 1 for an illustration.) When the metabolic rate decreases, the thyroid gland is stimulated to secrete more thyroxine. As thyroxine increases the rate of cell respiration and raises the metabolic rate, a negative feedback mechanism inhibits further secretion until metabolic rate decreases again. Thus, thyroxine is secreted whenever there is a need for increased cell respiration and is probably the most important regulator of day-to-day energy production.
2. In stress situations, **epinephrine** and norepinephrine are secreted by the adrenal medulla, and the **sympathetic** nervous system becomes more active. Epinephrine increases the rate of cell respiration, especially in organs such as the heart, skeletal muscles, and liver. Sympathetic stimulation also increases the activity of these organs. The increased production of ATP to meet the demands of the stress situation also means that more heat will be produced.
3. Organs that are normally active (producing ATP) are significant sources of heat when the body is at rest. The skeletal muscles, for example, are usually in a state of slight contraction called muscle tone. Because even slight contraction requires ATP, the muscles are also producing heat. This amounts to about 25% of the total body heat at rest and much more during exercise, when more ATP is produced.

   The liver is another organ that is continually active, producing ATP to supply energy for its many functions. As a result, the liver produces as much as 20% of the total body heat at rest. The heat produced by these active organs is dispersed throughout the body by the blood. As the relatively cooler blood flows through organs such as the muscles and liver, the heat they produce is transferred to the blood, warming it. The warmed blood circulates to other areas of the body, distributing this heat.
4. The intake of food also increases heat production because the metabolic activity of the digestive tract is increased. Heat is generated as the digestive organs produce ATP for peristalsis and for the synthesis of digestive enzymes.
5. Changes in body temperature also have an effect on metabolic rate and heat production. This becomes clinically important when a person has a **fever**, an abnormally high body temperature. The higher temperature increases the metabolic rate, which increases heat production and elevates body temperature further.

Thus, a high fever may trigger a vicious cycle of ever-increasing heat production. Fever is discussed later in this chapter.

The factors that affect heat production are summarized in Table 17–1.

HEAT LOSS

The pathways of heat loss from the body are the skin, the respiratory tract, and, to a lesser extent, the urinary and digestive tracts.

Heat Loss through the Skin

Because the skin covers the body, most body heat is lost from the skin to the environment. When the environment is cooler than body temperature (as it usually is), heat loss is unavoidable. The amount of heat that is lost is determined by blood flow through the skin and by the activity of sweat glands.

Blood flow through the skin influences the amount of heat lost by the processes of radiation, conduction, and convection. **Radiation** means that heat from the body is transferred to cooler objects not touching the skin, much as a radiator warms the contents of a room (radiation starts to become less effective when the environmental temperature rises above 88°F). **Conduction** is the loss of heat to cooler air or objects, such as clothing, that touch the skin. **Convection** means that air currents move the warmer air away from the skin surface and facilitate the loss of heat; this is why a fan makes us feel cooler on hot days. Loss of heat by convection also gives us the "wind chill factor" we hear about in winter. A cold day that is windy will feel colder than a cold day when the air is still, because the wind blows the slightly warmer air surrounding the body away, replacing it with colder air.

As you may recall from Chapter 5, the temperature of the skin and the subsequent loss of heat are determined by blood flow through the skin. The arterioles in the dermis may constrict or dilate to decrease or increase blood flow. In a cold environment, **vasoconstriction** decreases blood flow through the dermis and thereby decreases heat loss. In a warm environment, **vasodilation** in the dermis increases blood flow to the body surface and loss of heat to the environment.

The other mechanism by which heat is lost from the skin is sweating. The **eccrine sweat glands** secrete sweat (water) onto the skin surface, and excess body heat evaporates the sweat. Think of running water into a hot frying pan; the pan is rapidly cooled as its heat vaporizes the water. Although sweating is not quite as dramatic (no visible formation of steam), the principle is just the same.

Sweating is most efficient when the humidity of the surrounding air is low. Humidity is the percentage of the maximum amount of water vapor the atmosphere can contain. A humidity reading of 90% means that the air is already 90% saturated with water vapor and can hold little more. In such a situation, sweat does not readily evaporate, but instead remains on the skin even as more sweat

Table 17–1 | FACTORS THAT AFFECT HEAT PRODUCTION

FACTOR	EFFECT
Thyroxine	The most important regulator of day-to-day metabolism; increases use of foods for ATP production, thereby increasing heat production
Epinephrine and sympathetic stimulation	Important in stress situations; increases the metabolic activity of many organs; increases ATP and heat production
Skeletal muscles	Normal muscle tone requires ATP; the heat produced is about 25% of the total body heat at rest
Liver	Always metabolically active; produces as much as 20% of total body heat at rest
Food intake	Increases activity of the GI tract; increases ATP and heat production
Higher body temperature	Increases metabolic rate, which increases heat production, which further increases metabolic rate and heat production; may become detrimental during high fevers

is secreted. If the humidity is 40%, however, the air can hold a great deal more water vapor, and sweat evaporates quickly from the skin surface, removing excess body heat. In air that is completely dry, a person who remains well hydrated may tolerate a temperature of 200°F for nearly 1 hour.

Although sweating is a very effective mechanism of heat loss, it does have a disadvantage in that it requires the loss of water in order to also lose heat. Water loss during sweating may rapidly lead to dehydration, and the water lost must be replaced by drinking fluids (see Box 17–1: Heat-Related Disorders).

Small amounts of heat are also lost in what is called "insensible water loss." Because the skin is not like a plastic bag, but is somewhat permeable to water, a small amount of water diffuses through the skin and is evaporated by body heat. Compared with sweating, however, insensible water loss is a minor source of heat loss.

Heat Loss through the Respiratory Tract

Heat is lost from the respiratory tract as the warmth of the respiratory mucosa evaporates some water from the living epithelial surface. The water vapor formed is exhaled, and a small amount of heat is lost.

Animals such as dogs that do not have numerous sweat glands often pant in warm weather. Panting is the rapid movement of air into and out of the upper respiratory passages, where the warm surfaces evaporate large amounts of water. In this way the animal may lose large amounts of heat.

Heat Loss through the Urinary and Digestive Tracts

When excreted, urine and feces are at body temperature, and their elimination results in a very small amount of heat loss.

The pathways of heat loss are summarized in Table 17–2.

REGULATION OF BODY TEMPERATURE

The **hypothalamus** is responsible for the regulation of body temperature and is considered the "thermostat" of the body. As the thermostat, the hypothalamus maintains the "setting" of body temperature by balancing heat production and heat loss to keep the body at the set temperature.

To do this, the hypothalamus must receive information about the temperature within the body and about the environmental temperature. Specialized neurons of the hypothalamus detect changes in the temperature of the blood that flows through the brain. The temperature receptors in the skin provide information about the external temperature changes to which the body is exposed. The hypothalamus then integrates this sensory information and promotes the necessary responses to maintain body temperature within the normal range.

Box 17–1 | HEAT-RELATED DISORDERS

Heat exhaustion is caused by excessive sweating with loss of water and salts, especially NaCl. The affected person feels very weak, and the skin is usually cool and clammy (moist). Body temperature is normal or slightly below normal, the pulse is often rapid and weak, and blood pressure may be low because of fluid loss. Other symptoms may include dizziness, vomiting, and muscle cramps. Treatment involves rest and consumption of salty fluids or fruit juices (in small amounts at frequent intervals).

Heat stroke is a life-threatening condition that may affect elderly or chronically ill people on hot, humid days, or otherwise healthy people who exercise too strenuously during such weather. High humidity makes sweating an ineffective mechanism of heat loss, but in high heat the sweating process continues. As fluid loss increases, sweating stops to preserve body fluid, and body temperature rises rapidly (above 105°F, possibly as high as 110°F).

The classic symptom of heat stroke is hot, dry skin. The affected person often loses consciousness, reflecting the destructive effect of such a high body temperature on the brain. Treatment should involve hospitalization so that IV fluids may be administered and body temperature lowered under medical supervision. A first-aid measure would be the application of cool (not ice cold) water to as much of the skin as possible. Fluids should never be forced on an unconscious person because the fluid may be aspirated into the respiratory tract.

Table 17–2 | PATHWAYS OF HEAT LOSS

PATHWAY	MECHANISM(S)
Skin (major pathway)	Radiation and conduction—heat is lost from the body to cooler air or objects. Convection—air currents move warm air away from the skin. Sweating—excess body heat evaporates sweat on the skin surface.
Respiratory tract (secondary pathway)	Evaporation—body heat evaporates water from the respiratory mucosa, and water vapor is exhaled.
Urinary tract (minor pathway)	Urination—urine is at body temperature when eliminated.
Digestive tract (minor pathway)	Defecation—feces are at body temperature when eliminated.

Mechanisms to Increase Heat Loss

In a warm environment or during exercise, the body temperature tends to rise, and greater heat loss is needed. This is accomplished by vasodilation in the dermis and an increase in sweating. Vasodilation brings more warm blood close to the body surface, and heat is lost to the environment. However, if the environmental temperature is close to or higher than body temperature, this mechanism becomes ineffective. The second mechanism is increased sweating, in which excess body heat evaporates the sweat on the skin surface. As mentioned previously, sweating becomes inefficient when the atmospheric humidity is high.

On hot days, heat production may also be decreased by a decrease in muscle tone. This is why we may feel very sluggish on hot days; our muscles are even less slightly contracted than usual and are slower to respond.

Mechanisms to Conserve Heat

In a cold environment, heat loss from the body is unavoidable but may be reduced to some extent. Vasoconstriction in the dermis shunts blood away from the body surface so that more heat is kept in the core of the body. Sweating decreases and will stop completely if the temperature of the hypothalamus falls below about 98.6°F. (Remember that the internal temperature of the brain is higher than an oral temperature and is less subject to any changes in environmental temperature.)

If these mechanisms are not enough to prevent the body temperature from dropping, more heat may be produced by increasing muscle tone. When the core temperature (in the liver, for example) approaches 97°F, this greater muscle tone becomes noticeable as shivering. Shivering may increase heat production by as much as five times the normal.

People also have behavioral responses to cold. Such things as putting on a sweater or going indoors reflect our awareness of the discomfort of being cold. For people (we do not have thick fur as do some other mammals), these voluntary activities are important to prevent excessive heat loss when it is very cold (see Box 17–2: Cold-Related Disorders).

FEVER

A fever is an abnormally high body temperature and may accompany infectious diseases, extensive physical trauma, cancer, or damage to the CNS. The substances that may cause a fever are called **pyrogens**. Pyrogens include bacteria, foreign proteins, and chemicals released during inflammation. The inflammatory chemicals are called **endogenous pyrogens**. *Endogenous* means "generated from within." It is believed that pyrogens chemically affect the hypothalamus and "raise the setting" of the hypothalamic thermostat. The hypothalamus will then stimulate responses by the body to raise body temperature to this higher setting.

Let us use as a specific example a child who has strep throat. The bacterial and endogenous pyrogens reset the hypothalamic thermostat upward, to 102°F. At first, the body is "colder" than the setting of the hypothalamus, and the heat conservation and production mechanisms are activated. The child feels cold and begins to shiver (chills). Eventually, sufficient heat is produced to raise the body temperature to the hypothalamic setting of 102°F. At this time, the child will feel neither too warm nor too cold because the body temperature is what the hypothalamus wants.

Box 17–2 | COLD-RELATED DISORDERS

Frostbite is the freezing of part of the body. Fingers, toes, the nose, and ears are most often affected by prolonged exposure to cold because these areas have little volume in proportion to their surface.

At first the skin tingles, then becomes numb. If body fluids freeze, ice crystals may destroy capillaries and tissues (because water expands when it freezes), and blisters form. In the most severe cases gangrene develops; that is, tissue dies because of lack of oxygen.

Treatment of frostbite includes rewarming the affected area. If skin damage is apparent, it should be treated as if it were a burn injury.

Hypothermia is an abnormally low body temperature (below 95°F) that is most often the result of prolonged exposure to cold. Although the affected person certainly feels cold at first, this sensation may pass and be replaced by confusion, slurred speech, drowsiness, and lack of coordination. At this stage, people often do not realize the seriousness of their condition, and if outdoors (ice skating or skiing) may not seek a warmer environment. In progressive hypothermia, breathing and heart rate slow, and coma and death follow.

Other people at greater risk for hypothermia include the elderly, whose temperature-regulating mechanisms are no longer effective, and quadriplegics, who have no sensation of cold in the body. For both of these groups, heat production is or may be low because of inactivity of skeletal muscles.

Artificial hypothermia may be induced during some types of cardiovascular or neurologic surgery. This carefully controlled lowering of body temperature decreases the metabolic rate and need for oxygen and makes possible prolonged surgery without causing extensive tissue death in the patient.

As the effects of the pyrogens diminish, the hypothalamic setting decreases, perhaps close to normal again, 99°F. Now the child will feel warm, and the heat loss mechanisms will be activated. Vasodilation in the skin and sweating will occur until the body temperature drops to the new hypothalamic setting. This is sometimes referred to as the "crisis," but actually the crisis has passed, because sweating indicates that the body temperature is returning to normal. The sequence of temperature changes during a fever is shown in Fig. 17–1.

You may be wondering if a fever serves a useful purpose. For low fevers that are the result of infection, the answer is yes. White blood cells increase their activity at moderately elevated temperatures, and the metabolism of some pathogens is inhibited. Thus, a fever may be beneficial in that it may shorten the duration of an infection by accelerating the destruction of the pathogen.

High fevers, however, may have serious consequences. A fever increases the metabolic rate, which increases heat production, which in turn raises body temperature even more. This is a positive feedback mechanism that will continue until an external event (such as aspirin or death of the pathogens) acts as a brake (see Fig. 1–3 in Chapter 1). When the body temperature rises above 106°F, the hypothalamus begins to lose its ability to regulate temperature. The proteins of cells, especially the enzymes, are also damaged by such high temperatures. Enzymes become denatured, that is, lose their shape and do not catalyze the reactions necessary within cells (see Fig. 2–9 in Chapter 2). As a result, cells begin to die. This is most serious in the brain because neurons cannot be replaced, or certainly not quickly. Cellular death is the cause of brain damage that may follow a prolonged high fever. The effects of changes in body temperature on the hypothalamus are shown in Fig. 17–2.

A medication such as aspirin is called an **antipyretic** because it lowers a fever, probably by affecting the hypothalamic thermostat. To help lower a high fever, the body may be cooled by sponging it with cool water. The excessive body heat will cause this external water to evaporate, thus reducing temperature. A very high fever requires medical attention.

METABOLISM

The term **metabolism** encompasses all of the reactions that take place in the body. Everything that happens within us is part of our metabolism. The reactions of metabolism may be divided into two major categories: anabolism and catabolism.

Anabolism means synthesis or "formation" reactions, the bonding together of smaller molecules to form larger

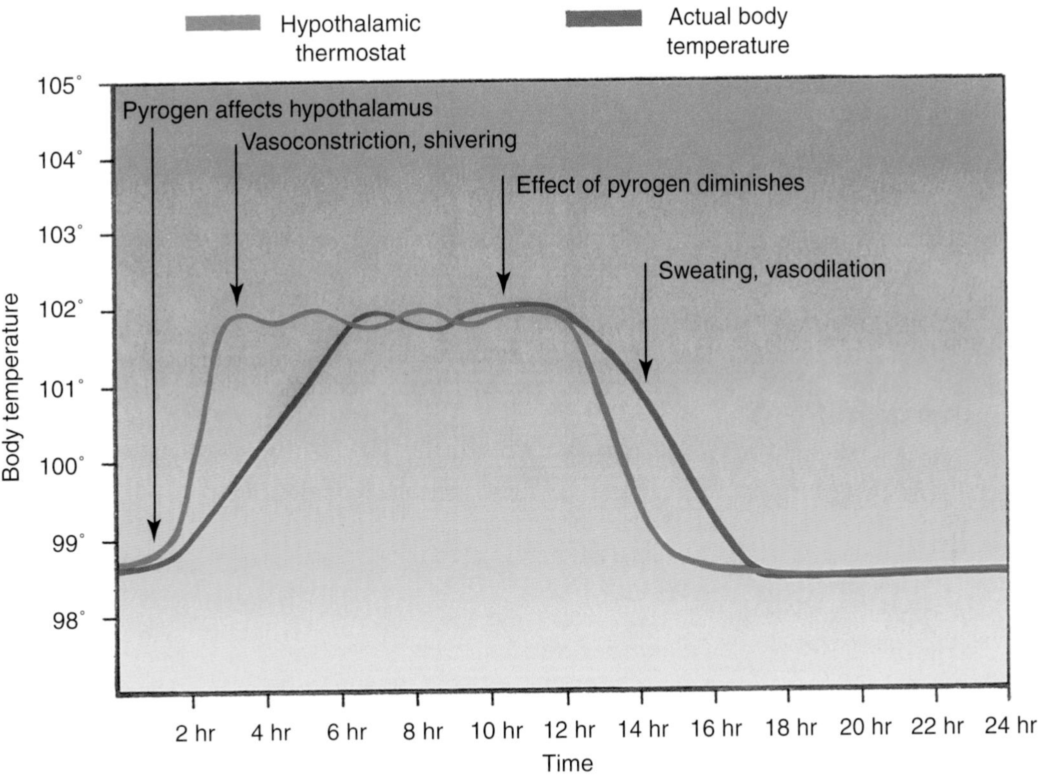

Figure 17–1 Changes in body temperature during an episode of fever. The body temperature changes (purple line) lag behind the changes in the hypothalamic thermostat (blue line) but eventually reach whatever the thermostat has called for.

QUESTION: In this cycle of fever, why do sweating and vasodilation occur when they do?

ones. The synthesis of hemoglobin by cells of the red bone marrow, synthesis of bone matrix by osteoblasts, synthesis of glycogen by liver cells, and synthesis of fat to be stored in adipose tissue are all examples of anabolism. Such reactions require energy, usually in the form of ATP.

Catabolism means decomposition, the breaking of bonds of larger molecules to form smaller molecules. Cell respiration is a series of catabolic reactions that break down food molecules to carbon dioxide and water. During catabolism, energy is often released and used to synthesize ATP (the heat energy released was discussed in the previous section). The ATP formed during catabolism is then used for energy-requiring anabolic reactions such as the DNA replication that precedes mitosis.

Most of our anabolic and catabolic reactions are catalyzed by enzymes. Enzymes are proteins that enable reactions to take place rapidly at body temperature. Recall from Chapter 2 the active site theory, which states that the shapes of an enzyme and the substrate molecules will determine the function of the enzyme. The body has thousands of enzymes, and each is specific, that is, it will catalyze only one type of reaction. As you read the discussions that follow, keep in mind the essential role of enzymes.

CELL RESPIRATION

You are already familiar with the summary reaction of cell respiration,

$$\underset{\text{(glucose)}}{C_6H_{12}O_6} + O_2 \rightarrow CO_2 + H_2O + \text{ATP} + \text{Heat}$$

the purpose of which is to produce ATP. Glucose contains potential energy, and when it is broken down to CO_2 and H_2O, this energy is released in the forms of ATP and heat. The oxygen that is required comes from breathing, and the CO_2 formed is circulated to the lungs to be exhaled. The water formed is called metabolic water and

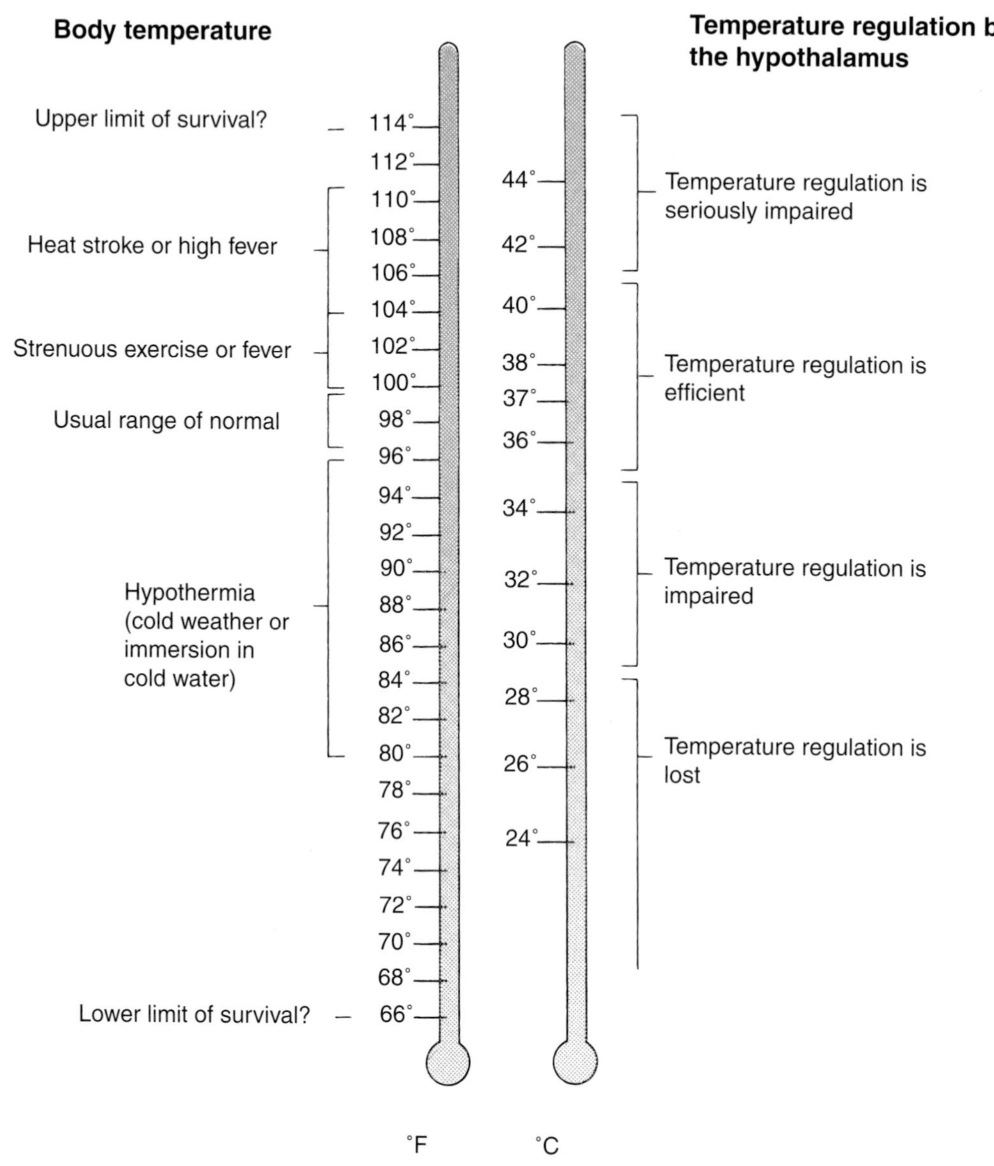

Figure 17–2 Effects of changes in body temperature on the temperature-regulating ability of the hypothalamus. Body temperature is shown in degrees Fahrenheit and degrees Celsius.

QUESTION: Give a range of temperature that an average person would probably survive.

helps to meet our daily need for water. Energy in the form of heat gives us a body temperature, and the ATP formed is used for energy-requiring reactions. Synthesis of ATP means that energy is used to bond a free phosphate molecule to ADP (adenosine diphosphate). ADP and free phosphates are present in cells after ATP has been broken down for energy-requiring processes (see Fig. 2–11 in Chapter 2).

The breakdown of glucose summarized here is not quite that simple, however, and involves a complex series of reactions. Glucose is taken apart "piece by piece," with the removal of hydrogens and the splitting of carbon–carbon bonds. This releases the energy of glucose gradually so that a significant portion (about 40%) is available to synthesize ATP.

Cell respiration of glucose involves three major stages: glycolysis, the Krebs citric acid cycle, and the cytochrome (or electron) transport system. Although the details of each stage are beyond the scope of this book, we will summarize the most important aspects of each, and then relate to them the use of amino acids and fats for energy. This simple summary is depicted in Fig. 17–3. The three major food types and their end products of digestion are shown at the top of the picture; the arrows pointing down lead to the stages of cell respiration.

Glycolysis

The enzymes for the reactions of **glycolysis** are found in the cytoplasm of cells, and oxygen is not required (glycolysis is an anaerobic process). Refer now to Fig. 17–3 as you read the following. In glycolysis, a six-carbon glucose molecule is broken down to two three-carbon molecules of pyruvic acid. Two molecules of ATP are necessary to start the process. The energy they supply is called energy of activation and is necessary to make glucose unstable enough to begin to break down. As a result of these reactions, enough energy is released to synthesize four molecules of ATP, for a net gain of two ATP molecules per glucose molecule. Also during glycolysis, two pairs of hydrogens are removed by NAD, a carrier molecule that contains the vitamin **niacin**. Two NAD molecules thus become $2NADH_2$, and these attached hydrogen pairs will be transported to the cytochrome transport system (stage 3).

If no oxygen is present in the cell, as may happen in muscle cells during exercise, pyruvic acid is converted to lactic acid, which contributes to muscle fatigue. If oxygen *is* present, however, pyruvic acid continues into the next stage, the Krebs citric acid cycle (or, more simply, the Krebs cycle).

Krebs Citric Acid Cycle

The enzymes for the **Krebs cycle** (or **citric acid cycle**) are located in the mitochondria of cells. This second stage of cell respiration is aerobic, meaning that oxygen is required. In a series of reactions, a pyruvic acid molecule is "taken apart," and its carbons are converted to CO_2. The first CO_2 molecule is removed by an enzyme that contains the vitamin **thiamine**. This leaves a two-carbon molecule called an acetyl group, which combines with a molecule called coenzyme A to form acetyl coenzyme A (acetyl CoA). As acetyl CoA continues in the Krebs cycle, two more carbons are removed as CO_2, and more pairs of hydrogens are picked up by NAD and FAD (another carrier molecule that contains the vitamin **riboflavin**). $NADH_2$ and $FADH_2$ will carry their hydrogens to the cytochrome transport system.

During the Krebs cycle, a small amount of energy is released, enough to synthesize one molecule of ATP (two per glucose). Notice also that a four-carbon molecule (oxaloacetic acid) is regenerated after the formation of CO_2. This molecule will react with the next acetyl CoA, which is what makes the Krebs cycle truly a self-perpetuating cycle. The results of the stages of cell respiration are listed in Table 17–3. Before you continue, you may wish to look at that table to see just where the process has gotten thus far.

Cytochrome (Electron) Transport System

Cytochromes are proteins that contain either **iron** or **copper** and are found on the inner membrane of the mitochondria of cells. The pairs of hydrogens that were once part of glucose are brought to the cytochromes by the carrier molecules NAD and FAD. Each hydrogen atom is then split into its proton (H^+ ion) and its electron. The electrons of the hydrogens are passed from one cytochrome to the next, and finally to oxygen. The H^+ ions accumulate and create a concentration gradient. They flow through an enzyme called ATP synthase to an area of lesser concentration. Think of the turbines in a large dam that spin as river water passes through and generate electricity. So, too, is ATP synthase "turned" by the flow of H^+ ions (protons), and enough energy is released to synthesize 25 molecules of ATP. As you can see, most of the ATP produced in cell respiration comes from this third stage.

Finally, and very importantly, each oxygen atom that has gained two electrons (from the cytochromes) reacts with two of the H^+ ions to form water. The formation of metabolic water contributes to the necessary intracellular fluid and also prevents acidosis. If H^+ ions accumulated, they would rapidly lower the pH of the cell. This does not happen, however, because the H^+ ions react with oxygen to form water, and a decrease in pH is prevented.

The summary of the three stages of cell respiration in Table 17–3 also includes the vitamins and minerals that are essential for this process. An important overall concept is the relationship between eating and breathing. Eating provides us with a potential energy source (often glucose) and with necessary vitamins and minerals. However, to release the energy from food, we must breathe. This is *why* we breathe. The oxygen we inhale is essential for the

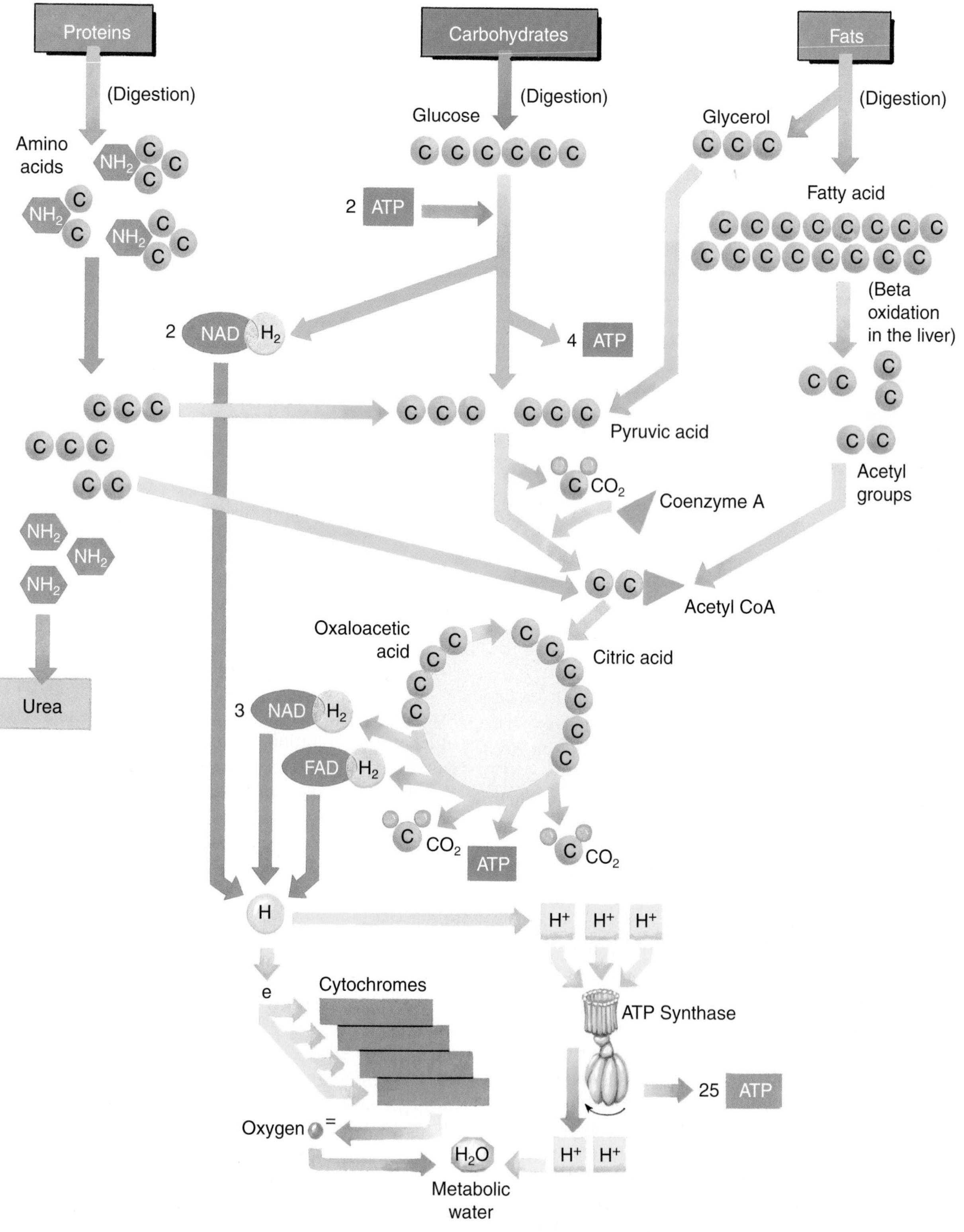

Figure 17–3 Schematic representation of cell respiration. The breakdown of glucose is shown in the center, amino acids on the left and fatty acids and glycerol on the right. See text for description.

QUESTION: To which two molecules can all three food types be converted to enter the citric acid cycle?

Table 17–3 | SUMMARY OF CELL RESPIRATION

STAGE (LOCATION)	MOLECULES THAT ENTER THE PROCESS	RESULTS	VITAMINS OR MINERALS NEEDED
Glycolysis (cytoplasm)	Glucose—ATP needed as energy of activation	■ 2 ATP (net) ■ 2 $NADH_2$ (to cytochrome transport system) ■ 2 pyruvic acid (aerobic: to Krebs cycle; anaerobic: lactic acid formation)	Niacin (part of NAD)
Krebs citric acid cycle (mitochondria)	Pyruvic acid—from glucose or glycerol or excess amino acids *Or* Acetyl CoA—from fatty acids or excess amino acids	■ CO_2 (exhaled) ■ ATP (2 per glucose) ■ 3 $NADH_2$ and 1 $FADH_2$ (to cytochrome transport system) ■ A 4-carbon molecule is regenerated for the next cycle	■ Thiamine (for removal of CO_2) ■ Niacin (part of NAD) ■ Riboflavin (part of FAD) ■ Pantothenic acid (part of coenzyme A)
Cytochrome or electron transport system (mitochondria)	$NADH_2$ and $FADH_2$—from glycolysis or the Krebs cycle	■ 25 ATP ■ Metabolic water	■ Iron and copper (part of some cytochromes)

completion of cell respiration, and the CO_2 produced is exhaled.

Proteins and Fats as Energy Sources

Although glucose is the preferred energy source for cells, proteins and fats also contain potential energy and are alternative energy sources in certain situations.

As you know, proteins are made of the smaller molecules called **amino acids**, and the primary use for the amino acids we obtain from food is the synthesis of new proteins. Excess amino acids, however—those not needed immediately for protein synthesis—may be used for energy production. In the liver, excess amino acids are **deaminated**, that is, the amino group (NH_2) is removed. The remaining portion is converted to a molecule that will fit into the Krebs cycle. For example, a deaminated amino acid may be changed to a three-carbon pyruvic acid or to a two-carbon acetyl group. When these molecules enter the Krebs cycle, the results are just the same as if they had come from glucose. This is diagrammed in Fig. 17–3.

Fats are made of glycerol and fatty acids, which are the end products of fat digestion. These molecules may also be changed to ones that will take part in the Krebs cycle, and the reactions that change them usually take place in the liver. Glycerol is a three-carbon molecule that can be converted to the three-carbon pyruvic acid, which enters the Krebs cycle. In the process of beta-oxidation, the long carbon chains of fatty acids are split into two-carbon acetyl groups, which enter a later step in the Krebs cycle (see Fig. 17–3).

Both amino acids and fatty acids may be converted by the liver to **ketones**, which are two- or four-carbon molecules such as acetone and acetoacetic acid. Although body cells can use ketones in cell respiration, they do so slowly. In situations in which fats or amino acids have become the primary energy sources, a state called **ketosis** may develop; this is described in Box 17–3: Ketosis. Excess amino acids may also be converted to glucose; this is important to supply the brain when dietary intake of carbohydrates is low. The effects of hormones on the metabolism of food are summarized in Table 17–4.

Energy Available from the Three Nutrient Types

The potential energy in food is measured in units called **Calories** or **kilocalories**. A calorie (lowercase "c") is the

Box 17–3 | KETOSIS

When fats and amino acids are to be used for energy, they are often converted by the liver to ketones. Ketones are organic molecules such as acetone that may be changed to acetyl CoA and enter the Krebs cycle. Other cells are able to use ketones as an energy source, but they do so slowly. When ketones are produced in small amounts, as they usually are between meals, the blood level does not rise sharply.

A state of **ketosis** exists when fats and proteins become the primary energy sources, and ketones accumulate in the blood faster than cells can utilize them. Because ketones are organic acids, they lower the pH of the blood. As the blood ketone level rises, the kidneys excrete ketones, but they must also excrete more water as a solvent, which leads to dehydration.

Ketosis is clinically important in diabetes mellitus, starvation, and eating disorders such as anorexia nervosa. Diabetics whose disease is poorly controlled may progress to **ketoacidosis**, a form of metabolic acidosis that may lead to confusion, coma, and death. Reversal of this state requires a carbohydrate energy source and the insulin necessary to utilize it.

Table 17–4 | HORMONES THAT REGULATE METABOLISM

HORMONE (GLAND)	EFFECTS
Thyroxine (thyroid gland)	■ Increases use of all three food types for energy (glucose, fats, amino acids) ■ Increases protein synthesis
Growth hormone (anterior pituitary)	■ Increases amino acid transport into cells ■ Increases protein synthesis ■ Increases use of fats for energy
Insulin (pancreas)	■ Increases glucose transport into cells and use for energy ■ Increases conversion of glucose to glycogen in liver and muscles ■ Increases transport of amino acids and fatty acids into cells to be used for synthesis (*not* energy production)
Glucagon (pancreas)	■ Increases conversion of glycogen to glucose ■ Increases use of amino acids and fats for energy
Cortisol (adrenal cortex)	■ Increases conversion of glucose to glycogen in liver ■ Increases use of amino acids and fats for energy ■ Decreases protein synthesis except in liver and GI tract
Epinephrine (adrenal medulla)	■ Increases conversion of glycogen to glucose ■ Increases use of fats for energy

amount of energy needed to raise the temperature of 1 gram of water 1°C. A kilocalorie or Calorie (capital "C") is 1000 times that amount of energy.

One gram of carbohydrate yields about 4 kilocalories. A gram of protein also yields about 4 kilocalories. A gram of fat, however, yields 9 kilocalories, and a gram of alcohol yields 7 kilocalories. This is why a diet high in fat is more likely to result in weight gain if the calories are not expended in energy-requiring activities: A particular weight, say the 8 grams of fat in a serving of potato chips, has twice as many calories as the same weight of sugars (or starches) in a cookie.

You may have heard the phrase "empty calories" applied to candy or soft drinks. "Empty" in this sense does not mean "zero" or "nothing"; it means "without usefulness." The 150 calories of sugar in a soft drink, for example, may certainly be used for energy production, but the sugar has no other uses for which it is needed in abundance—and calories in excess of energy needs will be changed to fat and stored.

The calorie content is part of the nutritional information on food labels. On such labels the term *calorie* actually means Calorie or kilocalories but is used for the sake of simplicity.

SYNTHESIS USES OF FOODS

Besides being available for energy production, each of the three food types is used in anabolic reactions to synthesize necessary materials for cells and tissues. A simple summary of these reactions is shown in Fig. 17–4. The three food types and their end products of digestion are at the

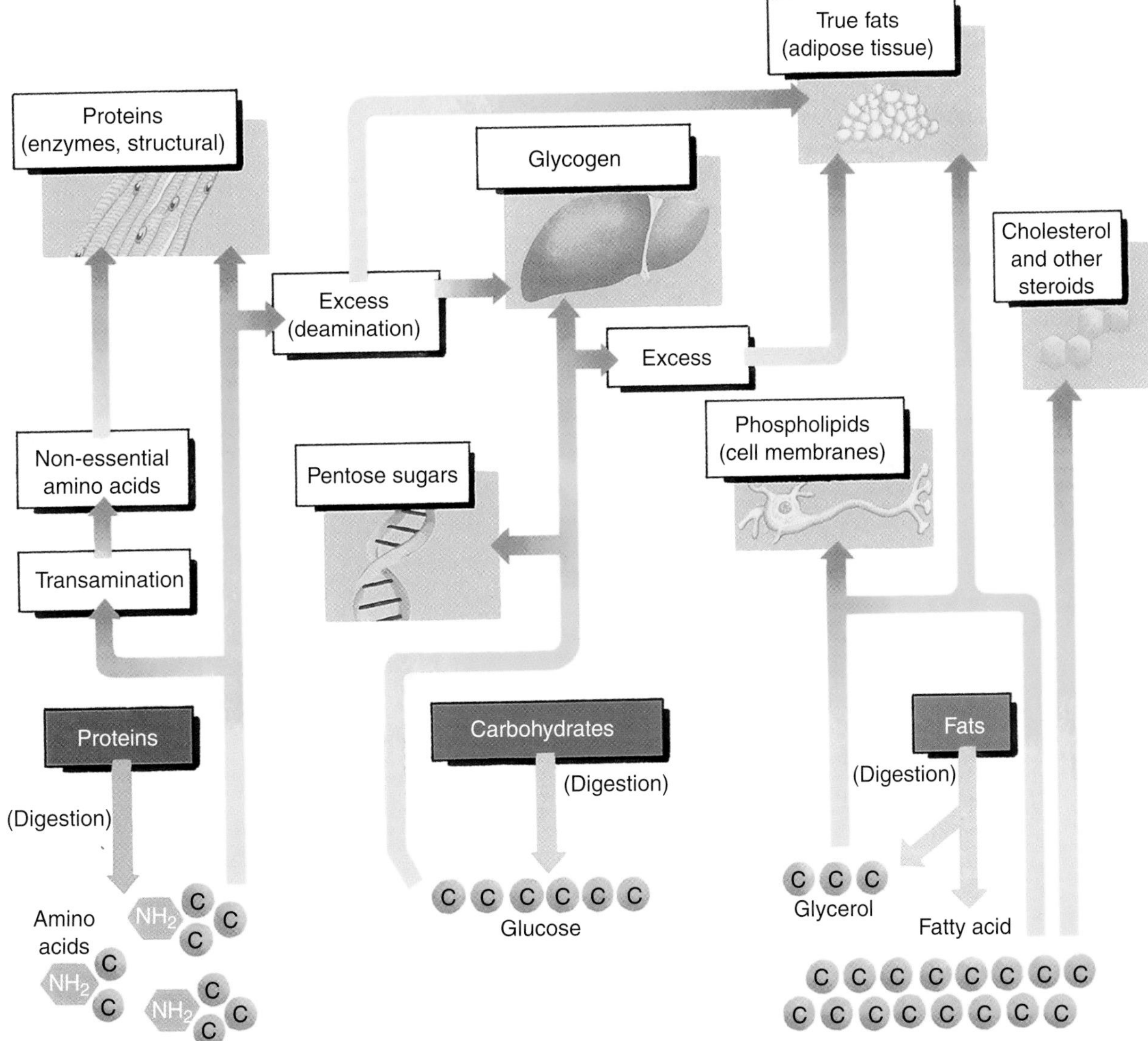

Figure 17–4 Synthesis uses of foods. See text for description.

QUESTION: Excess amino acids can be used to synthesize carbohydrates or fats. Can any other food be used to synthesize proteins?

bottom of the picture, and the arrows going upward indicate synthesis and lead to the products formed. You may want to refer to Fig. 17–4 as you read the next sections.

Glucose

Glucose is the raw material for the synthesis of another important monosaccharide, the **pentose sugars** that are part of nucleic acids. Deoxyribose is the five-carbon sugar found in DNA, and ribose is found in RNA. This function of glucose is very important, for without the pentose sugars our cells could neither produce new chromosomes for cell division nor carry out the process of protein synthesis.

Any glucose in excess of immediate energy needs or the need for pentose sugars is converted to **glycogen** in the liver and skeletal muscles. Glycogen is then an energy source during states of hypoglycemia or during exercise. If still more glucose is present, it will be changed to fat and stored in adipose tissue.

Amino Acids

As mentioned previously, the primary uses for amino acids are the synthesis of the **non-essential amino acids** by the liver and the synthesis of new **proteins** in all tissues. By way of review, we can mention some proteins with which you are already familiar: keratin and melanin in the epidermis; collagen in the dermis, tendons, and ligaments; myosin, actin, and myoglobin in muscle cells; hemoglobin in RBCs; antibodies produced by WBCs; prothrombin and fibrinogen for clotting; albumin to maintain blood volume; pepsin and amylase for digestion; growth hormone and insulin; and the thousands of enzymes needed to catalyze reactions within the body.

The amino acids we obtain from the proteins in our food are used by our cells to synthesize all of these proteins in the amounts needed by the body. Only when the body's needs for new proteins have been met are amino acids used for energy production. But notice in Fig. 17–4 what happens to excess amino acids; they will be deaminated and converted to simple carbohydrates and contribute to glycogen storage or they may be changed to fat and stored in adipose tissue.

Fatty Acids and Glycerol

The end products of fat digestion that are not needed immediately for energy production may be stored as fat (triglycerides) in **adipose tissue**. Most adipose tissue is found subcutaneously and is potential energy for times when food intake decreases. Notice in Table 17–4 that insulin promotes fat synthesis and storage. One theory of weight gain proposes that a diet high in sugars and starches stimulates the secretion of so much insulin that fat can only be stored, not taken out of storage and used for energy.

Fatty acids and glycerol are also used for the synthesis of **phospholipids**, which are essential components of all cell membranes. Myelin, for example, is a phospholipid of the membranes of Schwann cells, which form the myelin sheath of peripheral neurons.

The liver can synthesize most of the fatty acids needed by the body. Two exceptions are linoleic acid and linolenic acid, which are **essential fatty acids** and must be obtained from the diet. Linoleic acid is part of lecithin, which in turn is part of all cell membranes. Vegetable oils are good sources of these essential fatty acids.

When fatty acids are broken down in the process of beta-oxidation, the resulting acetyl groups may also be used for the synthesis of **cholesterol**, a steroid. This takes place primarily in the liver, although all cells are capable of synthesizing cholesterol for their cell membranes. The liver uses cholesterol to synthesize bile salts for the emulsification of fats in digestion. The **steroid hormones** are also synthesized from cholesterol. Cortisol and aldosterone are produced by the adrenal cortex, estrogen and progesterone by the ovaries, and testosterone by the testes.

VITAMINS AND MINERALS

Vitamins are organic molecules needed in very small amounts for normal body functioning. Some vitamins are **coenzymes**; that is, they are necessary for the functioning of certain enzymes. Others are antioxidant vitamins, including vitamins C, E, and beta-carotene (a precursor for vitamin A). Antioxidants prevent damage from **free radicals**, which are molecules that contain an unpaired electron and are highly reactive. The reactions of free radicals can damage DNA, cell membranes, and the cell organelles. Free radicals are formed during some normal body reactions, but smoking and exposure to pollution will increase their formation. Antioxidant vitamins combine with free radicals before they can react with cellular components. Plant foods are good sources of these vitamins. Table 17–5 summarizes some important metabolic and nutritional aspects of the vitamins we need.

Deficiencies of vitamins often result in disease: vitamin C deficiency and scurvy, for example (see Box 4–2 in Chapter 4). Other deficiency diseases that have been known for decades include pellagra (lack of niacin), beri-beri (riboflavin), pernicious anemia (B_{12}), and

Table 17–5 | VITAMINS

VITAMIN	FUNCTIONS	FOOD SOURCES	COMMENT
WATER SOLUBLE			
Thiamine (B_1)	■ Conversion of pyruvic acid to acetyl CoA in cell respiration ■ Synthesis of pentose sugars ■ Synthesis of acetylcholine	Meat, eggs, legumes, green leafy vegetables, grains	Rapidly destroyed by heat
Riboflavin (B_2)	■ Part of FAD in cell respiration	Meat, milk, cheese, grains	Small amounts produced by GI bacteria
Niacin (nicotinamide)	■ Part of NAD in cell respiration ■ Metabolism of fat for energy	Meat, fish, grains, eggs, legumes	Can be synthesized from the amino acid tryptophan
Pyridoxine (B_6)	■ Part of enzymes needed for amino acid metabolism and protein synthesis, nucleic acid synthesis, synthesis of antibodies	Meat, fish, grains, yeast, yogurt	Small amounts produced by GI bacteria
B_{12} (cyanocobalamin)	■ Synthesis of DNA, especially in RBC production ■ Metabolism of amino acids for energy ■ Synthesis of myelin sheath, especially in the CNS	Liver, meat, fish, eggs, milk, cheese	Contains cobalt; intrinsic factor from gastric parietal cells required for absorption
Biotin	■ Synthesis of nucleic acids ■ Metabolism of fatty acids and amino acids	Yeast, liver, eggs	Small amounts produced by GI bacteria
Folic acid (folacin)	■ Synthesis of DNA, especially in blood cell production ■ Contributes to development of fetal CNS	Liver, grains, legumes, leafy green vegetables	Small amounts produced by GI bacteria
Pantothenic acid	■ Part of coenzyme A in cell respiration, use of amino acids and fats for energy	Meat, fish, grains, legumes, vegetables	Small amounts produced by GI bacteria
Vitamin C (ascorbic acid)	■ Synthesis of collagen, especially for wound healing ■ Metabolism of amino acids ■ Absorption of iron ■ An antioxidant—prevents cellular damage from free radicals	Citrus fruits, tomatoes, potatoes	Rapidly destroyed by heat

Continued

Table 17–5 | VITAMINS—cont'd

VITAMIN	FUNCTIONS	FOOD SOURCES	COMMENT
FAT SOLUBLE			
Vitamin A	■ Synthesis of rhodopsin ■ Calcification of growing bones ■ Maintenance of epithelial tissues	Yellow and green vegetables, liver, milk, eggs	Stored in liver; bile salts required for absorption
Vitamin D	■ Absorption of calcium and phosphorus in the small intestine ■ Contributes to immune responses, action of insulin, and preservation of muscle mass and strength	Fortified milk, egg yolks, fish liver oils	Produced in skin exposed to UV rays; stored in liver; bile salts required for absorption
Vitamin E	■ An antioxidant—prevents destruction of cell membranes ■ Contributes to wound healing and detoxifying ability of the liver	Nuts, wheat germ, seed oils	Stored in liver and adipose tissue; bile salts required for absorption
Vitamin K	■ Synthesis of prothrombin and other clotting factors	Liver, spinach, cabbage	Produced by GI bacteria; bile salts needed for absorption; stored in liver

rickets (D). More recently the importance of folic acid (folacin) for the development of the fetal central nervous system has been recognized. Adequate folic acid during pregnancy can significantly decrease the chance of spina bifida (open spinal column) and anencephaly (absence of the cerebrum, always fatal) in a fetus.

Minerals are simple inorganic chemicals and have a variety of functions, many of which you are already familiar with from our discussion of the trace elements in Chapter 2. Table 17–6 lists some important aspects of minerals. You will see that some functions are structural, such as calcium in bone matrix or chlorine as part of hydrochloric acid, and other functions are part of a process, such as calcium in blood clotting and chlorine in osmosis. We will return to the minerals as part of our study of fluid–electrolyte balance in Chapter 19.

METABOLIC RATE

Although the term **metabolism** is used to describe all of the chemical reactions that take place within the body, **metabolic rate** is usually expressed as an amount of heat production. This is because many body processes that utilize ATP also produce heat. These processes include the contraction of skeletal muscle, the pumping of the heart, and the normal breakdown of cellular components. Therefore, it is possible to quantify heat production as a measure of metabolic activity.

As mentioned previously, the energy available from food is measured in kilocalories (kcal). Kilocalories are also the units used to measure the energy expended by the body. During sleep, for example, energy expended by a 150-pound person is about 60 to 70 kcal per hour. Getting up and preparing breakfast increases energy expenditure to 80 to 90 kcal per hour. For mothers with several small children, this value may be significantly higher. Clearly, greater activity results in greater energy expenditure.

The energy required for merely living (lying quietly in bed) is the **basal metabolic rate** (BMR). See Box 17–4: Metabolic Rate for a formula to estimate your own

Table 17–6 | **MINERALS**

MINERAL	FUNCTIONS	FOOD SOURCES	COMMENT
Calcium	■ Formation of bones and teeth ■ Neuron and muscle functioning ■ Blood clotting	Milk, cheese, yogurt, shellfish, leafy green vegetables	Vitamin D required for absorption; stored in bones
Phosphorus	■ Formation of bones and teeth ■ Part of DNA, RNA, ATP, and phospholipids ■ Part of phosphate buffer system	Milk, cheese, fish, meat	Vitamin D required for absorption; stored in bones
Sodium	■ Contributes to osmotic pressure of body fluids ■ Nerve impulse transmission and muscle contraction ■ Part of bicarbonate buffer system	Table salt, almost all foods	Most abundant cation (+) in extracellular fluid
Potassium	■ Contributes to osmotic pressure of body fluids ■ Nerve impulse transmission and muscle contraction	Virtually all foods	Most abundant cation (+) in intracellular fluid
Chlorine	■ Contributes to osmotic pressure of body fluids ■ Part of HCl in gastric juice	Table salt	Most abundant anion (–) in extracellular fluid
Iron	■ Part of hemoglobin and myoglobin ■ Part of some cytochromes in cell respiration	Meat, shellfish, dried apricots, legumes, eggs	Stored in liver
Iodine	■ Part of thyroxine and T_3	Iodized salt, seafood	Crucial for the mental development of children
Sulfur	■ Part of some amino acids ■ Part of thiamine and biotin	Meat, eggs	Insulin and keratin require sulfur
Magnesium	■ Formation of bone ■ Metabolism of ATP–ADP	Green vegetables, legumes, seafood, milk	Part of chlorophyll in green plants
Manganese	■ Formation of urea ■ Synthesis of fatty acids and cholesterol	Legumes, grains, nuts, leafy green vegetables	Some stored in liver
Copper	■ Synthesis of hemoglobin ■ Part of some cytochromes in cell respiration ■ Synthesis of melanin	Liver, seafood, grains, nuts, legumes	Stored in liver
Cobalt	■ Part of vitamin B_{12}	Liver, meat, fish	Vitamin B_{12} stored in liver
Zinc	■ Part of carbonic anhydrase needed for CO_2 transport ■ Part of peptidases needed for protein digestion ■ Necessary for normal taste sensation ■ Involved in wound healing	Meat, seafood, grains, legumes	Excess interferes with copper metabolism and may impair sense of smell

Box 17–4 | METABOLIC RATE

To estimate basal metabolic rate (BMR), calculate kilocalories (kcal) used per hour as follows:

For women: use the factor of 0.9 kcal per kilogram (kg) of body weight
For men: use the factor of 1.0 kcal per kg of body weight
Then multiply kcal/hour by 24 hours to determine kcal per day.

Example: **A 120-pound woman:**

1. Change pounds to kilograms:
   120 lb at 2.2 lb/kg = 55 kg
2. Multiply kg weight by the BMR factor:
   55 kg × 0.9 kcal/kg/hr = 49.5 kcal/hr
3. Multiply kcal/hr by 24:
   49.5 kcal/hr × 24 = 1188 kcal/day
   (BMR about 1200 kcal/day)

Example: **A 160-pound man:**

1. 160 lb at 2.2 lb/kg = 73 kg
2. 73 kg × 1.0 kcal/kg/hr = 73 kcal/hr
3. 73 kcal/hr × 24 = 1752 kcal/day

To approximate the amount of energy actually expended during an average day (24 hours), the following percentages may be used:

Sedentary activity: add 40% to 50% of the BMR to the BMR
Light activity: add 50% to 65% of the BMR to the BMR
Moderate activity: add 65% to 75% of the BMR to the BMR
Strenuous activity: add 75% to 100% of the BMR to the BMR

Using our example of the 120-pound woman with a BMR of 1200 kcal/day:

Sedentary: 1680 to 1800 kcal/day
Light: 1800 to 1980 kcal/day
Moderate: 1980 to 2100 kcal/day
Strenuous: 2100 to 2400 kcal/day

metabolic rate. A number of factors affect the metabolic rate of an active person:

1. Exercise—Contraction of skeletal muscle increases energy expenditure and raises metabolic rate (see Box 17–5: Weight Loss).
2. Age—Metabolic rate is highest in young children and decreases with age. The energy requirements for growth and the greater heat loss by a smaller body contribute to the higher rate in children. After growth has stopped, metabolic rate decreases about 2% per decade. If a person becomes less active, the total decrease is almost 5% per decade.
3. Body configuration of adults—Tall, thin people usually have higher metabolic rates than do short, stocky people of the same weight. This is so because the tall, thin person has a larger surface area (proportional to weight) through which heat is continuously lost. The metabolic rate, therefore, is slightly higher to compensate for the greater heat loss. The variance of surface-to-weight ratios for different body configurations is illustrated in Fig. 17–5.
4. Sex hormones—Testosterone increases metabolic activity to a greater degree than does estrogen, giving men a slightly higher metabolic rate than women. Also, men tend to have more muscle, an active tissue, whereas women tend to have more fat, a relatively inactive tissue.
5. Sympathetic stimulation—In stress situations, the metabolic rate of many body cells is increased. Also contributing to this are the hormones epinephrine and norepinephrine.
6. Decreased food intake—If the intake of food decreases for a prolonged period of time, metabolic rate also begins to decrease. It is as if the body's metabolism is "slowing down" to conserve whatever energy sources may still be available. (See also Box 17–6: Leptin and Body-Mass Index.)
7. Climate—People who live in cold climates may have metabolic rates 10% to 20% higher than people who

Box 17–5 | WEIGHT LOSS

Losing weight depends on one simple fact: calorie expenditure in activity must exceed calorie intake in food (the term **calorie** here will be used to mean kilocalorie).

To lose 1 pound of body fat, which consists of fat, water, and protein, 3500 calories of energy must be expended. Although any form of exercise uses calories, the more strenuous the exercise, the more calories expended. Some examples are shown in the accompanying table.

Most food packaging contains nutritional information, including calories per serving. Keeping track of daily caloric intake is an important part of trying to lose weight. It is also important to remember that sustained loss of fat usually does not exceed 1 to 2 pounds per week. In part this is so because as calorie intake decreases, the metabolic rate decreases. Exercise is very important.

A sensible weight-loss diet will include carbohydrates to supply energy needs, will have sufficient protein (40 to 45 grams per day), and will be low in animal fat. Including vegetables and fruits will supply vitamins, minerals, and fiber.

Activity	Average calories per 10 minutes	Activity	Average calories per 10 minutes
Walking briskly	45	Running (8 mph)	120
Walking up stairs	170	Cycling (10 mph)	70
Dancing (slow)	40	Cycling (15 mph)	115
Dancing (fast)	65	Swimming	100

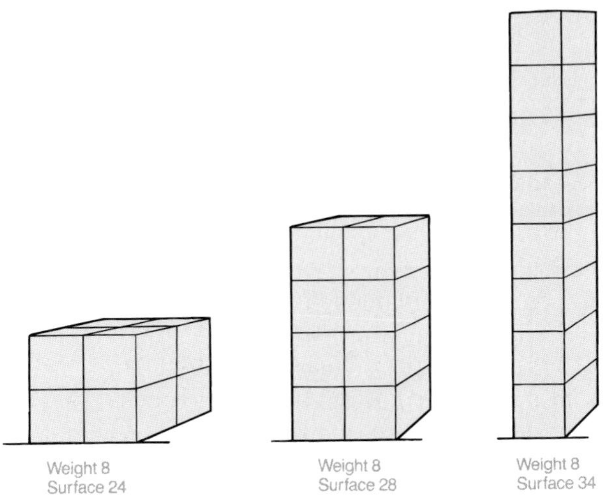

Figure 17–5 Surface-to-weight ratios. Imagine that the three shapes are people who all weigh the same amount. The "tall, thin person" on the right has about 50% more surface area than does the "short, stocky person" on the left. The more surface area (where heat is lost), the higher the metabolic rate.

QUESTION: Which of these ratios best represents an infant? (Rather than weight, think of inside-outside proportion.)

live in tropical regions. This is believed to be due to variations in the secretion of thyroxine, the hormone most responsible for regulation of metabolic rate. In a cold climate, the necessity for greater heat production brings about an increased secretion of thyroxine and a higher metabolic rate.

AGING AND METABOLISM

As mentioned in the previous section, metabolic rate decreases with age. Elderly people who remain active, however, can easily maintain energy production adequate for their needs as long as their general health is good. Some elderly people subject to physical or emotional disability, however, may be at risk for malnutrition. Caregivers may assess such a risk by asking how often the person eats every day; if appetite is good, fair, or poor; and how the food tastes. These simple questions may help ensure adequate nutrition.

Sensitivity to external temperature changes may decrease with age, and the regulation of body temperature is no longer as precise. Sweat glands are not as active, and prolonged high environmental temperatures are a real danger for elderly people. In August 2003, in Europe, an

Box 17–6 | LEPTIN AND BODY MASS INDEX

Leptin is a peptide produced by fat cells, a hormone that signals the hypothalamus to suppress appetite. It informs the brain of how much stored fat the body has and is involved in the regulation of body weight (along with many other chemicals, some still unknown).

Leptin also contributes to the onset of puberty, especially in females. Girls who are very thin, with little body fat, tend to have a later first menstrual period than girls with average body fat, and a certain level of body fat is necessary for continued ovulation. Leptin is a chemical mediator of this information.

Leptin also works with osteocalcin produced by osteoblasts to decrease fat storage in cells (and use it for energy) and to improve the efficiency of the pancreatic cells that produce insulin.

One measure of leanness or fatness is the **body mass index**. To calculate:

Multiple weight in pounds by 703.
Divide by height in inches.
Divide again by height in inches = body mass index

Example: A person five foot six (66 inches) weighing 130 pounds.

$$130 \times 703 = 91{,}390$$
$$91{,}390 \div 66 = 1385$$
$$1385 \div 66 = 20.98$$

The optimal body-mass index is considered to be 21. An index over 25 is considered overweight.

unusually long and severe heat wave was the cause of at least 25,000 deaths. Most of those who died were elderly.

SUMMARY

Food is needed for the synthesis of new cells and tissues and to produce the energy required for such synthesis reactions. As a consequence of metabolism, heat energy provides a constant body temperature and permits the continuation of metabolic activity. The metabolic pathways described in this chapter are a small portion of the body's total metabolism. Even this simple presentation, however, suggests the great chemical complexity of the functioning human being.

STUDY OUTLINE

Body Temperature

1. Normal range is 96.5° to 99.5°F (36° to 38°C), with an average of 98.6°F (37°C).
2. Normal fluctuation in 24 hours is 1° to 2°F.
3. Temperature regulation in infants and the elderly is not as precise as it is at other ages.

Heat Production

Heat is one of the energy products of cell respiration. Many factors affect the total heat actually produced (see Table 17–1).

1. Thyroxine from the thyroid gland—the most important regulator of daily heat production. As metabolic rate decreases, more thyroxine is secreted to increase the rate of cell respiration.
2. Stress—sympathetic impulses and epinephrine and norepinephrine increase the metabolic activity of many organs, increasing the production of ATP and heat.
3. Active organs continuously produce heat. Skeletal muscle tone produces 25% of the total body heat at rest. The liver provides up to 20% of the resting body heat.
4. Food intake increases the activity of the digestive organs and increases heat production.
5. Changes in body temperature affect metabolic rate. A fever increases the metabolic rate, and more heat is produced; this may become detrimental during very high fevers.

Heat Loss (see Table 17–2)

1. Most heat is lost through the skin.
2. Blood flow through the dermis determines the amount of heat that is lost by radiation, conduction, and convection.
3. Vasodilation in the dermis increases blood flow and heat loss; radiation and conduction are effective only if the environment is cooler than the body.
4. Vasoconstriction in the dermis decreases blood flow and conserves heat in the core of the body.
5. Sweating is a very effective heat loss mechanism; excess body heat evaporates sweat on the skin surface; sweating is most effective when the atmospheric humidity is low.
6. Sweating also has a disadvantage in that water is lost and must be replaced to prevent serious dehydration.
7. Heat is lost from the respiratory tract by the evaporation of water from the warm respiratory mucosa; water vapor is part of exhaled air.
8. A very small amount of heat is lost as urine and feces are excreted at body temperature.

Regulation of Body Temperature

1. The hypothalamus is the thermostat of the body and regulates body temperature by balancing heat production and heat loss.
2. The hypothalamus receives information from its own neurons (blood temperature) and from the temperature receptors in the dermis.
3. Mechanisms to increase heat loss are vasodilation in the dermis and increased sweating. Decreased muscle tone will decrease heat production.
4. Mechanisms to conserve heat are vasoconstriction in the dermis and decreased sweating. Increased muscle tone (shivering) will increase heat production.

Fever—an abnormally elevated body temperature

1. Pyrogens are substances that cause a fever: bacteria, foreign proteins, or chemicals released during inflammation (endogenous pyrogens).
2. Pyrogens raise the setting of the hypothalamic thermostat; the person feels cold and begins to shiver to produce heat.
3. When the pyrogen has been eliminated, the hypothalamic setting returns to normal; the person feels warm, and sweating begins to lose heat to lower the body temperature.
4. A low fever may be beneficial because it increases the activity of WBCs and inhibits the activity of some pathogens.
5. A high fever may be detrimental because enzymes are denatured at high temperatures. This is most critical in the brain, where cells that die cannot be replaced.

Metabolism—all the reactions within the body

1. Anabolism—synthesis reactions that usually require energy in the form of ATP.
2. Catabolism—decomposition reactions that often release energy in the form of ATP.
3. Enzymes catalyze most anabolic and catabolic reactions.

Cell Respiration—the breakdown of food molecules to release their potential energy and synthesize ATP (Fig. 17–3)

1. Glucose + oxygen yields CO_2 + H_2O + ATP + heat.
2. The breakdown of glucose involves three stages: glycolysis, the Krebs cycle, and the cytochrome (electron) transport system (see also Table 17–3).
3. The oxygen necessary comes from breathing.
4. The water formed becomes part of intracellular fluid; CO_2 is exhaled; ATP is used for energy-requiring reactions; heat provides a body temperature.

Proteins and Fats—as energy sources (see Table 17–4 for hormonal regulation)

1. Excess amino acids are deaminated in the liver and converted to pyruvic acid or acetyl groups to enter the Krebs cycle. Amino acids may also be converted to glucose to supply the brain (Fig. 17–3).
2. Glycerol is converted to pyruvic acid to enter the Krebs cycle.
3. Fatty acids, in the process of beta-oxidation in the liver, are split into acetyl groups to enter the Krebs cycle; ketones are formed for transport to other cells (see Fig. 17–3).

Energy Available from Food

1. Energy is measured in kilocalories (Calories): kcal.

2. There are 4 kcal per gram of carbohydrate, 4 kcal per gram of protein, 9 kcal per gram of fat. With reference to food, kilocalories may be called calories.

Synthesis Uses of Foods (Fig. 17–4)

1. Glucose—used to synthesize the pentose sugars for DNA and RNA; used to synthesize glycogen to store energy in liver and muscles.
2. Amino acids—used to synthesize new proteins and the non-essential amino acids; essential amino acids must be obtained in the diet.
3. Fatty acids and glycerol—used to synthesize phospholipids for cell membranes, triglycerides for fat storage in adipose tissue, and cholesterol and other steroids; essential fatty acids must be obtained in the diet.
4. Any food eaten in excess will be changed to fat and stored.
5. Vitamins and minerals—see Tables 17–5 and 17–6.

Metabolic Rate—heat production by the body; measured in kcal

1. Basal metabolic rate (BMR) is the energy required to maintain life (see Box 17–4). Exercise increases metabolic rate, and several other factors influence the metabolic rate of an active person.
   a. Age—metabolic rate is highest in young children and decreases with age.
   b. Body configuration—more surface area proportional to weight (tall and thin) means a higher metabolic rate.
   c. Sex hormones—men usually have a higher metabolic rate than do women; men have more muscle proportional to fat than do women.
   d. Sympathetic stimulation—metabolic activity increases in stress situations.
   e. Decreased food intake—metabolic rate decreases to conserve available energy sources.
   f. Climate—people who live in cold climates usually have higher metabolic rates because of a greater need for heat production.

REVIEW QUESTIONS

1. State the normal range of human body temperature in °F and °C. (p. 438)
2. State the summary equation of cell respiration, and state what happens to (or the purpose of) each of the products. (p. 443)
3. Describe the role of each in heat production: thyroxine, skeletal muscles, stress situations, and the liver. (p. 438)
4. Describe the two mechanisms of heat loss through the skin, and explain the role of blood flow. Describe how heat is lost through the respiratory tract. (pp. 439–440)
5. Explain the circumstances that exist when sweating and vasodilation in the dermis are not effective mechanisms of heat loss. (p. 439)
6. Name the part of the brain that regulates body temperature, and explain what is meant by a thermostat. (p. 440)
7. Describe the responses by the body to a warm environment and to a cold environment. (p. 441)
8. Explain how pyrogens are believed to cause a fever, and give two examples of pyrogens. (p. 441)
9. Define metabolism, anabolism, catabolism, kilocalorie, and metabolic rate. (pp. 442–443, 447, 452)
10. Name the three stages of the cell respiration of glucose and state where in the cell each takes place and whether or not oxygen is required. (p. 445)
11. For each, state the molecules that enter the process and the results of the process: glycolysis, Krebs cycle, and cytochrome (electron) transport system. (pp. 445, 447)
12. Explain how fatty acids, glycerol, and excess amino acids are used for energy production in cell respiration. (p. 447)
13. Describe the synthesis uses for glucose, amino acids, and fatty acids. (p. 450)
14. Describe four factors that affect the metabolic rate of an active person. (p. 454)
15. If lunch consists of 60 grams of carbohydrate, 15 grams of protein, and 10 grams of fat, how many kilocalories are provided? (p. 448)

FOR FURTHER THOUGHT

1. Fourteen-year-old Donna has just decided that she will be a vegetarian. What difficulties are there with such a diet; that is, what nutrients may be lacking? How may they be obtained?
2. Studies with animals have shown that caloric restriction may prolong life by delaying some effects of aging. The animals' diet was about half their usual calories. For people, 1250 to 1500 calories per day would be restrictive (compared with the 2000 calories or more that many of us in North America consume). Would it be worth it for a life span of 110 years? Describe the problems with such a diet.
3. Every summer small children are left in cars "just for a few minutes," while a parent does an errand. The result may be severe brain damage or death of the child from heat stroke. Explain why small children are so susceptible to heat.
4. Remember the *Titanic*, which sank in April of 1912? There were not enough lifeboats for everyone, and many people were in the water of the North Atlantic. They did have life jackets and did not drown, but many were dead within half an hour. Explain why.
5. An elderly person and a quadriplegic person may each have difficulties during cold weather. Explain how the problem is a little different for each.
6. Question Figure 17–A depicts the regulation of body temperature. On the left (# 2-4) are the body's responses to hot weather. On the right (# 6-8) are the responses to cold. Label each response. What is indicated by # 1, and what is meant by the arrows (# 5 and 9) returning to it?

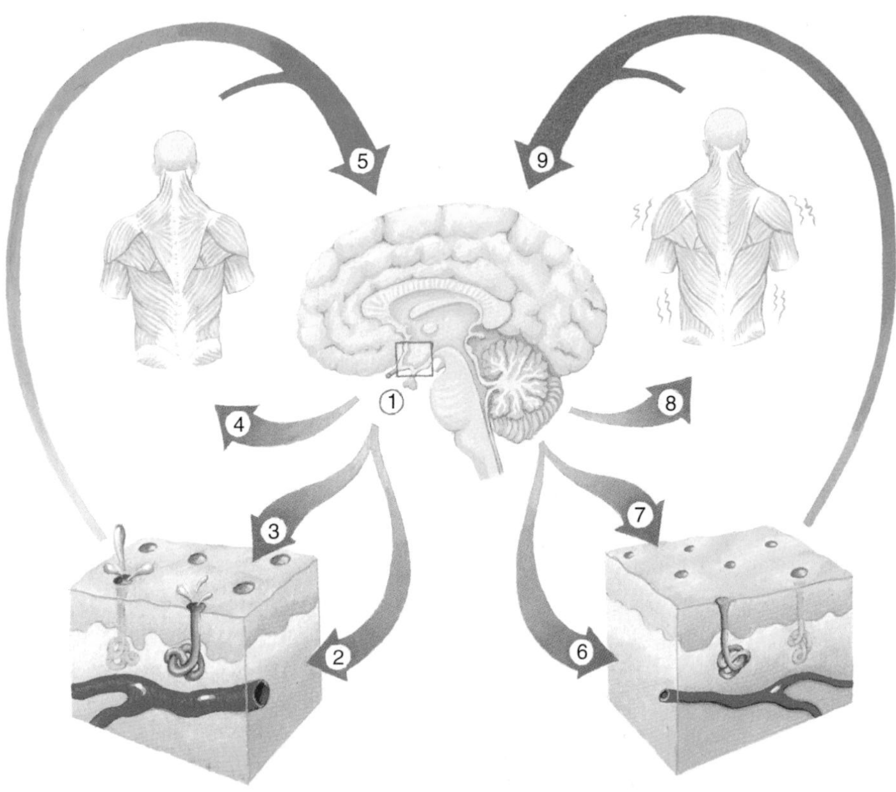

QUESTION FIGURE 17–A: Regulation of Body Temperature

CHAPTER

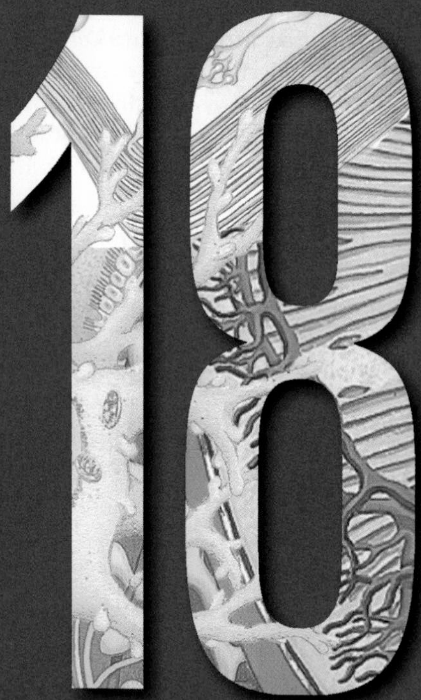

The Urinary System

STUDENT OBJECTIVES

- Describe the location and general function of each organ of the urinary system.
- Name the parts of a nephron and the important blood vessels associated with them.
- Explain how the following are involved in urine formation: glomerular filtration, tubular reabsorption, tubular secretion, and blood flow through the kidney.
- Describe the mechanisms of tubular reabsorption, and explain the importance of tubular secretion.
- Describe how the kidneys help maintain normal blood volume and blood pressure.
- Name and state the functions of the hormones that affect the kidneys.
- Describe how the kidneys help maintain normal pH of blood and tissue fluid.
- Describe the urination reflex, and explain how voluntary control is possible.
- Describe the characteristics of normal urine.

CHAPTER OUTLINE

NEW TERMINOLOGY

Bowman's capsule *(**BOW**-manz **KAP**-suhl)*
Detrusor muscle *(de-**TROO**-ser)*
External urethral sphincter *(yoo-**REE**-thruhl **SFINK**-ter)*
Glomerular filtration rate *(gloh-**MER**-yoo-ler fill-**TRAY**-shun RAYT)*
Glomerulus *(gloh-**MER**-yoo-lus)*
Internal urethral sphincter *(yoo-**REE**-thruhl **SFINK**-ter)*
Juxtaglomerular cells *(JUKS-tah-gloh-**MER**-yoo-ler SELLS)*
Micturition *(MIK-tyoo-**RISH**-un)*
Nephron *(**NEFF**-ron)*
Nitrogenous wastes *(nigh-**TRAH**-jen-us)*
Peritubular capillaries *(PER-ee-**TOO**-byoo-ler)*
Renal corpuscle *(**REE**-nuhl **KOR**-pus'l)*
Renal filtrate *(**REE**-nuhl **FILL**-trayt)*
Renal tubule *(**REE**-nuhl **TOO**-byoo'l)*
Retroperitoneal *(RE-troh-PER-i-toh-**NEE**-uhl)*
Specific gravity *(spe-**SIF**-ik **GRA**-vi-tee)*
Threshold level *(**THRESH**-hold **LE**-vuhl)*
Trigone *(**TRY**-gohn)*
Ureter *(**YOOR**-uh-ter)*
Urethra *(yoo-**REE**-thrah)*
Urinary bladder *(**YOOR**-i-NAR-ee **BLA**-der)*

RELATED CLINICAL TERMINOLOGY

Cystitis *(sis-**TIGH**-tis)*
Dysuria *(dis-**YOO**-ree-ah)*
Hemodialysis *(HEE-moh-dye-**AL**-i-sis)*
Nephritis *(ne-**FRY**-tis)*
Oliguria *(AH-li-**GYOO**-ree-ah)*
Polyuria *(PAH-li-**YOO**-ree-ah)*
Renal calculi *(**REE**-nuhl **KAL**-kew-lye)*
Renal failure *(**REE**-nuhl **FAYL**-yer)*
Rhabdomyolysis *(RAB-doh-my-**AHL**-i-sis)*
Uremia *(yoo-**REE**-me-ah)*

*Terms that appear in **bold type** in the chapter text are defined in the glossary, which begins on page 603.*

The first successful human organ transplant was a kidney transplant performed in 1953. Because the donor and recipient were identical twins, rejection of the kidney by the recipient was not a problem. Thousands of kidney transplants have been performed since then, and the development of more effective immunosuppressive medications has permitted many people to live normal lives with donated kidneys. Although a person usually has two kidneys, one kidney is sufficient to carry out the complex work required to maintain homeostasis of the body fluids.

The **urinary system** consists of two kidneys, two ureters, the urinary bladder, and the urethra (Fig. 18-1). The formation of urine is the function of the kidneys, and the rest of the system is responsible for eliminating the urine.

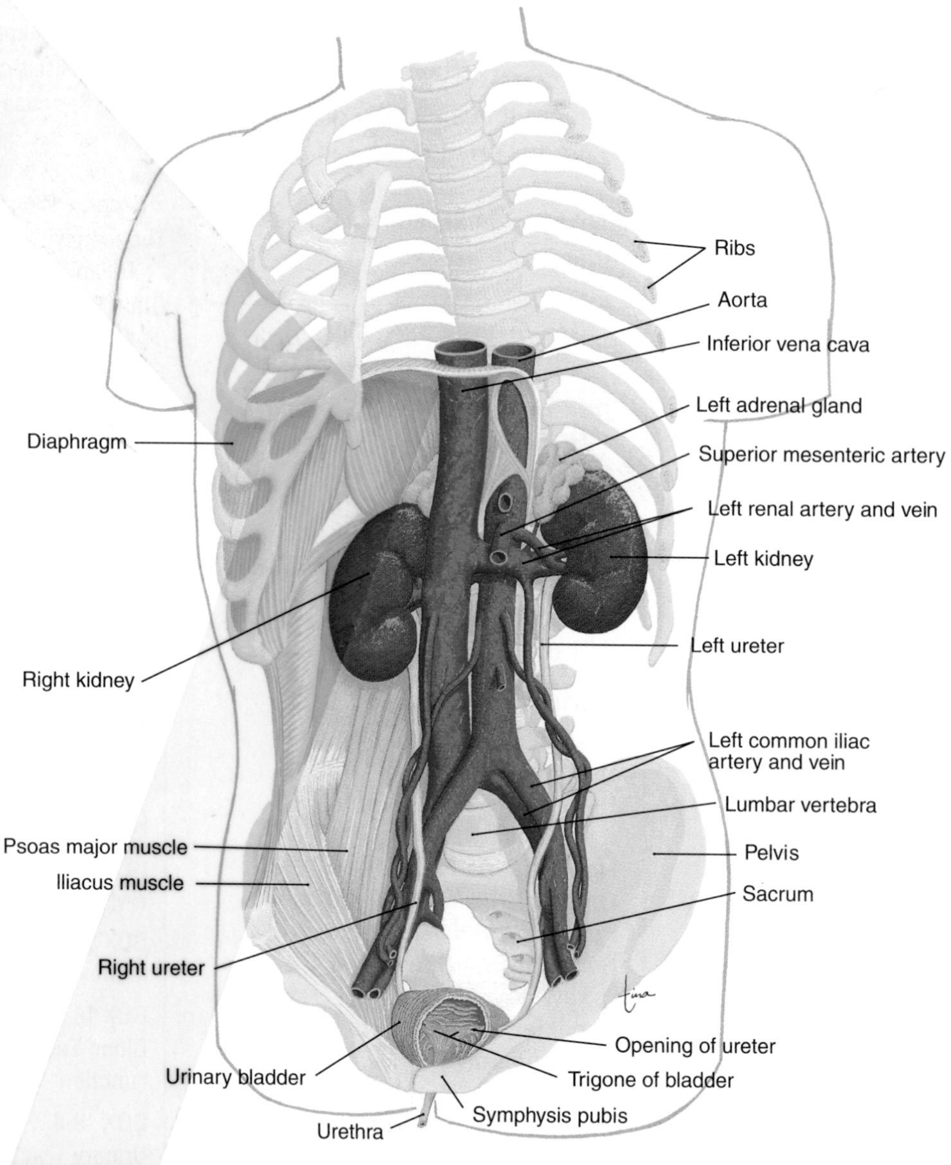

Figure 18-1 The urinary system shown in anterior view.

QUESTION: Why is blood pressure relatively high in the kidneys? What do you see that would suggest this?

Body cells produce waste products such as urea, creatinine, and ammonia, which must be removed from the blood before they accumulate to toxic levels. The foods we eat and the medications we take are also metabolized and may form chemicals that are of no use to the body and may even be harmful. As the kidneys form urine to excrete these waste products, they also accomplish several other important functions:

1. Regulation of the volume of blood by excretion or conservation of water
2. Regulation of the electrolyte content of the blood by the excretion or conservation of minerals
3. Regulation of the acid-base balance of the blood by excretion or conservation of ions such as H^+ ions or HCO_3^- ions
4. Regulation of all of the above in tissue fluid

The process of urine formation, therefore, helps maintain the normal composition, volume, and pH of both blood and tissue fluid by removing those substances that would upset the normal constancy and balance of these extracellular fluids.

KIDNEYS

The two **kidneys** are located in the upper abdominal cavity on either side of the vertebral column, behind the peritoneum (**retroperitoneal**). The upper portions of the kidneys rest on the lower surface of the diaphragm and are enclosed and protected by the lower rib cage (see Fig. 18-1). You can see in Fig. 18-1 that the left kidney is slightly higher than the right one. The right kidney is lower because of the presence of the liver in the upper right abdominal quadrant. The kidneys are embedded in adipose tissue that acts as a cushion and is in turn covered by a fibrous connective tissue membrane called the **renal fascia**, which helps hold the kidneys in place (see Box 18-1: Floating Kidney).

Each kidney has an indentation called the **hilus** on its medial side. At the hilus, the renal artery enters the kidney, and the renal vein and ureter emerge. The renal artery is a branch of the abdominal aorta, and the renal vein returns blood to the inferior vena cava (see Fig. 18-1). The ureter carries urine from the kidney to the urinary bladder.

INTERNAL STRUCTURE OF THE KIDNEY

In a coronal or frontal section of the kidney, three areas can be distinguished (Fig. 18-2). The lateral and middle areas are tissue layers, and the medial area at the hilus is a cavity. The outer tissue layer is called the **renal cortex**; it is made of renal corpuscles and convoluted tubules. These are parts of the nephron and are described in the next section. The inner tissue layer is the **renal medulla**, which is made of loops of Henle and collecting tubules (also parts of the nephron). The renal medulla consists of wedge-shaped pieces called **renal pyramids**. The tip of each pyramid is its apex or papilla.

The third area is the **renal pelvis**; this is not a layer of tissues, but rather a cavity formed by the expansion of the ureter within the kidney at the hilus. Funnel-shaped extensions of the renal pelvis, called **calyces** (singular: **calyx**), enclose the papillae of the renal pyramids. Urine flows from the renal pyramids into the calyces, then to the renal pelvis and out into the ureter.

THE NEPHRON

The **nephron** is the structural and functional unit of the kidney. Each kidney contains approximately 1 million nephrons. It is in the nephrons, with their associated blood vessels, that urine is formed. Each nephron has two major portions: a renal corpuscle and a renal tubule. Each of

Box 18–1 | FLOATING KIDNEY

A floating kidney is one that has moved out of its normal position. This may happen in very thin people whose renal cushion of adipose tissue is thin, or it may be the result of a sharp blow to the back that dislodges a kidney.

A kidney can function in any position; the problem with a floating kidney is that the ureter may become twisted or kinked. If urine cannot flow through the ureter, the urine backs up and collects in the renal pelvis. Incoming urine from the renal tubules then backs up as well. If the renal filtrate cannot flow out of Bowman's capsules, the pressure within Bowman's capsules increases, opposing the blood pressure in the glomeruli. Glomerular filtration then cannot take place efficiently. If uncorrected, this may lead to permanent kidney damage.

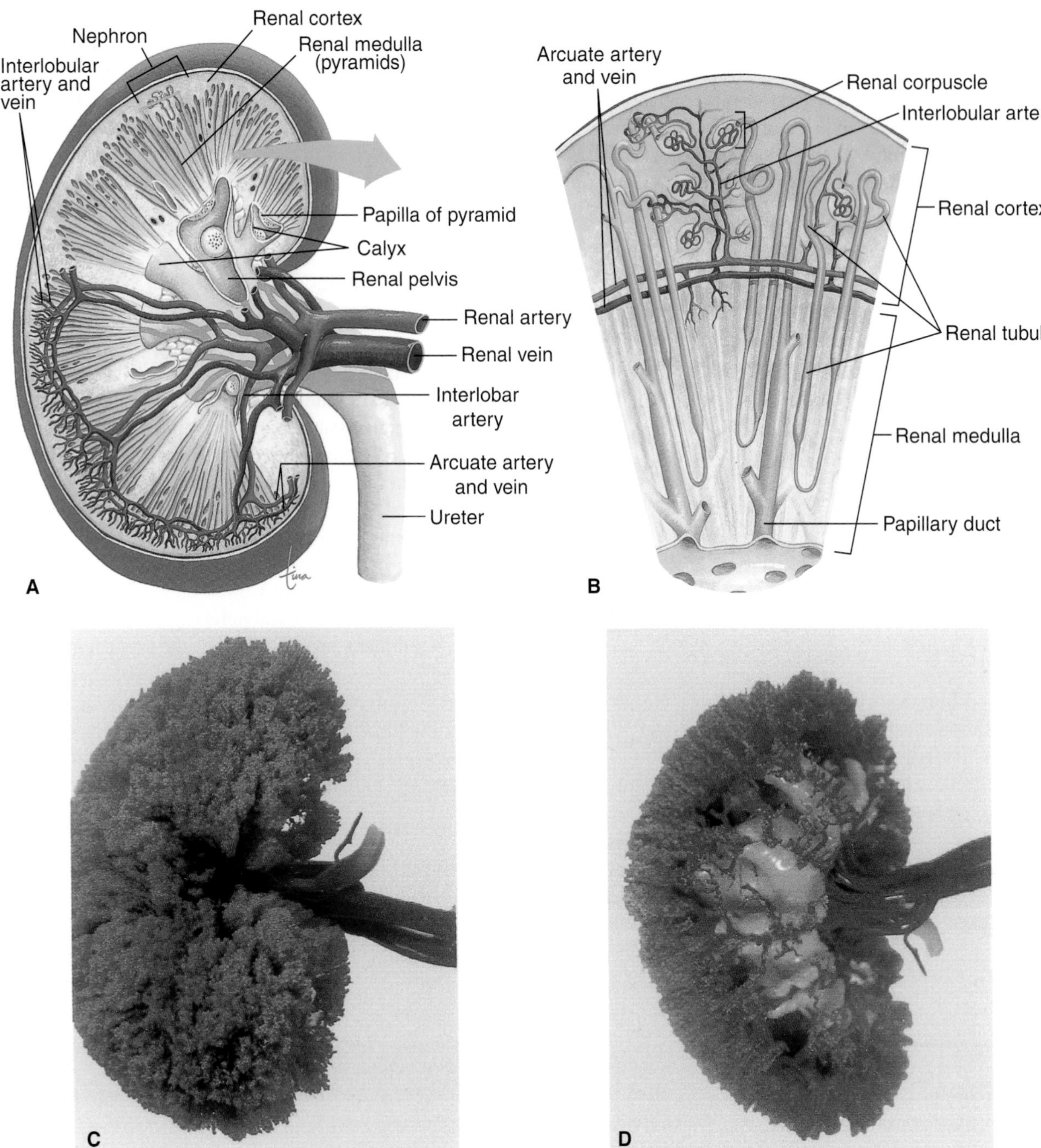

Figure 18-2 (**A**) Frontal section of the right kidney showing internal structure and blood vessels. (**B**) The magnified section of the kidney shows several nephrons. (**C**) Vascular cast of a kidney in lateral view. Red plastic fills the blood vessels. (**D**) Vascular cast in medial view. Blood vessels have been removed; yellow plastic fills the renal pelvis and ureter. (Photographs C and D by Dan Kaufman.)

QUESTION: Which main parts of a nephron are found in the renal cortex? Which areas of a kidney have many blood vessels?

these major parts has further subdivisions, which are shown with their blood vessels in Fig. 18-3.

Renal Corpuscle

A **renal corpuscle** consists of a glomerulus surrounded by a Bowman's capsule. The **glomerulus** is a capillary network that arises from an **afferent arteriole** and empties into an **efferent arteriole**. The diameter of the efferent arteriole is smaller than that of the afferent arteriole, which helps maintain a fairly high blood pressure in the glomerulus.

Bowman's capsule (or glomerular capsule) is the expanded end of a renal tubule; it encloses the glomerulus. The inner layer of Bowman's capsule is made of **podocytes**; the name means "foot cells," and the "feet" of the podocytes are on the surface of the glomerular capillaries (see Fig. 18-3). The arrangement of podocytes creates pores, slits between adjacent "feet," which make this layer very permeable. The outer layer of Bowman's capsule has no pores and is not permeable. The space between the inner and outer layers of Bowman's capsule contains renal filtrate, the fluid that is formed from the blood in the glomerulus and will eventually become urine.

Renal Tubule

The **renal tubule** continues from Bowman's capsule and consists of the following parts: **proximal convoluted tubule** (in the renal cortex), **loop of Henle** (or loop of the nephron, in the renal medulla), and **distal convoluted tubule** (in the renal cortex). The distal convoluted tubules from several nephrons empty into a **collecting tubule**. Several collecting tubules then unite to form a papillary duct that empties urine into a calyx of the renal pelvis.

Cross-sections of the parts of the renal tubule are shown in Fig. 18-3. Notice how thin the walls of the tubule are, as well as the microvilli in the proximal convoluted tubule. These anatomic characteristics provide for efficient exchanges of materials, as you will see.

All parts of the renal tubule are surrounded by **peritubular capillaries**, which arise from the efferent arteriole. The peritubular capillaries will receive the materials reabsorbed by the renal tubules; this is described in the section on urine formation.

BLOOD VESSELS OF THE KIDNEY

The pathway of blood flow through the kidney is an essential part of the process of urine formation. Blood from the abdominal aorta enters the **renal artery**, which branches within the kidney into several interlobar arteries (between the renal pyramids). Each interlobar artery becomes an arcuate artery (arches over a pyramid), which branches into many interlobular arteries that enter the renal cortex (see Fig. 18-2). The interlobular arteries give rise to afferent arterioles in the renal cortex (see Fig. 18-3). From the afferent arterioles, blood flows into the glomeruli (capillaries), to efferent arterioles, to peritubular capillaries, and to a series of veins with the same names (interlobular and arcuate) as their neighboring arteries. The interlobar veins all unite at the hilus to form the **renal vein**, which empties blood into the inferior vena cava. Notice that this pathway has two sets of capillaries, and recall that it is in capillaries that exchanges take place between the blood and surrounding tissues. Therefore, in the kidneys there are two sites of exchange. The exchanges that take place between the nephrons and the capillaries of the kidneys will form urine from blood plasma.

Figure 18-2 also shows two views of a vascular cast of a kidney; the shape of the blood vessels has been preserved in red plastic. You can see how dense the vasculature of a kidney is, and most of these vessels are capillaries.

FORMATION OF URINE

The formation of urine involves three major processes. The first is glomerular filtration, which takes place in the renal corpuscles. The second and third are tubular reabsorption and tubular secretion, which take place in the renal tubules.

GLOMERULAR FILTRATION

You may recall that filtration is the process in which blood pressure forces plasma and dissolved material out of capillaries. In **glomerular filtration**, blood pressure forces plasma, dissolved substances, and small proteins out of the glomeruli and into Bowman's capsules. This fluid is no longer plasma but is called **renal filtrate**.

The blood pressure in the glomeruli, compared with that in other capillaries, is relatively high, about 60 mm Hg. The pressure in Bowman's capsule is very low, and its inner, podocyte layer is very permeable, so that approximately 20% to 25% of the blood that enters glomeruli becomes renal filtrate in Bowman's capsules. The blood cells and larger proteins are too large to be forced out of the glomeruli, so they remain in the blood. Waste products are dissolved in blood plasma, so they pass into the renal filtrate. Useful materials such as nutrients and minerals are also dissolved in plasma and are also present in renal filtrate. Filtration is not selective with respect to usefulness; it is selective only with respect to size.

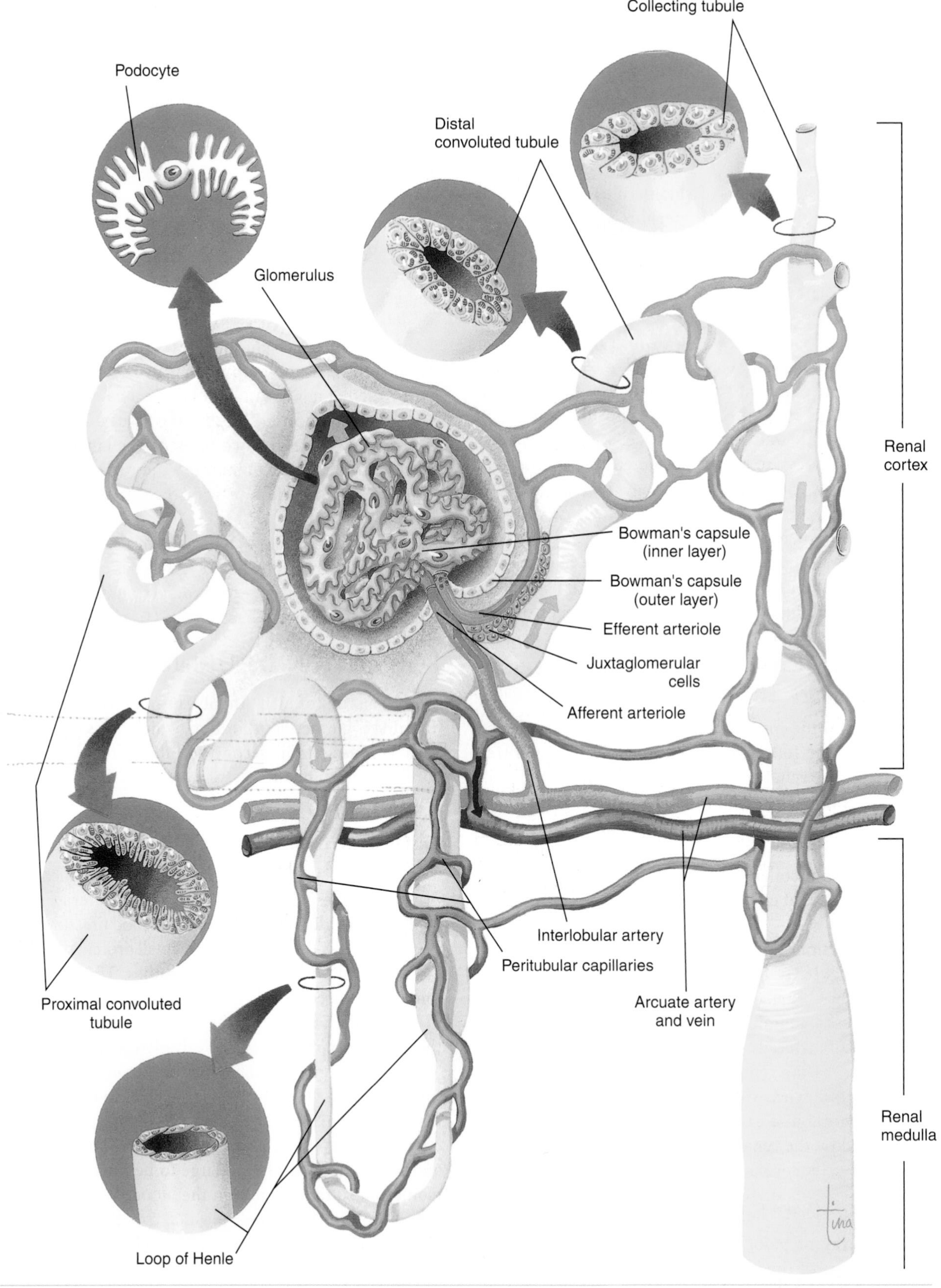

Figure 18-3 A nephron with its associated blood vessels. Portions of the nephron have been magnified. The arrows indicate the direction of blood flow and flow of renal filtrate. See text for description.

QUESTION: How does the shape of a podocyte contribute to its function? How is the lining of the proximal convoluted tubule specialized?

Therefore, renal filtrate is very much like blood plasma, except that there is far less protein and no blood cells are present.

The **glomerular filtration rate** (GFR) is the amount of renal filtrate formed by the kidneys in 1 minute and averages 100 to 125 mL per minute. GFR may be altered if the rate of blood flow through the kidneys changes. If blood flow increases, the GFR increases, and more filtrate is formed. If blood flow decreases (as may happen following a severe hemorrhage), the GFR decreases, less filtrate is formed, and urinary output decreases (see Box 18-2: Renal Failure and Hemodialysis).

Box 18–2 | RENAL FAILURE AND HEMODIALYSIS

Renal failure, the inability of the kidneys to function properly, may be the result of three general causes, which may be called prerenal, intrinsic renal, and postrenal.

"Prerenal" means that the problem is "before" the kidneys, that is, in the blood flow to the kidneys. Any condition that decreases blood flow to the kidneys may result in renal damage and failure. Examples are severe hemorrhage or very low blood pressure following a heart attack (MI) or fluid loss because of severe diarrhea or vomiting.

"Intrinsic renal" (or intrarenal) means that the problem is in the kidneys themselves. Diabetes and hypertension damage the blood vessels of the kidneys and are the causes of 70% of all cases of end-stage renal failure. Bacterial infections of the kidneys or exposure to chemicals (certain antibiotics) may cause damage to the nephrons. **Rhabdomyolysis** is the result of damage to skeletal muscle tissue; large molecules such as myoglobin leak from the damaged cells into the blood and may clog the kidney tubules. This potentially fatal condition may be caused by extensive crush injuries (as in car accidents) or electrical shock. Polycystic kidney disease is a genetic disorder in which the kidney tubules dilate and become nonfunctional. Severe damage may not be apparent until age 40 to 60 years but may then progress to renal failure.

"Postrenal" means that the problem is "after" the kidneys, somewhere in the rest of the urinary tract. Obstruction of urine flow may be caused by kidney stones in a ureter, a twisted ureter, or prostatic hypertrophy that impairs emptying of the bladder.

Treatment of renal failure involves correcting the specific cause, if possible. If not possible, and kidney damage is permanent, the person is said to have chronic renal failure. **Hemodialysis** is the use of an artificial kidney machine to do what the patient's nephrons can no longer do. The patient's blood is passed through minute tubes surrounded by fluid (dialysate) with the same chemical composition as plasma. Waste products and excess minerals diffuse out of the patient's blood into the fluid of the machine.

Although hemodialysis does prolong life for those with chronic renal failure, it does not fully take the place of functioning kidneys. The increasing success rate of kidney transplants, however, does indeed provide the possibility of a normal life for people with chronic renal failure.

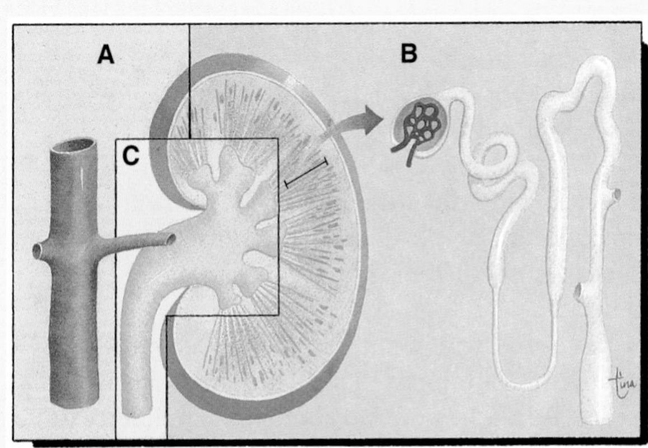

Box Figure 18–A Causes of renal failure. (**A**) Prerenal. (**B**) Intrinsic renal. (**C**) Postrenal.

TUBULAR REABSORPTION

Tubular reabsorption takes place from the renal tubules into the peritubular capillaries. In a 24-hour period, the kidneys form from 150 to 180 liters of filtrate, and normal urinary output in that time is 1 to 2 liters. Imagine that you have on your desk 150 pennies. That is quite a few pennies and represents how many liters of filtrate your kidneys form each day. If you are the kidneys, how many pennies will you have to give away to represent daily urinary output? Right, only one or two; the rest you will keep. Therefore, you can see that most of the renal filtrate is kept in the body, returned to the blood, and does not become urine. In fact, approximately 99% of the filtrate is reabsorbed back into the blood in the peritubular capillaries. Only about 1% of the filtrate will enter the renal pelvis as urine.

Most reabsorption and secretion (about 65%) take place in the proximal convoluted tubules, whose cells have **microvilli** that greatly increase their surface area. The distal convoluted tubules and collecting tubules are also important sites for the reabsorption of water (Fig. 18-4).

Mechanisms of Reabsorption

1. **Active transport**—the cells of the renal tubule use ATP to transport most of the useful materials from the filtrate to the blood. These useful materials include glucose, amino acids, vitamins, and positive ions.

   For many of these substances, the renal tubules have a **threshold level** of reabsorption. This means that there is a limit to how much the tubules can remove from the filtrate. For example, if the filtrate level of glucose is normal (reflecting a normal blood glucose level), the tubules will reabsorb all of the glucose, and none will be found in the urine. What happens is this: The number of glucose transporter molecules in the membranes of the tubule cells is sufficient to take in the number of glucose molecules passing by in the filtrate. If, however, the blood glucose level is above normal, the amount of glucose in the filtrate will also be above normal and will exceed the threshold level of reabsorption. The number of glucose molecules to be reabsorbed is more than the number of the transporter molecules available to do so. In this situation, therefore, some glucose will remain in the filtrate and be present in urine.

   The reabsorption of Ca^{+2} ions is increased by parathyroid hormone (PTH). The parathyroid glands secrete PTH when the blood calcium level decreases. The reabsorption of Ca^{+2} ions by the kidneys is one of the mechanisms by which the blood calcium level is raised back to normal.

   The hormone aldosterone, secreted by the adrenal cortex, increases the reabsorption of Na^+ ions and the excretion of K^+ ions. Besides regulating the blood levels of sodium and potassium, aldosterone also affects the volume of blood.

2. **Passive transport**—many of the negative ions that are returned to the blood are reabsorbed following the reabsorption of positive ions, because unlike charges attract.
3. **Osmosis**—the reabsorption of water follows the reabsorption of minerals, especially sodium ions. The hormones that affect reabsorption of water are discussed in the next section.
4. **Pinocytosis**—small proteins are too large to be reabsorbed by active transport. They become adsorbed to the membranes of the cells of the proximal convoluted tubules. The cell membrane then sinks inward and folds around the protein to take it in (see Fig. 3-3 in Chapter 3 for depictions of this and the other transport mechanisms). Normally all proteins in the filtrate are reabsorbed; none are found in urine.

TUBULAR SECRETION

This mechanism also changes the composition of urine. In **tubular secretion**, however, substances are actively secreted from the blood in the peritubular capillaries into the filtrate in the renal tubules (the opposite of tubular reabsorption). Waste products, such as ammonia and some creatinine, and the metabolic products of medications may be secreted into the filtrate to be eliminated in urine. The walls of the collecting tubules have **intercalated cells** that contain proton pumps in the membranes of their free surfaces. These pumps can secrete hydrogen ions (H^+) into the renal filtrate, even against a very high concentration gradient, to help maintain the normal pH of blood. This is why the pH of urine can be much more acidic than the pH of the blood from which it was made.

HORMONES THAT INFLUENCE REABSORPTION OF WATER

Aldosterone is secreted by the adrenal cortex in response to a high blood potassium level, to a low blood sodium level, or to a decrease in blood pressure. When aldosterone stimulates the reabsorption of Na^+ ions, water follows from the filtrate back to the blood. This helps maintain normal blood volume and blood pressure.

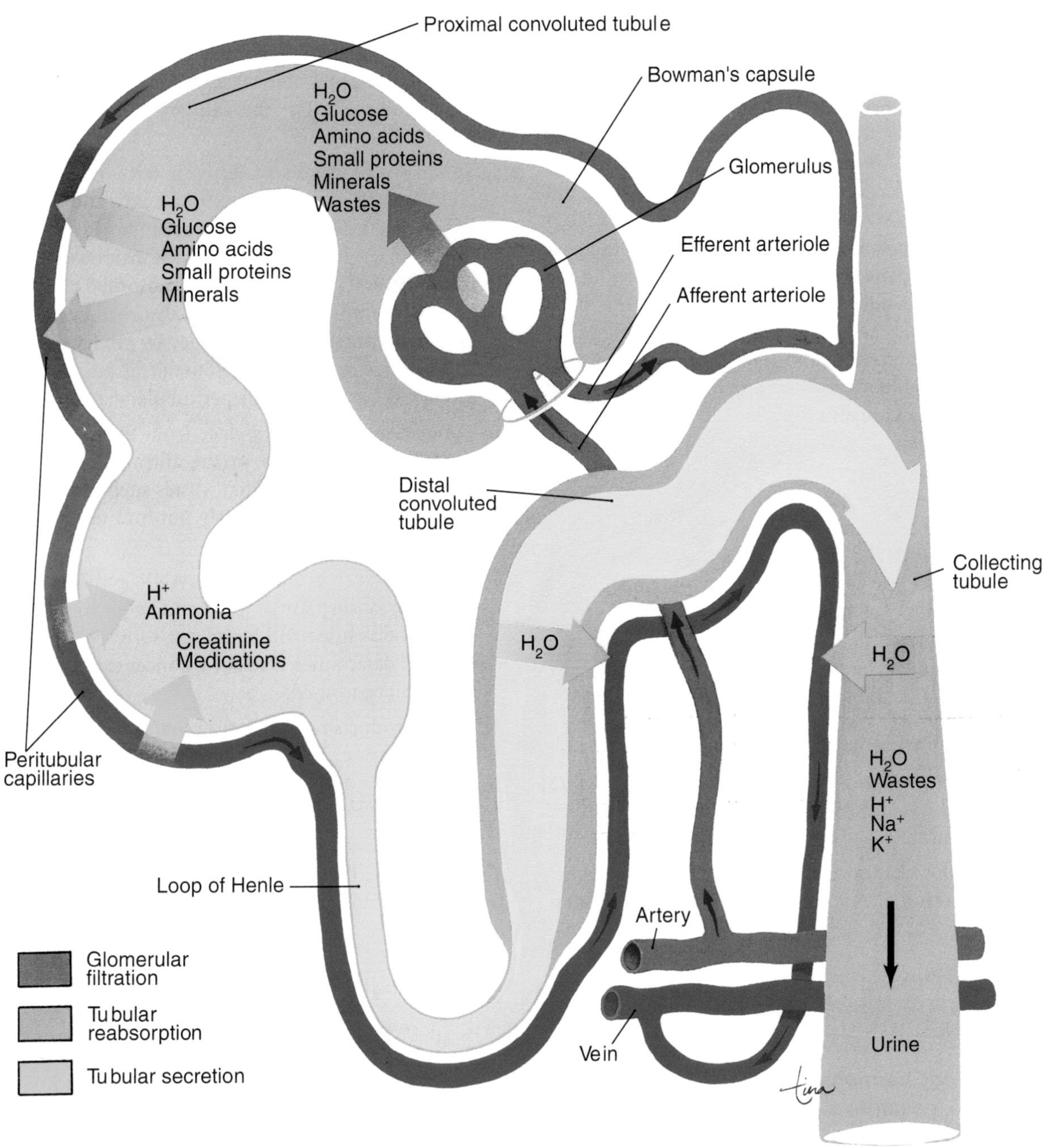

Figure 18-4 Schematic representation of glomerular filtration, tubular reabsorption, and tubular secretion. The renal tubule has been uncoiled, and the peritubular capillaries are shown adjacent to the tubule.

QUESTION: Describe tubular secretion; that is, it goes from where to where? What substances may be secreted?

You may recall that the antagonist to aldosterone is **atrial natriuretic peptide** (ANP, one of a group of these cardiac peptides), which is secreted by the atria of the heart when the atrial walls are stretched by high blood pressure or greater blood volume. ANP decreases the reabsorption of Na^+ ions by the kidneys; these remain in the filtrate, as does water, and are excreted. By increasing the elimination of sodium and water, ANP lowers blood volume and blood pressure.

Antidiuretic hormone (ADH) is released by the posterior pituitary gland when the amount of water in the body decreases. Under the influence of ADH, the distal convoluted tubules and collecting tubules are able to reabsorb more water from the renal filtrate. This helps maintain normal blood volume and blood pressure and also permits the kidneys to produce urine that is more concentrated than body fluids. Producing a concentrated urine is essential to prevent excessive water loss while still excreting all the substances that must be eliminated.

If the amount of water in the body increases, however, the secretion of ADH diminishes, and the kidneys will reabsorb less water. Urine then becomes dilute, and water is eliminated until its concentration in the body returns to normal. This may occur following ingestion of excessive quantities of fluids. The effects of hormones on the kidneys are summarized in Table 18-1 and illustrated in Fig. 18-5.

SUMMARY OF URINE FORMATION

1. The kidneys form urine from blood plasma. Blood flow through the kidneys is a major factor in determining urinary output.
2. Glomerular filtration is the first step in urine formation. Filtration is not selective in terms of usefulness of materials; it is selective only in terms of size. The relatively high blood pressure in the glomeruli forces plasma, dissolved materials, and small proteins into Bowman's capsules; the fluid is now called renal filtrate.
3. Tubular reabsorption is selective in terms of usefulness. Nutrients such as glucose, amino acids, and vitamins are reabsorbed by active transport and may have renal threshold levels. Positive ions are reabsorbed by active transport, and negative ions are reabsorbed most often by passive transport. Water is reabsorbed by osmosis, and small proteins are reabsorbed by pinocytosis.

   Reabsorption takes place from the filtrate in the renal tubules to the blood in the peritubular capillaries.
4. Tubular secretion takes place from the blood in the peritubular capillaries to the filtrate in the renal tubules and can ensure that wastes such as creatinine or excess H^+ ions are actively put into the filtrate to be excreted.
5. Hormones such as aldosterone, ANP, and ADH influence the reabsorption of water and help maintain normal blood volume and blood pressure. The secretion of ADH determines whether a concentrated or dilute urine will be formed.
6. Waste products remain in the renal filtrate and are excreted in urine.

THE KIDNEYS AND ACID-BASE BALANCE

The kidneys are the organs most responsible for maintaining the pH of blood and tissue fluid within normal ranges.

Table 18–1 | **EFFECTS OF HORMONES ON THE KIDNEYS**

HORMONE (GLAND)	FUNCTION
Antidiuretic hormone (ADH) (posterior pituitary)	Increases reabsorption of water from the filtrate to the blood. (Urinary output decreases.)
Parathyroid hormone (PTH) (parathyroid glands)	Increases reabsorption of Ca^{+2} ions from filtrate to the blood and excretion of phosphate ions into the filtrate.
Aldosterone (adrenal cortex)	Increases reabsorption of Na^+ ions from the filtrate to the blood and excretion of K^+ ions into the filtrate. Water is reabsorbed following the reabsorption of sodium. (Urinary output decreases.)
Atrial natriuretic peptide (ANP) (atria of heart)	Decreases reabsorption of Na^+ ions, which remain in the filtrate. More sodium and water are eliminated in urine. (Urinary output increases.)

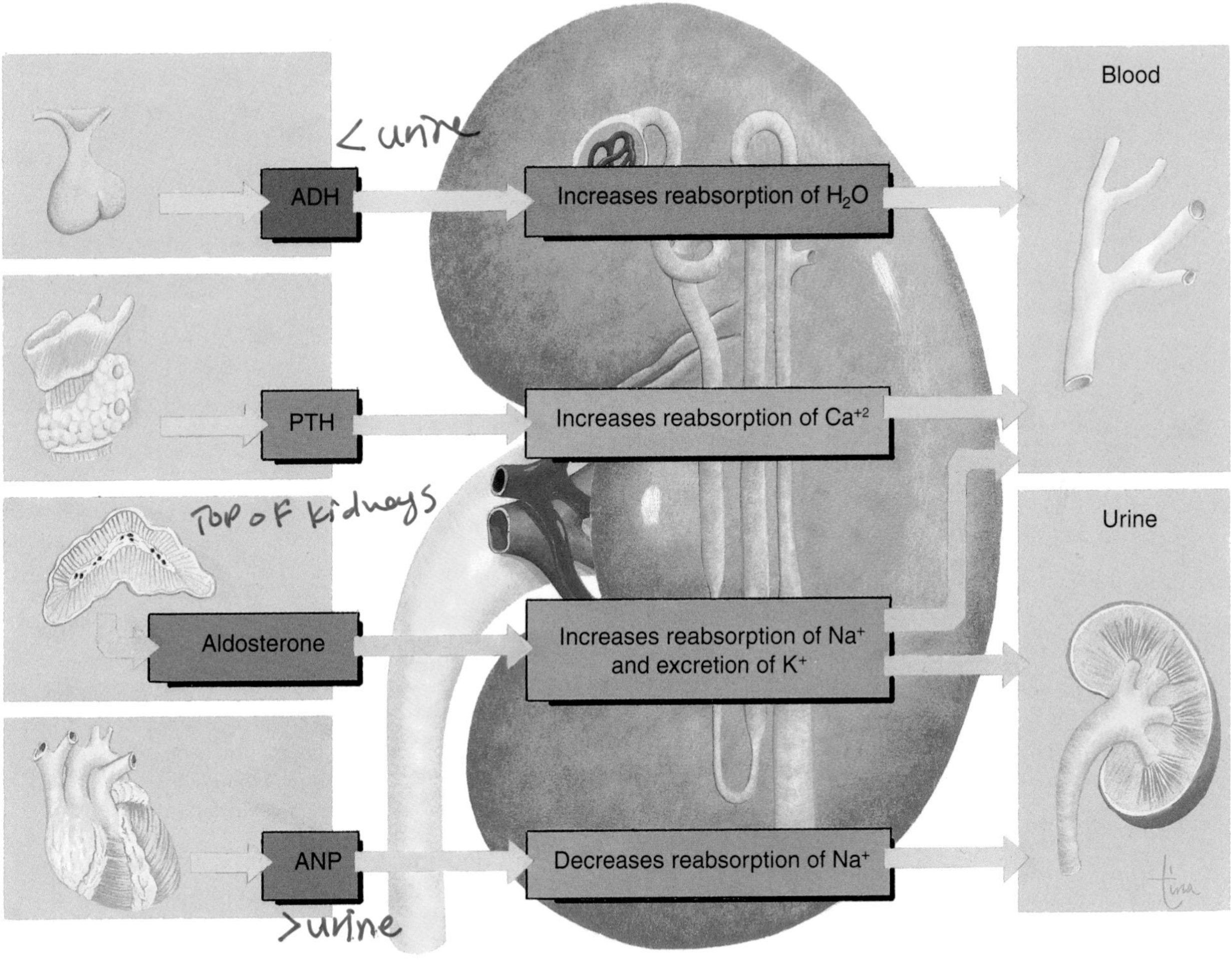

Figure 18-5 Effects of hormones on the kidneys.

QUESTION: Do any of these hormones affect both reabsorption and secretion? If so, how?

They have the greatest ability to compensate for the pH changes that are a normal part of body metabolism or the result of disease and to make the necessary corrections.

This regulatory function of the kidneys is complex, but at its simplest it may be described as follows. If body fluids are becoming too acidic, the kidneys will secrete more H^+ ions into the renal filtrate and will return more HCO_3^- ions to the blood. This will help raise the pH of the blood back to normal. The reactions involved in such a mechanism are shown in Fig. 18-6, to which we will return later. First, however, let us briefly consider how the kidneys will compensate for body fluids that are becoming too alkaline. You might expect the kidneys to do the opposite of what was just described, and that is precisely what happens. The kidneys will return H^+ ions to the blood and excrete HCO_3^- ions in urine. This will help lower the pH of the blood back to normal.

Because the natural tendency is for body fluids to become more acidic, let us look at the pH-raising mechanism in more detail (see Fig. 18-6). The cells of the renal tubules can secrete H^+ ions or ammonia in exchange for Na^+ ions and, by doing so, influence the reabsorption of other ions. Hydrogen ions and bicarbonate ions are obtained from the reaction of CO_2 and water (or other processes). An amine group from an amino acid is combined with an H^+ ion to form ammonia.

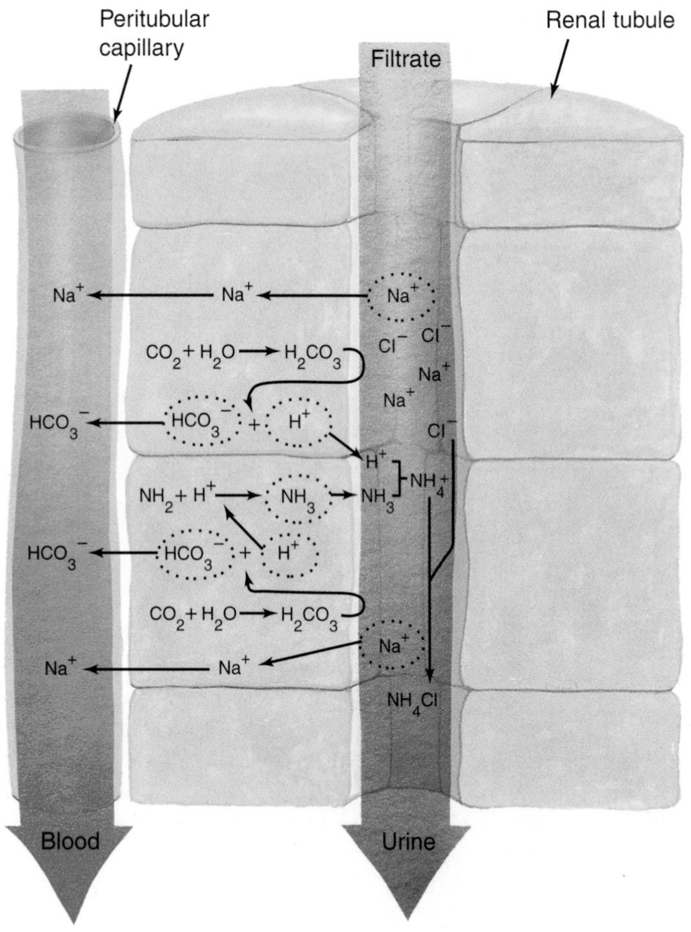

Figure 18-6 Renal regulation of acid-base balance. The cells of the renal tubule secrete H^+ ions and ammonia into the filtrate and return Na^+ ions and HCO_3^- ions to the blood in the peritubular capillaries. See text for further description.

QUESTION: The cells of the renal tubule make good use of CO_2. What do the cells use CO_2 for?

The tubule cell secretes the H^+ ion and the ammonia into the renal filtrate, and two Na^+ ions are reabsorbed in exchange. In the filtrate, the H^+ ion and ammonia form NH_4^+ (an ammonium radical), which reacts with a chloride ion (Cl^-) to form NH_4Cl (ammonium chloride) that is excreted in urine.

As the Na^+ ions are returned to the blood in the peritubular capillaries, the HCO_3^- ions that were generated in the tubule cell follow. Notice what has happened: Two H^+ ions have been excreted in urine, and two Na^+ ions and two HCO_3^- ions have been returned to the blood. As reactions like these take place, the body fluids are prevented from becoming too acidic. The kidneys are the only organs that can eliminate H^+ ions from the body to correct a decreasing pH.

Another mechanism used by the cells of the kidney tubules to regulate pH is the phosphate buffer system, which is based on the same principle: the creation of H^+ ions and HCO_3^- ions to excrete or retain. This mechanism is described and illustrated in Chapter 19.

OTHER FUNCTIONS OF THE KIDNEYS

In addition to the functions described thus far, the kidneys have other functions, some of which are not directly related to the formation of urine. These functions are secretion of renin (which does influence urine formation), production of erythropoietin, and activation of vitamin D.

1. **Secretion of renin**—When blood pressure decreases, the **juxtaglomerular** (*juxta* means "next to") **cells** in the walls of the afferent arterioles secrete the enzyme **renin**. Renin then initiates the renin-angiotensin mechanism to raise blood pressure. This was first described in Chapter 13, and the sequence of events is presented in Table 18-2. The end product of this mechanism is

Table 18–2 | THE RENIN-ANGIOTENSIN MECHANISM

SEQUENCE

1. Decreased blood pressure stimulates the kidneys to secrete renin.
2. Renin splits the plasma protein angiotensinogen (synthesized by the liver) to angiotensin I.
3. Angiotensin I is converted to angiotensin II by an enzyme found in lung tissue and vascular endothelium.
4. Angiotensin II causes vasoconstriction and stimulates the adrenal cortex to secrete aldosterone.

angiotensin II, which causes vasoconstriction and increases the secretion of aldosterone, both of which help raise blood pressure.

A normal blood pressure is essential to normal body functioning. Perhaps the most serious change is a sudden, drastic decrease in blood pressure, such as would follow a severe hemorrhage. In response to such a decrease, the kidneys will decrease filtration and urinary output and will initiate the formation of angiotensin II. In these ways the kidneys help ensure that the heart has enough blood to pump to maintain cardiac output and blood pressure.

2. **Secretion of erythropoietin**—This hormone is secreted whenever the blood oxygen level decreases (hypoxemia). Erythropoietin stimulates the red bone marrow to increase the rate of RBC production. With more RBCs in circulation, the oxygen-carrying capacity of the blood is greater, and the hypoxic state may be corrected (see also Box 18-3: Erythropoietin).
3. **Activation of vitamin D**—Recall that vitamin D is formed from cholesterol in the skin when the skin is exposed to ultraviolet rays. This vitamin exists in several structural forms that are converted to vitamin D_3 (calcitriol) by the kidneys. Vitamin D_3 is the most active form of vitamin D, which increases the absorption of calcium and phosphate in the small intestine and has other metabolic functions (see Chapter 17, Table 17-5).

ELIMINATION OF URINE

The ureters, urinary bladder, and urethra do not change the composition or amount of urine but are responsible for the periodic elimination of urine.

URETERS

Each **ureter** extends from the hilus of a kidney to the lower, posterior side of the urinary bladder (see Fig. 18-1). Like the kidneys, the ureters are retroperitoneal, that is, behind the peritoneum of the dorsal abdominal cavity. A cross-section of a ureter is shown in Fig. 18-7. Notice how thick the smooth muscle layer is. Notice also how small the lumen (cavity) is. The lining of the ureter has wide, deep folds that reduce the size of the lumen.

The smooth muscle in the wall of the ureter contracts in peristaltic waves to propel urine toward the urinary bladder. As the bladder fills, it expands and compresses the lower ends of the ureters to prevent backflow of urine.

URINARY BLADDER

The **urinary bladder** is a muscular sac below the peritoneum and behind the pubic bones. In women, the

Box 18–3 | ERYTHROPOIETIN

Anemia is one of the most debilitating consequences of renal failure, one that hemodialysis cannot reverse. Diseased kidneys stop producing erythropoietin, a natural stimulus for RBC production. Erythropoietin can be produced by genetic engineering and is available for hemodialysis patients. In the past, their anemia could be treated only with transfusions, which exposed these patients to possible immunologic complications as a result of repeated exposure to donated blood or to viral diseases. The synthetic erythropoietin eliminates such risks.

Caution is advised, however, because some clinical studies have shown that recipients of artificial erythropoietin were more likely to die sooner than those patients who did not receive the drug. Some researchers suggest that the synthetic erythropoietin may act as a growth stimulator for certain cancer tumors.

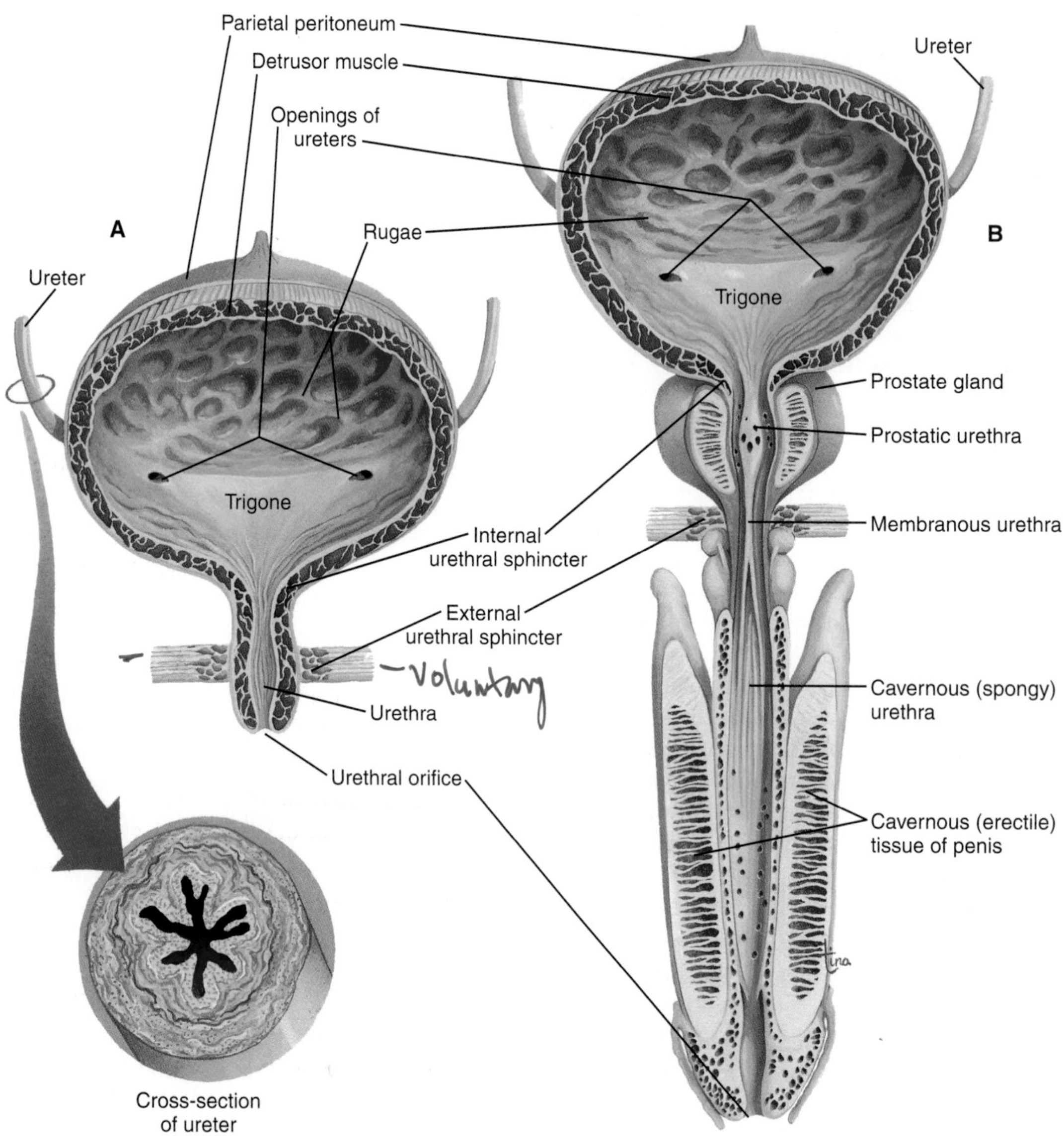

Figure 18-7 (**A**) Frontal section of female urinary bladder and urethra; a cross-section of the ureter is also shown. (**B**) Frontal section of male urinary bladder and urethra.

QUESTION: Name the sphincters of the urinary system and state whether each is voluntary or involuntary.

bladder is inferior to the uterus; in men, the bladder is superior to the prostate gland. The bladder is a reservoir for accumulating urine, and it contracts to eliminate urine.

The mucosa of the bladder is **transitional epithelium**, which permits expansion without tearing the lining. When the bladder is empty, the mucosa appears wrinkled; these folds are **rugae**, which also permit expansion. On the floor of the bladder is a triangular area called the **trigone**, which has no rugae and does not expand. The points of the triangle are the openings of the two ureters and that of the urethra (Fig. 18-7).

The smooth muscle layer in the wall of the bladder is called the **detrusor muscle**. It is a muscle in the form of a sphere; when it contracts it becomes a smaller sphere, and its volume diminishes. Around the opening of the urethra the muscle fibers of the detrusor form the **internal urethral sphincter** (or sphincter of the bladder), which is involuntary.

URETHRA

The **urethra** (see Fig. 18-7) carries urine from the bladder to the exterior. The **external urethral sphincter** is made of the surrounding skeletal (striated) muscle of the pelvic floor and is under voluntary control.

In women, the urethra is 1 to 1.5 inches (2.5 to 4 cm) long and is anterior to the vagina. In men, the urethra is 7 to 8 inches (17 to 20 cm) long. The first part just outside the bladder is called the prostatic urethra because it is surrounded by the prostate gland. The next inch is the membranous urethra, around which is the external urethral sphincter. The longest portion is the cavernous urethra (or spongy or penile urethra), which passes through the cavernous (or erectile) tissue of the penis. The male urethra carries semen and urine.

THE URINATION REFLEX

Urination may also be called **micturition** or **voiding**. This reflex is a spinal cord reflex over which voluntary control may be exerted. The stimulus for the reflex is stretching of the detrusor muscle of the bladder. The bladder can hold as much as 800 mL of urine, or even more, but the reflex is activated long before the maximum is reached.

When urine volume reaches 200 to 400 mL, the stretching is sufficient to generate sensory impulses that travel to the sacral spinal cord. Motor impulses return along parasympathetic nerves to the detrusor muscle, causing contraction. At the same time, the internal urethral sphincter relaxes. If the external urethral sphincter is voluntarily relaxed, urine flows into the urethra, and the bladder is emptied.

Urination can be prevented by voluntary contraction of the external urethral sphincter. However, if the bladder continues to fill and be stretched, voluntary control is eventually no longer possible.

CHARACTERISTICS OF URINE

The characteristics of urine include physical and chemical aspects that are often evaluated as part of a urinalysis. Some of these are described here (see also Appendix D: Normal Values for Some Commonly Used Urine Tests).

Amount—normal urinary output per 24 hours is 1 to 2 liters. Many factors can significantly change output. Excessive sweating or loss of fluid through diarrhea will decrease urinary output (**oliguria**) to conserve body water. Excessive fluid intake will increase urinary output (**polyuria**). Consumption of alcohol will also increase output because alcohol inhibits the secretion of ADH, and the kidneys will reabsorb less water.

Color—the typical yellow color of urine (from urochrome, a breakdown product of bile) is often called "straw" or "amber." Concentrated urine is a deeper yellow (amber) than is dilute urine. Freshly voided urine is clear, not cloudy.

Specific gravity—the normal range is 1.010 to 1.025; this is a measure of the dissolved materials in urine. The specific gravity of distilled water is 1.000, meaning that there are no solutes present. Therefore, the higher the specific gravity number, the more dissolved material is present. Someone who has been exercising strenuously and has lost body water in sweat will usually produce less urine, which will be more concentrated and have a higher specific gravity.

The specific gravity of the urine is an indicator of concentrating ability: The kidneys must excrete, in as little water as possible, the waste products that are constantly formed.

pH—the pH range of urine is between 4.6 and 8.0, with an average value of 6.0. Diet has the greatest influence on urine pH. A vegetarian diet will result in a more alkaline urine, whereas a high-protein diet will result in a more acidic urine.

Constituents—urine is approximately 95% water, which is the solvent for waste products and salts. Salts are not considered true waste products because they may well be utilized by the body when needed, but excess amounts will be excreted in urine (see Box 18-4: Kidney Stones).

Nitrogenous wastes—as their name indicates, all of these wastes contain nitrogen. Urea is formed by liver cells when excess amino acids are deaminated to be used for energy production. Creatinine comes from the metabolism of creatine phosphate, an energy source in muscles. Uric acid comes from the metabolism of nucleic acids, that is, the breakdown of DNA and RNA. Although these are waste products, there is always a certain amount of each in the blood. Box 18-5: Blood Tests and Kidney Function describes the relationship between blood levels of these waste products and kidney function.

Other non-nitrogenous waste products include small amounts of urobilin from the hemoglobin of old

Box 18-4 | KIDNEY STONES

Kidney stones, or **renal calculi**, are crystals of the salts that are normally present in urine. A very high concentration of salts in urine may trigger precipitation of the salt and formation of crystals, which can range in size from microscopic to 10 to 20 mm in diameter. The most common type of kidney stone is made of calcium salts; a less common type is made of uric acid.

Kidney stones are most likely to form in the renal pelvis. Predisposing factors include decreased fluid intake or overingestion of minerals (as in mineral supplements), both of which lead to the formation of a very concentrated urine.

The entry of a kidney stone into a ureter may cause intense pain (renal colic) and bleeding. Obstruction of a ureter by a stone may cause backup of urine and possible kidney damage. Treatments include surgery to remove the stone, or lithotripsy, the use of shock waves to crush the stone into pieces small enough to be eliminated without damage to the urinary tract.

Box 18-5 | BLOOD TESTS AND KIDNEY FUNCTION

Waste products are normally present in the blood, and the concentration of each varies within a normal range. As part of the standard lab work called blood chemistry, the levels of the three nitrogenous waste products are determined (urea, creatinine, and uric acid).

If blood levels of these three substances are within normal ranges, it may be concluded that the kidneys are excreting these wastes at normal rates. If, however, these blood levels are elevated, one possible cause is that kidney function has been impaired. Of the three, the creatinine level is probably the most reliable indicator of kidney functioning. Blood urea nitrogen (BUN) may vary considerably in certain situations not directly related to the kidneys. For example, BUN may be elevated as a consequence of a high-protein diet or of starvation when body protein is being broken down at a faster rate than normal. Uric acid levels may also vary according to diet. However, elevated blood levels of all three nitrogenous wastes usually indicate impaired glomerular filtration.

Uremia is a general term for an elevated blood urea level. Some clinicians think the term is inaccurate, that other waste products cause the toxicity. However, because the term is still used, we should be aware of its meaning.

RBCs (see Fig. 11-4 in Chapter 11) and may include the metabolic products of medications. Table 18-3 summarizes the characteristics of urine.

When a substance not normally found in urine does appear there, there is a reason for it. The reason may be quite specific or more general. Table 18-4 lists some abnormal constituents of urine and possible reasons for each (see also Box 18-6: Urinary Tract Infections).

AGING AND THE URINARY SYSTEM

With age, the number of nephrons in the kidneys decreases, often to half the original number by the age of 70 to 80, and the kidneys lose some of their concentrating ability. The glomerular filtration rate also decreases, partly as a consequence of arteriosclerosis and diminished renal blood flow. Despite these changes, excretion of nitrogenous wastes usually remains adequate.

The urinary bladder decreases in size, and the tone of the detrusor muscle decreases. These changes may lead to a need to urinate more frequently. Urinary incontinence (the inability to control voiding) is *not* an inevitable consequence of aging and can be prevented or minimized. Elderly people are, however, more at risk for infections of the urinary tract, especially if voiding leaves residual urine in the bladder.

Table 18–3 | CHARACTERISTICS OF NORMAL URINE

CHARACTERISTIC	DESCRIPTION
Amount	1-2 liters per 24 hours; highly variable depending on fluid intake and water loss through the skin and GI tract
Color	Straw or amber; darker means more concentrated; should be clear, not cloudy
Specific gravity	1.010-1.025; a measure of the dissolved material in urine; the lower the value, the more dilute the urine
pH	Average 6; range 4.6-8.0; diet has the greatest effect on urine pH
Composition	95% water; 5% salts and waste products
Nitrogenous wastes	Urea—from amino acid metabolism Creatinine—from muscle metabolism Uric acid—from nucleic acid metabolism

Table 18–4 | ABNORMAL CONSTITUENTS IN URINE

CHARACTERISTIC	REASON(S)
Glycosuria (presence of glucose)	As long as blood glucose levels are within normal limits, filtrate levels will also be normal and will not exceed the threshold level for reabsorption. In an untreated diabetic, for example, blood glucose is too high; therefore the filtrate glucose level is too high. The kidneys reabsorb glucose up to their threshold level, but the excess remains in the filtrate and is excreted in urine.
Proteinuria (presence of protein)	Most plasma proteins are too large to be forced out of the glomeruli, and the small proteins that enter the filtrate are reabsorbed by pinocytosis. The presence of protein in the urine indicates that the glomeruli have become too permeable, as occurs in some types of kidney disease.
Hematuria (presence of blood—RBCs)	The presence of RBCs in urine may also indicate that the glomeruli have become too permeable. Another possible cause might be bleeding somewhere in the urinary tract. Pinpointing the site of bleeding would require specific diagnostic tests.
Bacteriuria (presence of bacteria)	Bacteria give urine a cloudy rather than clear appearance; WBCs may be present also. The presence of bacteria means that there is an infection somewhere in the urinary tract. Further diagnostic tests would be needed to determine the precise location.
Ketonuria (presence of ketones)	Ketones are formed from fats and proteins that are used for energy production. A trace of ketones in urine is normal. Higher levels of ketones indicate an increased use of fats and proteins for energy. This may be the result of malfunctioning carbohydrate metabolism (as in diabetes mellitus) or simply the result of a high-protein diet.

Box 18-6 | URINARY TRACT INFECTIONS

Infections may occur anywhere in the urinary tract and are most often caused by the microbial agents of sexually transmitted diseases (see Chapter 20) or by the bacteria that are part of the normal flora of the colon. In women especially, the urinary and anal openings are in close proximity, and colon bacteria on the skin of the perineum may invade the urinary tract. The use of urinary catheters in hospitalized or bedridden patients may also be a factor if sterile technique is not carefully followed.

Cystitis is inflammation of the urinary bladder. Symptoms include frequency of urination, painful voiding, and low back pain. **Nephritis** (or pyelonephritis) is inflammation of the kidneys. Although this may be the result of a systemic bacterial infection, nephritis is a common complication of untreated lower urinary tract infections such as cystitis. Possible symptoms are fever and flank pain (in the area of the kidneys). Untreated nephritis may result in severe damage to nephrons and progress to renal failure.

SUMMARY

The kidneys are the principal regulators of the internal environment of the body. The composition of all body fluids is either directly or indirectly regulated by the kidneys as they form urine from blood plasma. The kidneys are also of great importance in the regulation of the pH of the body fluids. These topics are the subject of the next chapter.

STUDY OUTLINE

The urinary system consists of two kidneys, two ureters, the urinary bladder, and the urethra.

1. The kidneys form urine to excrete waste products and to regulate the volume, electrolytes, and pH of blood and tissue fluid.
2. The other organs of the system are concerned with elimination of urine.

Kidneys (see Fig. 18-1)

1. Retroperitoneal on either side of the backbone in the upper abdominal cavity; partially protected by the lower rib cage.
2. Adipose tissue and the renal fascia cushion the kidneys and help hold them in place.
3. Hilus—an indentation on the medial side; renal artery enters, renal vein and ureter emerge.

Kidney—internal structure (see Fig. 18-2)

1. Renal cortex—outer tissue layer, made of renal corpuscles and convoluted tubules.
2. Renal medulla (pyramids)—inner tissue layer, made of loops of Henle and collecting tubules.
3. Renal pelvis—a cavity formed by the expanded end of the ureter within the kidney at the hilus; extensions around the papillae of the pyramids are called calyces, which collect urine.

The Nephron—the functional unit of the kidney (see Fig. 18-3); 1 million per kidney

1. Renal corpuscle—consists of a glomerulus surrounded by a Bowman's capsule.
   a. Glomerulus—a capillary network between an afferent arteriole and an efferent arteriole.
   b. Bowman's capsule—the expanded end of a renal tubule that encloses the glomerulus; inner layer is made of podocytes, has pores, and is very permeable; contains renal filtrate (potential urine).
2. Renal tubule—consists of the proximal convoluted tubule, loop of Henle, distal convoluted tubule, and collecting tubule. Collecting tubules unite to form papillary ducts that empty urine into the calyces of the renal pelvis.
   a. Peritubular capillaries—arise from the efferent arteriole and surround all parts of the renal tubule.

Blood Vessels of the Kidney (see Figs. 18-1, 18-2, and 18-3)

1. Pathway: abdominal aorta → renal artery → interlobar arteries → arcuate arteries → interlobular arteries → afferent arterioles → glomeruli → efferent arterioles → peritubular capillaries → interlobular veins → arcuate veins → interlobar veins → renal vein → inferior vena cava.
2. Two sets of capillaries provide for two sites of exchanges between the blood and tissues in the process of urine formation.

Formation of Urine (see Fig. 18-4)

1. Glomerular filtration—takes place from the glomerulus to Bowman's capsule. High blood pressure (60 mm Hg) in the glomerulus forces plasma, dissolved materials, and small proteins out of the blood and into Bowman's capsule. The fluid is now called filtrate. Filtration is selective only in terms of size; blood cells and large proteins remain in the blood.
2. GFR is 100 to 125 mL per minute. Increased blood flow to the kidney increases GFR; decreased blood flow decreases GFR.
3. Tubular reabsorption—takes place from the filtrate in the renal tubule to the blood in the peritubular capillaries; 99% of the filtrate is reabsorbed; only 1% becomes urine.
   a. Active transport—reabsorption of glucose, amino acids, vitamins, and positive ions; threshold level is a limit to the quantity that can be reabsorbed.
   b. Passive transport—most negative ions follow the reabsorption of positive ions.
   c. Osmosis—water follows the reabsorption of minerals, especially sodium.
   d. Pinocytosis—small proteins are engulfed by proximal tubule cells.
4. Tubular secretion—takes place from the blood in the peritubular capillaries to the filtrate in the renal tubule; creatinine and other waste products may be secreted into the filtrate to be excreted in urine. Body fluids naturally tend to become more acidic; secretion of H^+ ions helps maintain pH of blood.
5. Hormones that affect reabsorption—aldosterone, atrial natriuretic peptide, antidiuretic hormone, and parathyroid hormone—see Table 18-1 and Fig. 18-5.

The Kidneys and Acid-Base Balance

1. The kidneys have the greatest capacity to compensate for normal and abnormal pH changes.
2. If the body fluids are becoming too acidic, the kidneys excrete H^+ ions and return HCO_3^- ions to the blood (see Fig. 18-6).
3. If the body fluids are becoming too alkaline, the kidneys return H^+ ions to the blood and excrete HCO_3^- ions.

Other Functions of the Kidneys

1. Secretion of renin by juxtaglomerular cells when blood pressure decreases (see Table 18-2). Angiotensin II causes vasoconstriction and increases secretion of aldosterone.
2. Secretion of erythropoietin in response to hypoxia; stimulates red bone marrow to increase rate of RBC production.
3. Activation of vitamin D—conversion of inactive forms to the active form, D_3.

Elimination of Urine—the function of the ureters, urinary bladder, and urethra

Ureters (see Figs. 18-1 and 18-7)

1. Each extends from the hilus of a kidney to the lower posterior side of the urinary bladder.
2. Peristalsis of smooth muscle layer propels urine toward bladder.

Urinary Bladder (see Figs. 18-1 and 18-7)

1. A muscular sac below the peritoneum and behind the pubic bones; in women, below the uterus; in men, above the prostate gland.
2. Mucosa—transitional epithelial tissue folded into rugae; permit expansion without tearing.
3. Trigone—triangular area on bladder floor; no rugae, does not expand; bounded by openings of ureters and urethra.
4. Detrusor muscle—the smooth muscle layer, a spherical muscle; contracts to expel urine (reflex).
5. Internal urethral sphincter—involuntary; formed by detrusor muscle fibers around the opening of the urethra.

Urethra—takes urine from the bladder to the exterior (see Fig. 18-7)

1. In women—1 to 1.5 inches long; anterior to vagina.
2. In men—7 to 8 inches long; passes through the prostate gland and penis.
3. Has the external urethral sphincter: skeletal muscle of pelvic floor (voluntary).

The Urination Reflex—also called micturition or voiding

1. Stimulus: stretching of the detrusor muscle by accumulating urine.
2. Sensory impulses to spinal cord, motor impulses (parasympathetic) return to detrusor muscle, which contracts; internal urethral sphincter relaxes.
3. The external urethral sphincter provides voluntary control.

Characteristics of Urine (see Table 18-3)

Abnormal Constituents of Urine (see Table 18-4)

REVIEW QUESTIONS

1. Describe the location of the kidneys, ureters, urinary bladder, and urethra. (pp. 463, 473–475)
2. Name the three areas of the kidney, and state what each consists of. (p. 463)
3. Name the two major parts of a nephron. State the general function of nephrons. (p. 465)
4. Name the parts of a renal corpuscle. What process takes place here? Name the parts of a renal tubule. What processes take place here? (pp. 465, 468)
5. Explain what is meant by a threshold level of reabsorption, and state the mechanism of tubular reabsorption of each of the following: (p. 468)
   a. Water
   b. Glucose
   c. Small proteins
   d. Positive ions
   e. Negative ions
   f. Amino acids
   g. Vitamins
6. Explain the importance of tubular secretion. (p. 468)
7. Describe the pathway of blood flow through the kidney from the abdominal aorta to the inferior vena cava. (p. 465)
8. Name the two sets of capillaries in the kidney, and state the processes that take place in each. (pp. 465, 468)
9. Name the hormone that has each of these effects on the kidneys: (pp. 468, 470)
   a. Promotes reabsorption of Na^+ ions
   b. Promotes direct reabsorption of water
   c. Promotes reabsorption of Ca^{+2} ions
   d. Promotes excretion of K^+ ions
   e. Decreases reabsorption of Na^+ ions
10. In what circumstances will the kidneys excrete H^+ ions? What ions will be returned to the blood? How will this affect the pH of blood? (p. 471)
11. In what circumstances do the kidneys secrete renin, and what is its purpose? (pp. 472–473)
12. In what circumstances do the kidneys secrete erythropoietin, and what is its purpose? (p. 473)
13. Describe the function of the ureters and that of the urethra. (pp. 473, 475)
14. Describe the function of rugae and the detrusor muscle of the urinary bladder. (p. 474)
15. Describe the urination reflex in terms of stimulus, part of the CNS involved, effector muscle, internal urethral sphincter, and voluntary control. (p. 475)
16. Describe the characteristics of normal urine in terms of appearance, amount, pH, specific gravity, and composition. (p. 475)
17. State the source of each of the nitrogenous waste products: creatinine, uric acid, and urea. (p. 475)

FOR FURTHER THOUGHT

1. The functioning of the kidneys may be likened to cleaning your room by throwing everything out the window, then going outside to retrieve what you wish to keep, such as jammies and slippers. Imagine the contents of a room, liken them to the materials in the blood (you yourself are a kidney), and describe what happens to each, and why.
2. Explain why fatty acids are not found in urine. Under what circumstances are water-soluble vitamins (such as vitamin C) found in urine?
3. Explain how a spinal cord transection at the level of T11 will affect the urination reflex.
4. As part of his physical for the college football team, Patrick has a urinalysis, which shows a high level of ketones. He is not diabetic and not ill. What might cause the high urine level of ketones? What blood chemistry test (for nitrogenous wastes) would help confirm this?
5. A patient with possible food poisoning has a blood pH of 7.33, a urine pH of 4.5, and a respiratory rate of 28 per minute. What kind of pH imbalance is this? Explain your reasoning step by step.
6. Erythropoietin, called EPO, has become a drug used illegally by some athletes. Which athletes use EPO, that is, in what kind of sports? What benefits are they hoping for? What part of a CBC would indicate that an athlete is taking EPO? Explain.
7. After a 4-hour workout on a hot June day, the high school track coach tells her group to keep drinking plenty of water. The girls assure their coach that they will know just how to determine if they are sufficiently hydrated that evening, that they have their color scheme memorized. What do they mean?
8. Question Figure 18-A is a schematic of blood flow through a kidney. Sections 3, 4, 9, and 10 have been labeled with the names of the blood vessels. Can you label the other numbered sections?

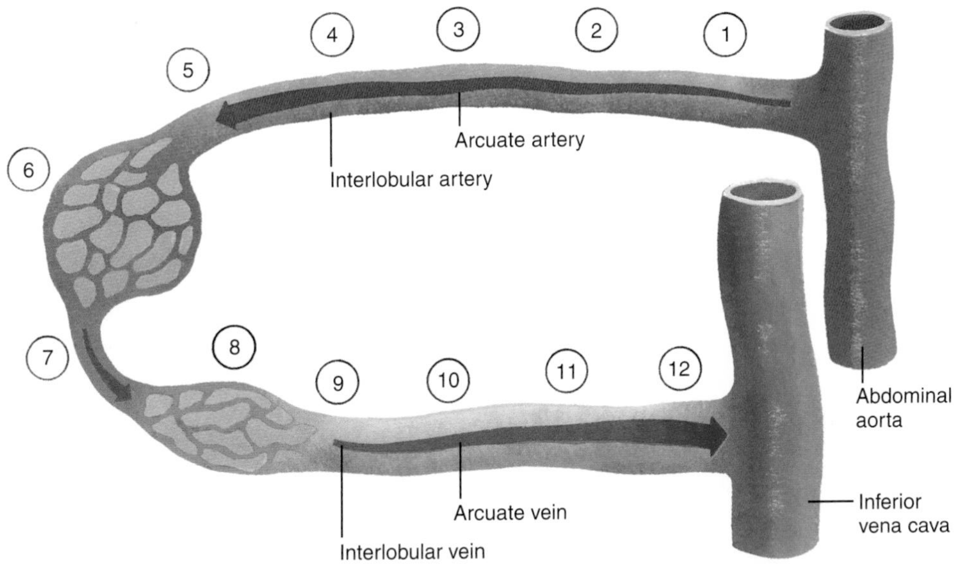

QUESTION FIGURE 18-A: Schematic pathway of blood flow through the kidney.

CHAPTER

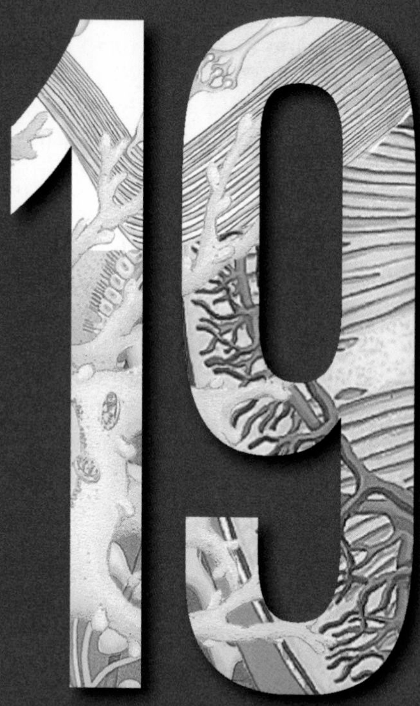

Fluid—Electrolyte and Acid—Base Balance

STUDENT OBJECTIVES

- Describe the water compartments and the name for the water in each.
- Explain how water moves between compartments.
- Explain the regulation of the intake and output of water.
- Name the major electrolytes in body fluids, and state their functions.
- Explain the regulation of the intake and output of electrolytes.
- Describe the three buffer systems in body fluids.
- Explain why the respiratory system has an effect on pH, and describe respiratory compensating mechanisms.
- Explain the renal mechanisms for pH regulation of extracellular fluid.
- Describe the effects of acidosis and alkalosis.

NEW TERMINOLOGY

Amine group *(ah-**MEEN**)*
Anions *(**AN**-eye-ons)*
Carboxyl group *(kar-**BAHK**-sul)*
Cations *(**KAT**-eye-ons)*
Electrolytes *(ee-**LEK**-troh-lites)*
Osmolarity *(ahs-moh-**LAR**-i-tee)*
Osmoreceptors *(AHS-moh-re-**SEP**-ters)*

RELATED CLINICAL TERMINOLOGY

Edema *(uh-**DEE**-muh)*
Hypercalcemia *(HIGH-per-kal-**SEE**-me-ah)*
Hyperkalemia *(HIGH-per-kuh-**LEE**-me-ah)*
Hypernatremia *(HIGH-per-nuh-**TREE**-me-ah)*
Hypocalcemia *(HIGH-poh-kal-**SEE**-me-ah)*
Hypokalemia *(HIGH-poh-kuh-**LEE**-me-ah)*
Hyponatremia *(HIGH-poh-nuh-**TREE**-me-ah)*

CHAPTER OUTLINE

*Terms that appear in **bold type** in the chapter text are defined in the glossary, which begins on page 603.*

People are watery creatures. More precisely, we are salt-watery creatures, though not as salty as the oceans. Water, the fluid medium of the human body, makes up 55% to 70% of the total body weight. Infants are more watery than adults, and adult men are more watery than women.

Electrolytes are the positive and negative ions present in body fluids. In previous chapters we have called these salts or, in some cases, trace elements. Many of these ions are minerals that are already familiar to you. They each have specific functions in body fluids, and some of them are also involved in the maintenance of the normal pH of the body fluids. In this chapter we will first discuss fluid–electrolyte balance, then review and summarize the mechanisms involved in acid–base balance.

WATER COMPARTMENTS

Most of the water of the body, about two-thirds of the total water volume, is found within individual cells and is called **intracellular fluid** (ICF). The remaining third is called **extracellular fluid** (ECF) and includes blood plasma, lymph, tissue fluid, and the specialized fluids such as cerebrospinal fluid, synovial fluid, aqueous humor, and serous fluid.

Water constantly moves from one fluid site in the body to another by the processes of filtration and **osmosis**. These fluid sites are called **water compartments** (Fig. 19–1). The chambers of the heart and all of the blood vessels form one compartment, and the water within is called plasma. By the process of filtration in capillaries, some plasma is forced out into tissue spaces (another compartment) and is then called tissue fluid. When tissue fluid enters cells by the process of osmosis, it has moved to still another compartment and is called intracellular fluid. The tissue fluid that enters lymph capillaries is in yet another compartment and is called lymph.

The other process (besides filtration) by which water moves from one compartment to another is osmosis, which, you may recall, is the diffusion of water through a semi-permeable membrane. Water will move through cell membranes from the area of its greater concentration to the area of its lesser concentration. Another way of expressing this is to say that water will diffuse to an area with a greater concentration of dissolved material. The concentration of electrolytes present in the various water compartments determines just how osmosis will take place. Therefore, if water is in balance in all of the compartments, the electrolytes are also in balance.

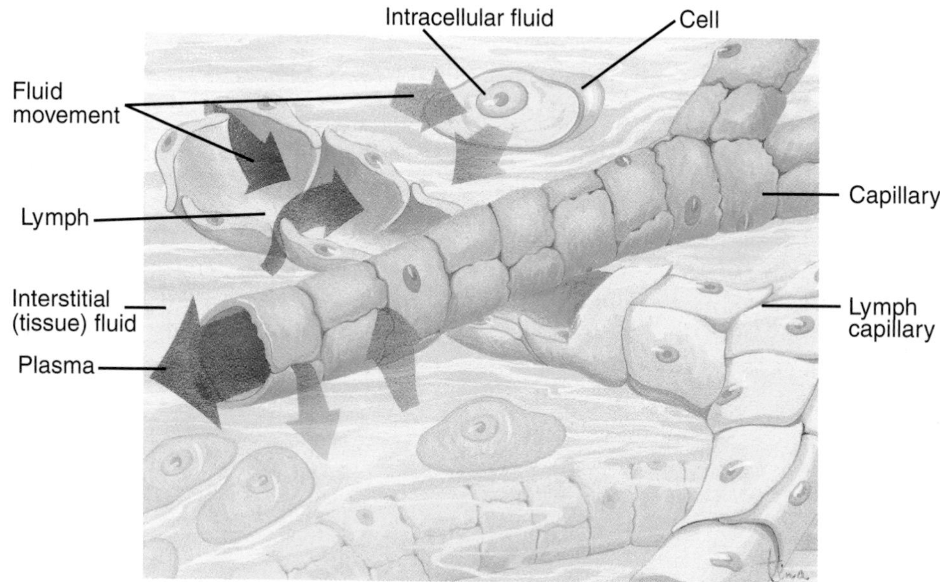

Figure 19–1 Water compartments. The name given to water in each of its locations is indicated.

QUESTION: Name two specialized fluids that are similar to tissue fluid.

Although water and ions are constantly moving, their relative proportions in the compartments remain constant; this is fluid–electrolyte homeostasis, and its maintenance is essential for life (see Box 19–1: Edema).

WATER INTAKE AND OUTPUT

Most of the water the body requires comes from the ingestion of liquids; this amount averages 1600 mL per day. The food we eat also contains water. Even foods we think of as somewhat dry, such as bread, contain significant amounts of water. The daily water total from food averages 700 mL. The last source of water, about 200 mL per day, is the metabolic water that is a product of cell respiration. The total intake of water per day, therefore, is about 2500 mL, or 2.5 liters.

Most of the water lost from the body is in the form of urine produced by the kidneys; this averages 1500 mL per day. About 500 mL per day is lost in the form of sweat, another 300 mL per day is in the form of water vapor in exhaled air, and another 200 mL per day is lost in feces. The total output of water is thus about 2500 mL per day.

Naturally, any increase in water output must be compensated for by an increase in intake. Someone who exercises strenuously, for example, may lose 1 to 2 liters of water in sweat and must replace that water by drinking more fluids. In a healthy individual, water intake equals water output, even though the amounts of each may vary greatly from the averages just mentioned (Fig. 19–2 and Table 19–1).

REGULATION OF WATER INTAKE AND OUTPUT

The hypothalamus in the brain contains **osmoreceptors** that detect changes in the osmolarity of body fluids. **Osmolarity** is the concentration of dissolved materials present in a fluid. Dehydration raises the osmolarity of the blood; that is, there is less water in proportion to the amount of dissolved materials. Another way to express this is to simply say that the blood is now a more concentrated solution. When dehydrated, we feel the sensation of thirst, characterized by dryness of the mouth and throat, as less saliva is produced. Thirst is an uncomfortable sensation, and we drink fluids to relieve it. The water we drink is readily absorbed by the mucosa of the stomach and small intestine and has the effect of decreasing the osmolarity of the blood. In other words, we can say that the water we just drank is causing the blood to become a more dilute solution, and, as the serum osmolarity returns to normal, the sensation of thirst diminishes.

As you may recall, the hypothalamus is also involved in water balance because of its production of antidiuretic hormone (ADH), which is stored in the posterior pituitary

Box 19–1 | EDEMA

Edema is an abnormal increase in the amount of tissue fluid, which may be localized or systemic. Sometimes edema is inapparent, and sometimes it is apparent as swelling.

Localized edema follows injury and inflammation of a body part. Spraining an ankle, for example, damages tissues that then release histamine. Histamine increases the permeability of capillaries, and more tissue fluid is formed. As tissue fluid accumulates, the ankle may become swollen.

Systemic edema is the result of an imbalance between the movement of water out of and into capillaries, that is, between filtration and osmosis. Excessive filtration will occur when capillary pressure rises. This may be caused by venous obstruction due to blood clots or by congestive heart failure. Edema of this type is often apparent in the lower extremities (pulmonary edema was described in Chapter 15).

Systemic bacterial infections may increase capillary permeability, and loss of plasma to tissue spaces is one aspect of septicemia. In this situation, however, the edema is of secondary importance to the hypotension, which may be life-threatening.

Insufficient osmosis, the return of tissue fluid into capillaries, is a consequence of a decrease in plasma proteins, especially albumin. This may occur in severe liver diseases such as cirrhosis, kidney disease involving loss of protein in urine, malnutrition, or severe burn injuries.

Because edema is a symptom rather than a disease, treatment is aimed at correcting the specific cause. If that is not possible, the volume of tissue fluid may be diminished by a low-salt diet and the use of diuretics.

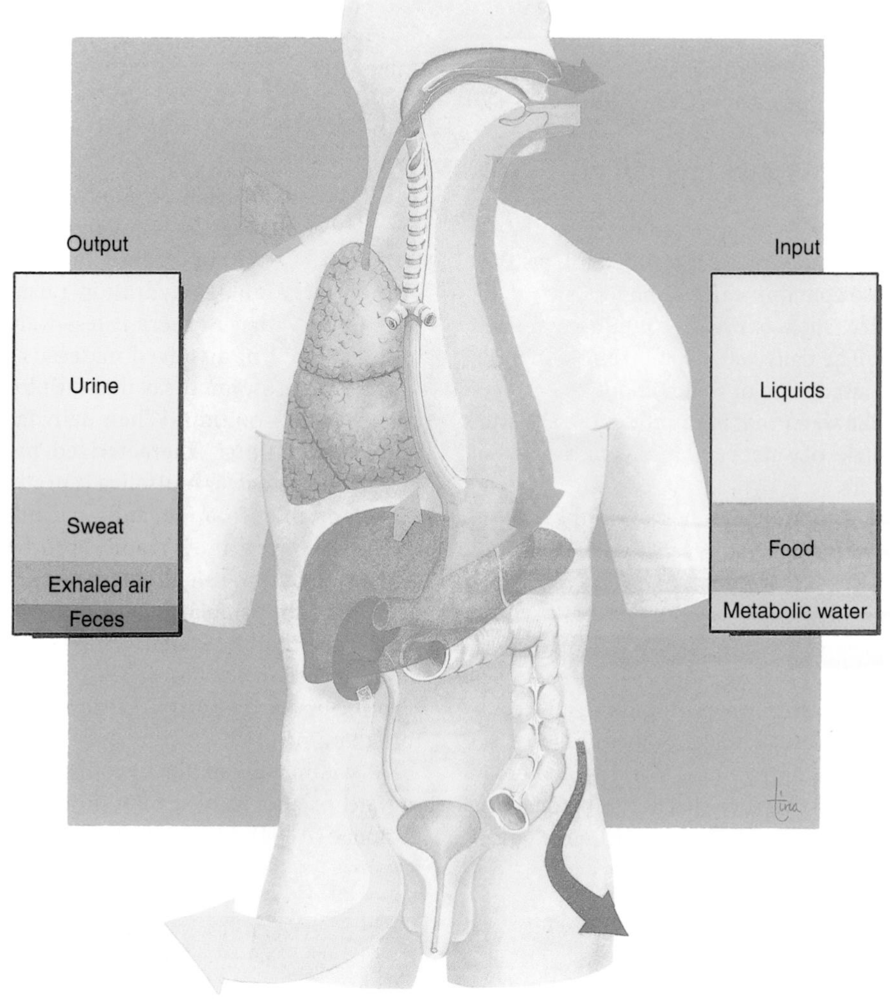

Figure 19–2 Water intake and output. See text and Table 19–1 for description.

QUESTION: On a very hot day, how might the output volumes change?

gland. In a state of dehydration, the hypothalamus stimulates the release of ADH from the posterior pituitary. Antidiuretic hormone then increases the reabsorption of water by the kidney tubules. Water is returned to the blood to preserve blood volume, and urinary output decreases.

The hormone aldosterone, from the adrenal cortex, also helps regulate water output. Aldosterone increases the reabsorption of Na^+ ions by the kidney tubules, and water from the renal filtrate follows the Na^+ ions back to the blood. Aldosterone is secreted when the Na^+ ion concentration of the blood decreases or whenever there is a significant decrease in blood pressure (the renin-angiotensin mechanism).

Several other factors may also contribute to water loss. These include excessive sweating, hemorrhage, diarrhea or vomiting, severe burns, and fever. In these circumstances, the kidneys will conserve water, but water must also be replaced by increased consumption. Following hemorrhage or during certain disease states, fluids may also be replaced by intravenous administration.

A less common occurrence is overhydration, the presence of too much water in the body. This may happen

Table 19–1 | WATER INTAKE AND OUTPUT

FORM	AVERAGE AMOUNT PER 24 HOURS (ML)
INTAKE	
Liquids	1600
Food	700
Metabolic water	200
OUTPUT	
Urine	1500
Sweat (and insensible water loss)	500
Exhaled air (water vapor)	300
Feces	200

following overconsumption of fluids. The osmolarity of the blood decreases, and there is too much water in proportion to electrolytes (or the blood is too dilute). This condition may become symptomatic and is called water intoxication. Symptoms are dizziness, abdominal cramps, nausea, and lethargy. Convulsions are possible in severe cases, and fluids must be restricted until the kidneys can excrete the excess water. A hormone that will contribute to that is atrial natriuretic peptide (ANP), which is secreted by the atria when blood volume or blood pressure increases. ANP then decreases the reabsorption of Na^+ ions by the kidneys, which increases urinary output of sodium and water. Also, secretion of ADH will diminish, which will contribute to a greater urinary output that will return the blood osmolarity to normal.

ELECTROLYTES

Electrolytes are chemicals that dissolve in water and dissociate into their positive and negative ions. Most electrolytes are the inorganic salts, acids, and bases found in all body fluids.

Most organic compounds are non-electrolytes; that is, they do not ionize when in solution. Glucose, for example, dissolves in water but does not ionize; it remains as intact glucose molecules. Some proteins, however, do form ionic bonds and when in solution dissociate into ions.

Positive ions are called **cations**. Examples are Na^+, K^+, Ca^{+2}, Mg^{+2}, Fe^{+2}, and H^+. Negative ions are called **anions**, and examples are Cl^-, HCO_3^-, SO_4^{-2} (sulfate), HPO_4^{-2} (phosphate), and protein anions.

Electrolytes help create the osmolarity of body fluids and, therefore, help regulate the osmosis of water between water compartments. Some electrolytes are involved in acid–base regulatory mechanisms, or they are part of structural components of tissues or part of enzymes. Some electrolytes can be stored in the body: calcium, phosphorus, and magnesium in bones and iron and copper in the liver.

ELECTROLYTES IN BODY FLUIDS

The three principal fluids in the body are intracellular fluid and the extracellular fluids plasma and tissue fluid. The relative concentrations of the most important electrolytes in these fluids are depicted in Fig. 19–3. The major differences may be summarized as follows. In intracellular fluid, the most abundant cation is K^+, the most abundant anion is HPO_4^{-2}, and protein anions are also abundant. In both tissue fluid and plasma, the most abundant cation is Na^+, and the most abundant anion is Cl^-. Protein anions form a significant part of plasma but not of tissue fluid. The functions of the major electrolytes are described in Table 19–2.

INTAKE, OUTPUT, AND REGULATION

Electrolytes are part of the food and beverages we consume, are absorbed by the gastrointestinal tract into the blood, and become part of body fluids. Hormones regulate the ECF concentrations of some electrolytes. Aldosterone increases the reabsorption of Na^+ ions and the excretion of K^+ ions by the kidneys. The blood sodium level is thereby raised, and the blood potassium level is lowered. ANP increases the excretion of Na^+ ions by the kidneys and lowers the blood sodium level. Parathyroid hormone (PTH) and calcitonin regulate the blood levels of calcium and phosphate. PTH increases the reabsorption of these minerals from bones and increases their absorption from food in the small intestine (vitamin D is also necessary). Calcitonin promotes the removal of calcium and phosphate from the blood to form bone matrix.

Electrolytes are lost in urine, sweat, and feces. Urine contains the electrolytes that are not reabsorbed by the kidney tubules; the major one of these is Na^+ ions. Other electrolytes are present in urine when their concentrations in the blood exceed the body's need for them.

The most abundant electrolytes in sweat are Na^+ ions and Cl^- ions. Electrolytes lost in feces are those that are not absorbed in either the small intestine or colon.

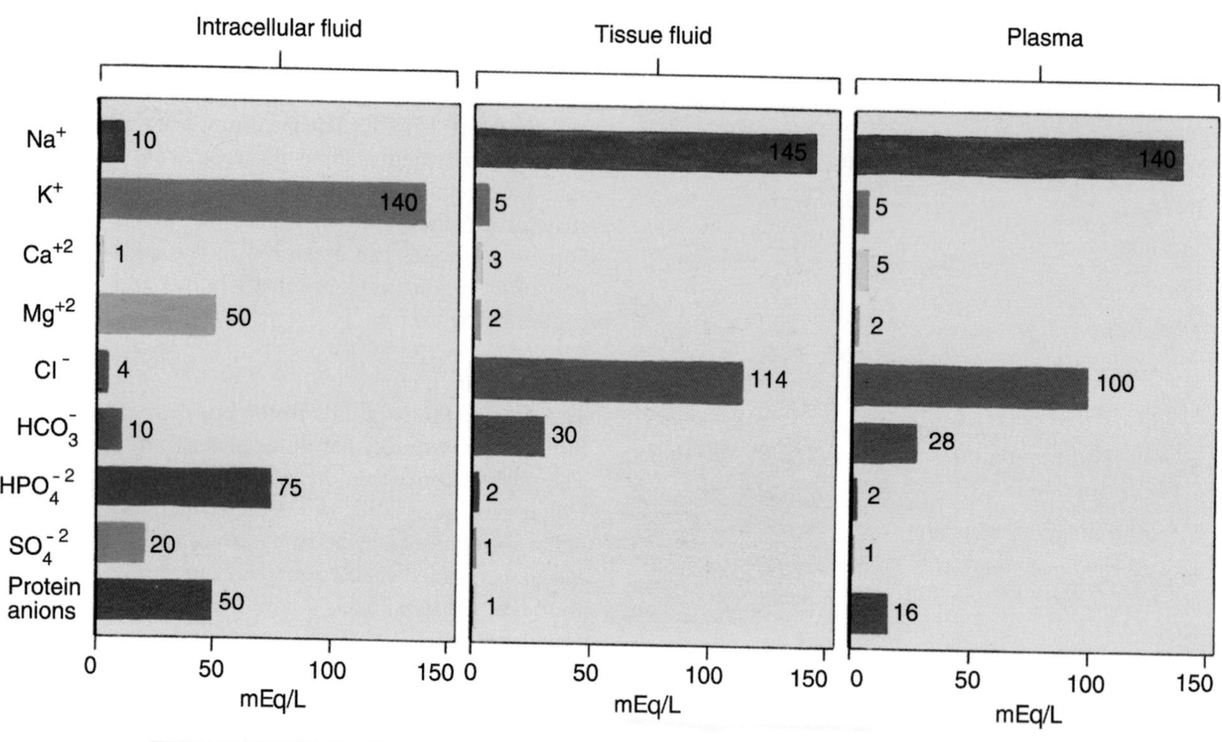

Figure 19–3 Electrolyte concentrations in intracellular fluid, tissue fluid, and plasma. Concentrations are expressed in milliequivalents per liter. See text for summary of major differences among these fluids.

QUESTION: Tissue fluid is most like which of the other fluids? Why did you already know this?

Table 19–2 | **MAJOR ELECTROLYTES**

ELECTROLYTE	PLASMA LEVEL mEq/L*	ICF LEVEL mEq/L	FUNCTIONS
Sodium (Na^+)	136–142	10	■ Creates much of the osmotic pressure of ECF; the most abundant cation in ECF ■ Essential for electrical activity of neurons and muscle cells
Potassium (K^+)	3.8–5.0	141	■ Creates much of the osmotic pressure in ICF; the most abundant cation in ICF ■ Essential for electrical activity of neurons and muscle cells
Calcium (Ca^{+2})	4.6–5.5	1	■ Most (98%) is found in bones and teeth ■ Maintains normal excitability of neurons and muscle cells ■ Essential for blood clotting
Magnesium (Mg^{+2})	1.3–2.1	58	■ Most (50%) is found in bone ■ More abundant in ICF than in ECF ■ Essential for ATP production and activity of neurons and muscle cells

Table 19–2 | MAJOR ELECTROLYTES—cont'd

ELECTROLYTE	PLASMA LEVEL mEq/L*	ICF LEVEL mEq/L	FUNCTIONS
Chloride (Cl^-)	95–103	4	■ Most abundant anion in ECF; diffuses easily into and out of cells; helps regulate osmotic pressure ■ Part of HCl in gastric juice
Bicarbonate (HCO_3^-)	28	10	■ Part of the bicarbonate buffer system
Phosphate (HPO_4^{-2})	1.7–2.6	75	■ Most (85%) is found in bones and teeth ■ Primarily an ICF anion ■ Part of DNA, RNA, ATP, phospholipids ■ Part of phosphate buffer system
Sulfate (SO_4^{-2})	1	2	■ Part of some amino acids and proteins

*The concentration of an ion is often expressed in milliequivalents per liter, abbreviated mEq/L, which is the number of electrical charges in each liter of solution.

Some of the major imbalances of electrolyte levels are described in Box 19–2: Electrolyte Imbalances.

ACID–BASE BALANCE

You have already learned quite a bit about the regulation of the pH of body fluids in the chapters on chemistry (see Chapter 2 for the pH scale), the respiratory system, and the urinary system. In this section, we will put all of that information together.

The normal pH range of blood is 7.35 to 7.45. The pH of tissue fluid is similar but can vary slightly above or below this range. The intracellular fluid has a pH range of 6.8 to 7.0. Notice that these ranges of pH are quite narrow; they must be maintained in order for enzymatic reactions and other processes to proceed normally.

Maintenance of acid–base homeostasis is accomplished by the buffer systems in body fluids, the rate and depth of respiration, and the kidneys.

BUFFER SYSTEMS

The purpose of a **buffer system** is to prevent drastic changes in the pH of body fluids by chemically reacting with strong acids or bases that would otherwise greatly

Box 19–2 | ELECTROLYTE IMBALANCES

IMBALANCES OF SODIUM

Hyponatremia—a consequence of excessive sweating, diarrhea, or vomiting. Characterized by dizziness, confusion, weakness, low BP, shock.

Hypernatremia—a consequence of excessive water loss or sodium ingestion. Characterized by loss of ICF and extreme thirst and agitation.

IMBALANCES OF POTASSIUM

Hypokalemia—a consequence of vomiting, diarrhea, or kidney disease. Characterized by fatigue, confusion, possible cardiac failure.

Hyperkalemia—a consequence of acute renal failure or Addison's disease. Characterized by weakness, abnormal sensations, cardiac arrhythmias, and possible cardiac arrest.

IMBALANCES OF CALCIUM

Hypocalcemia—a consequence of hypoparathyroidism or decreased calcium intake. Characterized by muscle spasms leading to tetany.

Hypercalcemia—a consequence of hyperparathyroidism. Characterized by muscle weakness, bone fragility, and possible kidney stones.

change the pH. A buffer system consists of a weak acid and a weak base. These molecules react with strong acids or bases that may be produced and change them to substances that do not have a great effect on pH.

Bicarbonate Buffer System

The two components of this buffer system are carbonic acid (H_2CO_3), a weak acid, and sodium bicarbonate ($NaHCO_3$), a weak base. Each of these molecules participates in a specific type of reaction.

If a potential pH change is created by a strong acid, the following reaction takes place:

$$\underset{\text{(strong acid)}}{HCl} + NaHCO_3 \rightarrow NaCl + \underset{\text{(weak acid)}}{H_2CO_3}$$

The strong acid has reacted with the sodium bicarbonate to produce a salt (NaCl) that has no effect on pH and a weak acid that has little effect on pH.

If a potential pH change is created by a strong base, the following reaction takes place:

$$\underset{\text{(strong base)}}{NaOH} + H_2CO_3 \rightarrow H_2O + \underset{\text{(weak base)}}{NaHCO_3}$$

The strong base has reacted with the carbonic acid to produce water, which has no effect on pH, and a weak base that has little effect on pH.

The bicarbonate buffer system is important in both the blood and tissue fluid. During normal metabolism, these fluids tend to become more acidic, so more sodium bicarbonate than carbonic acid is needed. The usual ratio of these molecules to each other is about 20:1 ($NaHCO_3$ to H_2CO_3).

Phosphate Buffer System

The two components of this buffer system are sodium dihydrogen phosphate (NaH_2PO_4), a weak acid, and sodium monohydrogen phosphate (Na_2HPO_4), a weak base. Let us use specific reactions to show how this buffer system works.

If a potential pH change is created by a strong acid, the following reaction takes place:

$$\underset{\text{(strong acid)}}{HCl} + Na_2HPO_4 \rightarrow NaCl + \underset{\text{(weak acid)}}{NaH_2PO_4}$$

The strong acid has reacted with the sodium monohydrogen phosphate to produce a salt that has no effect on pH and a weak acid that has little effect on pH.

If a potential pH change is created by a strong base, the following reaction takes place:

$$\underset{\text{(strong base)}}{NaOH} + NaH_2PO_4 \rightarrow H_2O + \underset{\text{(weak base)}}{Na_2HPO_4}$$

The strong base has reacted with the sodium dihydrogen phosphate to form water, which has no effect on pH, and a weak base that has little effect on pH.

The phosphate buffer system is important in the regulation of the pH of the blood by the kidneys (see Fig. 19–4). The cells of the kidney tubules can remove excess hydrogen ions by forming NaH_2PO_4, which is excreted in urine. The retained Na^+ ions are returned to the blood in the peritubular capillaries, along with bicarbonate ions. These are new bicarbonate ions that the renal cells synthesize from carbon dioxide and water.

Protein Buffer System

This buffer system is the most important one in the intracellular fluid. You may recall from Chapter 15 that hemoglobin buffers the hydrogen ions formed during CO_2 transport. The amino acids that make up proteins each have a **carboxyl group** (COOH) and an **amine** (or amino) **group** (NH_2) and may act as either acids or bases.

The carboxyl group may act as an acid because it can donate a hydrogen ion (H^+) to the fluid to counteract increasing alkalinity:

$$NH_2-\overset{\overset{\large H}{|}}{\underset{\underset{\large R}{|}}{C}}-COOH \rightarrow NH_2-\overset{\overset{\large H}{|}}{\underset{\underset{\large R}{|}}{C}}-COO^- + H^+$$

The amine group may act as a base because it can pick up an excess hydrogen ion from the fluid to counteract increasing acidity:

$$COOH-\overset{\overset{\large H}{|}}{\underset{\underset{\large R}{|}}{C}}-NH_2 \rightarrow COOH-\overset{\overset{\large H}{|}}{\underset{\underset{\large R}{|}}{C}}-NH_3^+$$

The buffer systems react within a fraction of a second to prevent drastic pH changes. However, they have the least capacity to prevent great changes in pH because a limited number of molecules of these buffers are present in body fluids. When an ongoing cause is disrupting the normal pH, the respiratory and renal mechanisms will also be needed.

RESPIRATORY MECHANISMS

The respiratory system affects pH because it regulates the amount of CO_2 present in body fluids. As you know, the respiratory system may be the cause of a pH imbalance

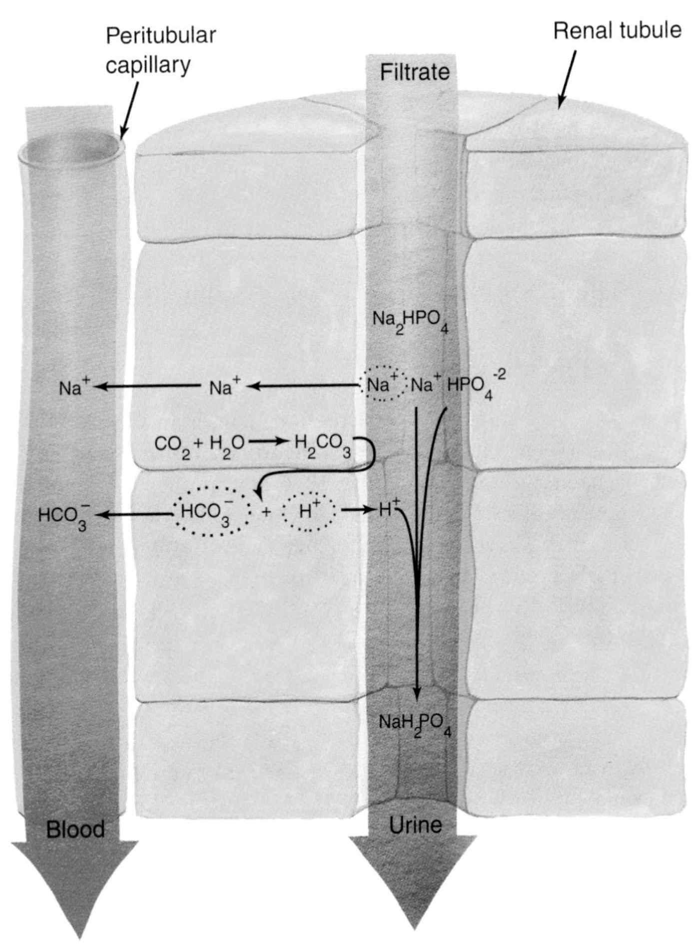

Figure 19–4 The phosphate buffer system. The reactions are shown in a kidney tubule. See text for description.

QUESTION: From where does the kidney tubule cell get a hydrogen ion to excrete?

or may help correct a pH imbalance from some other cause.

Respiratory Acidosis and Alkalosis

Respiratory acidosis is caused by anything that decreases the rate or efficiency of respiration. Severe pulmonary diseases are possible causes of respiratory acidosis. When CO_2 cannot be exhaled as fast as it is formed during cell respiration, excess CO_2 results in the formation of excess H^+ ions, as shown in this reaction:

$$CO_2 + H_2O \rightarrow H_2CO_3 \rightarrow H^+ + HCO_3^-$$

The excess H^+ ions lower the pH of body fluids.

Respiratory alkalosis is far less common but is the result of breathing more rapidly, which increases the amount of CO_2 exhaled. Because there are fewer CO_2 molecules in the body fluids, fewer H^+ ions are formed and pH tends to rise.

Respiratory Compensation for Metabolic pH Changes

Changes in pH caused by other than a respiratory disorder are called metabolic acidosis or alkalosis. In either case, the respiratory system may help prevent a drastic change in pH.

Metabolic acidosis may be caused by kidney disease, uncontrolled diabetes mellitus, excessive diarrhea or vomiting, or the use of some diuretics. When excess H^+ ions are present in body fluids, pH begins to decrease, and this stimulates the respiratory centers in the medulla. The response is to increase the rate of breathing to exhale more CO_2 to decrease H^+ ion formation. This helps raise the pH back toward the normal range.

Metabolic alkalosis is not common but may be caused by the overuse of antacid medications or the vomiting of stomach contents only. As the pH of body fluids begins to rise, breathing slows and decreases the amount of

CO_2 exhaled. The CO_2 retained within the body increases the formation of H^+ ions, which will help lower the pH back toward the normal range.

The respiratory system responds quickly to prevent drastic changes in pH, usually within 1 to 3 minutes. For an ongoing metabolic pH imbalance, however, the respiratory mechanism does not have the capacity to fully compensate. In such cases, respiratory compensation is only 50% to 75% effective.

RENAL MECHANISMS

As just discussed in Chapter 18, the kidneys help regulate the pH of extracellular fluid by excreting or conserving H^+ ions and by reabsorbing (or not) Na^+ ions and HCO_3^- ions. One mechanism was depicted in Fig. 18–6, and another, involving the phosphate buffer system, is shown in Fig. 19–4.

The kidneys have the greatest capacity to buffer an ongoing pH change. Although the renal mechanisms do not become fully functional for several hours to days, once they do they continue to be effective far longer than respiratory mechanisms. We will look more closely at why this is so in a moment, but first let us use as an example a patient with untreated diabetes mellitus who is in ketoacidosis, a metabolic acidosis. As acidic ketones accumulate in the blood, the capacity of the extracellular fluid (ECF) buffer systems is quickly exhausted. Breathing rate then increases, and more CO_2 is exhaled to decrease H^+ ion formation and raise the pH of ECF. There is, however, a limit to how much the respiratory rate can increase, but the renal buffering mechanisms will then become effective. At this time it is the kidneys that are keeping the patient alive by preventing acidosis from reaching a fatal level.

The kidneys have the greatest capacity to prevent fatal acidosis because the kidneys are able to remove H^+ ions from the body fluids and excrete them in urine. The buffer systems do not remove H^+ ions from the body, but keep them sequestered in molecules that do not ionize readily. The respiratory system can increase exhalations to prevent more H^+ ion formation from CO_2 but cannot get rid of H^+ ions from other sources (such as ketones). Only the kidneys can actually remove H^+ ions from body fluids, as well as create new bicarbonate ions to put into the blood. Even the kidneys have limits, however, and the cause of the acidosis must be corrected to prevent death.

In the case of an alkalosis, the kidney tubule cells will synthesize H^+ ions and HCO_3^- ions from CO_2 and water (as in Fig. 19–4). But the ions to be retained and returned to the blood are the H^+ ions, and the ions excreted in urine are the bicarbonate ions; this will lower the blood pH toward the normal range.

A summary of acid–base regulation is depicted in Fig. 19–5. Part A compares the speed and capacity of the buffer systems, respirations, and the kidneys. Part B depicts the compensating mechanisms for pH changes.

EFFECTS OF PH CHANGES

A state of **acidosis** is most detrimental to the central nervous system, causing depression of impulse transmission at synapses. A person in acidosis becomes confused and disoriented, then lapses into a coma.

Alkalosis has the opposite effect and affects both the central and peripheral nervous systems. Increased synaptic transmission, even without stimuli, is first indicated by irritability and muscle twitches. Progressive alkalosis is characterized by severe muscle spasms and convulsions.

The types of pH changes are summarized in Table 19–3.

AGING AND FLUID AND PH REGULATION

Changes in fluid balance or pH in elderly people are often the result of disease or damage to particular organs. A weak heart (congestive heart failure) that cannot pump efficiently allows blood to back up in circulation. In turn, this may cause edema, an abnormal collection of fluid. Edema may be systemic (often apparent in the lower legs) if the right ventricle is weak or pulmonary if the left ventricle is failing.

The sense of thirst may not be as acute in elderly people, who may become severely dehydrated before they begin to feel thirsty. An important behavioral consideration is that elderly people who fear urinary incontinence may decrease their intake of fluids.

Deficiencies of minerals in elderly people may be the result of poor nutrition or a side effect of some medications, especially those for hypertension that increase urinary output. Disturbances in pH may be caused by chronic pulmonary disease, diabetes, or kidney disease.

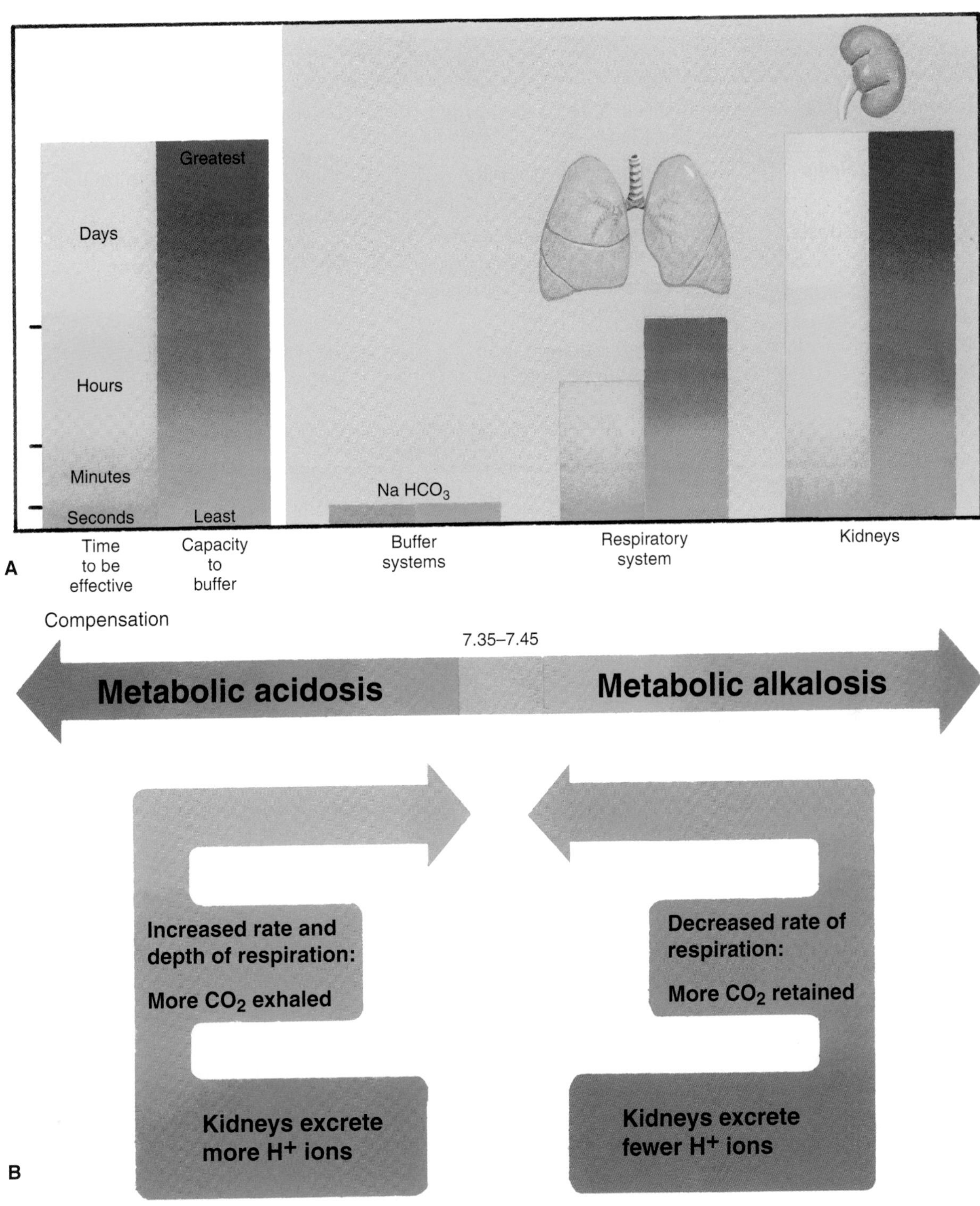

Figure 19–5 Summary of acid–base regulation. (**A**) Acid–base regulatory mechanisms compared with respect to time needed to become effective and capacity to buffer an ongoing pH change. (**B**) Compensation for metabolic acidosis or alkalosis. The respiratory and renal mechanisms contribute to returning the blood pH to its normal range.

QUESTION: In part B, why are the compensating mechanisms on the right side colored red and those on the left side colored blue?

Table 19–3 | PH CHANGES

CHANGE	POSSIBLE CAUSES	COMPENSATION
Metabolic acidosis	Kidney disease, ketosis, diarrhea, or vomiting	Increased respirations to exhale CO_2
Metabolic alkalosis	Overingestion of bicarbonate medications, gastric suctioning	Decreased respirations to retain CO_2
Respiratory acidosis	Decreased rate or efficiency of respiration: emphysema, asthma, pneumonia, paralysis of respiratory muscles	Kidneys excrete H^+ ions and reabsorb Na^+ ions and HCO_3^- ions
Respiratory alkalosis	Increased rate of respiration: anxiety, high altitude	Kidneys retain H^+ ions and excrete Na^+ ions and HCO_3^- ions

STUDY OUTLINE

Fluid–Electrolyte Balance

1. Water makes up 55% to 70% of the total body weight.
2. Electrolytes are the ions found in body fluids; most are minerals.

Water Compartments (see Fig. 19–1)

1. Intracellular fluid (ICF)—water within cells; about two-thirds of total body water.
2. Extracellular fluid (ECF)—water outside cells; includes plasma, lymph, tissue fluid, and specialized fluids.
3. Water constantly moves from one compartment to another. Filtration: plasma becomes tissue fluid. Osmosis: tissue fluid becomes plasma, lymph, or ICF.
4. Osmosis is regulated by the concentration of electrolytes in body fluids (osmolarity). Water will diffuse through membranes to areas of greater electrolyte concentration.

Water Intake (see Fig. 19–2)

1. Fluids, food, metabolic water—see Table 19–1.

Water Output (see Fig. 19–2)

1. Urine, sweat, exhaled air, feces—see Table 19–1.
2. Any variation in output must be compensated for by a change in input.

Regulation of Water Intake and Output

1. Hypothalamus contains osmoreceptors that detect changes in osmolarity of body fluids.
2. Dehydration stimulates the sensation of thirst, and fluids are consumed to relieve it.
3. ADH released from the posterior pituitary increases the reabsorption of water by the kidneys.
4. Aldosterone secreted by the adrenal cortex increases the reabsorption of Na^+ ions by the kidneys; water is then reabsorbed by osmosis.
5. If there is too much water in the body (overhydration caused by overconsumption), secretion of ADH decreases and urinary output increases.
6. If blood volume increases, ANP promotes loss of Na^+ ions and water in urine.

Electrolytes

1. Chemicals that dissolve in water and dissociate into ions; most are inorganic.
2. Cations are positive ions such as Na^+ and K^+.
3. Anions are negative ions such as Cl^- and HCO_3^-.
4. By creating osmotic pressure, electrolytes regulate the osmosis of water between compartments.
5. Calcium, phosphorus, and magnesium are stored in bones; iron and copper are stored in the liver.

Electrolytes in Body Fluids (see Fig. 19–3 and Table 19–2)

1. ICF—principal cation is K^+; principal anion is HPO_4^{-2}; protein anions are also abundant.
2. Plasma—principal cation is Na^+; principal anion is Cl^-; protein anions are significant.
3. Tissue fluid—same as plasma except that protein anions are insignificant.

Intake, Output, and Regulation

1. Intake—electrolytes are part of food and beverages.
2. Output—urine, sweat, feces.
3. Hormones involved: aldosterone—Na^+ and K^+; ANP—Na^+; PTH and calcitonin—Ca^{+2} and HPO_4^{-2}.

Acid–Base Balance

1. Normal pH ranges—blood: 7.35 to 7.45; ICF: 6.8 to 7.0; tissue fluid: similar to blood.
2. Normal pH of body fluids is maintained by buffer systems, respirations, and the kidneys.

Buffer Systems

1. Each consists of a weak acid and a weak base; react with strong acids or bases to change them to substances that do not greatly affect pH. React within a fraction of a second, but have the least capacity to prevent pH changes.
2. Bicarbonate buffer system—see text for reactions; important in both blood and tissue fluid; base to acid ratio is 20:1.
3. Phosphate buffer system—see Fig. 19–4 and text for reactions; important in ICF and in the kidneys.
4. Protein buffer system—amino acids may act as either acids or bases. See text for reactions; important in ICF.

Respiratory Mechanisms

1. The respiratory system affects pH because it regulates the amount of CO_2 in body fluids.
2. May be the cause of a pH change or help compensate for a metabolic pH change—see Table 19–3.
3. Respiratory compensation is rapidly effective (within a few minutes), but limited in capacity if the pH imbalance is ongoing.

Renal Mechanisms

1. The kidneys have the greatest capacity to buffer pH changes, but they may take several hours to days to become effective (see Table 19–3).
2. Reactions: see Figs. 18–6 and 19–4.
3. Summary of reactions: in response to acidosis, the kidneys will excrete H^+ ions and retain Na^+ ions and HCO_3^- ions; in response to alkalosis, the kidneys will retain H^+ ions and excrete Na^+ ions and HCO_3^- ions (see also Fig. 19–5).
4. Only the kidneys are able to remove excess H^+ ions from the body to counteract an ongoing acidosis, as well as to create new bicarbonate ions to retain or excrete as the pH situation requires.

Effects of pH Changes

1. Acidosis—depresses synaptic transmission in the CNS; result is confusion, coma, and death.
2. Alkalosis—increases synaptic transmission in the CNS and PNS; result is irritability, muscle spasms, and convulsions.

REVIEW QUESTIONS

1. Name the major water compartments and the name for water in each of them. Name three specialized body fluids and state the location of each. (p. 484)
2. Explain how water moves between compartments; name the processes. (p. 484)
3. Describe the three sources of water for the body and the relative amounts of each. (p. 485)
4. Describe the pathways of water output. Which is the most important? What kinds of variations are possible in water output? (p. 485)
5. Name the hormones that affect fluid volume, and state the function of each. (pp. 485–486)
6. Define *electrolyte, cation, anion, osmosis,* and *osmolarity.* (pp. 485, 487)
7. Name the major electrolytes in plasma, tissue fluid, and intracellular fluid, and state their functions. (pp. 487–489)
8. Explain how the bicarbonate buffer system will react to buffer a strong acid. (p. 490)
9. Explain how the phosphate buffer system will react to buffer a strong acid. (p. 490)
10. Explain why an amino acid may act as either an acid or a base. (p. 490)
11. Describe the respiratory compensation for metabolic acidosis and for metabolic alkalosis. (p. 491)
12. If the body fluids are becoming too acidic, what ions will the kidneys excrete? What ions will the kidneys return to the blood? (p. 492)
13. Which of the pH regulatory mechanisms works most rapidly? Most slowly? Which of these mechanisms has the greatest capacity to buffer an ongoing pH change? Which mechanism has the least capacity? (pp. 490, 492)
14. Describe the effects of acidosis and alkalosis. (p. 492)

FOR FURTHER THOUGHT

1. Men tend to be more watery than women. The reason has to do with two tissues, one of which is more watery than the other. What are these tissues that are usually present in different proportions in men and women? Explain your answer.
2. Mrs. T, age 82, tells her visiting nurse that she has trouble walking around her house because her feet and ankles are swollen. The nurse makes a doctor's appointment for Mrs. T and says the problem may be her heart. Explain.
3. Ms. H, age 18, is on a diet that advises eight 8-ounce glasses of water a day. Ms. H thinks that if eight glasses are good, perhaps 12 glasses would be better, because "water is good for you." What can you tell her? Is water always good?

4. Mr. C has what he calls "acid indigestion" and takes chewable tablets to try to relieve it. He admits that the fruit flavors of the tablets often have him "popping them like candy" all day. He is visiting his doctor because he says his muscles feel "jumpy." What would you expect to find for blood pH, respirations per minute, and urine pH? Explain your answers.
5. Look at Question Figure 19–A. This is a graph of the pH values of extracellular fluid that might be expected in certain situations: severe asphyxiation, severe diabetes, intense hyperventilation, overingestion of antacids, and vomiting of intestinal contents. Can you match the pH values with the correct situation? (Note that two are very close; you just have to get the proper pair.)

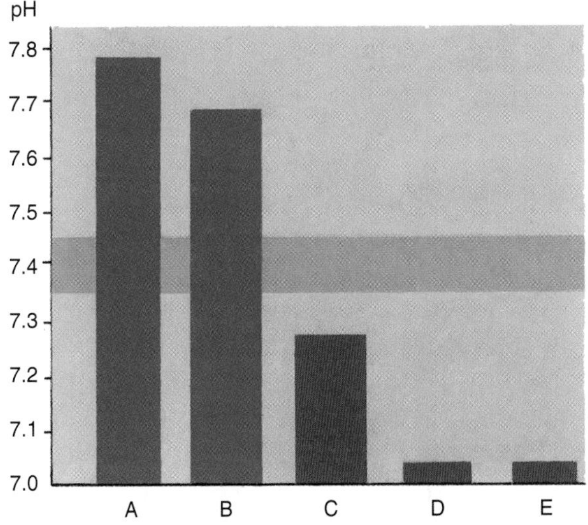

QUESTION FIGURE 19–A: Situational pH values of extracellular fluid.

CHAPTER

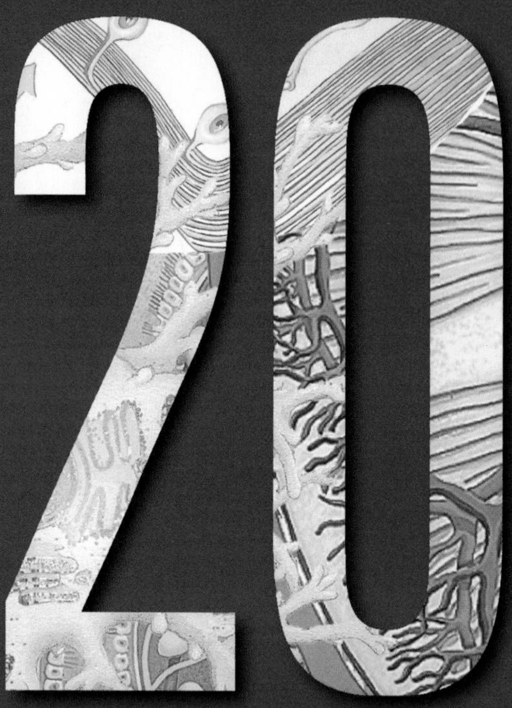

The Reproductive Systems

STUDENT OBJECTIVES

- Describe the process of meiosis. Define *diploid* and *haploid*.
- Describe the differences between spermatogenesis and oogenesis.
- Name the hormones necessary for the formation of gametes, and state the function of each.
- Describe the location and functions of the testes.
- Explain the functions of the epididymis, ductus deferens, ejaculatory duct, and urethra.
- Explain the functions of the seminal vesicles, prostate gland, and bulbourethral glands.
- Describe the composition of semen, and explain why its pH must be a lkaline.
- Name the parts of a sperm cell, and state the function of each.
- Describe the functions of the ovaries, fallopian tubes, uterus, and vagina.
- Describe the structure and function of the myometrium and endometrium.
- Describe the structure of the mammary glands and the functions of the hormones involved in lactation.
- Describe the menstrual cycle in terms of the hormones involved and the changes in the ovaries and endometrium.

CHAPTER OUTLINE

NEW TERMINOLOGY

Cervix *(**SIR**-viks)*
Ductus deferens *(**DUK**-tus **DEF**-er-enz)*
Endometrium *(EN-doh-**MEE**-tree-uhm)*
Fallopian tube *(fuh-**LOH**-pee-an TOOB)*
Graafian follicle *(**GRAF**-ee-uhn **FAH**-li-kuhl)*
Inguinal canal *(**IN**-gwi-nuhl ka-**NAL**)*
Menopause *(**MEN**-ah-paws)*
Menstrual cycle *(**MEN**-stroo-uhl **SIGH**-kuhl)*
Myometrium *(MY-oh-**MEE**-tree-uhm)*
Oogenesis *(OH-oh-**JEN**-e-sis)*
Prostate gland *(**PRAHS**-tayt)*
Seminiferous tubules *(sem-i-**NIFF**-er-us)*
Spermatogenesis *(SPER-ma-toh-**JEN**-e-sis)*
Vulva *(**VUHL**-vah)*
Zygote *(**ZYE**-goht)*

RELATED CLINICAL TERMINOLOGY

Amenorrhea *(ay-MEN-uh-**REE**-ah)*
Down syndrome *(DOWN **SIN**-drohm)*
Ectopic pregnancy *(ek-**TOP**-ik **PREG**-nun-see)*
In vitro fertilization *(IN **VEE**-troh FER-ti-li-**ZAY**-shun)*
Mammography *(mah-**MOG**-rah-fee)*
Prostatic hypertrophy *(prahs-**TAT**-ik high-**PER**-truh-fee)*
Trisomy *(**TRY**-suh-mee)*
Tubal ligation *(**TOO**-buhl lye-**GAY**-shun)*
Vasectomy *(va-**SEK**-tuh-me)*

*Terms that appear in **bold type** in the chapter text are defined in the glossary, which begins on page 603.*

The purpose of the male and female **reproductive systems** is to continue the human species by the production of offspring. How dry and impersonal that sounds, until we remember that each of us is a continuation of our species and that many of us in turn will have our own children. Although some other animals care for their offspring in organized families or societies, the human species is unique, because of cultural influences, in the attention we give to reproduction and to family life.

Yet like other animals, the actual production and growth of offspring is a matter of our anatomy and physiology. The male and female reproductive systems produce **gametes**, that is, sperm and egg cells, and ensure the union of gametes in fertilization following sexual intercourse. In women, the uterus provides the site for the developing embryo-fetus until it is sufficiently developed to survive outside the womb.

This chapter will describe the organs of reproduction and the role of each in the creation of new life or the functioning of the reproductive system as a whole. First, however, we will discuss the formation of gametes.

MEIOSIS

The cell division process of **meiosis** produces the gametes—sperm or egg cells. In meiosis, one cell with the diploid number of chromosomes (46 for humans) divides twice to form four cells, each with the haploid number of chromosomes. *Haploid* means half the usual diploid number, so for humans the haploid number is 23. Although the process of meiosis is essentially the same in men and women, there are some important differences.

SPERMATOGENESIS

Spermatogenesis is the process of meiosis as it takes place in the testes, the site of sperm production. Within each testis are **seminiferous tubules** that contain spermatogonia, which are stem cells that generate sperm. A spermatogonium divides by mitosis to form two cells, one of which will remain in place as a stem cell, while the other differentiates (specializes) to become a primary spermatocyte that will undergo meiosis (Fig. 20–1). As you may recall from Chapter 10, gamete formation is regulated by hormones. The hypothalamus secretes gonadotropin-releasing hormone (GnRH), which stimulates the anterior pituitary gland to secrete follicle-stimulating hormone (FSH) and luteinizing hormone (LH). FSH initiates sperm production, and testosterone, secreted by the testes when stimulated by LH, promotes the maturation of sperm. Inhibin, also produced by the testes, decreases the secretion of FSH. As you can see in Fig. 20–1, for each primary spermatocyte that undergoes meiosis, four functional sperm cells are produced.

Sperm production begins at **puberty** (10 to 14 years of age), and millions of sperm are formed each day in the testes. Although sperm production diminishes with advancing age, there is usually no complete cessation, as there is of egg production in women at menopause.

OOGENESIS

Oogenesis is the process of meiosis for egg cell formation; it begins in the ovaries and is also regulated by hormones. GnRH from the hypothalamus stimulates secretion of FSH by the anterior pituitary gland. FSH initiates the growth of **ovarian follicles**, each of which contains an oogonium, a stem cell for egg cell production (Fig. 20–2). This hormone also stimulates the follicle cells to secrete estrogen, which promotes the maturation of the ovum. Notice that for each primary oocyte that undergoes meiosis, only one functional egg cell is produced. The other three cells produced are called polar bodies. They have no function and will simply deteriorate. A mature ovarian follicle actually contains the secondary oocyte; the second meiotic division will take place if and when the egg is fertilized.

The production of ova begins at puberty (10 to 14 years of age) and continues until **menopause** (45 to 55 years of age), when the ovaries atrophy and no longer respond to pituitary hormones. During this 30- to 40-year span, egg production is cyclical, with a mature ovum being produced approximately every 28 days (the menstrual cycle is discussed later in this chapter). Actually, several follicles usually begin to develop during each cycle. However, the rupturing (ovulation) of the first follicle to mature stops the growth of the others.

The process of meiosis is like other human processes in that "mistakes" may sometimes occur. One of these, trisomy, is discussed in Box 20–1: Trisomy and Down Syndrome.

The haploid egg and sperm cells produced by meiosis each have 23 chromosomes. When fertilization occurs, the nuclei of the egg and sperm merge, and the fertilized egg (**zygote**) has 46 chromosomes, the diploid number. Thus, meiosis maintains the diploid number of the human species by reducing the number of chromosomes by half in the formation of gametes.

MALE REPRODUCTIVE SYSTEM

The male reproductive system consists of the testes and a series of ducts and glands. Sperm are produced in the testes and are transported through the reproductive

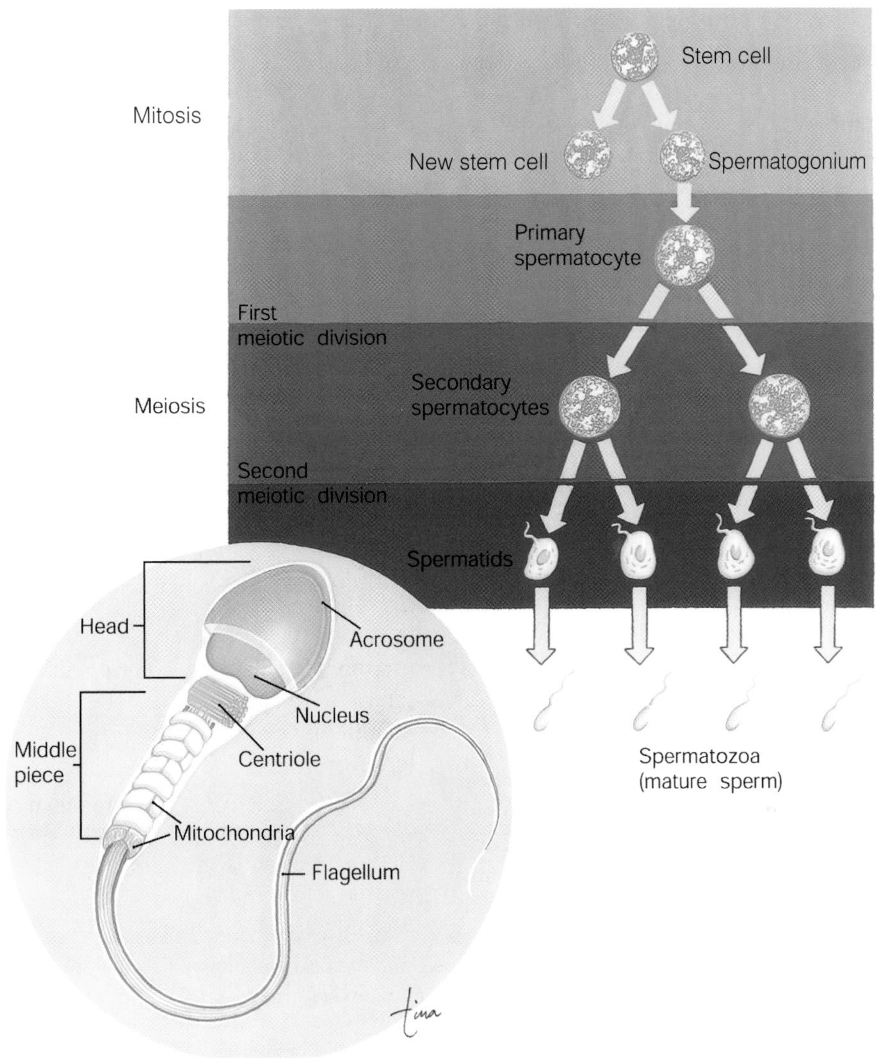

Figure 20–1 Spermatogenesis. The processes of mitosis and meiosis are shown. For each primary spermatocyte that undergoes meiosis, four functional sperm cells are formed. The structure of a mature sperm cell is also shown.

QUESTION: How many chromosomes does a sperm cell have, and where are they located?

ducts: epididymis, ductus deferens, ejaculatory duct, and urethra (Fig. 20–3). The reproductive glands produce secretions that become part of semen, the fluid that is ejaculated from the urethra. These glands are the seminal vesicles, prostate gland, and bulbourethral glands.

TESTES

The **testes** are located in the **scrotum**, a sac of skin between the upper thighs. The temperature within the scrotum is about 96°F, slightly lower than body temperature, which is necessary for the production of viable sperm. In the male fetus, the testes develop near the kidneys, then descend into the scrotum just before birth. **Cryptorchidism** is the condition in which the testes fail to descend, and the result is sterility unless the testes are surgically placed in the scrotum.

Each testis is about 1.5 inches long by 1 inch wide (4 cm by 2.5 cm) and is divided internally into lobes (Fig. 20–4).

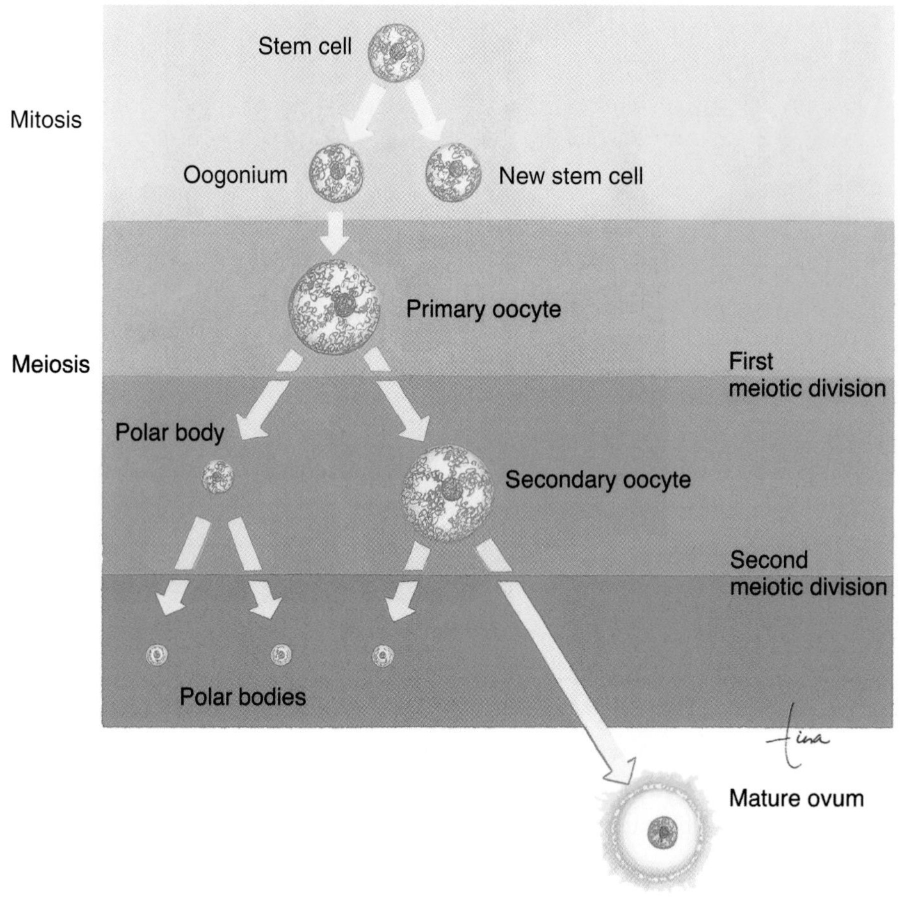

Figure 20–2 Oogenesis. The processes of mitosis and meiosis are shown. For each primary oocyte that undergoes meiosis, only one functional ovum is formed.

QUESTION: When does the secondary oocyte begin the second meiotic division?

Box 20–1 | TRISOMY AND DOWN SYNDROME

Trisomy means the presence of three (rather than the normal two) of a particular chromosome in the cells of an individual. This may occur because of nondisjunction (nonseparation) of a chromosome pair during the second meiotic division, usually (but not always) in an egg cell. The egg cell has two of a particular chromosome, and if fertilized by a sperm, will then contain three of that chromosome and a total of 47 chromosomes.

Most trisomies are probably lethal; that is, the affected embryo will quickly die, even before the woman realizes she is pregnant. When an embryo-fetus survives and a child is born with a trisomy, developmental defects are always present.

The severity of trisomies may be seen in two of the more rarely occurring ones: Trisomy 13 and Trisomy 18, each of which occurs about once for every 5000 live births. Both of these trisomies are characterized by severe mental and

Box 20–1 | TRISOMY AND DOWN SYNDROME *(Continued)*

physical retardation, heart defects, deafness, and bone abnormalities. Affected infants usually die within their first year.

Down syndrome (Trisomy 21) is the most common trisomy, with a frequency of about one per 750 live births. Children with Down syndrome have cognitive impairment, but there is a great range of mental ability in this group. Physical characteristics include a skin fold above each eye, short stature, poor muscle tone, and heart defects. Again, the degree of severity is highly variable.

Women older than the age of 35 are believed to be at greater risk of having a child with Down syndrome. The reason may be that as egg cells age, the process of meiosis is more likely to proceed incorrectly.

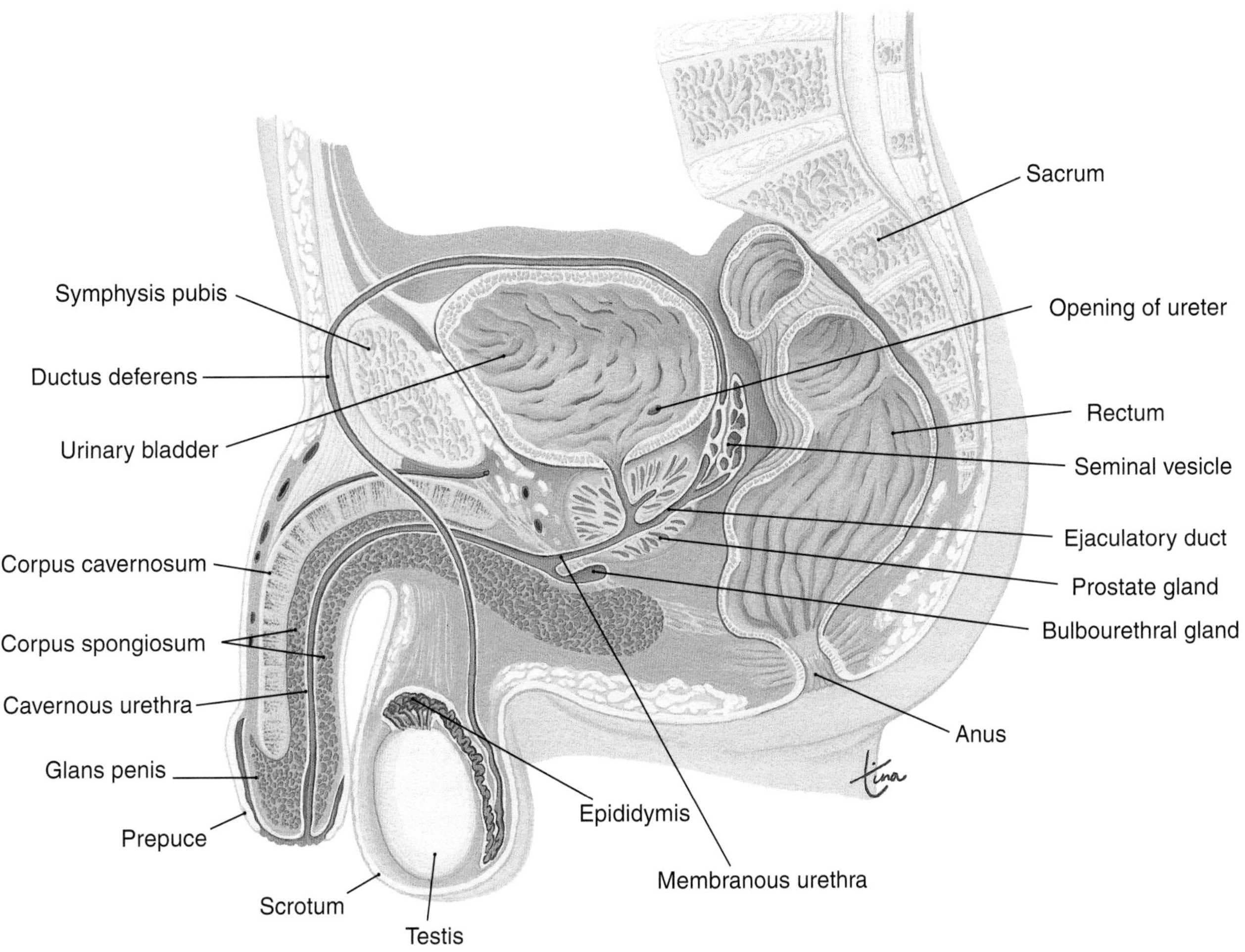

Figure 20–3 Male reproductive system shown in a midsagittal section through the pelvic cavity.

QUESTION: Name the duct that carries sperm into the pelvic cavity.

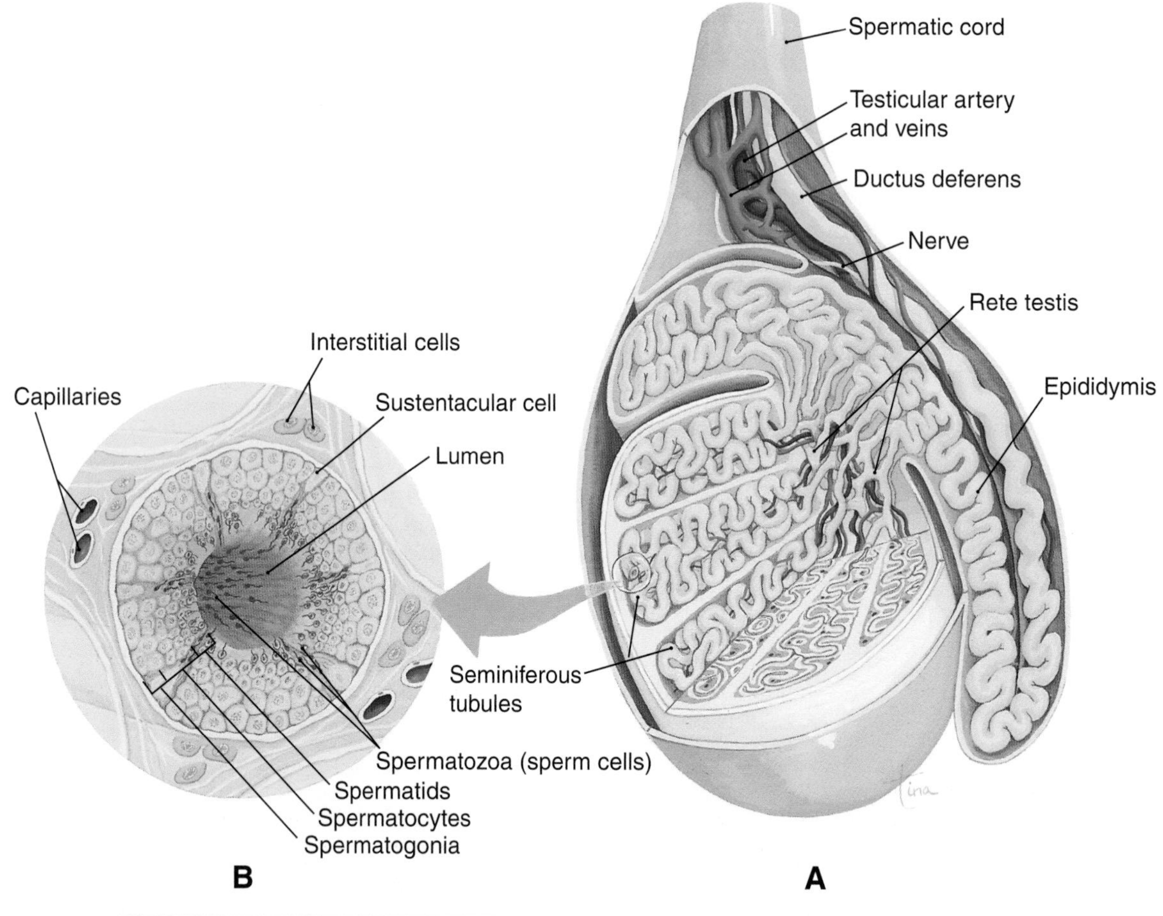

Figure 20–4 (**A**) Midsagittal section of portion of a testis; the epididymis is on the posterior side of the testis. (**B**) Cross-section through a seminiferous tubule showing development of sperm.

QUESTION: Trace the pathway of sperm from their formation to the ductus deferens.

Each lobe contains several **seminiferous tubules**, in which spermatogenesis takes place. Among the spermatogonia of the seminiferous tubules are **sustentacular** (**Sertoli**) **cells**, which produce the hormone **inhibin** when stimulated by testosterone. Between the loops of the seminiferous tubules are **interstitial cells**, which produce **testosterone** when stimulated by luteinizing hormone (LH) from the anterior pituitary gland. Besides its role in the maturation of sperm, testosterone is also responsible for the male secondary sex characteristics, which begin to develop at puberty (Table 20–1).

A sperm cell consists of several parts, which are shown in Fig. 20–1. The head contains the 23 chromosomes. On the tip of the head is the **acrosome**, which is similar to a lysosome and contains enzymes to digest the membrane of an egg cell. Within the middle piece are mitochondria that produce ATP. The **flagellum** provides motility, the capability of the sperm cell to move. It is the beating of the flagellum that requires energy from ATP.

Sperm from the seminiferous tubules enter a tubular network called the rete testis, then enter the epididymis, the first of the reproductive ducts.

EPIDIDYMIS

The **epididymis** (plural: epididymides) is a tube about 20 feet (6 m) long that is coiled on the posterior surface of each testis (see Fig. 20–4). Within the epididymis the sperm complete their maturation, and their flagella

Table 20–1 | HORMONES OF MALE REPRODUCTION

HORMONE	SECRETED BY	FUNCTIONS
FSH	Anterior pituitary	■ Initiates production of sperm in the testes
LH (ICSH)	Anterior pituitary	■ Stimulates secretion of testosterone by the testes
Testosterone*	Testes (interstitial cells)	■ Promotes maturation of sperm ■ Initiates development of the secondary sex characteristics: — growth of the reproductive organs — growth of the larynx — growth of facial and body hair — increased protein synthesis, especially in skeletal muscles
Inhibin	Testes (sustentacular cells)	■ Decreases secretion of FSH to maintain constant rate of spermatogenesis

*In both sexes, testosterone (from the adrenal cortex in women) contributes to sex drive and muscle-protein synthesis.

become functional. Smooth muscle in the wall of the epididymis propels the sperm into the ductus deferens.

DUCTUS DEFERENS

Also called the **vas deferens**, the **ductus deferens** extends from the epididymis in the scrotum on its own side into the abdominal cavity through the **inguinal canal**. This canal is an opening in the abdominal wall for the **spermatic cord**, a connective tissue sheath that contains the ductus deferens, testicular blood vessels, and nerves. Because the inguinal canal is an opening in a muscular wall, it is a natural "weak spot," and it is the most common site of hernia formation in men.

Once inside the abdominal cavity, the ductus deferens extends upward over the urinary bladder, then down the posterior side to join the ejaculatory duct on its own side (see Fig. 20–3). The smooth muscle layer of the ductus deferens contracts in waves of peristalsis as part of ejaculation (see Box 20–2: Contraception).

EJACULATORY DUCTS

Each of the two **ejaculatory ducts** receives sperm from the ductus deferens and the secretion of the seminal vesicle on its own side. Both ejaculatory ducts empty into the single urethra (see Fig. 20–3).

SEMINAL VESICLES

The paired **seminal vesicles** are posterior to the urinary bladder (see Fig. 20–3). Their secretion contains fructose to provide an energy source for sperm and is alkaline to enhance sperm motility. The duct of each seminal vesicle joins the ductus deferens on that side to form the ejaculatory duct.

PROSTATE GLAND

A muscular gland just below the urinary bladder, the **prostate gland** is about 1.2 inches high by 1.6 inches wide by 0.8 inch deep (3 cm by 4 cm by 2 cm; about the size of a walnut). It surrounds the first inch of the urethra as it emerges from the bladder (see Fig. 20–3). The glandular tissue of the prostate secretes a slightly acidic fluid that contains an antimicrobial chemical and citric acid for energy production (in the mitochondria of sperm cells). The smooth muscle of the prostate gland contracts during **ejaculation** to contribute to the expulsion of semen from the urethra (see Box 20–3: Prostatic Hypertrophy).

BULBOURETHRAL GLANDS

Also called Cowper's glands, the **bulbourethral glands** are about the size of peas and are located below the prostate gland; they empty into the urethra. Their alkaline secretion coats the interior of the urethra just before ejaculation, which neutralizes any acidic urine that might be present.

You have probably noticed that the secretions of two of the three male reproductive glands are alkaline. This is important because the cavity of the female vagina has an acidic pH created by the normal flora, the natural bacterial population of the vagina. The alkalinity of seminal fluid helps neutralize the acidic vaginal pH and permits

Box 20–2 | CONTRACEPTION

There are several methods of contraception, or birth control; some are more effective than others. The only method that is 100 percent effective is abstinence.

Sterilization—Sterilization in men involves a relatively simple procedure called a **vasectomy**. The ductus (vas) deferens is accessible in the scrotum, in which a small incision is made on either side. The ductus is then sutured and cut. Although sperm are still produced in the testes, they cannot pass the break in the ductus, and they simply die and are reabsorbed.

Sterilization in women is usually accomplished by **tubal ligation**, the suturing and severing of the fallopian tubes. Usually this can be done by way of a small incision in the abdominal wall. Ova cannot pass the break in the tube, nor can sperm pass from the uterine side to fertilize an ovum.

When done properly, these forms of surgical sterilization are virtually 100 percent effective.

Oral contraceptives ("the pill")—Birth control pills contain progesterone and estrogen in varying proportions. They prevent ovulation by inhibiting the secretion of FSH and LH from the anterior pituitary gland. When taken according to schedule, birth control pills are about 98 percent effective. Some women report side effects such as headaches, weight gain, and nausea. Women who use this method of contraception should not smoke because smoking seems to be associated with abnormal clotting and a greater risk of heart attack or stroke.

Barrier methods—These include the condom, diaphragm, and cervical cap, which prevent sperm from reaching the uterus and fallopian tubes. The use of a spermicide (sperm-killing chemical) increases the effectiveness of these methods. A condom is a latex or rubber sheath that covers the penis and collects and contains ejaculated semen. Leakage is possible, however, and the condom is considered 80 to 90 percent effective. This is the only contraceptive method that decreases the spread of sexually transmitted diseases.

The diaphragm and cervical cap are plastic structures that are inserted into the vagina to cover the cervix. They are about 80 percent effective. These methods should not be used, however, by women with vaginal infections or abnormal Pap smears or by those who have had toxic shock syndrome.

Box 20–3 | PROSTATIC HYPERTROPHY

Prostatic hypertrophy is enlargement of the prostate gland. Benign prostatic hypertrophy is a common occurrence in men over age 60. The enlarged prostate compresses the urethra within it and may make urination difficult or result in urinary retention. A prostatectomy is the surgical removal of part or all of the prostate. A possible consequence is that ejaculation may be impaired. Newer surgical procedures may preserve sexual function, however, and medications are available to shrink enlarged prostate tissue.

Cancer of the prostate is the second most common cancer among men (lung cancer is first). Most cases occur in men older than age 50. Treatment may include surgery to remove the prostate, radiation therapy, or hormone therapy to reduce the patient's level of testosterone.

sperm motility in what might otherwise be an unfavorable environment.

URETHRA—PENIS

The **urethra** is the last of the ducts through which semen travels, and its longest portion is enclosed within the penis. The **penis** is an external genital organ; its distal end is called the glans penis and is covered with a fold of skin called the prepuce or foreskin. **Circumcision** is the surgical removal of the foreskin. This is a common procedure performed on male infants, and though there is considerable medical debate as to whether circumcision has a useful purpose, research studies have found fewer cases of HIV infection among circumcised men, compared with men who are uncircumcised.

Within the penis are three masses of cavernous (erectile) tissue (see Fig. 20–3). Each consists of a framework of smooth muscle and connective tissue that contains blood sinuses, which are large, irregular vascular channels.

When blood flow through these sinuses is minimal, the penis is flaccid. During sexual stimulation, the arteries to the penis dilate, the sinuses fill with blood, and the penis becomes erect and firm. The dilation of penile arteries and the resulting erection are brought about by the localized release of nitric oxide (NO) and by parasympathetic impulses. The erect penis is capable of penetrating the female vagina to deposit sperm. The culmination of sexual stimulation is ejaculation, a sympathetic response that is brought about by peristalsis of all of the reproductive ducts and contraction of the prostate gland and the muscles of the pelvic floor.

SEMEN

Semen consists of sperm and the secretions of the seminal vesicles, prostate gland, and bulbourethral glands; its average pH is about 7.4. During ejaculation, approximately 2 to 4 mL of semen is expelled. Each milliliter of semen contains about 100 million sperm cells.

FEMALE REPRODUCTIVE SYSTEM

The female reproductive system consists of the paired ovaries and fallopian tubes, the single uterus and vagina, and the external genital structures (Fig. 20–5). Egg cells (ova) are produced in the ovaries and travel through the fallopian tubes to the uterus. The uterus is the site for the growth of the embryo-fetus.

OVARIES

The **ovaries** are a pair of oval structures about 1.5 inches (4 cm) long on either side of the uterus in the pelvic cavity (Fig. 20–6). The ovarian ligament extends from the medial side of an ovary to the uterine wall, and the broad ligament is a fold of the peritoneum that covers the ovaries. These ligaments help keep the ovaries in place.

Within an ovary are several hundred thousand **primary follicles**, which are present at birth. During a woman's childbearing years, only 300 to 400 of these follicles will produce mature ova. As with sperm production in men, the supply of potential gametes far exceeds what is actually needed, but this helps ensure the continuation of the human species.

Each primary ovarian follicle contains an oocyte, a potential ovum or egg cell. Surrounding the oocyte are the follicle cells, which secrete estrogen. Maturation of a follicle, requiring FSH and estrogen, was described previously in the section on oogenesis. A mature follicle may also be called a **graafian follicle**, and the hormone LH from the anterior pituitary gland causes ovulation, that is, rupture of the mature follicle with release of the ovum. At this time, other developing follicles begin to deteriorate; these are called **atretic follicles** and have no further purpose. Under the influence of LH, the ruptured follicle becomes the **corpus luteum** and begins to secrete progesterone, as well as estrogen. Hormones produced in smaller amounts by the corpus luteum are inhibin and relaxin.

FALLOPIAN TUBES

There are two **fallopian tubes** (also called uterine tubes or oviducts); each is about 4 inches (10 cm) long. The lateral end of a fallopian tube encloses an ovary, and the medial end opens into the uterus. The end of the tube that encloses the ovary has **fimbriae**, fringelike projections that create currents in the fluid surrounding the ovary to pull the ovum into the fallopian tube.

Because the ovum has no means of self-locomotion (as do sperm), the structure of the fallopian tube ensures that the ovum will be kept moving toward the uterus. The smooth muscle layer of the tube contracts in peristaltic waves that help propel the ovum (or zygote, as you will see in a moment). The lining (mucosa) is extensively folded and is made of ciliated epithelial tissue. The sweeping action of the cilia also moves the ovum toward the uterus. A cross-section of a fallopian tube is shown in Fig. 20–6.

Fertilization usually takes place in the fallopian tube. If not fertilized, an ovum dies within 24 to 48 hours and disintegrates, either in the tube or the uterus. If fertilized, the ovum becomes a zygote and is swept into the uterus; this takes about 4 to 5 days (see Box 20–4: *In Vitro* Fertilization).

In 1% to 2% of all pregnancies, the zygote will not reach the uterus but will still continue to develop. This is called an **ectopic pregnancy**; *ectopic* means "in an abnormal site." The developing embryo may become implanted in the fallopian tube, the ovary itself, or even elsewhere in the abdominal cavity. An ectopic pregnancy usually does not progress for very long because these other sites are not specialized to provide a placenta or to expand to accommodate the growth of a fetus, as the uterus is. The spontaneous termination of an ectopic pregnancy is usually the result of bleeding in the mother, and surgery may be necessary to prevent maternal death from circulatory shock. In the United States, better diagnosis has reduced the mortality rate to 1 death per 2000

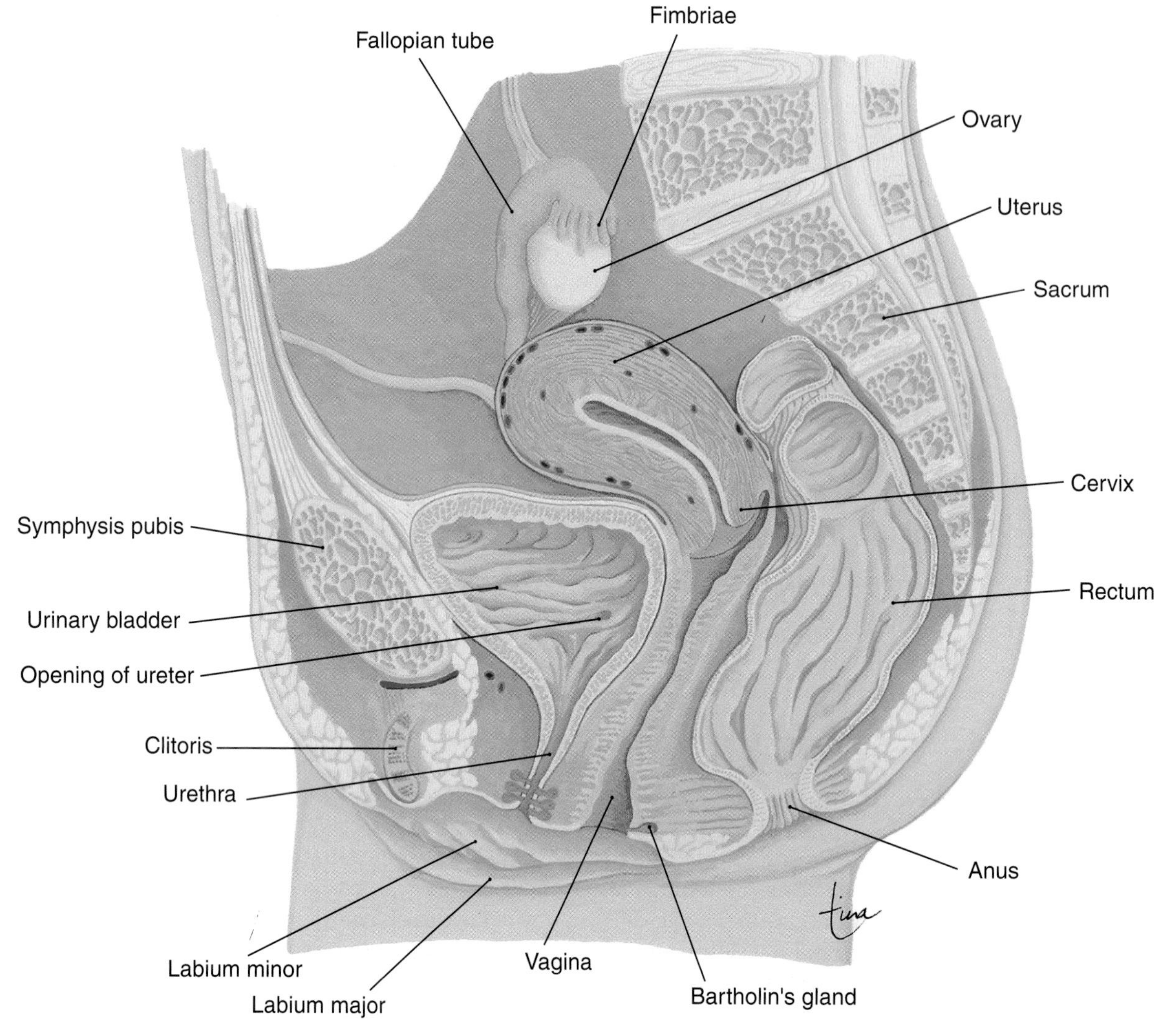

Figure 20–5 Female reproductive system shown in a midsagittal section through the pelvic cavity.

QUESTION: Where is the uterus with respect to the urinary bladder, and why is this important?

pregnancies; in many developing nations, the maternal mortality rate is much higher. Occasionally an ectopic pregnancy does go to full term and produces a healthy baby; such an event is a credit to the adaptability of the human body and to the advances of medical science.

UTERUS

The **uterus** is shaped like an upside-down pear, about 3 inches long by 2 inches wide by 1 inch deep (7.5 cm by 5 cm by 2.5 cm), superior to the urinary bladder and between the two ovaries in the pelvic cavity (see Fig. 20–5). In addition to covering the ovaries, the broad ligament also covers the uterus (see Fig. 20–6). During pregnancy the uterus increases greatly in size, contains the placenta to nourish the embryo-fetus, and expels the baby at the end of gestation.

The parts and layers of the uterus are shown in Fig. 20–6. The **fundus** is the upper portion above the entry of the fallopian tubes, and the **body** is the large central portion. The narrow, lower end of the uterus is the **cervix**, which opens into the vagina.

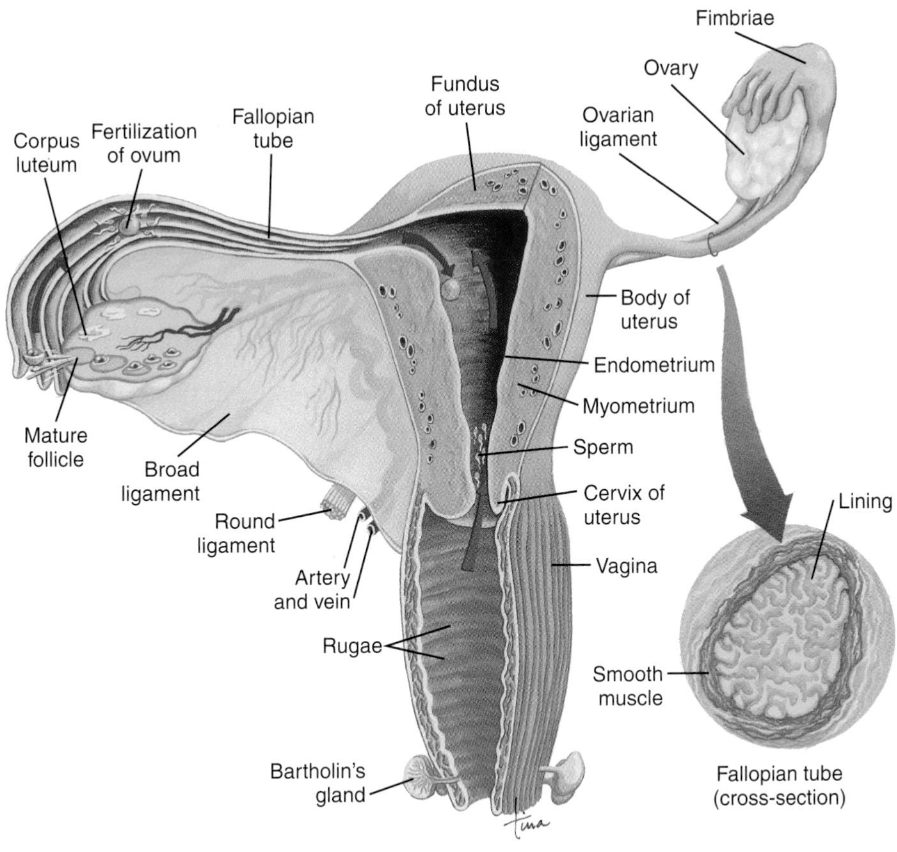

Figure 20–6 Female reproductive system shown in anterior view. The ovary at the left of the illustration has been sectioned to show the developing follicles. The fallopian tube at the left of the illustration has been sectioned to show fertilization. A cross-section of the right fallopian tube depicts its internal structure. The uterus and vagina have been sectioned to show internal structures. Arrows indicate the movement of the ovum toward the uterus and the movement of sperm from the vagina toward the fallopian tube.

QUESTION: Which layer of the uterine wall is thicker? What tissue is it made of?

Box 20–4 | *IN VITRO* FERTILIZATION

***In vitro* fertilization** (IVF) is fertilization outside the body, usually in a glass dish. A woman who wishes to conceive by this method is given FSH to stimulate the simultaneous development of several ovarian follicles. LH may then be given to stimulate simultaneous ovulation. The ova are removed by way of a small incision in the abdominal wall and are placed in a solution containing the sperm of the woman's partner (or an anonymous donor). After fertilization and the first mitotic divisions of cleavage, the very early embryo is placed in the woman's uterus.

It is also possible to mix the removed ova with sperm and return them almost immediately to the woman's fallopian tube. Development then proceeds as if the ova had been fertilized naturally.

Since the birth of the first "test tube baby" in 1978, many thousands of babies have been born

Continued

Box 20–4 | *IN VITRO* FERTILIZATION *(Continued)*

following *in vitro* fertilization. The techniques are not always successful, and repeated attempts can be very expensive.

As an adjunct to IVF, pre-implantation genetic diagnosis may be done, to test for genetic diseases and chromosome abnormalities such as the trisomies described in Box 20–1. This may be especially useful for older women trying to conceive and for couples with a family history of a genetic disease such as sickle-cell anemia or cystic fibrosis.

The outermost layer of the uterus, the serosa or epimetrium, is a fold of the peritoneum. The **myometrium** is the smooth muscle layer; during pregnancy these cells increase in size to accommodate the growing fetus and contract for labor and delivery at the end of pregnancy.

The lining of the uterus is the **endometrium**, which itself consists of two layers. The **basilar layer**, adjacent to the myometrium, is vascular but very thin and is a permanent layer. The **functional layer** is regenerated and lost during each menstrual cycle. Under the influence of estrogen and progesterone from the ovaries, the growth of blood vessels thickens the functional layer in preparation for a possible embryo. If fertilization does not occur, the functional layer sloughs off in menstruation. During pregnancy, the endometrium forms the maternal portion of the placenta.

VAGINA

The **vagina** is a muscular tube about 4 inches (10 cm) long that extends from the cervix to the vaginal orifice in the **perineum** (pelvic floor). It is posterior to the urethra and anterior to the rectum (see Fig. 20–5). The vaginal opening is usually partially covered by a thin membrane called the **hymen**, which is ruptured by the first sexual intercourse or by the use of tampons during the menstrual period.

The functions of the vagina are to receive sperm from the penis during sexual intercourse, to provide the exit for menstrual blood flow, and to become the birth canal at the end of pregnancy.

The vaginal mucosa after puberty is stratified squamous epithelium, which is relatively resistant to pathogens. The normal flora (microbiota) of the vagina creates an acidic pH that helps inhibit the growth of pathogens, especially yeasts. An antibiotic taken for an infection elsewhere in the body, however, may diminish the resident vaginal bacteria, which raises the pH of the vaginal microbiome, and makes it a more favorable environment for the rapid growth of any yeast present (see Box 20–5: Sexually Transmitted Diseases).

Box 20–5 | SEXUALLY TRANSMITTED DISEASES

Sexually transmitted diseases (STDs) are those in which the pathogen is acquired during sexual activity. Most are caused by bacteria or viruses.

Gonorrhea—caused by the bacterium *Neisseria gonorrhoeae*. Infected men have urethritis with painful and frequent urination and pus in the urine. Women are often asymptomatic, and the bacteria may spread from the cervix to other reproductive organs (pelvic inflammatory disease [PID]). The use of antibiotics in the eyes of all newborns has virtually eliminated neonatal conjunctivitis acquired from an infected mother. Gonorrhea can be treated with antibiotics, but resistant strains of the bacteria complicate treatment.

Syphilis—caused by the bacterium *Treponema pallidum*. Although syphilis can be cured with penicillin, it is a disease that may be ignored by the person who has it because the symptoms may seem minor and often do not last long. If untreated, however, syphilis may cause severe or even fatal damage to the nervous system and heart. In the last few years the number of reported cases of syphilis has been decreasing, and the

Box 20–5 | SEXUALLY TRANSMITTED DISEASES *(Continued)*

Centers for Disease Control and Prevention has hopes of eradicating syphilis in the United States.

Chlamydial infection—caused by the very simple bacterium *Chlamydia trachomatis*. Infected men may have urethritis or epididymitis. Women often have no symptoms at first but may develop PID, which increases the risk of ectopic pregnancy. Infants born to infected women may develop conjunctivitis or pneumonia. Chlamydial infection can be treated successfully with antibiotics.

Genital herpes—caused by the virus herpes simplex (usually type 2). Painful lesions in the genital area are the primary symptom. Although the lesions heal within 5 to 9 days, recurrences are possible, perhaps triggered by physiological stresses such as illness. Although herpes is not curable at present, medications have proved useful in suppressing recurrences.

Neonatal herpes is an infection acquired by a newborn during passage through the birth canal. The infant's immune system is too immature to control the herpes virus, and the infection may be fatal or cause brain damage. A pregnant woman with a history of genital herpes may choose to have the baby delivered by cesarean section to avoid this possible outcome.

Human papilloma virus (HPV)—more than 100 types of HPV exist, some of which cause genital warts. Several stimulate abnormal growth of cells and cause cervical cancer in women; others may cause throat or oral cancers in both sexes. As with other virus diseases, a cure is not yet possible, but a vaccine is available for the two types that cause approximately 70% of all cervical cancers, and the two types that most frequently cause genital warts. The vaccine is recommended for both boys and girls at the age of 11 to 12.

EXTERNAL GENITALS

The female external genital structures may also be called the **vulva** (Fig. 20–7) and include the clitoris, labia majora and minora, and the Bartholin's glands (see Fig. 20–5).

The **clitoris** is a small mass of erectile tissue anterior to the urethral orifice. The only function of the clitoris is sensory; it responds to sexual stimulation, and its vascular sinuses become filled with blood.

The mons pubis is a pad of fat over the pubic symphysis, covered with skin and pubic hair. Extending posteriorly from the mons are the **labia majora** (lateral) and **labia minora** (medial), which are paired folds of skin. The area between the labia minora is called the vestibule and contains the openings of the urethra and vagina. The labia cover these openings and prevent drying of their mucous membranes.

Bartholin's glands, also called vestibular glands (see Figs. 20–5 and 20–6), are within the floor of the vestibule;

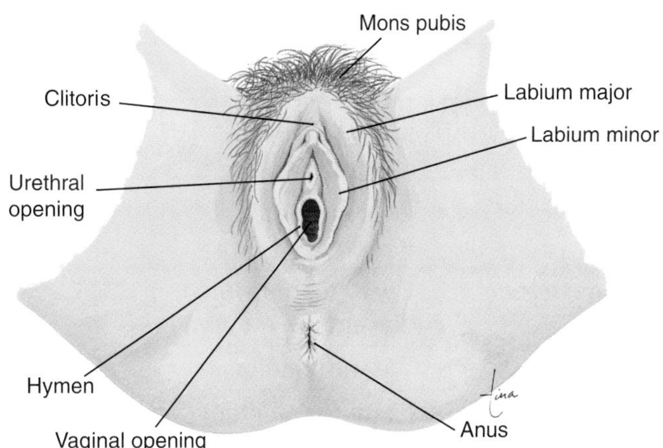

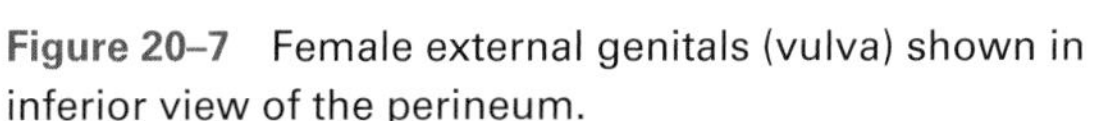

Figure 20–7 Female external genitals (vulva) shown in inferior view of the perineum.

QUESTION: What is the function of the labia majora and minora?

their ducts open onto the mucosa at the vaginal orifice. The secretion of these glands keeps the mucosa moist and lubricates the vagina during sexual intercourse.

MAMMARY GLANDS

The **mammary glands** are structurally related to the skin but functionally related to the reproductive system because they produce milk for the nourishment of offspring. Enclosed within the breasts, the mammary glands are anterior to the pectoralis major muscles; their structure is shown in Fig. 20–8.

The glandular tissue is surrounded by adipose tissue. The **alveolar glands** produce milk after pregnancy; the milk enters lactiferous ducts that converge at the nipple. The skin around the nipple is a pigmented area called the areola.

The formation of milk is under hormonal control. During pregnancy, high levels of estrogen and progesterone prepare the glands for milk production. **Prolactin** from the anterior pituitary gland causes the actual synthesis of milk after pregnancy. The sucking of the infant on the nipple stimulates the hypothalamus to send nerve impulses to the posterior pituitary gland, which secretes **oxytocin** to cause the release of milk. The effects of these hormones on the mammary glands are summarized in Table 20–2.

Human milk is mostly water, with lactose, fatty acids, proteins, and minerals to nourish the infant. The oligosaccharides present are for the nourishment of the baby's developing intestinal microbiota, the bacteria that help establish mucosal immunity and suppress excessive inflammation. Also of great importance for the infant are the maternal antibodies in milk, the IgA molecules. Infants who are breastfed receive passive immunity to the same diseases their mothers are immune to. As you recall from Chapter 14, such immunity is temporary but may persist for up to 6 months after breast feeding is stopped (see also Box 20–6: Mammography).

THE MENSTRUAL CYCLE

The **menstrual cycle** includes the activity of the hormones of the ovaries and anterior pituitary gland and the resultant

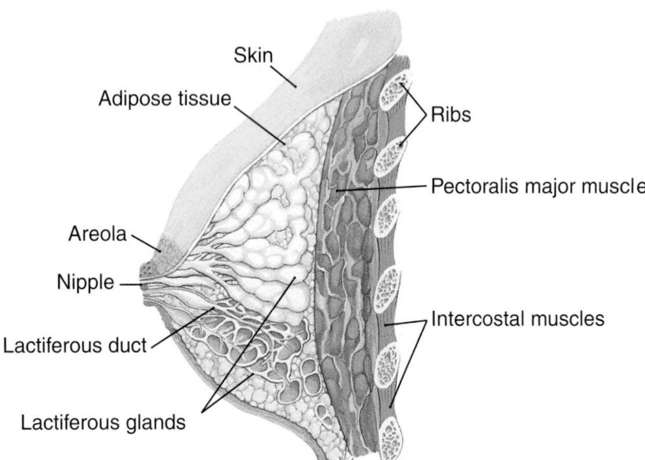

Figure 20–8 Mammary gland shown in a midsagittal section.

QUESTION: Name the hormones that stimulate the production of milk and release of milk.

Table 20–2 | HORMONE EFFECTS ON THE MAMMARY GLANDS

HORMONE	SECRETED BY	FUNCTIONS
Estrogen	Ovary (follicle) Placenta	■ Promotes growth of duct system
Progesterone	Ovary (corpus luteum) Placenta	■ Promotes growth of secretory cells
Prolactin	Anterior pituitary	■ Promotes production of milk after birth
Oxytocin	Posterior pituitary (hypothalamus)	■ Promotes release of milk

Box 20–6 | MAMMOGRAPHY

Mammography is an x-ray technique that is used to evaluate breast tissue for abnormalities. By far the most frequent usage is to detect breast cancer, which is one of the most common malignancies in women. If detected early, breast cancer may be cured through a combination of surgery, radiation, and chemotherapy. Women should practice breast self-examination monthly, but mammography can detect lumps that are too small to be felt manually. Women in their 30s may have a mammogram done to serve as a comparison for mammograms later in life.

changes in the ovaries (ovarian cycle) and uterus (uterine cycle). These are all incorporated into Fig. 20–9, which may look complicated at first, but refer to it as you read the following.

Notice first the four hormones involved: **FSH** and **LH** from the anterior pituitary gland, **estrogen** from the ovarian follicle, and **progesterone** from the corpus luteum. The fluctuations of these hormones are shown as they would occur in an average 28-day cycle. A cycle may be described in terms of three phases: menstrual phase, follicular phase, and luteal phase.

1. **Menstrual phase**—The loss of the functional layer of the endometrium is called **menstruation** or the menses. Although this is actually the end of a menstrual cycle, the onset of menstruation is easily pinpointed and is, therefore, a useful starting point. Menstruation may last 2 to 8 days, with an average of 3 to 6 days. At this time, secretion of FSH is increasing, and several ovarian follicles begin to develop.
2. **Follicular phase**—FSH stimulates growth of ovarian follicles and secretion of estrogen by the follicle cells. The secretion of LH is also increasing, but more slowly. FSH and estrogen promote the growth and maturation of the ovum, and estrogen stimulates the growth of blood vessels in the endometrium to regenerate the functional layer.

   This phase ends with ovulation, when a sharp increase in LH causes rupture of a mature ovarian follicle.
3. **Luteal phase**—Under the influence of LH, the ruptured follicle becomes the corpus luteum and begins to secrete progesterone, as well as estrogen. Progesterone promotes successful implantation of the 5- to 8-day-old embryo in the endometrium, perhaps by inhibiting inflammation at the site. It also stimulates further growth of blood vessels in the functional layer of the endometrium and promotes the storage of nutrients such as glycogen.

   As progesterone secretion increases, LH secretion decreases, and if the ovum is not fertilized, the secretion of progesterone also begins to decrease. Without progesterone, the endometrium cannot be maintained and begins to slough off in menstruation. FSH secretion begins to increase (as estrogen and progesterone decrease), and the cycle begins again.

Also secreted by the corpus luteum during a cycle are the hormones inhibin and relaxin. **Inhibin** inhibits the secretion of FSH, and perhaps LH as well, from the anterior pituitary gland. **Relaxin** is believed to inhibit contractions of the myometrium (as does progesterone), which would help make implantation of the early embryo successful.

The 28-day cycle shown in Fig. 20–9 is average. Women may have cycles of anywhere from 23 to 35 days, the normal range. Women who engage in strenuous exercise over prolonged periods of time may experience **amenorrhea**, that is, cessation of menses. This seems to be related to reduction of body fat. The reproductive cycle ceases if a woman does not have sufficient reserves of energy for herself and a developing fetus. The exact mechanism by which this happens is not completely understood but is believed to involve leptin, a hormone of adipose tissue that signals the hypothalamus about changes in the level of subcutaneous fat reserves (see Box 17–6 in Chapter 17). Amenorrhea may also accompany states of physical or emotional stress, anorexia nervosa, or various endocrine disorders.

The functions of the hormones of female reproduction are summarized in Table 20–3.

AGING AND THE REPRODUCTIVE SYSTEMS

Women experience a definite end to reproductive capability; this is called the menopause and usually occurs between the ages of 45 and 55. Estrogen secretion decreases; ovulation and menstrual cycles become irregular and finally cease. The decrease in estrogen has other

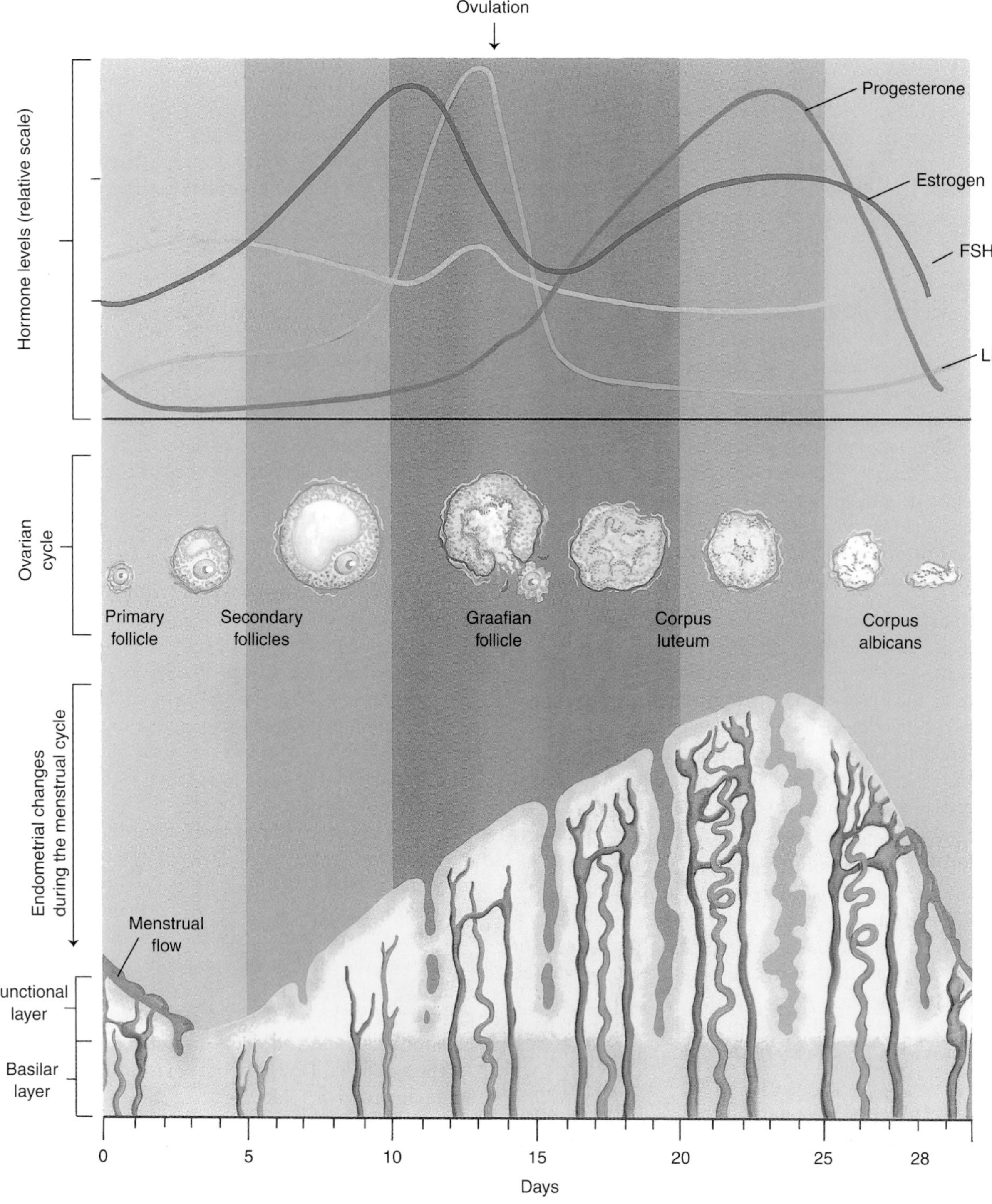

Figure 20–9 The menstrual cycle. The levels of the important hormones are shown relative to one another throughout the cycle. Changes in the ovarian follicle are depicted. The relative thickness of the endometrium is also shown.

QUESTION: Which hormone triggers ovulation? What else does this hormone do to the follicle?

Table 20–3 | HORMONES OF FEMALE REPRODUCTION

HORMONE	SECRETED BY	FUNCTIONS
FSH	Anterior pituitary	■ Initiates development of ovarian follicles ■ Stimulates secretion of estrogen by follicle cells
LH	Anterior pituitary	■ Causes ovulation ■ Converts the ruptured ovarian follicle into the corpus luteum ■ Stimulates secretion of progesterone by the corpus luteum
Estrogen*	Ovary (follicle) Placenta during pregnancy	■ Promotes maturation of ovarian follicles ■ Promotes growth of blood vessels in the endometrium ■ Initiates development of the secondary sex characteristics: — growth of the uterus and other reproductive organs — growth of the mammary ducts and fat deposition in the breasts — broadening of the pelvic bone — subcutaneous fat deposition in hips and thighs
Progesterone	Ovary (corpus luteum) Placenta during pregnancy	■ Promotes successful implantation of the embryo in the endometrium ■ Promotes further growth of blood vessels in the endometrium and storage of nutrients ■ Inhibits contractions of the myometrium
Inhibin	Ovary (corpus luteum)	■ Inhibits secretion of FSH
Relaxin	Ovary (corpus luteum) Placenta during pregnancy	■ Inhibits contractions of the myometrium to facilitate implantation ■ Promotes stretching of ligaments of the pubic symphysis

*Estrogen has effects on adipose tissue and organs such as bones and blood vessels in both men and women. Estrogen is produced in adipose tissue in the breasts and hips. In men, testosterone is converted to estrogen in the brain.

effects as well. Loss of bone matrix may lead to osteoporosis and fractures; an increase in blood cholesterol makes women more likely to develop coronary artery disease; and drying of the vaginal mucosa increases susceptibility to vaginal infections. Estrogen replacement therapy may delay some of these consequences of menopause, but it does involve risks, and women should be fully informed of them before starting such therapy. The likelihood of breast cancer also increases with age, and women older than age 50 should consider having a mammogram to serve as a baseline and consult with a medical professional about the timing of further ones.

For most men, testosterone secretion continues throughout life, as does sperm production, though both diminish with advancing age. Perhaps the most common reproductive problem for older men is prostatic hypertrophy, enlargement of the prostate gland. As the urethra is compressed by the growing prostate gland, urination becomes difficult and residual urine in the bladder increases the chance of urinary tract infection. Prostate hypertrophy is usually benign, but cancer of the prostate is one of the more common cancers in elderly men.

SUMMARY

The production of male or female gametes is a process that is regulated by hormones. When fertilization of an ovum by a sperm cell takes place, the zygote, or fertilized egg, has the potential to become a new human being. The development of the zygote to embryo-fetus to newborn infant is also dependent on hormones and is the subject of our next chapter.

STUDY OUTLINE

Reproductive Systems—purpose is to produce gametes (egg and sperm), to ensure fertilization, and in women to provide a site for the embryo-fetus

Meiosis—the cell division process that produces gametes

1. One cell with the diploid number of chromosomes (46) divides twice to form four cells, each with the haploid number of chromosomes (23).
2. Spermatogenesis takes place in the testes; a continuous process from puberty throughout life; each primary spermatocyte produces four functional sperm (see Fig. 20–1). FSH and testosterone are directly necessary (see Table 20–1).
3. Oogenesis takes place in the ovaries; the process is cyclical (every 28 days) from puberty until menopause; each primary oocyte produces one functional ovum and three nonfunctional polar bodies (see Fig. 20–2). FSH, LH, and estrogen are necessary (see Table 20–3).

Male Reproductive System—consists of the testes and the ducts and glands that contribute to the formation of semen (see Fig. 20–3)

1. Testes (paired)—located in the scrotum between the upper thighs; temperature in the scrotum is 96°F to permit production of viable sperm. Sperm are produced in seminiferous tubules (see Fig. 20–4 and Table 20–1). A sperm cell consists of the head, which contains 23 chromosomes; the middle piece, which contains mitochondria; the flagellum for motility; and the acrosome on the tip of the head to digest the membrane of the egg cell (see Fig. 20–1).
2. Epididymis (paired)—a long coiled tube on the posterior surface of each testis (see Fig. 20–4). Sperm complete their maturation here.
3. Ductus deferens (paired)—extends from the epididymis into the abdominal cavity through the inguinal canal, over and down behind the urinary bladder to join the ejaculatory duct (see Fig. 20–3). Smooth muscle in the wall contracts in waves of peristalsis.
4. Ejaculatory ducts (paired)—receive sperm from the ductus deferens and the secretions from the seminal vesicles (see Fig. 20–3); empty into the urethra.
5. Seminal vesicles (paired)—posterior to urinary bladder; duct of each opens into ejaculatory duct (see Fig. 20–3). Secretion contains fructose to nourish sperm and is alkaline to enhance sperm motility.
6. Prostate gland (single)—below the urinary bladder, encloses the first inch of the urethra (see Fig. 20–3); secretion contains citric acid for energy production by sperm; smooth muscle contributes to the force required for ejaculation.
7. Bulbourethral glands (paired)—below the prostate gland; empty into the urethra (see Fig. 20–3); secretion is alkaline to line the urethra prior to ejaculation and enhance sperm motility.
8. Urethra (single)—within the penis; carries semen to exterior (see Fig. 20–3). The penis contains three masses of erectile tissue that have blood sinuses. Sexual stimulation and parasympathetic impulses cause dilation of the penile arteries and an erection. Ejaculation of semen involves peristalsis of all male ducts and contraction of the prostate gland and pelvic floor.
9. Semen—composed of sperm and the secretions of the seminal vesicles, prostate gland, and bulbourethral glands. The alkaline pH (7.4) neutralizes the acidic pH of the female vagina.

Female Reproductive System—consists of the ovaries, fallopian tubes, uterus, vagina, and external genitals

1. Ovaries (paired)—located on either side of the uterus (see Fig. 20–6). Egg cells are produced in ovarian follicles; each ovum contains 23 chromosomes. Ovulation of a graafian follicle is stimulated by LH (see Table 20–3).

2. Fallopian tubes (paired)—each extends from an ovary to the uterus (see Fig. 20–6); fimbriae sweep the ovum into the tube; ciliated epithelial tissue and peristalsis of smooth muscle propel the ovum toward the uterus; fertilization usually takes place in the fallopian tube.
3. Uterus (single)—superior to the urinary bladder and between the two ovaries (see Fig. 20–5). Myometrium is the smooth muscle layer that contracts for delivery (see Fig. 20–6). Endometrium is the lining that may become the placenta; basilar layer is permanent; functional layer is lost in menstruation and regenerated. Parts: upper fundus, central body, and lower cervix.
4. Vagina (single)—extends from the cervix to the vaginal orifice (see Figs. 20–5 and 20–6). Receives sperm during intercourse; serves as exit for menstrual blood and as the birth canal during delivery. Normal flora provide an acidic pH that inhibits the growth of pathogens.
5. External genitals (see Figs. 20–5 and 20–7)—also called the vulva. The clitoris is a small mass of erectile tissue that responds to sexual stimulation; labia majora and minora are paired folds of skin that enclose the vestibule and cover the urethral and vaginal openings; Bartholin's glands open into the vaginal orifice and secrete mucus.

Mammary Glands—anterior to the pectoralis major muscles, surrounded by adipose tissue (see Fig. 20–8)

1. Alveolar glands produce milk; lactiferous ducts converge at the nipple.
2. Hormonal regulation—see Table 20–2.
3. Breast milk contains lactose, fatty acids, and protein for nutrition, antibodies for passive immunity, and oligosaccharides to encourage the growth of the baby's intestinal microbiota.

The Menstrual Cycle—average is 28 days; includes the hormones FSH, LH, estrogen, and progesterone, and changes in the ovaries and endometrium (see Fig. 20–9 and Table 20–3)

1. Menstrual phase—loss of the endometrium.
2. Follicular phase—several ovarian follicles develop; ovulation is the rupture of a mature follicle; blood vessels grow in the endometrium.
3. Luteal phase—the ruptured follicle becomes the corpus luteum; the endometrium continues to develop.
4. If fertilization does not occur, decreased progesterone results in the loss of the endometrium in menstruation.

REVIEW QUESTIONS

1. Describe spermatogenesis and oogenesis in terms of site, number of functional cells produced by each cell that undergoes meiosis, and timing of the process. (p. 500)
2. Describe the functions of FSH, LH, inhibin, and testosterone in spermatogenesis. Describe the functions of FSH and estrogen in oogenesis. (p. 500)
3. Describe the locations of the testes and epididymides, and explain their functions. (pp. 501, 504)
4. Name all the ducts, in order, that sperm travel through from the testes to the urethra. (pp. 504–505)
5. Name the male reproductive glands, and state how each contributes to the formation of semen. (p. 505)
6. Explain how the structure of cavernous tissue permits erection of the penis. Name the structures that bring about ejaculation. (p. 507)
7. State the function of each part of a sperm cell: head, middle piece, flagellum, and acrosome. (p. 504)
8. Describe the location of the ovaries, and name the hormones produced by the ovaries. (p. 507)
9. Explain how an ovum or zygote is kept moving through the fallopian tube. (p. 507)
10. Describe the function of the myometrium, the basilar layer of the endometrium, and the functional layer of the endometrium. Name the hormones necessary for growth of the endometrium. (p. 510)
11. State the functions of the vagina, labia majora and minora, and Bartholin's glands. (pp. 510–512)
12. Name the parts of the mammary glands, and state the function of each. (p. 512)
13. Name the hormone that has each of these effects on the mammary glands: (p. 512)
    a. Causes release of milk
    b. Promotes growth of the ducts
    c. Promotes growth of the secretory cells
    d. Stimulates milk production
14. Name the phase of the menstrual cycle in which each of these actions takes place: (p. 513)
    a. Rupture of a mature follicle
    b. Loss of the endometrium
    c. Final development of the endometrium
    d. Development of the corpus luteum
    e. Development of several ovarian follicles

FOR FURTHER THOUGHT

1. Compare meiosis with mitosis in terms of number of divisions, number of cells produced, number of chromosomes in each cell, and purpose of the cells produced.
2. An ovum is released by a mature ovarian follicle, but the subsequent corpus luteum does not secrete progesterone. If the ovum is fertilized, is implantation possible? Is a full-term pregnancy possible? Explain your answers.
3. A sexually transmitted disease such as gonorrhea is usually symptomatic for men, but quite often women do not have symptoms. Explain the consequences of this, and to whom those consequences apply.
4. Some textbooks or articles speak of the genitourinary system or the urogenital system. Is this terminology correct for everyone? For anyone? If it is correct for some, describe what the two systems share anatomically.
5. The reproductive system may seem a bit isolated from other body systems in that its purpose is to create new life and not to maintain existing life, but of course there are many connections. Question Figure 20–A depicts the relationships of the reproductive systems (represented by the ovary and testis in the center) to other body systems. The blue arrows represent contributions to the reproductive systems; briefly describe each. The orange arrows represent the influence of the reproductive hormones on other body systems; briefly describe each.

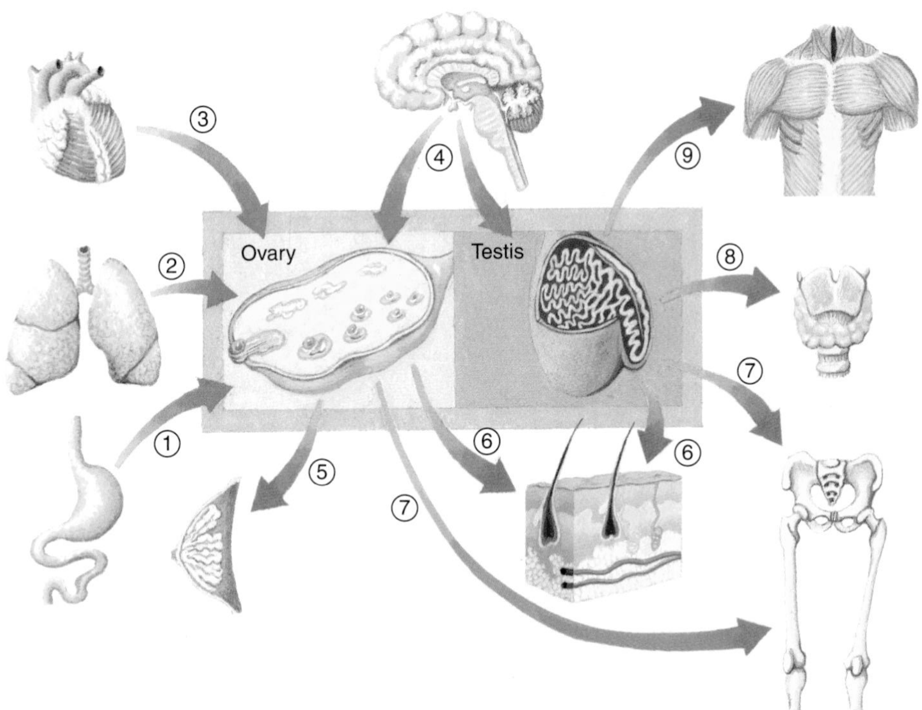

QUESTION FIGURE 20–A: Relationships between the reproductive systems and other body systems.

CHAPTER

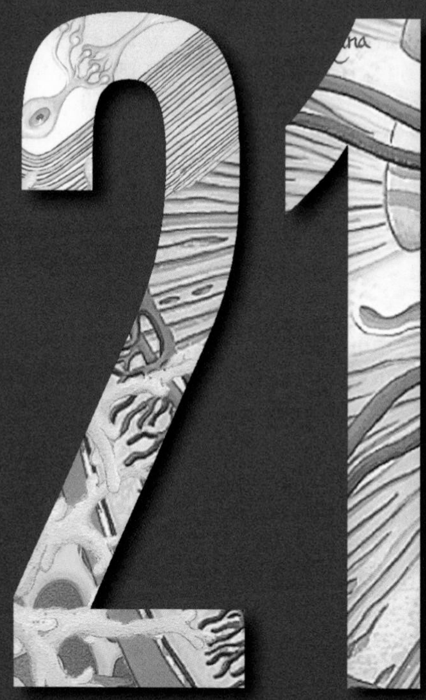

Human Development and Genetics

STUDENT OBJECTIVES

- Describe the process of fertilization and cleavage to the blastocyst stage.
- Explain when, where, and how implantation of the embryo occurs.
- Describe the functions of the embryonic membranes.
- Describe the structure and functions of the placenta and umbilical cord.
- Name and explain the functions of the placental hormones.
- State the length of the average gestation period, and describe the stages of labor.
- Describe the major changes in the infant at birth.
- Describe some important maternal changes during pregnancy.
- Explain homologous chromosomes, autosomes, sex chromosomes, and genes.
- Define alleles, genotype, phenotype, homozygous, and heterozygous.
- Explain the following patterns of inheritance: dominant–recessive, multiple alleles, and sex-linked traits.

NEW TERMINOLOGY

Alleles *(uh-**LEELZ**)*
Amnion *(**AM**-nee-on)*
Amniotic fluid *(**AM**-nee-AH-tik **FLOO**-id)*
Autosomes *(**AW**-toh-sohms)*
Cleavage *(**KLEE**-vije)*
Embryo *(**EM**-bree-oh)*
Genotype *(**JEE**-noh-type)*
Gestation *(jes-**TAY**-shun)*
Heterozygous *(HET-er-oh-**ZYE**-gus)*
Homologous pair *(hoh-**MAHL**-ah-gus PAYR)*
Homozygous *(HOH-moh-**ZYE**-gus)*
Implantation *(IM-plan-**TAY**-shun)*
Labor *(**LAY**-ber)*
Parturition *(PAR-tyoo-**RISH**-uhn)*
Phenotype *(**FEE**-noh-type)*
Sex chromosome *(SEKS **KROH**-muh-sohm)*

RELATED CLINICAL TERMINOLOGY

Amniocentesis *(AM-nee-oh-sen-**TEE**-sis)*
APGAR score *(**APP**-gar SKOR)*
Cesarean section *(se-**SAR**-ee-an **SEK**-shun)*
Chorionic villus sampling *(KOR-ee-**ON**-ik **VILL**-us)*
Congenital *(kon-**JEN**-i-tuhl)*
Fetal alcohol syndrome *(**FEE**-tuhl **AL**-koh-hol)*
Teratogen *(te-**RAH**-toh-jen)*

*Terms that appear in **bold type** in the chapter text are defined in the glossary, which begins on page 603.*

CHAPTER OUTLINE

How often have we heard comments such as "She has her mother's eyes" or "That nose is just like his father's"—because people cannot resist comparing a newborn with his or her parents. Although a child may not resemble either parent, there is a sound basis for such comparisons, because the genetic makeup and many of the traits of a child are the result of the chromosomes inherited from mother and father.

In this chapter, we will cover some of the fundamentals of genetics and inheritance. First, however, we will look at the development of a fertilized egg into a functioning human being.

HUMAN DEVELOPMENT

During the 40 weeks of **gestation**, the embryo-fetus is protected and nourished in the uterus of the mother. A human being begins life as one cell, a fertilized egg called a zygote, which develops into an individual human being consisting of billions of cells organized into the body systems with whose functions you are now quite familiar.

FERTILIZATION

Although millions of sperm are deposited in the vagina during sexual intercourse, only one will fertilize an ovum. As the sperm swim through the fluid of the uterus and fallopian tube, they undergo a final metabolic change, called **capacitation**. This change involves the **acrosome**, which becomes more fragile. When sperm and egg make contact, the acrosomal enzymes will digest the layers of cells and membrane around an ovum.

Once a sperm nucleus enters the ovum, changes in the egg cell membrane block the entry of other sperm. The nucleus of the ovum completes the second meiotic division, and the nuclei of ovum and sperm fuse, restoring the diploid number of chromosomes in the zygote.

The human diploid number of 46 chromosomes is actually 23 pairs of chromosomes: 23 from the sperm and 23 from the egg. These 23 pairs consist of 22 pairs of **autosomes** (designated by the numerals 1 through 22) and one pair of **sex chromosomes**. Women have the sex chromosomes XX, and men have the sex chromosomes XY. Figure 21–1 shows the inheritance of gender. The Y chromosome has a gene that triggers the development of male gonads in the embryo. In the absence of the Y chromosome, the embryo will develop as a female.

IMPLANTATION

Fertilization usually takes place within the fallopian tube, and the zygote begins to divide even as it is being swept toward the uterus. These are mitotic divisions and are called **cleavage**. Refer to Fig. 21–2 as you read the following.

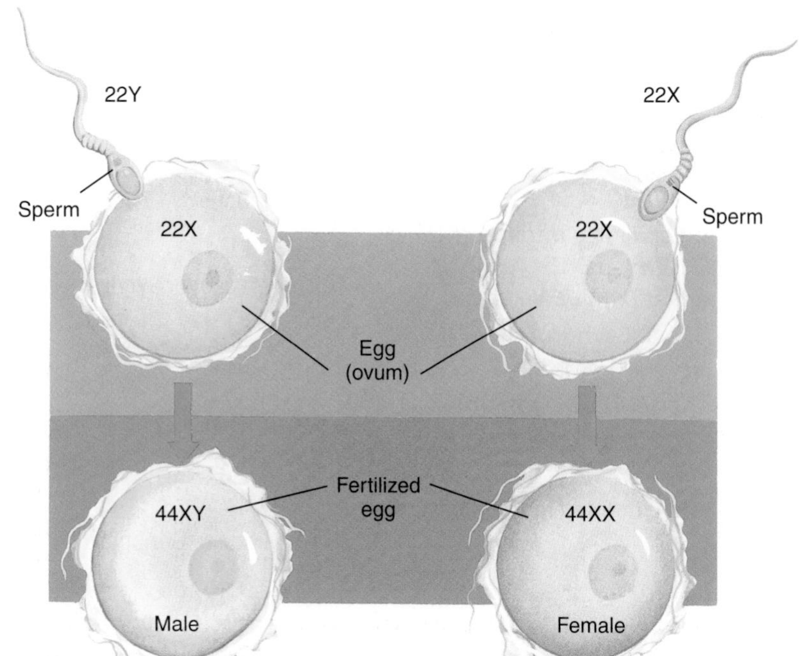

Figure 21–1 Inheritance of gender. Each ovum contains 22 autosomes and an X chromosome. Each sperm contains 22 autosomes and either an X chromosome or a Y chromosome.

QUESTION: Which parent determines the sex of the embryo-fetus?

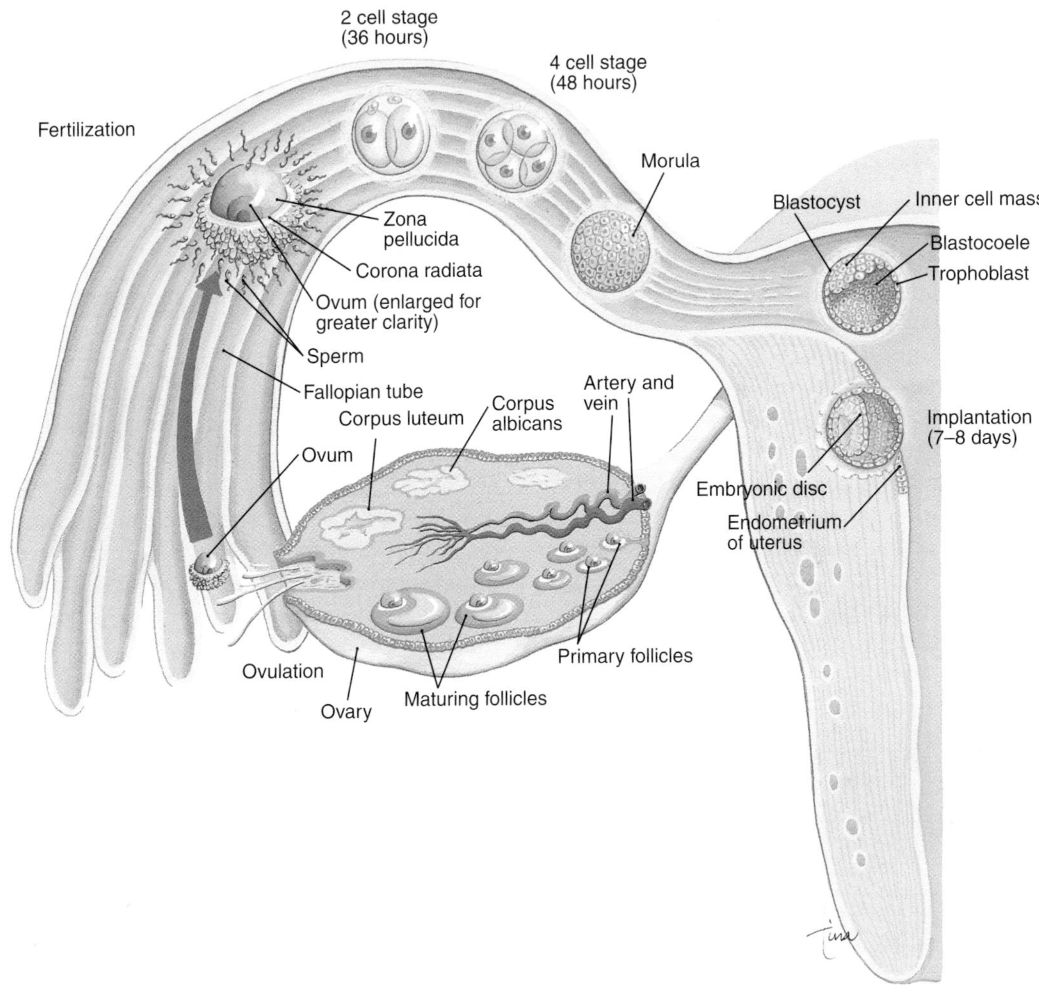

Figure 21–2 Ovulation, fertilization, and early embryonic development. Fertilization takes place in the fallopian tube, and the embryo has reached the blastocyst stage when it becomes implanted in the endometrium of the uterus.

QUESTION: Find the blastocyst stage. What is the inner cell mass? What kind of cells make it up?

The single-cell zygote divides into a two-cell stage, four-cell stage, eight-cell stage, and so on. Three days after fertilization there are 16 cells, which continue to divide to form a solid sphere of cells called a **morula** (see Box 21–1: Twins). As mitosis proceeds, this sphere becomes hollow and is called a **blastocyst**, which is still about the same size as the original zygote.

A fluid-filled blastocyst consists of an outer layer of cells called the **trophoblast** and an **inner cell mass** (or **embryoblast**) that contains the potential embryo. It is the blastocyst stage that becomes **implanted** in the uterine wall, about 5 to 8 days after fertilization.

Successful implantation is not simply a matter of the blastocyst contacting the uterine lining. The endometrium produces carbohydrate "docking" molecules toward the end of the uterine cycle, and the blastocyst has a surface protein that fits the docking sites. Once this "fit" is made, the trophoblast secretes enzymes to digest the surface of the endometrium, creating a small crater into which the blastocyst sinks. The hormone progesterone is believed to

Box 21–1 | TWINS

Fraternal twins are the result of two separate ova fertilized by separate sperm (see Box Figure 21–A, part A). This may occur when two ovarian follicles reach maturity and rupture at the same time. Fraternal twins may be of the same sex or different sexes. Even if of the same sex, however, they are as genetically different as any siblings might be.

Identical twins are the result of the splitting of the very early embryo before the cells start to become specialized (usually within 8 days after fertilization). For example, if a 16-cell stage becomes separated into two groups of 8 cells each (see part B of the figure), each group will usually continue to develop in the usual way. Also possible is the splitting of the early inner cell mass within the blastocyst. This, too, is before significant specialization has taken place, and each new inner cell mass may develop into a complete individual. Twins of this type may be called monozygotic, meaning that they have come from one fertilized egg. Identical twins are always of the same sex, are very much alike in appearance, and are genetically identical in other respects.

Conjoined twins are believed to result most often from a split embryo within a blastocyst partially reuniting (see part C: if the two embryos remain separate, they will be identical twins; if the two embryos partially fuse, resembling an hourglass, they will be conjoined twins). The name *Siamese twins* refers to Chang and Eng (1811–1874), famous Chinese brothers born in Siam, now Thailand. Conjoined twins may share superficial parts such as skin and muscle (as in part C, at the hip), or they may share a vital organ such as a liver. Advances in microsurgery and reparative surgery have permitted the separation of many sets of conjoined twins.

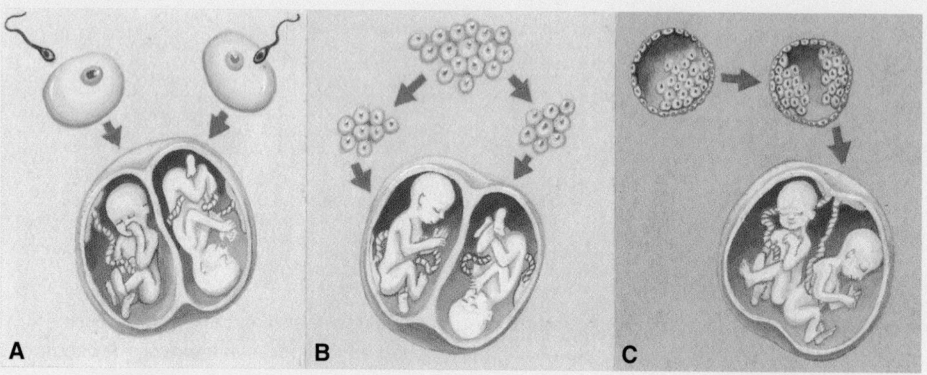

Box Figure 18–A Types of twins. (**A**) Fraternal twins. (**B**) Identical twins. (**C**) Conjoined twins.

prevent the inflammation that might arise from even this tiny bit of damage, inflammation that would destroy the embryo. With implantation successful, the trophoblast will become the **chorion**, the embryonic membrane that will form the fetal portion of the placenta. Following implantation, the inner cell mass will grow to become the embryo and other membranes.

The cells of the inner cell mass are embryonic stem cells. In these cells, all of the DNA has the potential for being switched on, that is, the potential exists for a cell to develop into any of the 200 kinds of human cells that will be present at birth. As the cells continue to divide and become more numerous, some DNA will be chemically switched off in each cell, genes will become inactive, and the possibilities for the specialization of each cell will be narrowed down.

EMBRYO AND EMBRYONIC MEMBRANES

An **embryo** is the developing human individual from the time of fertilization until the eighth week of gestation. Several stages of early embryonic development are shown in

Fig. 21–3. At approximately 12 days, the **embryonic disc** (the potential person) is simply a plate of cells within the blastocyst. As cells keep dividing, the plate of cells begins to fold. At 14 days twinning is believed to be no longer possible.

Very soon thereafter, three primary layers, or germ layers, begin to develop: the **ectoderm**, **mesoderm**, and **endoderm**. This is a major step in the specialization of the embryo cells because different sets of genes are switched off for each of the three layers, while the genes appropriate

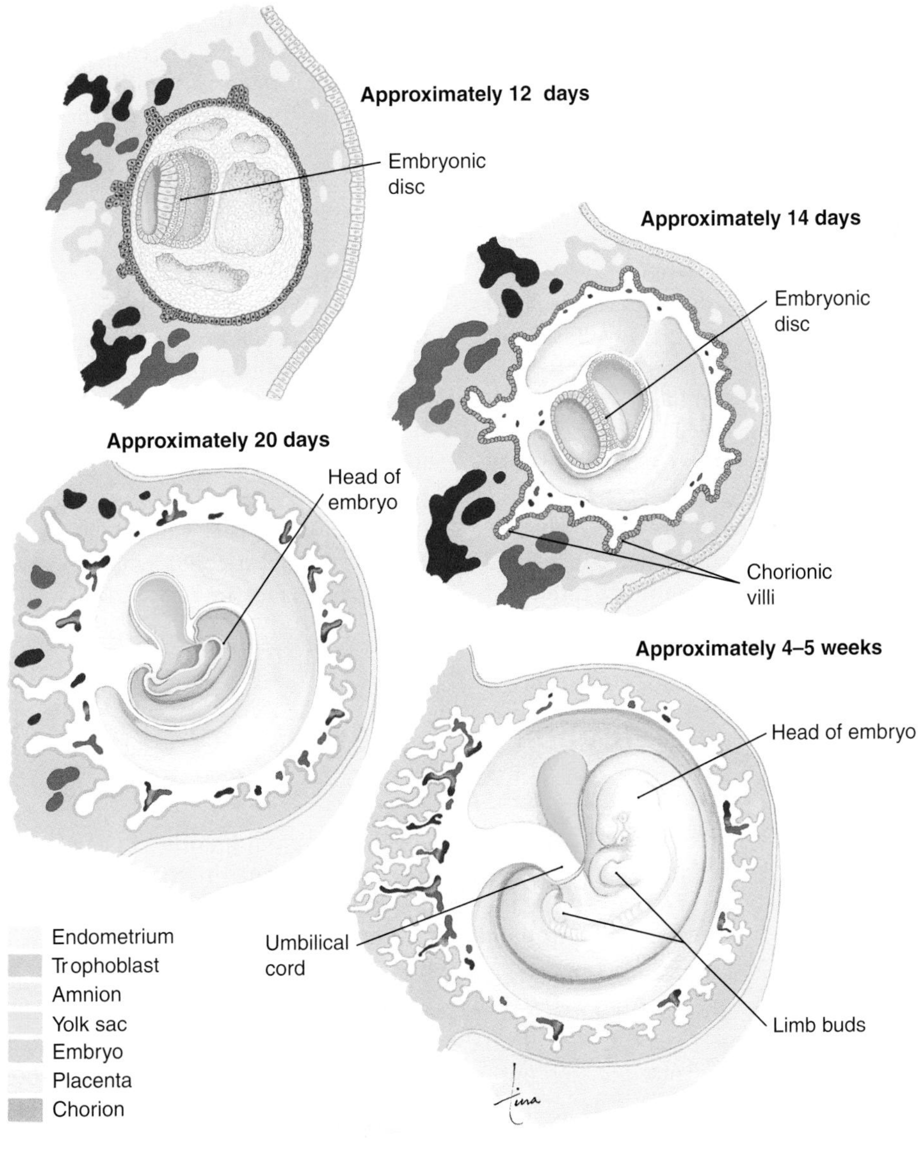

Figure 21–3 Embryonic development at 12 days (after fertilization), 14 days, 20 days, and 4 to 5 weeks. By 5 weeks, the embryo has distinct parts but does not yet look definitely human. See text for description of embryonic membranes.

QUESTION: At 14 days, what structures shown will become the fetal portion of the placenta?

for the layer remain switched on. Each cell is now committed to a particular layer and can no longer "go back," that is, become a cell of either of the other two layers.

Each primary layer develops further; its cells become more specialized as more and more genes in each cell are switched off. With the active genes, those that remain switched on, the cells in each layer are thereby committed to develop into specific organs or parts of organs. *Ecto* means "outer"; the epidermis is derived from ectoderm, and in some of these cells the gene for producing keratin is active. *Meso* means "middle"; the skeletal muscles develop from mesoderm, and in these cells the genes for producing myosin and actin are active. *Endo* means "inner"; the stomach lining is derived from endoderm, and in these cells, the gene for producing pepsinogen is active. Table 21–1 lists some other structures derived from each of the primary germ layers.

At 20 days, the **embryonic membranes** can be clearly distinguished from the embryo itself. The **yolk sac** does not contain nutrient yolk, as it does for bird and reptile embryos. It is, however, the site for the formation of the first blood cells and the cells that will become spermatogonia or oogonia. As the embryo grows, the yolk sac membrane is incorporated into the umbilical cord and blood cell production is taken over first by the liver.

The **amnion** is a thin membrane that eventually surrounds the embryo and contains **amniotic fluid**. This fluid provides a cushion for the fetus against mechanical injury as the mother moves. When the fetal kidneys become functional, they excrete urine into the amniotic fluid. Also in this fluid are cells that have sloughed off the fetus; this is clinically important in the procedure called amniocentesis (see Box 21–2: Fetal Diagnosis). The rupture of the amnion (sometimes called the "bag of waters") is usually an indication that labor has begun.

The **chorion** is the name given to the trophoblast as it develops further. Once the embryo has become implanted in the uterus, small projections called **chorionic villi** begin to grow into the endometrium. These will contain the fetal blood vessels that become the fetal portion of the placenta.

At about 4 to 5 weeks of development, the embryo shows definite form. The head is apparent, the heart is beating, and limb buds are visible. The period of embryonic growth continues until the 8th week. At this time, the embryo is about 1.5 inches (3 cm) long, 1 gram in weight, and all of the organ systems have been established. The systems will continue to grow and mature until the end of gestation. The period of fetal growth extends from the 9th through the 40th week. Table 21–2 lists some of the major aspects of development in the growth of the embryo-fetus. The fetus at 16 weeks is depicted in Fig. 21–4. (See also Box 21–3: Congenital Fetal Infections and Box 21–4: Fetal Alcohol Syndrome.) Maternal changes during pregnancy are summarized in Table 21–3.

Table 21–1 | STRUCTURES DERIVED FROM THE PRIMARY GERM LAYERS

LAYER	STRUCTURES DERIVED*
Ectoderm	■ Epidermis; hair and nail follicles; sweat glands ■ Nervous system; pituitary gland; adrenal medulla ■ Lens and cornea; internal ear ■ Mucosa of oral and nasal cavities; salivary glands
Mesoderm	■ Dermis; bone and cartilage ■ Skeletal muscles; cardiac muscle; most smooth muscle ■ Kidneys and adrenal cortex ■ Bone marrow and blood; lymphatic tissue; lining of blood vessels
Endoderm	■ Mucosa of esophagus, stomach, and intestines ■ Epithelium of respiratory tract, including lungs ■ Liver and mucosa of gallbladder ■ Thyroid gland; pancreas

*These are representative lists, not all-inclusive ones. Keep in mind also that most organs are combinations of tissues from each of the three germ layers. Related structures are grouped together.

Box 21–2 | FETAL DIAGNOSIS

Several procedures are currently available to determine certain kinds of abnormalities in a fetus or to monitor development.

ULTRASOUND (OR FETAL ULTRASONOGRAPHY)

This is a noninvasive procedure; high-frequency sound waves are transmitted through the abdominal wall into the uterus. The reflected sound waves are converted into an image called a sonogram. This method is used to confirm multiple pregnancies, to determine fetal age or position, or to detect fetal heart defects or malformations of other organs.

AMNIOCENTESIS

This procedure can be performed between 16 and 20 weeks of gestation. A hypodermic needle is inserted through the wall of the abdomen into the amniotic sac, and about 10 to 20 mL of amniotic fluid is removed. Within this fluid are fetal cells, which can be cultured so that their chromosomes may be examined. Through such examination and biochemical tests, a number of genetic diseases or chromosome abnormalities may be detected. Because women over the age of 35 years are believed to have a greater chance of having a child with Down syndrome, amniocentesis is often recommended for this age group. A family history of certain genetic diseases is another reason a pregnant woman may want to have this procedure.

CHORIONIC VILLUS SAMPLING (CVS)

In this procedure, a biopsy catheter is inserted through the vagina and cervix to collect a small portion of the chorionic villi. These cells are derived from the fetus but are not part of the fetus itself. The information obtained is the same as that for amniocentesis, but CVS may be performed earlier in pregnancy, between 8 and 11 weeks. Although there is a risk that the procedure may cause a miscarriage, CVS is considered comparable in safety to amniocentesis. It is important to remember that no invasive procedure is without risks.

MATERNAL BLOOD TESTS

Alpha-fetoprotein (AFP) is produced by the fetus and is found in maternal circulation. The level reaches a peak between 12 and 15 weeks of gestation and should then decrease. If AFP is still high after 16 to 18 weeks, there is a 95% chance that the fetus has spina bifida or anencephaly, malformations of the central nervous system. Recall from Chapter 17 that sufficient folic acid during pregnancy will greatly reduce the risk to the fetus.

The newest tests evaluate the fragments of fetal DNA (from the placenta) that have entered maternal blood and can be done at the end of the first trimester. Such a test is accurate for many genetic and chromosomal disorders but is still considered a screening test, with results to be confirmed by amniocentesis or CVS.

Table 21–2 | GROWTH OF THE EMBRYO-FETUS

MONTH OF GESTATION (END)	ASPECTS OF DEVELOPMENT	APPROXIMATE OVERALL SIZE IN INCHES
1	■ Heart begins to beat; limb buds form; backbone forms; facial features not distinct	0.25
2	■ Calcification of bones begins; fingers and toes are apparent on limbs; facial features more distinct; body systems are established	1.25–1.5
3	■ Facial features distinct but eyes are still closed; nails develop on fingers and toes; ossification of skeleton continues; fetus is distinguishable as male or female	3

Continued

Table 21–2 | **GROWTH OF THE EMBRYO-FETUS—cont'd**

MONTH OF GESTATION (END)	ASPECTS OF DEVELOPMENT	APPROXIMATE OVERALL SIZE IN INCHES
4	■ Head still quite large in proportion to body, but the arms and legs lengthen; hair appears on head; body systems continue to develop	5–7
5	■ Skeletal muscles become active ("quickening" may be felt by the mother); body grows more rapidly than head; body is covered with fine hair (lanugo)	10–12
6	■ Eyelashes and eyebrows form; eyelids open; skin is quite wrinkled; pulmonary surfactant is first produced	11–14
7	■ Head and body approach normal infant proportions; deposition of subcutaneous fat makes skin less wrinkled	13–17
8	■ Testes of male fetus descend into scrotum; more subcutaneous fat is deposited; production of pulmonary surfactant is sufficient to permit breathing if birth is premature	16–18
9	■ Lanugo is shed; nails are fully developed; cranial bones are ossified with fontanels present; lungs are more mature	19–21

Table 21–3 | **MATERNAL CHANGES DURING PREGNANCY**

ASPECT	CHANGE
Weight	■ Gain of 2–3 pounds for each month of gestation
Uterus	■ Enlarges considerably and displaces abdominal organs upward
Thyroid gland	■ Increases secretion of thyroxine, which increases metabolic rate
Skin	■ Appearance of striae (stretch marks) on abdomen
Circulatory system	■ Heart rate increases, as do stroke volume and cardiac output; blood volume increases; varicose veins may develop in the legs and anal canal
Digestive system	■ Nausea and vomiting may occur in early pregnancy (morning sickness); constipation may occur in later pregnancy
Urinary system	■ Kidney activity increases; frequency of urination often increases in later pregnancy (bladder is compressed by uterus)
Respiratory system	■ Respiratory rate increases; lung capacity decreases as diaphragm is forced upward by compressed abdominal organs in later pregnancy
Skeletal system	■ Lordosis may occur with increased weight at front of abdomen; sacroiliac joints and pubic symphysis become more flexible prior to birth

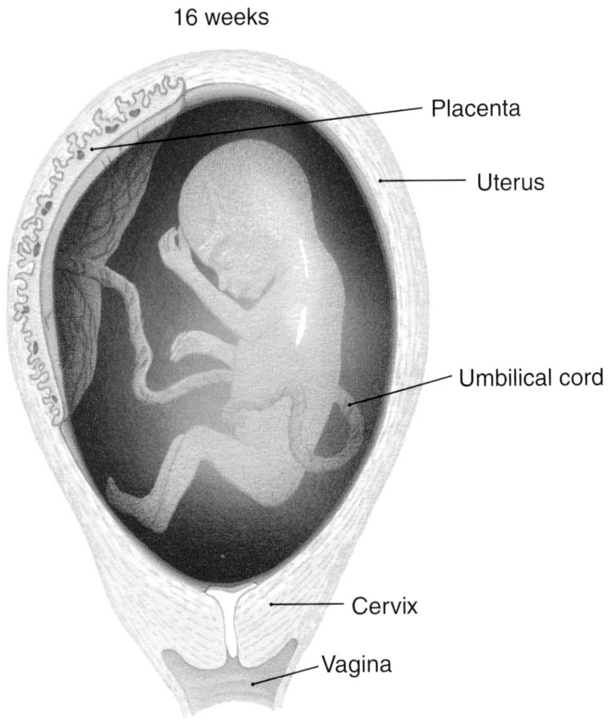

Figure 21–4 Fetal development at 16 weeks.

QUESTION: Name the fluid that surrounds the fetus, and state its function.

PLACENTA AND UMBILICAL CORD

The **placenta** is made of both fetal and maternal tissue. The chorion of the embryo and the endometrium of the uterus contribute, and the placenta is formed by the third month of gestation (12 weeks). The mature placenta is a flat disc about 7 inches (17 to 18 cm) in diameter.

The structure of a small portion of the placenta is shown in Fig. 21–5. Notice that the fetal blood vessels are within maternal blood sinuses, but there is no direct connection between fetal and maternal vessels. Though some fetal cells may cross into maternal circulation, normally, the blood of the fetus does not mix with that of the mother. The placenta has two functions: to be the site of exchanges between maternal and fetal blood and to produce hormones to maintain pregnancy. We will consider the exchanges first.

The fetus is dependent upon the mother for oxygen and nutrients and for the removal of waste products. The **umbilical cord** connects the fetus to the placenta and grows to about 20 inches (50 cm) long. Within the cord are two umbilical arteries that carry blood from the fetus to the placenta and one umbilical vein that returns blood from the placenta to the fetus.

The surface area for the fetal-maternal exchanges within the placenta (if all of the capillaries were opened and flattened out) is estimated to be at least 100 square feet, and a healthy placenta easily supplies fetal needs.

Box 21–3 | CONGENITAL FETAL INFECTIONS

A **teratogen** is anything that may cause developmental abnormalities in an embryo-fetus. Several infectious microorganisms are known to be teratogenic; they may cross the placenta from maternal blood to fetal blood and damage the fetus.

Congenital rubella syndrome—the virus of German measles (rubella) is perhaps the best known of the infectious teratogens. If a woman acquires rubella during pregnancy, there is a 20% chance that her fetus will be affected. Consequences for the fetus may be death (stillbirth), heart defects, deafness, or mental retardation. Use of the rubella vaccine has made this syndrome rare in the United States, but many developing nations do not have extensive vaccination programs.

Congenital varicella syndrome—chickenpox (herpes zoster) is a viral disease that many people have during childhood. If a pregnant woman acquires chickenpox, however, the virus may cross the placenta. Consequences for the fetus include malformed limbs, cutaneous scars, blindness, and mental retardation. This is not a common congenital syndrome, and the success of the chickenpox vaccine should make it truly rare.

Congenital syphilis—syphilis is a sexually transmitted disease caused by a bacterium (*Treponema pallidum*). These bacteria may cross the placenta after the fourth month of gestation. Consequences of early infection of the fetus are death, malformations of bones and teeth, or cataracts. If infection occurs toward the end of gestation, the child may be born with syphilis. This is most often apparent as a rash on the skin and mucous membranes. Syphilis in adults can be cured by penicillin; prevention of congenital

Continued

Box 21–3 | CONGENITAL FETAL INFECTIONS (Continued)

syphilis depends upon good prenatal care for women who may be infected.

Congenital toxoplasmosis—caused by the protozoan parasite *Toxoplasma gondii.* For most healthy people, toxoplasmosis has no symptoms; it is a harmless infection. Because cats and some other mammals are hosts for this parasite, pregnant women may acquire infection from contact with cat feces or by eating rare beef or lamb. Consequences for the fetus are death, mental retardation, or blindness. Prevention depends upon education of pregnant women to avoid potential sources of infection.

Box 21–4 | FETAL ALCOHOL SYNDROME

Fetal alcohol syndrome is the group of characteristics present in infants who were exposed to alcohol during their fetal life. Alcohol is a toxin for adults and even more so for fetal tissues that are immature and growing rapidly. Either alcohol or its toxic intermediate product (acetaldehyde) may pass from maternal to fetal circulation and impair fetal development.

Consequences for infants include low birth weight, small head with facial abnormalities, heart defects, malformation of other organs, and irritability and agitation. The infant often grows slowly, both physically and mentally.

Because such damage cannot be reversed, prevention by means of education is very important; women should be aware of the consequences their consumption of alcohol may have for a fetus.

When blood in the umbilical arteries enters the placenta, CO_2 and waste products in the fetal capillaries diffuse into the maternal blood sinuses. Oxygen diffuses from the maternal blood sinuses into the fetal capillaries; nutrients enter the fetal blood by diffusion and active transport mechanisms. This oxygen- and nutrient-rich blood then flows through the umbilical vein back to the fetus. Circulation within the fetus was described in Chapter 13.

When the baby is delivered at the end of gestation, the umbilical cord is cut. The placenta then detaches from the uterine wall and is delivered, with the rest of the umbilical cord, as the **afterbirth**. Sometimes during pregnancy, for reasons that cannot be determined, a part of the placenta becomes detached too soon. With even a small detachment, the oxygen supply to the fetus will be diminished, and such a decrease, even if not fatal, may cause brain damage. For the mother, the loss of blood may be small at first, but has the potential to become greater very rapidly, which will endanger her and the fetus.

The umbilical cord is also part of the afterbirth. The fetal blood in the remnant of the umbilical cord contains abundant stem cells, and their potential to become different kinds of cells is somewhere between that of embryonic stem cells (which can become any human cell) and adult stem cells (which are more limited). Umbilical cord stem cells do have an advantage over embryonic stem cells, however, in that cord stem cells do not have the propensity to form tumors, as do embryonic stem cells. Umbilical cord stem cells have already been used to treat newborns with infantile Krabbe's disease, a neurologic disorder that is fatal by the age of 2 years. Such treatment depends on genetic testing and having suitable donated cord stem cells available at birth. Banks of cord blood have been established by many medical centers (because such donated blood can be frozen and stored), and the use of cord stem cells can, in certain cases, take the place of a bone marrow transplant from an adult donor.

Placental Hormones

The first hormone secreted by the placenta is **human chorionic gonadotropin** (hCG), which is produced by the chorion of the early embryo. The function of hCG is to stimulate the corpus luteum in the maternal ovary so that it will continue to secrete estrogen and progesterone. The secretion of progesterone is particularly important to prevent contractions of the myometrium, which would

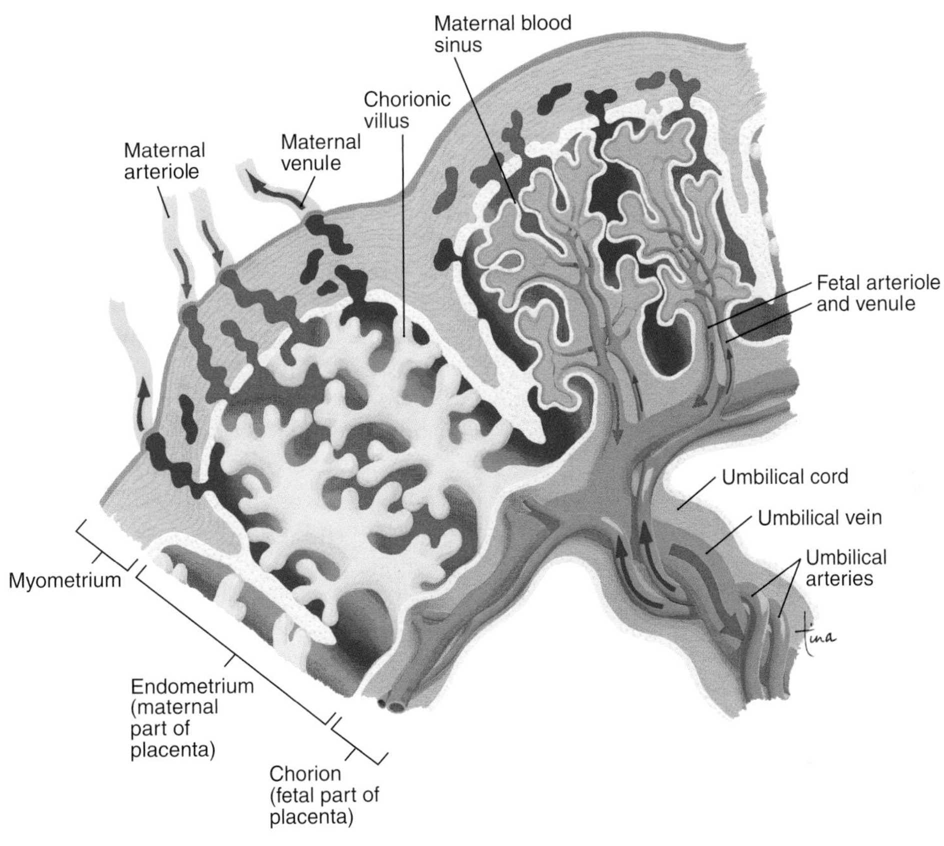

Figure 21–5 Placenta and umbilical cord. The fetal capillaries in chorionic villi are within the maternal blood sinuses. Arrows indicate the direction of blood flow in maternal and fetal vessels.

QUESTION: What substances move from maternal blood to fetal blood?

otherwise result in miscarriage of the embryo. Once hCG enters maternal circulation, it is excreted in urine, which is the basis for many pregnancy tests. Tests for hCG in maternal blood are even more precise and can determine whether a pregnancy has occurred even before a menstrual period is missed.

The corpus luteum is a small structure, however, and cannot secrete sufficient amounts of estrogen and progesterone to maintain a full-term pregnancy. The placenta itself begins to secrete **estrogen** and **progesterone** within a few weeks, and the levels of these hormones increase until shortly before birth. As the placenta takes over, the secretion of hCG decreases and the corpus luteum becomes nonfunctional. During pregnancy, estrogen and progesterone inhibit the anterior pituitary secretion of FSH and LH, so no other ovarian follicles develop. These placental hormones also prepare the mammary glands for lactation.

The placenta also secretes **relaxin**, which helps inhibit contractions of the myometrium. Relaxin also permits stretching of the ligaments of the pubic symphysis so that this joint will give a little, if necessary, during birth.

PARTURITION AND LABOR

Parturition is the rather formal term for birth, and **labor** is the sequence of events that occur during birth. The average gestation period is 40 weeks (280 days), with a range of 37 to 42 weeks (see Box 21–5: Premature Birth). Toward the end of gestation, the placental secretion of progesterone decreases while the estrogen level remains high, and the myometrium begins to contract weakly at irregular intervals. At this time the fetus is often oriented head

Box 21–5 | PREMATURE BIRTH

A premature birth is the spontaneous delivery of an infant before the end of the gestation period, or the intentional delivery (for reasons concerning the health of the mother or fetus) before that time. A premature infant may also be defined as one who weighs less than 2500 grams (5.5 pounds), though gestation time is more important than birth weight.

The March of Dimes estimates that 13 million premature births occur each year worldwide. Most of these are in Africa and Asia. Of the 13 million premature babies, about 1 million die soon after birth.

In terms of gestation time, an 8-month infant has a very good chance of surviving if good medical care is available. Infants of 7-months gestation or less often have respiratory distress because their lungs have not yet produced enough surfactant to permit inflation of the alveoli.

Infants as young as 23 (in a few cases, 22) weeks of gestation have been successfully treated and eventually sent home with their parents. Whether there will be any long-term detrimental effects of their very premature births will only be known in time. The newborn nervous system is especially vulnerable to lack of oxygen.

Medical science may have reached its maximum capability in this area. In a fetus of 20 weeks, the cells of the alveoli and the cells of the pulmonary capillaries are just not close enough to each other to permit gas exchange. At present there is no medical intervention that can overcome this anatomic fact.

The lowest birth weight with subsequent survival is believed to be 244 grams (8.6 oz) in September 2004. The little girl had a gestational age of 26 weeks.

down within the uterus (Fig. 21–6). Labor itself may be divided into three stages:

First stage—dilation of the cervix. As the uterus contracts, the amniotic sac is forced into the cervix, which dilates (widens) the cervical opening. At the end of this stage, the amniotic sac breaks (rupture of the "bag of waters") and the fluid leaves through the vagina, which may now be called the **birth canal**. This stage lasts an average of 8 to 12 hours but may vary considerably.

Second stage—delivery of the infant. More powerful contractions of the uterus are brought about by **oxytocin** released by the posterior pituitary gland and perhaps by the placenta itself. This stage may be prolonged by several factors. If the fetus is positioned other than head down, delivery may be difficult. This is called a breech birth and may necessitate a **cesarean section** (C-section), which is delivery of the fetus through a surgical incision in the abdominal wall and uterus. For some women, the central opening in the pelvic bone may be too small to permit a vaginal delivery. Fetal distress, as determined by fetal monitoring of heartbeat, for example, may also require a cesarean section.

Third stage—delivery of the placenta (afterbirth). Continued contractions of the uterus expel the placenta and membranes, usually within 10 minutes after delivery of the infant. There is some bleeding at this time, but the uterus rapidly decreases in size, and the contractions compress the endometrium to close the ruptured blood vessels at the former site of the placenta. This is important to prevent severe maternal hemorrhage.

THE INFANT AT BIRTH

Immediately after delivery, the umbilical cord is clamped and cut, and the infant's nose and mouth are aspirated to remove any fluid that might interfere with breathing (see Box 21–6: APGAR Score). Now the infant is independent of the mother, and the most rapid changes occur in the respiratory and circulatory systems.

As the level of CO_2 in the baby's blood increases, the respiratory center in the medulla is stimulated and brings about inhalation to expand and inflate the lungs. Full expansion of the lungs may take up to 7 days following birth, and the infant's respiratory rate may be very rapid at this time, as high as 40 respirations per minute.

Breathing promotes greater pulmonary circulation, and the increased amount of blood returning to the left atrium closes the flap of the **foramen ovale**. The **ductus arteriosus** begins to constrict, apparently in response to the higher blood oxygen level. Full closure of the ductus arteriosus may take up to 3 months.

The **ductus venosus** no longer receives blood from the umbilical vein and begins to constrict within a few minutes

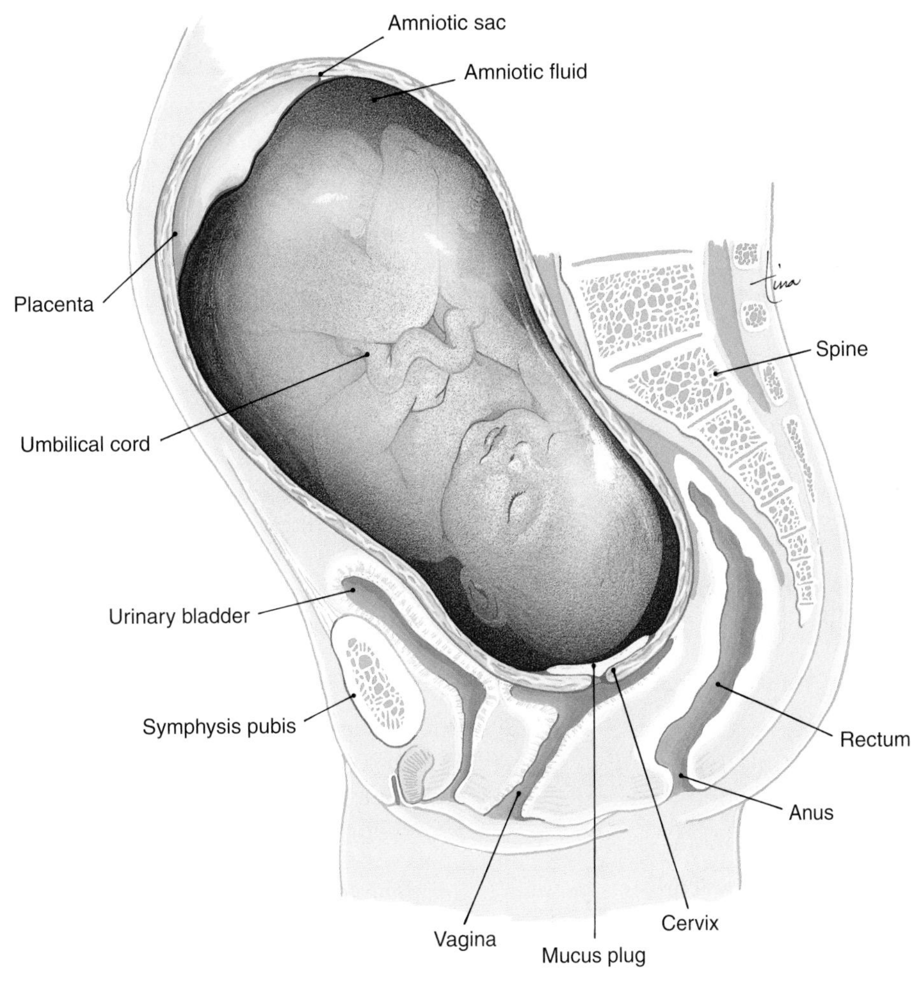

Figure 21–6 Full-term fetus positioned head down within the uterus.

QUESTION: Why is it beneficial for the fetus to be positioned head down?

after birth. Within a few weeks the ductus venosus becomes a nonfunctional ligament.

The infant's liver is not fully mature at birth and may be unable to excrete bilirubin efficiently. This may result in jaundice, which may occur in as many as half of all newborns. Such jaundice is not considered serious unless there is another possible cause, such as Rh incompatibility (see Chapter 11).

GENETICS

Genetics is the study of inheritance. Most, if not virtually all, human characteristics are regulated at least partially by genes. We will first look at what genes are, then describe some patterns of inheritance.

CHROMOSOMES AND GENES

Each of the cells of an individual (except mature red blood cells and egg and sperm cells) contains 46 chromosomes, the diploid number. These chromosomes are in 23 pairs called **homologous pairs**. One member of each pair has come from the egg and is called maternal, and the other member has come from the sperm and is called paternal. The autosomes are the chromosome pairs designated 1 to 22. The sex chromosomes form the remaining pair. In women these are designated XX and in men XY.

Chromosomes are made of DNA and protein; the DNA is the hereditary material. Recall from Chapter 3 that the sequence of bases in the DNA of chromosomes is the

Box 21–6 | APGAR SCORE

The APGAR score is an overall assessment of an infant and is usually made 1 minute after birth (repeated at 5 minutes if the first score is low). The highest score is 10. Infants who score less than 5 require immediate medical attention.

Characteristic	Description	Score
Heartbeat	• Over 100 bpm • Below 100 bpm • No heartbeat	2 1 0
Respiration	• Strong, vigorous cry • Weak cry • No respiratory effort	2 1 0
Muscle tone	• Spontaneous, active motion • Some motion • No muscle tone	2 1 0
Reflex response to stimulation of sole of the foot	• A cry in response • A grimace in response • No response	2 1 0
Color	• Healthy coloration • Cyanotic extremities • Cyanosis of trunk and extremities	2 1 0

genetic code for proteins, structural proteins, as well as enzymes. The DNA code for one protein is called a gene. Our genes have been "mapped," that is, we know the precise location of each gene on a particular chromosome. For example, a specific region of the DNA of chromosome 11 is the code for the beta chain of hemoglobin. Because an individual has two of chromosome 11, he or she will have two genes for this protein, a maternal gene inherited from the mother and a paternal gene inherited from the father. This is true for virtually all of the 22,000 genes estimated to be found in our chromosomes. In our **genome**, or complete genetic makeup, each of us has two genes for each protein.

GENOTYPE AND PHENOTYPE

For each gene of a pair, there may be two or more versions of it, possibilities for its "expression"; that is, how it will appear or how it will affect the individual. These possibilities are called **alleles**. A person, therefore, may be said to have two alleles for each protein or trait; the alleles may be the same or may be different.

If the two alleles are the same, the person is said to be **homozygous** for the trait. If the two alleles are different, the person is said to be **heterozygous** for the trait.

The **genotype** is the actual genetic makeup, that is, the alleles present. The **phenotype** is the appearance, or how the alleles are expressed. When a gene has two or more alleles, one allele may be **dominant** over the other, which is called **recessive**. For a person who is heterozygous for a trait, the dominant allele (or gene) is the one that will appear in the phenotype. The recessive allele (or gene) is hidden but not lost and may be passed to children. For a recessive trait to be expressed in the phenotype, the person must be homozygous recessive, that is, have two recessive alleles (genes) for the trait.

An example will be helpful here to put all this together and is illustrated in Fig. 21–7. When doing genetics problems, a **Punnett square** is used to show the possible combinations of genes in the egg and sperm for a particular set of parents and the possible combinations, or outcomes, for their children. Remember that an egg or sperm has only 23 chromosomes and, therefore, has only one gene for each trait.

In this example, the inheritance of eye color has been simplified. Although eye color is determined by many pairs of genes, with many possible phenotypes, one pair is considered the principal pair, with brown eyes dominant over blue eyes. A dominant gene is usually represented by

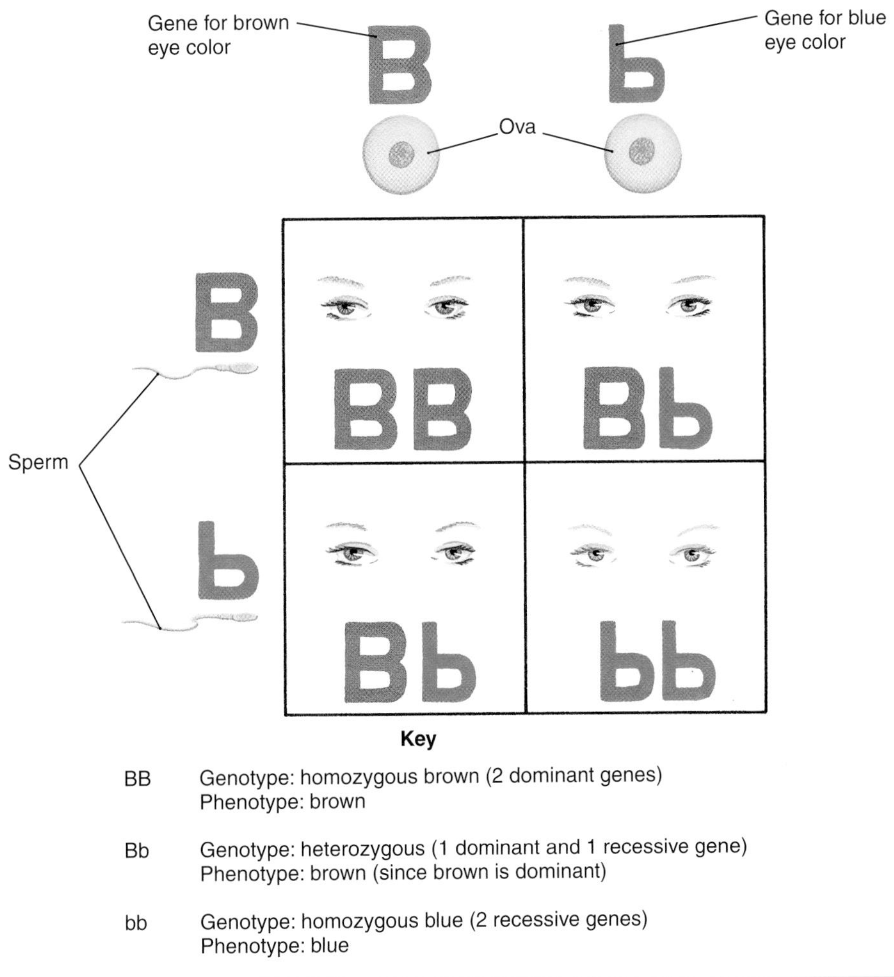

Figure 21–7 Inheritance of eye color. Both mother and father are heterozygous for brown eyes. The Punnett square shows the possible combinations of genes for eye color for each child of these parents. See text for further description.

QUESTION: If Dad is heterozygous for brown eyes and Mom has blue eyes, what will be the four possible combinations?

a capital letter, and the corresponding recessive gene is represented by the same letter, but lowercase. The parents in Fig. 21–7 are both heterozygous for eye color. Their genotype consists of a gene for brown eyes and a gene for blue eyes, but their phenotype is brown eyes.

Each egg produced by the mother has a 50% chance of containing the gene for brown eyes, or an equal 50% chance of containing the gene for blue eyes. Similarly, each sperm produced by the father has a 50% chance of containing the gene for brown eyes and a 50% chance of containing the gene for blue eyes.

Now look at the boxes of the Punnett square; these represent the possibilities for the genetic makeup of each child. For eye color there are three possibilities: a 25% (one of four) chance for homozygous brown eyes, a 50% (two of four) chance for heterozygous brown eyes, and a 25% (one of four) chance for homozygous blue eyes. Notice that BB and Bb have the same phenotype (brown eyes) despite their different genotypes, and that the phenotype of blue eyes is possible only with the genotype bb. Can brown-eyed parents have a blue-eyed child? Yes; if each parent is heterozygous for brown eyes, each child has a 25% chance of inheriting blue eyes. Could these parents have four children with blue eyes? What is the probability or chance of this happening? The answers to these questions will be found in Box 21–7: Solution to Genetics Question.

INHERITANCE: DOMINANT–RECESSIVE

The inheritance of eye color just described is an example of a trait determined by a pair of alleles, one of which may dominate the other. Another example is sickle-cell anemia, which was discussed in Chapter 11. The gene for the beta chain of hemoglobin is on chromosome 11; an allele for normal hemoglobin is dominant, and an allele for sickle-cell hemoglobin is recessive. An individual who is heterozygous is said to have sickle-cell trait; an individual who is homozygous recessive will have sickle-cell anemia. The Punnett square in Fig. 21–8 shows that if both parents are heterozygous, each child has a 25% chance (1 of 4) of inheriting the two recessive genes. Table 21–4 lists some other human genetic diseases and their patterns of inheritance.

It is important to remember that in the terminology of genetics, *dominant* does not mean "common" or "frequent." It simply means that one gene is sufficient for the characteristic to appear in the phenotype. Think back to the ABO blood types. Which type is the most common in a population? Type O is most common, followed by type A, then type B. Type AB is the least common. Here is an instance in which the recessive trait, type O, is most frequent in a group of people. Why is type AB the least common, even though A and B alleles are dominant over an O allele? Because there are not many B alleles to be found in a population, not many people have a B allele. If you look at Table 21–6 later in this chapter, you will certainly be able to find other dominant traits that are rare.

INHERITANCE: MULTIPLE ALLELES

The best example of this pattern of inheritance is the human blood type of the ABO group. For each gene of this blood type, there are three possible alleles: A, B, or O. A person will have only two of these alleles, which may be the same or different. O is the recessive allele; A and B are co-dominant alleles, that is, dominant over O but not over each other.

You already know that in this blood group there are four possible blood types: O, AB, A, and B. Table 21–5 shows the combinations of alleles for each type. Notice that for types O and AB there is only one possible genotype. For types A and B, however, there are two possible genotypes because both A and B alleles are dominant over an O allele.

Let us now use a problem to illustrate the inheritance of blood type. The Punnett square in Fig. 21–9 shows that Mom has type O blood and Dad has type AB blood. The boxes of the square show the possible blood types for each child. Each child has a 50% chance of having type A blood and a 50% chance of having type B blood. The genotype, however, will always be heterozygous. Notice that in this example, the blood types of the children will not be the same as those of

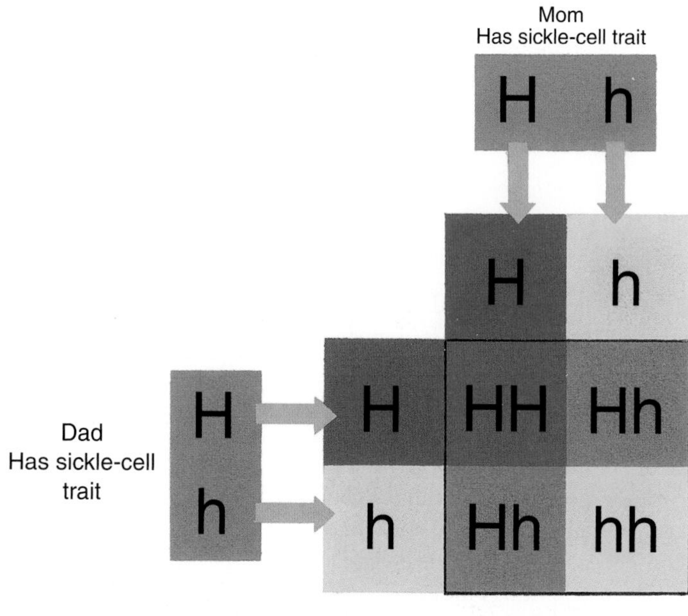

Figure 21–8 Inheritance of sickle-cell anemia (dominant–recessive pattern). See text for description.

QUESTION: If Dad has sickle-cell trait and Mom is homozygous for normal hemoglobin, can a child of theirs have sickle-cell anemia?

Table 21–4 | **HUMAN GENETIC DISEASES**

DISEASE (PATTERN OF INHERITANCE)	DESCRIPTION
Sickle-cell anemia (R)	The most common genetic disease among people of African ancestry. Sickle-cell hemoglobin forms rigid crystals that distort and disrupt RBCs; oxygen-carrying capacity of the blood is diminished.
Cystic fibrosis (R)	The most common genetic disease among people of European ancestry. Production of thick mucus clogs the bronchial tree and pancreatic ducts. Most severe effects are chronic respiratory infections and pulmonary failure.
Tay-Sachs disease (R)	The most common (though now rare) genetic disease among people of Jewish ancestry. Degeneration of neurons and the nervous system results in death by the age of 2 years.
Phenylketonuria or PKU (R)	Lack of an enzyme to metabolize the amino acid phenylalanine leads to severe mental and physical retardation. These effects may be prevented by the use of a diet (beginning at birth) that limits phenylalanine.
Huntington's disease (D)	Uncontrollable muscle contractions begin between the ages of 30 and 50 years, followed by loss of memory and personality. There is no treatment that can delay mental deterioration.
Hemophilia (X-linked)	Lack of Factor 8 impairs chemical clotting; may be controlled with Factor 8 from donated blood.
Duchenne's muscular dystrophy (X-linked)	Replacement of muscle by adipose or scar tissue, with progressive loss of muscle function; often fatal before age 20 years due to involvement of cardiac muscle.

R = recessive; D = dominant.

the parents. (The Rh factor is inherited independently of the ABO type and is of the dominant–recessive pattern. Rh positive is dominant and Rh negative is recessive.)

Table 21–6 lists some other human genetic traits, with the dominant and recessive phenotype for each.

INHERITANCE: SEX-LINKED TRAITS

Sex-linked traits may also be called X-linked traits because the genes for them are located only on the X chromosome. The Y does not have corresponding genes for many of the genes on the X chromosome. (The Y chromosome is very small and has only about 20 genes. Some of these genes are active only in the testes and contribute to spermatogenesis. Others are active in many body cells, but their functions are not yet known with certainty.)

The genes for sex-linked traits are recessive, but because there are no corresponding genes on the Y chromosome to mask them, a man needs only one gene to express one of these traits in his phenotype. A woman who has one of these recessive genes on one X chromosome and a dominant gene for normal function on the other X chromosome will not express this trait. She is called a carrier, however, because the gene is part of her genotype and may be passed to children.

Let us use as an example, red-green color blindness. The Punnett square in Fig. 21–10 shows that Mom is carrier of this trait and that Dad has normal color vision. A Punnett square for a sex-linked trait uses the X and Y chromosomes with a lowercase letter on the X to indicate the presence of the recessive gene. The possibilities for each child are divided equally into daughters and sons. In this example, each

Table 21–5 | **ABO BLOOD TYPES: GENOTYPES**

BLOOD TYPE	POSSIBLE GENOTYPES
O	OO
AB	AB
A	AA or OA
B	BB or OB

daughter has a 50% chance of being a carrier and a 50% chance of not being a carrier. In either case, a daughter will have normal color vision. Each son has a 50% chance of being red-green color blind and a 50% chance of having normal color vision. Men can never be carriers of a trait such as this; they either have it or do not have it.

The inheritance of other characteristics is often not as easily depicted as are the examples just discussed. Height, for example, is a multiple gene characteristic, meaning that many pairs of genes contribute. Many pairs of genes result in many possible combinations for genotype and many possible phenotypes. In addition, height is a trait that is influenced by environmental factors such as nutrition. These kinds of circumstances or influences are certainly important in many other human characteristics.

Although the human genome has been decoded, much work remains to be done. The focus now is on learning what each of our genes is for; that is, what protein the gene codes for and the function of that protein.

Clinical work is continuing on attempts to cure genetic diseases by inserting correct copies of malfunctioning genes into the cells of affected individuals. Certain immune deficiencies (which previously would have been fatal) seem to have been reversed in several children, and the ongoing damage of a severe eye disorder seems to have been stopped in other children. But these successes must be replicated; replication of results is an essential part of the scientific method. And when results fall short of expectations, researchers and clinicians must reevaluate the underlying principles of their work and the methods they have chosen, decide what changes are necessary, and try again. Because human beings are the subjects of this gene therapy, research must proceed slowly and potential risks must be assessed and reduced.

Other diseases that may eventually be cured or controlled with gene therapy include cystic fibrosis and hemophilia (for both of which clinical trials are continuing), Parkinson's disease, diabetes, muscular dystrophy, and sickle-cell anemia. Much more research and careful experimentation remain to be done before gene replacement becomes the standard treatment available to everyone with these genetic diseases.

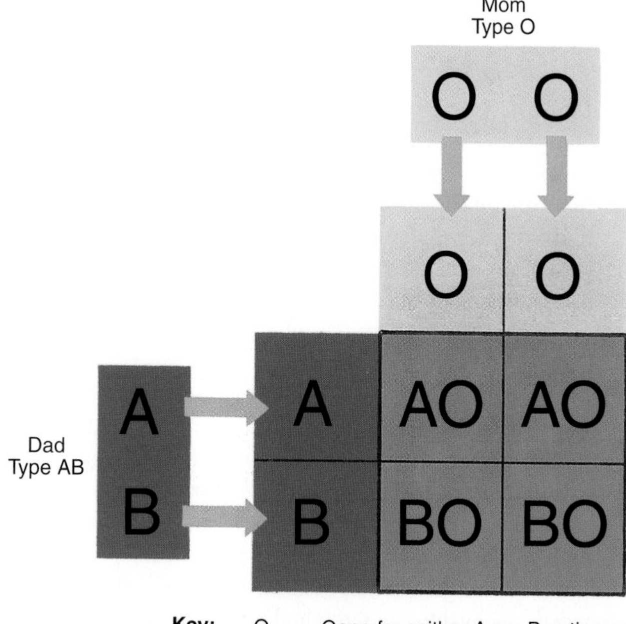

Figure 21–9 Inheritance of blood type (multiple alleles pattern). See text for description.

QUESTION: If Dad has type AB blood and Mom is heterozygous for type A, can a child of theirs have a blood type that is different from that of both parents?

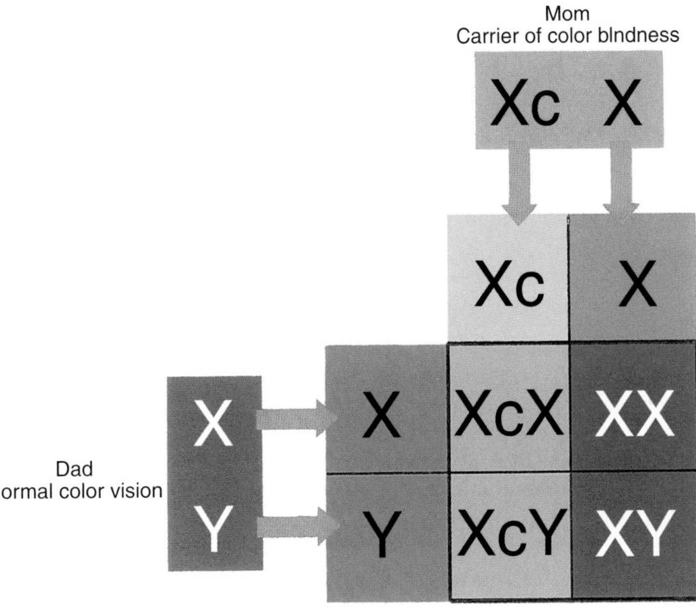

Figure 21–10 Inheritance of red-green color blindness (sex-linked pattern). See text for description.

QUESTION: If Dad is color blind and Mom is not a carrier, what are the possible outcomes for daughters and for sons?

Table 21–6 | **HUMAN GENETIC TRAITS**

TRAIT	DOMINANT PHENOTYPE	RECESSIVE PHENOTYPE
ABO blood type	AB, A, B	O
Rh blood type	Rh positive	Rh negative
Hair color	Dark	Light (blond or red)
Change in hair color	Premature gray	Gray later in life
Hair texture	Curly	Straight
Hairline	Widow's peak	Straight
Eye color	Dark	Light
Color vision	Normal	Color blind
Visual acuity	Nearsighted or farsighted	Normal
Skin color	Dark	Light
Freckles	Abundant	Few
Dimples	Present	Absent
Cleft chin	Present	Absent
Ear lobes	Unattached	Attached
Number of fingers/toes	Polydactyly (more than 5 digits)	5 per hand or foot
Mid-digital hair	Present	Absent
Double-jointed thumb	Present	Absent
Bent little finger	Present	Absent
Ability to roll tongue sides up	Able	Unable

Box 21–7 | SOLUTION TO GENETICS QUESTION

Question: Can parents who are both heterozygous for brown eyes have four children with blue eyes? What is the probability or chance of this happening?

Answer: Yes. For each child, the probability or chance of having blue eyes is 1 in 4 (or 25%). To calculate the probability of all four children having blue eyes, multiply the probability for each child separately:

1st child		2nd child		3rd child		4th child		
$\frac{1}{4}$	×	$\frac{1}{4}$	×	$\frac{1}{4}$	×	$\frac{1}{4}$	=	$\frac{1}{256}$

The probability is 1 in 256 (or 0.4%).

STUDY OUTLINE

Human Development—growth of a fertilized egg into a human individual

Fertilization—the union of the nuclei of egg and sperm; usually takes place in the fallopian tube

1. Sperm undergo final maturation (capacitation) within the female reproductive tract; the acrosome contains enzymes to digest the membrane of the ovum.
2. The 23 chromosomes of the sperm join with the 23 chromosomes of the egg to restore the diploid number of 46 in the zygote.
3. A zygote has 22 pairs of autosomes and one pair of sex chromosomes; XX in females, XY in males (see Fig. 21–1).

Implantation (see Fig. 21–2)—5 to 8 days after fertilization

1. Within the fallopian tube, the zygote begins mitotic divisions called cleavage to form two-cell, four-cell, eight-cell stages, and so on.
2. A morula is a solid sphere of cells that divides further to form a hollow sphere called a blastocyst.
3. A blastocyst consists of an outer layer of cells called the trophoblast and an inner cell mass that contains the potential embryo; the cells are stem cells, not yet specialized. The trophoblast secretes enzymes to form a crater in the endometrium into which the blastocyst sinks. Progesterone prevents inflammation at the site and is necessary for successful implantation.

Embryo—from zygote through 8 weeks of gestation (see Fig. 21–3)

1. In the embryonic disc, three primary germ layers develop: ectoderm, mesoderm, and endoderm (see Table 21–1).
2. By the eighth week of gestation (end of 2 months), all organ systems are formed (see Table 21–2).

Embryonic Membranes (see Fig. 21–3)

1. The yolk sac forms the first blood cells and the cells that become spermatogonia or oogonia.
2. The amnion surrounds the fetus and contains amniotic fluid; this fluid absorbs shock around the fetus.
3. The chorion develops chorionic villi that will contain blood vessels that form the fetal portion of the placenta.

Fetus—weeks 9 through 40 of gestation (see Table 21–2)

1. The organ systems grow and mature.
2. The growing fetus brings about structural and functional changes in the mother (see Table 21–3).

Placenta and Umbilical Cord

1. The placenta is formed by the chorion of the embryo and the endometrium of the uterus; the umbilical cord connects the fetus to the placenta.

2. Fetal blood does not mix with maternal blood; fetal capillaries are within maternal blood sinuses (see Fig. 21–5); this is the site of exchanges between maternal and fetal blood.
3. Two umbilical arteries carry blood from the fetus to the placenta; fetal CO_2 and waste products diffuse into maternal blood; oxygen and nutrients enter fetal blood.
4. Umbilical vein returns blood from placenta to fetus.
5. The placenta is delivered after the baby and is called the afterbirth.

Placental Hormones

1. hCG—secreted by the chorion; maintains the corpus luteum so that it secretes estrogen and progesterone during the first few months of gestation. The corpus luteum is too small to secrete sufficient hormones to maintain a full-term pregnancy.
2. Estrogen and progesterone secretion begins within 4 to 6 weeks and continues until birth in amounts great enough to sustain pregnancy.
3. Estrogen and progesterone inhibit FSH and LH secretion during pregnancy and prepare the mammary glands for lactation.
4. Progesterone inhibits contractions of the myometrium until just before birth, when progesterone secretion begins to decrease.
5. Relaxin inhibits contractions of the myometrium and permits stretching of the pubic symphysis.

Parturition and Labor

1. Gestation period ranges from 37 to 42 weeks; the average is 40 weeks.
2. Labor: first stage—dilation of the cervix; uterine contractions force the amniotic sac into the cervix; amniotic sac ruptures and fluid escapes.
3. Labor: second stage—delivery of the infant; oxytocin causes more powerful contractions of the myometrium. If a vaginal delivery is not possible, a cesarean section may be performed.
4. Labor: third stage—delivery of the placenta; the uterus continues to contract to expel the placenta, then contracts further, decreases in size, and compresses endometrial blood vessels.

The Infant at Birth (see Box 21–6)

1. Umbilical cord is clamped and severed; increased CO_2 stimulates breathing, and lungs are inflated.
2. Foramen ovale closes, and ductus arteriosus constricts; ductus venosus constricts; normal circulatory pathways are established.
3. Jaundice may be present if the infant's immature liver cannot rapidly excrete bilirubin.

Genetics—the study of inheritance; chromosomes—46 per human cell, in 23 homologous pairs

1. A homologous pair consists of a maternal and a paternal chromosome of the same type (designated #1, #2, etc.).
2. There are 22 pairs of autosomes and one pair of sex chromosomes (XX or XY).
3. DNA—the hereditary material of chromosomes.
4. Gene—the genetic code for one protein; an individual has two genes for each protein or trait, one maternal and one paternal.
5. Alleles—the versions of a gene, the possibilities for how a gene may be expressed.
6. Genotype—the alleles present in the genetic makeup
   a. Homozygous—having two similar alleles (genes).
   b. Heterozygous—having two different alleles.
7. Phenotype—the appearance or expression of the alleles present
   a. Depends on the dominance or recessiveness of alleles or the pattern of inheritance involved.

Inheritance—dominant–recessive

1. A dominant gene will appear in the phenotype of a heterozygous individual (who has only one dominant gene). A recessive gene will appear in the phenotype only if the individual is homozygous, that is, has two recessive genes.
2. See Figs. 21–7 and 21–8 for Punnett squares.

Inheritance—multiple alleles

1. More than two possible alleles for each gene: human ABO blood type.
2. An individual will have only two of the alleles (same or different). See Table 21–5 and Fig. 21–9.

Inheritance—sex-linked traits

1. Genes are recessive and found only on the X chromosome; there are no corresponding genes on the Y chromosome.
2. Women with one gene (and one gene for normal functioning) are called carriers of the trait.
3. Men cannot be carriers; they either have the trait or do not have it. See Fig. 21–10.

REVIEW QUESTIONS

1. Where does fertilization usually take place? How many chromosomes are present in a human zygote? Explain what happens during cleavage, and describe the blastocyst stage. (pp. 522–523)
2. Describe the process of implantation, and state where this takes place. (pp. 522–523)
3. How long is the period of embryonic growth? How long is the period of fetal growth? (p. 526)
4. Name two body structures derived from ectoderm, mesoderm, and endoderm. (p. 526)
5. Name the embryonic membrane with each of these functions: (p. 526)
   a. Forms the fetal portion of the placenta
   b. Contains fluid to cushion the embryo
   c. Forms the first blood cells for the embryo
6. Explain the function of: placenta, umbilical arteries, and umbilical vein. (pp. 529–530)
7. Explain the functions of the placental hormones: hCG, progesterone, and estrogen and progesterone (together). (pp. 530–531)
8. Describe the three stages of labor, and name the important hormone. (p. 532)
9. Describe the major pulmonary and circulatory changes that occur in the infant after birth. (pp. 532–533)
10. What is the genetic material of chromosomes? Explain what a gene is. Explain why a person has two genes for each protein or trait. (p. 533)
11. Define *homologous pairs, autosomes,* and *sex chromosomes*. (p. 533)
12. Define *allele, homozygous, heterozygous, genotype,* and *phenotype*. (p. 534)
13. Genetics Problem: Mom is heterozygous for brown eyes, and Dad has blue eyes. What is the percent chance that a child will have blue eyes? Brown eyes? (p. 535)
14. Genetics Problem: Mom is homozygous for type A blood, and Dad is heterozygous for type B blood. What is the percent chance that a child will have type AB blood? Type A? Type B? Type O? (pp. 537–538)
15. Genetics Problem: Mom is red-green color blind, and Dad has normal color vision. What is the percent chance that a son will be color blind? That a daughter will be color blind? That a daughter will be a carrier? (p. 538)

FOR FURTHER THOUGHT

1. Women who smoke cigarettes should make the effort to stop if they want to have children, in part because nicotine causes vasoconstriction. Describe how maternal smoking would affect a fetus.
2. The use of fertility drugs may lead to multiple fertilizations and embryos. With six embryos, or even five, what problems will there be in the maternal uterus?
3. Mr. and Mrs. Brown want to have children, but Mr. Brown is hesitant. He had an older brother who died of Duchenne's muscular dystrophy, and he is worried that he may have a gene that can be passed on. "It's recessive," he tells you, "and doesn't always show up; it can skip a generation." What can you tell the Browns?
4. Mr. and Mrs. Gray have six children: three have type A blood and three have type B blood. Can we say with certainty what the two blood types of the parents are? Can we list possible pairs? Can we say with certainty what the parents' blood types are not? (For example, Mr. and Mrs. Gray cannot both be type O.) Make a list of possible pairs and a list of pairs that are not possible.
5. Your friends, the Kalliomaa family, are of Finnish descent, and they are having a family reunion. Another friend asks you how all of these people in three generations can have blond hair and blue eyes, because these are recessive traits, and dark hair and eyes are dominant. What can you tell your friend to explain this?
6. Question Figure 21–A is a graph that depicts the relative levels of the three most important placental hormones in maternal blood throughout the 40 weeks of gestation. Name these hormones and match each with its line on the graph.

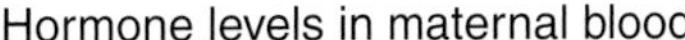

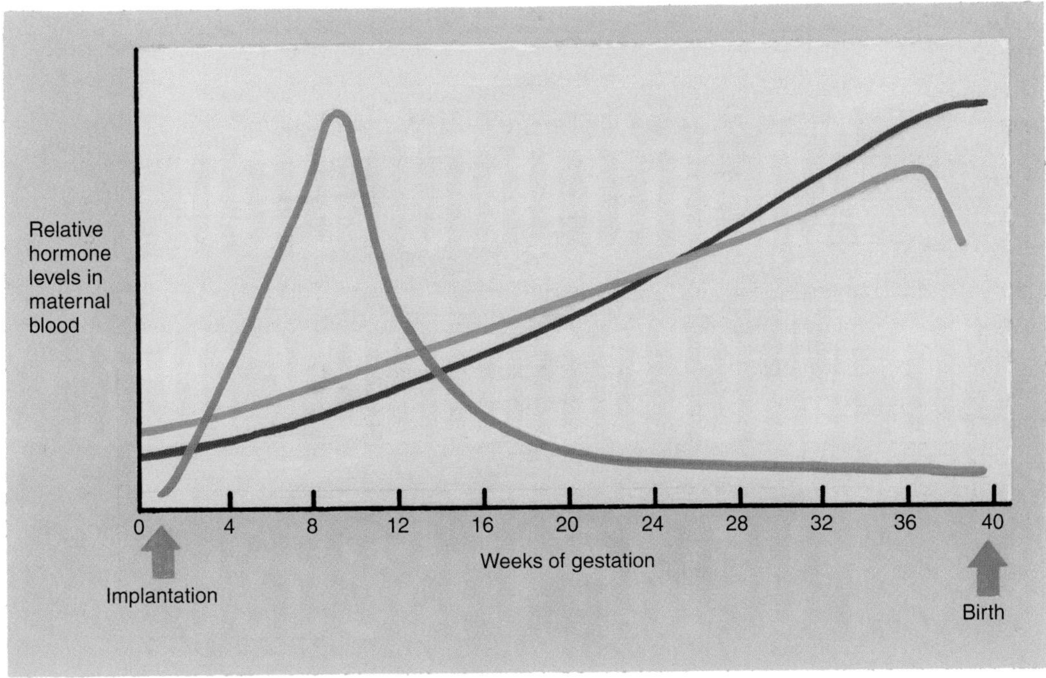

QUESTION FIGURE 21-A: Hormone levels in maternal blood.

CHAPTER

An Introduction to Microbiology and Human Disease

STUDENT OBJECTIVES

- Explain how microorganisms are classified and named.
- Describe the distribution of and benefits provided by normal flora.
- Explain what is meant by an infectious disease, and describe the different types of infection.
- Describe the ways in which infectious diseases may be spread.
- Explain how the growth of microorganisms may be controlled and the importance of this to public health.
- Describe the general structure of bacteria, viruses, fungi, and protozoa and the diseases they cause.
- Name the common worm infestations, and name the arthropods that are vectors of disease.

NEW TERMINOLOGY

Bacillus *(buh-**SILL**-us)*
Coccus *(**KOK**-us)*
Communicable *(kuhm-**YOO**-ni-kah-b'l)*
Contagious *(kun-**TAY**-jus)*
Epidemiology *(EP-i-DEE-mee-**AH**-luh-jee)*
Gram stain (GRAM STAYN)
Infestation *(in-fess-**TAY**-shun)*
Mycosis *(my-**KOH**-sis)*
Noncommunicable *(NON-kuhm-**YOO**-ni-kah-b'l)*
Portal of entry *(**POR**-tuhl of **EN**-tree)*
Portal of exit *(**POR**-tuhl of **EG**-zit)*
Reservoir *(**REZ**-er-vwor)*
Spirillum *(spih-**RILL**-uhm)*
Spirochete *(**SPY**-roh-keet)*
Vector *(**VEK**-ter)*
Zoonoses *(ZOH-oh-**NOH**-seez)*

*Terms that appear in **bold type** in the chapter text are defined in the glossary, which begins on page 603.*

CHAPTER OUTLINE

RELATED CLINICAL TERMINOLOGY

Antitoxin *(AN-tee-**TAHK**-sin)*
Broad spectrum *(BRAWD **SPEK**-trum)*
Culture and sensitivity testing *(**KUL**-chur and SEN-si-**TIV**-i-tee)*
Endotoxin *(EN-doh-**TAHK**-sin)*
Incubation period *(IN-kew-**BAY**-shun)*
Narrow spectrum *(**NAR**-oh **SPEK**-trum)*
Nosocomial infection *(no-zoh-**KOH**-mee-uhl)*
Opportunistic infection *(OP-er-too-**NIS**-tik)*
Secondary infection *(**SEK**-un-dery)*
Subclinical infection *(sub-**KLIN**-i-kuhl)*

Awakening with sniffles and a runny nose . . . a moldy surprise in the refrigerator behind the milk carton . . . wondering if that milk has gone sour. No matter that we cannot see them, the microbes, including viruses, fungi, and bacteria, are always with us.

Microbiology is the study of microorganisms (microbes) and of their place or role in their environment. Sometimes, the environment of microbes is people, and that will be our focus. We will concentrate on the microorganisms that affect the functioning of the human body. These microbes include our normal flora (microbiota) and those that are capable of causing human disease. Many diseases are not caused by microorganisms, but those that are may be called infectious diseases. The microorganisms that cause infectious diseases are called pathogens.

Pathogens may also be called parasites, that is, they live on another living organism called a host and cause harm to the host. Some parasites cause diseases that are fatal to the host, but many others live in a more balanced way with their hosts. These cause illnesses from which the host recovers, and the parasite often survives long enough to be spread to other hosts.

Our introduction to microbiology will begin with a brief description of the classification and naming of microorganisms, followed by a discussion of normal flora. We will then consider infectious diseases, types of infection, and the spread and control of infection. Last, we will describe the types of pathogens in more detail and include the methods we have to treat and control the diseases they cause. For a historical perspective on microbiology, see Box 22–1: The Golden Age of Microbiology and Box 22–2: Microbiology in the 20th Century.

CLASSIFICATION OF MICROORGANISMS

Bacteria are very simple, single-celled organisms that are found virtually everywhere. The natural habitats of bacteria include freshwater, saltwater, soil, and other living organisms. Most bacteria are not harmful to us, and within their normal environments they have the vital role of decomposing dead organic material and recycling their nutrients. However, a number of bacteria cause human diseases, including strep throat, pneumonia, and meningitis.

Viruses are not cells; they are even smaller and simpler in structure than the bacteria. All viruses are parasites because they can reproduce only within the living cells of a host. Therefore, all viruses cause disease. Common human viral diseases are influenza, the common cold, and chickenpox.

Protozoa are single-celled animals such as amoebas. Most protozoa are free living in freshwater or saltwater, where they consume bacteria, fungi, and one another. Human protozoan parasites include those that cause malaria, amebic dysentery, and giardiasis, another intestinal infection.

Fungi may be unicellular or multicellular. Molds and mushrooms are familiar fungi. They decompose organic matter in the soil and freshwater and help recycle nutrients. Fungal diseases of people include yeast infections, ringworm, and more serious diseases such as a type of meningitis.

Worms are multicellular animals. Most are free living; within the soil they consume dead organic matter or smaller living things. Worm infestations of people include trichinosis, hookworms, and tapeworms.

Box 22–1 | THE GOLDEN AGE OF MICROBIOLOGY

Microorganisms were first seen in the 17th century when simple microscopes were developed. Their roles, however, especially in relation to disease, remained largely unknown for another two centuries. The years between 1875 and 1900 are called "The Golden Age of Microbiology" because of the number and significance of the discoveries that were made during this time. The following is a partial list.

1877 Robert Koch proves that anthrax is caused by a bacterium.

1878 Joseph Lister first grows bacteria in pure culture.

The oil immersion lens for microscopes is developed.

1880 Louis Pasteur develops a vaccine for chicken cholera.

1881 Discovery that staphylococci cause infections.

1882 The cause of tuberculosis is found to be a bacterium.

1883 Diphtheria is found to be caused by a bacterium.

1884 The bacteria that cause tetanus, typhoid fever, and cholera are each isolated.

The first description of phagocytosis by white blood cells is published.

1885 Louis Pasteur first uses his vaccine for rabies.

1890 Development of antitoxins to treat tetanus and diphtheria.

1892 Discovery and demonstration of a virus.

1894 The bacterium that causes plague is discovered.

1897 Discovery of the cause of botulism.

Rat fleas are found to be vectors of plague.

1900 Walter Reed and his associates demonstrate that yellow fever is caused by a virus and that the vector is a mosquito.

Box 22–2 | MICROBIOLOGY IN THE 20TH CENTURY

Just a few of the advances made in microbiology during the 20th century are listed below. Many of them concerned infectious diseases, and some involved the new genetic technologies.

1928 Discovery of penicillin by Alexander Fleming.

1935 The first of the sulfa drugs is found to be effective against staphylococcal infections.

1938 Penicillin is purified and produced in large quantities.

1941 The fluorescent antibody test is developed.

1943 Streptomycin is discovered and is the first effective drug in the treatment of tuberculosis.

1953 Watson and Crick describe the structure of DNA.

1955 The Salk polio vaccine is first used.

1957 Interferon is discovered.

1959 A vaccine for whooping cough is available.

1962 The Sabin polio vaccine is created.

1963 The measles vaccine becomes available.

1969 A vaccine for rubella is developed.

1976 Legionnaire's disease is described.

1980 Genetically engineered bacteria produce the hormone insulin.

1981 The first cases of AIDS are described.

1982 The first vaccine for hepatitis B is licensed.

1986 Genetically engineered yeast are used to produce a more effective vaccine for hepatitis B.

Genetically engineered bacteria produce human growth hormone.

1997 Avian flu H5N1 infects 18 people in Hong Kong; then the virus seems to disappear until 2003.

1999 West Nile encephalitis virus is first reported in North America, in New York City.

Arthropods (the name means "jointed legs") are multicellular animals such as lobsters, shrimp, the insects, ticks, and mites. Some insects (such as mosquitoes and fleas) are **vectors** of disease; that is, they spread pathogens from host to host when they bite to obtain blood. Ticks are also vectors of certain diseases, and some mites may cause infestations of the skin.

BINOMIAL NOMENCLATURE

We can refer to bacteria and all other living things with scientific names. A scientific name has two parts (binomial nomenclature), the genus and the species. The genus name is first, is capitalized, and is the larger category. The species name is second, is not capitalized, and is the smaller category. Let us use as examples *Staphylococcus aureus* and *Staphylococcus epidermidis.* These two bacteria are in the same genus, *Staphylococcus,* which tells us that they are related or similar to one another. Yet they are different enough to be given their own species names: *aureus* or *epidermidis.* It may be helpful here to think of our own names. Each of us has a family name, which indicates that we are related to other members of our families, and each of us has a first name indicating that we are individuals in this related group. If we wrote our own names using the form of binomial nomenclature, we would write Smith Mary and Smith John.

In scientific articles and books, for the sake of convenience, the genus name is often abbreviated with its first letter. We might read of *S. aureus* as a cause of a food poisoning outbreak or see *E. coli* (*E.* for *Escherichia*) on a lab report as the cause of a urinary tract infection. Therefore, it is important to learn both genus and species names of important pathogens.

NORMAL FLORA–MICROBIOTA

Each of us has a natural population of microorganisms living on and within us: our normal flora or microbiota. These microbes may be further categorized as residents or transients. **Resident flora** are those species that live on or in nearly everyone almost all the time. These species live in specific sites, called microbiomes; we provide favorable environments for them. Some, such as *Staphylococcus epidermidis,* live on the skin. Others, such as *E. coli,* live in the intestines. When in their natural sites, resident flora do not cause harm to healthy tissue, and some are even beneficial to us. However, residents may become pathogenic if they are introduced into abnormal sites. If *E. coli,* for example, gains access to the urinary bladder, it causes an infection called cystitis. In this situation, *E. coli* is considered an **opportunist**, which is a normally harmless species that has become a pathogen in special circumstances.

Transient flora are those species that are found periodically on or in the body; they are not as well adapted to us as are the resident flora. *Streptococcus pneumoniae,* for example, is a transient in the upper respiratory tract, where it usually does not cause harm in healthy people. However, transients may become pathogenic when the host's resistance is lowered. In an elderly person with influenza, *S. pneumoniae* may invade the lower respiratory tract and cause a serious or even fatal pneumonia.

The distribution of our microbiota is summarized in Table 22–1. You can see that an important function of normal flora is to inhibit the growth of pathogens in the oral cavity, intestines, and in women, the vagina. The resident bacteria are believed to do this by producing antibacterial chemicals but also by simply being there and providing competition that makes it difficult for pathogens to establish themselves. Recall from Chapter 16 (Box 16–4) infant botulism. Infants may acquire botulism by ingesting the spores of the bacteria on foods such as honey or raw vegetables. The infant's colon flora is not yet abundant, and the botulism spores may germinate into active cells that produce toxin. For older people, botulism spores are harmless if ingested because the normal colon flora prevents the growth of these bacteria.

Research suggests that some intestinal microbiota are important in other ways. Various species are believed to contribute to the normal development of certain aspects of the human immune system, such as production of normal T cells by the thymus gland and the proper functioning of the spleen. Others are believed to help keep the intestinal lining intact and healthy. We have much more to learn.

Resident flora may be diminished by the use of antibiotics to treat bacterial infections. An antibiotic does not distinguish between the pathogen and the resident bacteria. In such circumstances, without the usual competition, yeasts or pathogenic bacteria may be able to overgrow and create new infections. This is most likely to occur on mucous membranes such as those of the oral cavity and vagina.

INFECTIOUS DISEASE

An infectious disease is one that is caused by microorganisms or by the products (toxins) of microorganisms. To cause an infection, a microorganism must enter and establish itself in a host and begin reproducing.

Several factors determine whether a person will develop an infection when exposed to a pathogen. These include the virulence of the pathogen and the resistance of

Table 22-1 | **DISTRIBUTION OF NORMAL FLORA—MICROBIOTA—IN THE HUMAN BODY**

BODY SITE	DESCRIPTION OF FLORA
Skin	Exposed to the environment; therefore has a large bacterial population and small numbers of fungi, especially where the skin is often moist. Harmful flora are kept in check by the resident microbiota and continual loss of dead cells from the stratum corneum.
Nasal cavities	Bacteria, mold spores, and viruses constantly enter with inhaled air; the ciliated epithelium limits the microbial population by continuously sweeping mucus and trapped pathogens to the pharynx, where they are swallowed.
Trachea, bronchi, and lungs	The cilia of the trachea and large bronchial tubes sweep mucus and microbes upward toward the pharynx, where they are swallowed. Very few pathogens reach the lungs, and most of these are destroyed by alveolar macrophages.
Oral cavity	Large bacterial population and small numbers of yeasts and protozoa. Kept in check by lysozyme, the enzyme in saliva that inhibits bacterial reproduction. The resident flora help prevent the growth of pathogens.
Esophagus	Contains the microorganisms swallowed with saliva or food.
Stomach	The hydrochloric acid in gastric juice kills most bacteria. This may not be effective if large numbers of a pathogen or bacterial toxins are present in contaminated food.
Small intestine	The ileum, adjacent to the colon, has the largest bacterial population. The duodenum, adjacent to the stomach, has the smallest.
Large intestine	Contains an enormous population of bacteria, which inhibits the growth of pathogens and produces vitamins. The vitamins are absorbed as the colon absorbs water. Vitamin K is obtained in amounts usually sufficient to meet a person's daily need. Smaller amounts of folic acid, riboflavin, and other vitamins are also obtained from colon flora.
Urinary bladder	Is virtually free of bacteria, as is the upper urethra. The lower urethra, especially in women, has a flora similar to that of the skin.
Vagina	A large bacterial population creates an acidic pH that inhibits the growth of pathogens.
Tissue fluid	Small numbers of bacteria and viruses penetrate mucous membranes or get through breaks in the skin. Most are destroyed in lymph nodules or lymph nodes or by wandering macrophages in tissue fluid.
Blood	Should be free of microorganisms.

the host. **Virulence** is the ability of the pathogen to cause disease. Host **resistance** is the total of the body's defenses against pathogens. Our defenses include aspects of innate immunity such as intact skin and mucous membranes and the sweeping of cilia in the respiratory tract, as well as adequate nutrition and the adaptive immune responses of our lymphocytes and macrophages (Chapter 14).

To illustrate these concepts, let us compare the measles virus and rhinoviruses (common cold). The measles virus has at least a 90% infectivity rate, meaning that for every 100 non-immune people exposed, at least 90 will develop clinical measles. Thus, the measles virus is considered highly virulent. However, people who have recovered from measles or who have received the measles vaccine have developed an active immunity that increases their resistance to measles. Even if exposed many times, they probably will not develop clinical measles.

In contrast, the rhinoviruses are not considered virulent because healthy people may have them in their upper respiratory tracts without developing illness. However, fatigue, malnutrition, and other physiological stresses may lower a person's resistance and increase the likelihood of developing a cold upon exposure to these viruses.

Once infected, a person may have a **clinical** (**apparent** or **symptomatic**) infection, in which symptoms appear. **Symptoms** are observable or measurable changes that indicate illness. For some diseases, **subclinical** (**inapparent** or **asymptomatic**) infections are possible, in which the person shows no symptoms. Women with the sexually transmitted disease gonorrhea, for example, may have subclinical infections, that is, no symptoms at all. It is important to remember that such people are still **reservoirs** (sources) of the pathogen for others, who may then develop clinical infections.

COURSE OF AN INFECTIOUS DISEASE

When a pathogen establishes itself in a host, there is a period of time before symptoms appear. This is called the **incubation period**. Most infectious diseases have rather specific incubation periods (Table 22–2). Some diseases, however, have more variable incubation periods (see hepatitis in Table 22–2), which may make it difficult to predict the onset of illness after exposure or to trace outbreaks of a disease.

A short time called the prodromal period may follow the incubation period. During this time, vague, non-specific symptoms may begin. These include generalized muscle aches, lethargy, and fatigue, or a feeling that "I'm coming down with something."

During the invasion period, the specific symptoms of the illness appear. These might include a high fever, rash, swollen lymph nodes, cough, diarrhea, or such things as the gradual paralysis of botulism. The acme is the worst stage of the disease, and this is followed by the recovery or death of the host.

Some diseases are **self-limiting**; that is, they typically last a certain length of time and are usually followed by recovery. The common cold, chickenpox, and mumps are considered self-limiting.

TYPES OF INFECTION

The terminology of infection may refer to the location of the pathogens in the body, to the general nature of the disease, or to how or where the pathogen was acquired.

Table 22–2 | **INCUBATION PERIODS OF SOME INFECTIOUS DISEASES**

DISEASE	INCUBATION PERIOD
Chickenpox	14–16 days
Cholera	1–3 days
Diphtheria	2–6 days
Gas gangrene	1–5 days
Gonorrhea	3–5 days
Hepatitis A	2 weeks–2 months
Hepatitis B	6 weeks–6 months
Hepatitis C	2 weeks–6 months
Herpes simplex	4 days
Influenza	1–3 days
Leprosy	3 months–20+ years
Measles	10–12 days
Meningitis (bacterial)	1–7 days
Mumps	2–3 weeks
Pertussis	5 days–3 weeks
Pinworm	2–6 weeks
Plague	2–6 days
Polio	7–14 days
Rabies	2 weeks–2 months (up to 1 year)
Salmonella food poisoning	12–72 hours
Staphylococcus food poisoning	1–8 hours
Syphilis	10 days–3 months
Tetanus	3 days–5 weeks
Tuberculosis	2–10 weeks

A **localized** infection is one that is confined to one area of the body. Examples are the common cold of the upper respiratory tract, boils of the skin, and salmonella food poisoning that affects the intestines.

In a **systemic** infection, the pathogen is spread throughout the body by way of the lymph or blood. Typhoid fever, for example, begins as an intestinal infection, but the bacteria eventually spread to the liver, gallbladder, kidneys, and other organs. Bubonic plague is an infection that begins in lymph nodes, but again the bacteria are carried throughout the body, and fatal plague is the result of pneumonia.

Bacteremia and **septicemia** are terms that are often used interchangeably in clinical practice, although technically they have different meanings. Bacteremia means that bacteria are present in the blood; septicemia means that the bacteria present are multiplying rapidly. Septicemia is always serious because it means that the immune defenses have been completely overwhelmed and are unable to stop the spread of the pathogen.

With respect to timing and duration, some infections may be called acute or chronic. An **acute** infection is one that usually begins abruptly and is severe. In contrast, a **chronic** infection often progresses slowly and may last for a long time.

A **secondary infection** is one that is made possible by a primary infection that has lowered the host's resistance. Influenza in an elderly person, for example, may be followed by bacterial pneumonia. This secondary bacterial infection might not have occurred had not the person first been ill with the flu.

Nosocomial infections are those that are acquired in hospitals or institutions such as nursing homes. The hospital population includes newborns, the elderly, postoperative patients, people with chronic diseases, cancer patients receiving chemotherapy, and others whose resistance to disease is lowered. Some hospital-acquired pathogens, such as *Staphylococcus aureus,* are spread from patient to patient by healthy hospital personnel. These staff members are reservoirs for *S. aureus* and carry it on their skin or in their nasal passages.

Other nosocomial infections, however, are caused by the patient's own normal flora that has been inadvertently introduced into an abnormal body site. Such infections may be called **endogenous**, which literally means "generated from within." Intestinal bacilli such as *E. coli* are also an important cause of nosocomial infections. Without very careful aseptic technique (and sometimes in spite of it), the patient's own intestinal bacteria may contaminate urinary catheters, decubitus ulcers, surgical incisions, and intravenous lines. Such infections are a significant problem in hospitals, and all those involved in any aspect of patient care should be aware of this.

EPIDEMIOLOGY

Epidemiology is the study of the patterns and spread of disease within a population. This term is related to **epidemic**, which is an outbreak of disease, that is, more than the usual number of cases in a given time period. An **endemic** disease is one that is present in a population, with an expected or usual number of cases in a given time. Influenza, for example, is endemic in large cities during the winter, and public health personnel expect a certain number of cases. In some winters, however, the number of cases of influenza increases, often markedly, and this is an epidemic.

A **pandemic** is an epidemic that has spread throughout several countries. The bubonic plague pandemic of the 14th century affected nearly all of Europe and killed one-fourth of the population. Just after World War I, from 1918 to 1920, an especially virulent strain of the influenza virus spread around the world and caused at least 40 million deaths. More recently, central Africa has had an ongoing pandemic of meningococcal meningitis, with tens of thousands of cases every year (in contrast, the United States has about four thousand or fewer cases each year). Keep in mind, however, that use of the word *pandemic* is not related to the severity of the disease. Influenza usually has a low fatality rate but often causes pandemics.

To understand the epidemiology of a disease, we must know several things about the pathogen. These include where it lives in a host, the kinds of hosts it can infect, and whether it can survive outside of hosts.

PORTALS OF ENTRY AND EXIT

The **portal of entry** is the way the pathogen enters a host (Fig. 22–1). Breaks in the skin, even very small ones, are potential portals of entry, as are the natural body openings. Pathogens may be inhaled, consumed with food and water, or acquired during sexual activity. Most pathogens that enter the body by way of these natural routes are destroyed by the white blood cells found in and below the skin and mucous membranes, but some may be able to establish themselves and cause disease. You may wonder if the eye can be a portal of entry for other than eye infections, or you may already know that it is a portal for many respiratory viruses. People may pick up cold or flu viruses on their hands and then rub their eyes; the viruses are then washed by tears into the nasal cavities, their preferred site of infection.

Insects such as mosquitoes and fleas, and other arthropods, such as ticks, are **vectors** of disease. They spread pathogens when they bite to obtain a host's blood. Mosquitoes, for example, are vectors of malaria, yellow fever, and encephalitis. Ticks are vectors of Lyme disease and Rocky Mountain spotted fever.

As mentioned previously, it is important to keep in mind that many hospital procedures may provide portals

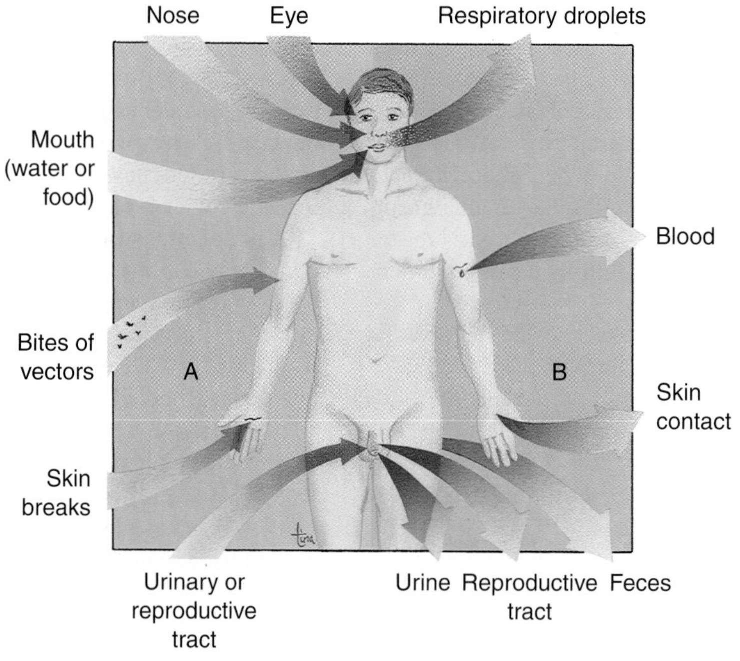

Figure 22–1 (**A**) Portals of entry. (**B**) Portals of exit.

QUESTION: Are there any portals of entry that are unlikely portals of exit?

of entry for pathogens. Any invasive procedure, whether it involves the skin or the mucous membranes, may allow pathogens to enter the body.

The **portal of exit** (see Fig. 22–1) is the way the pathogen leaves the body or is shed from the host. Skin lesions, such as those of chickenpox, contain viruses that may be passed to others by cutaneous contact. Intestinal pathogens such as the hepatitis A virus and the cholera bacteria are excreted in the host's feces, which may contaminate food or water and be ingested by another host (the fecal–oral route of transmission). Respiratory pathogens such as influenza and measles viruses are shed in respiratory droplets from the mouth and nose and may be inhaled by others. The pathogens of the reproductive tract, such as the bacteria that cause syphilis and gonorrhea, are spread to others by sexual contact. Notice that with respect to epidemiology, the pathogen travels from one host's portal of exit to another host's portal of entry.

RESERVOIRS OF INFECTION

Some pathogens cause disease only in people. Measles, whooping cough, syphilis, and bacterial meningitis are strictly human diseases. To acquire such a disease, a person must be exposed to someone who has the illness.

Also of importance is that upon recovery from some diseases, the host may continue to harbor the pathogen and thus be a reservoir of it for others. Such a person is called a **carrier**. Diseases for which the carrier state is possible include typhoid, diphtheria, and hepatitis B.

Many other diseases, however, are really animal diseases that people acquire in certain circumstances. These diseases are called **zoonoses** (singular: **zoonosis**) and include plague, Lyme disease, encephalitis, and Rocky Mountain spotted fever, which are spread from animal to person by vectors such as ticks or fleas. Human rabies is rare in the United States; the few cases each year are acquired by contact with infected saliva or tissue of wild animals such as bats, the virus entering the new host through breaks in the skin. In Africa and Asia, where pet vaccination is rare, more than 50,000 cases occur every year, most acquired from dogs. Salmonellosis is a type of food poisoning caused by the intestinal bacilli of animals that contaminate meats such as chicken and turkey. Prevention of such diseases depends upon knowledge of how they are spread. For example, people who live in areas where Lyme disease is endemic should be aware that the disease is acquired by way of a tick bite. If children and pets are examined for ticks after they have been out of doors, the chance of acquiring Lyme disease is greatly diminished.

Some bacteria are pathogenic only by accident, for their natural habitat is soil or water, where they act as decomposers. The bacteria that cause gas gangrene, tetanus, and botulism are normal soil flora and cause disease when they (or their toxins) contaminate a skin wound, or, in the case of botulism, the toxin is present in food.

SPREAD OF INFECTION

On the basis of our knowledge thus far, we can classify infectious diseases as noncommunicable or communicable. A **noncommunicable** disease is one in which a resident species causes disease under certain conditions or in which a non-resident species causes disease when it enters the body. Such diseases cannot be transmitted directly or indirectly from host to host. Cystitis caused by *E. coli* in a hospital patient, for example, is not communicable to the nurses who care for that patient. Similarly, a nurse caring for a patient with tetanus or botulism need not worry about acquiring these diseases; both are noncommunicable.

A **communicable** disease is one in which the pathogen may be transmitted directly or indirectly from host to host. Direct spread of infection is by way of cutaneous contact (including sexual contact), respiratory droplets, contaminated blood, or placental transmission from mother to fetus. Indirect spread is by way of contaminated food or water, or vectors, or **fomites**, which are inanimate objects that carry the pathogen. Influenza and cold viruses, for example, can survive outside their hosts for a time, so that objects such as eating utensils, door knobs, or children's toys may be vehicles of transmission for these pathogens.

Some communicable diseases may also be called **contagious**, which means that they are easily spread from person to person by casual cutaneous contact or by respiratory droplets. Chickenpox, measles, and influenza are contagious diseases. In contrast, AIDS is not contagious because sexual contact, blood contact, or placental transmission is necessary to acquire the virus (HIV). HIV is not spread by cutaneous contact or by respiratory droplets.

METHODS OF CONTROL OF MICROBES

Microorganisms are everywhere in our environment, and although we need not always be aware of their presence, there are times when we must try to diminish or even eliminate them. These situations include the use of chemicals for disinfection, especially in hospitals, and the protection of our food and water supplies.

ANTISEPTICS, DISINFECTANTS, AND STERILIZATION

We are all familiar with the practice of applying iodine, hydrogen peroxide, or alcohol to minor cuts in the skin, and we know the purpose of this: to prevent bacterial infection. The use of such chemicals does indeed destroy many harmful bacteria, although it has no effect on bacterial spores. The chemicals used to prevent infection may be called antiseptics or disinfectants. An **antiseptic** (anti = against; septic = infection) is a chemical that destroys bacteria or inhibits their growth on a living being. The chemicals named earlier are antiseptics on skin surfaces. A **disinfectant** is a chemical that is used on inanimate objects. Chemicals with antibacterial effects may be further classified as bactericidal or bacteriostatic. **Bactericides** kill bacteria by disrupting important metabolic processes. **Bacteriostatic** chemicals do not destroy bacteria but rather inhibit their reproduction and slow their growth. Alcohol, for example, is a bactericide that is both an antiseptic and a disinfectant, depending upon the particular surface on which it is used.

Some chemicals are not suitable for use on human skin because they are damaging, but they may be used as disinfectants. Bleach, such as Clorox, and cresols, such as Lysol, may be used in bathrooms, on floors or countertops, and even on dishes (if rinsed thoroughly). These bactericides will also destroy certain viruses, such as those that cause influenza. A dilute (10%) bleach solution will inactivate HIV, the virus that causes AIDS.

In hospitals, environmental surfaces are disinfected, but materials such as surgical instruments, sutures, and dressings must be sterilized. **Sterilization** is a process that destroys all living organisms. Most medical and laboratory products are sterilized by autoclaving. An **autoclave** is a chamber in which steam is generated under pressure. This pressurized steam penetrates the contents of the chamber and kills all microorganisms present, including bacterial spores.

Materials such as disposable plastics that might be damaged by autoclaving are often sterilized by exposure to radiation. Foods such as meats may also be sterilized by this method. Such food has a very long shelf life (equivalent to canned food), and this procedure is used for preparing some military field rations.

PUBLIC HEALTH MEASURES

Each of us is rightfully concerned with our own health and the health of our families. People who work in the public health professions, however, consider the health of all of us, that is, the health of a population. Two traditional aspects of public health are ensuring safe food and safe drinking water. Two more recent aspects are tracking and learning about emerging diseases, as well as preparing defenses against the possible use of biological weapons.

Food

The safety of our food depends on a number of factors. Most cities have certain standards and practices that must be followed by supermarkets and restaurants, and inspections are conducted on a regular basis.

Food companies prepare their products using specific methods to prevent the growth of microorganisms. Naturally, it is in the best interests of these companies to do so, for they would soon be out of business if their products made people ill. Also of importance is the willingness of companies to recall products that are suspected of being contaminated. For example, since 1925 in the United States, only five fatal cases of botulism have been traced to commercially canned food. If we consider that billions of cans of food have been consumed during this time, we can appreciate the standards the food industry has maintained.

Milk and milk products provide ideal environments for the growth of bacteria because they contain both protein and sugar (lactose) as food sources. For this reason, milk must be **pasteurized**, that is, heated to 145°F (62.9°C) for 30 minutes. Newer methods of pasteurization use higher temperatures for shorter periods of time, but the result is the same: The pathogens that may be present in milk are killed, although not all bacteria are totally destroyed. Milk products such as cheese and ice cream are also pasteurized or made from pasteurized milk.

When a food-related outbreak of disease does take place, public health workers try to trace the outbreak to its source. This stops the immediate spread of disease by preventing access to the contaminated food, and the ensuing publicity on television, the Internet, or in newspapers may help remind everyone of the need for careful monitoring of food preparation.

Some foods meant to be eaten raw or briefly cooked, such as fruit or rare beef, do carry a small risk. Consumers should realize that food is not sterile, that meat, for example, is contaminated with the animals' intestinal bacteria during slaughtering. Meat should be thoroughly cooked. Fruit and vegetables should be washed or peeled before being eaten raw. (Food-borne diseases are included in the tables of diseases at the end of this chapter.)

Finally, the safety of our food may depend on something we often take for granted: our refrigerators. For example, a Thanksgiving turkey that was carved for dinner at 3 p.m. and left on the kitchen counter until midnight probably should not be used for turkey sandwiches the next day. Although we have to rely on others to ensure that commercially prepared food will be safe, once food reaches our homes, all we really need (besides the refrigerator) is our common sense.

Water

When we turn on a faucet to get a glass of water, we usually do not wonder whether the water is safe to drink. It usually is. Having a reliable supply of clean drinking water depends on two things: diverting human sewage away from water supplies and chlorinating water intended for human consumption.

Large cities have sewer systems for the collection of wastewater and its subsequent treatment in sewage plants. Once treated, however, the sludge (solid, particulate matter) from these plants must be disposed of. This is becoming more of a problem simply because there is so much sewage sludge (because there are so many of us). Although the sludge is largely free of pathogens, it ought not to be put in landfills, and because ocean dumping is being prohibited in many coastal areas, this is a problem that will be with us for a long time.

Drinking water for cities and towns is usually chlorinated. The added chlorine kills virtually all bacteria that may be present. The importance of chlorination is shown by a 1978 outbreak of enteritis (diarrhea) in a Vermont town of 10,000 people. The chlorination process malfunctioned for 2 days, and 2,000 of the town's inhabitants became ill. (The bacterium was *Campylobacter*, a common intestinal inhabitant of animals.)

You may now be wondering if all those bottled spring waters are safe to drink. The answer, in general, is yes, because the bottling companies do not wish to make people ill and put themselves out of business. Some bottled waters, however, do have higher mold spore counts than does chlorinated tap water. Usually these molds are not harmful when ingested; they are destroyed by the hydrochloric acid in gastric juice.

In much of North America, nearly everyone has easy access to safe drinking water. We might remind ourselves once in a while that our water will not give us typhoid, dysentery, or cholera. These diseases are still very common in other parts of the world, where the nearest river or stream is the laundry, the sewer, and the source of drinking water. The World Health Organization (WHO) estimates that more than 2.5 billion people do not have basic sanitation, and more than 1 billion do not have dependable access to clean water to drink.

Emerging Diseases and Biological Weapons

The term *emerging diseases* may be a bit misleading because some of the pathogens are not really new. What has happened is that we have become aware of them. A good example of this is Lyme disease. Lyme disease in the United States was named for the town in Connecticut where a cluster of cases was discovered in the 1970s. When the causative bacteria were later found and the disease fully characterized, health officials realized that the disease had been described in Scandinavia in the early years of the 20th century. Lyme disease was not a new disease after all, merely a newly encountered disease for Americans.

Other emerging diseases are those caused by the Ebola and Marburg viruses, Hantavirus, West Nile virus, the MERS (Middle East respiratory syndrome) coronavirus, certain strains of *E. coli,* and antibiotic-resistant strains of enterococci. The tasks of public health officials are to keep track of all cases of these diseases and to educate medical personnel about them.

Anthrax is no longer in the news, as it was in the autumn of 2001 when spores were sent through the U.S. mail. Research in vaccine production that was spurred by the use of anthrax as a weapon has been applied to emerging diseases as well. Vaccines for new influenza viruses can be produced more quickly.

You may recall hearing about avian influenza (several types), or "bird flu," that is truly an emerging disease. Each virus is a natural parasite of wild birds but has infected domestic flocks in Asia, Europe, and Africa. Although not a frequent event, people have caught the virus from infected chickens or ducks, and the human mortality rate has been as high as 50%. The great concern is that the virus will mutate and become contagious for people, that is, easily transmissible from person to person. By way of plane travel, the virus could be spread throughout the world in a matter of weeks. Because this would be a "new" disease for people, it is possible that no group of people will have evolved any kind of resistance to it. Bird flu may be for us what measles was to the Hawaiian islanders in the 18th and 19th centuries. The measles virus was brought to the islands by Europeans (for whom it was usually not fatal, reflecting thousands of years of coexistence) and nearly wiped out the native population, for whom it was a new virus.

However, this is by no means certain. It may be that milder cases of human avian flu have been overlooked thus far, that these viruses cause a wide spectrum of disease in people, from mild to fatal. Some human cases may even be asymptomatic (antibody studies would be needed to determine that).

The novel H1N1 influenza virus of 2009 was also a new virus, a hybrid with genes from avian, swine, and human flu viruses. It was believed that older people who were exposed as children to other H1N1 flu viruses had some natural protection. Many of the deaths were children and young adults, which is unusual for influenza viruses. It is not possible to predict if the virus will cause more serious illness when it returns, but it is expected to return periodically for several years. By then we may even have another "new flu." (See also Box 22–3: Microbiology in the 21st Century.)

THE PATHOGENS

In the sections that follow, each group of pathogens will be described with a summary of important characteristics and examples of specific pathogens. Tables of human diseases caused by each group of pathogens are at the end of this chapter.

BACTERIA (see table 22–3)

Bacteria are very simple unicellular organisms. All are microscopic in size, and a magnification of 1000 times is usually necessary to see them clearly. A bacterial cell consists of watery cytoplasm and a single chromosome (made of DNA) surrounded by a cell membrane. Enclosing all of these structures is a cell wall, which is strong and often rigid, giving the bacterium its characteristic shape.

Based on shape, bacteria are classified as one of three groups: coccus, bacillus, or spirillum (Fig. 22–2). A **coccus** (plural: **cocci**) is a sphere; under the microscope, cocci appear round. Certain prefixes may be used to describe the arrangement of spheres. **Staphylo** means clusters, **strepto** refers to chains of cells, and **diplo** means pairs of cells.

A **bacillus** (plural: **bacilli**) is a rod-shaped bacterium; rods may vary in length depending on the genus. A **spirillum** (plural: **spirilla**) is a long cell with one or more curves or coils. Some spirilla, such as those that cause syphilis and Lyme disease, are called **spirochetes**. Many of the bacilli and spirilla are capable of movement because they have **flagella**. These are long, threadlike structures that project from the cell and beat rhythmically.

Bacteria reproduce by the process of **binary fission**, in which the chromosome duplicates itself, and the original cell divides into two identical cells. The presence or absence of oxygen may be important for bacterial reproduction. **Aerobic** bacteria can reproduce only in the presence of oxygen, and **anaerobic** bacteria can reproduce only in the absence of oxygen. **Facultatively anaerobic** bacteria are not inhibited in either situation; they are able to reproduce in either the presence or absence of oxygen. This is obviously

Box 22–3 | MICROBIOLOGY IN THE 21ST CENTURY

The 21st century has just begun; here is a microbiological perspective.

2001 In sub-Saharan Africa, more than 25 million people have AIDS or are HIV positive.
Anthrax spores are sent through the U.S. mail, causing 22 cases of the disease, with 5 fatalities.

2002 In China, the number of AIDS cases increases ever more rapidly.
Multidrug-resistant strains of *Mycobacterium tuberculosis* proliferate throughout the world.
A strain of *Staphylococcus aureus* is found that is fully resistant to the antibiotic vancomycin.

2003 Cases of SARS are reported by China, and the disease spreads to Europe and North America, affecting more than 8000 people.
The first cases of mad cow disease are reported in North America.
Donated blood and organs are screened for the West Nile virus.

2004 SARS vaccines are tested, but the human SARS virus seems to disappear.
Avian influenza A (H5N1) causes sporadic cases in people in East Asia.
A vaccine for the human papilloma viruses that cause most cases of cervical cancer proves to be effective.

2005 A U.S. teenager becomes the first person to survive rabies without having received the rabies vaccine.
Vaccines for the Ebola and Marburg viruses are successful in monkeys.
A vaccine for shingles is effective in adults.

2009 A novel H1N1 flu virus is discovered in April and spreads around the world. Vaccines are available by October.

2010 Cholera becomes epidemic in Haiti.

2012 Middle East Respiratory Syndrome (MERS) coronavirus is discovered in Saudi Arabia.

2013 Outbreaks of polio occur in Somalia and Syria.

an advantage for the bacteria, and many pathogens and potential pathogens are facultative anaerobes.

The Gram Stain

On the basis of the chemicals in their cell walls, most bacteria can be put into one of two groups, called **gram positive** or **gram negative**. A simple laboratory procedure called the **Gram stain** (see Fig. 22–2) shows us the shape of the bacteria and their gram reactions. Gram-positive bacteria appear purple or blue, and gram-negative bacteria appear pink or red. Some bacteria do not stain with the Gram method (many spirilla and spirochetes do not), but for those that do, each genus is either gram positive or gram negative. This does not change, just as the characteristic shape of the bacteria does not change. The genus *Streptococcus,* for example, is always a gram-positive coccus; the genus *Escherichia* is always a gram-negative bacillus. If a Gram stain is done on a sputum specimen from a patient with pneumonia, and a gram-positive coccus is found, this eliminates all of the gram-negative cocci and bacilli that may also cause pneumonia. The Gram stain, therefore, is often an important first step in the identification of the pathogen that is causing a particular infection. In Table 22–3 (at the end of this chapter), the gram reaction (where applicable) and shape are included for each pathogen.

Special Characteristics

Although bacteria are simple cells, many have special structural or functional characteristics that help them to survive. Some bacilli and cocci have capsules (see Fig. 22–2); a **capsule** is a gelatinous sheath that encloses the entire cell. Capsules are beneficial to the bacteria because they inhibit phagocytosis by the host's white blood cells. This gives the bacteria time to reproduce and possibly establish themselves in the host. This is *not* beneficial from our point of view (remember that we are the hosts), but bacterial capsules are also **antigenic**, which means that they stimulate antibody production by our lymphocytes. This starts the destruction of bacteria by our immune responses. We take advantage of this by using bacterial capsules in some of our vaccines, such as those used to prevent pneumonia and meningitis.

Some bacilli are able to survive unfavorable environments by forming spores. A **spore** is a dormant (inactive) stage that consists of the chromosome and a small amount

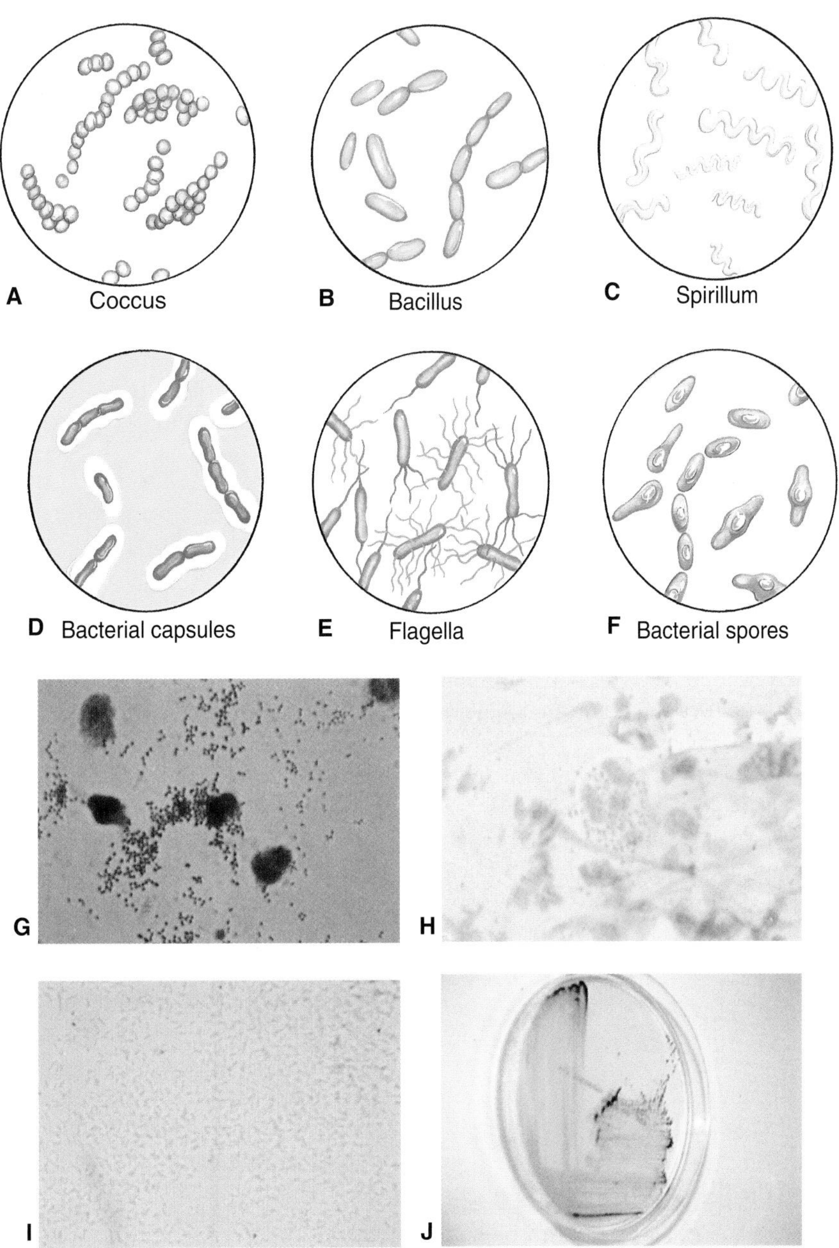

Figure 22–2 (**A–F**) Bacterial shapes and specialized structures (magnification ×2000) (**G**) Gram-positive *Staphylococcus aureus* (×1000). (**H**) Gram-negative *Neisseria gonorrhoeae* in WBCs (×1000). (**I**) Gram-negative *Campylobacter jejuni* (×1000). (**J**) *Salmonella enteritidis* growing on agar in a Petri dish. The black colonies indicate production of hydrogen sulfide gas. (G–J from Sacher, RA, and McPherson, RA: Widmann's Clinical Interpretation of Laboratory Tests. ed 11, FA Davis, Philadelphia, 2000, color plates 58, 59, 60 and 92, with permission.)

QUESTION: In parts A–F, most of the bacteria are blue or pink. What do these colors indicate? The spirillum, C, is neither color. What does this tell us?

of cytoplasm surrounded by a thick wall. Spores can survive conditions such as heat (even boiling), freezing, or dehydration, which would kill the vegetative (active) forms of the bacterial cells. Fortunately for us, most pathogens are unable to form spores, but some that do are the causative agents of gas gangrene, botulism, tetanus, and anthrax. These bacteria are decomposers in the soil environment, and their spore-forming ability enables them to survive the extremes of temperature and lack of water that may occur in the soil.

Many bacteria cause disease because they produce **toxins**, which are chemicals that are harmful to host tissues. Often these toxins are the equivalent of our digestive enzymes, which break down the food we eat. Some bacterial toxins such as hemolysins and proteases literally digest host tissues such as red blood cells and proteins. The bacteria then absorb the digested nutrients.

The toxins of other bacteria have very specific effects on certain cells of the host. Botulism and tetanus toxins, for example, are **neurotoxins** that disrupt the functioning of nerve cells, leading to the characteristic symptoms of each disease (see Box 7–2). The diphtheria toxin causes heart failure, the pertussis (whooping cough) toxin immobilizes the cilia of the respiratory tract, and the cholera enterotoxin causes diarrhea.

The cell walls of gram-negative bacteria are made of chemicals called endotoxins. **Endotoxins** all have the same effects on the host: They cause fever and circulatory shock (low blood pressure and heart failure). **Endotoxin shock** (also called **gram-negative shock**) is a life-threatening condition that may accompany any serious infection with gram-negative bacteria.

Rickettsias and Chlamydias

These two groups of bacteria differ from most other bacteria in that they are obligate intracellular parasites. This means that they can reproduce only within the living cells of a host.

The rickettsias (also: rickettsiae) are parasites of mammals (including people) and are often spread by arthropod vectors. In the United States, the most common rickettsial disease is Rocky Mountain spotted fever, which is spread by ticks. In other parts of the world, epidemic typhus, which is spread by body lice, is still an important disease. From a historical perspective, until World War I, more people died of epidemic typhus during times of war than were killed by weapons.

The chlamydias (also: chlamydiae) cause several human diseases, including ornithosis (parrot fever) and trachoma, which is the leading cause of blindness throughout the world. In the United States, sexually transmitted chlamydial infection is much more common than trachoma.

Both rickettsial and chlamydial infections can be treated with antibiotics.

Antibiotics

Antibiotics are chemicals that are used to treat bacterial infections. A **broad-spectrum** antibiotic is one that affects many different kinds of bacteria; a **narrow-spectrum** antibiotic affects just a few kinds of bacteria.

The use of antibiotics is based on a very simple principle: Certain chemicals can disrupt or inhibit the chemical reactions that bacteria must carry out to survive. An antibiotic such as penicillin blocks the formation of bacterial cell walls; without their cell walls, bacteria will die. Other antibiotics inhibit DNA synthesis or protein synthesis. These are vital activities for the bacteria, and without them bacteria cannot reproduce and will die.

It is very important to remember that our own cells carry out chemical reactions that are very similar to some of those found in bacteria. For this reason, our own cells may be damaged by antibiotics. This is why some antibiotics have harmful side effects. The most serious side effects are liver and kidney damage or depression of the red bone marrow. The liver is responsible for detoxifying the medication, which may accumulate and damage liver cells. Similar damage may occur in the kidneys, which are responsible for excreting the medication. The red bone marrow is a very active tissue, with constant mitosis and protein synthesis to produce RBCs, WBCs, and platelets. Any antibiotic that interferes with these processes may decrease production of all of these blood cells. Patients who are receiving any of the potentially toxic antibiotics should be monitored with periodic tests of liver and kidney function or with blood counts to assess the state of the red bone marrow.

Another problem with the use of antibiotics is that bacteria may become resistant to them, and so be unaffected. Bacterial **resistance** means that the bacteria are able to produce an enzyme that destroys the antibiotic, rendering it useless. This is a genetic capability on the part of bacteria, and it is, therefore, passed to new generations of bacterial cells.

Let us use an example with small numbers and say that, of 1000 bacterial cells, 998 are killed by a certain antibiotic. The remaining two bacteria have the gene for an enzyme that breaks the antibiotic molecule, so they survive. What will these two bacteria do? Each will divide by binary fission, becoming two cells, four cells, eight cells, and so on. At the end of 20 divisions (which under optimum conditions may take less than 24 hours) each bacterium has become more than a million bacteria. And what is true of all of these bacteria? They all have the gene for resistance to that particular antibiotic.

This is exactly what has happened with *Staphylococcus aureus*, first becoming resistant to penicillin, and some strains are now resistant to most other antibiotics as well. Most of the gram-negative intestinal bacilli are resistant to a great variety of antibiotics. This is why **culture and sensitivity testing** is so important before an antibiotic is chosen to treat these infections.

Education is also important, and healthcare personnel must help educate the general public not to demand antibiotics for colds or the flu. These are viral diseases for which antibiotics are useless. What happens is that the antibiotic kills all susceptible bacteria (even beneficial ones) and leaves resistant bacteria to become the most numerous, perhaps to cause serious disease in the future.

To counteract bacterial resistance, new antibiotics are produced that are not inactivated by the destructive bacterial enzymes. Within a few years, however, the usefulness of these new antibiotics will probably diminish as bacteria mutate and develop resistance. This is not a battle that we can ever truly win because bacteria are living organisms that evolve as their environment changes. We must never underestimate the ability of bacteria to evolve ways to neutralize the antibiotics we use to kill them. The development of new antibiotics is crucial if we are to stay a step ahead of these remarkably adaptable microorganisms.

Antibiotics have changed our lives, although we may not always realize that. A child's strep throat will probably not progress to meningitis, and bacterial pneumonia does not have the very high fatality rate that it once did. But, we must keep in mind that antibiotics are not a "cure" for any disease. A serious infection means that the immune system has been overwhelmed by the pathogen. An antibiotic diminishes the number of bacteria to a level with which the immune system can cope. Ultimately, however, the body's own white blood cells must eliminate the very last of the bacteria.

VIRUSES (see table 22–4)

Viruses are not cells; their structure is even simpler than that of bacteria, which are the simplest cells. A virus consists of either DNA or RNA surrounded by a protein shell called a **capsid**. The capsid has a shape that is characteristic for each virus (Fig. 22–3). There are no enzymes, cytoplasm, cell membranes, or cell walls in viruses, and they can reproduce only when inside the living cells of a host. Therefore, all viruses are obligate intracellular parasites, and they cause disease when they reproduce inside cells. When a virus enters a host cell, it

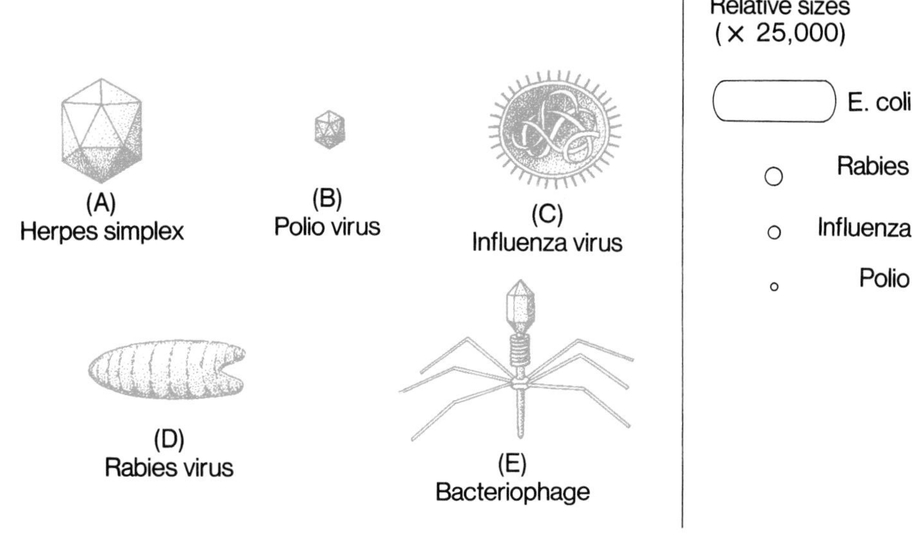

Figure 22–3 Viruses: representative shapes and relative sizes.

QUESTION: The influenza virus shows the two parts of a virus. What are these two parts?

uses the cell's chromosomes, RNA, and enzymes to make new viruses. Several hundred new viruses may be produced from just one virus. The host cell ruptures and dies, releasing the new viruses, which then enter other cells and reproduce.

The severity of a viral disease depends upon the types of cells infected. If the virus affects skin cells, for example, the disease is usually mild and self-limiting, such as chickenpox. Small numbers of skin cells are not crucial to our survival, and these cells can be replaced by mitosis. If, however, the virus affects nerve cells, the disease is more serious and may be fatal. Rabies is such a disease. Neurons are much more vital to us, and they cannot be replaced once they die.

Some viruses, such as those that cause German measles (rubella) and chickenpox, are able to cross the placenta, that is, pass from maternal circulation to fetal circulation. Although the disease may be very mild for the pregnant woman, the virus may severely damage developing fetal organs and cause congenital birth defects such as blindness, heart malformations, and brain damage. In the most serious cases, fetal infection may result in miscarriage or stillbirth.

Some viruses cause an initial infection, become dormant, then are reactivated, causing another infection months or years later. The herpes viruses that cause cold sores "hide out" in nerves of the face following the initial skin lesion. At some later time when the host's resistance is lowered, the viruses emerge from the nerves and cause another cold sore. The chickenpox virus, most often acquired in childhood, is a herpes virus that may become dormant in nerves for years, and then be reactivated and cause shingles in adults.

A few human viruses are known to be tumor viruses, that is, they cause cells to develop abnormally and form tumors. The Epstein-Barr virus, which causes mononucleosis in North America, is associated with Burkitt's lymphoma in Africa and with nasopharyngeal carcinoma in China. There are environmental factors, as yet unknown, that contribute to the development of these cancers in specific parts of the world. Several of the human papillomaviruses have also been associated with cancers of the mouth or larynx, and three of these viruses are found in 90% of cervical carcinomas in women.

Important viral diseases are described in Table 22–4 at the end of this chapter.

Antiviral Medications

The treatment of viral diseases with chemicals poses some formidable challenges. First, viruses are active (reproducing) only within cells, so the medication must be able to enter infected cells to be effective. Second, viruses are such simple structures that the choice of which of their chemical processes to attempt to disrupt is limited. Third, viruses use the host cell's DNA and enzymes for self-replication, and a medication that interferes with DNA or enzymes may kill the host cell even as it kills the virus.

These problems are illustrated by zidovudine (AZT), the first medication that was effective against HIV, the virus that causes AIDS. Zidovudine works by interfering with DNA synthesis, which the virus must carry out to reproduce. The side effects of zidovudine, which are experienced by a significant number of AIDS patients, are caused by the disruption of DNA synthesis in the person's own cells.

Despite these obstacles, some useful antiviral drugs have been developed. We must be aware, however, that many viruses undergo frequent mutations. Influenza viruses do (this is why we need a new flu vaccine every year), and it was perhaps inevitable that flu virus mutations would provide them with resistance to antiviral medications. This happened in 2006–2009: most strains of influenza A virus prevalent those winters were resistant to previously successful medications. Mutations occur for reasons we cannot explain, and vaccination, wherever possible, remains of greatest importance, prevention rather than need for treatment.

FUNGI (see table 22–5)

Fungi may be unicellular, such as yeasts, or multicellular, such as the familiar molds and mushrooms. Most fungi are **saprophytes** (or **saprobes**); that is, they live on dead organic matter and decompose it to recycle the chemicals as nutrients. The pathogenic fungi cause infections that are called **mycoses** (singular: **mycosis**), which may be superficial or systemic.

Yeasts (Fig. 22–4) have been used by people for thousands of years in baking and brewing. In small numbers, yeasts such as *Candida albicans* are part of the resident flora of the skin, mouth, intestines, and vagina. In larger numbers, however, yeasts may cause superficial infections of mucous membranes or the skin or very serious systemic infections of internal organs. An all-too-common trigger for oral or vaginal yeast infections is the use of an antibiotic to treat a bacterial infection. The antibiotic diminishes the normal bacterial flora, thereby removing competition for the yeasts, which are then able to overgrow. Yeasts may also cause skin infections in diabetics or in obese people who have skin folds that are always moist. In recent years, *Candida* has become an important cause of nosocomial infections. The resistance of hospital patients is often lowered because of their diseases or treatments, and they

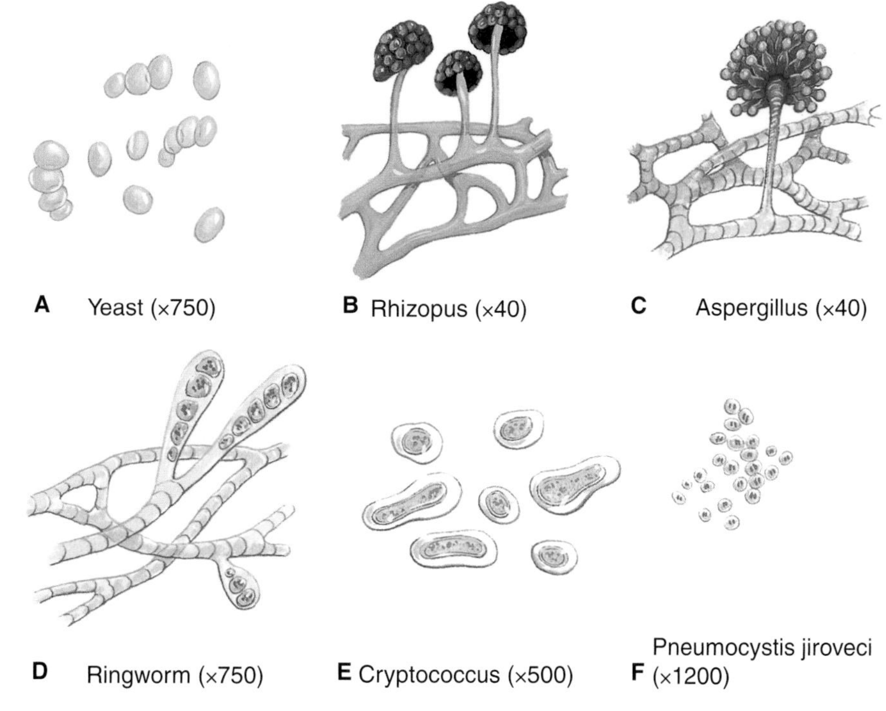

Figure 22–4 Fungi.

QUESTION: Which of the fungi shown have a mycelium?

are more susceptible to systemic yeast infections in the form of pneumonia or endocarditis.

Another superficial mycosis is ringworm (tinea), which may be caused by several species of fungi (see Table 22–5). The name *ringworm* is misleading because there are no worms involved. It is believed to have come from the appearance of the lesions: circular, scaly patches with reddened edges; the center clears as the lesion grows. Athlete's foot, which is probably a bacterial-fungal infection, is perhaps the most common form of ringworm.

The systemic mycoses are more serious diseases that occur when spores of some fungi gain access to the interior of the body. Most of these fungi grow in a moldlike pattern. The molds we sometimes see on stale bread or overripe fruit look fluffy or fuzzy. The fluff is called a mycelium and is made of many threadlike cellular structures called hyphae. The sporangia (spore cases) give the mold color (see Fig. 22–4). Each spore may be carried by the air to another site, where it germinates and forms another mycelium.

Because spores of these fungi are common in the environment, they are often inhaled. The immune responses are usually able to prevent infection and healthy people are usually not susceptible to systemic mycoses. Elderly people and those with chronic pulmonary diseases are much more susceptible, however, and they may develop lung infections. The importance of the immune system is clearly evident if we consider people with AIDS. Without the normal immune responses, AIDS patients are very susceptible to invasive fungal diseases, including meningitis caused by *Cryptococcus*. *Pneumocystis jiroveci* (formerly *P. carinii* and classified with the protozoa, its DNA sequences suggest it is closer to the fungi) is an important cause of pneumonia in people with AIDS. This species is usually not pathogenic because the healthy immune system can easily control it. For AIDS patients, however, this form of pneumonia may be the cause of death.

Antifungal Medications

One of the most effective drugs used to treat serious, systemic mycoses, amphotericin B, has great potential to cause serious side effects. Patients receiving this medication should have periodic tests of liver and kidney function.

Newer medications are less toxic to the recipient and may prove to be as effective as amphotericin B.

Superficial mycoses such as ringworm may be treated with certain oral medications. Taken orally, the drug is incorporated into living epidermal cells. When these cells die and reach the stratum corneum, they are resistant to the digestive action of the ringworm fungi. Topical drugs may not be as effective, especially for infections of nails.

There are several effective medications for mucosal yeast infections, but it is important that the trigger for the infection (such as antibiotic therapy) be resolved as well. If it is not, the yeast infection may recur when the medication is stopped.

PROTOZOA (see table 22–6)

Protozoa are unicellular animals, single cells that are adapted to life in freshwater (including soil) and saltwater. Some are human pathogens and are able to form cysts. Cysts are dormant cells that are resistant to heat, cold, or drying out, and are thus able to survive passage from host to host.

Intestinal protozoan parasites of people include *Entamoeba histolytica*, which causes amebic dysentery, and *Giardia lamblia*, which causes diarrhea called giardiasis (Fig. 22–5 and Table 22–6). People acquire these by ingesting food or water contaminated with the cysts of these species. Giardiasis can become a problem in daycare centers if the staff is not careful concerning hand washing and food preparation.

Leishmaniasis is caused by the genus *Leishmania* (they resemble the *Trypanosoma* shown in Fig. 22–5). This protozoan is spread by the bite of female sandflies and may cause cutaneous lesions that military personnel in Iraq and Afghanistan have named "Baghdad boil." The less common but more serious visceral infection is kala-azar (black fever), which may have an incubation period of several months to a year and not appear until a soldier has returned home. These protozoa are not endemic to North America or Europe, but medical professionals should be familiar with them.

Plasmodium species cause malaria, affect hundreds of millions of people throughout the world, and are probably the most important protozoan parasite. They are becoming increasingly resistant to the standard antimalarial drugs, which are used to prevent disease and treat it. Clinical trials are being conducted for several malaria vaccines, some of which have shown promise.

Medications are available that can treat most protozoan infections.

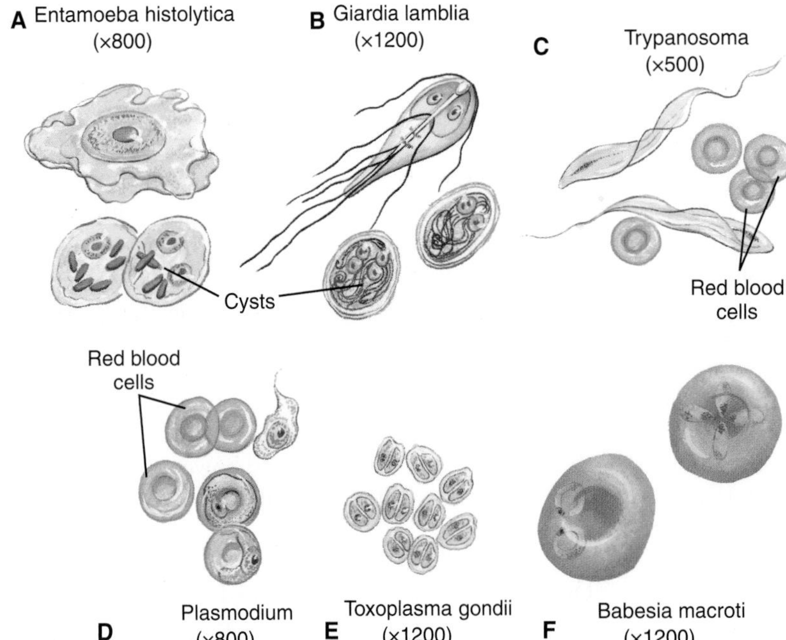

FIGURE 22–5 Protozoa.

QUESTION: QUESTION: In which human organ system do *Entamoeba* and *Giardia* live?

WORMS (HELMINTHS) (see table 22–7)

Most worms are simple multicellular animals. The parasitic worms are even simpler than the familiar earthworm because they live within hosts and use the host's blood or nutrients as food. Many of the parasitic worms have complex life cycles that involve two or more different host species.

The flukes are flatworms that are rare in most of North America but very common in parts of Africa and Asia. People acquire these species by eating aquatic plants or raw fish in which the larval worms have encysted. Within the person, each species lives in a specific site: the intestine, bile ducts, or certain veins. Although rarely fatal, these chronic infestations are often debilitating, and the host person is a source of the eggs of the fluke, which may then infect others.

Tapeworms are also flatworms (Fig. 22–6). Some are 10 to 15 feet long, and the fish tapeworm can grow to 60 feet. They are as flat as a ribbon, however, and one could easily be folded and held in the palm of the hand. The tapeworm holds on to the lining of a host's small intestine with the suckers and hooks on its scolex (front end). The segments, called proglottids, are produced continuously in most species and absorb nutrients from the host's digested food. The only function of the proglottids is reproduction: Eggs in one segment are fertilized by sperm from another segment. Mature proglottids containing fertilized eggs break off and are excreted in the host's feces. An intermediate host such as a cow or pig eats food contaminated with human feces; the eggs hatch within this animal and grow into larval worms that encyst in the animal's muscle tissue. People become infected by eating poorly cooked beef or pork that contains cysts.

Parasitic roundworms of people include hookworm, pinworm, *Ascaris*, and *Trichinella* (see Table 22–7 at the end of this chapter). Medications are available that can eliminate worm infestations. In endemic areas, however, reinfestation is quite common.

ARTHROPODS (see table 22–8)

Arthropods such as the scabies mite and head lice are **ectoparasites** that live on the surface of the body. The infestations they cause are very itchy and uncomfortable but not debilitating or life threatening (Fig. 22–7). Of greater importance are the arthropods that are vectors of disease. These are listed in Table 22–8. Mosquitoes, fleas, lice, and flies are all insects. Ticks and mites are not insects but are more closely related to spiders.

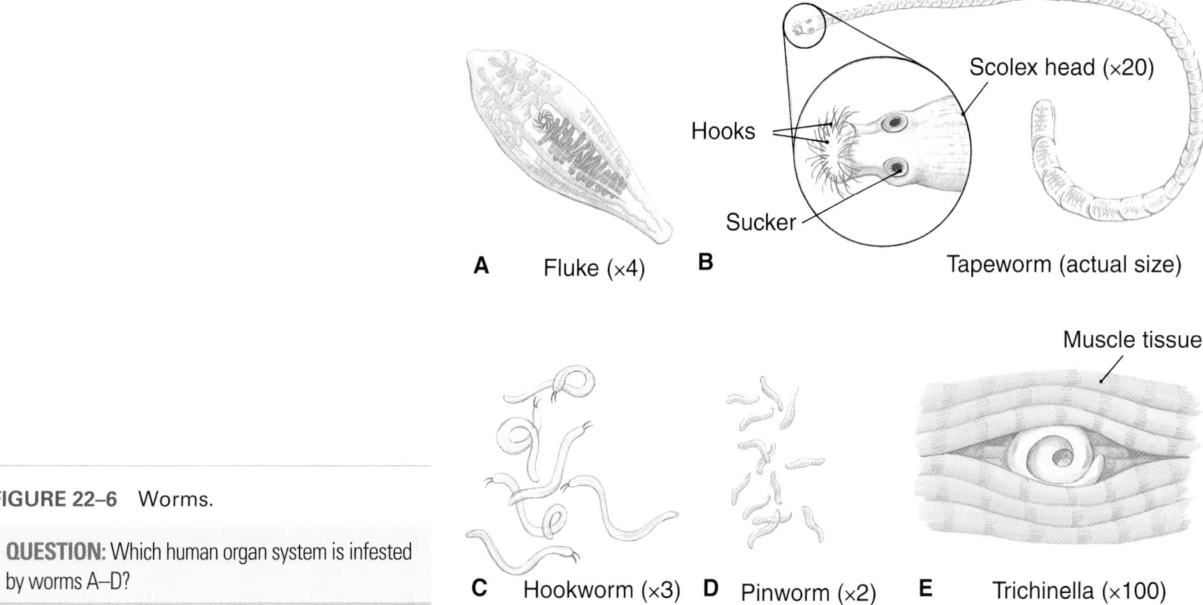

FIGURE 22–6 Worms.

QUESTION: Which human organ system is infested by worms A–D?

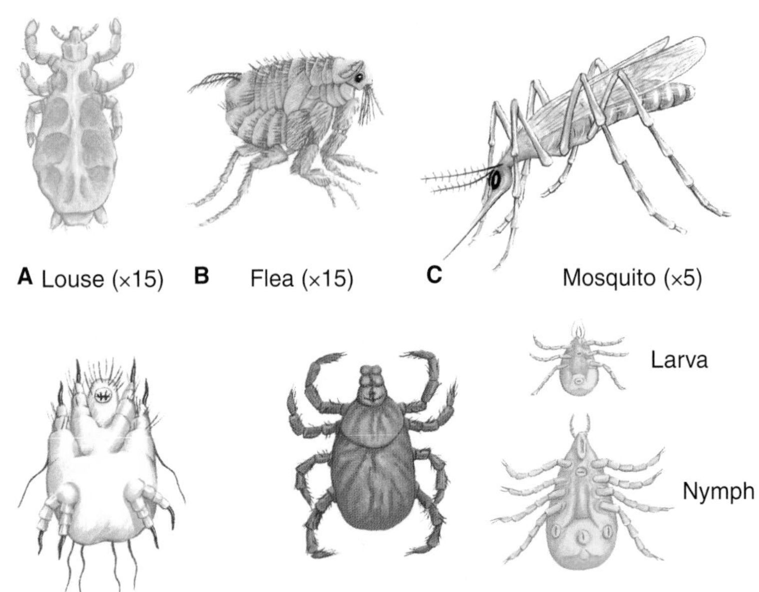

FIGURE 22–7 Arthropods.

QUESTION: Which of these arthropods are not insects (an old name for insects is hexapods)?

SUMMARY

The preceding discussion is an introduction to microorganisms and human disease and is only part of the story. The rest of this story is the remarkable ability of the human body to resist infection. Although we are surrounded and invaded by potential pathogens, most of us remain healthy most of the time. The immune responses that destroy pathogens and enable us to remain healthy are described in Chapter 14. Also in that chapter are discussions of vaccines. The development of vaccines represents the practical application of our knowledge of pathogens and of immunity, and it enables us to prevent many diseases. The availability of specific vaccines is noted in the tables of bacterial and viral diseases that follow.

Table 22–3 | **DISEASES CAUSED BY BACTERIA**

BACTERIAL SPECIES	DISCUSSION/DISEASE(S) CAUSED
Staphylococcus aureus gram (+) coccus	Skin infections such as boils, pneumonia, toxic shock syndrome, osteomyelitis, septicemia. Most strains resistant to penicillin and many strains to related antibiotics as well. An important cause of nosocomial infections, carried on the hands or in the nasal cavities of healthcare personnel. Food poisoning characterized by rapid onset (1–8 hours) and vomiting. No vaccine.
Staphylococcus epidermidis gram (+) coccus	Normal skin flora; potential pathogen for those with artificial internal prostheses such as heart valves and joints.
Streptococcus pyogenes **(Group A streptococci)** gram (+) coccus	Strep throat, otitis media, scarlet fever, endocarditis, puerperal sepsis; possible immunologic complications are rheumatic fever (transient arthritis and permanent damage to heart valves) and glomerulonephritis (transient kidney damage, usually with complete recovery). Rare strains cause necrotizing fasciitis, a potentially fatal hemolytic gangrene. Several vaccines are in the testing stages.

Table 22–3 | **DISEASES CAUSED BY BACTERIA—cont'd**

BACTERIAL SPECIES	DISCUSSION/DISEASE(S) CAUSED
***Streptococcus* Group B** gram (+) coccus	An important cause of neonatal infection, the bacteria are acquired from the mother during childbirth; risk factors are premature birth and intrapartum fever. May result in pneumonia, meningitis, or septicemia. May be prevented by testing pregnant women for Group B strep colonization and, if present, administering ampicillin. No vaccine.
Streptococcus pneumoniae gram (+) coccus	Pneumonia: accumulation of fluids and white blood cells in the alveoli. The vaccine contains capsules of the most common strains; recommended for the elderly and infants to prevent invasive disease. Possible cause of meningitis in adults with predisposing factors such as sickle-cell anemia, alcoholism, asplenism, or head trauma.
Enterococcus faecalis and other species gram (+) coccus	Normal colon flora. Has become an important cause of nosocomial infections of the urinary tract. No vaccine. Other species *(E. faecium)* may be acquired from animals. Some strains are resistant to many antibiotics.
Neisseria gonorrhoeae gram (−) coccus	Gonorrhea: inflammation of the mucous membranes of the reproductive and urinary tracts. May cause scarring of reproductive ducts and subsequent sterility; in women may cause pelvic inflammatory disease. Infants of infected women may acquire the bacteria during birth; this is termed *ophthalmia neonatorum* and is prevented by antibiotic eyedrops. No vaccine.
Neisseria meningitidis gram (−) coccus	Meningitis: inflammation and edema of the meninges; pressure on the brain may cause death or permanent brain damage. Also causes internal hemorrhages, DIC, and gangrene. Most common in older children and young adults, many of whom are asymptomatic carriers. Most cases are sporadic, not part of epidemics. The vaccine is given to military recruits and is strongly recommended for children ages 11–12, summer campers, high school freshman, and college freshmen living in dorms; the vaccine also prevents the carrier state. Post-exposure prophylaxis (prevention) requires antibiotics.
Moraxella catarrhalis gram (+) coccobacillus	Otitis media and upper respiratory infection in children; pneumonia in adults, especially the immunocompromised or elderly. No vaccine.
Bacillus anthracis gram (+) bacillus (spore-forming)	Anthrax: spores in soil may be acquired by cattle or sheep. People acquire disease from these animals or from animal products such as wool or leather. The three forms are pulmonary, cutaneous, and gastrointestinal, reflecting the portal of entry. The toxin causes death of tissue, and the pulmonary form may be fatal. Rare in the U.S. because grazing animals are vaccinated. The vaccine for people was reserved for the military but has been offered to people thought to be exposed to spores. Anthrax is a potential biological weapon.

Continued

Table 22–3 | **DISEASES CAUSED BY BACTERIA—cont'd**

BACTERIAL SPECIES	DISCUSSION/DISEASE(S) CAUSED
Clostridium perfringens and other species gram (+) bacillus (spore-forming)	Gas gangrene: normal soil flora may contaminate wounds; spores require anaerobic environment (dead tissue); toxins destroy more tissue, permitting the bacteria to spread; gas produced collects as bubbles in dead tissue. Food poisoning: from contaminated meat, self-limiting diarrhea. Some species have contaminated human tissue (ligament, tendon) used for transplants. No vaccine.
Clostridium tetani gram (+) bacillus (spore-forming)	Tetanus: normal soil flora may contaminate wounds; spores require anaerobic conditions. The toxin prevents muscle relaxation, resulting in muscle spasms. May be fatal if respiratory muscles are affected. The vaccine contains the toxoid (inactivated toxin) and has made this a rare disease in the U.S. Boosters are strongly recommended for older adults.
Clostridium botulinum gram (+) bacillus (spore-forming)	Botulism: normal soil flora; spores present in anaerobic food containers germinate and produce the toxin, which causes paralysis. Respiratory paralysis may be fatal without assisted ventilation. May cause infant botulism in children younger than 2 years of age who have ingested spores. No vaccine. Treatment is antitoxin (antibodies).
Clostridium difficile gram (+) bacillus (spore-forming)	Diarrhea: the most common identifiable cause of antibiotic-associated diarrhea (pseudomembranous enterocolitis); has become a significant nosocomial pathogen. A vaccine is in the testing stage.
Corynebacterium diphtheriae gram (+) bacillus	Diphtheria: toxin causes heart failure and paralysis; a pseudomembrane that grows in the pharynx may cover the larynx and cause suffocation. Vaccination of infants (DTP) has made this a very rare disease in the U.S. Older adults should receive boosters (combined with tetanus: DT).
Listeria monocytogenes gram (+) bacillus	Listeriosis: septicemia and meningitis in the elderly, infants, and unborn; may cause miscarriage or stillbirth. The bacteria are found in soil and in animals such as cattle. In the U.S., food poisoning outbreaks traced to contaminated milk or milk products. Sporadic cases traced to undercooked hot dogs or chicken or to cold cuts from delicatessen counters. No vaccine.
Salmonella typhi gram (−) bacillus	Typhoid fever: intestinal infection with erosion and septicemia; subsequent infection of liver, gallbladder, or kidneys. Upon recovery, the carrier state (bacteria in gallbladder) may occur. Rare in the U.S. because of chlorination of drinking water. The vaccine is used in endemic areas of the world such as Asia.
Salmonella enteritidis and other species gram (−) bacillus	Salmonellosis: food poisoning following consumption of contaminated animal products such as poultry or eggs. Diarrhea is usually self-limiting, but it may be fatal for the elderly. In the U.S. estimates are 4 million cases per year. No vaccine.

Table 22–3 | **DISEASES CAUSED BY BACTERIA—cont'd**

BACTERIAL SPECIES	DISCUSSION/DISEASE(S) CAUSED
Shigella species gram (−) bacillus	Bacillary dysentery: mild to severe diarrhea; may be fatal because of dehydration and circulatory shock. Usually transmitted by food prepared by people with mild cases. No vaccine. An important cause of illness in daycare centers.
Escherichia coli, Serratia marcescens, Proteus vulgaris and other genera of gram (−) bacilli	Normal colon flora; cause opportunistic infections when introduced into any other part of the body. This group is one of the most common causes of nosocomial infections (urinary tract, pneumonia, skin infections).
Escherichia coli 0157:H7 gram (−) bacillus	Hemorrhagic colitis and hemolytic uremic syndrome, potentially fatal. The bacteria may survive in undercooked meat, especially ground beef. A vaccine is in the research stage.
Pseudomonas aeruginosa gram (−) bacillus	Normal soil and water flora; also transient in human intestines. A serious potential pathogen for patients with severe burns, cystic fibrosis (causes pneumonia), or cancer. May even survive in disinfectant solutions. No vaccine.
Burkholderia cepacia gram (−) bacillus	Pneumonia: especially in people with cystic fibrosis or those with compromised immune systems. No vaccine. (Former genus name: *Pseudomonas.*)
Yersinia pestis gram (−) bacillus	Bubonic plague: swollen lymph nodes, septicemia, and hemorrhagic pneumonia; often fatal. Animal reservoirs are prairie dogs, ground squirrels, and other rodents. Rats and people are infected by fleas (the vector). In the U.S., the few cases each year occur in the Southwest. The vaccine is no longer available.
Francisella tularensis gram (−) bacillus	Tularemia (rabbit fever): septicemia and pneumonia; not often fatal but very debilitating. Reservoirs are wild animals and birds. People are infected by vectors (ticks, lice, and biting flies), by ingestion of contaminated animal meat, or by inhalation. No vaccine. Tularemia is a potential biological weapon.
Brucella species gram (−) bacillus	Brucellosis (undulant fever): extreme weakness and fatigue, anorexia, a fever that rises and falls. Reservoirs are cattle, sheep, goats, and pigs; people acquire infection by contact with contaminated animal products. In the U.S., this is an occupational disease: meat processing workers, vets, farmers. Vaccines are available for animals.
Haemophilus influenzae gram (−) bacillus	Meningitis in children, especially those younger than 2 years of age. Older people may have mild upper respiratory infections or a potentially fatal epiglottitis. The vaccine (Hib) contains the capsules of the bacteria and is recommended for infants beginning at age 2 months. This was the most common cause of meningitis in the U.S., approximately 20,000 cases per year. The vaccine has provided a 90% reduction.

Continued

Table 22–3 | **DISEASES CAUSED BY BACTERIA—cont'd**

BACTERIAL SPECIES	DISCUSSION/DISEASE(S) CAUSED
Haemophilus aegyptius gram (−) bacillus	Conjunctivitis: painful inflammation of the conjunctiva; spread by direct contact or fomites; may occur in epidemics among groups of children. No vaccine.
Bordetella pertussis gram (−) bacillus	Whooping cough (pertussis): paroxysms of violent coughing that may last for several weeks. Adults may have less severe coughing and go undiagnosed. Pneumonia is a complication that may be fatal, especially for children younger than 1 year of age. People are the only host. Concern about the safety of the original vaccine has prompted the development of newer vaccines, but in the U.S. the number of cases has increased sharply, in part because of parental complacency.
Vibrio cholerae gram (−) bacillus (comma shaped)	Cholera: profuse watery diarrhea; infection ranges from mild to fatal. Spread of infection is usually by way of water contaminated with human feces. Rare in the U.S.; epidemic in Asia, Africa, and South America. The oral vaccine seems effective.
Vibrio parahaemolyticus gram (−) bacillus (comma shaped)	Enteritis: diarrhea and nausea. Acquired by ingestion of raw or lightly cooked seafood; usually self-limiting. No vaccine.
Vibrio vulnificus gram (−) bacillus (comma shaped)	Gangrene and septicemia: acquired from ocean water that contaminates a wound or by the ingestion of raw shellfish. Illness is often severe and protracted and may be fatal, especially for people who are immunosuppressed or who have liver disease. No vaccine.
Campylobacter jejuni gram (−) helical bacillus	Enteritis: diarrhea that is often self-limiting but may be severe in the elderly or very young. Reservoirs are animals such as poultry; people acquire infection from contaminated meat. In the U.S., estimates are 2 million cases per year. No vaccine.
Helicobacter pylori gram (−) helical bacillus	Gastric ulcers: most are caused by *H. pylori*, which has also been implicated in cancer of the stomach. No vaccine.
Legionella pneumophila gram (−) bacillus	Legionellosis, which occurs in two forms: Legionnaire's disease is a pneumonia that may be fatal; Pontiac fever is a mild upper respiratory infection that is usually self-limiting. The bacteria are found in natural water and soil and may contaminate air conditioning systems or water supplies. Person-to-person transmission does not occur. An important cause of nosocomial pneumonia. No vaccine.
Mycobacterium tuberculosis acid-fast bacillus	Tuberculosis (TB): formation of tubercles containing bacteria and white blood cells, usually in the lung. Lung tissue is destroyed (caseation necrosis) and is removed by macrophages, leaving large cavities. The bacteria are spread by respiratory droplets from people with active cases. Many people acquire a primary infection that becomes dormant and is without symptoms yet may be triggered later into an active

Table 22–3 | **DISEASES CAUSED BY BACTERIA—cont'd**

BACTERIAL SPECIES	DISCUSSION/DISEASE(S) CAUSED
	secondary infection. The BCG vaccine is not used in the U.S., but is in other parts of the world. In the U.S., TB cases are frequent among homeless people, those with AIDS, and in closed populations such as prisons. Worldwide, the WHO estimates that there are 7–8 million new infections each year and 3 million deaths; 30% of the world's people are infected with active or latent TB. Strains of the bacteria resistant to the standard TB medications are becoming much more common and pose a difficult treatment problem. New vaccines are being tested.
Mycobacterium avium and other species acid-fast bacillus	Atypical mycobacterial infections: clinically similar to TB; usually in the lungs. These bacteria are pathogenic for people with AIDS or other forms of immunosuppression and for those with chronic pulmonary diseases.
Mycobacterium leprae acid-fast bacillus	Leprosy (Hansen's disease): chronic disease characterized by disfiguring skin lesions and nerve damage that may cause paralysis or loss of sensation. The bacteria are acquired by cutaneous contact or respiratory droplets. The incubation period may be several years; children develop clinical disease more rapidly than do adults. A vaccine is in the testing stage.
Treponema pallidum spirochete	Syphilis: a sexually transmitted disease that progresses in three stages. Primary syphilis: a painless, hard chancre at the site of entry on skin or mucous membrane. Secondary syphilis: a rash on the skin and mucous membranes (indicates systemic infection). Tertiary syphilis (5–40 years later): necrotic lesions (gummas) in the brain, heart valves, aorta, spinal cord, skin, or other organs. Congenital syphilis (the bacteria can cross the placenta) may cause bone and teeth defects and mental retardation. The WHO estimates that more than 12 million new cases occur worldwide every year, a serious public health problem. No vaccine.
Leptospira interrogans spirochete	Leptospirosis: a disease of wild or domestic animals that excrete the bacteria in urine. People acquire the bacteria by contact with contaminated water. Disease is usually mild, resembling intestinal virus infection. Weil's disease is the serious form, with hemorrhages in the liver and kidneys, and jaundice always present, indicating severe liver damage. A vaccine is available for dogs.
Borrelia burgdorferi spirochete	Lyme disease: begins as a flu-like illness, perhaps with a bull's-eye rash at the site of the tick bite. May be followed by cardiac arrhythmias, self-limiting meningitis, or arthritis. Animal reservoirs are deer and field mice; the vector is the deer tick (genus *Ixodes*). The vaccine was taken off the market because of poor sales.

Continued

Table 22–3 | **DISEASES CAUSED BY BACTERIA—cont'd**

BACTERIAL SPECIES	DISCUSSION/DISEASE(S) CAUSED
Borrelia vincentii spirochete	Trench mouth (Vincent's gingivitis): ulcerations of the gums and pharynx caused by overgrowth of *Borrelia* and other oral flora. Triggered by poor oral hygiene or infection, which must be corrected to make antibiotics effective.
Rickettsia prowazekii rickettsia	Epidemic typhus: high fever and delirium, hemorrhagic rash; 40% fatality rate. Vector is the human body louse. Very rare in the U.S. but still endemic in other parts of the world. No vaccine.
Rickettsia typhi rickettsia	Endemic typhus: similar to epidemic typhus but milder; 2% fatality rate. Reservoirs are rats and wild rodents; vectors are fleas. The few cases in the U.S. each year usually occur in the Southeast. No vaccine.
Rickettsia rickettsii rickettsia	Rocky Mountain spotted fever (RMSF): high fever, hemorrhagic rash, and pneumonia; 20% fatality rate. Reservoirs are wild rodents and dogs; vectors are ticks. Despite its name, RMSF in the U.S. is most prevalent in Southeast coastal states (North and South Carolina) and in Oklahoma. No vaccine.
Chlamydia trachomatis (serogroups D–K) chlamydia	Genitourinary infection: in men, urethritis or epididymitis; in women, cervicitis, although many women are asymptomatic. Complications in women include pelvic inflammatory disease, ectopic pregnancy, and miscarriage. Newborns of infected women may develop conjunctivitis or pneumonia. No vaccine.
Chlamydia trachomatis (serogroups A–C) chlamydia	Trachoma: conjunctivitis with papillae and vascular invasion of the cornea leading to scarring and blindness. Spread by direct contact. The leading cause of blindness throughout the world, especially in dry, dusty environments. No vaccine.
Chlamydia pneumoniae chlamydia	Pneumonia, usually community-acquired and mild enough to be called "walking pneumonia," with fever, cough, and hoarseness. No vaccine.
Chlamydia psittaci chlamydia	Psittacosis, also called ornithosis or parrot fever. Reservoirs are wild and domestic birds; pathogen shed in feces. Acquired by inhalation of fecal dust; disease ranges from mild upper respiratory infection to serious pneumonia. No vaccine.

Table 22–4 | **DISEASES CAUSED BY VIRUSES**

VIRUS	DISCUSSION/DISEASE(S) CAUSED
Herpes simplex	Type 1: fever blisters (cold sores) on the lip or in oral cavity; the virus is dormant in nerves of the face between attacks. Spread in saliva; may cause eye infections (self-inoculation). Type 2: genital herpes; painful lesions in the genital area; a sexually transmitted disease. Many people have few or no symptoms but may still spread the virus to sexual partners. Several vaccines are being tested.

Table 22–4 | DISEASES CAUSED BY VIRUSES—cont'd

VIRUS	DISCUSSION/DISEASE(S) CAUSED
	Either type may be oral or genital and may cause systemic infection and herpes encephalitis in newborns, whose immune systems cannot contain the virus.
Herpes varicella-zoster	Chickenpox: the disease of the first exposure; vesicular rash; pneumonia is a possible complication, especially in adults. The virus then becomes dormant in nerves. Shingles: painful, raised lesions on the skin above the affected nerves following reactivation of the dormant virus. Usually occurs in adults. The (HVZ) chickenpox vaccine is recommended for children. A shingles vaccine is available for adults.
Epstein-Barr virus (EBV)	Mononucleosis: swollen lymph nodes, fatigue, fever, possible spleen or liver enlargement. Spread by saliva. Has been statistically implicated as a contributing factor to the onset of multiple sclerosis. EBV is linked to Burkitt's lymphoma in Africa and to nasopharyngeal carcinoma in China. No vaccine.
Cytomegalovirus (CMV)	Most people have asymptomatic infection; the virus does no harm but remains in the body. Fetal infection may result in mental retardation, blindness, or deafness. CMV is the most frequent viral infection following organ transplants and may cause a serious pneumonia. A cause of blindness in people with AIDS. No vaccine.
Human herpesvirus 6 (HHV-6)	Sixth disease (the 6th childhood illness that includes a rash, also called roseola or exanthema subitum): high fever and a rash predominantly on the trunk. Most common in infants, and most infections are mild. The virus remains dormant in T lymphocytes, may be reactivated and spread by saliva. No vaccine.
Human herpesvirus 8 (HHV-8)	Kaposi's sarcoma: a malignancy of blood vessels often seen in people with AIDS; the virus is sexually transmitted. No vaccine.
Human papillomaviruses (HPVs)	More than 100 types, some cause genital warts. Several cause cervical cancer in women. A vaccine for HPV-6, 11, 16, and 18 (the causes of most cancers) is available. The vaccine must be administered before a person becomes sexually active.
Adenoviruses	Many different types: some cause acute respiratory disease (ARD) similar to the common cold; others cause pharyngoconjunctival fever and may occur in epidemics related to swimming pools. The ARD vaccine is used only in the military.
Rhinoviruses	More than 100 types. Common cold: sore throat, runny nose, low fever; usually self-limiting. No vaccine.
Influenza viruses	Influenza: muscle aches, fever, fatigue, spread in respiratory droplets. Three types: A, B, and C. Type A is responsible for most epidemics. These are mutating viruses, and new vaccines are needed as the virus changes. The most serious

Continued

Table 22–4 | **DISEASES CAUSED BY VIRUSES—cont'd**

VIRUS	DISCUSSION/DISEASE(S) CAUSED
	complications are secondary bacterial pneumonia and a "cytokine storm" if the immune system overresponds to the virus.
Respiratory syncytial virus (RSV)	Pneumonia: at high risk are infants and young children, especially. those who must be hospitalized. Decades of work have yet to produce an effective vaccine.
Human meta-pneumovirus	Lower respiratory tract infection: bronchiolitis and pneumonia, especially in infants and probably in elderly adults. Most infections occur during the winter. This is a newly discovered pathogen, related to RSV, and much remains to be learned. No vaccine.
Hantaviruses	Hantavirus pulmonary syndrome: fever, cough, pulmonary edema, hypotension. Mortality rate is 40%–50%. Acquired by contact with rodent feces or urine, or inhalation of virus in rodent-infested areas. No vaccine.
Measles virus	Measles (rubeola): fever, sore throat, Koplik's spots (white) on lining of mouth, rash. Complications are ear infections, pneumonia, and measles encephalitis, which may be fatal. The vaccine is given to infants (MMR: with mumps and rubella).
Rubella virus	German measles: mild upper respiratory symptoms; a rash may be present. The virus may cross the placenta and cause congenital rubella syndrome (CRS): blindness, deafness, heart defects, mental retardation, or miscarriage. CRS is most likely if the fetus is infected during the first trimester. The vaccine is given to infants (MMR).
Parvovirus B19	Fifth disease: a childhood illness characterized by a rash on the cheeks and limbs. Adults may develop transitory arthritis; anemia may occur in immunocompromised people or those with sickle-cell anemia. The virus can cross the placenta and may cause miscarriage or severe damage to the fetal liver. No vaccine yet for human disease (as there are for animal parvoviruses) because development of one is not seen as commercially profitable.
Mumps virus	Mumps: fever, swelling of the parotid salivary glands or the others (asymptomatic infections do occur); the virus is spread in saliva. Complications are rare in children but include pancreatitis, nerve deafness, and mumps encephalitis. Adult men may develop orchitis, inflammation of the testes. Adult women may develop oophoritis, inflammation of the ovaries. The vaccine is given to infants.
Polio viruses	Polio: most infections are asymptomatic or mild; major infection may result in paralysis. Two vaccines: IPV (Salk) contains a killed virus and cannot cause polio; booster injections are needed. OPV (Sabin) contains an attenuated virus, is given orally, and carries a very small risk of causing polio. In the U.S., polio cases are vaccine related; polio is still endemic in other parts of the world. Eradication is still a goal for the WHO.

Table 22–4 | **DISEASES CAUSED BY VIRUSES—cont'd**

VIRUS	DISCUSSION/DISEASE(S) CAUSED
Coxsackie viruses (29 types)	Hand, foot, and mouth disease: fever, blisters on the palms, soles, tongue, and throat; most common among children. May also cause conjunctivitis, myositis, and myocarditis. Highly contagious, spread by the fecal–oral route and by respiratory droplets. No vaccine.
Rabies virus	Rabies: headache, nausea, fever, spasms of the swallowing muscles; seizures; virtually 100% fatal, with respiratory or heart failure. Reservoirs are wild animals; the virus is in their saliva. Postexposure prevention requires human rabies immune globulin (HRIG-antibodies) and the rabies vaccine.
Encephalitis viruses	Encephalitis: most infections are mild; CNS involvement is indicated by confusion, lethargy, or coma. Several types of these viruses occur in the U.S. Reservoirs are wild birds and small mammals; vectors are mosquitoes. Vaccines are available for horses and for people whose occupations put them at risk.
West Nile virus	West Nile encephalitis: first found in North America in New York City in 1999 (well known in Africa and the Middle East). Natural reservoirs are birds; several species of mosquitoes are vectors. Symptoms include headache and confusion, but most infections are mild or asymptomatic; fatalities are not common. No vaccine.
Dengue virus (4 serotypes)	Dengue fever: an influenza-like illness (break-bone fever) and dengue hemorrhagic fever characterized by vascular leakage and defective clotting. Vectors are mosquitos in the genus *Aedes*. Endemic in the tropics and subtropics, with an estimated 100 million cases per year and 25,000 fatalities, and is moving north. Vaccines are in the testing stages.
Rotaviruses	Enteritis: worldwide the leading cause of diarrhea and potentially fatal dehydration in infants and children. A new vaccine seems to be effective.
Noroviruses (formerly Norwalk viruses)	Gastroenteritis: vomiting; called by many "stomach flu." Acquired from food such as shellfish, or from food handled by people with mild cases. No vaccine.
Ebola and **Marburg viruses**	Hemorrhagic fever: high fever, systemic hemorrhages, necrosis of the liver; mortality rate 25%–90%. The viruses also affect monkeys, which may be reservoirs of infection. Vaccines are in the testing stage.
Yellow fever virus	Yellow fever: hemorrhages in the liver, spleen, kidneys, and other organs. The vector is a mosquito. The vaccine is recommended for travelers to endemic areas: Central and South America and Africa.
Hepatitis viruses types A,B, and C	Hepatitis: anorexia, nausea, fatigue, jaundice (may not be present in mild cases). HAV is spread by the fecal–oral route; contaminated shellfish or food prepared by people with mild cases. No carriers after recovery. HBV is spread by sexual activity or contact with blood or other body fluids. Carrier state is possible; may lead to

Continued

Table 22–4 | **DISEASES CAUSED BY VIRUSES—cont'd**

VIRUS	DISCUSSION/DISEASE(S) CAUSED
	liver cancer or cirrhosis. HCV transmission is similar to that of HBV. Carrier state is possible. There are vaccines for hepatitis A and B. Other hepatitis viruses are designated D, E, F, and G.
Human immunodeficiency virus (HIV)	AIDS: destruction of helper T cells and suppression of the immune system; opportunistic infections; invariably fatal, often after many years. HIV is spread by sexual activity, contact with blood, or placental transmission. No vaccine.
Variola major	Smallpox: declared eradicated by the WHO in 1980. Is a potential biological weapon. Contagious, characterized by a hemorrhagic rash and internal hemorrhages. Fatality rate is 30%–50%. In the U.S., childhood vaccination was stopped in 1982.
SARS virus	Severe acute respiratory syndrome: a pneumonia in which the lungs fill with fluid; 10% fatality rate. The reservoir is the horseshoe bat of China. The first cases were in China in 2002; in 2004, the human form of the virus disappeared. Vaccines are in the development stage.

Table 22–5 | **DISEASES CAUSED BY FUNGI**

FUNGUS GENUS	DISCUSSION/DISEASE(S) CAUSED
Microsporum, Trichophyton, Epidermophyton	Ringworm (tinea): scaly red patches on the skin or scalp; loss of hair. Tinea pedis is athlete's foot. May also infect damaged nails. Spores of these fungi are acquired from people or animals.
Candida albicans (and other species)	Yeast infections: mucosal infections are called thrush; may be oral or vaginal; yeasts have come from resident flora. Systemic infections include pneumonia and endocarditis. Important nosocomial pathogens.
Cryptococcus	Cryptococcosis: pulmonary infection that may progress to meningitis, especially in AIDS patients. Spores are carried in the air from soil or pigeon droppings.
Histoplasma	Histoplasmosis: pulmonary infection that is often self-limiting. Progressive disease involves ulcerations of the liver, spleen, and lymph nodes; usually fatal. Spores are carried by the air from soil.
Coccidioides	Coccidioidomycosis (valley fever): pulmonary infection that is often self-limiting. Progressive disease involves the meninges, bones, skin, and other organs; high mortality rate. Spores are carried by the air.
Rhizopus	Common bread mold that is harmless to most people but may cause invasive disease in those with compromised immune systems or poorly controlled diabetes. The spores may be

Table 22–5 | DISEASES CAUSED BY FUNGI—cont'd

FUNGUS GENUS	DISCUSSION/DISEASE(S) CAUSED
	inhaled or ingested, leading to systemic infection characterized by clotting and necrosis.
Aspergillus	A common mold found on fruits, harmless to healthy people. In those who are immunocompromised it may cause sinusitis, otitis, pneumonia, or more invasive disease.
Pneumocystis jiroveci	Pneumonia: only in very debilitated or immunosuppressed persons, such as people with AIDS. Although its antibiotic susceptibility is that of a protozoan, its DNA sequences are more similar to those of fungi. Many people become infected during childhood, but a normal immune system prevents any damage. Such a latent infection may become symptomatic and very serious when cell-mediated immunity is impaired.

Table 22–6 | DISEASES CAUSED BY PROTOZOA

PROTOZOAN	DISCUSSION/DISEASE(S) CAUSED
Entamoeba histolytica	Amebic dysentery; ulcerative lesions in the colon, bloody diarrhea; abscesses may form in the liver, lungs, or brain. Cysts are spread by the fecal–oral route in water or food. No vaccine.
Naegleria species	Amebic meningoencephalitis: inflammation of the meninges and brain; uncommon in the U.S. but almost always fatal. Amoebas in fresh water are acquired when swimmers sniff water into the nasal cavities; the amoebas move along the olfactory nerves into the brain.
Balantidium coli	Balantidiasis: abdominal discomfort and diarrhea; often mild. Reservoirs are pigs and other domestic animals; spread by the fecal–oral route. No vaccine.
Giardia lamblia	Giardiasis: fatty diarrhea; may be mild. Reservoirs are wild and domestic animals and people. Spread by the fecal–oral route (cysts) in water or food prepared by people with mild cases. An important cause of diarrhea in daycare centers. No vaccine.
Trichomonas vaginalis	Trichomoniasis: a sexually transmitted disease. Women: causes cervicitis and vaginitis; men are often asymptomatic. No vaccine.
Trypanosoma species	African sleeping sickness: lethargy progressing to coma and death. Reservoirs are wild and domestic animals; vector is the tsetse fly. No vaccine.
Leishmania major and other species	Leishmaniasis: cutaneous lesions ("Baghdad boil") or the more serious visceral infection kala-azar; vector is the female sandfly; endemic in southwest and central Asia. No vaccine.

Continued

Table 22–6 | **DISEASES CAUSED BY PROTOZOA—cont'd**

PROTOZOAN	DISCUSSION/DISEASE(S) CAUSED
Plasmodium species	Malaria: the protozoa reproduce in red blood cells, causing hemolysis and anemia. The vector is the *Anopheles* mosquito. Cerebral malaria is the most severe form, and it is often fatal for children. The WHO estimates 200 million new cases each year, with 1 million deaths. Several vaccines are in the testing stages.
Toxoplasma gondii	Toxoplasmosis: asymptomatic infection in healthy people. Congenital infection: miscarriage or mental retardation, blindness. Reservoirs are cats and grazing animals. Pregnant women may acquire cysts from cat feces or from ingestion of rare beef or lamb.
Cryptosporidium species	Diarrhea: ranges from mild to severe; spread by the fecal–oral route. An important cause of diarrhea in daycare centers and in AIDS patients. Is very resistant to chlorine, may contaminate municipal water supplies or swimming pools and cause extensive epidemics.
Babesia microti and other species	Babesiosis: first symptoms similar to influenza; the protozoa reproduce in and destroy RBCs; can cross the placenta. In severe cases the hemolytic anemia may lead to renal failure. The vectors are *Ixodes* ticks. No vaccine.

Table 22–7 | **INFESTATIONS CAUSED BY WORMS**

WORM (*GENUS*)	DISCUSSION/DISEASE(S) CAUSED
Chinese liver fluke (*Clonorchis*)	Abdominal discomfort; cirrhosis after many years. Adult worms (½ inch) live in bile ducts. Acquired by people from ingestion of raw fish that contains worm cysts.
Tapeworms (*Taenia, Diphyllobothrium*)	Bloating and abdominal discomfort; constipation or diarrhea. People acquire the worms by eating poorly cooked beef, pork, or fish (the alternate hosts) that contain worm cysts.
Pinworm (*Enterobius*)	Adult worms (⅛ inch) live in colon; females lay eggs on perianal skin while host is asleep, causing irritation and itching of skin. Eggs are spread to family members on hands and bed linens. In the U.S., this is probably the most common worm infestation.
Hookworm (*Necator*)	Adult worms (½ inch) live in the small intestine; their food is blood. Heavy infestations cause anemia and fatigue. Eggs are excreted in feces; larval worms burrow through the skin of a bare foot and migrate to the intestine. Worldwide, in tropical and subtropical regions, an estimated 800 million people are infested. Hookworm is now rare in North America.

Table 22–7 | INFESTATIONS CAUSED BY WORMS—cont'd

WORM (*GENUS*)	DISCUSSION/DISEASE(S) CAUSED
Ascaris	Adults are 10–12 inches long and live in the small intestine. Large numbers of worms may cause intestinal obstruction. Eggs are excreted in feces and are spread to others on hands or vegetation contaminated by human feces.
Trichinella spiralis	Trichinosis: severe muscle pain as migrating worms form cysts that become calcified. Acquired by eating poorly cooked pork (or wild animals) that contains cysts.

Table 22–8 | ARTHROPOD VECTORS AND PESTS

ARTHROPOD	DISEASE (TYPE OF PATHOGEN)*	COMMENT
Mosquito	Malaria (protozoan) Encephalitis (many viruses) Yellow fever (virus)	Eggs are laid and larvae develop in water; denying breeding sites and use of netting while sleeping are simple and effective preventive measures.
Flea	Plague (bacterium) Endemic typhus (rickettsia)	Fleas are wingless but are able to hop from host to host (as far as 8 inches); the worm-like larvae hatch from eggs laid in a host's fur.
Body louse	Epidemic typhus (rickettsia) Tularemia (bacterium) Relapsing fever (bacterium)	Body lice live on clothing and move to the skin only to feed; they have no wings and move slowly.
Tick	Lyme disease (bacterium) Rocky Mountain spotted fever (rickettsia) Tularemia (bacterium)	Ticks move slowly on clothing or the skin and climb upward; tick checks after being in wooded or grassy areas are an effective preventive measure.
Tsetse fly	African sleeping sickness (protozoan)	Bites are painful.
Deer fly, horse fly	Tularemia (bacterium)	Large, aggressive blood-sucking flies; bites are painful.
Sandfly	Leishmaniasis (protozoan)	The female flies are one-fourth the size of a house fly.
Head louse	Not a vector of disease	Eggs (nits) are glued to hair shafts.
Bedbug	Not a vector of disease	Bedbugs are nocturnal feeders and often very numerous; by day they hide in bedding or in room crevices.
Scabies mite	Not a vector of disease	Female mites tunnel into the skin to lay their eggs; itching is intense, especially at night.

*These diseases are described in previous tables.

STUDY OUTLINE

Classification of Microorganisms

1. Bacteria—unicellular; some are pathogens.
2. Viruses—not cells; all are parasites.
3. Protozoa—unicellular animals; some are pathogens.
4. Fungi—unicellular (yeasts) or multicellular (molds); most are decomposers.
5. Worms—multicellular animals; a few are parasites.
6. Arthropods—insects, ticks, or mites that are vectors of disease or cause infestations.
   a. Binomial nomenclature—the genus and species names.

Normal Flora—Microbiota—see Table 22–1

1. Resident flora—the microorganisms that live on or in nearly everyone, in specific body sites; cause no harm when in their usual sites.
2. Transient flora—the microorganisms that periodically inhabit the body and usually cause no harm unless the host's resistance is lowered.

Infectious Disease

1. Caused by microorganisms or their toxins.
2. Clinical infections are characterized by symptoms; in a subclinical infection, the person shows no symptoms.
3. Course of an infectious disease: Incubation period—the time between the entry of the pathogen and the onset of symptoms. The acme is the worst stage of the disease, followed by recovery or death. A self-limiting disease typically lasts a certain period of time and is followed by recovery.
4. Types of Infection
   a. Localized—the pathogen is in one area of the body.
   b. Systemic—the pathogen is spread throughout the body by the blood or lymph.
   c. Septicemia (bacteremia)—bacteria in the blood.
   d. Acute—usually severe or of abrupt onset.
   e. Chronic—progresses slowly or is prolonged.
   f. Secondary—made possible by a primary infection that lowered host resistance.
   g. Nosocomial—a hospital-acquired infection.
   h. Endogenous—caused by the person's own normal flora in an abnormal site.

Epidemiology—see Fig. 22–1

1. The study of the patterns and spread of disease.
   a. Endemic—the disease is present in a population.
   b. Epidemic—more cases than is usual in a given time.
   c. Pandemic—an epidemic that affects several countries.
2. Portal of entry—the way a pathogen enters a host.
3. Portal of exit—the way a pathogen leaves a host.
4. Reservoirs—persons with the disease, carriers after recovery, or animal hosts (for zoonoses).
5. Noncommunicable disease—cannot be directly or indirectly transmitted from host to host.
6. Communicable disease—may be transmitted directly from host to host by respiratory droplets, cutaneous or sexual contact, placental transmission, or blood contact. May be transmitted indirectly by food or water, vectors, or fomites.

7. Contagious disease—easily spread from person to person by casual cutaneous contact or respiratory droplets.

Methods of Control of Microbes

1. Antiseptics—chemicals that destroy or inhibit bacteria on a living being.
2. Disinfectants—chemicals that destroy or inhibit bacteria on inanimate objects.
3. Sterilization—a process that destroys all living organisms.
4. Public health measures include laws and regulations to ensure safe food and water.

Bacteria—see Fig. 22–2

1. Shapes: coccus, bacillus, and spirillum.
2. Flagella provide motility for some bacilli and spirilla.
3. Aerobes require oxygen; anaerobes are inhibited by oxygen; facultative anaerobes grow in the presence or absence of oxygen.
4. The gram reaction (positive or negative) is based on the chemistry of the cell wall. The Gram stain is a laboratory procedure used in the identification of bacteria.
5. Capsules inhibit phagocytosis by white blood cells. Spores are dormant forms that are resistant to environmental extremes.
6. Toxins are chemicals produced by bacteria that are poisonous to host cells.
7. Rickettsias and chlamydias differ from other bacteria in that they must be inside living cells to reproduce.
8. Antibiotics are chemicals used in the treatment of bacterial diseases. Broad-spectrum: affects many kinds of bacteria. Narrow-spectrum: affects only a few kinds of bacteria.
9. Bacteria may become resistant to certain antibiotics, which are then of no use in treatment. Resistance is a genetic trait and will be passed to future generations. Culture and sensitivity testing may be necessary before an antibiotic is chosen to treat an infection.
10. Diseases—see Table 22–3.

Viruses—see Fig. 22–3

1. Not cells; a virus consists of either DNA or RNA surrounded by a protein shell.
2. Must be inside living cells to reproduce, which causes death of the host cell.
3. Severity of disease depends on the types of cells infected; some viruses may cross the placenta and infect a fetus.
4. Antiviral medications must interfere with viral reproduction without harming host cells.
5. Diseases—see Table 22–4.

Fungi—see Fig. 22–4

1. Most are saprophytes, decomposers of dead organic matter. May be unicellular yeasts or multicellular molds.
2. Mycoses may be superficial, involving the skin or mucous membranes, or systemic, involving internal organs such as the lungs or meninges.
3. Effective antifungal medications are available, but some are highly toxic.
4. Diseases—see Table 22–5.

Protozoa—see Fig. 22–5

1. Unicellular animals; some are pathogens.
2. Some are spread by vectors, others by fecal contamination of food or water.
3. Effective medications are available for most diseases.
4. Diseases—see Table 22–6.

Worms—see Fig. 22–6

1. Simple multicellular animals; the parasites are flukes, tapeworms, and some roundworms.
2. May have life cycles that involve other animal hosts and people.
3. Effective medications are available for most worm infestations.
4. Diseases—see Table 22–7.

Arthropods—see Fig. 22–7

1. Some cause superficial infestations (ectoparasites).
2. Others are vectors of disease—see Table 22–8.

REVIEW QUESTIONS

1. Define resident flora (microbiota), and explain its importance. (p. 548)
2. State the term described by each statement: (pp. 550–552)
   a. An infection in which the person shows no symptoms
   b. Bacteria that are inhibited by oxygen
   c. A disease that lasts a certain length of time and is followed by recovery
   d. A disease that is usually present in a given population
   e. The presence of bacteria in the blood
   f. An infection made possible by a primary infection that lowers host resistance
   g. A disease of animals that may be acquired by people
   h. Bacteria that are spherical in shape
3. Name these parts of bacterial cell: (pp. 555–558)
   a. Inhibits phagocytosis by white blood cells
   b. Provides motility
   c. The basis for the gram reaction or Gram stain
   d. A form resistant to heat and drying
   e. Chemicals produced that are poisonous to host cells
4. Explain what is meant by a nosocomial infection, and describe the two general kinds with respect to sources of the pathogen. (p. 551)
5. Name five potential portals of entry for pathogens. (p. 551)
6. Name five potential portals of exit for pathogens. (p. 552)
7. Explain the difference between a communicable disease and a contagious disease. (p. 553)
8. Explain the difference between pasteurization and sterilization. (pp. 553–554)
9. Describe the structure of a virus, and explain how viruses cause disease. (pp. 559–560)
10. Describe the differences between yeasts and molds. (p. 560)
11. Describe the difference between superficial and systemic mycoses. (pp. 560–562)
12. Name some diseases spread by vectors, and name the vector for each. (pp. 575–577)

FOR FURTHER THOUGHT

1. Smallpox has been eradicated (in the wild). Polio is the next target of world health officials, then measles. What characteristics must a disease or its pathogen have that would allow us even to consider trying to eradicate it? Try to think of five.
2. To understand the epidemiology of a disease, we must know several things about the disease or its agent (pathogen). Again, try to think of five.
3. Many working mothers depend on daycare centers to care for their children. What pathogens are likely to flourish in a daycare center if proper precautions are not taken? There are two general kinds. Besides being sure that all children have the proper vaccinations, what do you think is the most important proper precaution (think: lunchtime)?
4. We're still at the daycare center. Name three diseases that all 2-year-olds should have been vaccinated against. There may be a 6-month-old child in the group who has not yet received certain vaccinations, yet this child may be protected by what we call "herd immunity." Describe what is meant by herd immunity.
5. Explain why leptospirosis may be misdiagnosed as hepatitis (compare the descriptions in the tables of pathogens). Explain the consequences for the patient (notice what kind of pathogen causes each). What does this suggest to us about rare diseases, or the study of rare diseases?
6. Ms. D has had second thoughts about her eyebrow ring, so she has taken it out and now wants the hole to close. She comes to the clinic on campus because the pierced site is not healing and has become inflamed, red, and painful. Ms. D claims that she keeps the site very clean by applying hydrogen peroxide several times a day. What do you tell her to do?
7. West Nile virus encephalitis was new to North America in 1999. Less than a year later, public health officials could say that most infections were asymptomatic or mild, and only a very small percentage were serious or fatal. How do you think they discovered this?
8. Question Figure 22–A depicts a bacterial culture (in a Petri dish) with disks of four different antibiotics. Which antibiotic would be the best one to prescribe if this bacterium were the cause of an infection? Which one should not even be considered?

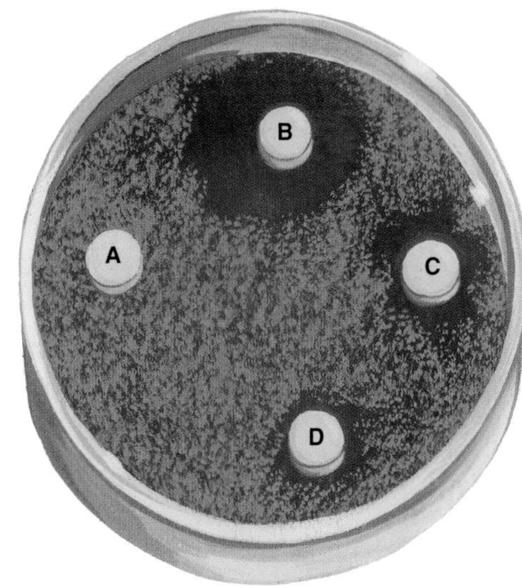

QUESTION FIGURE 22–A Bacterial culture with antibiotic disks for sensitivity testing.

APPENDIX A

Units of Measure

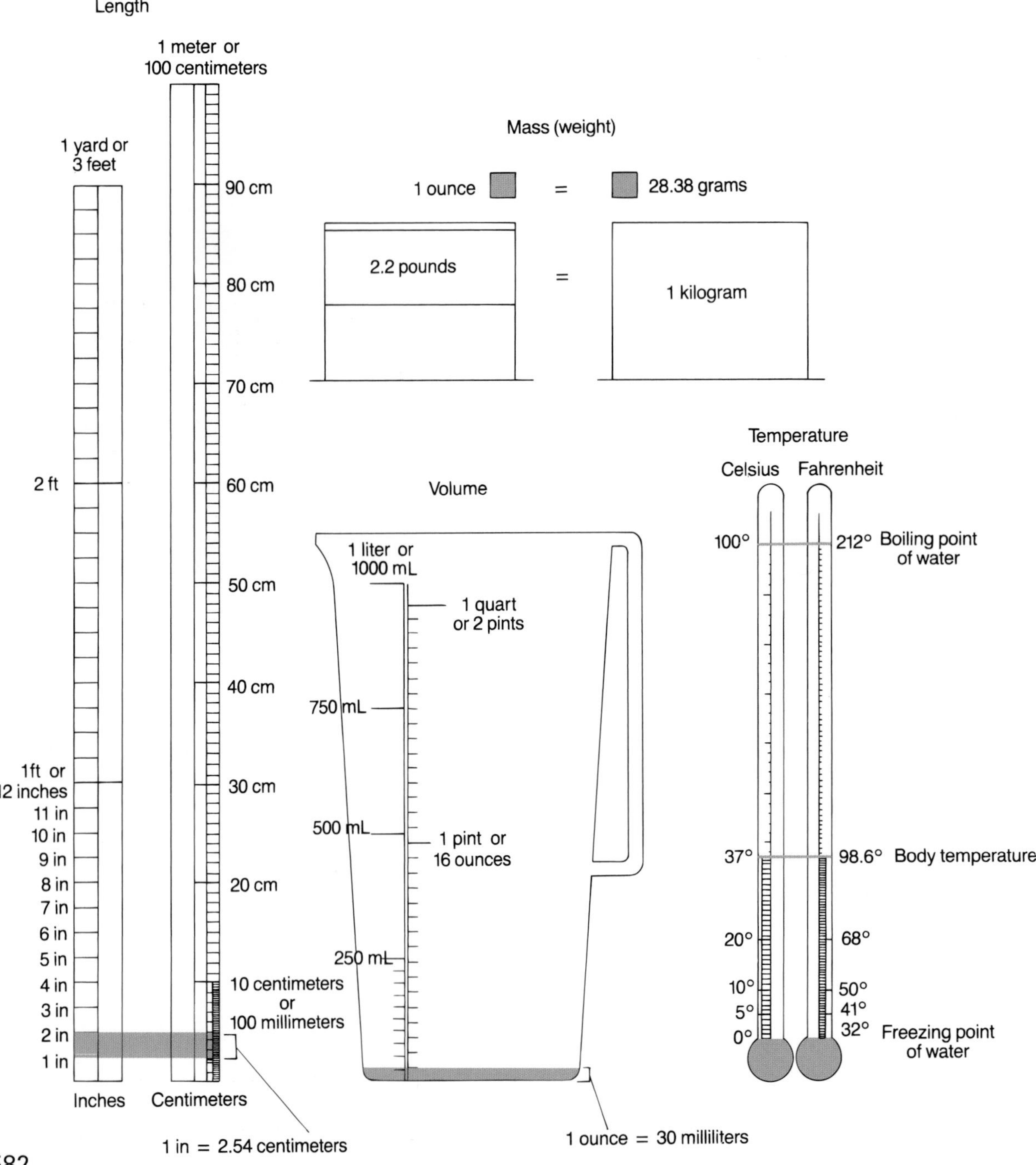

UNITS OF LENGTH

		mm	cm	in.	ft	yd	m
1 millimeter	=	1.0	0.1	0.04	0.003	0.001	0.001
1 centimeter	=	10.0	1.0	0.39	0.032	0.011	0.01
1 inch	=	25.4	2.54	1.0	0.083	0.028	0.025
1 foot	=	304.8	30.48	12.0	1.0	0.33	0.305
1 yard	=	914.4	91.44	36.0	3.0	1.0	0.914
1 meter	=	1000.0	100.0	39.37	3.28	1.09	1.0

1 μ = 1 mu = 1 micrometer (micron) = 0.001 mm = 0.00004 in.
mm = millimeters; cm = centimeters; in. = inches; ft = feet; yd = yards; m = meters.

UNITS OF WEIGHT

		mg	g	oz	lb	kg
1 milligram	=	1.0	0.001	0.00004	0.000002	0.000001
1 gram	=	1000.0	1.0	0.035	0.002	0.001
1 ounce	=	28,380	28.4	1.0	0.06	0.028
1 pound	=	454,000	454.0	16.0	1.0	0.454
1 kilogram	=	1,000,000	1000.0	35.2	2.2	1.0

mg = milligrams; g = grams; oz = ounces; lb = pounds; kg = kilograms.

UNITS OF VOLUME

		mL	in.^{3}	oz	qt	L
1 milliliter	=	1.0	0.06	0.034	0.001	0.001
1 cubic inch	=	16.4	1.0	0.55	0.017	0.016
1 ounce	=	29.6	1.8	1.0	0.03	0.029
1 quart	=	946.3	57.8	32.0	1.0	0.946
1 liter	=	1000.0	61.0	33.8	1.06	1.0

mL = milliliters; in.^{3} = cubic inches; oz = ounces; qt = quarts; L = liters.

TEMPERATURE: CELSIUS AND FAHRENHEIT

°C	= °F	°C	= °F	°C	= °F	°C	= °F	°C	= °F	°C	= °F
0°C	32°F	10°C	50°F	20°C	68°F	30°C	86°F	40°C	104°F	50°C	122°F
5°C	41°F	15°C	59°F	25°C	77°F	35°C	95°F	45°C	113°F	55°C	131°F

APPENDIX B

Abbreviations

The use of abbreviations for medical and scientific terms is time-saving and often standard practice. Some of the most frequently used abbreviations have been listed here. Notice that some have more than one meaning or interpretation. It is important to know the abbreviations approved by your institution, use only those, and *never* make up your own abbreviations. If there is any chance of confusion, write out the words.

ABC	airway, breathing, circulation
ABG	arterial blood gas
ABX	antibiotics
ACh	acetylcholine
ACTH	adrenocorticotropic hormone
AD	Alzheimer's disease
ADH	antidiuretic hormone
AIDS	acquired immunodeficiency syndrome
ALS	amyotrophic lateral sclerosis
ANS	autonomic nervous system
ARDS	acute respiratory distress syndrome
ARF	acute renal failure (acute respiratory failure)
ATP	adenosine triphosphate
AV	atrioventricular
BAL	blood alcohol level
BBB	blood-brain barrier
BMR	basal metabolic rate
BP	blood pressure
BPH	benign prostatic hypertrophy (hyperplasia)
BPM	beats per minute
BS	blood sugar (bowel sounds, breath sounds)
BUN	blood urea nitrogen
CA	cancer
CAD	coronary artery disease
CAPD	continuous ambulatory peritoneal dialysis
CBC	complete blood count
CC	creatinine clearance (critical condition, chief complaint)
CCCC	closed-chest cardiac compression
CF	cystic fibrosis (cardiac failure)
CHD	coronary heart disease (congenital heart disease)
CHF	congestive heart failure
CI	cardiac insufficiency (cerebral infarction)
CNS	central nervous system
CO	cardiac output (carbon monoxide)
COPD	chronic obstructive pulmonary disease
CP	cerebral palsy
CPR	cardiopulmonary resuscitation
CRF	chronic renal failure
C-section	cesarean section
CSF	cerebrospinal fluid
CT (CAT)	computed (axial) tomography
CVA	cerebrovascular accident
CVP	central venous pressure
CVS	chorionic villus sampling
D&C	dilation and curettage
DM	diabetes mellitus (diastolic murmur)
DMD	Duchenne's muscular dystrophy
DNA	deoxyribonucleic acid
DNR	do not resuscitate
DOA	date of admission (dead on arrival)
DRG	diagnosis-related group
Dx	diagnosis
EBV	Epstein-Barr virus
ECF	extracellular fluid (extended care facility)
ECG (EKG)	electrocardiogram
EDV	end-diastolic volume
EEG	electroencephalogram
EFM	electronic fetal monitoring
EP	ectopic pregnancy
ER	endoplasmic reticulum

ERT	estrogen replacement therapy
ESR	erythrocyte sedimentation rate
ESRD	end-stage renal disease
ESV	end-systolic volume
FAS	fetal alcohol syndrome
FBG	fasting blood glucose
FOBT	fecal occult blood testing
FSH	follicle-stimulating hormone
FUO	fever of unknown origin
Fx	fracture
GB	gallbladder
GFR	glomerular filtration rate
GH	growth hormone
GI	gastrointestinal
HAV	hepatitis A virus
Hb	hemoglobin
HBV	hepatitis B virus
HCG	human chorionic gonadotropin
Hct	hematocrit
HCV	hepatitis C virus
HDL	high-density lipoprotein
HLA	human leukocyte antigen
HR	heart rate
HRT	hormone replacement therapy
HSV	herpes simplex virus
HTN	hypertension
Hx	history
IBD	inflammatory bowel disease
IBS	irritable bowel syndrome
ICF	intracellular fluid
ICP	intracranial pressure
ICU	intensive care unit
ID	intradermal
IDDM	insulin-dependent diabetes mellitus
Ig	immunoglobulin
IM	intramuscular
IV	intravenous
LA	left atrium
LDL	low-density lipoprotein
LH	luteinizing hormone
LLQ	left lower quadrant
LUQ	left upper quadrant
LV	left ventricle
mEq/L	milliequivalents per liter
MG	myasthenia gravis
MHC	major histocompatibility complex
MI	myocardial infarction
mL	milliliter
mm^3	cubic millimeter
mm Hg	millimeters of mercury
MRI	magnetic resonance imaging
MS	multiple sclerosis
MSOF	multisystem organ failure
MVP	mitral valve prolapse
NGU	non-gonococcal urethritis
NIDDM	non-insulin-dependent diabetes mellitus
NPN	non-protein nitrogen
OC	oral contraceptive
OTC	over the counter
PE	pulmonary embolism
PET	positron emission tomography
PG	prostaglandin
PID	pelvic inflammatory disease
PKU	phenylketonuria
PMN	polymorphonuclear leukocyte
PMS	premenstrual syndrome
PNS	peripheral nervous system
PT	prothrombin time (patient, patient teaching, physical therapy)
PTH	parathyroid hormone
PTT	partial thromboplastin time
PVC	premature ventricular contraction
RA	right atrium
RBC	red blood cell
RBM	red bone marrow
RDA	recommended daily allowance
RDS	respiratory distress syndrome
REM	rapid eye movement
RE(S)	reticuloendothelial (system)
Rh	*Rhesus*
RIA	radioimmunoassay
RLQ	right lower quadrant
RNA	ribonucleic acid
RUQ	right upper quadrant
RV	right ventricle
Rx	prescription

SA	sinoatrial
SaO_2	oxygen-hemoglobin saturation
SC	subcutaneous
SCID	severe combined immunodeficiency
SF	synovial fluid
SIDS	sudden infant death syndrome
SLE	systemic lupus erythematosus
SPF	sun protection factor
S/S (sx)	signs and symptoms
STD	sexually transmitted disease
SV	stroke volume
T_3	triiodothyronine
T_4	thyroxine
TIA	transient ischemic attack
TMJ	temporomandibular joint
t-PA	tissue plasminogen activator
TPN	total parenteral nutrition
TSH	thyroid-stimulating hormone
TSS	toxic shock syndrome
Tx	treatment
UA	urinalysis
URI	upper respiratory infection
US	ultrasound
UTI	urinary tract infection
UV	ultraviolet
VPC	ventricular premature contraction
VD	venereal disease
VS	vital signs
WBC	white blood cell
WNL	within normal limits

APPENDIX C

Normal Values for Some Commonly Used Blood Tests

TEST	NORMAL VALUE	CLINICAL SIGNIFICANCE OF VARIATIONS
Albumin	3.5–5.5 g/100 mL	■ Decreases: kidney disease, severe burns
Bilirubin—Total	0.3–1.4 mg/100 mL	■ Increases: liver disease, rapid RBC destruction, biliary obstruction
Direct	0.1–0.4 mg/100 mL	
Indirect	0.2–1.0 mg/100 mL	
Calcium	4.3–5.3 mEq/L	■ Increases: hyperparathyroidism ■ Decreases: hypoparathyroidism, severe diarrhea, malnutrition
Chloride	95–108 mEq/L	■ Decreases: severe diarrhea, severe burns, ketoacidosis
Cholesterol	140–199 mg/100 mL	■ Increases: hypothyroidism, diabetes mellitus
HDL cholesterol	29–77 mg/100 mL	
LDL cholesterol	<130 mg/100 mL	
Clotting time	5–10 minutes	■ Increases: liver disease
Creatinine	0.6–1.5 mg/100 mL	■ Increases: kidney disease
Globulins	2.3–3.5 g/100 mL	■ Increases: chronic infections
Glucose	70–110 mg/100 mL	■ Increases: diabetes mellitus, liver disease, hyperthyroidism, pregnancy
Hematocrit	38%–48%	■ Increases: dehydration, polycythemia ■ Decreases: anemia, hemorrhage
Hemoglobin	12–18 g/100 mL	■ Increases: polycythemia, high altitude, chronic pulmonary disease ■ Decreases: anemia, hemorrhage
P_{CO_2}	35–45 mm Hg	■ Increases: pulmonary disease ■ Decreases: acidosis, diarrhea, kidney disease

Continued

TEST	NORMAL VALUE	CLINICAL SIGNIFICANCE OF VARIATIONS
pH	7.35–7.45	■ Increases: hyperventilation, metabolic alkalosis ■ Decreases: ketoacidosis, severe diarrhea, hypoventilation
Po_2	75–100 mm Hg	■ Decreases: anemia, pulmonary disease
Phosphorus	1.8–4.1 mEq/L	■ Increases: kidney disease, hypoparathyroidism ■ Decreases: hyperparathyroidism
Platelet count	150,000–300,000/μL	■ Decreases: leukemia, aplastic anemia
Potassium	3.5–5.0 mEq/L	■ Increases: severe cellular destruction ■ Decreases: diarrhea, kidney disease
Prothrombin time	11–15 seconds	■ Increases: liver disease, vitamin K deficiency
Red blood cell count	4.5–6.0 million/μL	■ Increases: polycythemia, dehydration ■ Decreases: anemia, hemorrhage, leukemia
Reticulocyte count	0.5%–1.5%	■ Increases: anemia, following hemorrhage
Sodium	136–142 mEq/L	■ Increases: dehydration ■ Decreases: kidney disease, diarrhea, severe burns
Urea nitrogen (BUN)	8–25 mg/100 mL	■ Increases: kidney disease, high-protein diet
Uric acid	3.0–7.0 mg/100 mL	■ Increases: kidney disease, gout, leukemia
White blood cell count	5,000–10,000/μL	■ Increases: acute infection, leukemia ■ Decreases: aplastic anemia, radiation sickness

APPENDIX D

Normal Values for Some Commonly Used Urine Tests

TEST	NORMAL VALUE	CLINICAL SIGNIFICANCE OF VARIATIONS
Acetone and acetoacetic acid (ketones)	0	■ Increases: ketoacidosis, starvation
Albumin	0–trace	■ Increases: kidney disease, hypertension
Bilirubin	0	■ Increases: biliary obstruction
Calcium	< 250 mg/24 hr	■ Increases: hyperparathyroidism ■ Decreases: hypoparathyroidism
Creatinine	1.0–2.0 g/24 hr	■ Increases: infection ■ Decreases: kidney disease, muscle atrophy
Glucose	0	■ Increases: diabetes mellitus
pH	4.5–8.0	■ Increases: urinary tract infection, alkalosis, vegetarian diet ■ Decreases: acidosis, starvation, high-protein diet
Protein	0	■ Increases: kidney disease, extensive trauma, hypertension
Specific gravity	1.010–1.025	■ Increases: dehydration ■ Decreases: excessive fluid intake, alcohol intake, severe kidney damage
Urea	25–35 g/24 hr	■ Increases: high-protein diet; excessive tissue breakdown ■ Decreases: kidney disease
Uric acid	0.4–1.0 g/24 hr	■ Increases: gout, liver disease ■ Decreases: kidney disease
Urobilinogen	0–4 mg/24 hr	■ Increases: liver disease, hemolytic anemia

APPENDIX E

Eponymous Terms

An eponym is a person for whom something is named, and an eponymous term is a term that uses that name or eponym. For example, *fallopian tube* is named for Gabriele Fallopio, an Italian anatomist of the 16th century.

In recent years it has been suggested that eponymous terms be avoided because they are not descriptive and that they be replaced with more informative terms. Such changes, however, occur slowly, because the older terms are so familiar to those of us who teach. Some of us may even use them as opportunities to impart a little history, also known as "telling stories."

In this edition, the most familiar eponymous terms have been retained, with the newer term in parentheses after the first usages. The list below is provided to show the extent of reclassification of eponymous terms as related to basic anatomy and physiology.

Eponymous Term	New Term
Achilles reflex	plantar reflex
Achilles tendon	calcaneal tendon
Adam's apple	thyroid cartilage
ampulla of Vater	hepatopancreatic ampulla
aqueduct of Sylvius	cerebral aqueduct
Auerbach's plexus	myenteric plexus
Bartholin's glands	greater vestibular glands
Bowman's capsule	glomerular capsule
Broca's area	Broca's speech area
Brunner's glands	duodenal submucosal glands
bundle of His	atrioventricular bundle
canal of Schlemm	scleral venous sinus
circle of Willis	cerebral arterial circle
Cowper's glands	bulbourethral glands
crypts of Lieberkuhn	intestinal glands
duct of Santorini	accessory pancreatic duct
duct of Wirsung	pancreatic duct
eustachian tube	auditory tube
fallopian tube	uterine tube
fissure of Rolando	central sulcus
fissure of Sylvius	lateral cerebral sulcus
graafian follicle	vesicular ovarian follicle
Graves' disease	hyperthyroidism
haversian canal	central canal
haversian system	osteon
Heimlich maneuver	abdominal thrust maneuver

Eponymous Term	New Term
islet of Langerhans	pancreatic islet
Krebs cycle	citric acid cycle
Kupffer cells	stellate reticuloendothelial cells
Langerhans cell	non-pigmented granular dendrocyte
Leydig cells	interstitial cells
loop of Henle	loop of the nephron
Meissner's corpuscles	tactile corpuscles
Meissner's plexus	submucosal plexus
nodes of Ranvier	neurofibril nodes
organ of Corti	spiral organ
Pacinian corpuscle	lamellated corpuscle
Peyer's patches	aggregated lymph nodules
Purkinje fibers	cardiac conducting myofibers
Schwann cell	neurolemmocyte
Sertoli cells	sustentacular cells
sphincter of Boyden	sphincter of the common bile duct
sphincter of Oddi	sphincter of the hepatopancreatic ampulla
Stensen's ducts	parotid ducts
Volkmann's canal	perforating canal, nutrient canal
Wernicke's area	posterior speech area
Wharton's duct	submandibular duct
Wormian bone	sutural bone

APPENDIX F

Prefixes, Combining Word Roots, and Suffixes Used in Medical Terminology

PREFIXES AND COMBINING WORD ROOTS

a-, an- absent, without (amenorrhea: absence of menstruation)
ab- away from (abduct: move away from the midline)
abdomin/o- abdomen (abdominal aorta: the portion of the aorta in the abdomen)
acou- hearing (acoustic nerve: the cranial nerve for hearing)
ad- toward, near, to (adduct: move toward the midline)
aden/o- gland (adenohypophysis: the glandular part of the pituitary gland)
af- to, toward (afferent: toward a center)
alba- white (albino: an animal lacking coloration)
alg- pain (myalgia: muscle pain)
ana- up, back (anabolism: the constructive phase of metabolism)
angi/o- vessel (angiogram: imaging of blood vessels, as in the heart)
ante- before (antenatal: before birth)
anti- against (antiemetic: an agent that prevents vomiting)
arthr/o- joint (arthritis: inflammation of a joint)
atel- imperfect, incomplete (atelectasis: incomplete expansion of a lung)
auto- self (autoimmune disease: a disease in which immune reactions are directed against part of one's own body)
bi- two, twice (biconcave: concave on each side, as a red blood cell)
bio- life (biochemistry: the chemistry of living organisms)
blasto- growth, budding (blastocyst: a rapidly growing embryonic stage)
brachi/o- arm (brachial artery: the artery that passes through the upper arm)
brachy- short (brachydactyly: abnormally short fingers or toes)
brady- slow (bradycardia: slow heart rate)
bronch- air passage (bronchioles: small air passages in the lungs)
carcin/o- cancer (carcinogen: cancer-causing substance)
cardi/o- heart (cardiopathy: heart disease)
carp/o- wrist (carpals: bones of the wrist)
cata- down (catabolism: the breaking down phase of metabolism)
caud- tail (cauda equina: the spinal nerves that hang below the end of the spinal cord and resemble a horse's tail)
celi/o- abdomen (celiac artery: a large artery that supplies abdominal organs)
cephal/o- head (cephaledema: swelling of the head)
cerebr/o- brain (cerebrum: the largest part of the human brain)
cervic- neck (cervical nerves: the spinal nerves from the neck portion of the spinal cord)
chem/o- chemical (chemotherapy: the use of chemicals to treat disease)
chondr/o- cartilage (chondrocyte: cartilage cell)
circum- around (circumoral: around the mouth)
co-, com- with, together (congenital: born with)
con-, contra- opposite, against (contraception: the prevention of conception)
cost/o- ribs (intercostal muscles: muscles between the ribs)
crani/o- skull, head (cranial nerves: the nerves that arise from the brain)
cut- skin (cutaneous: pertaining to the skin)
cyan/o- blue (cyanosis: bluish discoloration of the skin due to lack of oxygen)
cyst- bladder, sac (cystic duct: duct of the gallbladder)
cyt/o- cell (hepatocyte: cell of the liver)

dactyl/o- digits, fingers or toes (polydactyly: more than five fingers or toes)
de- down, from (dehydration: loss of water)
derm- skin (dermatologist: a specialist in diseases of the skin)
di- two, twice (disaccharide: a sugar made of two monosaccharides)
diplo- double (diplopia: double vision)
dis- apart, away from (dissect: to cut apart)
duct- lead, conduct (ductus arteriosus: a fetal artery)
dys- difficult, diseased (dyspnea: difficult breathing)
ecto- outside (ectoparasite: a parasite that lives on the body surface)
edem- swelling (edematous: affected with swelling)
endo- within (endocardium: the innermost layer of the heart wall)
enter/o- intestine (enterotoxin: a toxin that affects the intestine and causes diarrhea)
epi- on, over, upon (epidermis: the outer layer of the skin)
erythr/o- red (erythrocyte: red blood cell)
eu- normal, good (eupnea: normal breathing)
ex- out of (excise: to cut out or remove surgically)
exo- without, outside of (exophthalmia: protrusion of the eyeballs)
extra- outside of, in addition to, beyond (extraembryonic membranes: the membranes that surround the embryo-fetus)
fasci- band (fascia: a fibrous connective tissue membrane)
fore- before, in front (forehead: the front of the head)
gastro/o- stomach (gastric juice: the digestive secretions of the stomach lining)
gluco-, glyco- sugar (glycosuria: glucose in the urine)
gyn/o-, gyne/co- woman, female (gynecology: study of the female reproductive organs)
haplo- single, simple (haploid: a single set, as of chromosomes)
hema-, hemato-, hemo- blood (hemoglobin: the protein of red blood cells)
hemi- half (cerebral hemisphere: the right or left half of the cerebrum)
hepat/o- liver (hepatic duct: the duct that takes bile out of the liver)
hetero- different (heterozygous: having two different genes for a trait)
hist/o- tissue (histology: the study of tissues)
homeo- unchanged (homeostasis: the state of body stability)
homo- same (homozygous: having two similar genes for a trait)
hydr/o- water (hydrophobia: fear of water)
hyper- excessive, above (hyperglycemia: high blood glucose level)
hypo- beneath, under, deficient (hypodermic: below the skin)
idio- distinct, peculiar to the individual (idiopathic: of unknown cause, as a disease)
inter- between, among (interventricular septum: the wall between the ventricles of the heart)
intra- within (intracellular: within cells)
is/o- equal, the same (isothermal: having the same temperature)
kinesi/o- movement (kinesthetic sense: muscle sense)
labi- lip (herpes labialis: cold sores of the lips)
lacri- tears (lacrimal glands: tear-producing glands)
lact/o- milk (lactation: milk production)
leuc/o, leuk/o- white (leukocyte: white blood cell)
lip/o- fat (liposuction: removal of fat with a suctioning instrument)
macr/o- large (macromolecule: a large molecule such as a protein)
mal- poor, bad (malnutrition: poor nutrition)
medi- middle (mediastinum: a middle cavity, as in the chest)
mega- large (megacolon: abnormally dilated colon)
meta- next to, beyond (metatarsal: bone of the foot next to the ankle)
micr/o- small (microcephaly: small head)
mon/o- one (monozygotic twins: identical twins, from one egg)
morph/o- shape, form (amorphous: without definite shape)
multi- many (multicellular: made of many cells)
my/o- muscle (myocardium: heart muscle)
narco- sleep (narcotic: a drug that produces sleep)
nat/a- birth (neonate: a newborn infant)
neo- new (neoplasty: surgical restoration of parts)
nephr/o- kidney (nephrectomy: removal of a kidney)
neur/o- nerve (neuron: nerve cell)
non- not (non-communicable: unable to spread)
ocul/o- eye (oculomotor nerve: a cranial nerve for eye movement)
olig/o- few, scanty (oliguria: diminished amount of urine)
oo- egg (oogenesis: production of an egg cell)
ophthalmo- eye (ophthalmoscope: instrument to examine the eye)
orth/o- straight, normal, correct (orthostatic: related to standing upright)
oste/o- bone (osteocyte: bone cell)
ot/o- ear (otitis media: inflammation of the middle ear)

ovi-, ovo- egg (oviduct: duct for passage of an egg cell, fallopian tube)
path/o- disease (pathology: the study of disease)
ped/ia- child (pediatric: concerning the care of children)
per- through (permeate: to pass through)
peri- around (pericardium: membranes that surround the heart)
phag/o- eat (phagocyte: a cell that engulfs particulate matter)
phleb/o- vein (phlebitis: inflammation of a vein)
pleuro-, pleura- rib (pleurisy: inflammation of the pleural membranes of the chest cavity)
pneumo- lung (pneumonia: lung infection)
pod- foot (pseudopod: false foot, as in ameboid movement)
poly- many (polysaccharide: a carbohydrate made of many monosaccharides)
post- after (postpartum: after delivery of a baby)
pre- before (precancerous: a growth that probably will become malignant)
pro- before, in front of (progeria: premature old age, before its time)
pseudo- false (pseudomembrane: false membrane)
py/o- pus (pyogenic: pus producing)
pyel/o- renal pelvis (pyelogram: an x-ray of the renal pelvis and ureter)
quadr/i- four (quadriceps femoris: a thigh muscle with four parts)
retro- behind, backward (retroperitoneal: located behind the peritoneum)
rhin/o- nose (rhinoviruses that cause the common cold)
salping/o- fallopian tube (salpingitis: inflammation of a fallopian tube)
sarc/o- flesh, muscle (sarcolemma: membrane of a muscle cell)
sclero- hard (sclerosis: deterioration of tissue with loss of function)
semi- half (semilunar valve: a valve shaped like a half-moon)
steno- narrow (aortic stenosis: narrowing of the aorta)
sub- below, beneath (subcutaneous: below the skin)
supra- above (suprarenal gland: gland above the kidney, the adrenal gland)
sym- together (symphysis: a joint where two bones meet)
syn- together (synapse: the space between two nerve cells)
tachy- fast (tachycardia: rapid heart rate)
thorac/o- chest (thoracic cavity: chest cavity)
thromb/o- clot (thrombosis: formation of a blood clot)
tox- poison (toxicology: the study of poisons)
trans- across (transmural: across the wall of an organ)
tri- three (trigone: a three-sided area on the floor of the urinary bladder)
ultra- excessive, extreme (ultrasonic: sound waves beyond the normal hearing range)
un/i- one (unicellular: made of one cell)
uria-, uro- urine (urinary calculi: stones in the urine)
vas/o- vessel (vasodilation: dilation of a blood vessel)
viscera-, viscero- organ (visceral pleura: the pleural membrane that covers the lungs)

SUFFIXES

-ac pertaining to (cardiac: pertaining to the heart)
-al pertaining to (intestinal: pertaining to the intestine)
-an, -ian characteristic of, pertaining to, belonging to (ovarian cyst: a cyst of the ovary)
-ar relating to (muscular: relating to muscles)
-ary relating to, connected with (salivary: relating to saliva)
-ase enzyme (sucrase: an enzyme that digests sucrose)
-atresia abnormal closure (biliary atresia: closure or absence of bile ducts)
-blast grow, produce (osteoblast: a bone-producing cell)
-cele swelling, tumor (meningocele: a hernia of the meninges)
-centesis puncture of a cavity (thoracocentesis: puncture of the chest cavity to remove fluid)
-cide kill (bactericide: a chemical that kills bacteria)
-clast destroy, break down (osteoclast: a bone-reabsorbing cell)
-desis binding, stabilizing, fusion (arthrodesis: the surgical immobilization of a joint)
-dipsia thirst (polydipsia: excessive thirst)
-dynia pain (gastrodynia: stomach pain)
-ectasia, -ectasis expansion (atelectasis: without expansion)
-ectomy excision, cutting out (thyroidectomy: removal of the thyroid)
-emia pertaining to blood (hypokalemia: low blood potassium level)
-form structure (spongiform: resembling a sponge)
-gen producing (carcinogen: a substance that produces cancer)
-genesis production of, origin of (spermatogenesis: production of sperm)
-globin protein (myoglobin: a muscle protein)
-gram record, writing (electroencephalogram: a record of the electrical activity of the brain)
-graph an instrument for making records (ultrasonography: the use of ultrasound to produce an image)
-ia condition (pneumonia: condition of inflammation of the lungs)

-iasis diseased condition (cholelithiasis: gallstones)
-ic pertaining to (atomic: pertaining to atoms)
-ile having qualities of (febrile: feverish)
-ism condition, process (alcoholism: condition of being dependent on alcohol)
-ist practitioner, specialist (neurologist: a specialist in diseases of the nervous system)
-itis inflammation (hepatitis: inflammation of the liver)
-lepsy seizure (narcolepsy: a sudden onset of sleep)
-lith stone, crystal (otoliths: stones in the inner ear)
-logy study of (virology: the study of viruses)
-lysis break down (hemolysis: rupture of red blood cells)
-megaly enlargement (splenomegaly: enlargement of the spleen)
-meter a measuring instrument (spirometer: an instrument to measure pulmonary volumes)
-ness state of, quality (illness: state of being ill)
-oid the appearance of (ovoid: resembling an oval or egg)
-ole small, little (arteriole: small artery)
-oma tumor (carcinoma: malignant tumor)
-opia eye (hyperopia: farsightedness)
-ory pertaining to (regulatory: pertaining to regulation)
-ose having qualities of (comatose: having qualities of a coma)
-osis state, condition, action, process (keratosis: abnormal growth of the skin)
-ostomy creation of an opening (colostomy: creation of an opening between the intestine and the abdominal wall)
-otomy cut into (tracheotomy: cut into the trachea)
-ous pertaining to (nervous: pertaining to nerves)
-pathy disease (retinopathy: disease of the retina)
-penia lack of, deficiency (leukopenia: lack of white blood cells)
-philia love of, tendency (hemophilia: a clotting disorder; "love of blood")
-phobia an abnormal fear (acrophobia: fear of heights)
-plasia growth (hyperplasia: excessive growth)
-plasty formation, repair (rhinoplasty: plastic surgery on the nose)
-plegia paralysis (hemiplegia: paralysis of the right or left half of the body)
-poiesis production (erythropoiesis: production of red blood cells)
-ptosis dropping, falling (hysteroptosis: falling of the uterus)
-rrhage burst forth (hemorrhage: loss of blood from blood vessels)
-rrhea discharge, flow (diarrhea: frequent discharge of feces)
-scope instrument to examine (microscope: instrument to examine small objects)
-spasm involuntary contraction (blepharospasm: twitch of the eyelid)
-stasis to be still, control, stop (hemostasis: to stop loss of blood)
-sthenia strength (myasthenia: loss of muscle strength)
-stomy surgical opening (colostomy: a surgical opening in the colon)
-taxia muscle coordination (ataxia: loss of coordination)
-tension pressure (hypertension: high blood pressure)
-tic pertaining to (paralytic: pertaining to paralysis)
-tomy incision, cut into (phlebotomy: incision into a vein)
-tripsy crush (lithotripsy: crushing of stone such as gallstones)
-trophic related to nutrition or growth (autotrophic: capable of making its own food, such as a green plant)
-tropic turning toward (chemotropic: turning toward a chemical)
-ula, -ule small, little (venule: small vein)
-uria urine (hematuria: blood in the urine)
-y condition, process (healthy: condition of health)

APPENDIX G

Answers to Illustration Questions

CHAPTER 1

1-1: The circulatory system works directly with the urinary system. Notice the red artery and blue vein entering the left kidney.

1-2: See Table 1–1.

1-3: For the negative feedback mechanism, the brake is in the cycle itself: the rise in metabolic rate that inhibits the hypothalamus and pituitary gland. For the positive feedback mechanism, the brake is outside the cycle: the white blood cells destroying the bacteria.

1-4: The femoral area contains the femur, the patellar area the patella, the frontal area the frontal bone, the temporal area the temporal bone; there are others.

1-5: The cranial, vertebral (spinal), and thoracic cavities are surrounded by bone. (Let's go a step further: Name the organs in these cavities that are protected by bone.)

1-6: Any tubular organ would have similar sections: an artery, a vein, the esophagus, or the trachea.

1-7: The small and large intestines are in all four quadrants.

CHAPTER 2

2-1: The charge of this atom is neutral because the number of protons equals the number of electrons (all atoms are neutral).

2-2: The sodium ion has 10 electrons (it lost one) but still has 11 protons; therefore, it has a charge of +1.

2-3: The bond of the oxygen molecule is a double covalent bond: two pairs of shared electrons. (Let's go a step further: Which atom is able to form four covalent bonds?)

2-4: Plasma, tissue fluid, and lymph are extracellular fluids.

2-5: The pH range of blood is very narrow and slightly alkaline. The pH range of urine is much greater, from slightly alkaline to moderately acidic.

2-6: The chemical formula for glucose is $C_6H_{12}O_6$. (A step further: What is a disaccharide made of? A polysaccharide?)

2-7: A diglyceride consists of a glycerol with two fatty acid chains.

2-8: Myoglobin contains iron; iron enables myoglobin to store oxygen. (This information was in Tables 2–2 and 2–5.)

2-9: Picture D; excess hydrogen ions would block the active site just as a heavy metal ion would.

2-10: Adenine paired with guanine would be too wide to fit between the uprights of the DNA ladder, and hydrogen bonds would not form between them. (A step further: State two structural differences between DNA and RNA.)

2-11: The energy from ATP may be used for cell division, for growth or repair, for movement, or for synthesis of new proteins or other molecules.

CHAPTER 3

3-1: The receptor site is probably a protein; a cell has many different protein receptor sites on its membrane.

3-2: Cilia project through the cell membrane and have an anchor inside; microvilli are folds of the cell membrane. (Let's go a step further: What are the functions of motile cilia and microvilli?)

3-3: Filtration depends on blood pressure. Phagocytosis depends on the movement of WBCs. (A step further: What does diffusion depend on, and what does active transport depend on?)

3-4: One tRNA attachment site bonds to a specific amino acid. The other site is the anticodon that will bond to a complementary codon on the mRNA.

3-5: A pair of identical chromatids is made of the original DNA molecule and its copy (which was synthesized during interphase). (A step further: When do the chromatids separate and become individual chromosomes?)

CHAPTER 4

4-1: Simple squamous epithelium is best for diffusion because it is the thinnest. (Let's go a step further: Where is simple squamous epithelium found?)

4-2: Stratified squamous epithelium and transitional epithelium are most similar structurally because both have several layers.

4-3: The cilia of the trachea sweep mucus and foreign material upward toward the pharynx.

4-4: The matrix of blood is plasma. Triglycerides are stored in adipocytes.

4-5: Collagen fibers are the matrix of fibrous CT; calcium salts and collagen fibers form the matrix of bone.

4-6: Skeletal muscle cells and cardiac muscle cells have striations, which result from the arrangement of the cells' contraction proteins. (A step further: Which type of muscle tissue may be called "voluntary"?)

4-7: The central neuron has eight processes, which look alike, but one would be an axon and the other seven dendrites. (A step further: Where is the nucleus of the neuron located?)

4-8: The mesentery covers the small and large intestines, the stomach, and the liver.

CHAPTER 5

5-1: Blood vessels are found in the dermis and subcutaneous tissue.

5-2: The Langerhans cell can pick up foreign material, such as a bacterium, and transport it to a lymph node. (Let's go a step further: What do melanocytes produce, and what is its function?)

5-3: A hair shaft is made of keratin. (A step further: What other human structures are made mostly of keratin?)

5-4: The nail bed consists of living layers of the epidermis and the dermis.

CHAPTER 6

6-1: The osteocytes are living cells and need a good blood supply, with oxygen and nutrients.

6-2: The frontal bone forms in two parts, which in the infant skull are still separate. The two parts will eventually grow together (with no suture).

6-3: In a closed epiphyseal disc, all of the cartilage has been replaced by bone. (Let's go a step further: Name the cells that produce bone, that reabsorb bone, and that maintain the bone matrix.)

6-4: The vertebrae and facial bones are irregular bones. (A step further: Name the other bone categories and give examples of each.)

6-5:
6-6: The openings at the back of the eye sockets permit passage of the optic nerve and blood vessels of the eye.

6-7: The foramen magnum is the opening through which the spinal cord merges with the brain.

6-8: The olfactory foramina are the openings for the olfactory nerves (sense of smell).

6-9: "Sinus headache" pain is usually from the frontal sinus and the maxillary sinuses.

6-10: The lumbar vertebra is larger and bulkier than the thoracic vertebra; the lumbar vertebrae support more weight. (A step further: What kind of joint is found between vertebrae?)

6-11: All of the ribs articulate posteriorly with the thoracic vertebrae.

6-12: The joints of the arm are (from the top): ball-and-socket joint at the shoulder, hinge joint at the elbow, pivot joint in the forearm, gliding joints at the wrist, hinge joints in the fingers, and a saddle joint at the base of the thumb.

6-13: The female pelvic inlet is much larger than the male pelvic inlet; this is an adaptation for childbirth.

6-14: There is no pivot joint between the tibia and fibula, and no saddle joint in the big toe.

6-15: The ball-and-socket joint is the most movable; the symphysis is the least movable.

6-16: These two bones are long bones because each has an epiphysis. Examples are the joints between phalanges or between the femur and tibia.

CHAPTER 7

7-1: When a muscle contracts it shortens and exerts a pulling force.

7-2: The fitting of an acetylcholine molecule into an ACh receptor opens a sodium channel in the sarcolemma. (Let's go a step further: What causes a motor neuron to release acetylcholine?)

7-3: The unit of contraction of skeletal muscle is a sarcomere, shown in part D. (A step further: Name the contracting proteins in a sarcomere.)

7-4: Sodium ions enter the cell during depolarization; potassium ions leave the cell during repolarization.

7-5: The myosin filaments pull the actin filaments toward the center of the sarcomere. (A step further: Name the proteins that inhibit the sliding of myosin and actin, as well as the ion that takes them out of the way.)

7-6: The muscular, circulatory, respiratory, and integumentary systems all respond to exercise.

7-7: Crossing the arm in front of the chest is flexion of the arm.

7-8: Shape: trapezius (trapezoid), deltoid (the Greek letter delta)

Size: pectoralis major, gluteus maximus

Location: rectus abdominis, biceps brachii, latissimus dorsi

A bone: tibialis anterior, biceps femoris, sternocleidomastoid, brachioradialis

Function: adductor longus

7-9: Both orbicularis muscles are circular muscles that regulate the size of an opening.

7-10: The pectoralis major, latissimus dorsi, and teres major all move the arm. They are on the trunk because the sternum and vertebrae provide strong anchors (origins).

7-11: Flexor muscles of the fingers are on the anterior side of the forearm. You knew because of the names *flexor* and *digitorum*, or you followed the tendons from the fingers and saw that they led to these muscles.

7-12: The gastrocnemius is much larger than the tibialis anterior. The gastrocnemius extends the foot, as when standing on tiptoes or pushing off to walk. In either case, it must be strong enough (large enough) to support the entire body.

7-13: The muscles of the female pelvic floor support the urinary bladder and uterus.

CHAPTER 8

8-1: The axon terminal of the motor neuron would be found at muscle tissues and glands.

Table Fig. 8–A: The oligodendrocytes produce the myelin sheath for CNS neurons, as do the Schwann cells for PNS neurons.

8-2: This is an excitatory synapse because sodium ions enter the postsynaptic neuron, causing depolarization. At an inhibitory synapse, potassium ions leave the postsynaptic neuron, causing hyperpolarization.

8-3: An ascending tract carries sensory impulses to the brain; a descending tract carries motor impulses from the brain. (Let's go a step further: Where are the cell bodies of sensory and motor neurons located?)

8-4: The spinal cord ends between the first and second lumbar vertebrae. This is important for a lumbar puncture: The needle must be inserted into the meningeal sac below the end of the spinal cord.

8-5: The receptor is a stretch receptor, and the muscle that is stretched contracts.

8-6: The corpus callosum connects the cerebral hemispheres, so that each knows what the other is doing. It is a flat though slightly arched band of nerve fibers (white matter) extending left and right. (A step further: What parts of a neuron make up white matter?)

8-7: A lateral ventricle extends from the frontal lobe back through the parietal and occipital lobes, and forward and down into the temporal lobe.

8-8: The general sensory area in the parietal lobe feels and interprets the cutaneous senses and muscle sense.

8-9: The spinal dura mater is a single layer. The cranial dura mater is a double layer, and at intervals it contains the cranial venous sinuses.

8-10: Cerebrospinal fluid is reabsorbed from the cranial subarachnoid space, through the arachnoid villi, into the blood in the cranial venous sinuses. (A step further: Why is CSF considered tissue fluid?)

8-11: Secretion of saliva is mediated by the facial and glossopharyngeal nerves; gastrointestinal secretions are mediated by the vagus nerves.

8-12: The parasympathetic neuron emerges from the brain stem (if you said "medulla," bonus points for you) and is part of the vagus (10th cranial) nerve.

8-13: Both ANS divisions supply the heart and have opposite functions. Sympathetic impulses increase the heart rate, and parasympathetic impulses decrease the rate.

CHAPTER 9

9-1: Most cutaneous receptors are in the dermis; some are in subcutaneous tissue. (Let's go a step further: Which cutaneous receptors are free nerve endings, and which are encapsulated nerve endings?)

9-2: Visceral pain may be referred to a limb from the heart, kidney, and urinary bladder in particular, and to a lesser extent from the esophagus or liver-gallbladder.

9-3: The air we inhale (with vapor molecules) goes down the pharynx and passes the back of the tongue (with taste buds).

9-4: Tears end up in the nasal cavities.

9-5: The inferior rectus muscle pulls the eyeball downward, as if you were looking at the floor.

9-6: The iris changes the size of the pupil. (A step further: Which set of iris muscles constricts the pupil and which dilates it? One more step: Which nerves are involved? Think ANS.)

9-7: The ganglion neurons form the optic nerve. The rods and cones are the photoreceptors.

9-8: If the right visual area were to become nonfunctional, the left half of the visual field would no longer be perceived.

9-9: The first structure to vibrate is the tympanic membrane, and second is the malleus. (A step further: Be sure you can complete the pathway of vibrations for hearing.)

9-10: The vibrations of the sound waves cause the round window to bulge out, preventing damaging pressure in the cochlea.

9-11: The canals and cochlear duct contain fluid. The receptors are the hair cells below the tectorial membrane. (A step further: Name the cranial nerve and lobe of the cerebral cortex concerned with hearing.)

9-12: In part A: Gravity pulls on the otoliths and bends the hair cells. In part B: Movement of the head causes the hair cells to sway. (A step further: Name the cranial nerve and parts of the brain concerned with equilibrium.)

CHAPTER 10

10-1: The thyroid hormones are carried by the blood throughout the body (true of all hormones) to their target organs.

10-2: ACTH, TSH, FSH, and LH all affect other endocrine glands.

10-3: In part A: ADH and oxytocin are stored in the posterior pituitary. In part B: Releasing hormones from the hypothalamus stimulate secretion of anterior pituitary hormones. (Let's go a step further: What kind of feedback mechanism stimulates the anterior pituitary gland?)

10-4: Growth hormone increases mitosis and protein synthesis, both of which directly contribute to growth.

10-5: Both the increase in protein synthesis and the production of energy from all types of foods contribute to growth and maintenance of bones and muscles. (These functions of thyroxine and T_3 are necessary for other organs as well.)

10-6: Calcitonin promotes calcium retention in bones. PTH contributes to the activation of vitamin D in the kidneys. (A step further: What is the stimulus for secretion of each of these hormones?)

10-7: Bones are a reservoir for calcium.

10-8: Insulin enables cells to take in glucose. The stimulus for insulin secretion is hyperglycemia, such as after a meal.

10-9: Epinephrine causes vasodilation and increases cell respiration in skeletal muscles; norepinephrine causes vasoconstriction. (A step further: How does epinephrine increase blood pressure?)

10-10: Aldosterone directly increases the reabsorption of sodium ions and the excretion of potassium ions by the kidneys. (A step further: What are the indirect effects of these functions of aldosterone?)

10-11: Under the stimulus of cortisol, most tissues will use fats and excess amino acids for energy production, and glucose will be stored as glycogen in the liver.

10-12: A target cell must have a specific receptor for the hormone, either in the cell membrane (protein hormones) or in the cytoplasm (steroid hormones).

CHAPTER 11

11-1: Blood plasma is mostly water (91.5%); RBCs are the most numerous cells.

11-2: Normoblasts and reticulocytes are usually found in the red bone marrow because they are immature stages of RBC development. (Let's go a step further: Which cell shown here is an immature WBC?)

11-3: The center of an RBC is pale because it is thinner than the edge; this is where the nucleus was.

11-4: Iron and amino acids are recycled; the heme of the hemoglobin is excreted as bilirubin. (A step further: Where can iron be stored?)

11-5: Answers will vary, but if you are type O you can donate to types A, B, and AB, as well as type O. If you are type A you can donate to type A or AB, and so on.

11-6: The diameter of the arteriole is much larger than that of the capillary, and platelet plugs would be washed away before they could cover the opening. Once a fibrin mesh forms, the platelets are trapped, as are RBCs. (A step further: What other mechanism of hemostasis also works in arterioles, and why?)

11-7: The liver is a vital organ because it produces many of the protein clotting factors.

CHAPTER 12

12-1: Intercalated discs are folds of the cell membrane, as are microvilli, and their general purpose is the same: to increase surface area.

12-2: Serous fluid is found between the serous pericardial layers; it prevents friction as the heart beats.

12-3: The blue arrows represent blood that is low in oxygen, returning to the RA from the body by way of the caval veins. (Let's go a step further: What do the red arrows in the left atrium represent?)

12-4: The mitral and tricuspid valves close when the ventricles contract, to prevent backflow of blood from the ventricles to the atria. (A step further: When do the arterial semilunar valves close, and why is this important?)

12-5: The coronary vessels circulate blood throughout the myocardium.

12-6: The onset of ventricular contraction (systole) makes the AV valves close and the semilunar valves open.

12-7: The SA node is the pacemaker of the heart; it depolarizes 60 to 80 times per minute, that is, the normal resting heart rate. (A step further: Define bradycardia and tachycardia.)

12-8: Sympathetic impulses increase the heart rate and force of contraction. (A step further: Name the parasympathetic nerves to the heart, and name their neurotransmitter.)

CHAPTER 13

13-1: The tunica media is made of smooth muscle and is thicker in an artery because it is needed to help regulate blood pressure. (Let's go a step further: What structure found in veins is not found in arteries, and why not?)

13-2: The highest pressure is BP at the arterial end of the capillary network; it brings about the process of filtration. (A step further: By what process are gases exchanged?)

13-3: Many possible answers. For bones: radial, ulnar, femoral, tibial, iliac, subclavian, occipital. For organs: renal, celiac, hepatic, splenic.

13-4: Many possible answers: subclavian, axillary, brachial, iliac, femoral, popliteal, tibial, renal, splenic, intercostal.

13-5: The internal jugular vein is the counterpart of the common carotid artery.

13-6: The brain is always active and needs a large supply of blood.

13-7: The blood in the portal vein is going to the liver. The blood is coming from the capillaries of the digestive organs and spleen.

13-8: Blood flows through the foramen ovale from the RA to the LA, to bypass the fetal lungs. (A step further: What other fetal structure helps blood bypass the fetal lungs?)

13-9: As cross-sectional area increases, velocity of blood flow decreases. Blood velocity is slowest in the capillaries. (A step further: Why is this slow flow important?)

13-10: Aldosterone increases the reabsorption of sodium ions by the kidneys and ANP increases the excretion of sodium ions. In both cases water follows sodium to increase (aldosterone) or decrease (ANP) blood volume and BP.

13-11: The skeletal muscles have the greatest increase in blood flow, followed by the skin and heart. The GI tract and kidneys have the greatest decrease.

13-12: The kidneys produce renin when BP decreases. Angiotensin II causes vasoconstriction and increases the secretion of aldosterone.

13-13: Changes in BP are the sensory information used to keep BP within normal limits. The pressoreceptors are located in the carotid and aortic sinuses.

CHAPTER 14

14-1: Lymph is returned to the subclavian veins. Return of lymph to the blood is important to maintain normal blood volume and BP.

14-2: Before becoming lymph, the water is tissue fluid.

14-3: Major paired groups of lymph nodes are the cervical, axillary, and inguinal. (Let's go a step further: Why are these locations so important?)

14-4: Plasma cells produce antibodies.

14-5: T cells (T lymphocytes) mature in the thymus.

14-6: There are many connections. Lysozyme is a chemical, yet is found in some mucous membranes; defensins are chemicals produced by the epidermis. WBCs are part of each aspect: barriers, cells, and chemicals. Langerhans cells are part of the epidermis but are mobile.

14-7: Basophils and mast cells are part of subcutaneous tissue and produce histamine and leukotrienes that contribute to inflammation.

14-8: Memory B cells and T cells provide memory; each cell remembers one specific foreign antigen.

14-9: The attached antibodies change the shape of the toxin, and it cannot fit where it might produce harmful effects. (A step further: What happens to a virus?)

14-10: After a second exposure, IgG production is faster and in greater quantity. (A step further: Explain how a vaccine could be part of this illustration.)

CHAPTER 15

15-1: The conchae resemble curled shelves or scrolls; they increase the surface area of the nasal mucosa. (Let's go a step further: What are the functions of the nasal mucosa?)

15-2: The epiglottis covers the larynx during swallowing, like a lid or trap door.

15-3: Exhaled air makes the vocal cords vibrate.

15-4: The right and left primary bronchi have C-shaped cartilages to keep them open, and they are lined with ciliated epithelium.

15-5: The cell of the alveolus and the cell of the capillary are part of the respiratory membrane. Alveolar type II cells secrete pulmonary surfactant. Alveolar macrophages phagocytize pathogens and dust.

15-6: During a normal exhalation, the diaphragm and external intercostal muscles are relaxing (not contracting as they do for inhalation). (A step further: Which muscles are involved in a forced exhalation?)

15-7: Tidal volume + inspiratory reserve + expiratory reserve = vital capacity. Residual volume cannot be measured with a spirometer. (A step further: Why is residual volume important?)

15-8: In external respiration, oxygen moves from the air in the alveoli to the blood in the pulmonary capillaries. In internal respiration, CO_2 moves from the tissues (cells) to the blood in the systemic capillaries.

15-9: The inspiratory center in the medulla directly stimulates inhalation: The red arrows go directly from the center to the respiratory muscles. (A step further: What other part of the brain contains respiratory centers?)

15-10: Increased rate and depth of breathing will correct both imbalances, by taking in more O_2 or exhaling more CO_2.

CHAPTER 16

16-1: Digestion takes place in the oral cavity, stomach, and small intestine.

16-2: The pulp cavity (with blood vessels and nerves) and the dentin (similar to bone) are living. Another way of knowing that parts of a tooth are living is that a cavity that has eroded through the enamel causes pain.

16-3: The salivary glands are exocrine glands because they have ducts. Saliva is made *from* blood plasma. (Let's go a step further: What is saliva made *of*?)

Table Fig. 16–A: Start at the protein box and follow the arrows backward to the stomach, pancreas, and small intestine. (A step further: Be sure you can do the same for carbohydrates and fats.)

16-4: The external muscle layer contracts locally for mechanical digestion and in waves for peristalsis.

16-5: The pyloric sphincter prevents backup of food from the duodenum to the stomach.

16-6: Blood flows from the hepatic artery and portal vein through the sinusoids to the central vein of the lobule and to the hepatic vein. (A step further: What is found in the blood from the portal vein?)

16-7: The acini secrete the pancreatic enzymes and bicarbonates.

16-8: The villi increase the surface area for the absorption of end products of digestion, as do the microvilli and plica circulares.

16-9: The ileocecal valve prevents backflow of fecal material from the cecum to the ileum.

16-10: The internal anal sphincter is a continuation of the circular muscle layer of the rectum.

CHAPTER 17

17-1: The cooling responses occur because the body temperature is higher than that of the hypothalamic thermostat; the fever has broken.

17-2: Most of us would probably survive a range of 88° to 105°F (31° to 41°C).

17-3: If you follow the arrows from all of the end products of digestion, you will see that they converge at pyruvic acid and acetyl CoA.

17-4: No. Only amino acids in the diet (or from transamination) can be used to synthesize proteins. Notice that no other arrows go to proteins.

17-5: The one on the right has more surface area in proportion to weight. Or put another way: a small interior with a large surface—which would be true for an infant.

CHAPTER 18

18-1: You can see that the left renal artery is short (so is the right one) and is a direct branch of the abdominal aorta, where BP is relatively high because it is close to the left ventricle.

18-2: Renal corpuscles and convoluted tubules are found in the renal cortex. The renal cortex and medulla have blood vessels (the renal pelvis is a space).

18-3: The podocyte's many "feet" contribute to the filter for blood. The lining of the proximal convoluted tubule has microvilli, which increase the surface area for reabsorption. (Let's go a step further: What is meant by a threshold level for reabsorption?)

18-4: Tubular secretion takes place from the blood in the peritubular capillaries to the filtrate in the renal tubule. Hydrogen ions, creatinine, and ammonia are secreted, as are the metabolic products of medications.

18-5: Aldosterone affects both: It increases the reabsorption of sodium ions and the excretion of potassium ions.

18-6: Carbon dioxide is used to make carbonic acid, which then yields a hydrogen ion to be excreted and a bicarbonate ion to be retained.

18-7: The internal urethral sphincter is involuntary; the external urethral sphincter is voluntary. (A step further: What kind of muscle tissue is the detrusor muscle, and is it voluntary or involuntary?)

CHAPTER 19

19-1: Cerebrospinal fluid and aqueous humor are the tissue fluid of the CNS and eye, respectively.

19-2: On a hot day urine volume might decrease and sweat volume might increase. Loss of water vapor in exhaled air might also increase.

19-3: Tissue fluid is most like blood plasma, and you knew this because you knew that tissue fluid is made directly from plasma by filtration, a process that would not greatly affect electrolytes.

19-4: A kidney tubule cell obtains a hydrogen ion from the reaction of carbon dioxide and water to form carbonic acid, which ionizes (also yielding a bicarbonate ion to be retained).

19-5: The compensations on the right are red because they are acidifying mechanisms to counteract increased alkalinity. Those on the left are blue because they are alkalizing mechanisms to counteract increased acidity.

CHAPTER 20

20-1: The 23 chromosomes are found in the head of the sperm.

20-2: The secondary oocyte completes meiosis when (if) the ovum is fertilized.

20-3: The ductus deferens carries sperm from the epididymis to the urethra.

20-4: Seminiferous tubule (site of formation) to the rete testis to the epididymis to the ductus deferens. (Let's go a step further: What is the function of the interstitial cells and the sustentacular cells of the testis?)

20-5: The uterus is above the urinary bladder, and during pregnancy it will not displace the bladder (though it will compress the bladder).

20-6: The myometrium is thicker in this view; it is made of smooth muscle. (A step further: Which uterine layer regularly changes in thickness?)

20-7: The labia cover the urethral and vaginal openings to prevent drying of their mucous membranes.

20-8: Prolactin stimulates milk production and oxytocin stimulates release of milk. (A step further: Which hormones contribute to the growth of the mammary glands?)

20-9: LH triggers ovulation, and then transforms the ruptured follicle into the corpus luteum. (A step further: Which hormones are secreted by the corpus luteum?)

CHAPTER 21

21-1: The father, because the sperm cell will have either an X or a Y chromosome. (The egg cell will always have an X chromosome.)

21-2: The inner cell mass will become the embryo; it is made of embryonic stem cells.

21-3: The chorionic villi will become the fetal portion of the placenta. (Let's go a step further: Which cells are first produced by the yolk sac?)

21-4: The amniotic fluid is a cushion or shock absorber for the fetus.

21-5: Oxygen and nutrients move from maternal to fetal blood.

21-6: The head of a fetus is the largest part, so if the head emerges first from the birth canal, the limbs are usually in position to emerge easily.

21-7: With Bb and bb for the parents, the four possibilities are Bb, Bb, bb, and bb.

21-8: No. With Hh and HH for the parents, the four possibilities are HH, HH, Hh, and Hh.

21-9: Yes. With AB and AO for the parents, the four possibilities are AA, AO, AB, and BO. A child may have type B blood.

21-10: With XcY and XX for the parents, the two possibilities for daughters are XcX and XcX; any daughter will be a carrier. The two possibilities for sons are XY and XY; any son will have normal color vision.

CHAPTER 22

22-1: The eyes; tears are an unlikely (though we cannot say impossible) portal of exit.

22-2: The blue and pink colors indicate the Gram reaction, positive or negative. Spirilla are neither color because they do not stain with the Gram method.

22-3: The two parts of a virus are the protein shell (capsid) and the internal nucleic acid (in this case RNA).

22-4: *Rhizopus, Aspergillus,* and ringworm have mycelia, masses of threadlike hyphae.

22-5: *Entamoeba* and *Giardia* live in the digestive system of a host.

22-6: The human digestive system is home to these parasitic worms.

22-7: The mite and both ticks have eight legs (in all but the most immature forms) and are not insects, which have six legs.

PRONUNCIATION GUIDE

This pronunciation guide is intended to help you pronounce the words that appear in the Glossary. Although it is not a true phonetic key, it does help to suggest the necessary sounds by spelling the sounds of the syllables of frequently encountered words and then using these familiar combinations to "spell out" a pronunciation of the new word being defined in the Glossary.

VOWELS

Long vowel sounds: ay, ee, eye or igh, oh or ow, yoo

The sound spelled as ...	Is pronounced as it appears in ...
ay	a as in face
a	a as in atom
aw	au as in cause
	o as in frost
ah	o as in proper
ee	e as in beat
e	e as in ten
i	i as in it
u	u as in up

CONSONANTS

Consonants are pronounced just as they look, with *g* pronounced as it is in gone.

ACCENTS WITHIN WORDS

One accent: boldface capital letters

Two accents: primary accent is in boldface capital letters; secondary accent is in capital letters

A

Abdomen (**AB**-doh-men) Portion of the body between the diaphragm and the pelvis (Chapter 1).

Abdominal cavity (ab-**DAHM**-in-uhl **KAV**-i-tee) The body cavity inferior to the diaphragm and above the pelvic cavity (Chapter 1).

Abducens nerves (ab-**DEW**-senz) Cranial nerve pair VI. Motor to an extrinsic muscle of the eye (Chapter 8).

Abduction (ab-**DUK**-shun) Movement of a body part away from the midline of the body (Chapter 7).

ABO group (A-B-O GROOP) The red blood cell types determined by the presence or absence of A and B antigens on the red blood cell membrane; the four types are A, B, AB, and O (Chapter 11).

Absorption (ab-**ZORB**-shun) The taking in of materials by cells or tissues (Chapter 3).

Accessory nerves (ak-**SES**-suh-ree) Cranial nerve pair XI. Motor to the larynx and shoulder muscles (Chapter 8).

Accessory organs (ak-**SES**-suh-ree) The digestive organs that contribute to the process of digestion, although digestion does not take place within them; consist of the teeth, tongue, salivary glands, liver, gallbladder, and pancreas (Chapter 16).

Acetabulum (ASS-uh-**TAB**-yoo-lum) The deep socket in the hip bone that articulates with the head of the femur (from the Latin "little vinegar cup") (Chapter 6).

Acetylcholine (as-**SEE**-tull-KOH-leen) A chemical neurotransmitter released at neuromuscular junctions, as well as by neurons in the central and peripheral nervous systems (Chapter 7).

Acid (**ASS**-id) A hydrogen ion (H^+) donor; when in solution has a pH less than 7 (Chapter 2).

Acidosis (ASS-i-**DOH**-sis) The condition in which the pH of the blood falls below 7.35 (Chapter 2).

Acne (**AK**-nee) Inflammation of the sebaceous glands and hair follicles (Chapter 5).

Acoustic nerves (uh-**KOO**-stik) Cranial nerve pair VIII. Sensory for hearing and equilibrium (Chapter 8).

Acquired immunity (uh-**KWHY**-erd im-**YOO**-ni-tee) The immunity obtained upon exposure to a pathogen or a vaccine or upon reception of antibodies for a particular pathogen (Chapter 14).

Acromegaly (AK-roh-**MEG**-ah-lee) Hypersecretion of growth hormone in an adult, resulting in excessive growth of the bones of the face, hands, and feet (Chapter 10).

Acrosome (**AK**-roh-sohm) The tip of the head of a sperm cell, a modified lysosome; contains enzymes to digest the membrane of the ovum (Chapter 20).

Actin (**AK**-tin) A contractile protein in the sarcomeres of muscle fibers; is pulled by myosin; also forms the cytoskeleton in most cells (Chapter 3).

Action potential (**AK**-shun poh-**TEN**-shul) The changes in electrical charges on either side of a cell membrane in response to a stimulus; depolarization followed by repolarization (Chapter 7).

Active immunity (**AK**-tiv im-**YOO**-ni-tee) The immunity provided by the production of antibodies after exposure to a foreign antigen; may be natural (recovery from disease) or artificial (reception of a vaccine) (Chapter 14).

Active site theory (**AK**-tiv SITE **THEER**-ree) The process by which an enzyme catalyzes a specific reaction; depends on the shapes of the enzyme and the substrate molecules (Chapter 2).

Active transport (**AK**-tiv **TRANS**-port) The process in which there is movement of molecules against a concentration gradient; that is, from an area of lesser concentration to an area of greater concentration. Requires energy (Chapter 3).

Acute (ah-**KEWT**) 1. Characterized by rapid onset. 2. Sharp or severe, with respect to symptoms; not chronic (Chapter 22).

Adaptation (A-dap-**TAY**-shun) The characteristic of sensations in which awareness of the sensation diminishes despite a continuing stimulus (Chapter 9).

Addison's disease (**ADD**-i-sonz) Hyposecretion of the hormones of the adrenal cortex, characterized by low blood pressure, dehydration, muscle weakness, and mental lethargy (Chapter 10).

Adduction (ad-**DUK**-shun) The movement of a body part toward the midline of the body (Chapter 7).

Adenohypophysis (uh-DEN-oh-high-**POFF**-e-sis) The anterior pituitary gland (Chapter 10).

Adhesion (add-**HEE**-zhun) The tendency for unlike molecules to be attracted to one another, as are water molecules to a glass surface (Chapter 2).

Adipocyte (**ADD**-i-poh-site) A cell of adipose tissue, specialized to store fat (white fat) or metabolize fat for heat (brown fat) (Chapter 4).

Adipose tissue (**ADD**-i-pohz **TISH**-yoo) A connective tissue composed primarily of adipocytes; may be called white fat; function is fat storage as a source of potential energy. Brown fat is thermogenic (Chapter 4).

Adrenal cortex (uh-**DREE**-nuhl **KOR**-teks) The outer layer of the adrenal glands, which secretes cortisol and aldosterone (Chapter 10).

Adrenal glands (uh-**DREE**-nuhl) The endocrine glands located on the top of the kidneys; each consists of an adrenal cortex, which secretes cortisol and aldosterone, and an adrenal medulla, which secretes epinephrine and norepinephrine (Syn.—suprarenal glands) (Chapter 10).

Adrenal medulla (uh-**DREE**-nuhl muh-**DEW**-lah) The inner layer of the adrenal glands; secretes epinephrine and norepinephrine (Chapter 10).

Adrenocorticotropic hormone (**ACTH**) (uh-DREE-no-KOR-ti-koh-**TROH**-pik) A hormone produced by the anterior pituitary gland that stimulates the adrenal cortex to secrete cortisol (Chapter 10).

Aerobic (air-**ROH**-bik) Requiring oxygen (Chapter 3).

Afferent (**AFF**-er-rent) To carry toward a center or main part (Chapter 8).

Afferent arteriole (**AFF**-er-ent ar-**TIR**-ee-ohl) The arteriole that takes blood from the renal artery into a glomerulus; within its wall are juxtaglomerular cells that secrete renin (Chapter 18).

Afterbirth (**AFF**-ter-berth) The placenta and umbilical cord delivered shortly after delivery of the infant (Chapter 21).

After-image (**AFF**-ter-IM-ije) The characteristic of sensations in which a sensation remains in the consciousness even after the stimulus has stopped (Chapter 9).

Age-related macular degeneration (**AMD**) (**MAK**-yoo-lar dee-jen-e-**RAY**-shun) Loss of central vision because of the growth of abnormal blood vessels or bleeding in the retina (Chapter 9).

Agglutination (uh-GLOO-ti-**NAY**-shun) Clumping of blood cells or microorganisms; the result of an antigen–antibody reaction (Chapter 11).

AIDS (AYDS) Acquired immunodeficiency syndrome; caused by a virus (HIV) that infects helper T cells and depresses immune responses (Chapter 14).

Albumin (al-**BYOO**-min) A protein synthesized by the liver; circulates in blood plasma and contributes to the colloid osmotic pressure of the blood (Chapter 11).

Aldosterone (al-**DAH**-ster-ohn) A hormone (mineralocorticoid) secreted by the adrenal cortex that increases the reabsorption of sodium and the excretion of potassium by the kidneys (Chapter 10).

Alimentary tube (AL-i-**MEN**-tah-ree TOOB) The series of digestive organs that extends from the mouth to the anus; consists of the oral cavity, pharynx, esophagus, stomach, small intestine, and large intestine (Chapter 16).

Allele (uh-**LEEL**) One of two or more different genes for a particular characteristic (Chapter 21).

Allergen (**AL**-er-jen) A substance capable of stimulating an allergic response (Chapter 14).

Allergy (**AL**-er-jee) A hypersensitivity to a foreign antigen that usually does not stimulate an immune response in people; the immune response serves no useful purpose (Chapter 14).

Alopecia (AL-oh-**PEE**-she-ah) Loss of hair, especially that of the scalp (Chapter 5).

Alpha cells (**AL**-fah SELLS) The cells of the islets of Langerhans of the pancreas that secrete the hormone glucagon (Chapter 10).

Alveolar type I cell (al-**VEE**-oh-lar TIGHP WON SELL) The simple squamous epithelial cell that forms the walls of the alveoli of the lungs (Chapter 15).

Alveolar type II cell (al-**VEE**-oh-lar TIGHP TOO SELL) The septal cell in the lungs that produces pulmonary surfactant (Chapter 15).

Alveolar ventilation (al-**VEE**-oh-lar VEN-ti-**LAY**-shun) The amount of inhaled air that reaches the alveoli and participates in gas exchange; about 350–400 mL of a 500-mL tidal volume (Chapter 15).

Alveoli (al-**VEE**-oh-lye) The air sacs of the lungs, made of simple squamous epithelium, in which gas exchange takes place (Chapter 15).

Alzheimer's disease (**ALZ**-high-mers) A progressive brain disease, of unknown cause, resulting in loss of memory, intellectual ability, speech, and motor control (Chapter 8).

Amblyopia (AM-blee-**OH**-pee-ah) Impaired vision without apparent damage to an eye; often the result of lazy eye because the brain ignores the image from the lazy eye and the eye stops focusing (Chapter 9).

Amenorrhea (ay-MEN-uh-**REE**-ah) Absence of menstruation (Chapter 20).

Amine/amino group (ah-**MEEN**/ah-**MEE**-noh) The NH_2 portion of a molecule such as an amino acid (Chapter 12).

Amino acid (ah-**MEE**-noh **ASS**-id) An organic compound that contains an amino, or amine, group (NH_2) and a carboxyl group (COOH). Twenty different amino acids are the subunit molecules of which human proteins are made (Chapter 2).

Amniocentesis (AM-nee-oh-sen-**TEE**-sis) A diagnostic procedure in which amniotic fluid is obtained for culture of fetal cells; used to detect genetic diseases or other abnormalities in the fetus (Chapter 21).

Amnion (**AM**-nee-on) An embryonic membrane that holds the fetus suspended in amniotic fluid; fuses with the chorion by the end of the third month of gestation (Chapter 21).

Amniotic fluid (AM-nee-**AH**-tik **FLOO**-id) The fluid contained within the amnion; cushions the fetus and absorbs shock (Chapter 21).

Amphiarthrosis (AM-fee-ar-**THROH**-sis) A slightly movable joint, such as a symphysis (Chapter 6).

Amylase (**AM**-i-lays) A digestive enzyme that breaks down starch to maltose; secreted by the salivary glands and the pancreas (Chapter 16).

Anabolic steroid (AN-ah-**BAHL**-lik **STEER**-oyds) A chemical similar in structure and action to the male hormone testosterone; increases protein synthesis, especially in muscles (Chapter 7).

Anabolism (an-**NAB**-uh-lizm) Synthesis reactions, in which smaller molecules are bonded together to form larger molecules; require energy (ATP) and are catalyzed by enzymes (Chapter 17).

Anaerobic (AN-air-**ROH**-bik) 1. In the absence of oxygen. 2. Not requiring oxygen (Chapter 7).

Anaphase (**AN**-ah-fayz) The third stage of mitosis, in which the separate sets of chromosomes move toward opposite poles of the cell (Chapter 3).

Anaphylactic shock (AN-uh-fi-**LAK**-tik SHAHK) A type of circulatory shock that is the result of a massive allergic reaction (from the Greek "unguarded") (Chapter 13).

Anastomosis (a-NAS-ti-**MOH**-sis) A connection or joining, especially of blood vessels (Chapter 13).

Anatomic position (AN-uh-**TOM**-ik pa-**ZI**-shun) The position of the body used in anatomic descriptions: The body is erect and facing forward, the arms are at the sides with the palms facing forward (Chapter 1).

Anatomy (uh-**NAT**-uh-mee) The study of the structure of the body and the relationships among the parts (Chapter 1).

Anemia (uh-**NEE**-mee-yah) A deficiency of red blood cells or hemoglobin (Chapter 11).

Anencephaly (an-en-**SEFF**-ah-lee) A congenital nervous system defect in which the cerebrum has not developed; is always fatal (Chapter 17).

Aneurysm (**AN**-yur-izm) A localized sac or bubble that forms in a weak spot in the wall of a blood vessel, usually an artery (Chapter 13).

Angiotensin II (AN-jee-oh-**TEN**-sin TOO) The final product of the renin–angiotensin mechanism; stimulates vasoconstriction and increased secretion of aldosterone, both of which help raise blood pressure (Chapter 13).

Anion (**AN**-eye-on) An ion with a negative charge (Chapter 2).

Antagonistic muscles (an-**TAG**-on-ISS-tik **MUSS**-uhls) Muscles that have opposite functions with respect to the movement of a joint (Chapter 7).

Anterior (an-**TEER**-ee-your) Toward the front (Syn.—ventral) (Chapter 1).
Antibiotic (AN-ti-bye-**AH**-tik) A chemical medication that stops or inhibits the growth of bacteria or fungi (Chapter 22).
Antibody (**AN**-ti-BAH-dee) A protein molecule produced by plasma cells that is specific for and will bond to a particular foreign antigen (Syn.—gamma globulin, immune globulin, immunoglobulin) (Chapter 14).
Antibody-mediated immunity (**AN**-ti-BAH-dee-**MEE**-dee-ay-ted im-**YOO**-ni-tee) The mechanism of adaptive immunity that involves antibody production and the destruction of foreign antigens by the activities of B cells, T cells, and macrophages (Syn.—humoral immunity) (Chapter 14).
Antibody titer (**AN**-ti-BAH-dee **TIGH**-ter) A diagnostic test that determines the level or amount of a particular antibody in blood or serum (Chapter 14).
Anticodon (**AN**-ti-KOH-don) A triplet of bases on tRNA that matches a codon on mRNA (Chapter 3).
Antidiuretic hormone (**ADH**) (AN-ti-DYE-yoo-**RET**-ik) A hormone produced by the hypothalamus and stored in the posterior pituitary gland; increases the reabsorption of water by the kidney tubules, and in large amounts causes vasoconstriction and is called vasopressin (Chapter 8).
Antigen (**AN**-ti-jen) A chemical marker that identifies cells of a particular species or individual. May be "self" or "foreign." Foreign antigens stimulate immune responses (Chapter 2).
Antigenic (AN-ti-**JEN**-ik) Capable of stimulating antibody production (Chapter 14).
Anti-inflammatory effect (AN-ti-in-**FLAM**-uh-tor-ee) To lessen the process of inflammation; cortisol is the hormone that has this effect (Chapter 10).
Antipyretic (AN-tigh-pye-**RET**-ik) A medication, such as aspirin, that lowers a fever (Chapter 17).
Antiseptic (AN-ti-**SEP**-tik) A chemical that destroys bacteria or inhibits their growth on a living being (Chapter 22).
Antithrombin (**AN**-ti-THROM-bin) A protein synthesized by the liver that inactivates excess thrombin to prevent abnormal clotting (Chapter 11).
Antitoxin (AN-tee-**TAHK**-sin) Antibodies specific for a bacterial toxin; used in treatment of diseases such as botulism or tetanus (Chapter 7).
Anus (**AY**-nus) The terminal opening of the alimentary tube for the elimination of feces; surrounded by the internal and external anal sphincters (Chapter 16).
Aorta (ay-**OR**-tah) The largest artery of the body; emerges from the left ventricle; has four parts: ascending aorta, aortic arch, thoracic aorta, and abdominal aorta (Chapter 13).
Aortic body (ay-OR-tik **BAH**-dee) The site of chemoreceptors in the wall of the aortic arch; detect changes in blood pH and the blood levels of oxygen and carbon dioxide (Chapter 9).
Aortic semilunar valve (ay-**OR**-tik SEM-ee-**LOO**-nar VALV) The valve at the junction of the left ventricle and the aorta; prevents backflow of blood from the aorta to the ventricle when the ventricle relaxes (Chapter 12).
Aortic sinus (ay-**OR**-tik **SIGH**-nus) The site of pressoreceptors in the wall of the aortic arch; detects changes in blood pressure (Chapter 9).
Apgar score (**APP**-gar SKOR) A system of evaluating an infant's condition 1 minute after birth; includes heart rate, respiration, muscle tone, response to stimuli, and color (Chapter 21).
Aphasia (ah-**FAY**-zhuh) Impairment or absence of the ability to communicate in speech, reading, or writing. May involve word deafness or word blindness (Chapter 8).
Aplastic anemia (ay-**PLAS**-tik uh-**NEE**-mee-yah) Failure of the red bone marrow resulting in decreased numbers of red blood cells, white blood cells, and platelets; may be a side effect of some medications (Chapter 11).
Apneustic center (ap-**NEW**-stik **SEN**-ter) The respiratory center in the pons that prolongs inhalation (Chapter 15).
Apocrine gland (**AP**-oh-krin) The type of sweat gland (exocrine) found primarily in the axillae and genital area; actually a modified scent gland (Chapter 5).
Aponeurosis (A-poh-new-**ROH**-sis) A flat tendon (Chapter 7).
Apoptosis (AP-oh-**TOH**-sis) A process by which a cell brings about its own death; part of the normal cell cycle for unnecessary or damaged cells; also called genetically programmed cell death (Chapter 3).
Apparent (uh-**PAR**-ent) 1. Readily seen or visible. 2. An infection in which the patient exhibits the symptoms of the disease (Chapter 22).
Appendicitis (uh-PEN-di-**SIGH**-tis) Inflammation of the appendix (Chapter 16).
Appendicular skeleton (AP-en-**DIK**-yoo-lar) The portion of the skeleton that consists of the shoulder and pelvic girdles and the bones of the arms and legs (Chapter 6).

Appendix (uh-**PEN**-diks) A small tubular organ that extends from the cecum; has no known function for people and is considered a vestigial organ (Chapter 16).

Aqueous (**AY**-kwee-us) Pertaining to water; used especially to refer to solutions (Chapter 2).

Aqueous humor (**AY**-kwee-us **HYOO**-mer) The tissue fluid of the eye within the anterior cavity of the eyeball; nourishes the lens and cornea (Chapter 9).

Arachnoid membrane (uh-**RAK**-noid) The middle layer of the meninges, made of web-like connective tissue (from the Greek "spider-like") (Chapter 8).

Arachnoid villi (uh-**RAK**-noid **VILL**-eye) Projections of the cranial arachnoid membrane into the cranial venous sinuses, through which cerebrospinal fluid is reabsorbed back into the blood (Chapter 8).

Areolar connective tissue (uh-**REE**-oh-lar) A tissue that consists of tissue fluid, fibroblasts, collagen and elastin fibers, and wandering WBCs; found in all mucous membranes and in subcutaneous tissue (Syn.—loose connective tissue) (Chapter 4).

Arrhythmia (uh-**RITH**-me-yah) An abnormal or irregular rhythm of the heart (Chapter 12).

Arteriole (ar-**TEER**-ee-ohl) A small artery (Chapter 5).

Arteriosclerosis (ar-TIR-ee-oh-skle-**ROH**-sis) Deterioration of arteries with loss of elasticity that is often a consequence of aging or hypertension; a contributing factor to aneurysm or stroke (Chapter 13).

Artery (**AR**-tuh-ree) A blood vessel that takes blood from the heart toward the capillaries (Chapter 13).

Arthropod (**AR**-throw-pod) Invertebrate animals characterized by an exoskeleton and jointed appendages; includes insects, spiders, ticks, mites, and crustaceans (Chapter 22).

Articular cartilage (ar-**TIK**-yoo-lar **KAR**-ti-lidj) The cartilage on the joint surfaces of a bone; provides a smooth surface (Chapter 6).

Articulation (ar-TIK-yoo-**LAY**-shun) A joint (Chapter 6).

Ascites (a-**SIGH**-teez) An abnormal accumulation of fluid in the peritoneal space (Chapter 15).

Asthma (**AZ**-mah) A respiratory disorder characterized by constriction of the bronchioles, excessive mucus production, and dyspnea; often caused by allergies (Chapter 15).

Astigmatism (uh-**STIG**-mah-TIZM) An error of refraction caused by an irregular curvature of the lens or cornea (Chapter 9).

Astrocyte (**ASS**-troh-site) A type of neuroglia that forms the blood–brain barrier to prevent potentially harmful substances from affecting brain neurons (Chapter 8).

Asymptomatic (AY-simp-toh-**MAT**-ik) Without symptoms (Chapter 22).

Atelectasis (AT-e-**LEK**-tah-sis) Collapsed or airless lung, without gas exchange (Chapter 15).

Atherosclerosis (ATH-er-oh-skle-**ROH**-sis) The abnormal accumulation of lipids and other materials in the walls of arteries; narrows the lumen of the vessel and may stimulate abnormal clot formation (Chapter 2).

Atlas (**AT**-las) An irregular bone, the first cervical vertebra; supports the skull (Chapter 6).

Atmospheric pressure (AT-mus-**FEER**-ik) The pressure exerted by the atmosphere on objects on the earth's surface; 760 mm Hg at sea level (Chapter 15).

Atom (**A**-tom) The unit of matter that is the smallest part of an element (Chapter 2).

Atomic number (a-**TOM**-ik) Number of protons in the nucleus of an atom (Chapter 2).

Atomic weight (a-**TOM**-ik WAYT) The weight of an atom determined by adding the number of protons and neutrons (Chapter 2).

ATP (**adenosine triphosphate**) A specialized nucleotide that traps and releases biologically useful energy (Chapter 2).

Atrial natriuretic peptide (**ANP**) (**AY**-tree-uhl NAY-tree-yu-**RET**-ik) One of a group of peptide hormones secreted by the heart when blood pressure or blood volume increases, upon exposure to cold, or with consistent exercise; increases loss of sodium ions and water by the kidneys, and promotes conversion of white (storage) adipocytes to brown (thermogenic) adipocytes (Syn.—atrial natriuretic hormone) (Chapter 12).

Atrioventricular (**AV**) **node** (AY-tree-oh-ven-**TRIK**-yoo-lar NOHD) The second part of the cardiac conduction pathway, located in the lower interatrial septum (Chapter 12).

Atrium (**AY**-tree-um) (Pl.—atria) One of the two upper chambers of the heart that receive venous blood from the lungs or the body (Chapter 12).

Atrophy (**AT**-ruh-fee) Decrease in size of a body part due to lack of use; a wasting (Chapter 7).

Attenuated (uh-**TEN**-yoo-AY-ted) Weakened, or less harmful; used to describe the microorganisms contained in vaccines, which have been treated to reduce their pathogenicity (Chapter 14).

Auditory bones (**AW**-di-tor-ee) The malleus, incus, and stapes in the middle ear (Chapter 6).

Auerbach's plexus (**OW**-er-baks **PLEK**-sus) The enteric nerve plexus in the external muscle layer of the organs of the alimentary tube; regulates the contractions of the external muscle layer (Syn.—myenteric plexus) (Chapter 16).

Auricle (**AW**-ri-kuhl) The portion of the outer ear external to the skull; made of cartilage covered with skin (Syn.—pinna) (Chapter 9).

Autoclave (**AW**-toh-clayve) A machine that uses steam under pressure for sterilization (Chapter 22).

Autoimmune disease (AW-toh-im-**YOON** di-**ZEEZ**) A condition in which the immune system produces antibodies to the person's own tissue (Chapter 6).

Autonomic nervous system (AW-toh-**NOM**-ik **NER**-vuhs) The portion of the peripheral nervous system that consists of visceral motor neurons to smooth muscle, cardiac muscle, and glands (Chapter 8).

Autophagy (aw-**TOFF**-uh-jee) A process of destruction and recycling of old or damaged cellular parts; these are digested by the enzymes of lysosomes (Chapter 3).

Autosomes (**AW**-toh-sohms) Chromosomes other than the sex chromosomes; for people there are 22 pairs of autosomes in each somatic cell (Chapter 3).

Axial skeleton (**AK**-see-uhl) The portion of the skeleton that consists of the skull, vertebral column, and rib cage (Chapter 6).

Axis (**AK**-sis) An irregular bone, the second cervical vertebra; forms a pivot joint with the atlas (Chapter 6).

Axon (**AK**-sahn) The cellular process of a neuron that carries impulses away from the cell body (Chapter 4).

Axon terminal (**AK**-sahn **TER**-mi-nuhl) The end of the axon of a motor neuron, part of the neuromuscular junction (Chapter 7).

Azotemia (AZ-oh-**TEE**-mee-ah) The presence of urea and other nitrogenous waste products in the blood (Chapter 18).

B

B cell (B SELL) A subgroup of lymphocytes, including memory B cells and plasma cells, both of which are involved in adaptive immune responses (Chapter 11).

Bacillus (buh-**SILL**-us) (Pl.—bacilli) A rod-shaped bacterium (Chapter 22).

Bacteremia (bak-tah-**REE**-mee-ah) The presence of bacteria in the blood, which is normally sterile (Chapter 22).

Bacteria (bak-**TEER**-ee-yuh) (Sing.—bacterium) The simple unicellular microorganisms of the class Schizomycetes; may be free living, saprophytic, or parasitic (Chapter 22).

Bactericide (bak-**TEER**-i-sigh'd) A chemical that kills bacteria (Chapter 22).

Bacteriostatic (bak-TEE-ree-oh-**STAT**-ik) Capable of inhibiting the reproduction of bacteria (Chapter 22).

Bacteruria (BAK-tur-**YOO**-ree-ah) The presence of large numbers of bacteria in urine (Chapter 18).

Ball-and-socket joint (BAWL and **SOK**-et) A diarthrosis that permits movement in all planes (Chapter 6).

Band cell (BAND SELL) An immature neutrophil with a nucleus that has not yet segmented (Chapter 11).

Bartholin's glands (**BAR**-toh-linz) The small glands in the wall of the vagina; secrete mucus into the vagina and vestibule (Syn.—vestibular glands) (Chapter 20).

Basal ganglia (**BAY**-zuhl **GANG**-lee-ah) Masses of gray matter within the white matter of the cerebral hemispheres; concerned with subconscious aspects of skeletal muscle activity, such as accessory movements (Chapter 8).

Basal metabolic rate (**BAY**-zuhl met-ah-**BAHL**-ik RAYT) The energy required to maintain the functioning of the body in a resting condition (Chapter 17).

Base (BAYS) A hydrogen ion (H^+) acceptor, or hydroxyl ion (OH^+) donor; when in solution, has a pH greater than 7 (Chapter 2).

Basilar layer (bah-**SILL**-ar **LAY**-er) The permanent vascular layer of the endometrium that is not lost in menstruation; regenerates the functional layer during each menstrual cycle (Chapter 20).

Basophil (**BAY**-so-fill) A type of white blood cell (granular); contains heparin and histamine (Chapter 11).

Benign (bee-**NINE**) Not malignant (Chapter 3).

Beta cells (**BAY**-tah SELLS) The cells of the islets of Langerhans of the pancreas that secrete the hormone insulin (Chapter 10).

Beta-oxidation (BAY-tah-AHK-si-**DAY**-shun) The process by which the long carbon chain of a fatty acid molecule is broken down into two-carbon acetyl groups to be used in cell respiration; takes place in the liver (Chapter 16).

Bile (BYL) The secretion of the liver that is stored in the gallbladder and passes to the duodenum; contains bile salts to emulsify fats; is the fluid in which bilirubin and excess cholesterol are excreted (Chapter 16).

Bile salts (BYL SAWLTS) The active components of bile that emulsify fats in the digestive process (Chapter 16).

Bilirubin (**BILL**-ee-roo-bin) The bile pigment produced from the heme portion of the hemoglobin of old red blood cells; excreted by the liver in bile (Chapter 11).

Binary fission (**BYE**-na-ree **FISH**-en) The asexual reproductive process in which one cell divides into two identical new cells (Chapter 22).

Binocular vision (bye-**NOK**-yoo-lur **VI**-zhun) Normal vision involving the use of both eyes; the ability of the brain to create one image from the slightly different images received from each eye (Chapter 9).

Biopsy (**BYE**-op-see) Removal of a small piece of living tissue for microscopic examination; a diagnostic procedure (Chapter 5).

Birth canal (BERTH ka-**NAL**) The vagina during delivery of an infant (Chapter 21).

Blastocyst (**BLAS**-toh-sist) The early stage of embryonic development that follows the morula; consists of the outer trophoblast and the internal inner cell mass and blastocoel (cavity) (Chapter 21).

Blister (**BLISS**-ter) A collection of fluid below or within the epidermis (Chapter 5).

Blood (BLUHD) The fluid that circulates in the heart and blood vessels; consists of blood cells and plasma (Chapter 4).

Blood–brain barrier (BLUHD BRAYN) The barrier between the circulating blood and brain tissue, formed by astrocytes and brain capillaries; prevents harmful substances in the blood from damaging brain neurons (Chapter 8).

Blood pressure (BLUHD **PRE**-shure) The force exerted by the blood against the walls of the blood vessels; measured in mm Hg (Chapter 13).

Body (**BAH**-dee) 1. The physical human being as a whole. 2. The supporting part of a vertebra. 3. The central portion of the sternum. 4. Any of a number of small structures, such as the cell body of a neuron or the sensory carotid body (Chapter 1).

Body-mass index (**BAH**-dee mass **IN**-deks) A measure of leanness using height and weight (Chapter 17).

Bond (BAHND) An attraction or force that holds atoms together in the formation of molecules (Chapter 2).

Bone (BOWNE) 1. A connective tissue made of osteocytes in a calcified matrix. 2. An organ that is an individual part of the skeleton (Chapter 4).

Botulism (**BAHT**-chu-lizm) A disease, characterized by muscle paralysis, caused by the bacterium *Clostridium botulinum* (Chapter 7).

Bowman's capsule (**BOW**-manz **KAP**-suhl) The expanded end of the renal tubule that encloses a glomerulus; receives filtrate from the glomerulus (Chapter 18).

Bradycardia (BRAY-dee-**KAR**-dee-yah) An abnormally slow heart rate; less than 60 beats per minute (Chapter 12).

Brain (BRAYN) The part of the central nervous system within the skull; regulates the activity of the rest of the nervous system (Chapter 8).

Brain stem (**BRAYN** stem) The portion of the brain that consists of the medulla, pons, and midbrain (Chapter 8).

Broad spectrum (BRAWD **SPEK**-trum) An antibiotic that is effective against a wide variety of bacteria (Chapter 22).

Bronchial tree (**BRONG**-kee-uhl TREE) The entire system of air passageways formed by the branching of the bronchial tubes within the lungs; the smallest bronchioles terminate in clusters of alveoli (Chapter 15).

Bronchioles (**BRONG**-kee-ohls) The smallest of the air passageways within the lungs (Chapter 15).

Brush border (BRUSH **BORE**-der) The collective name for the microvilli of the absorptive cells of the mucosa of the small intestine (Chapter 16).

Buffer system (**BUFF**-er **SIS**-tem) A pair of chemicals that prevents significant changes in the pH of a body fluid (Chapter 2).

Bulbourethral glands (BUHL-boh-yoo-**REE**-thruhl) The glands on either side of the prostate gland that open into the urethra; secrete an alkaline fluid that becomes part of semen (Syn.—Cowper's glands) (Chapter 20).

Bundle of His (**BUN**-duhl of HISS) The third part of the cardiac conduction pathway, located in the upper interventricular septum (Syn.—atrioventricular bundle) (Chapter 12).

Burn (BERN) Damage caused by heat, flames, chemicals, or electricity, especially to the skin; classified as first degree (minor), second degree (blisters), third degree (full skin thickness damage), or fourth degree (muscle or bone damage) (Chapter 5).

Bursa (**BURR**-sah) A sac of synovial fluid that decreases friction between a tendon and a bone (Chapter 6).

Bursitis (burr-**SIGH**-tiss) Inflammation of a bursa (Chapter 6).

C

Cadherins (kad-**HEER**-ins) Glycoproteins that form junctions between adjacent epithelial cells; especially important in capillaries and endothelium (Chapter 11).

Calcaneus (kal-**KAY**-nee-us) A short bone, the largest of the tarsals; the heel bone (Chapter 6).

Calcitonin (KAL-si-**TOH**-nin) A hormone secreted by the thyroid gland that decreases the reabsorption of calcium from bones (Chapter 10).

Calcitriol (kal-**SI**-tree-awl) The active form of vitamin D (Chapter 5).

Callus (**KAL**-us) Thickening of an area of epidermis (Chapter 5).

Calorie (**KAL**-oh-ree) 1. Lowercase "calorie": the amount of heat energy needed to change the temperature of 1 gram of water 1 degree centigrade. 2. Uppercase "Calorie": a kilocalorie, used to indicate the energy content of foods (Chapter 17).

Calyx (**KAY**-liks) (Pl.—calyces) A funnel-shaped extension of the renal pelvis that encloses the papilla of a renal pyramid and collects urine (Chapter 18).

Canal of Schlemm (ka-**NAL** of SHLEM) Small veins at the junction of the cornea and iris of the eye; the site of reabsorption of aqueous humor into the blood (Syn.—scleral venous sinus) (Chapter 9).

Canaliculi (KAN-a-**LIK**-yoo-lye) Small channels, such as those in bone matrix that permit contact between adjacent osteocytes (Chapter 6).

Cancer (**KAN**-ser) A malignant tumor or growth of cells (Chapter 3).

Capacitation (KAH-pas-i-**TAY**-shun) The maturation of sperm within the female reproductive tract; sperm become capable of fertilization (Chapter 21).

Capillary (**KAP**-i-lar-ee) A blood vessel that takes blood from an arteriole to a venule; walls are one cell in thickness to permit exchanges of materials (Chapter 4).

Capsid (**KAP**-sid) The protein shell of a virus (Chapter 22).

Capsule (**KAP**-suhl) 1. A membrane that encloses an organ such as a lymph node (Chapter 14). 2. A gelatinous layer located outside the cell wall of some bacteria; provides resistance to phagocytosis (Chapter 22).

Carbaminohemoglobin (KAR-buh-mee-noh-**HEE**-muh-glow-bin) The carbon dioxide–hemoglobin molecule; 10% to 20% of CO_2 transport (Chapter 15).

Carbohydrate (KAR-boh-**HIGH**-drayt) An organic compound that contains carbon, hydrogen, and oxygen; includes sugars, starches, and cellulose (Chapter 2).

Carbonic anhydrase (kar-**BAHN**-ik an-**HIGH**-drays) The enzyme present in red blood cells and other cells that catalyzes the reaction of carbon dioxide and water to form carbonic acid (Chapter 15).

Carboxyhemoglobin (Kar-BAHK-see-**HEE**-muh-glow-bin) The carbon monoxide–hemoglobin molecule; the bond is tenacious (Chapter 15).

Carboxyl group (kar-**BAHK**-sul) The COOH portion of a molecule such as an amino acid (Chapter 19).

Carcinogen (kar-**SIN**-oh-jen) A substance that increases the risk of developing cancer (Chapter 3).

Carcinoma (KAR-sin-**OH**-mah) A malignant tumor of epithelial tissue (Chapter 5).

Cardiac cycle (**KAR**-dee-yak **SIGH**-kuhl) The sequence of events in one heartbeat, in which simultaneous contraction of the atria is followed by simultaneous contraction of the ventricles (Chapter 12).

Cardiac muscle (**KAR**-dee-yak **MUSS**-uhl) The muscle tissue that forms the walls of the chambers of the heart (Chapter 4).

Cardiac output (**KAR**-dee-yak **OUT**-put) The amount of blood pumped by a ventricle in 1 minute; the resting average is 5 to 6 liters/min (Chapter 12).

Cardiac reserve (**KAR**-dee-yak ree-**ZERV**) The difference between resting cardiac output and maximum exercise cardiac output (Chapter 12).

Carotid body (kah-**RAH** tid **BAH**-dee) The site of chemoreceptors in the wall of the internal carotid artery; detects changes in blood pH and the levels of oxygen and carbon dioxide in the blood (Chapter 9).

Carotid sinus (kah-**RAH**-tid **SIGH**-nus) The site of pressoreceptors in the wall of the internal carotid artery; detect changes in blood pressure (Chapter 9).

Carpals (**KAR**-puhls) The eight short bones of each wrist (Chapter 6).

Carrier (**KAR**-ree-yur) 1. A person who recovers from a disease but continues to be a source of the pathogen and may infect others (Chapter 22). 2. In genetics, a woman with one gene for a sex-linked trait (Chapter 21).

Carrier enzyme (**KAR**-ree-yur **EN**-zime) An enzyme that is part of a cell membrane and carries out the process of facilitated diffusion of a specific substance (Syn.—transporter) (Chapter 3).

Cartilage (**KAR**-ti-lidj) A connective tissue made of chondrocytes in a protein matrix; is firm yet flexible (Chapter 4).

Catabolism (kuh-**TAB**-uh-lizm) Breakdown or degradation reactions, in which larger molecules are broken down to smaller molecules; often release energy (ATP) and are catalyzed by enzymes (Chapter 17).

Catalyst (**KAT**-ah-list) A chemical that affects the speed of a chemical reaction, while remaining itself unchanged; enzymes are catalysts (Chapter 2).

Cataract (**KAT**-uh-rackt) An eye disorder in which the lens becomes opaque and impairs vision (from the Latin "waterfall") (Chapter 9).

Catecholamines (KAT-e-**KOHL**-ah-meens) Epinephrine and norepinephrine, the hormones secreted by the adrenal medulla (Chapter 10).

Cathelicidin (KATH-i-**LISS**-i-din) An antimicrobial peptide (one of a group) produced by white blood cells; it punctures the outer covering of pathogens (Chapter 5).

Cation (**KAT**-eye-on) An ion with a positive charge (Chapter 2).

Cauda equina (**KAW**-dah ee-**KWHY**-nah) The lumbar and sacral spinal nerves that hang below the end of the spinal cord, before they exit from the vertebral canal (Chapter 8).

Cavity (**KAV**-i-tee) A hollow area inside the body; the principal cavities are the cranial, spinal, thoracic, abdominal, and pelvic cavities (Chapter 1).

Cecum (**SEE**-kum) The first part of the large intestine, the dead-end portion adjacent to the ileum (from the Latin "blindness") (Chapter 16).

Cell (SELL) The smallest living unit of structure and function of the body (Chapter 1).

Cell body (SELL **BAH**-dee) The part of a neuron that contains the nucleus (Chapter 4).

Cell-mediated immunity (SELL-**MEE**-dee-ay-ted im-**YOO**-ni-tee) The mechanism of adaptive immunity that does not involve antibody production, but rather the destruction of foreign antigens by the activities of T cells and macrophages (Chapter 14).

Cell (plasma) membrane (SELL **MEM**-brayn) The membrane made of phospholipids, protein, and cholesterol that forms the outer boundary of a cell and regulates passage of materials into and out of the cell (Chapter 2).

Cell respiration (SELL RES-pi-**RAY**-shun) A cellular process in which the energy of nutrients is released in the form of ATP and heat. Oxygen is required, and carbon dioxide and water are produced (Chapter 2).

Cellulose (**SELL**-yoo-lowse) A polysaccharide produced by plants for their cell walls; it is not digestible by humans but is important as roughage or fiber in the diet (Chapter 2).

Central (**SEN**-truhl) The main part; or in the middle of (Chapter 1).

Central canal (**SEN**-truhl ka-**NAL**) The hollow center of the spinal cord that contains cerebrospinal fluid (Chapter 8).

Central nervous system (**SEN**-tral **NER**-vuhs) The part of the nervous system that consists of the brain and spinal cord (Chapter 8).

Centrioles (**SEN**-tree-ohls) The cell organelles that organize the spindle fibers during cell division (Chapter 3).

Cerebellum (SER-e-**BELL**-uhm) The part of the brain posterior to the medulla and pons; responsible for many of the subconscious aspects of skeletal muscle functioning, such as coordination and muscle tone (Chapter 7).

Cerebral aqueduct (se-**REE**-bruhl **A**-kwi-dukt) A tunnel through the midbrain that permits cerebrospinal fluid to flow from the third to the fourth ventricle (Chapter 8).

Cerebral cortex (se-**REE**-bruhl **KOR**-teks) The gray matter on the surface of the cerebral hemispheres. Includes motor areas, sensory areas, auditory areas, visual areas, taste areas, olfactory areas, speech areas, and association areas (Chapter 8).

Cerebrospinal fluid (se-**REE**-broh-**SPY**-nuhl) The tissue fluid of the central nervous system; formed by choroid plexuses in the ventricles of the brain, circulates in and around the brain and spinal cord, and is reabsorbed into cranial venous sinuses (Chapter 8).

Cerebrovascular accident (se-**REE**-broh-**VAS**-kyoo-lur) A hemorrhagic or ischemic lesion in the brain, often the result of aneurysm, arteriosclerosis, atherosclerosis, or hypertension (Syn.—stroke) (Chapter 8).

Cerebrum (se-**REE**-bruhm) The largest part of the brain, consisting of the right and left cerebral hemispheres; its many functions include movement, sensation, learning, and memory (Chapter 8).

Cerumen (suh-**ROO**-men) The waxy secretion of ceruminous glands (Chapter 5).

Ceruminous gland (suh-**ROO**-mi-nus) An exocrine gland in the dermis of the ear canal that secretes cerumen (ear wax) (Chapter 5).

Cervical (**SIR**-vi-kuhl) Pertaining to the neck (Chapter 1).

Cervical vertebrae (**SIR**-vi-kuhl **VER**-te-bray) The seven vertebrae in the neck (Chapter 6).

Cervix (**SIR**-viks) The most inferior part of the uterus that projects into the vagina (Chapter 20).

Cesarean section (se-**SAR**-ee-an **SEK**-shun) Removal of the fetus by way of an incision through the abdominal wall and uterus (Chapter 21).

Chaperone (**SHA**-per-own) One of a large group of intracellular proteins that is responsible for the proper folding of new proteins and for the repair or disposal of damaged proteins (Chapter 3).

Chemical clotting (**KEM**-i-kuhl **KLAH**-ting) A series of chemical reactions, stimulated by a rough surface or a break in a blood vessel, that result in the formation of a fibrin clot (Chapter 11).

Chemical digestion (**KEM**-i-kuhl dye-**JES**-chun) The breakdown of food accomplished by digestive enzymes; complex organic molecules are broken down to simpler organic molecules (Chapter 16).

Chemoreceptors (KEE-moh-re-**SEP**-ters) 1. A sensory receptor that detects a chemical change. 2. Olfactory receptors, taste receptors, and the carotid and aortic chemoreceptors that detect changes in blood gases and blood pH (Chapter 9).

Chemotherapy (KEE-moh-**THER**-uh-pee) The use of chemicals (medications) to treat disease (Chapter 3).

Chief cells (CHEEF SELLS) The cells of the gastric pits of the stomach that secrete pepsinogen, the inactive form of the digestive enzyme pepsin (Chapter 16).

Chitin (**KY**-tin) A polysaccharide found in the cell walls of fungi and the exoskeletons of arthropods; insect chitin may be an allergen that triggers asthma (Chapter 15).

Chlamydia (kluh-**MID**-ee-ah) A group of simple bacteria; *Chlamydia trachomatis* is a sexually transmitted pathogen that may cause conjunctivitis or pneumonia in infants born to infected women (Chapter 20).

Cholecystokinin (KOH-lee-SIS-toh-**KYE**-nin) A hormone secreted by the duodenum when food enters; stimulates contraction of the gallbladder and secretion of enzyme pancreatic juice (Chapter 16).

Cholesterol (koh-**LESS**-ter-ohl) A steroid that is synthesized by the liver and is part of cell membranes (Chapter 2).

Cholinesterase (KOH-lin-**ESS**-ter-ays) The chemical inactivator of acetylcholine (Chapter 7).

Chondrocyte (**KON**-droh-sight) A cartilage cell (Chapter 4).

Chordae tendineae (**KOR**-day ten-**DIN**-ee-ay) Strands of connective tissue that connect the flaps of an atrioventricular valve to the papillary muscles (Chapter 12).

Chorion (**KOR**-ee-on) An embryonic membrane that is formed from the trophoblast of the blastocyst and will develop chorionic villi and become the fetal portion of the placenta (Chapter 21).

Chorionic villi (**KOR**-ee-ON-ik **VILL**-eye) Projections of the chorion that will develop the fetal blood vessels that will become part of the placenta (Chapter 21).

Chorionic villus sampling (KOR-ee-**ON**-ik **VILL**-us) A diagnostic procedure in which a biopsy of the chorionic villi is performed; used to detect genetic diseases or other abnormalities in the fetus (Chapter 21).

Choroid layer (**KOR**-oyd) The middle layer of the eyeball, contains a dark pigment derived from melanin that absorbs light and prevents glare within the eye (Chapter 9).

Choroid plexus (**KOR**-oyd **PLEK**-sus) A capillary network in a ventricle of the brain; forms cerebrospinal fluid (Chapter 8).

Chromatid (**KROH**-mah-tid) A potential chromosome formed by the replication of the DNA of a chromosome during interphase; two identical chromatids are formed and are attached at the centromere; they separate during cell division (Chapter 3).

Chromatin (**KROH**-mah-tin) The thread-like structure of the genetic material when a cell is not dividing; is not visible as individual chromosomes (Chapter 3).

Chromosomes (**KROH**-muh-sohms) Structures made of DNA and protein within the nucleus of a cell. A human cell has 46 chromosomes (Chapter 3).

Chronic (**KRAH**-nik) Characterized by long duration or slow progression (Chapter 22).

Chylomicron (KYE-loh-**MYE**-kron) A small fat globule formed by the small intestine from absorbed fatty acids and glycerol (Chapter 16).

Cilia (**SILLY**-ah) Thread-like structures that project through a cell membrane. 1. Motile cilia are found in groups and sweep materials across the epithelial cell surface. 2. A primary cilium (one per cell) is a sensory structure that may be involved in the cell's development or its mature functioning (Chapter 3).

Ciliary body (**SILLY**-air-ee BAH-dee) A circular muscle that surrounds the edge of the lens of the eye and changes the shape of the lens (Chapter 9).

Ciliated epithelium (**SILLY**-ay-ted) The tissue that has motile cilia on the free surface of the cells (Chapter 4).

Circle of Willis (**SIR**-kuhl of **WILL**-iss) An arterial anastomosis that encircles the pituitary gland and supplies the brain with blood; formed by the two internal carotid arteries and the basilar (two vertebral) artery (Chapter 13).

Circulatory shock (**SIR**-kew-lah-TOR-ee SHAHK) The condition in which decreased cardiac output deprives all tissues of oxygen and permits the accumulation of waste products (Chapter 5).

Cisterna chyli (sis-**TER**-nah **KYE**-lee) A large lymph vessel formed by the union of lymph vessels from the lower body; continues superiorly as the thoracic duct (Chapter 14).

Clavicle (**KLAV**-i-kuhl) The flat bone that articulates with the scapula and sternum (from the Latin "little key") (Syn.—collarbone) (Chapter 6).

Cleavage (**KLEE**-vije) The series of mitotic cell divisions that take place in a fertilized egg; forms the early multicellular embryonic stages (Chapter 21).

Cleft palate (KLEFT **PAL**-uht) A congenital disorder in which the bones of the hard palate do not fuse, leaving an opening between the oral and nasal cavities (Chapter 6).

Clinical infection (**KLIN**-i-kuhl) An infection in which the patient exhibits the symptoms of the disease (Syn.—apparent, symptomatic) (Chapter 22).

Clitoris (**KLIT**-uh-ris) An organ that is part of the vulva; a small mass of erectile tissue at the anterior junction of the labia minora; enlarges in response to sexual stimulation (Chapter 20).

Clot retraction (KLAHT ree-**TRAK**-shun) The shrinking of a blood clot shortly after it forms due to the folding of the fibrin strands; pulls the edges of the ruptured vessel closer together (Chapter 11).

Coccus (**KOK**-us) (Pl.—cocci) A spherical bacterium (Chapter 22).

Coccyx (**KOK**-siks) The last four to five very small vertebrae; attachment site for some muscles of the pelvic floor (Chapter 6).

Cochlea (**KOK**-lee-uh) The snail-shell-shaped portion of the inner ear that contains the receptors for hearing in the organ of Corti (Chapter 9).

Codon (**KOH**-don) The sequence of three bases in DNA or mRNA that is the code for one amino acid; also called a triplet code (Chapter 3).

Coenzyme (koh-**EN**-zime) A non-protein molecule that combines with an enzyme and is essential for the functioning of the enzyme; some vitamins and minerals are coenzymes (Chapter 17).

Cohesion (koh-**HEE**-zhun) The tendency for like molecules to be attracted to each other, as are water molecules with the formation of hydrogen bonds (Chapter 2).

Collagen (**KAH**-lah-jen) A protein that is found in the form of strong fibers in many types of connective tissue (Chapter 4).

Collecting tubule (kah-**LEK**-ting) The part of a renal tubule that extends from a distal convoluted tubule to a papillary duct (Chapter 18).

Colloid osmotic pressure (**KAH**-loyd ahs-**MAH**-tik) The force exerted by the presence of protein in a solution; water will move by osmosis to the area of greater protein concentration (Chapter 13).

Colon (**KOH**-lun) The large intestine (Chapter 16).

Color blindness (**KUHL**-or **BLIND**-ness) The inability to distinguish certain colors, a hereditary trait (Chapter 9).

Columnar (kuh-**LUM**-nar) Shaped like a column; height greater than width; used especially in reference to epithelial tissue (Chapter 4).

Common bile duct (**KOM**-mon BYL DUKT) The duct formed by the union of the hepatic duct from the liver and the cystic duct from the gallbladder, and joined by the main pancreatic duct; carries bile and pancreatic juice to the duodenum (Chapter 16).

Communicable disease (kuhm-**YOO**-ni-kah-b'l) A disease that may be transmitted from person to person by direct or indirect contact (Chapter 22).

Compact bone (**KOM**-pakt BOWNE) Bone tissue made of osteons (haversian systems); forms the diaphyses of long bones and covers the spongy bone of other bones (Chapter 6).

Complement (**KOM**-ple-ment) A group of plasma proteins that are activated by and bond to an antigen–antibody complex; complement fixation results in the lysis of cellular antigens (Chapter 14).

Complement fixation test (**KOM**-ple-ment fik-**SAY**-shun) A diagnostic test that determines the presence of a particular antibody in blood or serum (Chapter 14).

Compliance (pulmonary) (kum-**PLY**-ans) The expansibility of the lungs and thoracic wall, necessary for adequate alveolar ventilation (Chapter 15).

Computed tomography (CT) scan (kom-**PEW**-ted toh-**MAH**-grah-fee SKAN) A diagnostic imaging technique that uses x-rays integrated by computer (Chapter 1).

Concentration gradient (KON-sen-**TRAY**-shun **GRAY**-de-ent) The relative amounts of a substance on either side of a membrane; diffusion occurs with, or along, a concentration gradient, that is, from high concentration to low concentration (Chapter 3).

Conchae (**KONG**-chay) Three pairs of curved, shelflike bones that extend into the nasal cavities; they increase the surface area of the nasal mucosa (Chapter 6).

Conduction (kon-**DUK**-shun) 1. The heat loss process in which heat energy from the skin is transferred to cooler objects touching the skin (Chapter 17). 2. The transfer of any energy form from one substance to another; includes nerve and muscle impulses and the transmission of vibrations in the ear (Chapter 7).

Condyle (**KON**-dyel) A rounded projection on a bone (Chapter 6).

Condyloid joint (**KON**-di-loyd) A diarthrosis that permits movement in one plane and some lateral movement (Chapter 6).

Cones (KOHNES) The sensory receptors in the retina of the eye that detect colors (the different wavelengths of the visible spectrum of light) (Chapter 9).

Congenital (kon-**JEN**-i-tuhl) Present at birth (Chapter 21).

Conjunctiva (KON-junk-**TIGH**-vah) The mucous membrane that lines the eyelids and covers the white of the eye (Chapter 9).

Conjunctivitis (kon-JUNK-ti-**VIGH**-tis) Inflammation of the conjunctiva, most often due to an allergy or bacterial infection (Chapter 9).

Connective tissue (kah-**NEK**-tiv **TISH**-yoo) Tissue that connects, supports, transports, or stores materials. Consists of cells and matrix (Chapter 4).

Contagious disease (kun-**TAY**-jus) A disease that is easily transmitted from person to person by casual contact (Chapter 22).

Contraction, concentric (kon-**TRAK**-shun, kon-**SEN**-trik) The exertion of force as a muscle shortens (Chapter 7).

Contraction, eccentric (ek-**SEN**-trik) The exertion of force, often opposing gravity, as a muscle lengthens (Chapter 7).

Contrast (**KON**-trast) The characteristic of sensations in which a previous sensation affects the perception of a current sensation (Chapter 9).

Contusion (kon-**TOO**-zhun) A bruise; the skin is not broken but may be painful, swollen, and discolored (Chapter 5).

Convection (kon-**VEK**-shun) The heat loss process in which heat energy is moved away from the skin surface by means of air currents (Chapter 17).

Convolution (kon-voh-**LOO**-shun) A fold, coil, roll, or twist; the surface folds of the cerebral cortex (Syn.—gyrus) (Chapter 8).

Cornea (**KOR**-nee-ah) The transparent anterior portion of the sclera of the eye; the first structure that refracts light rays that enter the eye (Chapter 9).

Coronal (frontal) section (koh-**ROH**-nuhl **SEK**-shun) A plane or cut from side to side, separating front and back parts (Chapter 1).

Coronary vessels (**KOR**-ah-na-ree **VESS**-uhls) The blood vessels that circulate blood throughout the myocardium; emerge from the ascending aorta and empty into the right atrium (Chapter 12).

Corpus callosum (**KOR**-pus kuh-**LOH**-sum) The band of white matter that connects the cerebral hemispheres (Chapter 8).

Corpus luteum (**KOR**-pus **LOO**-tee-um) The temporary endocrine gland formed from an ovarian follicle that has released an ovum; secretes progesterone and estrogen (Chapter 10).

Cortex (**KOR**-teks) The outer layer of an organ, such as the cerebrum, kidney, or adrenal gland (Chapter 8).

Cortisol (**KOR**-ti-sawl) A hormone (glucocorticoid) secreted by the adrenal cortex that promotes the efficient use of nutrients in stressful situations and has an anti-inflammatory effect (Chapter 10).

Cough reflex (KAWF) A reflex integrated by the medulla that expels irritating substances from the pharynx, larynx, or trachea by means of an explosive exhalation (Chapter 15).

Covalent bond (ko-**VAY**-lent) A chemical bond formed by the sharing of electrons between atoms (Chapter 2).

Cranial cavity (**KRAY**-nee-uhl **KAV**-i-tee) The cavity formed by the cranial bones; contains the brain (Chapter 1).

Cranial nerves (**KRAY**-nee-uhl NERVS) The 12 pairs of nerves that emerge from the brain (Chapter 8).

Cranial venous sinuses (**KRAY**-nee-uhl **VEE**-nus **SIGH**-nuh-sez) Large veins between the two layers of the cranial dura mater; the site of reabsorption of cerebrospinal fluid (Chapter 8).

Cranium (**KRAY**-nee-um) The cranial bones or bones of the skull that enclose and protect the brain (Chapter 6).

Creatine phosphate (**KREE**-ah-tin **FOSS**-fate) An energy source in muscle fibers; the energy released is used to synthesize ATP (Chapter 7).

Creatinine (kree-**A**-ti-neen) A nitrogenous waste product produced when creatine phosphate is used for energy; excreted by the kidneys in urine (Chapter 7).

Crest (KREST) A bony ridge, such as the iliac crest (Chapter 6).

Cretinism (**KREE**-tin-izm) Hyposecretion of thyroxine in an infant; if uncorrected, the result is severe mental and physical retardation (Chapter 10).

Cross-section (KRAWS **SEK**-shun) A plane or cut perpendicular to the long axis of an organ (Chapter 1).

Crypts of Lieberkühn (KRIPTS of **LEE**-ber-koon) The digestive glands of the small intestine; secrete digestive enzymes (Chapter 16).

Cuboidal (kew-**BOY**-duhl) Shaped like a cube; used especially in reference to epithelial tissue (Chapter 4).

Culture and sensitivity testing (**KUL**-chur and SEN-si-**TIV**-i-tee) A laboratory procedure to determine the best antibiotic with which to treat a bacterial infection (Chapter 22).

Cushing's syndrome (**KOOSH**-ingz **SIN**-drohm) Hypersecretion of the glucocorticoids of the adrenal cortex, characterized by fragility of skin, poor wound healing, truncal fat deposition, and thin extremities (Chapter 10).

Cutaneous senses (kew-**TAY**-nee-us) The senses of the skin; the receptors are mainly in the dermis (Chapter 9).

Cyanosis (SIGH-uh-**NOH**-sis) A blue, gray, or purple discoloration of the skin caused by hypoxia and abnormal amounts of reduced hemoglobin in the blood (Chapter 15).

Cyclic AMP (**SIK**-lik) A chemical that is the second messenger in the two-messenger mechanism of hormone action; formed from ATP and stimulates characteristic cellular responses to the hormone (Chapter 10).

Cystic duct (**SIS**-tik DUKT) The duct that takes bile into and out of the gallbladder; unites with the hepatic duct of the liver to form the common bile duct (Chapter 16).

Cystitis (sis-**TIGH**-tis) Inflammation of the urinary bladder; most often the result of bacterial infection (Chapter 18).

Cytochrome transport system (**SIGH**-toh-krohm) The stage of cell respiration in which most ATP is formed. Cytochromes react with the electrons of the hydrogen atoms that were once part of a food molecule, and metabolic water is formed; aerobic; takes place in the mitochondria of cells (Syn.—electron transport system) (Chapter 17).

Cytokines (**SIGH**-toh-kines) Chemicals released by activated T cells that attract macrophages. Are also released by many cells and tissues as part of cellular communication. (Chapter 14).

Cytokinesis (SIGH-toh-ki-**NEE**-sis) The division of the cytoplasm of a cell following mitosis (Chapter 3).

Cytoplasm (**SIGH**-toh-plazm) The cellular material between the nucleus and the cell membrane (Chapter 3).

Cytoskeleton (SIGH-toh-**SKEL**-e-ton) The protein microfilaments, including actin, that give shape to a cell, support the cell membrane, and provide for movement (Chapter 3).

Cytosol (**SIGH**-toh-sawl) The water of cytoplasm (Chapter 3).

D

Dead space (DED SPAYSE) 1. Anatomic: air that is in the respiratory passages at the end of inhalation and does not participate in gas exchange. 2. Physiological: the volume of nonfunctioning alveoli that decrease gas exchange (Chapter 15).

Deafness (**DEFF**-ness) Impairment of normal hearing; may be caused by damage to the vibration conduction pathway (conduction), the acoustic nerve or cochlear receptors (nerve), or the auditory area in the temporal lobe (central) (Chapter 9).

Deamination (DEE-am-i-**NAY**-shun) The removal of an amino (NH_2) group from an amino acid; takes place in the liver when excess amino acids are used for energy production; the amino groups are converted to urea (Chapter 16).

Decomposition reaction (**DE**-com-poh-**ZI**-shun) A chemical reaction in which bonds in a large molecule are broken and the products are two or more smaller molecules (Chapter 2).

Decubitus ulcer (dee-**KEW**-bi-tuss **UL**-ser) The breakdown and death of skin tissue because of prolonged pressure that interrupts blood flow to the area (Syn.—pressure ulcer) (Chapter 5).

Defecation reflex (DEF-e-**KAY**-shun) The spinal cord reflex that eliminates feces from the colon (Chapter 16).

Defensins (deh-**FEN**-sins) Antimicrobial peptides produced by the keratinocytes of the epidermis (Chapter 5).

Dehydration (DEE-high-**DRAY**-shun) Excessive loss of water from the body (Chapter 5).

Deltoid (**DELL**-toyd) 1. The shoulder region. 2. The large muscle that covers the shoulder joint (Chapter 1).

Denature (dee-**NAY**-chur) To make a molecule biologically inactive, as when heat changes the shape of an enzyme (Chapter 2).

Dendrite (**DEN**-dright) The cellular process of a neuron that carries impulses toward the cell body (Chapter 4).

Dendritic cell (den-**DRIT**-ik SELL) A mobile cell that picks up foreign antigens in the skin (Langerhans cell) or mucous membranes and presents them to lymphocytes in lymph nodes (Chapter 5).

Dental caries (**DEN**-tuhl **KAIR**-eez) Erosion of the enamel and dentin of a tooth, often by bacterial acids (from the Latin "rottenness") (Chapter 16).

Dentin (**DEN**-tin) The bonelike substance that forms the inner crown and the roots of a tooth (Chapter 16).

Depolarization (DE-poh-lahr-i-**ZAY**-shun) The reversal of electrical charges on either side of a cell membrane in response to a stimulus; negative charge outside and positive charge inside; brought about by a rapid inflow of sodium ions (Chapter 7).

Dermatology (DER-muh-**TAH**-luh-jee) The study of the skin and skin diseases (Chapter 5).

Dermis (**DER**-miss) The inner layer of the skin, made of fibrous connective tissue (Chapter 5).

Detached retina (dee-**TACHD RET**-in-nah) The separation of the retina from the choroid layer of the eyeball (Chapter 9).

Detrusor muscle (de-**TROO**-ser) The smooth muscle layer of the wall of the urinary bladder; contracts as part of the urination reflex to eliminate urine (Chapter 18).

Diabetes mellitus (DYE-ah-**BEE**-tis mel-**LYE**-tus) Hyposecretion of insulin by the pancreas or the inability of insulin to exert its effects; characterized by hyperglycemia, increased urinary output with glycosuria, and thirst (Chapter 10).

Diagnosis (DYE-ag-**NOH**-sis) The procedures used to identify the cause and nature of a person's illness (Chapter 1).

Diaphragm (**DYE**-uh-fram) The dome-shaped skeletal muscle that separates the thoracic and abdominal cavities; moves downward when it contracts to enlarge the thoracic cavity to bring about inhalation (Chapter 1).

Diaphysis (dye-**AFF**-i-sis) The shaft of a long bone; contains a marrow canal filled with yellow bone marrow (Chapter 6).

Diarthrosis (DYE-ar-**THROH**-sis) A freely movable joint such as hinge, pivot, and ball-and-socket joints; all are considered synovial joints because synovial membrane is present (Chapter 6).

Diastole (dye-**AS**-tuh-lee) In the cardiac cycle, the relaxation of the myocardium (Chapter 12).

Differential WBC count (**DIFF**-er-EN-shul KOWNT) A laboratory test that determines the percentage of each of the five kinds of white blood cells present in the blood (Chapter 11).

Diffusion (di-**FEW**-zhun) The process in which there is movement of molecules from an area of greater concentration to an area of lesser concentration; occurs because of the free energy (natural movement) of molecules (Chapter 3).

Digestive system (dye-**JES**-tiv **SIS**-tem) The organ system that changes food into simpler organic and inorganic molecules that can be absorbed by the blood and lymph and used by cells; consists of the alimentary tube and accessory organs (Chapter 16).

Dimer (**DYE**-mer) A two-part molecule, as is the immunoglobulin IgA (Chapter 14).

Diploid number (**DIH**-ployd) The characteristic or usual number of chromosomes found in the somatic (body) cells of a species (human: 46) (Chapter 3).

Disaccharide (dye-**SAK**-ah-ride) A carbohydrate molecule that consists of two monosaccharides bonded together; includes sucrose, maltose, and lactose (Chapter 2).

Disease (di-**ZEEZ**) A disorder or disruption of normal body functioning (Chapter 1).

Disinfectant (DIS-in-**FEK**-tent) A chemical that destroys microorganisms or limits their growth on inanimate objects (Chapter 22).

Dissociation (dih-SOH-see-**AY**-shun) The separation of an inorganic salt, acid, or base into its ions when dissolved in water (Syn.—ionization) (Chapter 2).

Distal (**DIS**-tuhl) Farthest from the origin or point of attachment (Chapter 1).

Distal convoluted tubule (**DIS**-tuhl KON-voh-**LOO**-ted) The part of a renal tubule that extends from a loop of Henle to a collecting tubule (Chapter 18).

Disulfide bond (digh-**SUL**-fyed BAHND) A covalent bond between the sulfur atoms of two amino acids in a protein; helps maintain the three-dimensional shape of the protein (Syn.—disulfide bridge) (Chapter 2).

Diverticulitis (DYE-ver-tik-yoo-**LYE**-tis) Inflammation of diverticula in the intestinal tract (Chapter 16).

DNA (deoxyribonucleic acid) A nucleic acid in the shape of a double helix. Makes up the chromosomes of cells and is the genetic code for hereditary characteristics (Chapter 2).

DNA replication (REP-li-**KAY**-shun) The process by which a DNA molecule makes a duplicate of itself. Takes place before mitosis or meiosis, to produce two sets of chromatids (potential chromosomes) within a cell (Chapter 3).

Dominant (**DAH**-ma-nent) In genetics, a characteristic that will be expressed even if only one gene for it is present in the homologous pair of chromosomes (Chapter 21).

Dormant (**DOOR**-ment) Temporarily inactive; a state of little metabolic activity (Chapter 22).

Dorsal (**DOR**-suhl) Toward the back (Syn.—posterior) (Chapter 1).

Dorsal cavity (**DOR**-suhl **KAV**-i-tee) The previously used term for the collective cranial and spinal cavities.

Dorsal root (**DOR**-suhl ROOT) The sensory root of a spinal nerve (Chapter 8).

Dorsal root ganglion (**DOR**-suhl ROOT **GANG**-lee-on) An enlarged area of the dorsal root of a spinal nerve that contains the cell bodies of sensory neurons (Chapter 8).

Down syndrome (DOWN **SIN**-drohm) A trisomy in which three chromosomes of number 21 are present; characterized by moderate to severe mental retardation and certain physical malformations (Chapter 20).

Duct (DUKT) A tube or channel, especially one that carries the secretion of a gland (Chapter 4).

Ductus arteriosus (**DUK**-tus ar-TIR-ee-**OH**-sis) A short fetal blood vessel that takes most blood in the pulmonary artery to the aorta, bypassing the fetal lungs (Chapter 13).

Ductus deferens (**DUK**-tus **DEF**-eer-enz) The tubular organ that carries sperm from the epididymis to the ejaculatory duct (Syn.—vas deferens) (Chapter 20).

Ductus venosus (**DUK**-tus ve-**NOH**-sus) A short fetal blood vessel that takes blood from the umbilical vein to the inferior vena cava (Chapter 13).

Duodenum (dew-**AH**-den-um or DEW-oh-**DEE**-num) The first 10 inches of the small intestine; the common bile duct enters it. (Chapter 16).

Dura mater (**DEW**-rah **MAH**-ter) The outermost layer of the meninges, made of fibrous connective tissue (Chapter 8).

Dwarfism (**DWORF**-izm) The condition of being abnormally small, especially small of stature due to a hereditary or endocrine disorder; pituitary dwarfism is caused by a deficiency of growth hormone (Chapter 10).

Dyspnea (**DISP**-nee-ah or disp-**NEE**-ah) Difficult breathing (Chapter 15).

Dysuria (dis-**YOO**-ree-ah) Painful or difficult urination (Chapter 18).

E

Ear (EER) The organ that contains the sensory receptors for hearing and equilibrium; consists of the outer ear, middle ear, and inner ear (Chapter 9).

Eccrine gland (**EK**-rin) The type of sweat gland (exocrine) that produces watery sweat; important in maintenance of normal body temperature (Chapter 5).

Ectoderm (**EK**-toh-derm) The outer primary germ layer of cells of an embryo; gives rise to the epidermis and nervous system (Chapter 21).

Ectoparasite (EK-toh-**PAR**-uh-sight) A parasite that lives on the surface of the body (Chapter 22).

Ectopic focus (ek-**TOP**-ik **FOH**-kus) The initiation of a heartbeat by part of the myocardium other than the sinoatrial node (Chapter 12).

Ectopic pregnancy (ek-**TOP**-ik **PREG**-nun-see) Implantation of a fertilized ovum outside the uterus; usually occurs in the fallopian tube but may be in the ovary or abdominal cavity; often results in death of the embryo because a functional placenta cannot be formed in these abnormal sites (Chapter 20).

Eczema (**EK**-zuh-mah) An inflammatory condition of the skin that may include the formation of vesicles or pustules (Chapter 5).

Edema (uh-**DEE**-muh) An abnormal accumulation of tissue fluid; may be localized or systemic (Chapter 19).

Effector (e-**FEK**-tur) An organ such as a muscle or gland that produces a characteristic response after receiving a stimulus (Chapter 8).

Efferent (**EFF**-er-rent) To carry away from a center or main part (Chapter 8).

Efferent arteriole (**EFF**-er-ent ar-**TIR**-ee-ohl) The arteriole that takes blood from a glomerulus to the peritubular capillaries that surround the renal tubule (Chapter 18).

Ejaculation (ee-JAK-yoo-**LAY**-shun) The ejection of semen from the male urethra (Chapter 20).

Ejaculatory duct (ee-**JAK**-yoo-la-TOR-ee DUKT) The duct formed by the union of the ductus deferens and the duct of the seminal vesicle; carries sperm to the urethra (Chapter 20).

Ejection fraction (ee-**JEK**-shun **FRAK**-shun) The percent of blood in a ventricle that is pumped during systole; a measure of the strength of the heart (Chapter 12).

Elastin (eh-**LAS**-tin) The primary protein that is found in the elastic fibers in several types of connective tissue (Chapter 4).

Electrocardiogram (ECG or EKG) (ee-LEK-troh-**KAR**-dee-oh-GRAM) A recording of the electrical changes that accompany the cardiac cycle (Chapter 12).

Electrolytes (ee-**LEK**-troh-lites) Substances that, in solution, dissociate into their component ions; include acids, bases, and salts (Chapter 19).

Electron (e-**LEK**-trahn) A subatomic particle that has a negative electrical charge; found orbiting the nucleus of an atom (Chapter 2).

Element (**EL**-uh-ment) A substance that consists of only one type of atom; 92 elements occur in nature (Chapter 2).

Embolism (**EM**-boh-lizm) Obstruction of a blood vessel by a blood clot or foreign substance that has traveled to and lodged in that vessel (Chapter 11).

Embryo (**EM**-bree-oh) The developing human individual from the time of fertilization until the eighth week of gestation (Chapter 21).

Embryoblast (**EM**-bree-oh-blast) A synonym for inner cell mass (Chapter 21).

Embryonic disc (EM-bree-**ON**-ik DISK) The portion of the inner cell mass of the early embryo that will develop into the individual (Chapter 21).

Emphysema (EM-fi-**SEE**-mah) The deterioration of alveoli and loss of elasticity of the lungs; normal exhalation and gas exchange are impaired (Chapter 15).

Emulsify (e-**MULL**-si-fye) To physically break up fats into smaller fat globules; the function of bile salts in bile (Chapter 16).

Enamel (en-**AM**-uhl) The hard substance that covers the crowns of teeth and forms the chewing surface (Chapter 16).

Encapsulated nerve ending (en-**KAP**-sul-LAY-ted NERV **END**-ing) A sensory nerve ending enclosed in a specialized cellular structure; the cutaneous receptors for touch and pressure (Chapter 5).

Endemic (en-**DEM**-ik) A disease that occurs continuously or expectedly in a given population (Chapter 22).

Endocardium (EN-doh-**KAR**-dee-um) The simple squamous epithelial tissue that lines the chambers of the heart and covers the valves (Chapter 12).

Endocrine gland (**EN**-doh-krin) A ductless gland that secretes its product (hormone) directly into the blood (Chapter 4).

Endocrine system (**EN**-doh-krin **SIS**-tem) The organ system that consists of the endocrine glands that secrete hormones into the blood (Chapter 10).

Endocytosis (EN-doh-sigh-**TOH**-sis) The process by which a cell takes in particulate matter or a fluid, such as phagocytosis of bacteria by WBCs; the cell membrane conforms to the material taken in and forms an intracellular vesicle or vacuole (Chapter 3).

Endoderm (**EN**-doh-derm) The inner primary germ layer of cells of an embryo; gives rise to respiratory organs and the lining of the digestive tract (Chapter 21).

Endogenous (en-**DOJ**-en-us) Coming from or produced within the body (Chapter 17).

Endogenous infection (en-**DOJ**-en-us) An infection caused by a person's own normal flora that have been introduced into an abnormal body site (Chapter 22).

Endolymph (**EN**-doh-limf) The fluid in the membranous labyrinth of the inner ear (Chapter 9).

Endometrium (EN-doh-**MEE**-tree-um) The vascular lining of the uterus that forms the maternal portion of the placenta (Chapter 20).

Endoplasmic reticulum (ER) (EN-doh-**PLAZ**-mik re-**TIK**-yoo-lum) A cell organelle found in the cytoplasm; a network of membranous channels that transport materials within the cell and synthesize lipids (Chapter 3).

Endothelin (EN-doh-**THEEL**-in) A peptide produced by the endothelium of blood vessels; it promotes vasoconstriction (Chapter 13).

Endothelium (EN-doh-**THEE**-lee-um) The simple squamous epithelial lining of arteries and veins, continuing as the walls of capillaries; prevents abnormal clotting and secretes both vasodilator and vasoconstrictor chemicals (Chapter 13).

Endotoxin (EN-doh-**TAHK**-sin) The toxic portion of the cell walls of gram-negative bacteria; causes fever and shock (Chapter 22).

Endotoxin shock (EN-doh-**TAHK**-sin SHAHK) A state of circulatory shock caused by infection with gram-negative bacteria (Chapter 22).

Energy levels (EN-er-jee **LEV**-els) The position of electrons within an atom (Syn.—orbitals or shells) (Chapter 2).

Enteric nervous system (en-**TER**-ik) The nerve fibers and plexuses of the alimentary tube; regulates secretions and contractions; is able to function independently of the CNS (Chapter 16).

Enteroendocrine cell (EN-ter-oh-**EN**-doh-krin SELL) A cell of the alimentary tube that secretes hormones (Chapter 16).

Enzyme (**EN**-zime) A protein that affects the speed of a chemical reaction. Also called an organic catalyst (Chapter 2).

Eosinophil (EE-oh-**SIN**-oh-fill) A type of white blood cell (granular); active in allergic reactions and parasitic infections (Chapter 11).

Ependymal cell (e-**PEN**-di-muhl SELL) A ciliated glial cell that lines the ventricles of the brain and central canal of the spinal cord (Chapter 8).

Epicardium (EP-ee-**KAR**-dee-um) The serous membrane on the surface of the myocardium (Syn.—visceral pericardium) (Chapter 12).

Epidemic (EP-i-**DEM**-ik) A disease that affects many people in a given population in a given time with more than the usual or expected number of cases (Chapter 22).

Epidemiology (EP-i-DEE-mee-**AH**-luh-jee) The study of the spread of disease and the factors that determine disease frequency and distribution (Chapter 22).

Epidermis (EP-i-**DER**-miss) The outer layer of the skin, made of stratified squamous epithelium (Chapter 5).

Epididymis (EP-i-**DID**-i-mis) (Pl.—epididymides) The tubular organ coiled on the posterior side of a testis; sperm mature here and are carried to the ductus deferens (Chapter 20).

Epigenetics (EP-i-je-**NET**-iks) The change in gene expression brought about by chemical activity on the chromosomes without any change in the base sequence of the DNA genes (Chapter 3).

Epiglottis (EP-i-**GLAH**-tis) The uppermost cartilage of the larynx; covers the larynx during swallowing (Chapter 15).

Epinephrine (EP-i-**NEFF**-rin) A hormone secreted by the adrenal medulla that stimulates many responses that enable the body to react to a stressful situation (Syn.—adrenaline) (Chapter 10).

Epiphyseal disc (e-**PIFF**-i-se-al DISK) A plate of cartilage at the junction of an epiphysis with the diaphysis of a long bone; the site of growth of a long bone (Chapter 6).

Epiphysis (e-**PIFF**-i-sis) The end of a long bone (Chapter 6).

Epithelial tissue (EP-i-**THEE**-lee-uhl **TISH**-yoo) The tissue found on external and internal body surfaces and that forms glands (Chapter 4).

Equilibrium (E-kwe-**LIB**-ree-um) 1. A state of balance. 2. The ability to remain upright and be aware of the position of the body (Chapter 9).

Erythema (ER-i-**THEE**-mah) Redness of the skin (Chapter 5).

Erythroblastosis fetalis (e-RITH-roh-blass-**TOH**-sis fee-**TAL**-is) Hemolytic anemia of the newborn, characterized by anemia and jaundice; the result of an Rh incompatibility of fetal blood and maternal blood; also called Rh disease of the newborn (Chapter 11).

Erythrocyte (e-**RITH**-roh-sight) A red blood cell (Chapter 11).

Erythropoietin (e-RITH-roh-**POY**-e-tin) A hormone secreted by the kidneys in a state of hypoxia; stimulates the red bone marrow to increase the rate of red blood cell production (Chapter 11).

Esophagus (e-**SOF**-uh-guss) The organ of the alimentary tube that is a passageway for food from the pharynx to the stomach (Chapter 16).

Essential amino acids (e-**SEN**-shul ah-**MEE**-noh **ASS**-ids) The amino acids that cannot be synthesized by the liver and must be obtained from proteins in the diet (Chapter 16).

Essential fatty acids (e-**SEN**-shul **FA**-tee **ASS**-ids) The fatty acids that cannot be synthesized by the body and must be obtained from fats in the diet (Chapter 17).

Estrogen (**ES**-troh-jen) The sex hormone secreted by a developing ovarian follicle; contributes to the growth of the female reproductive organs and the secondary sex characteristics (Chapter 10).

Ethmoid bone (**ETH**-moyd) An irregular cranial bone that forms the upper part of the nasal cavities and a small part of the lower anterior braincase (Chapter 6).

Eustachian tube (yoo-**STAY**-shun TOOB) The air passage between the middle ear cavity and the nasopharynx (Syn.—auditory tube) (Chapter 9).

Eversion (i-**VER**-zhun) To turn the sole of the foot laterally (Chapter 7).

Exocrine gland (**EK**-so-krin) A gland that secretes its product into a duct to be taken to a cavity or surface (Chapter 4).

Exocytosis (EKS-oh-sigh-**TOH**-sis) The process by which material is ejected or secreted from a cell; characteristic of the Golgi apparatus, in which membrane-bound vesicles fuse with the cell membrane and release their contents (Chapter 3).

Expiration (EK-spi-**RAY**-shun) Exhalation; the output of air from the lungs (Chapter 15).

Expiratory reserve (ek-**SPYR**-ah-tor-ee ree-**ZERV**) The volume of air beyond tidal volume that can be exhaled with the most forceful exhalation; average: 1000–1500 mL (Chapter 15).

Extension (eks-**TEN**-shun) To increase the angle of a joint (Chapter 7).

External (eks-**TER**-nuhl) On the outside; toward the surface (Chapter 1).

External anal sphincter (eks-**TER**-nuhl **AY**-nuhl **SFINK**-ter) The circular skeletal muscle that surrounds the internal anal sphincter and provides voluntary control of defecation (Chapter 16).

External auditory meatus (eks-**TER**-nuhl **AW**-di-TOR-ee me-**AY**-tuss) The ear canal; the portion of the outer ear that is a tunnel in the temporal bone between the auricle and the eardrum (Chapter 9).

External respiration (eks-**TER**-nuhl RES-pi-**RAY**-shun) The exchange of gases between the air in the alveoli and the blood in the pulmonary capillaries (Chapter 15).

External urethral sphincter (eks-**TER**-nuhl yoo-**REE**-thruhl **SFINK**-ter) The skeletal muscle of the pelvic floor encircling the urethra; provides voluntary control of urination (Chapter 18).

Extracellular fluid (EKS-trah-**SELL**-yoo-ler **FLOO**-id) The water found outside cells; includes plasma, tissue fluid, lymph, and other fluids (Chapter 2).

Extrinsic factor (eks-**TRIN**-sik **FAK**-ter) Vitamin B_{12}, obtained from food and necessary for DNA synthesis, especially by stem cells in the red bone marrow (Chapter 11).

Extrinsic muscles (eks-**TRIN**-sik) The six muscles that move the eyeball (Chapter 9).

F

Facet (**FA**-sit) A smooth, relatively flat articular surface on a bone (from the Latin "little face") (Chapter 6).

Facial bones (**FAY**-shul) The 14 irregular bones of the face (Chapter 6).

Facial nerves (**FAY**-shul) Cranial nerve pair VII; sensory for taste, motor to facial muscles and the salivary glands (Chapter 8).

Facilitated diffusion (fuh-**SILL**-ah-tay-ted di-**FEW**-zhun) The process in which a substance is transported through a membrane in combination with a carrier or transporter molecule (Chapter 3).

Facultative anaerobe (**FAK**-uhl-tay-tive **AN**-air-robe) A bacterium that is able to reproduce either in the presence or absence of oxygen (Chapter 22).

Fallopian tube (fuh-**LOH**-pee-an TOOB) The tubular organ that propels an ovum from the ovary to the uterus by means of ciliated epithelium and peristalsis of its smooth muscle layer (Syn.—uterine tube) (Chapter 20).

Fascia (**FASH**-ee-ah) A fibrous connective tissue membrane that covers individual skeletal muscles and certain organs (Chapter 4).

Fatty acid (**FA**-tee **ASS**-id) A lipid molecule that consists of an even-numbered carbon chain of 12 to 24 carbons with hydrogens; may be saturated or unsaturated; an end product of the digestion of fats (Chapter 2).

Femur (**FEE**-mur) The long bone of the thigh (Chapter 6).

Fermentation (FER-men-**TAY**-shun) The process of the decomposition of complex organic molecules to simpler molecules in the absence of oxygen; the energy-producing process for many bacteria of the microbiota (Chapter 1).

Fertilization (FER-ti-li-**ZAY**-shun) The union of the nuclei of an ovum and a sperm cell; restores the diploid number (Chapter 3).

Fetal alcohol syndrome (**FEE**-tuhl **AL**-koh-hol) Birth defects or developmental abnormalities in infants born to women who chronically consumed alcohol during the gestation period (Chapter 21).

Fever (**FEE**-ver) An abnormally high body temperature, caused by pyrogens; may accompany an infectious disease or severe physical injury (Chapter 17).

Fever blister (**FEE**-ver **BLISS**-ter) An eruption of the skin caused by the herpes simplex virus (Syn.—cold sore) (Chapter 5).

Fiber (**FYE**-ber) Cellulose in the diet that provides exercise for the colon and helps prevent constipation (Chapter 2).

Fibrillation (fi-bri-**LAY**-shun) Very rapid and uncoordinated heartbeats; ventricular fibrillation is a life-threatening emergency due to ineffective pumping and decreased cardiac output (Chapter 12).

Fibrillin (fye-**BRILL**-in) A protein that stabilizes the bundles of elastin fibers in elastic connective tissue (Chapter 4).

Fibrin (**FYE**-brin) A thread-like protein formed by the action of thrombin on fibrinogen; the substance of which a blood clot is made (Chapter 11).

Fibrinogen (fye-**BRIN**-o-jen) A protein clotting factor produced by the liver; converted to fibrin by thrombin (Chapter 11).

Fibrinolysis (FYE-brin-**AHL**-e-sis) 1. The dissolving of a fibrin clot by natural enzymes, after the clot has served its purpose. 2. The clinical use of clot-dissolving enzymes to dissolve abnormal clots (Chapter 11).

Fibroblast (**FYE**-broh-blast) A connective tissue cell that produces collagen and elastin fibers (Chapter 4).

Fibrous connective tissue (**FYE**-brus) The tissue that consists primarily of collagen fibers (the cells are fibroblasts). Its most important physical characteristic is its strength (Chapter 4).

Fibrous skeleton of the heart (**FYE**-brus **SKEL**-e-tun) The fibrous connective tissue that encircles and anchors the edges of the heart valves and prevents stretching of their openings; it also electrically insulates the ventricles from the atria so that impulses for contraction follow only the normal conduction pathway (Chapter 12).

Fibula (**FIB**-yoo-lah) A long bone of the lower leg; on the lateral side, thinner than the tibia (Chapter 6).

Filtration (fill-**TRAY**-shun) The process in which water and dissolved materials move through a membrane from an area of higher pressure to an area of lower pressure (Chapter 3).

Fimbriae (**FIM**-bree-ay) Finger-like projections at the end of the fallopian tube that enclose the ovary (Chapter 20).

Fissure (**FISH**-er) A groove or furrow between parts of an organ such as the brain (Syn.—sulcus) (Chapter 8).

Flagellum (flah-**JELL**-um) (Pl.—flagella) A long, thread-like projection through a cell membrane; provides motility for the cell (Chapter 3).

Flexion (**FLEK**-shun) To decrease the angle of a joint (Chapter 7).

Flexor reflex (**FLEKS**-er **REE**-fleks) A spinal cord reflex in which a painful stimulus causes withdrawal of a body part (Chapter 8).

Fluorescent antibody test (floor-**ESS**-ent **AN**-ti-BAH-dee) A diagnostic test that uses fluorescently tagged antibodies to determine the presence of a particular pathogen in the blood or other tissue specimen (Chapter 14).

Flutter (**FLUH**-ter) A very rapid yet fairly regular heartbeat (Chapter 12).

Follicle-stimulating hormone (FSH) (**FAH**-li-kuhl) A gonadotropic hormone produced by the anterior pituitary gland that initiates the production of ova in the ovaries or sperm in the testes (Chapter 10).

Fomites (**FOH**-mights; **FOH**-mi-teez) Inanimate objects capable of transmitting infectious microorganisms from one host to another (Chapter 22).

Fontanel (FON-tah-**NELL**) An area of fibrous connective tissue membrane between the cranial bones of an infant's skull, where bone formation is not complete (Chapter 6).

Foramen (for-**RAY**-men) A hole or opening, as in a bone (from the Latin "to bore") (Chapter 6).

Foramen ovale (for-**RAY**-men oh-**VAHL**-ee) An opening in the interatrial septum of the fetal heart that permits blood to flow from the right atrium to the left atrium, bypassing the fetal lungs (Chapter 13).

Forced expiratory volume (ek-**SPYR**-ah-tor-ee **VAHL**-yoom) The maximum amount of air that can be exhaled in 1, 2, or 3 seconds (Chapter 15).

Fossa (**FAH**-sah) A shallow depression in a bone (from the Latin "ditch") (Chapter 6).

Fovea (**FOH**-vee-ah) A depression in the retina of the eye directly behind the lens; contains only cones and is the area of best color vision (Chapter 9).

Fracture (**FRAK**-chur) A break in a bone (Chapter 6).

Free nerve ending (FREE NERV **END**-ing) The end of a sensory neuron; the receptor for the sense of pain, itch, heat, or cold in the skin and pain in the viscera (Chapter 5).

Free radical (FREE **RA**-di-kuhl) A molecule with an unpaired electron that is very reactive; formed during normal metabolism and contributes to the natural deterioration (aging) of cells (Chapter 17).

Frontal bone (**FRUN**-tuhl) The flat cranial bone that forms the forehead (Chapter 6).

Frontal lobes (**FRUN**-tuhl LOWBS) The most anterior parts of the cerebrum; contain the motor areas for voluntary movement and the motor speech area (Chapter 8).

Frontal section (**FRUN**-tuhl **SEK**-shun) A plane separating the body into front and back portions (Syn.—coronal section) (Chapter 1).

Frostbite (**FRAWST**-bite) The freezing of part of the body, resulting in tissue damage or death (gangrene) (Chapter 17).

Fructose (**FRUHK**-tohs) A monosaccharide, a six-carbon sugar that is part of the sucrose in food; converted to glucose by the liver (Chapter 2).

Functional layer (**FUNK**-shun-ul **LAY**-er) The vascular layer of the endometrium that is lost in menstruation, then regenerated by the basilar layer (Chapter 20).

Fungus (**FUNG**-gus) Any of the organisms of the kingdom Fungi; they lack chlorophyll; may be unicellular or multicellular, saprophytic or parasitic; include yeasts, molds, and mushrooms (Chapter 22).

G

Galactose (guh-**LAK**-tohs) A monosaccharide, a six-carbon sugar that is part of the lactose in food; converted to glucose by the liver (Chapter 2).

Gallbladder (**GAWL**-bla-der) An accessory organ of digestion; a sac located on the undersurface of the liver; stores and concentrates bile (Chapter 16).

Gallstones (**GAWL**-stohns) Crystals formed in the gallbladder or bile ducts; the most common type is made of cholesterol (Chapter 16).

Gametes (**GAM**-eets) The male or female reproductive cells, sperm cells or ova, each with the haploid number of chromosomes (Chapter 3).

Gamma globulins (**GA**-mah **GLAH**-byoo-lins) Antibodies (Chapter 14).

Ganglion (**GANG**-lee-on) A group of neuron cell bodies located outside the CNS (Chapter 8).

Ganglion neurons (**GANG**-lee-on **NYOOR**-onz) The neurons that form the optic nerve; carry impulses from the retina to the brain (Chapter 9).

Gastric juice (**GAS**-trik **JOOSS**) The secretion of the gastric pits of the stomach; contains hydrochloric acid, pepsin, gastrin, and mucus (Chapter 16).

Gastric pits (**GAS**-trik PITS) The glands of the mucosa of the stomach; secrete gastric juice (Chapter 16).

Gastric ulcer (**GAS**-trik **UL**-ser) An erosion of the gastric mucosa and submucosa (Chapter 16).

Gastrin (**GAS**-trin) A hormone secreted by the G cells of the gastric mucosa when food enters the stomach; stimulates the secretion of gastric juice (Chapter 16).

Gene (JEEN) A segment of DNA that is the genetic code for a particular protein and is located in a definite position on a particular chromosome (Chapter 3).

Gene expression (JEEN ek-**SPRESH**-un) The transcription and translation of a DNA gene to mRNA and to a protein that gives a cell (or organ or entire organism) a particular characteristic (Chapter 3).

Genetic code (je-**NET**-ik KOHD) The DNA code for proteins that is shared by all living things; the sequence of bases of the DNA in the chromosomes of cells (Chapter 2).

Genetic disease (je-**NET**-ik di-**ZEEZ**) A hereditary disorder that is the result of an incorrect sequence of bases in the DNA (gene) of a particular chromosome. May be passed to offspring (Chapter 3).

Genetic immunity (je-**NET**-ik im-**YOO**-ni-tee) The immunity provided by the genetic makeup of a species; reflects the inability of certain pathogens to cause disease in certain host species (Chapter 14).

Genome (**JEE**-nohm) The total genetic information contained in the chromosomes of a cell of a species; the human genome is approximately 22,000 genes (Chapter 3).

Genotype (**JEE**-noh-type) The genetic makeup of an individual; the genes that are present (Chapter 21).

Gestation (jes-**TAY**-shun) The length of time from conception to birth; the human gestation period averages 280 days (Chapter 21).

Giantism (**JIGH**-an-tizm) Excessive growth of the body or its parts; may be the result of hypersecretion of growth hormone in childhood (Chapter 10).

Gingiva (jin-**JIGH**-vah) The gums; the tissue that covers the upper and lower jaws around the necks of the teeth (Chapter 16).

Gland (GLAND) A cell or group of epithelial cells that is specialized to secrete a substance (Chapter 4).

Glaucoma (glaw-**KOH**-mah) An eye disease often characterized by increased intraocular pressure due to excessive accumulation of aqueous humor; may result in optic nerve damage and blindness (Chapter 9).

Glial cells (**GLEE**-al SELLS) The neuroglia of the central nervous system (Chapter 4).

Gliding joint (**GLY**-ding) A diarthrosis that permits a sliding movement (Chapter 6).

Globulins (**GLAH**-byoo-lins) Proteins that circulate in blood plasma; alpha and beta globulins are synthesized by the liver; gamma globulins (antibodies) are synthesized by lymphocytes (Chapter 11).

Glomerular filtration (gloh-**MER**-yoo-ler fill-**TRAY**-shun) The first step in the formation of urine; blood pressure in the glomerulus forces plasma, dissolved materials, and small proteins into Bowman's capsule; this fluid is then called renal filtrate (Chapter 18).

Glomerular filtration rate (gloh-**MER**-yoo-ler fill-**TRAY**-shun RAYT) The total volume of renal filtrate that the kidneys form in 1 minute; average is 100–125 mL/minute (Chapter 18).

Glomerulus (gloh-**MER**-yoo-lus) A capillary network that is enclosed by Bowman's capsule; filtration takes place from the glomerulus to Bowman's capsule (from the Latin "little ball") (Chapter 18).

Glossopharyngeal nerves (GLAH-so-fuh-**RIN**-jee-uhl) Cranial nerve pair IX; sensory for taste and cardiovascular reflexes; motor to salivary glands (Chapter 8).

Glottis (**GLAH**-tis) The opening between the vocal cords; an air passageway (Chapter 15).

Glucagon (**GLOO**-kuh-gahn) A hormone secreted by the pancreas that increases the blood glucose level (Chapter 10).

Glucocorticoids (GLOO-koh-**KOR**-ti-koids) The hormones secreted by the adrenal cortex that affect the metabolism of nutrients; cortisol is the major hormone in this group (Chapter 10).

Gluconeogenesis (GLOO-koh-nee-oh-**JEN**-i-sis) The conversion of excess amino acids to simple carbohydrates or to glucose to be used for energy production (Chapter 10).

Glucose (**GLOO**-kos) A hexose monosaccharide that is the primary energy source for body cells (Chapter 2).

Glycerol (**GLISS**-er-ol) A three-carbon molecule that is one of the end products of the digestion of fats (Chapter 2).

Glycogen (**GLY**-ko-jen) A polysaccharide that is the storage form for excess glucose in the liver and muscles (Chapter 2).

Glycogenesis (GLY-koh-**JEN**-i-sis) The conversion of glucose to glycogen to be stored as potential energy (Chapter 10).

Glycogenolysis (GLY-koh-jen-**AHL**-i-sis) The conversion of stored glycogen to glucose to be used for energy production (Chapter 10).

Glycolysis (gly-**KAHL**-ah-sis) The first stage of the cell respiration of glucose, in which glucose is broken down into two molecules of pyruvic acid and ATP is formed; anaerobic; takes place in the cytoplasm of cells (Chapter 17).

Glycosuria (GLY-kos-**YOO**-ree-ah) The presence of glucose in urine; often an indication of diabetes mellitus (Chapter 18).

Goblet cell (**GAHB**-let) Unicellular glands that secrete mucus; found in the respiratory and GI mucosa (Chapter 4).

Goiter (**GOY**-ter) An enlargement of the thyroid gland, often due to a lack of dietary iodine (Chapter 10).

Golgi apparatus (**GOHL**-jee) A cell organelle found in the cytoplasm; synthesizes carbohydrates and packages materials for secretion from the cell (Chapter 3).

Gonadotropic hormone (GAH-nah-doh-**TROH**-pik) A hormone that has its effects on the ovaries or testes (gonads); FSH and LH (Chapter 10).

Gonorrhea (GAH-nuh-**REE**-ah) A sexually transmitted disease caused by the bacterium *Neisseria gonorrhoeae;* may also cause conjunctivitis in newborns of infected women (Chapter 20).

Graafian follicle (**GRAF**-ee-uhn **FAH**-li-kuhl) A mature ovarian follicle that releases an ovum (Chapter 20).

Gram negative (GRAM **NEG**-uh-tiv) Bacteria that appear red or pink after Gram staining (Chapter 22).

Gram positive (GRAM **PAHS**-uh-tiv) Bacteria that appear purple or blue after Gram staining (Chapter 22).

Gram stain (GRAM STAYN) A staining procedure for bacteria to make them visible microscopically and to determine their Gram reaction, which is important in the identification of bacteria (Chapter 22).

Graves' disease (GRAYVES) Hypersecretion of thyroxine, believed to be an autoimmune disease; symptoms reflect the elevated metabolic rate (Chapter 10).

Gray matter (GRAY) Nerve tissue within the central nervous system that consists of the cell bodies of neurons (Chapter 8).

Growth hormone (GH) (GROHTH **HOR**-mohn) A hormone secreted by the anterior pituitary gland that increases the rate of cell division and protein synthesis (Chapter 10).

Gyrus (**JIGH**-rus) A fold or ridge, as in the cerebral cortex (Syn.—convolution) (Chapter 8).

H

Hair (HAIR) An accessory skin structure produced in a hair follicle (Chapter 5).

Hair cells (HAIR SELLS) Cells with specialized microvilli (called stereocilia) found in the inner ear; the receptors for hearing (cochlea), static equilibrium (utricle and saccule), and motion equilibrium (semicircular canals) (Chapter 9).

Hair follicle (HAIR **FAH**-li-kuhl) The structure within the skin in which a hair grows (Chapter 5).

Hair root (HAIR ROOT) The site of mitosis at the base of a hair follicle; nourished by the capillaries of the dermal papilla; new cells become the hair shaft (Chapter 5).

Haploid number (**HA**-ployd) Half the usual number of chromosomes found in the cells of a species. Characteristic of the gametes of the species (human: 23) (Chapter 3).

Hard palate (HARD **PAL**-uht) The anterior portion of the palate formed by the maxillae and the palatine bones (Chapter 6).

Haustra (**HOWS**-trah) The pouches of the colon (Chapter 16).

Haversian system (ha-**VER**-zhun) The structural unit of compact bone, consisting of a central haversian canal surrounded by concentric rings of osteocytes within matrix (Syn.—osteon) (Chapter 4).

Heart murmur (HART **MUR**-mur) An abnormal heart sound heard during the cardiac cycle; often caused by a malfunctioning heart valve (Chapter 12).

Heat exhaustion (HEET ig-**ZAWS**-chun) A state of weakness and dehydration caused by excessive loss of body water and sodium chloride in sweat; the result of exposure to heat or of strenuous exercise (Chapter 17).

Heat stroke (HEET STROHK) An acute reaction to heat exposure in which there is failure of the temperature-regulating mechanisms; sweating ceases, and body temperature rises sharply (Chapter 17).

Heimlich maneuver (**HIGHM**-lik ma-**NEW**-ver) A procedure used to remove foreign material lodged in the pharynx, larynx, or trachea (Chapter 15).

Helix (**HEE**-liks) A coil or spiral. Double helix is the descriptive term used for the shape of a DNA molecule: two strands of nucleotides coiled around each other and resembling a twisted ladder (Chapter 2).

Hematocrit (hee-**MAT**-oh-krit) A laboratory test that determines the percentage of red blood cells in a given volume of blood; part of a complete blood count (Chapter 11).

Hematuria (HEM-uh-**TYOO**-ree-ah) The presence of blood (RBCs) in urine (Chapter 18).

Hemodialysis (HEE-moh-dye-**AL**-i-sis) A technique for providing the function of the kidneys by passing the blood through tubes surrounded by solutions that selectively remove waste products and excess minerals; may be lifesaving in cases of renal failure (Chapter 18).

Hemoglobin (**HEE**-muh-GLOW-bin) The protein in red blood cells that contains iron and transports oxygen in the blood (Chapter 7).

Hemolysis (he-**MAHL**-e-sis) Lysis or rupture of red blood cells; may be the result of an antigen–antibody reaction or of increased fragility of red blood cells in some types of anemia (Chapter 11).

Hemophilia (HEE-moh-**FILL**-ee-ah) A hereditary blood disorder characterized by the inability of the blood to clot normally; hemophilia A is caused by a lack of clotting Factor 8 (Chapter 11).

Hemopoietic tissue (HEE-moh-poy-**ET**-ik) A blood-forming tissue, primarily the red bone marrow; lymphatic tissue produces some lymphocytes (Chapter 4).

Hemorrhoids (**HEM**-uh-royds) Varicose veins of the anal canal (Chapter 13).

Hemostasis (HEE-moh-**STAY**-sis) Prevention of blood loss; the mechanisms are chemical clotting, vascular spasm, and platelet plug formation (Chapter 11).

Heparin (**HEP**-ar-in) A chemical that inhibits blood clotting, an anticoagulant; produced by basophils. Also used clinically to prevent abnormal clotting, such as following some types of surgery (Chapter 11).

Hepatic duct (hep-**PAT**-ik DUKT) The duct that takes bile out of the liver; joins the cystic duct of the gallbladder to form the common bile duct (Chapter 16).

Hepatic portal circulation (hep-**PAT**-ik **POOR**-tuhl) The pathway of systemic circulation in which venous blood from the digestive organs and the spleen circulates through the liver before returning to the heart (Chapter 13).

Hepatitis (HEP-uh-**TIGH**-tis) Inflammation of the liver, most often caused by the hepatitis viruses A, B, or C (Chapter 16).

Herniated disc (**HER**-nee-ay-ted DISK) Rupture of an intervertebral disc (Chapter 6).

Herpes simplex (**HER**-peez **SIM**-pleks) A virus that causes lesions in the skin or mucous membranes of the mouth (usually type 1) or genital area (usually type 2); either type may cause death or mental retardation of infants of infected women (Chapter 20).

Heterozygous (HET-er-oh-**ZYE**-gus) Having two different alleles for a trait (Chapter 21).

Hexose sugar (**HEKS**-ohs) A six-carbon sugar, such as glucose, that is an energy source (in the process of cell respiration) (Chapter 2).

Hilus (**HIGH**-lus) An indentation or depression on the surface of an organ such as a lung or kidney (Chapter 15).

Hinge joint (HINJ) A diarthrosis that permits movement in one plane (Chapter 6).

Hip bone (HIP BOWNE) The flat bone that forms half of the pelvic bone; consists of the upper ilium, the lower posterior ischium, and the lower anterior pubis (Chapter 6).

Hippocampus (hih-poh-**KAM**-pus) Part of the brain in the temporal lobe on the floor of the lateral ventricle; it is essential for the formation of new memories (Chapter 8).

Histamine (**HISS**-tah-meen) An inflammatory chemical released by damaged tissues as part of innate immunity; stimulates increased capillary permeability and vasodilation (Chapter 5).

Hives (HIGHVZ) A very itchy eruption of the skin, usually the result of an allergy (Chapter 5).

Hodgkin's disease (**HODJ**-kinz) A malignancy of the lymphatic tissue; a lymphoma (Chapter 14).

Homeostasis (HOH-mee-oh-**STAY**-sis) The state in which the internal environment of the body remains relatively stable by responding appropriately to changes (Chapter 1).

Homologous pair (hoh-**MAHL**-ah-gus) A pair of chromosomes, one maternal and one paternal, that contain genes for the same characteristics (Chapter 21).

Homozygous (HOH-moh-**ZYE**-gus) Having two similar alleles for a trait (Chapter 21).

Hormone (**HOR**-mohn) The secretion of an endocrine gland that has specific effects on particular target organs (Chapter 4).

Human leukocyte antigens (HLA) (**HYOO**-man **LOO**-koh-sight **AN**-ti-jens) The antigens on white blood cells that are representative of the antigens present on all the cells of the individual; the "self" antigens that are controlled by the MHC genes on chromosome number 6; the basis for tissue typing before an organ transplant is attempted (Chapter 11).

Humerus (**HYOO**-mer-us) The long bone of the upper arm (Chapter 6).

Humoral immunity (**HYOO**-mohr-uhl im-**YOO**-ni-tee) The mechanism of adaptive immunity that involves antibody production and the destruction of foreign antigens by the activities of B cells, T cells, and macrophages (Syn.—antibody-mediated immunity) (Chapter 14).

Hyaline membrane disease (**HIGH**-e-lin **MEM**-brayn di-**ZEEZ**) Respiratory distress syndrome of the newborn; occurs in premature infants whose lungs have not yet produced sufficient pulmonary surfactant to permit inflation of the alveoli (Chapter 15).

Hydrochloric acid (HIGH-droh-**KLOR**-ik **ASS**-id) An acid secreted by the parietal cells of the gastric pits of the stomach; activates pepsin and maintains a pH of 1 to 2 in the stomach (Chapter 16).

Hydrogen bond (**HIGH**-droh-jen BAHND) A weak bond that helps maintain the three-dimensional shape of proteins and nucleic acids (Chapter 2).

Hymen (**HIGH**-men) A thin fold of mucous membrane that partially covers the vaginal orifice (Chapter 20).

Hypercalcemia (HIGH-per-kal-**SEE**-mee-ah) A high blood calcium level (Chapter 10).

Hypercapnia (HIGH-per-**KAP**-nee-ah) A higher than normal blood level of carbon dioxide (usually 45–50 mm Hg) (Chapter 15).

Hyperglycemia (HIGH-per-gligh-**SEE**-mee-ah) A high blood glucose level (Chapter 10).

Hyperkalemia (HIGH-per-kuh-**LEE**-mee-ah) A high blood potassium level (Chapter 19).

Hypernatremia (HIGH-per-nuh-**TREE**-mee-ah) A high blood sodium level (Chapter 19).

Hyperopia (HIGH-per-**OH**-pee-ah) Farsightedness; an error of refraction in which only distant objects are seen clearly (Chapter 9).

Hypertension (HIGH-per-**TEN**-shun) An abnormally high blood pressure, consistently above 130/85 mm Hg (Chapter 13).

Hypertonic (HIGH-per-**TAHN**-ik) Having a greater concentration of dissolved materials than the solution used as a comparison (Chapter 3).

Hypertrophy (high-**PER**-troh-fee) Increase in size of a body part, especially of a muscle following long-term exercise or overuse (Chapter 7).

Hypocalcemia (HIGH-poh-kal-**SEE**-mee-ah) A low blood calcium level (Chapter 10).

Hypoglossal nerves (HIGH-poh-**GLAH**-suhl) Cranial nerve pair XII; motor to the tongue (Chapter 8).

Hypoglycemia (HIGH-poh-gligh-**SEE**-mee-ah) A low blood glucose level (Chapter 10).

Hypokalemia (HIGH-poh-kuh-**LEE**-mee-ah) A low blood potassium level (Chapter 19).

Hyponatremia (HIGH-poh-nuh-**TREE**-mee-ah) A low blood sodium level (Chapter 19).

Hypophyseal portal system (high-POFF-e-**SEE**-al **POR**-tuhl) The pathway of circulation in which releasing hormones from the hypothalamus circulate directly to the anterior pituitary gland (Chapter 10).

Hypophysis (high-**POFF**-e-sis) The pituitary gland (Chapter 10).

Hypotension (HIGH-poh-**TEN**-shun) An abnormally low blood pressure, consistently below 90/60 mm Hg (Chapter 13).

Hypothalamus (HIGH-poh-**THAL**-uh-muss) The part of the brain superior to the pituitary gland and inferior to the thalamus; its many functions include regulation of body temperature and regulation of the secretions of the pituitary gland (Chapter 8).

Hypothermia (HIGH-poh-**THER**-mee-ah) 1. The condition in which the body temperature is abnormally low due to excessive exposure to cold. 2. A procedure used during some types of surgery to lower body temperature to reduce the patient's need for oxygen (Chapter 17).

Hypotonic (HIGH-po-**TAHN**-ik) Having a lower concentration of dissolved materials than the solution used as a comparison (Chapter 3).

Hypovolemic shock (HIGH-poh-voh-**LEEM**-ik SHAHK) A type of circulatory shock caused by a decrease in blood volume (Chapter 13).

Hypoxemia (HIGH-pahk-**SEE**-mee-ah) A deficiency of oxygen in the blood (Chapter 2).

Hypoxia (high-**PAHK**-see-ah) A deficiency or lack of oxygen in tissues (Chapter 2).

I

Idiopathic (ID-ee-oh-**PATH**-ik) A disease or disorder of unknown cause (Chapter 11).

Ileocecal valve (ILL-ee-oh-**SEE**-kuhl VALV) The tissue of the ileum that extends into the cecum; a flap that acts as a sphincter and prevents the backup of fecal material into the small intestine (Chapter 16).

Ileum (**ILL**-ee-um) The third and last portion of the small intestine, about 11 feet long (Chapter 16).

Ilium (**ILL**-ee-um) The upper, flared portion of the hip bone (Chapter 6).

Immune globulin (Ig) (im-**MYOON GLAH**-byoo-lin) A synonym for antibody, as is immunoglobulin (Chapter 14).

Immunity (im-**MYOO**-ni-tee) The state of being protected from an infectious disease, usually by having been exposed to the infectious agent or a vaccine; human immunity has two major components: innate and adaptive. Innate immunity is nonspecific, has no memory, and consists of anatomic barriers, defensive cells, and chemicals. Adaptive immunity is specific, has memory, and may involve antibodies (Chapter 11).

Impetigo (IM-pe-**TYE**-go) A bacterial infection of the skin that occurs most often in children (Chapter 5).

Implantation (IM-plan-**TAY**-shun) Embedding of the embryonic blastocyst in the endometrium of the uterus 5 to 8 days after fertilization (Chapter 21).

In vitro fertilization (IN **VEE**-troh FER-ti-li-**ZAY**-shun) Fertilization outside the body, in which sperm and ova are mixed in laboratory glassware; early embryos may then be introduced into the uterus for implantation (Chapter 20).

Inactivator (in-**AK**-ti-vay-tur) A chemical that inactivates a neurotransmitter to prevent continuous impulses (Chapter 8).

Inapparent infection (**IN**-uh-PAR-ent) An infection without symptoms (Syn.—subclinical, asymptomatic) (Chapter 22).

Incubation period (IN-kew-**BAY**-shun) In the course of an infectious disease, the time between the entry of the pathogen and the onset of symptoms (Chapter 22).

Incus (**ING**-kuss) The second of the three auditory bones in the middle ear; transmits vibrations from the malleus to the stapes (Chapter 9).

Infarct (**IN**-farkt) An area of tissue that has died due to lack of a blood supply (Chapter 12).

Infection (in-**FEK**-shun) A disease process caused by the invasion and multiplication of a microorganism (Chapter 22).

Inferior (in-**FEER**-ee-your) Below or lower (Chapter 1).

Inferior vena cava (**VEE**-nah **KAY**-vah) The vein that returns blood from the lower body to the right atrium (Chapter 12).

Infestation (in-fess-**TAY**-shun) The harboring of parasites, especially worms or arthropods (Chapter 22).

Inflammation (in-fluh-**MAY**-shun) The reactions of tissue to injury (Chapter 5).

Inguinal canal (**IN**-gwi-nuhl ka-**NAL**) The opening in the lower abdominal wall that contains a spermatic cord in men and the round ligament of the uterus in women; a natural weak spot that may be the site of hernia formation (Chapter 20).

Inhibin (in-**HIB**-in) A protein hormone secreted by the sustentacular cells of the testes and by the ovaries; inhibits secretion of follicle-stimulating hormone (Chapter 10).

Inner cell mass (**IN**-er SELL MASS) In the early embryo, the group of cells within the blastocyst, enclosed by the trophoblast; will develop the three germ layers and become the embryo proper (Syn.—embryoblast) (Chapter 21).

Inorganic (**IN**-or-GAN-ik) A chemical compound that does not contain carbon–hydrogen covalent bonds; includes water, salts, and oxygen (Chapter 1).

Insertion (in-**SIR**-shun) The more movable attachment point of a muscle to a bone (Chapter 7).

Inspiration (in-spi-**RAY**-shun) Inhalation; the intake of air to the lungs (Chapter 15).

Inspiratory reserve (in-**SPYR**-ah-tor-ee ree-**ZERV**) The volume of air beyond tidal volume that can be inhaled with the deepest inhalation; average: 2000–3000 mL (Chapter 15).

Insulin (**IN**-syoo-lin) A protein hormone secreted by the pancreas that decreases the blood glucose level by increasing storage of glycogen and use of glucose by cells for energy production (Chapter 10).

Integumentary system (in-TEG-yoo-**MEN**-tah-ree) The organ system that consists of the skin and its accessory structures and the subcutaneous tissue (Chapter 5).

Intensity (in-**TEN**-si-tee) The degree to which a sensation is felt (Chapter 9).

Intercalated cell (**IN**-ter-kuh-lay-ted SELL) A cell of the collecting tubule of the nephron; its free surface membrane contains proton pumps to secrete excess H^+ ions into the renal filtrate (Chapter 18).

Intercalated disc (**IN**-ter-kuh-lay-ted DISK) A modification of the cell membrane of cardiac muscle cells; the end membranes of adjacent cells are folded and fit into one another; permits rapid transmission of the electrical impulses that bring about contraction (Chapter 4).

Intercostal muscles (IN-ter-**KAHS**-tuhl **MUSS**-uhls) The skeletal muscles between the ribs; the external intercostals pull the ribs up and out for inhalation; the internal intercostals pull the ribs down and in for a forced exhalation (Syn.—spareribs) (Chapter 15).

Intercostal nerves (IN-ter-**KAHS**-tuhl NERVS) The pairs of peripheral nerves that are motor to the intercostal muscles (Chapter 15).

Interferon (in-ter-**FEER**-on) A chemical produced by T cells or by cells infected with viruses; is part of innate immunity and prevents the reproduction of viruses (Chapter 14).

Internal (in-**TER**-nuhl) On the inside, or away from the surface (Chapter 1).

Internal anal sphincter (in-**TER**-nuhl **AY**-nuhl **SFINK**-ter) The circular smooth muscle that surrounds the anus; relaxes as part of the defecation reflex to permit defecation (Chapter 16).

Internal respiration (in-**TER**-nuhl RES-pi-**RAY**-shun) The exchange of gases between the blood in the systemic capillaries and the surrounding tissue fluid and cells (Chapter 15).

Internal urethral sphincter (yoo-**REE**-thruhl **SFINK**-ter) The smooth muscle sphincter at the junction of the urinary bladder and the urethra; relaxes as part of the urination reflex to permit urination (Chapter 18).

Interneuron (**IN**-ter-NYOOR-on) A nerve cell entirely within the central nervous system (Chapter 8).

Interphase (**IN**-ter-fayz) The period of time between mitotic divisions during which DNA replication takes place (Chapter 3).

Interstitial cells (in-ter-**STISH**-uhl SELLS) The cells in the testes that secrete testosterone when stimulated by LH (Chapter 20).

Intestinal glands (in-**TESS**-tin-uhl) 1. The glands of the small intestine that secrete digestive enzymes. 2. The glands of the large intestine that secrete mucus (Chapter 16).

Intracellular fluid (IN-trah-**SELL**-yoo-ler **FLOO**-id) The water found within cells (Chapter 2).

Intramuscular injection (in-trah-**MUSS**-kew-ler in-**JEK**-shun) An injection of a medication into a muscle (Chapter 7).

Intrapleural pressure (in-trah-**PLOOR**-uhl) The pressure within the potential pleural space; always slightly below atmospheric pressure, about 756 mm Hg (Chapter 15).

Intrapulmonic pressure (in-trah-pull-**MAHN**-ik) The air pressure within the bronchial tree and alveoli; fluctuates below and above atmospheric pressure during breathing (Chapter 15).

Intrinsic factor (in-**TRIN**-sik **FAK**-ter) A chemical produced by the parietal cells of the gastric mucosa; necessary for the absorption of vitamin B_{12} (Chapter 11).

Inversion (in-**VER**-zhun) To turn the sole of the foot medially (Chapter 7).

Involuntary muscle (in-**VAHL**-un-tary **MUSS**-uhl) Another name for smooth muscle tissue (Chapter 4).

Ion (**EYE**-on) An atom or group of atoms with an electrical charge (Chapter 2).

Ionic bond (eye-**ON**-ik) A chemical bond formed by the loss and gain of electrons between atoms (Chapter 2).

Iris (**EYE**-ris) The colored part of the eye, between the cornea and lens; made of two sets of smooth muscle fibers that regulate the size of the pupil, the opening in the center of the iris (from the Latin "rainbow") (Chapter 9).

Irisin (**EYE**-ris-in) A hormone produced by skeletal muscle cells that undergo regular exercise; it transforms white (storage) adipocytes into brown (thermogenic) fat cells. (Chapter 4).

Ischemic (iss-**SKEE**-mik) Lack of blood to a body part, often due to an obstruction in circulation (Chapter 12).

Ischium (**ISH**-ee-um) The lower posterior part of the hip bone (Chapter 6).

Islets of Langerhans (**EYE**-lets of **LAHNG**-er-hanz) The endocrine portions of the pancreas that secrete insulin and glucagon (Syn.—pancreatic islets) (Chapter 10).

Isometric exercise (EYE-so-**MEH**-trik) Contraction of muscles without movement of a body part (Chapter 7).

Isotonic (EYE-so-**TAHN**-ik) Having the same concentration of dissolved materials as the solution used as a comparison (Chapter 3).

Isotonic exercise (EYE-so-**TAHN**-ik) Contraction of muscles with movement of a body part (Chapter 7).

J

Jaundice (**JAWN**-diss) A condition characterized by a yellow color in the whites of the eyes and in light skin; caused by an elevated blood level of bilirubin. May be hepatic, prehepatic, or posthepatic in origin (Chapter 11).

Jejunum (je-**JOO**-num) The second portion of the small intestine, about 8 feet long (Chapter 16).

Joint capsule (JOYNT **KAP**-suhl) The fibrous connective tissue sheath that encloses a joint (Chapter 6).

Juxtaglomerular cells (JUKS-tah-gloh-**MER**-yoo-ler SELLS) Cells in the wall of the afferent arteriole that secrete renin when blood pressure decreases (Chapter 18).

K

Keratin (**KER**-uh-tin) A protein produced by epidermal cells; found in the epidermis, hair, and nails (from the Greek "horn") (Chapter 5).

Keratinocyte (KER-uh-**TIN**-oh-sight) A cell of the epidermis, produces keratin before dying (Chapter 5).

Ketoacidosis (KEY-toh-ass-i-**DOH**-sis) A metabolic acidosis that results from the accumulation of ketones in the blood when fats and proteins are used for energy production (Chapter 10).

Ketones (**KEY**-tohns) Organic acid molecules that are formed from fats or amino acids when these nutrients are used for energy production; include acetone and acetoacetic acid (Chapter 10).

Ketonuria (KEY-ton-**YOO**-ree-ah) The presence of ketones in urine (Chapter 18).

Kidneys (**KID**-nees) The two organs on either side of the vertebral column in the upper abdomen that produce urine to eliminate waste products and to regulate the volume, pH, and fluid–electrolyte balance of the blood (Chapter 5).

Kilocalorie (KILL-oh-**KAL**-oh-ree) A Calorie, which is 1000 calories; used to indicate the energy content of foods or the energy expended in activity (See: Calorie) (Chapter 17).

Kinesthetic sense (KIN-ess-**THET**-ik) Muscle sense (Chapter 9).

Krebs cycle (KREBS **SIGH**-kuhl) The stage of cell respiration consisting of a series of reactions in which pyruvic acid or acetyl CoA is broken down to carbon dioxide and ATP is formed; aerobic; takes place in the mitochondria of cells (Syn.—citric acid cycle) (Chapter 17).

Kupffer cells (**KUP**-fer SELLS) The macrophages of the liver; phagocytize pathogens and old red blood cells (Chapter 16).

Kyphosis (kye-**FOH**-sis) An exaggerated thoracic curvature of the vertebral column (Chapter 6).

L

Labia majora (**LAY**-bee-uh muh-**JOR**-ah) The outer folds of skin of the vulva; enclose the labia minora and the vestibule (Chapter 20).

Labia minora (**LAY**-bee-uh min-**OR**-ah) The inner folds of the vulva; enclose the vestibule (Chapter 20).

Labor (**LAY**-ber) The process by which a fetus is expelled from the uterus through the vagina to the exterior of the body (Chapter 21).

Labyrinth (**LAB**-i-rinth) 1. A maze; an interconnected series of passageways. 2. In the inner ear, the bony labyrinth is a series of tunnels in the temporal bone lined with membrane called the membranous labyrinth (Chapter 9).

Lacrimal glands (**LAK**-ri-muhl) The glands that secrete tears, located at the upper, outer corner of each eyeball (Chapter 9).

Lactase (**LAK**-tays) A digestive enzyme that breaks down lactose to glucose and galactose; secreted by the small intestine (Chapter 16).

Lacteals (lak-**TEELS**) The lymph capillaries in the villi of the small intestine, which absorb the fat-soluble end products of digestion (Chapter 14).

Lactic acid (**LAK**-tik **ASS**-id) The chemical end product of anaerobic cell respiration; lowers pH and contributes to fatigue in muscle cells (Chapter 7).

Lactose (**LAK**-tohs) A disaccharide made of one glucose and one galactose molecule (Syn.—milk sugar) (Chapter 2).

Lactose intolerance (**LAK**-tohs in-**TAHL**-er-ense) The inability to digest lactose due to a deficiency of the enzyme lactase; may be congenital or acquired (Chapter 16).

Langerhans cell (**LAHNG**-er-hanz SELL) A mobile, phagocytic cell of the epidermis (Syn.—dendritic cell) (Chapter 5).

Large intestine (LARJ in-**TESS**-tin) The organ of the alimentary tube that extends from the small intestine to the anus; absorbs water, minerals, and vitamins and eliminates undigested materials (Syn.—colon) (Chapter 16).

Laryngopharynx (la-RIN-goh-**FA**-rinks) The lower portion of the pharynx that opens into the larynx and the esophagus; a passageway for both air and food (Chapter 15).

Larynx (**LA**-rinks) The organ that is an airway between the pharynx and the trachea; contains the vocal cords for speech (Syn.—voice box) (Chapter 15).

Lateral (**LAT**-er-uhl) Away from the midline or at the side (Chapter 1).

Lens (LENZ) The oval structure of the eye posterior to the pupil, made of transparent protein; the only adjustable portion of the refraction pathway for the focusing of light rays (Chapter 9).

Lesion (**LEE**-zhun) An area of pathologically altered tissue; an injury or wound (Chapter 5).

Leukemia (loo-**KEE**-mee-ah) Malignancy of blood-forming tissues, in which large numbers of immature and non-functional white blood cells are produced (Chapter 11).

Leukocyte (**LOO**-koh-sight) A white blood cell; the five kinds are neutrophils, eosinophils, basophils, lymphocytes, and monocytes (Chapter 11).

Leukocytosis (LOO-koh-sigh-**TOH**-sis) An elevated white blood cell count, often an indication of infection (Chapter 11).

Leukopenia (LOO-koh-**PEE**-nee-ah) An abnormally low white blood cell count; may be the result of aplastic anemia or a side effect of some medications (Chapter 11).

Leukotrienes (LOO-koh-**TRY**-ens) Chemicals produced by basophils and mast cells from the phospholipids of their cell membranes; they increase capillary permeability and attract WBCs during inflammation (Chapter 14).

Ligament (**LIG**-uh-ment) A fibrous connective tissue structure that connects bone to bone (Chapter 6).

Lipase (**LYE**-pays) A digestive enzyme that breaks down emulsified fats to fatty acids and glycerol; secreted by the pancreas (Chapter 16).

Lipid (**LIP**-id) An organic chemical insoluble in water; includes true fats, phospholipids, and steroids (Chapter 2).

Lipoprotein (li-poh-**PRO**-teen) A large molecule that is a combination of proteins, triglycerides, and cholesterol; formed by the liver to circulate lipids in the blood (Chapter 16).

Lithotripsy (LITH-oh-**TRIP**-see) Crushing of gallstones or renal calculi by an instrument that uses ultrasonic waves applied to the exterior of the body (Chapter 16).

Liver (**LIV**-er) The organ in the upper right and center of the abdominal cavity; secretes bile for the emulsification of fats in digestion; has many other functions related to the metabolism of nutrients and the composition of blood (Chapter 16).

Liver lobule (**LIV**-er **LAH**-byool) The structural unit of the liver; a columnar hexagon of liver cells and sinusoids surrounding a central vein; includes the smallest bile ducts (Chapter 16).

Localized infection (**LOH**-kuhl-IZ'D) An infection confined to one body organ or site (Chapter 22).

Longitudinal section (LAWNJ-i-**TOO**-din-uhl **SEK**-shun) A plane or cut along the long axis of an organ or the body (Chapter 1).

Loop of Henle (LOOP of **HEN**-lee) The part of a renal tubule that extends from the proximal convoluted tubule to the distal convoluted tubule (Chapter 18).

Lordosis (lor-**DOH**-sis) An exaggerated lumbar curvature of the vertebral column (Chapter 6).

Lower esophageal sphincter (e-SOF-uh-**JEE**-uhl **SFINK**-ter) The circular smooth muscle at the lower end of the esophagus; prevents backup of stomach contents (Syn.—cardiac sphincter) (Chapter 16).

Lower respiratory tract (**LOH**-er **RES**-pi-rah-TOR-ee TRAKT) The respiratory organs located within the chest cavity (Chapter 15).

Lumbar puncture (**LUM**-bar **PUNK**-chur) A diagnostic procedure that involves removal of cerebrospinal fluid from the lumbar meningeal sac to assess the pressure and constituents of cerebrospinal fluid (Syn.—spinal tap) (Chapter 8).

Lumbar vertebrae (**LUM**-bar **VER**-te-bray) The five large vertebrae in the small of the back (Chapter 6).

Lumen (**LOO**-min) The cavity of a tubular or hollow organ such as an artery or intestine (Chapter 13).

Lungs (LUHNGS) The paired organs in the thoracic cavity in which gas exchange takes place between the air in the alveoli and the blood in the pulmonary capillaries (Chapter 15).

Luteinizing hormone (LH or ICSH) (LOO-tee-in-**EYE**-zing) A gonadotropic hormone produced by the anterior pituitary gland that, in men, stimulates secretion of testosterone by the testes or, in women, stimulates ovulation and secretion of progesterone by the corpus luteum in the ovary (Chapter 10).

Lymph (LIMF) The water found within lymphatic vessels (Chapter 2).

Lymph node (LIMF NOHD) A small mass of lymphatic tissue located along the pathway of a lymph vessel; produces some lymphocytes and destroys pathogens in the lymph (Chapter 14).

Lymph nodule (LIMF **NAHD**-yool) A small mass of lymphatic tissue located in a mucous membrane; destroys pathogens that penetrate mucous membranes (Chapter 14).

Lymphatic tissue (lim-**FAT**-ik **TISH**-yoo) A hemopoietic tissue that produces some lymphocytes and in which lymphocytes mature and are activated; found in the spleen and lymph nodes and nodules (Chapter 11).

Lymphocyte (**LIM**-foh-sight) A type of white blood cell (agranular); T cells and B cells are involved in the specific responses of adaptive immunity; natural killer cells are nonspecific and are part of innate immunity (Chapter 11).

Lysosome (**LYE**-soh-zome) A cell organelle found in the cytoplasm; contains enzymes that digest damaged cell parts or material ingested by the cell (Chapter 3).

Lysozyme (**LYE**-soh-zyme) An enzyme in tears and saliva that inhibits the growth of bacteria in these fluids (Chapter 9).

M

Macrophage (**MAK**-roh-fahj) A phagocytic cell derived from monocytes that contributes to both innate and adaptive immunity. Capable of phagocytosis of pathogens, dead or damaged cells, and old red blood cells; also involved in recognition of foreign antigens and activation of lymphocytes (Chapter 11).

Macula lutea (**MAK**-yoo-lah **LOO**-tee-ah) A spot in the center of the retina; contains the fovea (Chapter 9).

Magnetic resonance imaging (MRI) (mag-**NET**-ik **REZ**-uh-nanse **IM**-ah-jing) A diagnostic imaging technique that uses a magnetic field and a computer to integrate the images of internal organs (Chapter 1).

Major histocompatibility complex (MHC) (HISS-toh-kom-pat-e-**BILL**-e-tee **KOM**-pleks) The genes on chromosome 6 that are the code for the human leukocyte antigens, our "self" antigens (Chapter 11).

Malignant (muh-**LIG**-nunt) Tending to spread and become worse; used especially with reference to cancer (Chapter 3).

Malleus (**MAL**-ee-us) The first of the three auditory bones in the middle ear; transmits vibrations from the eardrum to the incus (Chapter 9).

Maltase (**MAWL**-tays) A digestive enzyme that breaks down maltose to glucose; secreted by the small intestine (Chapter 16).

Maltose (**MAWL**-tohs) A disaccharide made of two glucose molecules (Chapter 2).

Mammary glands (**MAM**-uh-ree) The glands of the female breasts that secrete milk; secretion and release of milk are under hormonal control (Chapter 20).

Mammography (mah-**MOG**-rah-fee) A diagnostic procedure that uses radiography to detect breast cancer (Chapter 20).

Mandible (**MAN**-di-buhl) The lower jaw bone (Chapter 6).

Manubrium (muh-**NOO**-bree-um) The upper part of the sternum (Chapter 6).

Marrow canal (**MA**-roh ka-**NAL**) The cavity within the diaphysis of a long bone; contains yellow bone marrow (Chapter 4).

Mast cell (MAST SELL) A connective tissue cell of the innate immune system; formed in the red bone marrow and found in connective tissue throughout the body; produces histamine and leukotrienes (Chapter 5).

Mastoid sinus (**MASS**-toyd) An air cavity within the mastoid process of the temporal bone (Chapter 6).

Matrix (**MAY**-triks) 1. The non-living intercellular material that is part of connective tissues. 2. The part of a hair root in which mitosis takes place (Chapter 4).

Matter (**MAT**-ter) Anything that occupies space; may be solid, liquid, or gas; may be living or non-living (Chapter 2).

Maxilla (mak-**SILL**-ah) The upper jaw bone (Chapter 6).

Mechanical digestion (muh-**KAN**-i-kuhl dye-**JES**-chun) The physical breakdown of food into smaller pieces, which increases the surface area for the action of digestive enzymes (Chapter 16).

Media, median, medius (**MEE**-dee-uh, **MEE**-dee-an, **MEE**-dee-us) In the middle, as a middle layer (Chapter 8).

Medial (**MEE**-dee-uhl) Toward the midline (Chapter 1).

Mediastinum (ME-dee-ah-**STYE**-num) The area or space between the lungs; contains the heart and great vessels (Chapter 12).

Medulla (muh-**DEW**-lah) (muh-**DULL**-ah) 1. The part of the brain superior to the spinal cord; regulates vital functions such as heart rate, respiration, and blood pressure. 2. The inner part of an organ, such as the renal medulla or the adrenal medulla (Chapter 8).

Megakaryocyte (MEH-ga-**KA**-ree-oh-sight) A cell in the red bone marrow that breaks up into small fragments called platelets, which then circulate in peripheral blood (Chapter 11).

Meiosis (my-**OH**-sis) The process of cell division in which one cell with the diploid number of chromosomes divides twice to form four cells, each with the haploid number of chromosomes; forms gametes (Chapter 3).

Meissner's plexus (**MIZE**-ners **PLEK**-sus) The enteric nerve plexus in the submucosa of the organs of the alimentary tube; regulates secretions of the glands in the mucosa of these organs (Syn.—submucosal plexus) (Chapter 16).

Melanin (**MEL**-uh-nin) A protein pigment produced by melanocytes. Absorbs ultraviolet light; gives color to the skin, hair, iris, and choroid layer of the eye (Chapter 5).

Melanocyte (muh-**LAN**-oh-sight) A cell in the lower epidermis that synthesizes the pigment melanin (Chapter 5).

Melanoma (MEL-ah-**NOH**-mah) Malignant pigmented mole or nevus (Chapter 5).

Melatonin (mel-ah-**TOH**-nin) A hormone produced by the pineal gland; influences sleep cycles (Chapter 10).

Membrane (**MEM**-brayn) A sheet of tissue; may be made of epithelial tissue or connective tissue (Chapter 4).

Meninges (me-**NIN**-jeez) The connective tissue membranes that line the cranial and spinal cavities and cover the brain and spinal cord (Chapter 1).

Meningitis (MEN-in-**JIGH**-tis) Inflammation of the meninges, most often the result of bacterial infection (Chapter 8).

Menopause (**MEN**-ah-paws) The period during life in which menstrual activity ceases; usually occurs between the ages of 45 and 55 years (Chapter 20).

Menstrual cycle (**MEN**-stroo-uhl **SIGH**-kuhl) The periodic series of changes that occur in the female reproductive tract; the average cycle is 28 days (Chapter 20).

Menstruation (MEN-stroo-**AY**-shun) The periodic discharge of a bloody fluid from the uterus that occurs at regular intervals from puberty to menopause (Chapter 20).

Mesentery (**MEZ**-en-TER-ee) The visceral peritoneum (serous) that covers the abdominal organs; a large fold attaches the small intestine to the posterior abdominal wall (Chapter 1).

Mesoderm (**MEZ**-oh-derm) The middle primary germ layer of cells of an embryo; gives rise to muscles, bones, and connective tissues (Chapter 21).

Metabolic acidosis (MET-uh-**BAH**-lik ass-i-**DOH**-sis) A condition in which the blood pH is lower than normal, caused by any disorder that increases the number of acidic molecules in the body or increases the loss of alkaline molecules (Chapter 15).

Metabolic alkalosis (MET-uh-**BAH**-lik al-kah-**LOH**-sis) A condition in which the blood pH is higher than normal, caused by any disorder that decreases the number of acidic molecules in the body or increases the number of alkaline molecules (Chapter 15).

Metabolism (muh-**TAB**-uh-lizm) All of the physical changes and chemical reactions that take place within the body; includes anabolism and catabolism (Chapter 1).

Metacarpals (MET-uh-**KAR**-puhls) The five long bones in the palm of the hand (Chapter 6).

Metaphase (**MET**-ah-fayz) The second stage of mitosis, in which the pairs of chromatids line up on the equator of the cell (Chapter 3).

Metastasis (muh-**TASS**-tuh-sis) The spread of disease from one part of the body to another (Chapter 3).

Metatarsals (MET-uh-**TAR**-suhls) The five long bones in the arch of the foot (Chapter 6).

Microbiome (MY-kroh-**BYE**-ohm) A community of microorganisms, an ecosystem, a specific environment, and all of its flora. Many such communities are on or in humans, such as the skin, oral cavity, or colon (Chapter 1).

Microbiota (MY-kroh-bye-**OH**-ta) The population of microorganisms (bacteria, viruses, fungi, and protozoa, in various proportions) that resides on or within every person and contributes to the normal functioning of human processes (Syn.—normal flora, resident flora) (Chapter 1).

Microglia (my-kroh-**GLEE**-ah) A type of neuroglia capable of movement and phagocytosis of pathogens (Chapter 8).

Micron (**MY**-kron) Old name for a micrometer (Chapter 3).

Micrometer (**MY**-kroh-mee-ter) A unit of linear measure equal to one thousandth of a millimeter (0.001 mm) (Chapter 3).

Microvilli (MY-kro-**VILL**-eye) Folds of the cell membrane on the free surface of an epithelial cell; increase the surface area for absorption (Chapter 3).

Micturition (MIK-tyoo-**RISH**-un) Urination; the voiding or elimination of urine from the urinary bladder (Chapter 18).

Midbrain (**MID**-brayn) The part of the brain between the pons and hypothalamus; regulates visual, auditory, and righting reflexes (Chapter 8).

Mineral (**MIN**-er-al) An inorganic element or compound; many are needed by the body for normal metabolism and growth (Chapter 17).

Mineralocorticoids (MIN-er-al-oh-**KOR**-ti-koidz) The hormones secreted by the adrenal cortex that affect fluid–electrolyte balance; aldosterone is the major hormone in this group (Chapter 10).

Minute respiratory volume (**MIN**-uht RES-pi-rah-**TOR**-ee **VAHL**-yoom) The volume of air inhaled and exhaled in 1 minute; calculated by multiplying tidal volume by number of respirations per minute (Chapter 15).

Mitochondria (MY-toh-**KAHN**-dree-ah) The cell organelles in which aerobic cell respiration takes place and energy (ATP) is produced; found in the cytoplasm of a cell (Chapter 3).

Mitosis (my-**TOH**-sis) The process of cell division in which one cell with the diploid number of chromosomes divides once to form two identical cells, each with the diploid number of chromosomes (Chapter 3).

Mitral valve (**MY**-truhl VALV) The left atrioventricular valve (bicuspid valve), which prevents backflow of blood from the left ventricle to the left atrium when the ventricle contracts (Chapter 12).

Mixed nerve (MIKSD NERV) A nerve that contains both sensory and motor neurons (Chapter 8).

Molecule (**MAHL**-e-kuhl) A chemical combination of two or more atoms (Chapter 2).

Monocyte (**MAH**-no-sight) A type of white blood cell (agranular); differentiates into a macrophage, which is capable of phagocytosis of pathogens and dead or damaged cells (Chapter 11).

Monomer (**MAH**-noh-mer) A one-part molecule, as is the immunoglobulin IgG (Chapter 14).

Monosaccharide (MAH-noh-**SAK**-ah-ride) A carbohydrate molecule that is a single sugar; includes the hexose and pentose sugars (Chapter 2).

Morula (**MOR**-yoo-lah) An early stage of embryonic development, a solid sphere of cells (Chapter 21).

Motility (moh-**TILL**-e-tee) The ability to move (Chapter 3).

Motion sickness (**MOH**-shun) Queasiness that accompanies repetitive or unexpected motion (Chapter 9).

Motor area (**MOH**-ter) Part of the cerebral cortex of the frontal lobe; generates the impulses necessary for voluntary movement (Chapter 7).

Motor neuron (**MOH**-ter **NYOOR**-on) A nerve cell that carries impulses from the central nervous system to an effector (Syn.—efferent neuron) (Chapter 8).

Motor unit (**MOH**-ter **YOO**-nit) A motor neuron and all of the muscle fibers its branched axon innervates (Chapter 7).

Mucosa (mew-**KOH**-suh) A mucous membrane, the epithelial lining of a body cavity that opens to the environment (Chapter 4).

Mucous membrane (**MEW**-kuss **MEM**-brayn) The epithelial tissue lining of a body tract that opens to the environment (Chapter 4).

Mucus (**MEW**-kuss) The thick fluid secreted by mucous membranes or mucous glands (Chapter 4).

Multicellular (MULL-tee-**SELL**-yoo-lar) Consisting of more than one cell; made of many cells (Chapter 4).

Multiple sclerosis (**MULL**-ti-puhl skle-**ROH**-sis) A progressive nervous system disorder, an autoimmune disease, characterized by the degeneration of the myelin sheaths of CNS neurons (Chapter 8).

Muscle fatigue (**MUSS**-uhl fah-**TEEG**) The state in which muscle fibers can no longer contract efficiently; may be the result of lack of oxygen and/or the accumulation of lactic acid (Chapter 7).

Muscle fiber (**MUSS**-uhl **FYE**-ber) A muscle cell (Chapter 7).

Muscle sense (**MUSS**-uhl SENSE) The conscious or unconscious awareness of where the muscles are, and their degree of contraction, without having to look at them (Chapter 7).

Muscle tissue (**MUSS**-uhl **TISH**-yoo) The tissue specialized for contraction and movement of parts of the body (Chapter 4).

Muscle tone (**MUSS**-uhl TONE) The state of slight contraction present in healthy muscles (Chapter 7).

Muscular dystrophy (**MUSS**-kyoo-ler **DIS**-truh-fee) A genetic disease characterized by the replacement of muscle tissue by fibrous connective tissue or adipose tissue, with progressive loss of muscle functioning; the most common form is Duchenne's muscular dystrophy (Chapter 7).

Muscular system (**MUSS**-kew-ler) The organ system that consists of the skeletal muscles and tendons; its functions are to move the skeleton and produce body heat (Chapter 7).

Mutation (mew-**TAY**-shun) A change in DNA; a genetic change that may be passed to offspring (Chapter 3).

Myalgia (my-**AL**-jee-ah) Pain or tenderness in a muscle (Chapter 7).

Myasthenia gravis (MY-ass-**THEE**-nee-yuh **GRAH**-viss) An autoimmune disease characterized by extreme muscle weakness and fatigue following minimal exertion (Chapter 7).

Mycosis (my-**KOH**-sis) (Pl.—mycoses) An infection caused by a pathogenic fungus (Chapter 22).

Myelin (**MY**-uh-lin) A phospholipid produced by Schwann cells and oligodendrocytes that forms the myelin sheath of axons and dendrites (Chapter 2).

Myelin sheath (**MY**-uh-lin SHEETH) The white, segmented, phospholipid sheath of most axons and dendrites; provides electrical insulation and increases the speed of impulse transmission (Chapter 4).

Myocardial infarction (MI) (MY-oh-**KAR**-dee-yuhl in-**FARK**-shun) Death of part of the heart muscle due to lack of oxygen; often the result of an obstruction in a coronary artery (Syn.—heart attack) (Chapter 12).

Myocardium (MY-oh-**KAR**-dee-um) The cardiac muscle tissue that forms the walls of the chambers of the heart (Chapter 4).

Myocyte (**MY**-oh-sight) A muscle cell; may be used for any of the three types of muscle (Chapter 4).

Myofibril (MY-oh-**FYE**-bril) A linear arrangement of sarcomeres within a muscle fiber (Chapter 7).

Myoglobin (**MY**-oh-GLOW-bin) The protein in muscle fibers that contains iron and stores oxygen in muscle fibers (Chapter 7).

Myometrium (MY-oh-**MEE**-tree-uhm) The smooth muscle layer of the uterus; contracts for labor and delivery of an infant (Chapter 20).

Myopathy (my-**AH**-puh-thee) A disease or abnormal condition of skeletal muscles (Chapter 7).

Myopia (my-**OH**-pee-ah) Nearsightedness; an error of refraction in which only near objects are seen clearly (Chapter 9).

Myosin (**MY**-oh-sin) A contractile protein in the sarcomeres of muscle fibers; pulls actin filaments (Chapter 7).

Myxedema (MIK-suh-**DEE**-mah) Hyposecretion of thyroxine in an adult; decreased metabolic rate results in physical and mental lethargy (Chapter 10).

N

Nail follicle (NAYL **FAH**-li-kuhl) The structure within the skin of a finger or toe in which a nail grows; mitosis takes place in the nail root (Chapter 5).

Narrow spectrum (**NAR**-oh **SPEK**-trum) An antibiotic that is effective against only a few kinds of bacteria (Chapter 22).

Nasal cavities (**NAY**-zuhl **KAV**-i-tees) The two air cavities within the skull through which air passes from the nostrils to the nasopharynx; separated by the nasal septum (Chapter 15).

Nasal mucosa (**NAY**-zuhl mew-**KOH**-sah) The lining of the nasal cavities; made of ciliated epithelium that warms and moistens the incoming air and sweeps mucus, dust, and pathogens toward the nasopharynx (Chapter 15).

Nasal septum (**NAY**-zuhl **SEP**-tum) The vertical plate made of bone and cartilage that separates the two nasal cavities (Chapter 15).

Nasolacrimal duct (NAY-zo-**LAK**-ri-muhl) A duct that carries tears from the lacrimal sac to the nasal cavity (Chapter 9).

Nasopharynx (NAY-zo-**FA**-rinks) The upper portion of the pharynx above the level of the soft palate; an air passageway (Chapter 15).

Natural killer cell (**NATCH**-er-al **KILL**-er SELL) A type of lymphocyte that is not specific and is part of innate immunity; kills pathogens and tumor cells by direct contact (Chapter 14).

Necrotizing fasciitis (**NEK**-roh-ty-zing FASH-ee-**EYE**-tis) An acute, fulminant, and potentially fatal infection of fasciae often caused by Group A streptococci (Chapter 5).

Negative feedback mechanism (**NEG**-ah-tiv **FEED**-bak) A control system in which a stimulus initiates a response that reverses or reduces the stimulus, thereby stopping the response until the stimulus occurs again and there is a need for the response (Chapter 1).

Neonatal herpes (**NEE**-oh-NAY-tal **HER**-peez) A herpes simplex infection in a newborn; may cause encephalitis and may be fatal (Chapter 20).

Nephritis (ne-**FRY**-tis) Inflammation of the kidney; may be caused by bacterial infection or toxic chemicals (Chapter 18).

Nephron (**NEFF**-ron) The structural and functional unit of the kidney that forms urine; consists of a renal corpuscle and a renal tubule (Chapter 18).

Nerve (NERV) A group of neurons, together with blood vessels and connective tissue (Chapter 8).

Nerve tissue (NERV **TISH**-yoo) The tissue specialized to generate and transmit electrochemical impulses that have many functions in the maintenance of homeostasis (Chapter 4).

Nerve tract (NERV TRAKT) A group of neurons that share a common function within the central nervous system; a tract may be ascending (sensory) or descending (motor) (Chapter 8).

Nervous system (**NERV**-us **SIS**-tem) The organ system that regulates body functions by means of electrochemical impulses; consists of the brain, spinal cord, cranial nerves, and spinal nerves (Chapter 8).

Neuralgia (new-**RAL**-juh) Sharp, severe pain along the course of a nerve (Chapter 8).

Neuritis (new-**RYE**-tis) Inflammation of a nerve (Chapter 8).

Neuroglia (new-**ROG**-lee-ah) The non-neuronal cells of the central nervous system; produce the myelin sheath and contribute to the blood–brain barrier, among other functions (Chapter 4).

Neurohypophysis (NEW-roo-high-**POFF**-e-sis) The posterior pituitary gland (Chapter 10).

Neurolemma (NEW-roh-**LEM**-ah) The sheath around peripheral axons and dendrites, formed by the cytoplasm and nuclei of Schwann cells; is essential for the regeneration of damaged peripheral neurons (Chapter 8).

Neuromuscular junction (NYOOR-oh-**MUSS**-kew-lar **JUNK**-shun) The termination of a motor neuron on the sarcolemma of a muscle fiber; the synapse is the microscopic space between the two structures (Chapter 7).

Neuron (**NYOOR**-on) A nerve cell; consists of a cell body, an axon, and dendrites (Chapter 4).

Neuropathy (new-**RAH**-puh-thee) Any disease or disorder of the nerves; may be primary, such as shingles or rabies, or secondary, such as diabetic neuropathy (Chapter 8).

Neurotoxin (NEW-roh-**TOK**-sin) A chemical that disrupts an aspect of the functioning of the nervous system (Chapter 7).

Neurotransmitter (NYOOR-oh-**TRANS**-mih-ter) A chemical released by the axon of a neuron, which crosses a synapse and affects the electrical activity of the postsynaptic membrane (neuron or muscle cell or gland) (Chapter 4).

Neutron (**NEW**-trahn) A subatomic particle that has no electrical charge; found in the nucleus of an atom (Chapter 2).

Neutrophil (**NEW**-troh-fill) A type of granular white blood cell; capable of phagocytosis of pathogens (Chapter 11).

Nevus (**NEE**-vus) A pigmented area of the skin; a mole (Chapter 5).

Night blindness (NIGHT **BLIND**-ness) The inability to see well in dim light or at night; may result from a vitamin A deficiency (Chapter 9).

Nine areas (NYNE) The subdivision of the abdomen into nine equal areas to facilitate the description of locations (Chapter 1).

Noncoding DNA (non-**KOH**-ding) The DNA of chromosomes that does not code for proteins but functions as switches to alter gene expression (Chapter 3).

Noncommunicable disease (NON-kuhm-**YOO**-ni-kah-b'l) A disease that cannot be directly or indirectly transmitted from host to host (Chapter 22).

Non-essential amino acids (NON-e-**SEN**-shul ah-**MEE**-noh **ASS**-ids) The amino acids that can be synthesized by the liver (Chapter 16).

Norepinephrine (NOR-ep-i-**NEFF**-rin) A hormone secreted by the adrenal medulla that causes vasoconstriction throughout the body, which raises blood pressure in stressful situations (Chapter 10).

Normal flora (**NOR**-muhl **FLOOR**-uh) 1. The population of microorganisms that is usually present in certain parts of the body. 2. In the intestines, the bacteria that produce vitamins, inhibit the growth of pathogens, and have other beneficial functions (Syn.—microbiota) (Chapter 1).

Normoblast (**NOR**-mow-blast) A red blood cell with a nucleus, an immature stage in red blood cell formation; usually found in the red bone marrow and not in the peripheral circulation (Chapter 11).

Nosocomial infection (no-zoh-**KOH**-mee-uhl) An infection acquired in a hospital or other health care institution (Chapter 22).

Nuclear membrane (**NEW**-klee-er **MEM**-brayn) The double-layer membrane that encloses the nucleus of a cell (Chapter 3).

Nucleic acid (new-**KLEE**-ik **ASS**-id) An organic chemical that is made of nucleotide subunits. Examples are DNA and RNA (Chapter 2).

Nucleolus (new-**KLEE**-oh-lus) A small structure made of DNA, RNA, and protein. Found in the nucleus of a cell; produces ribosomal RNA (Chapter 3).

Nucleotide (**NEW**-klee-oh-tide) An organic compound that consists of a pentose sugar, a phosphate group, and one of five nitrogenous bases (adenine, guanine, cytosine, thymine, or uracil); the subunits of DNA and RNA (Chapter 2).

Nucleus (**NEW**-klee-us) 1. The membrane-bound part of a cell that contains the hereditary material in chromosomes. 2. The central part of an atom containing protons and neutrons (Chapters 2, 3).

O

Occipital bone (ahk-**SIP**-i-tuhl) The flat bone that forms the back of the skull (Chapter 6).

Occipital lobes (ahk-**SIP**-i-tuhl LOWBS) The most posterior part of the cerebrum; contain the visual areas (Chapter 8).

Oculomotor nerves (AHK-yoo-loh-**MOH**-tur) Cranial nerve pair III; motor to the extrinsic muscles of the eye, the ciliary body, and the iris (Chapter 8).

Olfactory nerves (ohl-**FAK**-tuh-ree) Cranial nerve pair I; sensory for smell (Chapter 8).

Olfactory receptors (ohl-**FAK**-tuh-ree ree-**SEP**-ters) The sensory receptors in the upper nasal cavities that detect vaporized chemicals, providing a sense of smell (Chapter 9).

Oligodendrocyte (ah-li-goh-**DEN**-droh-sight) A type of neuroglia that produces the myelin sheath around neurons of the central nervous system (Chapter 8).

Oligosaccharide (ah-lig-oh-**SAK**-ah-ride) A carbohydrate molecule that consists of from 3 to 20 monosaccharides bonded together; form "self" antigens on cell membranes (Chapter 2).

Oliguria (AH-li-**GYOO**-ree-ah) Decreased urine formation and output (Chapter 18).

Oogenesis (Oh-oh-**JEN**-e-sis) The process of meiosis in the ovary to produce an ovum (Chapter 3).

Opportunistic infection (OP-er-too-**NIS**-tik) An infection caused by a microorganism that is usually a saprophyte but may become a parasite under certain conditions, such as lowered host resistance (Chapter 22).

Opsonization (OP-sah-ni-**ZAY**-shun) The action of antibodies or complement that upon binding to a foreign antigen attracts macrophages and facilitates phagocytosis (from the Greek "to purchase food") (Chapter 14).

Optic chiasma (**OP**-tik kye-**AS**-muh) The site of the crossing of the medial fibers of each optic nerve, anterior to the pituitary gland; important for binocular vision (Chapter 9).

Optic disc (**OP**-tik DISK) The portion of the retina where the optic nerve passes through; no rods or cones are present (Syn.—blind spot) (Chapter 9).

Optic nerves (**OP**-tik) Cranial nerve pair II; sensory for vision (Chapter 8).

Optic tracts (**OP**-tik TRAKTS) The neuron pathways from the optic chiasma to the thalamus, then to the visual areas in the occipital lobes (Chapter 9).

Oral cavity (**OR**-uhl **KAV**-i-tee) The cavity in the skull bounded by the hard palate, cheeks, and tongue (Chapter 16).

Orbit (**OR**-bit) The cavity in the skull that contains the eyeball (from the Latin "circle" or "world") (Syn.—eye socket) (Chapter 9).

Orbitofrontal cortex (OR-bih-toh-**FRUN**-tuhl) The part of the frontal lobe behind the eye; is concerned with appropriate emotions and behavior, as well as awareness of the future (Syn.—prefrontal cortex) (Chapter 8).

Organ (**OR**-gan) A structure with specific functions; made of two or more tissues (Chapter 1).

Organ of Corti (**KOR**-tee) (spiral organ) The structure in the cochlea of the inner ear that contains the receptors for hearing (Chapter 9).

Organ system (**OR**-gan **SIS**-tem) A group of related organs that work together to perform specific functions (Chapter 1).

Organelle (OR-gan-**ELL**) An intracellular structure that has a specific function (Chapter 3).

Organic (or-**GAN**-ik) A chemical compound that contains carbon–hydrogen covalent bonds; includes carbohydrates, lipids, proteins, and nucleic acids (Chapter 1).

Origin (**AHR**-i-jin) 1. The more stationary attachment point of a muscle to a bone. 2. The beginning (Chapter 7).

Oropharynx (OR-oh-**FA**-rinks) The middle portion of the pharynx behind the oral cavity; a passageway for both air and food (Chapter 15).

Osmolarity (ahs-moh-**LAR**-i-tee) The concentration of osmotically active particles in a solution (Chapter 19).

Osmoreceptors (AHS-moh-re-**SEP**-ters) Specialized cells in the hypothalamus that detect changes in the water content of the body (Chapter 10).

Osmosis (ahs-**MOH**-sis) The diffusion of water through a selectively permeable membrane (Chapter 3).

Osmotic pressure (ahs-**MAH**-tik) Pressure that develops when two solutions of different concentration are separated by a selectively permeable membrane. A hypertonic solution that would cause cells to shrivel has a higher osmotic pressure. A hypotonic solution that would cause cells to swell has a lower osmotic pressure (Chapter 3).

Ossification (AHS-i-fi-**KAY**-shun) The process of bone formation; bone matrix is produced by osteoblasts during the growth or repair of bones (Chapter 6).

Osteoarthritis (AHS-tee-oh-ar-**THRY**-tiss) The inflammation of a joint, especially a weight-bearing joint, that is most often a consequence of aging (Chapter 6).

Osteoblast (**AHS**-tee-oh-BLAST) A bone-producing cell; produces bone matrix for the growth or repair of bones (Chapter 6).

Osteocalcin (AHS-tee-oh-**KAL**-sin) A protein produced by osteoblasts; it increases insulin production by the pancreas and decreases fat storage by adipose tissue (Chapter 6).

Osteoclast (**AHS**-tee-oh-KLAST) A bone-destroying cell; reabsorbs bone matrix as part of the growth or repair of bones (Chapter 6).

Osteocyte (**AHS**-tee-oh-sight) A bone cell (Chapter 4).

Osteomyelitis (AHS-tee-oh-my-uh-**LYE**-tiss) Inflammation of a bone caused by a pathogenic microorganism (Chapter 6).

Osteon (**AHS**-tee-on) The structural unit of compact bone, consisting of a central (haversian) canal surrounded by concentric rings of osteocytes within matrix (Syn.—haversian system) (Chapter 4).

Osteoporosis (AHS-tee-oh-por-**OH**-sis) A condition in which bone matrix is lost and not replaced, resulting in weakened bones that are then more likely to fracture (Chapter 6).

Otitis media (oh-**TIGH**-tis **MEE**-dee-ah) Inflammation of the middle ear (Chapter 9).

Otoliths (**OH**-toh-liths) Microscopic crystals of calcium carbonate in the utricle and saccule of the inner ear; are pulled by gravity (Chapter 9).

Oval window (**OH**-vul **WIN**-doh) The membrane-covered opening through which the stapes transmits vibrations to the fluid in the inner ear (Chapter 9).

Ovary (**OH**-vuh-ree) The female gonad that produces ova; also an endocrine gland that produces the hormones estrogen and progesterone (Chapter 10).

Ovum (**OH**-vuhm) (Pl.—ova) An egg cell, produced by an ovary (Chapter 20).

Oxygen debt (**AHKS**-ah-jen DET) The state in which there is not enough oxygen to complete the process of aerobic cell respiration; lactic acid is formed, which contributes to muscle fatigue (Syn.—recovery oxygen uptake) (Chapter 7).

Oxytocin (AHK-si-**TOH**-sin) A hormone produced by the hypothalamus and stored in the posterior pituitary gland; stimulates contraction of the myometrium during labor and release of milk by the mammary glands (Chapter 8).

P

Palate (**PAL**-uht) The roof of the mouth, which separates the oral cavity from the nasal cavities (Chapter 6).

Palpitation (pal-pi-**TAY**-shun) An irregular heartbeat of which the person is aware (Chapter 12).

Pancreas (**PAN**-kree-us) 1. An endocrine gland located between the curve of the duodenum and the spleen; secretes insulin and glucagon. 2. An exocrine gland that secretes digestive enzymes for the digestion of starch, fats, and proteins (Chapter 10).

Pancreatic duct (PAN-kree-AT-ik DUKT) The duct that takes pancreatic juices to the common bile duct (Chapter 16).

Pandemic (pan-**DEM**-ik) An epidemic that affects several countries at the same time (Chapter 22).

Papillae (pah-**PILL**-ay) 1. Elevated, pointed projections. 2. On the tongue, the projections that contain taste buds (Chapter 16).

Papillary layer (**PAP**-i-lar-ee **LAY**-er) The uppermost layer of the dermis; contains capillaries to nourish the epidermis (Chapter 5).

Papillary muscles (**PAP**-i-lar-ee **MUSS**-uhls) Columns of myocardium that project from the floor of a ventricle and anchor the flaps of the atrioventricular valve by way of the chordae tendineae (Chapter 12).

Paradox (**PAR**-ah-dahks) Something that does not seem logical and that, therefore, should not be true, but is true. (Chapter 6)

Paralysis (pah-**RAL**-i-sis) Complete or partial loss of function, especially of a muscle (Chapter 7).

Paralytic ileus (**PAR**-uh-LIT-ik **ILL**-ee-us) Paralysis of the intestines that may occur following abdominal surgery (Chapter 16).

Paranasal sinus (PAR-uh-**NAY**-zuhl **SIGH**-nus) An air cavity in the frontal, maxilla, sphenoid, or ethmoid bones; opens into the nasal cavities (Chapter 6).

Paraplegia (PAR-ah-**PLEE**-gee-ah) Paralysis of the legs (Chapter 8).

Parasite (**PAR**-uh-sight) An organism that lives on or in another living organism, called a host, to which it causes harm (from the Greek for "to eat at another's table") (Chapter 22).

Parasympathetic (**PAR**-ah-SIM-puh-THET-ik) The division of the autonomic nervous system that dominates during non-stressful situations (Chapter 8).

Parathyroid glands (PAR-ah-**THIGH**-royd) The four endocrine glands located on the posterior side of the thyroid gland; secrete parathyroid hormone (Chapter 10).

Parathyroid hormone (PTH) (PAR-ah-**THIGH**-royd) A hormone secreted by the parathyroid glands; increases the reabsorption of calcium from bones and the absorption of calcium by the small intestine and kidneys (Chapter 10).

Parietal (puh-**RYE**-uh-tuhl) 1. Pertaining to the walls of a body cavity (Chapter 1). 2. The flat bone that forms the crown of the cranial cavity (from the Latin "wall") (Chapter 6).

Parietal cells (puh-**RYE**-uh-tuhl SELLS) The cells of the gastric pits of the stomach that secrete hydrochloric acid and the intrinsic factor (Chapter 16).

Parietal lobes (puh-**RYE**-uh-tuhl LOWBS) The parts of the cerebrum posterior to the frontal lobes; contain the sensory areas for cutaneous sensation and conscious muscle sense (Chapter 8).

Parkinson's disease (**PAR**-kin-sonz) A progressive disorder of the basal ganglia, characterized by tremor, muscle weakness and rigidity, and a peculiar gait (Chapter 8).

Parotid glands (pah-**RAH**-tid) The pair of salivary glands located just below and in front of the ears (Chapter 16).

Partial pressure (**PAR**-shul **PRES**-shur) 1. The pressure exerted by a gas in a mixture of gases. 2. The value used to measure oxygen and carbon dioxide concentrations in the blood or other body fluid (Chapter 15).

Parturition (PAR-tyoo-**RISH**-uhn) The act of giving birth (Chapter 21).

Passive immunity (**PASS**-iv im-**YOO**-ni-tee) The immunity provided by the reception of antibodies from another source; may be natural (placental, breast milk) or artificial (injection of gamma globulins) (Chapter 14).

Pasteurization (PAS-tyoor-i-**ZAY**-shun) The process of heating a fluid to moderate temperatures in order to destroy pathogenic bacteria (Chapter 22).

Patella (puh-**TELL**-ah) The kneecap, a short bone (from the Latin "flat dish") (Chapter 6).

Patellar reflex (puh-**TELL**-ar **REE**-fleks) A stretch reflex integrated in the spinal cord, in which a tap on the patellar tendon causes extension of the lower leg (Syn.—knee-jerk reflex) (Chapter 8).

Pathogen (**PATH**-oh-jen) A microorganism capable of producing disease; includes bacteria, viruses, fungi, protozoa, and worms (Chapters 14, 22).

Pathophysiology (PATH-oh-FIZZ-ee-**AH**-luh-jee) The study of diseases as they are related to functioning (Chapter 1).

Pelvic cavity (**PELL**-vik **KAV**-i-tee) The most inferior cavity of the trunk, below the abdominal cavity (Chapter 1).

Penis (**PEE**-nis) The male organ of copulation when the urethra serves as a passage for semen; an organ of elimination when the urethra serves as a passage for urine (Chapter 20).

Pentamer (**PEN**-tah-mer) A five-part molecule, as is the immunoglobulin IgM (Chapter 14).

Pentose sugar (**PEN**-tohs) A five-carbon sugar (monosaccharide) that is a structural part of the nucleic acids DNA, RNA, and ATP (Chapter 2).

Pepsin (**PEP**-sin) The enzyme found in gastric juice that begins protein digestion; secreted by chief cells (Chapter 16).

Peptidases (**PEP**-ti-day-ses) Digestive enzymes that break down polypeptides to amino acids; secreted by the small intestine (Chapter 16).

Peptide (**PEP**-tyde) A short chain of amino acids, a yet-to-be-completed protein or a molecule with a specific function; many antimicrobials and signaling molecules are peptides (Chapter 2).

Peptide bond (**PEP**-tyde BAHND) A chemical bond that links two amino acids in a protein molecule (Chapter 2).

Perfusion (purr-**FEW**-zhun) The circulation of blood to a body area or organ; for most organs, the most important part of blood is oxygen (Chapter 13).

Pericardium (PER-ee-**KAR**-dee-um) The three membranes that enclose the heart, consisting of an outer fibrous layer and two serous layers (Chapter 12).

Perichondrium (PER-ee-**KON**-dree-um) The fibrous connective tissue membrane that covers cartilage (Chapter 4).

Perilymph (**PER**-i-limf) The fluid in the bony labyrinth of the inner ear (Chapter 9).

Periodontal membrane (PER-ee-oh-**DON**-tal) The membrane that lines the tooth sockets in the upper and lower jaws; produces a bonelike cement to anchor the teeth (Chapter 16).

Periosteum (PER-ee-**AHS**-tee-um) The fibrous connective tissue membrane that covers bone; contains osteoblasts for bone growth or repair (Chapter 4).

Peripheral (puh-**RIFF**-uh-ruhl) Extending from a main part; closer to the surface (Chapter 1).

Peripheral nervous system (puh-**RIFF**-uh-ruhl **NERV**-vuhs) The part of the nervous system that consists of the cranial nerves and spinal nerves (Chapter 8).

Peripheral resistance (puh-**RIFF**-uh-ruhl ree-**ZIS**-tense) The resistance of the blood vessels to the flow of blood; changes in the diameter of arteries have effects on blood pressure (Chapter 13).

Peristalsis (per-i-**STALL**-sis) Waves of muscular contraction (one-way) that propel the contents through a hollow organ (Chapter 2).

Peritoneum (PER-i-toh-**NEE**-um) The serous membrane that lines the abdominal cavity (Chapter 1).

Peritonitis (per-i-toh-**NIGH**-tis) Inflammation of the peritoneum (Chapter 16).

Peritubular capillaries (PER-ee-**TOO**-byoo-ler) The capillaries that surround the renal tubule and receive the useful materials reabsorbed from the renal filtrate; carry blood from the efferent arteriole to the renal vein (Chapter 18).

Pernicious anemia (per-**NISH**-us uh-**NEE**-mee-yah) An anemia that is the result of a deficiency of vitamin B_{12} or the intrinsic factor (Chapter 11).

Peyer's patches (**PYE**-erz) The lymph nodules in the mucosa of the small intestine, especially in the ileum (Chapter 14).

pH A symbol of the measure of the concentration of hydrogen ions in a solution. The pH scale extends from 0 to 14, with a value of 7 being neutral. Values lower than 7 are acidic; values higher than 7 are alkaline (basic) (Chapter 2).

Phagocytosis (FAG-oh-sigh-**TOH**-sis) The process by which a moving cell engulfs a particle; especially, the ingestion of microorganisms by white blood cells (Chapter 3).

Phalanges (fuh-**LAN**-jees) (Sing.—phalanx) The long bones of the fingers and toes. There are 14 in each hand or foot (from the Latin "line of soldiers") (Chapter 6).

Phantom pain (**FAN**-tum PAYN) Pain following amputation of a limb that seems to come from the missing limb (Chapter 9).

Pharynx (**FA**-rinks) A muscular tube located behind the nasal and oral cavities; a passageway for air and food (Chapter 15).

Phenotype (**FEE**-noh-type) The appearance of the individual as related to genotype; the expression of the genes that are present (Chapter 21).

Phlebitis (fle-**BY**-tis) Inflammation of a vein (Chapter 13).

Phospholipid (**FOSS**-foh-LIP-id) An organic compound in the lipid group that is made of one glycerol, two fatty acids, and a phosphate molecule; forms the bilayer of cell membranes (Chapter 2).

Phrenic nerves (**FREN**-ik NERVZ) The pair of peripheral nerves that are motor to the diaphragm (Chapter 15).

Physiology (FIZZ-ee-**AH**-luh-jee) The study of the functioning of the body and its parts (Chapter 1).

Pia mater (**PEE**-ah **MAH**-ter) The innermost layer of the meninges, made of thin connective tissue on the surface of the brain and spinal cord (Chapter 8).

Pilomotor muscle (**PYE**-loh-MOH-ter) A smooth muscle attached to a hair follicle; contraction pulls the follicle upright, resulting in "goose bumps" (Syn.—arrector pili muscle) (Chapter 5).

Pineal gland (**PIN**-ee-uhl) An endocrine gland on the posterior wall of the third ventricle of the brain; secretes melatonin (Chapter 10).

Pinocytosis (PIN-oh-sigh-**TOH**-sis) The process by which a stationary cell ingests very small particles or a liquid (Chapter 3).

Pituitary gland (pi-**TOO**-i-TER-ee) An endocrine gland located below the hypothalamus, consisting of anterior and posterior lobes (Syn.—hypophysis) (Chapter 10).

Pivot joint (**PI**-vot) A diarthrosis that permits rotation (Chapter 6).

Placenta (pluh-**SEN**-tah) The organ formed in the uterus during pregnancy, made of both fetal and maternal tissue; the site of exchanges of materials between fetal blood and maternal blood (Chapter 13).

Plane (PLAYN) An imaginary flat surface that divides the body in a specific way (Chapter 1).

Plasma (**PLAZ**-mah) The water found within the blood vessels. Plasma is 52% to 62% of the total blood (Chapter 2).

Plasma cell (**PLAZ**-mah SELL) A cell derived from an activated B cell that produces antibodies to a specific antigen (Chapter 14).

Plasma proteins (**PLAZ**-mah **PRO**-teenz) The proteins that circulate in the liquid portion of the blood; include albumin, globulins, and clotting factors (Chapter 11).

Plasticity (pla-**STIS**-si-tee) The ability of a tissue to grow or change; used especially for the ability of the brain to adapt to changing needs and to recruit different neurons for certain functions, as may occur in recovery from a stroke (Chapter 8).

Platelets (**PLAYT**-lets) Blood cells that are fragments of larger cells (megakaryocytes) of the red bone marrow; involved in blood clotting and other mechanisms of hemostasis (Syn.—thrombocytes) (Chapter 4).

Pleural membranes (**PLOOR**-uhl **MEM**-braynz) The serous membranes of the thoracic cavity (Chapter 1).

Plica circulares (**PLEE**-ka SIR-kew-**LAR**-es) The circular folds of the mucosa and submucosa of the small intestine; increase the surface area for absorption (Chapter 16).

Pneumonia (new-**MOH**-nee-ah) Inflammation of the lungs caused by bacteria, viruses, or chemicals (Chapter 15).

Pneumotaxic center (NEW-moh-**TAK**-sik **SEN**-ter) The respiratory center in the pons that helps bring about exhalation (Chapter 15).

Pneumothorax (NEW-moh-**THAW**-raks) The accumulation of air in the potential pleural space, which increases intrapleural pressure and causes collapse of a lung (Chapter 15).

Podocytes (**POH**-doh-sights) The cells that form the inner layer of Bowman's capsule of the renal corpuscle; adjacent foot processes form pores that make the layer very permeable (Chapter 18).

Polarization (POH-lahr-i-**ZAY**-shun) The distribution of ions on either side of a membrane; in a resting neuron or muscle cell, sodium ions are more abundant outside the cell, and potassium and negative ions are more abundant inside the cell, giving the membrane a positive charge outside and a relative negative charge inside (Chapter 7).

Polypeptide (PAH-lee-**PEP**-tyde) A short chain of amino acids, not yet a specific protein (Chapter 2).

Polysaccharide (PAH-lee-**SAK**-ah-ryde) A carbohydrate molecule that consists of many monosaccharides (usually glucose) bonded together; includes glycogen, starch, and cellulose (Chapter 2).

Polyuria (PAH-li-**YOO**-ree-ah) Increased urine formation and output (Chapter 18).

Pons (PONZ) The part of the brain anterior and superior to the medulla; contributes to the regulation of respiration (from the Latin "bridge") (Chapter 8).

Pore (POR) An opening on a surface to permit the passage of materials (Chapter 3).

Portal of entry (**POR**-tuhl of **EN**-tree) The way a pathogen enters the body, such as natural body openings or breaks in the skin (Chapter 22).

Portal of exit (**POR**-tuhl of **EG**-zit) The way a pathogen leaves a host, such as in respiratory droplets, feces, or reproductive secretions (Chapter 22).

Positive feedback (**PAHS**-ah-tiv **FEED**-bak) A control system that requires an external event to stop or reverse the stimulus; may become a self-perpetuating cycle that causes harm (Chapter 1).

Positron emission tomography (PET) (**PAHS**-i-tron eh-**MISH**-shun toh-**MAH**-grah-fee) An imaging technique that depicts rate of metabolism or blood flow in organs or tissues (Chapter 1).

Posterior (poh-**STEER**-ee-your) Toward the back (Syn.—dorsal) (Chapter 1).

Postganglionic neuron (POST-gang-lee-**ON**-ik) In the autonomic nervous system, a neuron that extends from a ganglion to a visceral effector (Chapter 8).

Precapillary sphincter (pree-**KAP**-i-lar-ee **SFINK**-ter) A smooth muscle cell at the beginning of a capillary network that regulates the flow of blood through the network (Chapter 13).

Preganglionic neuron (PRE-gang-lee-**ON**-ik) In the autonomic nervous system, a neuron that extends from the CNS to a ganglion and synapses with a postganglionic neuron (Chapter 8).

Premotor area (pre-**MOH**-ter) The area of the frontal cerebral cortex anterior to the motor area; is concerned with learning sequential movements (Chapter 8).

Presbyopia (PREZ-bee-**OH**-pee-ah) Farsightedness that is a consequence of aging and the loss of elasticity of the lens (Chapter 9).

Pressoreceptors (**PRESS**-oh-ree-SEP-ters) The sensory receptors in the carotid sinuses and aortic sinus that detect changes in blood pressure (Chapter 9).

Primary bronchi (**PRY**-ma-ree **BRONG**-kye) The two branches of the lower end of the trachea; air passageways to the right and left lungs (Chapter 15).

Prime mover (PRYME **MOO**-ver) The muscle responsible for the main action when a joint is moved (Chapter 7).

Prions (**PREE**-ons) Proteinaceous infectious particles that are the cause of lethal disease of the nervous system in people and animals (Chapter 2).

Process (**PRAH**-sess) 1. An action or series of actions that has a predictable and specific outcome, such as the process of protein synthesis. 2. A cellular extension, such as the axon of a neuron. 3. A projection of a bone, often for muscle attachment, such as the spinous process of a vertebra (Chapter 1).

Progesterone (proh-**JESS**-tuh-rohn) The sex hormone secreted by the corpus luteum of the ovary and by the placenta; contributes to the growth of the endometrium and the maintenance of pregnancy (Chapter 10).

Projection (proh-**JEK**-shun) The characteristic of sensations in which the sensation is felt in the area where the receptors were stimulated (Chapter 9).

Prolactin (proh-**LAK**-tin) A hormone produced by the anterior pituitary gland that stimulates milk production by the mammary glands (Chapter 10).

Pronation (proh-**NAY**-shun) Turning the palm downward, or lying face down (Chapter 7).

Prophase (**PROH**-fayz) The first stage of mitosis, in which the pairs of chromatids become visible (Chapter 3).

Proprioception (PROH-pree-oh-**SEP**-shun) The sense of the body, of its place, position, and movement; includes muscle sense and equilibrium (from the Latin "one's own") (Chapter 7).

Proprioceptor (PROH-pree-oh-**SEP**-ter) A sensory receptor in a muscle that detects stretching of the muscle (Syn.—stretch receptor) (Chapter 7).

Prostaglandins (PRAHS-tah-**GLAND**-ins) Locally acting hormone-like substances produced by virtually all cells from the phospholipids of their cell membranes; the many types have many varied functions (Chapter 10).

Prostate gland (**PRAHS**-tayt) A muscular gland that surrounds the first inch of the male urethra; secretes fluid that becomes part of semen; its smooth muscle contributes to ejaculation (Chapter 20).

Prostatic hypertrophy (prahs-**TAT**-ik high-**PER**-truh-fee) Enlargement of the prostate gland; may be benign or malignant (Chapter 20).

Proteasome (**PROH**-tee-ah-sohm) A cytoplasmic cell organelle that destroys misfolded or damaged proteins; contains enzymes called proteases (Chapter 3).

Protein (**PROH**-teen) An organic compound made of amino acids linked by peptide bonds (Chapter 2).

Proteinuria (PROH-teen-**YOO**-ree-ah) The presence of protein in urine (Chapter 18).

Prothrombin (proh-**THROM**-bin) A clotting factor synthesized by the liver and released into the blood; converted to thrombin in the process of chemical clotting (Chapter 11).

Proton (**PROH**-tahn) A subatomic particle that has a positive electrical charge; found in the nucleus of an atom (Chapter 2).

Proton pump (**PROH**-tahn PUMP) An enzyme of the parietal cells of the stomach lining; secretes a hydrogen ion (in exchange for potassium), which unites with a chloride ion to form HCl in gastric juice; in the intercalated cells of the kidney tubules, proton pumps secrete H^+ ions into the filtrate (Chapter 16).

Protozoa (PROH-tuh-**ZOH**-ah) (Sing.— protozoan) The simplest animal-like microorganisms in the kingdom Protista; usually unicellular, some are colonial; may be free living or parasitic (Chapter 22).

Proximal (**PROK**-si-muhl) Closest to the origin or point of attachment (Chapter 1).

Proximal convoluted tubule (**PROK**-si-muhl KON-voh-**LOO**-ted) The part of a renal tubule that extends from Bowman's capsule to the loop of Henle (Chapter 18).

Pruritus (proo-**RYE**-tus) Severe itching (Chapter 5).

Puberty (**PEW**-ber-tee) The period during life in which members of both sexes become sexually mature and capable of reproduction; usually occurs between the ages of 10 and 14 years (Chapter 20).

Pubic symphysis (**PEW**-bik **SIM**-fi-sis) The joint between the right and left pubic bones, in which a disc of cartilage separates the two bones (Chapter 6).

Pubis (**PEW**-biss) The lower anterior part of the hip bone (Syn.—pubic bone) (Chapter 6).

Pulmonary artery (**PULL**-muh-NER-ee **AR**-tuh-ree) The artery that takes blood from the right ventricle to the lungs (Chapter 12).

Pulmonary edema (**PULL**-muh-NER-ee uh-**DEE**-muh) Accumulation of tissue fluid in the alveoli of the lungs (Chapter 15).

Pulmonary semilunar valve (**PULL**-muh-NER-ee SEM-ee-**LOO**-nar VALV) The valve at the junction of the right ventricle and the pulmonary artery; prevents backflow of blood from the artery to the ventricle when the ventricle relaxes (Chapter 12).

Pulmonary surfactant (**PULL**-muh-NER-ee sir-**FAK**-tent) A lipoprotein secreted by the alveoli in the lungs; reduces the surface tension within alveoli to permit inflation (Chapter 15).

Pulmonary veins (**PULL**-muh-NER-ee VAYNS) The four veins that return blood from the lungs to the left atrium (Chapter 12).

Pulp cavity (PUHLP) The innermost portion of a tooth that contains blood vessels and nerve endings (Chapter 16).

Pulse (PULS) The force of the heartbeat detected at an arterial site such as the radial artery (Chapter 12).

Pulse deficit (PULS **DEF**-i-sit) The condition in which the radial pulse count is lower than the rate of the heartbeat heard with a stethoscope; may occur in some types of heart disease in which the heartbeat is weak (Chapter 13).

Pulse pressure (PULS **PRES**-shur) The difference between systolic and diastolic blood pressure; averages about 40 mm Hg (Chapter 13).

Punnett square (**PUHN**-net SKWAIR) A diagram used to determine the possible combinations of genes in the offspring of a particular set of parents (Chapter 21).

Pupil (**PYOO**-pil) The opening in the center of the iris; light rays pass through the aqueous humor in the pupil (Chapter 9).

Purkinje fibers (purr-**KIN**-jee) Specialized cardiac muscle fibers that are part of the cardiac conduction pathway (Chapter 12).

Pyloric sphincter (pye-**LOR**-ik **SFINK**-ter) The circular smooth muscle at the junction of the stomach and the duodenum; prevents backup of intestinal contents into the stomach (from the Greek "gatekeeper") (Chapter 16).

Pyloric stenosis (pye-**LOR**-ik ste-**NOH**-sis) Narrowing of the opening between the stomach and duodenum caused by hypertrophy of the pyloric sphincter; a congenital disorder (Chapter 16).

Pyrogen (**PYE**-roh-jen) Any microorganism or substance that causes a fever; includes bacteria, viruses, or chemicals released during inflammation (called endogenous pyrogens); activates the heat production and conservation mechanisms regulated by the hypothalamus (Chapter 17).

Q

QRS wave The portion of an ECG that depicts depolarization of the ventricles (Chapter 12).

Quadrants (**KWAH**-drants) A division into four parts, used especially to divide the abdomen into four areas to facilitate description of locations (Chapter 1).

Quadriplegia (KWAH-dri-**PLEE**-jee-ah) Paralysis of all four limbs (Chapter 17).

R

Radiation (RAY-dee-**AY**-shun) 1. The heat loss process in which heat energy from the skin is emitted to the cooler surroundings. 2. The emissions of certain radioactive elements; may be used for diagnostic or therapeutic purposes (Chapter 17).

Radius (**RAY**-dee-us) The long bone of the forearm on the thumb side (from the Latin "a spoke") (Chapter 6).

Range-of-motion exercises (RANJE of **MOH**-shun) Movements of joints through their full range of motion; used to preserve mobility or to regain mobility following an injury (Chapter 7).

Receptor (ree-**SEP**-tur) A specialized cell or nerve ending that responds to a particular change such as light, sound, heat, touch, or pressure (Chapter 5).

Receptor site (ree-**SEP**-ter SIGHT) An arrangement of molecules, often part of the cell membrane, that will accept only molecules with a complementary shape (Chapter 3).

Recessive (ree-**SESS**-iv) In genetics, a characteristic that will be expressed only if two genes for it are present in the homologous pair of chromosomes (Chapter 21).

Recovery oxygen uptake (ree-**KOV**-e-ree **AHKS**-ah-jen **UP**-tayk) Oxygen debt (Chapter 7).

Red blood cells (RED BLUHD SELLS) The most numerous cells in the blood; carry oxygen bonded to the hemoglobin within them (Syn.—erythrocytes) (Chapter 4).

Red bone marrow (RED BOWN **MAR**-row) The primary hemopoietic tissue; found in flat and irregular bones; produces all the types of blood cells (Chapter 6).

Reduced hemoglobin (re-**DOOSD HEE**-muh-GLOW-bin) Hemoglobin that has released its oxygen in the systemic capillaries (Chapter 11).

Referred pain (ree-**FURRD** PAIN) Visceral pain that is projected and felt as cutaneous pain (Chapter 9).

Reflex (**REE**-fleks) An involuntary response to a stimulus (Chapter 8).

Reflex arc (**REE**-fleks ARK) The pathway nerve impulses follow when a reflex is stimulated (Chapter 8).

Refraction (ree-**FRAK**-shun) The bending of light rays as they pass through the eyeball; normal refraction focuses an image on the retina (Chapter 9).

Relaxin (ree-**LAKS**-in) A hormone produced by the corpus luteum and placenta; inhibits contractions of the myometrium (Chapter 20).

Releasing hormones (ree-**LEE**-sing **HOR**-mohns) Hormones released by the hypothalamus that stimulate secretion of hormones by the anterior pituitary gland (Syn.—releasing factors) (Chapter 10).

Remission (ree-**MISH**-uhn) Lessening of severity of symptoms (Chapter 8).

Remodeling (ree-**MAHD**-ling) The process by which older bone matrix is replaced by new bone matrix; is ongoing in response to environmental changes and calcium needs within the body (Chapter 6).

Renal artery (**REE**-nuhl **AR**-te-ree) The branch of the abdominal aorta that takes blood into a kidney (Chapter 18).

Renal calculi (**REE**-nuhl **KAL**-kew-lye) Kidney stones; made of precipitated minerals in the form of crystals (Chapter 18).

Renal corpuscle (**REE**-nuhl **KOR**-pus'l) The part of a nephron that consists of a glomerulus enclosed by a Bowman's capsule; the site of glomerular filtration (Chapter 18).

Renal cortex (**REE**-nuhl **KOR**-teks) The outermost tissue layer of the kidney; consists of renal corpuscles and convoluted tubules (Chapter 18).

Renal failure (**REE**-nuhl **FAYL**-yer) The inability of the kidneys to function properly and form urine; causes include severe hemorrhage, toxins, and obstruction of the urinary tract (Chapter 18).

Renal fascia (**REE**-nuhl **FASH**-ee-ah) The fibrous connective tissue membrane that covers the kidneys and the surrounding adipose tissue and helps keep the kidneys in place (Chapter 18).

Renal filtrate (**REE**-nuhl **FILL**-trayt) The fluid formed from blood plasma by the process of filtration in the renal corpuscles; flows from Bowman's capsules through the renal tubules where most is reabsorbed; the filtrate that enters the renal pelvis is called urine (Chapter 18).

Renal medulla (**REE**-nuhl muh-**DEW**-lah) The inner tissue layer of the kidney; consists of loops of Henle and collecting tubules; the triangular segments of the renal medulla are called renal pyramids (Chapter 18).

Renal pelvis (**REE**-nuhl **PELL**-vis) The most medial area of the kidney; a cavity formed by the expanded end of the ureter at the hilus of the kidney (Chapter 18).

Renal pyramids (**REE**-nuhl **PEER**-ah-mids) The triangular segments of the renal medulla; the papillae of the pyramids empty urine into the calyces of the renal pelvis (Chapter 18).

Renal tubule (**REE**-nuhl **TOO**-byool) The part of a nephron that consists of a proximal convoluted tubule, loop of Henle, distal convoluted tubule, and collecting tubule; the site of tubular reabsorption and tubular secretion (Chapter 18).

Renal vein (**REE**-nuhl VAYN) The vein that returns blood from a kidney to the inferior vena cava (Chapter 18).

Renin–angiotensin mechanism (**REE**-nin AN-jee-oh-**TEN**-sin) A series of chemical reactions initiated by a decrease in blood pressure that stimulates the kidneys to secrete the enzyme renin; culminates in the formation of angiotensin II (Chapter 10).

Repolarization (RE-pol-lahr-i-**ZAY**-shun) The restoration of electrical charges on either side of a cell membrane following depolarization; positive charge outside and a negative charge inside brought about by a rapid outflow of potassium ions (Chapter 7).

Reproductive system (REE-proh-**DUK**-tive **SIS**-tem) The male or female organ system that produces gametes, ensures fertilization, and in women, provides a site for the developing embryo-fetus (Chapter 20).

Reservoir (**REZ**-er-vwor) 1. A person or animal who harbors a pathogen and is a source of the pathogen for others (Chapter 22). 2. A storage site (Chapter 7).

Resident flora (**REZ**-i-dent **FLOOR**-uh) Part of normal flora; those microorganisms on or in nearly everyone in specific body sites nearly all the time (Chapter 22).

Residual air (ree-**ZID**-yoo-al AIR) The volume of air that remains in the lungs after the most forceful exhalation; important to provide for continuous gas exchange; average: 1000–1500 mL (Chapter 15).

Resistance (re-**ZIS**-tenss) The total of all of the body's defenses against pathogens; includes the non-specific aspects of innate immunity such as unbroken skin and the specific mechanisms of adaptive immunity such as antibody production (Chapter 22).

Resorption (ree-**ZORP**-shun) The process of removal by absorption, such as the removal of bone matrix by osteoclasts (Chapter 6).

Respiratory acidosis (**RES**-pi-rah-**TOR**-ee ass-i-**DOH**-sis) A condition in which the blood pH is lower than normal, caused by disorders that decrease the rate or efficiency of respiration and permit the accumulation of carbon dioxide (Chapter 15).

Respiratory alkalosis (**RES**-pi-rah-**TOR**-ee al-kah-**LOH**-sis) A condition in which the blood pH is higher than normal, caused by disorders that increase the rate of respiration and decrease the level of carbon dioxide in the blood (Chapter 15).

Respiratory pump (**RES**-pi-rah-**TOR**-ee) A mechanism that increases venous return; pressure changes during breathing compress the veins that pass through the thoracic cavity (Chapter 13).

Respiratory system (**RES**-pi-rah-TOR-ee **SIS**-tem) The organ system that moves air into and out of the lungs so that oxygen and carbon dioxide may be exchanged between the air and the blood (Chapter 15).

Resting potential (**RES**-ting poh-**TEN**-shul) The difference in electrical charges on either side of a cell membrane not transmitting an impulse; positive charge outside and a negative charge inside (Chapter 7).

Reticulocyte (re-**TIK**-yoo-loh-sight) A red blood cell that contains remnants of the endoplasmic reticulum, an immature stage in red blood cell formation; makes up about 1% of the red blood cells in peripheral circulation (Chapter 11).

Reticuloendothelial system (re-TIK-yoo-loh-en-doh-**THEE**-lee-al) Former name for the tissue macrophage system, the organs or tissues that contain macrophages (RE cells) that phagocytize old red blood cells; the liver, spleen, and red bone marrow (Chapter 11).

Retina (**RET**-i-nah) The innermost layer of the eyeball that contains the photoreceptors, the rods and cones (Chapter 9).

Retroperitoneal (RE-troh-PER-i-toh-**NEE**-uhl) Located behind the peritoneum (Chapter 18).

Reuptake (ree-**UP**-tayk) The reabsorption of a substance that was just secreted; used with respect to some neurotransmitters (Chapter 8).

Rhabdomyolysis (RAB-doh-my-**AHL**-i-sis) The destruction of skeletal muscle tissue with the release of intercellular components such as myoglobin that may clog kidney tubules and lead to renal failure (Chapter 18).

Rh factor (R-H **FAK**-ter) The red blood cell types determined by the presence or absence of the Rh (D) antigen on the red blood cell membranes; the two types are Rh positive and Rh negative (Chapter 11).

Rheumatoid arthritis (**ROO**-muh-toyd ar-**THRY**-tiss) An autoimmune disease characterized by severe inflammation of joints. The joint damage may progress to fusion and immobility of the joint (Chapter 6).

Rhodopsin (roh-**DOP**-sin) The chemical in the rods of the retina that breaks down when light waves strike it; this chemical change initiates a nerve impulse (Chapter 9).

RhoGAM (**ROH**-gam) The trade name for the Rh (D) antibody administered to an Rh-negative woman who has delivered an Rh-positive infant; it will destroy any fetal red blood cells that may have entered maternal circulation (Chapter 11).

Ribosome (**RYE**-boh-sohme) A cell organelle found in the cytoplasm; the site of protein synthesis (Chapter 3).

Ribozyme (**RYE**-boh-zime) Ribosomal RNA that acts as an enzyme to form peptide bonds during protein synthesis (Chapter 3).

Ribs (RIBZ) The 24 flat bones that, together with the sternum, form the rib cage. The first seven pairs are true ribs, the next three pairs are false ribs, and the last two pairs are floating ribs (Chapter 6).

Rickets (**RIK**-ets) A deficiency of vitamin D in children, resulting in poor and abnormal bone growth (Chapter 6).

RNA (ribonucleic acid) A nucleic acid that is a single strand of nucleotides; essential for protein synthesis within cells; messenger RNA (mRNA) is a copy of the genetic code of DNA; transfer RNA (tRNA) aligns amino acids in the proper sequence on the mRNA (Chapter 2).

Rods (RAHDZ) The sensory receptors in the retina of the eye that detect the presence of light (Chapter 9).

Round window (ROWND **WIN**-doh) The membrane-covered opening of the inner ear that bulges to prevent pressure damage to the organ of Corti (Chapter 9).

Rugae (**ROO**-gay) Folds of the mucosa of organs such as the stomach, urinary bladder, and vagina; permit expansion of these organs (Chapter 16).

S

Saccule (**SAK**-yool) A membranous sac in the vestibule of the inner ear that contains receptors for static equilibrium (Chapter 9).

Sacroiliac joint (SAY-kroh-**ILL**-ee-ak) The slightly movable joint between the sacrum and the ilium (Chapter 6).

Sacrum (**SAY**-krum) The five fused sacral vertebrae at the base of the spine (Chapter 6).

Saddle joint (**SA**-duhl) The carpometacarpal joint of the thumb, a diarthrosis (Chapter 6).

Sagittal section (**SAJ**-i-tuhl SEK-shun) A plane or cut from front to back, separating right and left parts (from the Latin "arrow") (Chapter 1).

Saliva (sah-**LYE**-vah) The secretion of the salivary glands; mostly water and containing the enzyme amylase (Chapter 16).

Salivary glands (**SAL**-i-va-ree) The three pairs of exocrine glands that secrete saliva into the oral cavity; parotid, submandibular, and sublingual pairs (Chapter 16).

Salt (SAWLT) A chemical compound that consists of a positive ion other than hydrogen and a negative ion other than hydroxyl (Chapter 2).

Saltatory conduction (**SAWL**-tah-taw-ree kon-**DUK**-shun) The rapid transmission of a nerve impulse from one node of Ranvier to the next; characteristic of myelinated neurons (Chapter 8).

Saprophyte (**SAP**-roh-fight) An organism that lives on dead organic matter; a decomposer (Syn.—saprobe) (Chapter 22).

Sarcolemma (SAR-koh-**LEM**-ah) The cell membrane of a muscle fiber (Chapter 7).

Sarcomere (**SAR**-koh-meer) The unit of contraction in a skeletal muscle fiber; a precise arrangement of myosin and actin filaments between two Z lines (Chapter 7).

Sarcoplasmic reticulum (SAR-koh-**PLAZ**-mik re-**TIK**-yoo-lum) The endoplasmic reticulum of a muscle fiber; is a reservoir for calcium ions (Chapter 7).

Saturated fat (**SAT**-uhr-ay-ted) A true fat that is often solid at room temperature and of animal origin; its fatty acids contain the maximum number of hydrogens (Chapter 2).

Scapula (**SKAP**-yoo-luh) The flat bone of the shoulder that articulates with the humerus (Syn.—shoulder blade) (Chapter 6).

Schwann cell (SHWAHN SELL) A cell of the peripheral nervous system that forms the myelin sheath and neurolemma of peripheral axons and dendrites (Chapter 4).

Sclera (**SKLER**-ah) The outermost layer of the eyeball, made of fibrous connective tissue; the anterior portion is the transparent cornea (Chapter 9).

Scoliosis (SKOH-lee-**OH**-sis) A lateral curvature of the vertebral column (Chapter 6).

Scrotum (SKROH-tum) The sac of skin between the upper thighs in males; contains the testes, epididymides, and part of the ductus deferens (Chapter 20).

Sebaceous gland (suh-**BAY**-shus) An exocrine gland in the dermis that produces sebum (Chapter 5).

Sebum (**SEE**-bum) The lipid (oil) secretion of sebaceous glands (Chapter 5).

Secondary infection (**SEK**-un-DAR-ee) An infection made possible by a primary infection that has lowered the host's resistance (Chapter 22).

Secondary sex characteristics (**SEK**-un-DAR-ee SEKS) The features that develop at puberty in males or females; they are under the influence of the sex hormones but are not directly involved in reproduction. Examples are growth of facial or body hair and growth of muscles (Chapter 20).

Secretin (se-**KREE**-tin) A hormone secreted by the duodenum when food enters; stimulates secretion of bile by the liver and secretion of bicarbonate pancreatic juice (Chapter 16).

Secretion (si-**KREE**-shun) The production and release of a cellular product with a useful purpose (Chapter 4).

Section (**SEK**-shun) The cutting of an organ or the body to make internal structures visible (Chapter 1).

Selectively permeable (se-**LEK**-tiv-lee **PER**-me-uh-buhl) A characteristic of cell membranes; permits the passage of some materials but not of others (Chapter 3).

Self-limiting disease (self-**LIM**-i-ting) A disease that typically lasts a certain period of time and is followed by recovery (Chapter 22).

Semen (**SEE**-men) The thick, alkaline fluid that contains sperm and the secretions of the seminal vesicles, prostate gland, and bulbourethral glands (Chapter 20).

Semicircular canals (SEM-eye-**SIR**-kyoo-lur) Three oval canals in the inner ear that contain the receptors that detect motion (Chapter 9).

Seminal vesicles (**SEM**-i-nuhl **VESS**-i-kulls) The glands located posterior to the prostate gland and inferior to the urinary bladder; secrete an alkaline fluid that enters the ejaculatory ducts and becomes part of semen (Chapter 20).

Seminiferous tubules (sem-i-**NIFF**-er-us) The site of spermatogenesis in the testes (Chapter 20).

Sensation (sen-**SAY**-shun) A feeling or awareness of conditions outside or inside the body, resulting from the stimulation of sensory receptors and interpretation by the brain (Chapter 9).

Sensory neuron (**SEN**-suh-ree **NYOOR**-on) A nerve cell that carries impulses from a receptor to the central nervous system. (Syn.—afferent neuron) (Chapter 8).

Septic shock (**SEP**-tik SHAHK) A type of circulatory shock that is a consequence of a bacterial infection (Chapter 13).

Septicemia (SEP-tih-**SEE**-mee-ah) The presence of bacteria in the blood (Chapter 5).

Septum (**SEP**-tum) A wall that separates two cavities, such as the nasal septum between the nasal cavities or the interventricular septum between the two ventricles of the heart (Chapter 12).

Serous fluid (**SEER**-us **FLOO**-id) A fluid that prevents friction between the two layers of a serous membrane (Chapter 4).

Serous membrane (**SEER**-us **MEM**-brayn) An epithelial membrane that lines a closed body cavity and covers the organs in that cavity (Chapter 4).

Sex chromosomes (SEKS **KROH**-muh-sohms) The pair of chromosomes that determines the gender of an individual; designated XX in females and XY in males (Chapter 21).

Sex-linked trait (**SEKS**-LINKED TRAYT) A genetic characteristic in which the gene is located on the X chromosome (Chapter 7).

Simple (**SIM**-puhl) Having only one layer, used especially to describe certain types of epithelial tissue (Chapter 4).

Sinoatrial (SA) node (**SIGH**-noh-AY-tree-al NOHD) The first part of the cardiac conduction pathway, located in the wall of the right atrium; initiates each heartbeat (Chapter 12).

Sinusoid (**SIGH**-nuh-soyd) A large, very permeable capillary; permits proteins or blood cells to enter or leave the blood (Chapter 13).

Skeletal muscle pump (**SKEL**-e-tuhl **MUSS**-uhl) A mechanism that increases venous return; contractions of the skeletal muscles compress the deep veins, especially those of the legs (Chapter 13).

Skeletal system (**SKEL**-e-tuhl) The organ system that consists of the bones, ligaments, and cartilage; supports the body and is a framework for muscle attachment (Chapter 6).

Skin (SKIN) An organ that is part of the integumentary system; consists of the outer epidermis and the inner dermis (Chapter 5).

Sliding filament mechanism (**SLY**-ding **FILL**-ah-ment) The sequence of events that occurs within sarcomeres when a muscle fiber contracts (Chapter 7).

Small intestine (SMAWL in-**TESS**-tin) The organ of the alimentary tube between the stomach and the large intestine; secretes enzymes that complete the digestive process and absorbs the end products of digestion (Chapter 16).

Smooth muscle (SMOOTH **MUSS**-uhl) The muscle tissue that forms the walls of hollow internal organs. Also called visceral or involuntary muscle (Chapter 4).

Sneeze reflex (SNEEZ) A reflex integrated by the medulla that expels irritating substances from the nasal cavities by means of an explosive exhalation (Chapter 15).

Sodium-potassium pumps (**SEW**-dee-um pa-**TASS**-ee-um) The active transport mechanisms that maintain a high sodium ion concentration outside the cell and a high potassium ion concentration inside the cell (Chapter 7).

Soft palate (SAWFT **PAL**-uht) The posterior portion of the palate that is elevated during swallowing to block the nasopharynx (Chapter 15).

Solute (**SAH**-loot) The substance that is dissolved in a solution (Chapter 2).

Solution (suh-**LOO**-shun) The dispersion of one or more compounds (solutes) in a liquid (solvent) (Chapter 2).

Solvent (**SAHL**-vent) A liquid in which substances (solutes) will dissolve (Chapter 2).

Somatic (soh-**MA**-tik) Pertaining to structures of the body wall, such as skeletal muscles and the skin (Chapter 8).

Somatostatin (SOH-mat-oh-**STAT**-in) 1. Growth hormone inhibiting hormone (GHIH); produced by the hypothalamus. 2. The hormone produced by the delta cells of the pancreas (Chapter 10).

Somatotropin (SOH-mat-oh-**TROH**-pin) Growth hormone (Chapter 10).

Specialized fluids (**SPEH**-shul-eyezd **FLOO**-ids) Specific compartments of extracellular fluid; include cerebrospinal fluid, synovial fluid, and aqueous humor in the eye (Chapter 2).

Spermatic cord (sper-**MAT**-ik KORD) The cord that suspends the testis; composed of the ductus deferens, blood vessels, and nerves (Chapter 20).

Spermatogenesis (SPER-ma-toh-**JEN**-e-sis) The process of meiosis in the testes to produce sperm cells (Chapter 3).

Spermatozoa (sper-MAT-oh-**ZOH**-ah) (Sing.—spermatozoon) Sperm cells; produced by the testes (Chapter 20).

Sphenoid bone (**SFEE**-noyd) The flat bone that forms part of the anterior floor of the cranial cavity and encloses the pituitary gland (Chapter 6).

Sphincter (**SFINK**-ter) A circular muscle that regulates the size of an opening (Chapter 7).

Spina bifida (**SPY**-nuh **BIF**-i-duh) A congenital malformation of the backbone in which the spinal cord and meninges may protrude; there are many variations and degrees of impairment (Chapter 17).

Spinal cavity (**SPY**-nuhl **KAV**-i-tee) The cavity within the vertebral column that contains the spinal cord and meninges; (Syn.—vertebral canal or cavity) (Chapter 1).

Spinal cord (**SPY**-nuhl KORD) The part of the central nervous system within the vertebral canal; transmits impulses to and from the brain (Chapter 8).

Spinal cord reflex (**SPY**-nuhl KORD **REE**-fleks) A reflex integrated in the spinal cord in which the brain is not directly involved (Chapter 8).

Spinal nerves (**SPY**-nuhl NERVS) The 31 pairs of nerves that emerge from the spinal cord (Chapter 8).

Spinal shock (**SPY**-nuhl SHAHK) The temporary or permanent loss of spinal cord reflexes following injury to the spinal cord (Chapter 8).

Spirillum (spih-**RILL**-uhm) (Pl.—spirilla) A bacterium with a spiral shape (Chapter 22).

Spirochete (**SPY**-roh-keet) Spiral bacteria of the order Spirochaetales (Chapter 22).

Spleen (SPLEEN) An organ located in the upper left abdominal quadrant behind the stomach; consists of lymphatic tissue that produces lymphocytes; also contains macrophages that phagocytize old red blood cells (Chapter 14).

Spongy bone (**SPUN**-jee BOWNE) Bone tissue not organized into haversian systems; forms most of the body's short, flat, and irregular bones and forms epiphyses of long bones (Chapter 6).

Spontaneous fracture (spahn-**TAY**-nee-us) A fracture that occurs without apparent trauma; often a consequence of osteoporosis (Syn.—pathologic fracture) (Chapter 6).

Spore (SPOOR) 1. A bacterial form that is dormant and highly resistant to environmental extremes such as heat. 2. A unicellular fungal reproductive form (Chapter 22).

Squamous (**SKWAY**-mus) Flat or scalelike; used especially in reference to epithelial tissue (Chapter 4).

Stapes (**STAY**-peez) The third of the auditory bones in the middle ear; transmits vibrations from the incus to the oval window of the inner ear (Chapter 9).

Starch (STARCH) A polysaccharide produced by plants; digested to glucose, a source of energy for cell respiration (Chapter 2).

Starling's law of the heart (**STAR**-lingz LAW) The force of contraction of cardiac muscle fibers is determined by the length of the fibers; the more cardiac muscle fibers are stretched, the more forcefully they contract (Chapter 12).

Stem cell (STEM SELL) 1. An embryonic cell capable of differentiating into any of the specialized cells of an organism (Chapter 3). 2. The unspecialized cell found in red bone marrow and lymphatic tissue that is the precursor cell for all types of blood cells (Chapter 11). 3. Any unspecialized cell with the potential to differentiate (Chapter 3).

Stenosis (ste-**NOH**-sis) An abnormal constriction or narrowing of an opening or duct (Chapter 12).

Sterilization (STIR-ill-i-**ZAY**-shun) The process of completely destroying all of the microorganisms on or in a substance or object (Chapter 22).

Sternum (**STIR**-num) The flat bone that forms part of the anterior rib cage; consists of the manubrium, body, and xiphoid process (Syn.—breastbone) (Chapter 6).

Steroid (**STEER**-oyd) An organic compound in the lipid group; includes cholesterol and the sex hormones (Chapter 2).

Stimulus (**STIM**-yoo-lus) A change, especially one that affects a sensory receptor or that brings about a response in a living organism (Chapter 9).

Stomach (**STUM**-uk) The sac-like organ of the alimentary tube between the esophagus and the small intestine; is a reservoir for food and secretes gastric juice to begin protein digestion (Chapter 16).

Strabismus (strah-**BIZ**-mis) An impairment of binocular vision, the optic axes of the eyes cannot be oriented properly on an object because of an imbalance in one set of extrinsic muscles; the "lazy eye" may drift medially or laterally (Chapter 9).

Stratified (**STRA**-ti-fyed) Having two or more layers (Chapter 4).

Stratum corneum (**STRA**-tum **KOR**-nee-um) The outermost layer of the epidermis, made of many layers of dead, keratinized cells (Chapter 5).

Stratum germinativum (**STRA**-tum JER-min-ah-**TEE**-vum) The innermost layer of the epidermis; the cells undergo mitosis to produce new epidermis (Syn.—stratum basale) (Chapter 5).

Streptokinase (STREP-toh-**KYE**-nase) An enzyme produced by bacteria of the genus *Streptococcus* that was used clinically to dissolve abnormal clots, such as those in coronary arteries (Chapter 11).

Stretch receptor (STRETCH ree-**SEP**-ter) A sensory receptor in a muscle that detects stretching of the muscle (Syn.—proprioceptor) (Chapter 7).

Stretch reflex (STRETCH **REE**-fleks) A spinal cord reflex in which a muscle that is stretched will contract (Chapter 8).

Striated muscle (**STRY**-ay-ted MUSS-uhl) The muscle tissue that forms the skeletal muscles that move bones (Syn.—voluntary muscle, skeletal muscle) (Chapter 4).

Stroke volume (STROHK **VAHL**-yoom) The amount of blood pumped by a ventricle in one beat; the resting average is 60–80 mL/beat (Chapter 12).

Subarachnoid space (SUB-uh-**RAK**-noid) The space between the arachnoid membrane and the pia mater; contains cerebrospinal fluid (Chapter 8).

Subclinical infection (sub-**KLIN**-i-kuhl) An infection in which the person shows no symptoms (Syn.—inapparent, asymptomatic) (Chapter 22).

Subcutaneous (SUB-kew-**TAY**-nee-us) Below the skin; the superficial fascia between the dermis and the muscles (Chapter 5).

Sublingual glands (sub-**LING**-gwal) The pair of salivary glands located below the floor of the mouth (Chapter 16).

Submandibular glands (SUB-man-**DIB**-yoo-lar) The pair of salivary glands located at the posterior corners of the mandible (Chapter 16).

Submucosa (SUB-mew-**KOH**-sah) The layer of connective tissue and blood vessels located below the mucosa (lining) of a mucous membrane (Chapter 16).

Substrates (**SUB**-strayts) Substances acted upon, as by enzymes (Chapter 2).

Sucrase (**SOO**-krays) A digestive enzyme that breaks down sucrose to glucose and fructose; secreted by the small intestine (Chapter 16).

Sucrose (**SOO**-krohs) A disaccharide made of one glucose and one fructose molecule (Syn.—cane sugar, table sugar) (Chapter 2).

Sulcus (**SUHL**-kus) A furrow or groove, as between the gyri of the cerebrum (Syn.—fissure) (Chapter 8).

Superficial (soo-per-**FISH**-uhl) Toward the surface (Chapter 1).

Superficial fascia (soo-per-**FISH**-uhl **FASH**-ee-ah) The subcutaneous tissue, between the dermis and the muscles. Consists of areolar connective tissue and adipose tissue (Chapter 4).

Superior (soo-**PEER**-ee-your) Above, or higher (Chapter 1).

Superior vena cava (**VEE**-nah **KAY**-vah) The vein that returns blood from the upper body to the right atrium (Chapter 12).

Supination (SOO-pi-**NAY**-shun) Turning the palm upward, or lying face up (Chapter 7).

Suspensory ligaments (suh-**SPEN**-suh-ree **LIG**-uh-ments) The strands of connective tissue that connect the ciliary body to the lens of the eye (Chapter 9).

Sustentacular cells (SUS-ten-**TAK**-yoo-lar SELLS) The cells of the testes that secrete inhibin (Chapter 20).

Suture (**SOO**-cher) A synarthrosis, an immovable joint between cranial bones or facial bones (from the Latin "seam") (Chapter 6).

Symbiosis (SIM-bee-**OH**-sis) A close relationship between two species, most often meaning one that is beneficial to both species (Chapter 16).

Sympathetic (SIM-puh-**THET**-ik) The division of the autonomic nervous system that dominates during stressful situations (Chapter 8).

Sympathomimetic (SIM-pah-tho-mi-**MET**-ik) Having the same effects as sympathetic impulses, as has epinephrine, a hormone of the adrenal medulla (Chapter 10).

Symphysis (**SIM**-fi-sis) An amphiarthrosis in which a disc of cartilage is found between two bones, as in the vertebral column (Chapter 6).

Symptomatic infection (**SIMP**-toh-MAT-ik) An infection in which the patient exhibits the symptoms of the disease (Chapter 22).

Synapse (**SIN**-aps) The space between the axon of one neuron and the cell body or dendrite of the next neuron or between the end of a motor neuron and an effector cell (Chapter 4).

Synaptic knob (si-**NAP**-tik NAHB) The end of an axon of a neuron that releases a neurotransmitter (Chapter 8).

Synarthrosis (SIN-ar-**THROH**-sis) An immovable joint, such as a suture (Chapter 6).

Synergistic muscles (SIN-er-**JIS**-tik **MUSS**-uhls) Muscles that have the same function, or a stabilizing function, with respect to the movement of a joint (Chapter 7).

Synovial fluid (sin-**OH**-vee-uhl **FLOO**-id) A thick slippery fluid that prevents friction within joint cavities (Chapter 6).

Synovial membrane (sin-**OH**-vee-uhl **MEM**-brayn) The connective tissue membrane that lines joint cavities and secretes synovial fluid (Chapter 4).

Synthesis (**SIN**-the-siss) The process of forming complex molecules or compounds from simpler compounds or elements (Chapter 2).

Syphilis (**SIFF**-i-lis) A sexually transmitted disease caused by the bacterium *Treponema pallidum;* may also cause congenital syphilis in newborns of infected women (Chapter 20).

Systemic infection (sis-**TEM**-ik) An infection that has spread throughout the body from an initial site (Chapter 22).

Systole (**SIS**-tuh-lee) In the cardiac cycle, the contraction of the myocardium; ventricular systole pumps blood into the arteries (Chapter 12).

T

T cells (T SELLS) A subgroup of lymphocytes; include helper T cells, cytotoxic T cells, regulatory T cells, and memory T cells, all of which are involved in adaptive immune responses (Chapter 11).

T tubule (TEE **TOO**-byool) A transverse tubule, a fold of the sarcolemma; carries the action potential to the interior of a muscle fiber (Chapter 7).

Tachycardia (TAK-ee-**KAR**-dee-yah) An abnormally rapid heart rate; more than 100 beats per minute (Chapter 12).

Taenia coli (**TAY**-nee-uh **KOH**-lye) The longitudinal muscle layer of the colon; three bands of smooth muscle fibers that extend from the cecum to the sigmoid colon (Chapter 16).

Talus (**TAL**-us) One of the tarsals; articulates with the tibia (Chapter 6).

Target organ (**TAR**-get **OR**-gan) The organ (or tissue) in which a hormone exerts its specific effects (Chapter 10).

Tarsals (**TAR**-suhls) The seven short bones in each ankle (Chapter 6).

Taste buds (TAYST BUDS) Structures on the papillae of the tongue that contain the chemoreceptors for the detection of chemicals (food) dissolved in saliva (Chapter 9).

Tears (TEERS) The watery secretion of the lacrimal glands; wash the anterior surface of the eyeball and keep it moist (Chapter 9).

Teeth (TEETH) Bony projections in the upper and lower jaws that function in chewing (Chapter 16).

Telomeres (**TEL**-oh-meers) The DNA sequences at the ends of a chromosome; may be a marker of the aging of cells, as a bit is lost with each cell division (Chapter 3).

Telophase (**TELL**-ah-fayz) The fourth stage of mitosis, in which two nuclei are re-formed (Chapter 3).

Temporal bone (**TEM**-puh-ruhl) The flat bone that forms the side of the cranial cavity and contains middle and inner ear structures (Chapter 6).

Temporal lobes (**TEM**-puh-ruhl LOWBS) The lateral parts of the cerebrum; contain the auditory, olfactory, and taste areas (Chapter 8).

Tendon (**TEN**-dun) A fibrous connective tissue structure that connects muscle to bone (Chapter 7).

Teratogen (te-**RAH**-toh-jen) Anything that causes developmental abnormalities in an embryo; may be a chemical or microorganism to which an embryo is exposed by way of the mother (Chapter 21).

Testes (**TES**-teez) (Sing.—testis) The male gonads that produce sperm cells; also endocrine glands that secrete the hormone testosterone (Chapter 10).

Testosterone (tes-**TAHS**-ter-ohn) The sex hormone secreted by the interstitial cells of the testes; responsible for the maturation of sperm, growth of the male reproductive organs, and the secondary sex characteristics (Chapter 10).

Tetanus (**TET**-uh-nus) 1. A sustained contraction of a muscle fiber in response to rapid nerve impulses; the basis for all useful movements. 2. A disease, characterized by severe muscle spasms, caused by the bacterium *Clostridium tetani* (Chapter 7).

Thalamus (**THAL**-uh-muss) The part of the brain superior to the hypothalamus; regulates subconscious aspects of sensation (Chapter 8).

Theory (**THEER**-ree) A statement that is the best explanation of all the available evidence on a particular process or mechanism. A theory is not a guess (Chapter 2).

Thermogenic (THER-moh-**JEN**-ik) Heat generating, as is brown fat tissue (Chapter 4).

Thoracic cavity (thaw-**RASS**-ik **KAV**-i-tee) The body cavity superior to the diaphragm (Chapter 1).

Thoracic duct (thaw-**RASS**-ik DUKT) The lymph vessel that empties lymph from the lower half and upper left quadrant of the body into the left subclavian vein (Chapter 14).

Thoracic vertebrae (thaw-**RASS**-ik **VER**-te-bray) The 12 vertebrae that articulate with the ribs (Chapter 6).

Threshold level–renal (**THRESH**-hold **LE**-vuhl) The concentration at which a substance in the blood *not* normally excreted by the kidneys begins to appear in the urine; for several substances, such as glucose, in the renal filtrate, there is a limit to how much the renal tubules can reabsorb (Chapter 18).

Thrombocyte (**THROM**-boh-sight) Platelet; a fragment of a megakaryocyte (Chapter 11).

Thrombocytopenia (**THROM**-boh-SIGH-toh-PEE-nee-ah) An abnormally low platelet count (Chapter 11).

Thrombopoietin (THROM-boh-**POY**-e-tin) A hormone produced by the liver that stimulates development of megakaryocytes in the red bone marrow (Chapter 11).

Thrombus (**THROM**-bus) A blood clot that obstructs blood flow through a blood vessel (Chapter 11).

Thymus (**THIGH**-mus) An organ made of lymphatic tissue located inferior to the thyroid gland; large in the fetus and child, and shrinks with age; produces T cells and hormones necessary for the maturation of the immune system (Chapter 14).

Thyroid cartilage (**THIGH**-roid **KAR**-ti-ledj) The largest and most anterior cartilage of the larynx; may be felt in the front of the neck (Chapter 15).

Thyroid gland (**THIGH**-roid) An endocrine gland on the anterior side of the trachea below the larynx; secretes thyroxine, triiodothyronine, and calcitonin (Chapter 10).

Thyroid-stimulating hormone (TSH) A hormone secreted by the anterior pituitary gland that causes the thyroid gland to secrete triiodothyronine and thyroxine (Chapter 10).

Thyroxine (T_4) (thigh-**ROK**-sin) A hormone secreted by the thyroid gland that increases energy production and protein synthesis (Chapter 10).

Tibia (**TIB**-ee-yuh) The larger long bone of the lower leg (Syn.—shinbone) (Chapter 6).

Tidal volume (**TIGH**-duhl **VAHL**-yoom) The volume of air in one normal inhalation and exhalation; average: 400–600 mL (Chapter 15).

Tinnitus (ti-**NYE**-tus or **TIN**-i-tus) An abnormal sound of buzzing, crackling, or ringing in the ears; has many causes, one of which is projection by the brain in an attempt to "fill in" what has been lost with partial deafness (Chapter 9).

Tissue (**TISH**-yoo) A group of cells with similar structure and function (Chapter 1).

Tissue fluid (**TISH**-yoo **FLOO**-id) The water found in intercellular spaces. Also called interstitial fluid (Chapter 2).

Tissue macrophage system (**TISH**-yoo **MAK**-roh-fayj) The organs or tissues that contain macrophages that phagocytize old red blood cells: the liver, spleen, and red bone marrow (Chapter 11).

Tissue typing (**TISH**-yoo **TIGH**-ping) A laboratory procedure that determines the HLA types of a donated organ, prior to an organ transplant (Chapter 11).

Titin (**TIGH**-tin) The protein in sarcomeres that anchors myosin filaments to the Z lines (Chapter 7).

Tongue (TUHNG) A muscular organ on the floor of the oral cavity; contributes to chewing and swallowing and contains taste buds (Chapter 16).

Tonsillectomy (TAHN-si-**LEK**-toh-mee) The surgical removal of the palatine tonsils and/or adenoid (Chapter 14).

Tonsils (**TAHN**-sills) The lymph nodules in the mucosa of the pharynx, the palatine tonsils, and the adenoid; also the lingual tonsils on the base of the tongue (Chapter 14).

Toxin (**TAHK**-sin) A chemical that is poisonous to cells (Chapter 22).

Toxoid (**TAHK**-soyd) An inactivated bacterial toxin that is no longer harmful yet is still antigenic; used as a vaccine (Chapter 14).

Trace element (TRAYS **EL**-uh-ment) Those elements (minerals) needed in very small amounts by the body for normal functioning (Chapter 2).

Trachea (**TRAY**-kee-ah) The organ that is the air passageway between the larynx and the primary bronchi (Syn.—windpipe) (Chapter 15).

Transamination (TRANS-am-i-**NAY**-shun) The transfer of an amino (NH_2) group from an amino acid to a carbon chain to form a non-essential amino acid; takes place in the liver (Chapter 16).

Transcription (tran-**SKRIP**-shun) The process by which a complementary copy, mRNA, is made of a DNA gene; will be followed by translation (Chapter 3).

Transient flora (**TRAN**-zee-ent **FLOOR**-uh) Part of normal flora; those microorganisms that may inhabit specific sites in the body for short periods of time (Chapter 22).

Transitional (trans-**ZI**-shun-uhl) Changing from one form to another (Chapter 4).

Transitional epithelium (tran-**ZI**-shun-uhl) A type of epithelium in which the surface cells change from rounded to flat as the organ changes shape (Chapter 4).

Translation (trans-**LAY**-shun) The process by which proteins are synthesized on the ribosomes of a cell; tRNA molecules line up amino acids according to the codons on the mRNA molecule (Chapter 3).

Transporter (trans-**POOR**-ter) A protein that is part of a cell membrane and necessary for the facilitated diffusion of a substance such as glucose (Chapter 3).

Transverse section (trans-**VERS SEK**-shun) A plane or cut from front to back, separating upper and lower parts (Chapter 1).

Tricuspid valve (try-**KUSS**-pid VALV) The right AV valve, which prevents backflow of blood from the right ventricle to the right atrium when the ventricle contracts (Chapter 12).

Trigeminal nerves (try-**JEM**-in-uhl) Cranial nerve pair V; sensory for the face and teeth; motor to chewing muscles (Chapter 8).

Triglyceride (try-**GLI**-si-ryde) An organic compound, a true fat, that is made of one glycerol and three fatty acids (Chapter 2).

Trigone (**TRY**-gohn) Triangular area on the floor of the urinary bladder bounded by the openings of the two ureters and the urethra (Chapter 18).

Triiodothyronine (T_3) (TRY-eye-oh-doh-**THIGH**-roh-neen) A hormone secreted by the thyroid gland that increases energy production and protein synthesis (Chapter 10).

Trisomy (**TRY**-suh-mee) In genetics, having three homologous chromosomes instead of the usual two (Chapter 20).

Trochlear nerves (**TROK**-lee-ur) Cranial nerve pair IV; motor to an extrinsic muscle of the eye (Chapter 8).

Trophoblast (**TROH**-foh-blast) The outermost layer of the embryonic blastocyst; will become the chorion, one of the embryonic membranes (Chapter 21).

Tropomyosin (TROH-poh-**MYE**-oh-sin) A protein that inhibits the contraction of sarcomeres in a muscle fiber (Chapter 7).

Troponin (**TROH**-poh-nin) A protein that inhibits the contraction of the sarcomeres in a muscle fiber (Chapter 7).

True fat (TROO FAT) An organic compound in the lipid group that is made of glycerol and fatty acids (Chapter 2).

Trypsin (**TRIP**-sin) A digestive enzyme that breaks down proteins into polypeptides; secreted by the pancreas (Chapter 16).

Tubal ligation (**TOO**-buhl lye-**GAY**-shun) A surgical procedure to remove or sever the fallopian tubes; usually done as a method of contraception in women (Chapter 20).

Tubular reabsorption (**TOO**-byoo-ler REE-ab-**SORP**-shun) The processes by which useful substances in the renal filtrate are returned to the blood in the peritubular capillaries (Chapter 18).

Tubular secretion (**TOO**-byoo-ler se-**KREE**-shun) The processes by which cells of the renal tubules secrete substances into the renal filtrate to be excreted in urine (Chapter 18).

Tunica (**TOO**-ni-kah) A layer or coat, as in the wall of an artery (Chapter 13).

Tympanic membrane (tim-**PAN**-ik) The eardrum, the membrane that is stretched across the end of the ear canal; vibrates when sound waves strike it (Chapter 9).

Typing and cross-matching (**TIGH**-ping and **KROSS**-match-ing) A laboratory test that determines whether or not donated blood is compatible, with respect to the red blood cell types (Chapter 11).

U

Ubiquitin (yoo-**BIK**-wi-tin) An intracellular protein that tags old, damaged, or misfolded proteins so that they may be destroyed by the enzymes of proteasomes (from the Latin "everywhere") (Chapter 3).

Ulna (**UHL**-nuh) The long bone of the forearm on the little finger side (Chapter 6).

Ultrasound (**UHL**-tra-sownd) 1. Inaudible sound. 2. A technique used in diagnosis in which ultrasound waves provide outlines of the shapes of organs or tissues (Chapter 21).

Umbilical arteries (uhm-**BILL**-i-kull **AR**-tuh-rees) The fetal blood vessels contained in the umbilical cord that carry deoxygenated blood from the fetus to the placenta (Chapter 13).

Umbilical cord (uhm-**BILL**-i-kull KORD) The structure that connects the fetus to the placenta; contains two umbilical arteries and one umbilical vein (Chapter 13).

Umbilical vein (uhm-**BILL**-i-kull VAYN) The fetal blood vessel contained in the umbilical cord that carries oxygenated blood from the placenta to the fetus (Chapter 13).

Unicellular (YOO-nee-**SELL**-yoo-lar) Composed of one cell (Chapter 4).

Unsaturated fat (un-**SAT**-uhr-ay-ted) A true fat that is often liquid at room temperature and of plant origin; its fatty acids contain less than the maximum number of hydrogens (Chapter 2).

Upper respiratory tract (**UH**-per **RES**-pi-rah-TOR-ee TRAKT) The respiratory organs located outside the chest cavity (Chapter 15).

Urea (yoo-**REE**-ah) A nitrogenous waste product formed in the liver from the deamination of amino acids or from ammonia (Chapter 5).

Uremia (yoo-**REE**-me-ah) The condition in which blood levels of nitrogenous waste products are elevated; caused by renal insufficiency or failure (Chapter 18).

Ureter (**YOOR**-uh-ter) The tubular organ that carries urine from the renal pelvis (kidney) to the urinary bladder (Chapter 18).

Urethra (yoo-**REE**-thrah) The tubular organ that carries urine from the urinary bladder to the exterior of the body (Chapter 18).

Urinary bladder (**YOOR**-i-NAR-ee **BLA**-der) The organ that stores urine temporarily and contracts to eliminate urine by way of the urethra (Chapter 18).

Urinary system (**YOOR**-i-NAR-ee **SIS**-tem) The organ system that produces and eliminates urine; consists of the kidneys, ureters, urinary bladder, and urethra (Chapter 18).

Urine (**YOOR**-in) The fluid formed by the kidneys from blood plasma (Chapter 18).

Uterus (**YOO**-ter-us) The organ of the female reproductive system in which the placenta is formed to nourish a developing embryo-fetus (Chapter 20).

Utricle (**YOO**-tri-kuhl) A membranous sac in the vestibule of the inner ear that contains receptors for static equilibrium (Chapter 9).

V

Vaccine (vak-**SEEN**) A preparation of a foreign antigen that is administered by injection or other means in order to stimulate an antibody response to provide immunity to a particular pathogen (Chapter 14).

Vagina (vuh-**JIGH**-nah) The muscular tube that extends from the cervix of the uterus to the vaginal orifice; serves as the birth canal (Chapter 20).

Vagus nerves (**VAY**-gus) Cranial nerve pair X; sensory for cardiovascular and respiratory reflexes; motor to larynx, bronchioles, stomach, and intestines (Chapter 8).

Valence (**VAY**-lens) The combining power of an atom when compared with a hydrogen atom; expressed as a positive or negative number (Chapter 2).

Valve (VALVE) A structure in a cavity or tube that closes upon, and thus prevents, backflow of the fluid therein (from the Latin "a leaf of a double door") (Chapter 12).

Varicose vein (**VAR**-i-kohs VAYN) An enlarged, abnormally dilated vein; most often occurs in the legs (Chapter 13).

Vasectomy (va-**SEK**-tuh-me) A surgical procedure to remove or sever the ductus deferens; usually done as a method of contraception in men (Chapter 20).

Vasoconstriction (VAY-zoh-kon-**STRIK**-shun) A decrease in the diameter of a blood vessel caused by contraction of the smooth muscle in the wall of the vessel (Chapter 5).

Vasodilation (VAY-zoh-dye-**LAY**-shun) An increase in the diameter of a blood vessel caused by relaxation of the smooth muscle in the wall of the vessel (Chapter 5).

Vasomotor center (VAY-zoh-**MOH**-ter) The part of the medulla that regulates the diameter of arteries and veins; contributes to normal blood pressure (Chapter 8).

Vasopressin (VAY-zoh-**PRESS**-in) Antidiuretic hormone (Chapter 8).

Vector (**VEK**-ter) An arthropod that transmits pathogens from host to host, usually when it bites to obtain blood (Chapter 22).

Vein (VAYN) A blood vessel that takes blood from capillaries back to the heart (Chapter 13).

Venous return (**VEE**-nus ree-**TURN**) The amount of blood returned by the veins to the heart; is directly related to cardiac output, which depends on adequate venous return (Chapter 12).

Ventilation (VEN-ti-**LAY**-shun) The movement of air into and out of the lungs (Chapter 15).

Ventral (**VEN**-truhl) Toward the front (Syn.—anterior) (Chapter 1).

Ventral cavity (**VEN**-truhl **KAV**-i-tee) Previously used term for the collective thoracic, abdominal, and pelvic cavities.

Ventral root (**VEN**-truhl ROOT) The motor root of a spinal nerve (Chapter 8).

Ventricle (**VEN**-tri-kul) 1. A cavity, such as the four ventricles of the brain that contain cerebrospinal fluid. 2. One of the two lower chambers of the heart that pump blood to the body or to the lungs (Chapter 8).

Venule (**VEN**-yool) A small vein (Chapter 13).

Vertebra (**VER**-te-brah) One of the bones of the spine or backbone (Chapter 6).

Vertebral canal (**VER**-te-brahl ka-**NAL**) The spinal cavity that contains and protects the spinal cord (Chapter 6).

Vertebral column (**VER**-te-brahl **KAH**-luhm) The spine or backbone (Chapter 6).

Vestibule (**VES**-ti-byool) 1. The bony chamber of the inner ear that contains the utricle and saccule (Chapter 9). 2. The female external genital area between the labia minor that contains the openings of the urethra, vagina, and Bartholin's glands (Chapter 20).

Vestigial organ (ves-**TIJ**-ee-uhl) An organ that is reduced in size and function when compared with that of evolutionary ancestors; includes the appendix, ear muscles that move the auricle, and wisdom teeth (Chapter 16).

Villi (**VILL**-eye) (Sing.—villus) 1. Folds of the mucosa of the small intestine that increase the surface area for absorption; each villus contains a capillary network and a lacteal (Chapter 16). 2. Projections of the chorion, an embryonic membrane that forms the fetal portion of the placenta (Chapter 21).

Virulence (**VIR**-yoo-lents) The ability of a microorganism to cause disease; the degree of pathogenicity (Chapter 22).

Virus (**VIGH**-rus) The simplest type of microorganism, consisting of either DNA or RNA within a protein shell; all are obligate intracellular parasites (Chapter 14).

Visceral (**VISS**-er-uhl) Pertaining to organs within a body cavity, especially thoracic and abdominal organs (Chapter 8).

Visceral effectors (**VISS**-er-uhl e-**FEK**-turs) Smooth muscle, cardiac muscle, and glands; receive motor nerve fibers of the autonomic nervous system; responses are involuntary (Chapter 8).

Visceral muscle (**VIS**-ser-uhl **MUSS**-uhl) Another name for smooth muscle tissue (Chapter 4).

Vital capacity (**VY**-tuhl kuh-**PASS**-i-tee) The volume of air involved in the deepest inhalation followed by the most forceful exhalation; average: 3500–5000 mL (Chapter 15).

Vitamin (**VY**-tah-min) An organic molecule needed in small amounts by the body for normal metabolism or growth (Chapter 17).

Vitreous humor (**VIT**-ree-us **HYOO**-mer) The semi-solid, gelatinous substance in the posterior cavity of the eyeball; helps keep the retina in place (Chapter 9).

Vocal cords (**VOH**-kul KORDS) The pair of folds within the larynx that is vibrated by the passage of air, producing sounds that may be turned into speech (Chapter 15).

Volatile (**VAHL**-i-till) Evaporating at moderate temperatures, as gasoline does at room temperature (Chapter 5).

Voluntary muscle (**VAHL**-un-tary **MUSS**-uhl) Another name for striated or skeletal muscle tissue (Chapter 4).

Vomer (**VOH**-mer) The flat bone that forms the lower, posterior portion of the nasal septum (from the Latin "plowshare") (Chapter 6).

Vomiting (**VAH**-mi-ting) Ejection through the mouth of stomach and intestinal contents (Chapter 16).

Vulva (**VUHL**-vah) The female external genital organs (Chapter 20).

W–X–Y–Z

Wart (WART) An elevated, benign skin lesion caused by a virus (Chapter 5).

White blood cells (WHITE BLUHD SELLS) The cells that destroy pathogens that enter the body and provide immunity to some diseases; the five kinds are neutrophils, eosinophils, basophils, lymphocytes, and monocytes (Syn.—leukocytes) (Chapter 4).

White matter (WHITE **MA**-TUR) Nerve tissue within the central nervous system that consists of myelinated axons and dendrites of interneurons (Chapter 8).

Worm (WURM) An elongated invertebrate; parasitic worms include tapeworms and hookworms (Chapter 22).

Xiphoid process (**ZYE**-foyd) The most inferior part of the sternum (from the Greek "sword-like") (Chapter 6).

Yellow bone marrow (**YELL**-oh BOWNE **MAR**-roh) Primarily adipose tissue, found in the marrow cavities of the diaphyses of long bones and in the spongy bone of the epiphyses of adult bones (Chapter 6).

Yolk sac (YOHK SAK) An embryonic membrane that forms the first blood cells for the developing embryo (Chapter 21).

Z line (ZEE LYEN) The lateral boundary of a sarcomere in muscle tissue; anchors myosin and actin filaments (Chapter 7).

Zoonoses (ZOH-oh-**NOH**-seez, or zoh-**ON**-uh-seez) (Sing.—zoonosis) Diseases of animals that may be transmitted to people under certain conditions (Chapter 22).

Zygote (**ZYE**-goht) A fertilized egg, formed by the union of the nuclei of egg and sperm; the diploid number of chromosomes (46 for people) is restored (Chapter 20).

INDEX

Note: Page numbers followed by f refer to figures; page numbers followed by t refer to tables; page numbers followed by b refer to boxes.

A

B

C

D

E

F

I

J

K

L

M

N

O

Q

R

S

T

U

V

W

X

Y

Z